CEREBROVASCULAR DISEASE: IMAGING AND INTERVENTIONAL TREATMENT OPTIONS

CEREBROVASCULAR DISEASE: IMAGING AND INTERVENTIONAL TREATMENT OPTIONS

Calvin L. Rumbaugh, M.D.
Professor Emeritus
Harvard Medical School
Boston, Massachusetts
Department of Radiology
Brigham and Women's Hospital
Boston, Massachusetts

Ay-Ming Wang, M.D.
Co-Chief, Neuroradiology
Department of Diagnostic Radiology
William Beaumont Hospital
Royal Oak, Michigan
Clinical Professor of Radiology
University of Missouri
Kansas City School of Medicine
Kansas City, Missouri

Fong Y. Tsai, M.D.
Professor and Chairman
Department of Radiology
University of Missouri
Kansas City School of Medicine
Kansas City, Missouri

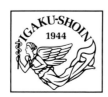

IGAKU-SHOIN   New York • Tokyo

Published and distributed by

IGAKU-SHOIN Medical Publishers, Inc.
One Madison Avenue, New York, New York 10010

IGAKU-SHOIN Ltd.,
5-24-3 Hongo, Bunkyo-ku, Tokyo 113-91

Library of Congress Cataloging-in-Publication Data

Cerebrovascular disease : imaging and interventional treatment options
  / [edited by] Calvin L. Rumbaugh, Ay-Ming Wang, Fong Y. Tsai.
     p.   cm.
    Includes bibliographical references and index.
    1. Cerebrovascular disease.   2. Cerebrovascular disease—Imaging.
3. Radiology, Interventional.   4. Radiology, Interventional—
methods.   I. Rumbaugh, Calvin L.   II. Wang, Ay-ming.   III. Tsai,
Fong Y.
    [DNLM: 1. Cerebrovascular Disorders—radiography.
2. Cerebrovascular Disorders—radionuclide imaging.
3. Cerebrovascular Disorders—therapy.   WL 355 C41342 1995]
RC388.5.C42   1995
616.8'1—dc20
DNLM/DLC
for Library of Congress   94-27327
                                                                    CIP

ISBN: 0-89640-259-2 (New York)
ISBN: 4-260-14259-3 (Tokyo)

Printed and bound in the U.S.A.
10 9 8 7 6 5 4 3 2 1

Dedication
To our wives, children, and friends
for their patience and support

Preface

Stroke is a major cause of death and disability in the United States, surpassed only by heart disease and cancer. The term *stroke* is defined as any sudden attack of disease or illness, but is usually restricted to the sudden onset of a neurological deficit secondary to disease or illness of the brain. Although the pathological process generally involves the cerebrovasculature, in 5–10% of cases the sudden neurological deficit is secondary to some other cause such as tumor, infection, or trauma.

For many years, much of the medical community has had a rather pessimistic attitude toward stroke, believing that little or nothing could be done for the patient, aside from observation. Others have felt that diagnostic studies should be pursued, but only after waiting for a few days or weeks until the patient's condition stabilized.

However, many neurosurgeons and neurologists have always maintained that the specific cause of the stroke should be diagnosed immediately if there is to be any hope of an increase in survival and improvement in the quality of life for the survivors.

With the enormous improvement in our diagnostic capabilities, especially diagnostic imaging, and with the exciting and encouraging improvements in the treatment of cerebrovascular disease, the advocates of immediate diagnostic evaluation have been proven correct. However, the time for action is critical; many authorities feel that there is only about a 6-hour window for effective treatment of central nervous system ischemia (i.e., the prognosis is best if treatment is initiated within 6 hours of onset of the neurological deficit). To initiate such early treatment, a definite diagnosis must be made first.

The old rule of waiting for 24 hours to see whether the patient's neurological deficit is a transient ischemic attack (TIA) or an infarct is obsolete. If the patient does have a TIA, early diagnosis of the cause is even more important. It should be possible to prevent a future impending stroke. Prevention of stroke is the big payoff in the future, and the potential for it exists now.

The purpose of this text is to provide in one reference source an introduction to some of the basic clinical and pathological apsects of cerebrovascular (CV) disease as well as to the various diagnostic imaging options available and some of the radiological interventional methods of treatment.

The neurosurgeons and the neurologists have made and continue to make major advances in the treatment of CV diseases. The radiology interventional groups also have made and continue to make major advances in the radiological interventional treatment of these diseases. The success of all of these impressive treatment advances depends upon the early and accurate diagnosis of the cause of the patient's clinical problem.

All of these successes in diagnosis and treatment are very expensive (the cutting edge of high-tech medicine). However, the cost is minimal compared with the expense to society resulting from the large number of deaths and the many disabled individuals suffering from stroke each year. Early diagnosis is critical!

It is the hope of the authors that this book will be helpful for any neuroscientist (basic or clinical) interested in CV diseases, their diagnosis, their treatment, and their prevention.

Calvin L. Rumbaugh, M.D.
Ay-Ming Wang, M.D.
Fong Y. Tsai, M.D.

Contributors

Abass Alavi, M.D.
Professor of Radiology
Director of Nuclear Medicine
University of Pennsylvania
Philadelphia, Pennsylvania

Kenneth Alfieri, M.D.
Assistant Professor of Radiology
University of Missouri
Kansas City School of Medicine
Kansas City, Missouri

Richard A. Baker, M.D.
Lecturer
Harvard Medical School
Chairman of Radiology
Lahey Clinic
Burlington, Massachusetts

Solomon Batnitzky, M.D.
Professor and Interim Chairman
Department of Radiology
University of Kansas Medical Center
Kansas City, Kansas

Hans J. Biersack, M.D.
Chairman and Professor
The Department of Nuclear Medicine
The University of Bonn
Bonn, Germany

John H. Bisese, M.D.
Neuroradiologist
Georgia Baptist Medical Center
Atlanta, Georgia

Edward M. Cohn, M.D.
Chief, Division of Neuro-Ophthalmology
Department of Ophthalmology
William Beaumont Hospital
Royal Oak, Michigan

Kenneth Dalen, M.D.
Radiologist
William Beaumont Hospital
Troy, Michigan

Christopher F. Dowd, M.D.
University of California, San Francisco
  Medical Center
Department of Radiology and Neurological
  Surgery
Interventional Neurovascular Radiology
  Division
San Francisco, California

Donald A. Eckard, M.D.
Associate Professor of Radiology
Department of Radiology
University of Kansas Medical Center
Kansas City, Kansas

Robert A. Ellwood, M.D.
Chief, Section Vascular/Interventional
   Radiology
Department of Diagnostic Radiology
William Beaumont Hospital
Royal Oak, Michigan

Kenneth Fraser, M.D.
Associate Professor of Radiology and
   Neurosurgery
Chief of Interventional Neuroradiology
University of Miami School of Medicine
Miami, Florida

**John Gilroy, M.D., P.C., FRCP
   (CAN)FACP**
Chairman, Neurology
William Beaumont Hospital
Royal Oak, Michigan
Clinical Professor of Neurology
Wayne State University
Detroit, Michigan

R. Gilberto González, M.D., Ph.D.
Director of MRI
Massachusetts General Hospital
Boston, Massachusetts

Charles R.G. Guttmann, M.D.
Instructor in Radiology
Department of Radiology
Brigham and Women's Hospital and Harvard
   Medical School
Boston, Massachusetts

Van V. Halbach, M.D.
University of California, San Francisco
   Medical Center
Department of Radiology and Neurological
   Surgery
Interventional Neurovascular Radiology
   Division
San Francisco, California

Tarek Hassan, M.D.
Senior Retina Fellow
Department of Ophthalmology
William Beaumont Hospital
Royal Oak, Michigan

Grant B. Hieshima, M.D.
University of California, San Francisco
   Medical Center
Department of Radiology and Neurological
   Surgery
Interventional Neurovascular Radiology
   Division
San Francisco, California

Randall T. Higashida, M.D.
Professor of Radiology and
   Neurological Surgery
Department of Radiology and Neurological
   Surgery
Interventional Neurovascular Radiology
   Division
University of California, San Francisco
   Medical Center
San Francisco, California

T. Edgar Huang, M.D.
Chief, Division of Neuropathology
Department of Anatomic Pathology
William Beaumont Hospital
Royal Oak, Michigan

John L. Johnson, CRP
Chief, Division of Ophthalmic Photography
Department of Ophthalmology
William Beaumont Hospital
Royal Oak, Michigan

Ferenc A. Jolesz, M.D.
Associate Professor of Radiology
Director of MRI
Department of Radiology
Brigham and Women's Hospital and Harvard
   Medical School
Boston, Masssachusetts

Daniel K. Kido, M.D.
Professor of Radiology
Director of Neuroradiology
Mallenkrodt Institute of Radiology
Washington University Medical School
St. Louis, Missouri

Matthias J. Kirsch, M.D.
Department of Diagnostic Radiology
William Beaumont Hospital
Royal Oak, Michigan

John E. Kirsch, Ph.D.
Assistant Professor, Diagnostic Radiology
Assistant Professor, Biomedical Engineering
Director of MRI Research
University of Kentucky Medical School
Lexington, Kentucky

Yukunori Korogi, M.D.
Assistant Professor of Radiology
Department of Radiology
Kumamoto University School of Medicine
Kumamoto, Japan

Graham K. Lee, M.D.
Clinical Associate Professor of Radiology
University of Missouri
Kansas City School of Medicine
Kansas City, Missouri

Jackson Ching-Tzer Lin, M.D., Ph.D.
Professor, Diagnostic Radiology and
   Neuroradiology
China Medical College
Taichung, Taiwan
Department of Radiology
MacKay Memorial Hospital
Taipei, Taiwan

Joseph F. Polak, M.D.
Associate Professor of Radiology
Harvard Medical School
Director of Noninvasive Imaging
Brigham and Women's Hospital
Boston, Massachusetts

Calvin L. Rumbaugh, M.D.
Professor Emeritus
Harvard Medical School
Department of Radiology
Brigham and Women's Hospital
Boston, Massachusetts

Richard B. Schwartz, M.D., Ph.D.
Assistant Professor of Radiology
Harvard Medical School
Assistant Director of Neuroradiology
Brigham and Women's Hospital
Boston, Massachusetts

Wei-Jen Shih, M.D.
Professor
The Department of Diagnostic Radiology
The Division of Nuclear Medicine
The University of Kentucky Medical School
Lexington, Kentucky
   and
Chief, Nuclear Medicine Service
The Department of Veterans Affairs Medical Center
Lexington, Kentucky

Anil N. Shetty, Ph.D.
Director of MRI Physics
Department of Diagnostic Radiology
William Beaumont Hospital
Royal Oak, Michigan

Edward L. Siegel, M.D.
Associate Professor of Radiology
Department of Radiology
University of Kansas Medical Center
Kansas City, Kansas

Mutsumasa Takahashi, M.D.
Professor and Chairman
Department of Radiology
Kumamoto University School of Medicine
Kumamoto, Japan

Fong Y. Tsai, M.D., FACR
Professor and Chairman
Department of Radiology
University of Missouri
Kansas City School of Medicine
Kansas City, Missouri

Benjamin M.W. Tsui, Ph.D.
Professor, Departments of Biomedical
   Engineering and Radiology
The University of North Carolina at Chapel Hill
Chapel Hill, North Carolina

Ay-Ming Wang, M.D.
Co-Chief, Neuroradiology
Department of Diagnostic Radiology
William Beaumont Hospital
Royal Oak, Michigan
Clinical Professor of Radiology
University of Missouri
Kansas City School of Medicine
Kansas City, Missouri

Jane Werner, M.D.
Chief, Division of Uveitis
Department of Ophthalmology
William Beaumont Hospital
Royal Oak, Michigan

William T.C. Yuh, M.D., MSEE
Professor of Radiology
University of Iowa
Director of MRI and Neuroradiology
University of Iowa Hospital and Clinics
Iowa City, Iowa

Amir A. Zamani, M.D.
Assistant Professor of Radiology
Harvard Medical School
Director of Neuroradiology
Brigham and Women's Hospital
Boston, Massachusetts

Contents

Section 1

Introduction

1

Clinical Applications and Introduction to Cerebrovascular Anatomy, Physiology, and Pathology

John Gilroy, M.D.

A *stroke* may be defined as death of tissue in the central nervous system owing to infarction or hemorrhage.

Cardiovascular disease, cancer, and stroke are the three leading causes of death in the United States, but stroke, the third leading cause of death, is the leading cause of disability. There are 500,000 new strokes each year; of these, 85% are thromboembolic and 15% hemorrhagic. The prevalence of stroke in the population at this time is over 2 million in the United States alone, with a mortality of 150,000 per year. As a consequence, stroke has a major impact on the patient, other family members, and the community. The commonly held conception that stroke is a disease of the elderly is not true, since one-third of the estimated 2 million stroke survivors are under the age of 65. Of these survivors, 30% require assistance, 20% need help with walking, and 15% are institutionalized. Furthermore, 70% have some impaired vocational capacity 7 years after their stroke.

DEFINITIONS

At the present time, the economic costs of stroke in terms of health care expenditures and lost productivity approach an estimated $15 billion per year in the United States.

A stroke may be considered under the heading of cerebral hemorrhage, which accounts for 10–15% of acute strokes, and cerebral infarction, which comprises the remaining 85%. Cerebral infarction may result from thrombosis of a cerebral artery, which accounts for 70% of cases, and from cerebral embolism in the remaining 30%. The diagnosis of cerebral embolism has increased steadily over the three decades because of improvement in screening techniques, and the figure may rise even further as stroke patients receive appropriate studies nationwide.

At the present time, a number of terms are used to define cases of cerebrovascular disease. The first, *transient ischemic attack (TIA)*, has been defined as an ischemic event lasting for less than 24 hr, without apparent permanent neurological deficit. It should be realized that the majority of TIAs are small strokes and that the original definition of TIA defined the period of neurological deficit as less than 20 min. Currently, it has been extended to 24 hr and the term needs to be analyzed in a more circumspect manner because it is becoming apparent that patients who have deficits of more than a few hours' duration have had small infarcts.

Another term, reversible ischemic neurologic deficit (*RIND*), was introduced to cover an individual with neurological deficits lasting more than 24 hr but less than 3 weeks. This is clearly an unnecessary term, since all of these patients have had a cerebral infarction.

The abolition of these terms and the recognition that focal ischemic events now labeled TIA or RIND are associated with infarction in most cases would do much to increase concern for patients with minor symptoms. It would also classify them as stroke victims rather than as persons experiencing some nebulous ischemic event with complete recovery.

INCIDENCE

The incidence of stroke in men is approximately 30% higher than in women, but the incidence increases sharply with age, regardless of sex. In patients over 55 years, the incidence of stroke doubles for each decade of life, remaining higher in men than in women up to the ninth decade, when the pattern is reversed. This gender difference is also reflected in age-adjusted stroke death rates when men are at higher risk of stroke and death than women and when African-American patients of either sex have almost a twofold higher risk of stroke than age- and sex-matched Caucasian patients.

The 30-day mortality has been studied in several countries; cerebral infarction shows a mortality of approximately 15% and intracerebral hemorrhage close to 80%. The 30-day mortality for stroke has declined in the past four decades, almost entirely as a result of the decline in mortality from cerebral infarction.

This decline has been attributed to improved medical care, primarily improved control of hypertension; however, this cannot be the only factor. Nevertheless, the decline in stroke mortality has slowed, and in fact may have been reversed in recent years, probably due to the increased incidence of stroke in the aging U.S. population.

RISK FACTORS

The major risk factors for thromboembolic stroke causing cerebral infarction are listed in Table 1-1. Hypertension is probably the most important risk factor for stroke at this time. The yearly incidence of ischemic stroke in men and women increases approximately threefold in patients with borderline hypertension (blood pressure above 140/90 but less than 160/96), and there is an eightfold increase in stroke incidence

TABLE 1-1 Risk Factors for Thromboembolic Stroke

Hypertension
Older age (65 + years)
Diabetes mellitus
Other metabolic abnormalities
  Hypothyroidism
  Hyperlipidemia
  Hyperuricemia
Obesity
Smoking
Alcohol abuse
Heart disease
Hypercoagulable state
  Primary—Protein C deficiency
         Protein S deficiency
         Antithrombin III deficiency
  Secondary—Antiphospholipid-positive arteritis
          Lupus anticoagulant use
          Homocystinuria
  Platelet hyperaggregability

in patients with definite hypertension (blood pressure above 160/96).

However, many patients with cerebral atherosclerosis are subject to marked fluctuations in blood pressure and may appear to be normotensive on casual blood pressure determinations. This gives the impression that an occasional reading in the hypertensive range is an anomaly and should not be treated. It is probably better to treat patients with occasional blood pressure readings in the definite hypertensive range as suffering from hypertension and to prescribe medication to ensure that the peaks of hypertension do not occur. Usually mild antihypertensive agents are effective in these cases.

Age is also an important factor in the incidence of stroke. The risk is about 5% in the 55- to 59-year age group but increases to 25% in the 80- to 84-year age group. This is observed in both men and women.

Diabetes mellitus is second in importance as a risk factor in the stroke population. Cerebral infarction is more common in the diabetic population, and the severity of infarction is increased when diabetics are compared to nondiabetics. The association of hypertension and diabetes mellitus is particularly pernicious.

The presence of hyperlipidemia is known to increase the risk of stroke. This includes both hypercholesterolemia and hypertriglyceridemia. The risk of stroke is increased in patients with familial hyperlipidemia.

Hyperuricemia has been rather neglected as a risk factor in the stroke population. In fact, it is a definite risk factor in cerebrovascular disease, just as it is in cardiovascular disease and peripheral vascular disease.

Hypothyroidism is present in a significant number of stroke patients and is believed to be an additional risk factor in the stroke-prone population.

Obesity appears to be an independent risk factor, and not only a condition predisposing to increased hypertension and diabetes.

Smoking has been shown to carry a significant risk in the stroke population, as has excessive consumption of alcohol.

The presence of heart disease in the stroke population is critical because there is a higher risk of dying from myocardial infarction than from a second stroke in patients who have had a stroke. This alone is cause for immediate concern in any patient who has suffered a stroke, indicating the need for full cardiac evaluation in all cases. In addition to the risk of myocardial infarction, there is an increased incidence of cerebral embolism in an individual with known heart disease. There have been several studies on atrial fibrillation in acute stroke indicating a significant risk in patients with atrial fibrillation compared to those with normal sinus rhythm. This risk factor appears to be approximately five to seven times normal in nonvalvular atrial fibrillation. However, when atrial fibrillation is studied in terms of valvular versus nonvalvular heart disease, the relative risk in patients with valvular heart disease increases 17-fold compared to the 5-fold increase in nonvalvular heart disease with atrial fibrillation. Cerebral embolism secondary to atrial fibrillation carries a 10% fatality rate, with severe neurological deficits occurring in approximately 50% of patients. The remainder have less severe residual signs.

The detection and treatment of a hypercoagulable state is of critical importance in children, adolescents, and young adults who have recurrent or familial cerebral thrombosis, with or without episodes of deep venous thrombosis. The syndrome is due to impairment of normal endothelial steady-state functions (primary hypercoagulable states) or endothelial activation with an increased thrombogenic propensity (secondary hypercoagulable states).

Primary hypercoagulable states include antithrombin III deficiency, protein C or protein S deficiency, fibrinolytic abnormalities, dysfibrinogenemia, hypoplasminogenemia, and homocystinuria.

Secondary hypercoagulable states occur in the antiphospholipid syndrome, hyperlipidemias, diabetes mellitus, increased levels of factor VII and fibrinogen, cancer, use of anticancer drugs, obesity, myeloproliferative disorders, and vasculitis.

Screening for a hypercoagulable state should include determination of antithrombin III, protein C, protein S, fibrinogen levels, and testing for homocystinuria for homozygous and heterozygous forms of the disease.

CLINICAL FEATURES

The symptoms and signs of stroke have been described traditionally in terms of the involved cerebral artery. This method has limitations, as described under collateral circulation (page 000), and may be of little value to a neuroradiologist who is accustomed to thinking in terms of neuroanatomy. For the clinician, one result of the traditional approach has been overemphasis on the carotid artery/middle cerebral artery territory and relative neglect of the vertebral basilar system. This leads to misdiagnosis and even inappropriate treatment since at least one-third of strokes are the result of infarction in the vertebral basilar territory. Emphasis on abnormal clinical signs related to the anatomical location of a stroke should facilitate diagnosis and direct the attention of those interpreting studies to the likely area of abnormality. Consequently, the following descriptions of the clinical features of a stroke generally emphasize location rather than putative vessel involvement. However, use of vascular terms is unavoidable in some cases.

Left frontal lobe (dominant hemisphere)	Aphasia or dysphasia
	Deviation of head and eyes to the left
	Right homonymous hemianopia
	Right facial paralysis, central type
	Right hemiparesis or hemiplegia
	Right hemihypalgesia
	Extensor plantar response on right side
Right frontal lobe (nondominant hemisphere)	Deviation of head and eyes to right
	Left homonymous hemianopia
	Left facial paralysis, central type
	Left hemiparesis or hemiplegia
	Left hemihypalgesia

	Extensor plantar response on left side
	Failure to recognize affected limb (autotopagnosia) or denial of involvement of affected side (anosognosia)
Medial aspect frontal lobe a. Paracentral lobule	Paralysis and sensory loss Contralateral lower limb
b. Anterior limb internal capsule	Contralateral paralysis of face and upper limb, with rigidity and dystonia if basal ganglia are involved
c. Medial aspect frontal lobe extending into corpus callosum	Contralateral hemiparesis and hemisensory loss, plus dyspraxia of the ipsilateral hand
Bilateral frontal lobe infarction	Coma and quadriparesis in the acute phase Survivors show minimal limb weakness Apathy Sucking, rooting, or grasp reflexes Indifference Bowel and bladder incontinence Memory impairment
Posterior limb internal capsule	Contralateral hemiplegia Transient contralateral hemisensory loss Visual field deficits, including contralateral hemianopia or quadrantanopia
Thalamus	Vomiting, stupor, and coma indicate hemorrhage, usually with intraventricular extension
a. Posterior thalamic infarction	Gaze palsies Contralateral hemiparesis Contralateral hemisensory loss Occasional pure sensory stroke or useless hand syndrome Dysphasia or aphasia Thalamic syndrome presenting as a severe hemisensory loss, with burning pain involving the contralateral limbs and trunk
b. Paramedian thalamic infarct	More likely to have gaze palsies Less likely to have contralateral hemiparesis and hemisensory loss
c. Dorsal thalamic infarct	Less likely to have gaze palsies Contralateral hemiparesis Less likely to have contralateral hemisensory loss Ataxia
d. Anterior thalamic infarct	Gaze palsies in one-third Contralateral hemiparesis Less likely to have hemisensory loss No ataxia
Parietal lobe (dominant hemisphere)	Contralateral hemisensory loss Contralateral hemisensory neglect Contralateral astereognosis Defective optokinetic nystagmus Dysphasia Dyslexia Agraphia
Parietal lobe (nondominant hemisphere)	Contralateral hemisensory loss Contralateral hemisensory neglect Contralateral astereognosis Autotopagnosia Anosognosia Defective optokinetic nystagmus Constructural apraxia Spatial disorientation Affective changes
Angular gyrus (dominant hemisphere)	Word blindness Agraphia Alexia Acalculia Right–left confusion Finger agnosia

Supramarginal gyrus (dominant hemisphere)	Difficulty comprehending language		Ipsilateral cerebellar ataxia
			Ipsilateral loss of pain and temperature sensation of face
Temporal lobe (dominant hemisphere)	Receptive dysphasia Jargon Dysphasia Dysnomia Contralateral upper homonymous hemianopia Impaired memory		Ipsilateral Horner's syndrome Contralateral loss of pain and temperature sensation of trunk and limbs
Temporal lobe (nondominant hemisphere)	Impaired memory Reduced discrimination of sounds, pitch, and tone Visual perceptual difficulties	Cerebellar infarction	Headache, nausea, vomiting, vertigo, dysarthria Gaze palsy toward affected side Nystagmus increasing toward affected side Ipsilateral dysdiadochokinesis Dysmetria and intention tremor
Occipital lobe infarction	Homonymous hemianopia or cortical blindness if there is bilateral involvement		
Midbrain infarction	Ipsilateral third nerve palsy with diplopia Ipsilateral cerebellar ataxia Contralateral hemiparesis	Cerebellar hemorrhage	Occipital headache, nausea, vomiting, vertigo, gait ataxia, truncal ataxia, ipsilateral dysdiadochokinesis, dysmetria, and intention tremor
Unilateral pontine infarction	Ipsilateral Horner's syndrome Cerebellar ataxia Contralateral corticospinal involvement with hemiparesis Dysarthria and dysphagia		Ipsilateral abducens and facial nerve palsies; gaze palsies with forced deviation of eyes or head toward unaffected side
Pontine hemorrhage	Coma Pinpoint pupils Quadriplegia		Brain stem involvement with coma
Bilateral pontine infarction	Coma Quadriplegia Locked-in syndrome on recovering consciousness		Ocular bobbing, pinpoint pupils and respiratory changes; carry a poor prognosis

DIAGNOSTIC PROCEDURES

Evaluation of the acute stroke due to thromboembolism should include all of the risk factors that have been outlined in Table 1-1. The evaluation then would include:

Medullary infarction	Acute onset with unilateral vomiting and facial pain Vertigo and ataxia in most cases Established cases showing dysarthria, dysphonia, dysphagia Nystagmus maximal on side of lesion

1. Full cardiac evaluation, including 24-hr cardiac monitoring, echocardiogram, and transesophageal

echocardiogram to detect embolism and to reduce the risk of myocardial infarction, the leading cause of death in patients who have had a stroke due to thromboembolism.

2. Adequate visualization of the ascending aorta by transesophageal echocardiogram to exclude ulcerative plaques as a source of embolism.
3. Real-time and Doppler ultrasonography of the carotid and vertebral arteries, with visualization of the intracranial extensions of these vessels, including the circle of Willis, middle cerebral artery, and basilar artery.
4. Monitoring for unpredictable hypertension.
5. Metabolic screening for diabetes mellitus, hypothyroidism, hyperlipidemia, and hyperuricemia.
6. Evaluation of swallowing within 24 hr in conscious patients to avoid aspiration when feeding.
7. Chest x-ray to exclude aspiration pneumonia.
8. Computed tomography (CT) scan of the head to rule out hemorrhage.
9. Magnetic resonance imaging (MRI) scan of the head to clearly delineate the extent of infarction when the CT scan is normal.
10. Check electrolytes at least once every 48 hr for sodium, potassium, calcium, magnesium, and phosphate.

TREATMENT OF ACUTE STROKE DUE TO THROMBOEMBOLISM

The treatment of an acute stroke should be directed toward (1) limiting damage to ischemic neurons which are located in the periphery of the infarcted area and have potential for survival; (2) reduction of cerebral edema; (3) prevention of a second event in patients with embolism; and (4) recognition that stroke is an event in an individual with generalized vascular and metabolic problems.

Consequently, a program may be instituted as follows:

1. Maintain blood pressure in the high normal or low hypertensive range because of the risk of interfering with autoregulatory mechanisms.
2. Heparinize patients with proven or suspected cerebral embolism (Table 1-2).
3. Control diabetes mellitus.

TABLE 1-2 Indications for Heparin/Warfarin Therapy

Atrial fibrillation
Recent myocardial infarction
Presence of a mural thrombus
Other cardiac dysrhythmias such as paroxysmal fibrillation
Presence of other structural cardiac abnormalities such as patent foramen ovale
Crescendo TIAs
Ulcerative carotid plaques, regardless of the degree of stenosis
Severe carotid stenosis (greater than 70%) awaiting surgery

4. Treat hypothyroidism.
5. Treat hyperuricemia.
6. Place a Foley catheter in bladder in obtunded, stuporous, or semicomatose and comatose patients.
7. Give intravenous fluids to maintain fluid and electrolyte balance.
8. Withhold oral fluids until the swallowing mechanism is assessed.
9. If the patient is conscious and the swallowing mechanism is intact, begin a light diet.
10. If swallowing is impaired, begin feeding by nasogastric tube after 24 hr, with the head kept in an elevated position.
11. Physical therapy with passive limb movements initially on the first day. The program may be modified according to the patient's progression and gradually extended to a more active state.
12. Treat any cardiac abnormalities which may be the source of embolism by anticoagulation. In addition, because of the high risk of myocardial infarction, the most common cause of death following stroke, all cardiac problems require treatment or follow-up.
13. A cerebral selective calcium channel blocking agent such as nimodipine, 60 mg every 4 hr by mouth or nasogastric tube, may be of benefit.
14. A hyperosmolar agent such as glycerol, 30 g every 6 hr by mouth or nasogastric tube, may reduce the extent of cerebral edema.
15. Treat hypercoagulable abnormalities in young patients with stroke.
16. Dietitian to see and prescribe diet for obese patients who are conscious and able to swallow.
17. Stop smoking.

SURGICAL TREATMENT OF CEREBRAL INFARCTION

Under certain circumstances, a stenosis of the internal carotid artery with more than 70% narrowing of the lumen is accepted as an indication for carotid endarterectomy. However, certain criteria should be met, including either the presence of an asymptomatic bruit or symptoms of a small stroke or major cerebral infarction on the affected side. The surgeon will usually elect to perform surgery within a few days of diagnosis in cases of an asymptomatic bruit or small infarction, but many surgeons prefer to wait at least 6 weeks before endarterectomy when there has been a major stroke. However, screening for risk factors should be performed in all cases and appropriate treatment prescribed prior to surgery to reduce the risk of complications during and after the procedure.

Carotid endarterectomy may also be indicated in patients with significant stenosis of the opposite carotid artery when the arterial supply to the affected hemisphere is blocked.

The presence of an ulcerative plaque which is the site of embolism is also an indication for endarterectomy, regardless of the degree of stenosis of the lumen.

SURGICAL TREATMENT OF INTRACEREBRAL HEMORRHAGE

Massive intracerebral hemorrhage may benefit from surgical removal of the blood clot in selected cases.

However, the condition is often catastrophic, and the clinical condition of the patient precludes surgical intervention in many cases. These patients require urgent control of blood pressure, as well as lowering of intracranial pressure by hyperventilation and the use of intravenous hyperosmolar agents such as mannitol. Intracranial pressure monitoring may be helpful to measure pressure changes and the response to treatment.

All cases of cerebellar hemorrhage should be evaluated by a neurosurgeon for possible evacuation of the hematoma. This may be a lifesaving procedure if performed before the hematoma causes acute hydrocephalus by pressure on the fourth ventricle or leads to rapid deterioration from pressure on the brain stem.

This brief introduction to cerebrovascular disease is intended to facilitate communication between the clinician, the neuroradiologist, and other specialists in the several neuroimaging techniques. The burgeoning of new methods of neuroimaging calls for correlation of clinical findings in all cases if the studies are to be appropriate, timely, and accurate. This cannot be accomplished in isolation, but it will be successful when communication is an accepted fact in the neurosciences and will be of most benefit to the patient when the clinician and the other neuroscientists have a basic understanding of each discipline in the field.

The following chapters will elaborate on the subjects mentioned in this introduction.

2

Normal Anatomy of the Cerebrovascular System

Daniel K. Kido, M.D., Calvin L. Rumbaugh, M.D., Richard A. Baker, M.D.

The cerebrovascular system is supplied by four arteries. In most individuals, the right common carotid artery and the right vertebral artery originate from the innominate artery, the left common carotid artery arises as a branch of the aortic arch, and the left vertebral artery originates from the left subclavian artery.[1,2]

However, in about 30% of individuals, there is a variation in the usual configuration.[1-3] One common variation is for the left common carotid artery to either share a common origin with the innominate artery or originate from the innominate artery close to the innominate artery's origin. A less common variation is for the left vertebral artery to arise directly from the aortic arch. Least common is an anomalous origin of the right subclavian artery from the aortic arch distal to the origin of the left subclavian artery.

INTERNAL CAROTID ARTERY

The common carotid artery usually bifurcates at the C3–4 or C4–5 level into the internal carotid and external carotid arteries. The internal carotid artery consists of five divisions: cervical, petrous, precavernous, intra-cavernous, and supraclinoid (Fig. 2-1). The petrous division has a small posterior branch (caroticotympanic artery) to the tympanic cavity, and a small anterior branch to the vidian canal which communicates with the internal maxillary artery.

Two major groups of small branches arise from the intracavernous division: the inferior cavernous sinus artery supplies the inferior cavernous sinus, the adjacent dura, and the dura in the middle cranial fossa; the meningohypophyseal trunk supplies the posterior pituitary gland and dura over the dorsum, clivis, and tentorial margins.[4,5] Occasionally, the meningohypophyseal trunk may arise from the precavernous division.

Three branches arise from the supraclinoid segment: the ophthalmic, posterior communicating, and anterior choroidal arteries. The ophthalmic artery supplies the globe, intraocular muscles, ethmoid and nasal mucosae, lacrimal gland, and part of the dura of the anterior fossa over the orbital roof (Fig. 2-2). The middle meningeal artery occasionally arises from the ophthalmic artery as a developmental variant.[6,7]

The posterior communicating artery connects the internal carotid and posterior cerebral arteries (Fig. 2-3). Sometimes it is quite large and appears as an extension

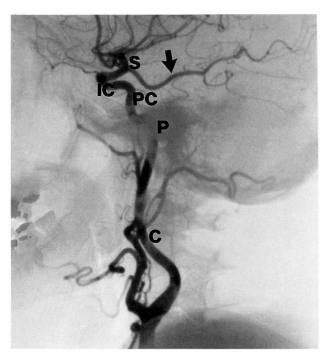

Fig. 2-1 Segments of the internal carotid artery: cervical (C), petrous (P), precavernous (PC), intracavernous (IC), and supraclinoid (S). Fetal posterior cerebral artery (arrow).

of the posterior cerebral artery (fetal posterior cerebral artery) (Fig. 2-1). At other times, it may be so small that it is difficult to identify. The junction of the posterior communicating artery with the internal carotid artery is often slightly dilated (infundibulum). If the infundibulum is larger than 3 mm in diameter, it is considered by some authors to be an aneurysm.[8] Small branches from the superior surface of the posterior communicating artery supply parts of the thalamus, hypothalamus, and internal capsule.

The anterior choroidal artery is the last branch of the internal carotid artery. It consists of two divisions: the cisternal segment, located in the crural cistern, supplies parts of the optic tract, internal capsule, basal ganglia, midbrain, uncus, and lateral geniculate body; the plexal segment supplies structures adjacent to the choroid fissure and the choroid plexus in the temporal horn (Fig. 2-4).

ANTERIOR CEREBRAL ARTERY

The anterior cerebral artery originates as the medial division of the internal carotid artery after its terminal bifurcation. The short horizontal segment of the ante-

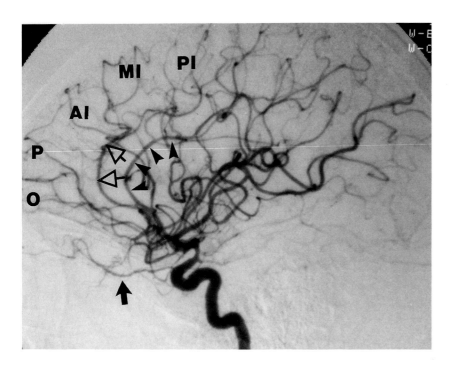

Fig. 2-2 The ophthalmic artery (arrow) is the first supraclinoid branch of the internal carotid artery. Cortical branches of the anterior cerebral artery include the orbitofrontal (O), frontopolar (P), anterior internal frontal (AI), middle internal frontal (MI), and posterior internal frontal (PI). Callosomarginal (open arrows) and pericallosal (arrowheads) arteries.

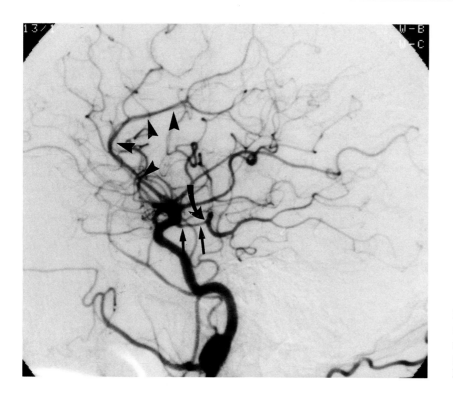

Fig. 2-3 Posterior communicating artery (arrows). Junction of the posterior communicating and posterior cerebral arteries (curved arrow). Pericallosal artery (arrowheads).

rior cerebral artery extends from the carotid bifurcation to its terminal branches, the anterior communicating artery and the pericallosal artery, and is often referred to as the A_1 segment (Fig. 2-5). Other branches of the anterior cerebral artery which arise from the A_1 segment are the medial lenticulostriate arteries (six to nine vessels) which supply parts of the optic nerve, optic chiasm, part of the hypothalamus and the midline structures around the foramen of Monro just superior to origin of these arteries. The recurrent artery of Heubner, which usually arises medial to the lenticulostriate arteries, runs laterally 2–3 cm, to supply portions of the anterior limb of the internal capsule and the inferior part of the head of the caudate nucleus and putamen.

The right and left A_1 segments communicate with each other via the anterior communicating artery. This communication completes the anterior portion of the circle of Willis. However, either the A_1 segment or the anterior communicating artery may be hypoplastic or aplastic. When one or more of these vessels is aplastic, the circle of Willis is incomplete and the collateral circulation system, which the circle of Willis helps to form, is compromised.[9] Magnetic resonance angiography (MRA) can demonstrate the entire circle of Willis without the use of a contrast medium (Fig. 2-6).

The pericallosal artery extends along the anterior (genu) and superior surfaces (body) of the corpus callosum and anastomoses with the posterior pericallosal artery near the posterior end (splenium) of the corpus callosum (Figs. 2-2 to 2-4). Occasionally, the proximal portions of both the right and left pericallosal arteries form a single trunk (azygous anterior cerebral artery). This anomaly is uncommon but, when present, may be associated with midline congenital defects, aneurysms, and arteriovenous malformations.[10] The cortical branches of the pericallosal artery supply the superior frontal gyrus, paracentral lobule, and precuneus. These branches are variable in their course. The largest branches are the orbitofrontal, frontopolar, internal frontal, and callosomarginal (Figs. 2-2 and 2-4). The callosomarginal artery courses posteriorly in the cingulate sulcus and is usually as large as or larger than the pericallosal artery.

MIDDLE CEREBRAL ARTERY

The middle cerebral artery originates as the lateral division of the internal carotid artery after its terminal bifurcation. The middle carotid artery is about 20% larger than the anterior cerebral artery[11] (Fig. 2-5).

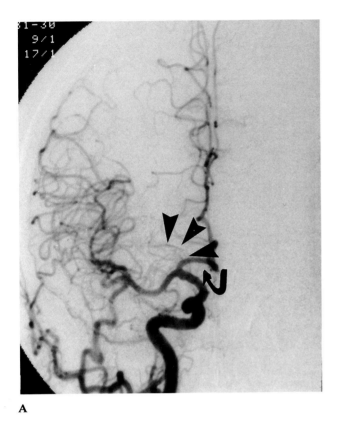

A

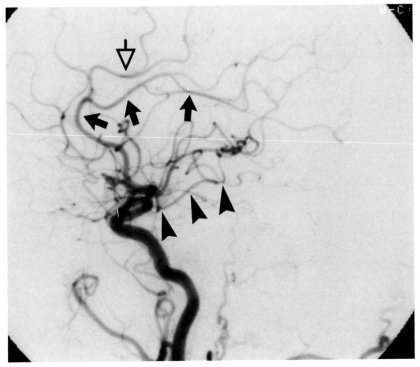

B

Fig. 2-4 AP (*A*) and lateral (*B*) view of the anterior choroidal artery (arrowheads). A_1 segment (curved arrows) of the anterior cerebral artery. The callosomarginal (open arrows) artery overlaps the pericallosal (arrow) artery in the midline on the AP views.

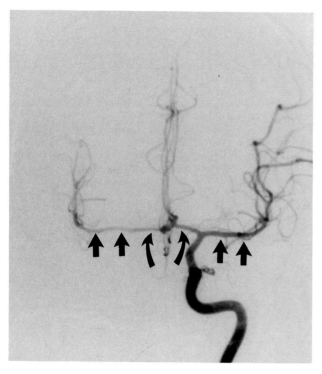

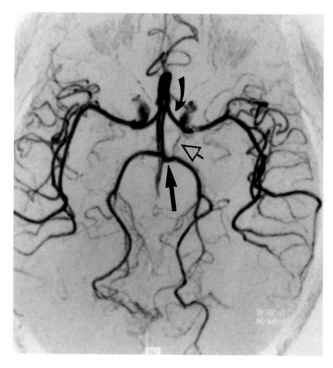

Fig. 2-5 Both the A₁ segments (curved arrows) and the M₁ segments (arrows) are opacified from a single left internal carotid injection.

Fig. 2-6 Circle of Willis demonstrated by MRA. The base view demonstrates the A₁ segment (curved arrow) of the anterior cerebral artery, the posterior communicating (open arrow) artery, and the proximal segment (arrow) of the posterior cerebral artery, which make up the left side of the circle of Willis.

The proximal few centimeters of the middle cerebral artery (M1 segment) extend horizontally and laterally to the sylvian fissure, where they abruptly turn posteriorly and superiorly (knee of the middle cerebral artery) over the surface of the insula (sylvian portion of the middle cerebral artery). The M1 segment gives rise to the lateral lenticulostriate branches (six to nine), which supply portions of the caudate nucleus, globus pallidus, putamen, and part of the anterior limb of the internal capsule (Fig. 2-7A). The M1 segment also gives rise to the anterior temporal artery, which supplies part of the anterior temporal lobe, and the orbitofrontal artery, which supplies the inferior and lateral surfaces of the frontal lobe.

From the sylvian portion of the middle cerebral artery arise four major cortical branches which fan out to supply the lateral surface of the cerebrum after exiting through the sylvian fissure. These major branches are the ascending frontal, posterior parietal, angular, and posterior temporal arteries (Fig. 2-7B). A smaller but

important branch is the artery to the central sulcus, which supplies the lateral surface of the motor and sensory cortices and is located between the ascending frontal and posterior parietal arteries.

POSTERIOR CEREBRAL ARTERIES

The posterior cerebral arteries usually arise from the basilar artery but commonly receive some blood from the internal carotid artery via the posterior communicating arteries. However, if the posterior cerebral arteries arise directly from the carotid arteries (fetal posterior cerebral artery), they will receive most or all of their blood from the carotid arteries (Fig. 2-1).

The major posterior cerebral artery branches are the thalamoperforating arteries (three to five vessels), which supply part of the thalamus and lateral geniculate bodies; the posterior medial choroidal artery,

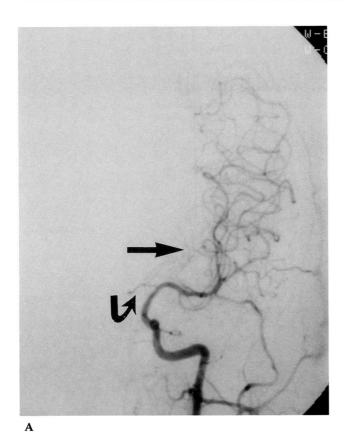

A

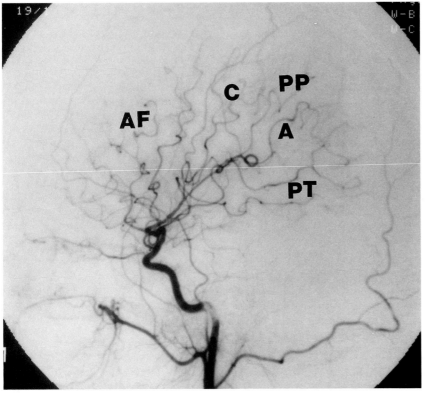

B

Fig. 2-7 Middle cerebral artery. (*A*) AP view. The lateral lenticulostriate arteries (arrow) are barely visible on this digital subtraction angiography (DSA) scan. These arteries were better seen on the original DSA scan. There is flash filling of the A_1 segment (curved arrow). (*B*) Lateral view. Ascending frontal (AF) artery, artery to the central sulcus (C), posterior parietal (PP), angular (A), and posterior temporal (PT) branches of the middle cerebral artery.

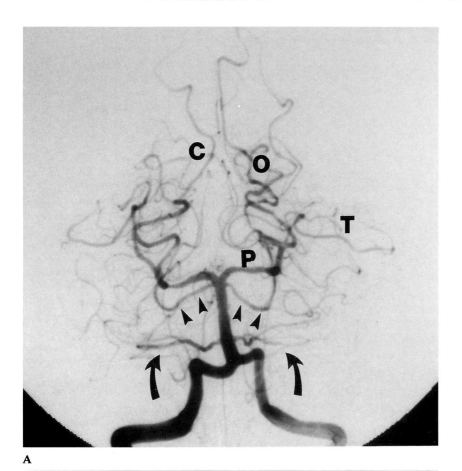

A

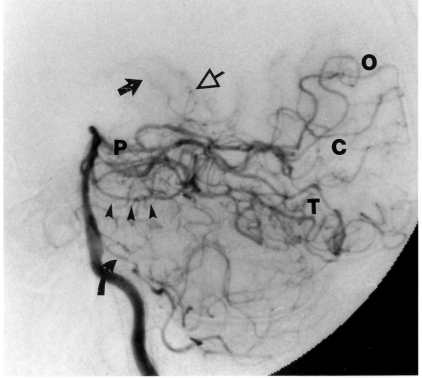

B

Fig. 2-8 Towne (*A*) and lateral (*B*) projections of the posterior cerebral (P) artery branches: posterior temporal artery (T), calcarine artery (C), and parieto-occipital artery (O). Posterior medial (arrow) and posterior lateral (open arrow) choroidal arteries. Anterior inferior (curved arrows) and superior (arrowheads) cerebellar arteries arise from the basilar artery.

which supplies the choroid plexus in the third ventricle; the posterolateral choroidal artery, which supplies portions of the choroid plexuses in the temporal horn, atrium, and body of the lateral ventricle; and lastly, the cortical branches (Fig. 2-8). The medial group of cortical branches supplies the medial surface of the occipital lobe and consists of the calcarine and parieto-occipital arteries (Fig. 2-8). The lateral group of cortical branches, consisting primarily of the posterior temporal artery, supplies part of the medial border of the hippocampus and the inferior surface of the temporal lobe (Fig. 2-8).

VERTEBRAL ARTERY

The medulla, inferior half of the cerebellum, and portions of the posterior fossa meninges are supplied by the two vertebral arteries. The posterior meningeal branch of the vertebral artery supplies the dura covering the occipital bone and adjacent falx and tentorium. The anterior meningeal artery supplies the dura at the skull base, including the condylar area.[12] Anastomoses often exists between these vertebral branches and the meningohypophyseal branch of the internal carotid artery, middle meningeal artery, ascending pharyngeal artery, and occipital branches of the external carotid artery.

The posterior inferior cerebellar arteries (PICA) are paired and are the last branches to originate from the vertebral arteries. They supply the medulla, tonsils, lower half of the vermis, and cerebellar hemispheres (Fig. 2-9). In 25% of cases the PICA is absent, and its territory is supplied by the anterior inferior cerebellar arteries (AICA).[13,14]

BASILAR ARTERY

The basilar artery is formed by the junction of the two vertebral arteries. It is often tortuous and has many small, perforating branches to the medulla and pons, as well as to two major branches which help supply the cerebellum, the anterior inferior cerebellar arteries (paired), and the superior cerebellar arteries (paired). The AICA supplies the anterior inferior surfaces of the cerebellum, the flocculus and the interior surface of the vermis (Fig. 2-8). The superior cerebellar arteries supply the superior surface of the vermis and the cerebellar hemispheres (Fig. 2-8).

VENOUS SYSTEM (SUPRATENTORIAL)

The supratentorial venous system consists of a superficial and a deep group. The superficial group of veins drains either superiorly toward the vertex of the skull or inferiorly toward the base of the skull. The veins located above the sylvian fissure, which drain the lateral cerebral convexity, consist of the anterior frontal, central, and parietal veins. These veins drain superiorly into the superior sagittal sinus. Immediately before their junction with the superior sagittal sinus, they receive veins from the medial surface of the cerebrum. Commonly, the largest of these draining surface veins is located in the parietal region and is called the *vein of Trolard* (Fig. 2-10). The sylvian fissure and the cerebrum adjacent to the fissure are drained by the superficial middle cerebral vein. This vein usually empties into the transverse sinus, but it may drain either anteriorly into the sphenoparietal sinus or medially into the deep middle cerebral vein. Veins on the lateral surface of the cerebrum beneath the sylvian fissure, as well as the inferior surfaces of the occipital and temporal lobes, drain directly into the transverse sinus. The largest of these lateral inferior surface veins is named the *vein of Labbe* (Fig. 2-10).

The deep venous system includes the internal cerebral veins (paired), basal veins of Rosenthal (paired), and thalamic veins (Fig. 2-11). They drain into the great vein of Galen (single, midline) and then into the straight sinus (single, midline). Medial and lateral subependymal veins in the walls of the lateral ventricles drain into the internal cerebral veins. The largest lateral subependymal vein (sometimes named the *thalamostriate vein*) defines the lateral wall of the lateral ventricle in its midportion. The anterior septal veins are medial subependymal veins in the frontal horns that drain into the internal cerebral veins. The basal veins of Rosenthal are formed in the medial portion of the lateral cerebral fissures, course around the superior aspect of the uncus, and pass posteriorly through the perimesencephalic cisterns to empty into the great vein of Galen (Fig. 2-11). Although drainage of the basal vein of Rosenthal is usually posteriorly into the vein of Galen, numerous alternative drainage routes are possible.

VENOUS SYSTEM (INFRATENTORIAL)

The posterior fossa venous system consists of three major groups. An anterior group drains into the petro-

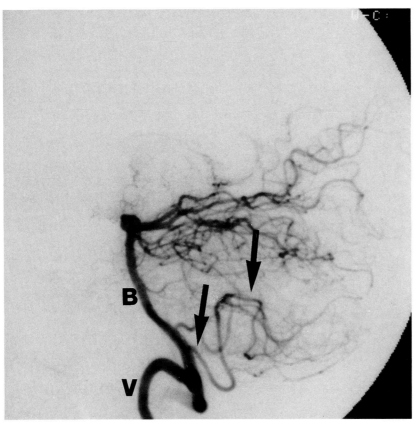

A

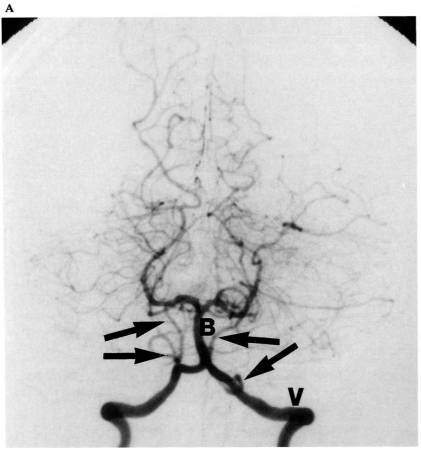

B

Fig. 2-9 Lateral (*A*) and Towne (*B*) projections of the vertebral (V) and basilar (B) arteries. Posterior inferior cerebellar arteries (arrows) arise from the vertebral arteries.

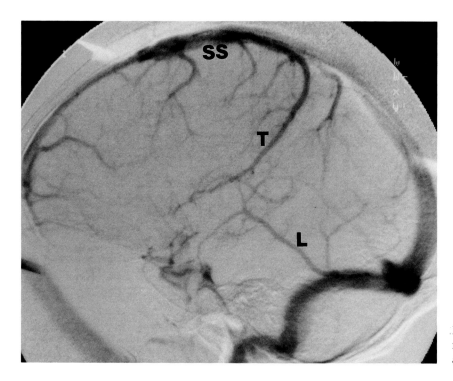

Fig. 2-10 Lateral view of the supratentorial venous system. Veins of Trolard (T) and Labbe (L). Superior sagittal sinus (SS).

sal sinus and consists of the anterior pontomesencephalic veins and the petrosal veins; a posterior group drains into the torcular Herophili and transverse sinuses and consists of the inferior vermian veins; and a superior group flows into the great vein of Galen and consists of the precentral cerebellar vein, the posterior mesencephalic veins, and the superior vermian veins (Fig. 2-12).

DURAL SINUSES

The superior sagittal sinus (SSS) lies within the dura at the attachment of the falx cerebri with the calvarium, at or close to the midline (Fig. 2-10). The venous lucunae, into which the arachnoid granulations drain, lies along the sides of the SSS and communicate with it. The SSS is variable in length but usually extends from the foramen cecum anteriorly to the torcular Herophili posteriorly. Sometimes the anterior origin of the SSS is located further posteriorly close to the coronal suture.[15] In about 30% of cases, the SSS may bypass the torcular Herophili and drain directly into one of the transverse sinuses, usually the right. In such a case the straight sinus empties into the left transverse sinus[16] (Fig. 2-11).

The cavernous sinus borders the sella turcica on both sides. It contains the carotid artery, as well as the third, fourth, sixth and third division of the fifth cranial nerves. Venous blood drains into it from the ophthalmic veins and sphenoparietal sinus. Blood flowing out of the cavernous sinus may drain into the superior petrosal sinus, inferior petrosal sinus, and/or pterygoid plexus.

CIRCULATION TIME AND SEQUENCE OF THE VENOUS SYSTEM

The average supratentorial circulation time is 3.43 ± 0.51 sec.[16,17] The infratentorial circulation time is about the same. The circulation time is influenced by the patient's age (younger patients have shorter circulation times than older patients), pH, blood pressure, blood volume, carbon dioxide and partial pressure (pCO_2). The resulting variability in circulation times decreases its value in calculating cerebral blood flow.

After an angiographic contrast injection, the superficial venous system fills from anterior to posterior. The frontal and middle cerebral veins usually fill first. The parietal veins usually fill after the frontal veins, and

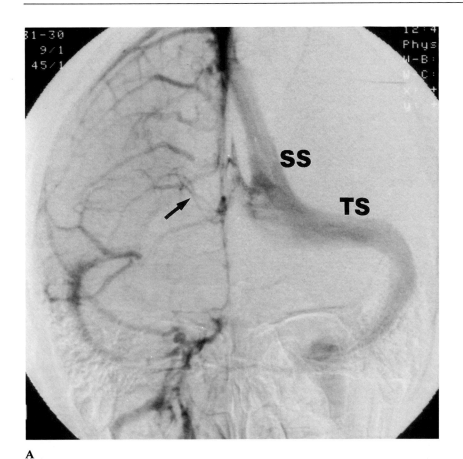

A

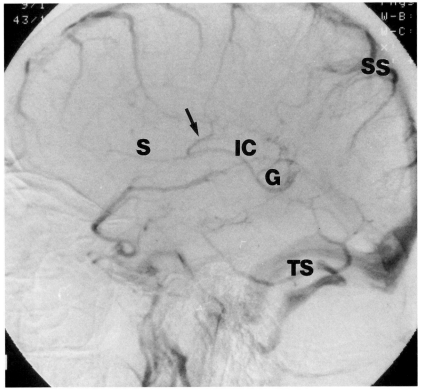

B

Fig. 2-11 Supratentorial venous system. (*A*) AP view. The superior sagittal sinus (SS) drains directly into the left transverse sinus (TS). Thalamostriate vein (arrow). (*B*) Lateral view. The deep system consists of the internal cerebral veins (IC) and the great vein of Galen (G), which drains into the straight sinus. The anterior septal (S) vein and the thalamostriate vein (arrow) drain into the internal cerebral vein.

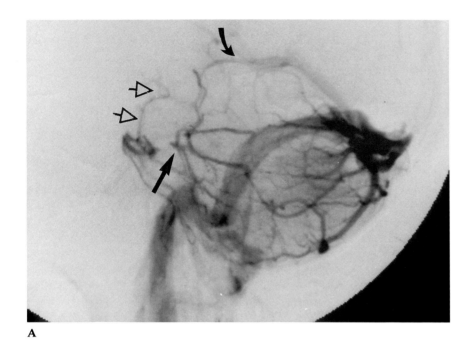

A

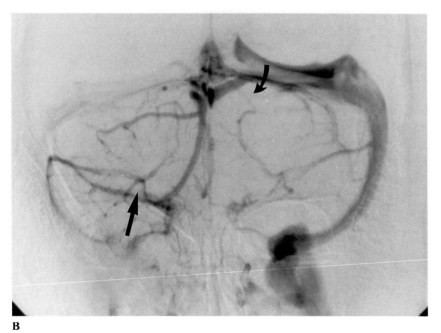

B

Fig. 2-12 Towne and lateral (*A*) and (*B*) views of the infratentorial venous systems. Anterior pontomesencephalic vein (open arrow). Petrosal vein (arrow). Posterior mesencephalic vein (curved arrow). Several hemispherical branches drain directly into the dural sinuses.

the occipital veins and veins of Labbe fill just before the vein of Trolard,[18] which usually is the last of the superficial veins to fill.

The blood flow in the deep system is slower because it drains mostly white matter (blood flow is slower in white matter). Consequently, the deep system opacifies later than the superficial system and continues to be opacified longer following a contrast injection. The sep-

tal vein drains only white matter; as a result, it is usually the last deep vein to opacify.

REFERENCES

1. Bosniak MA. An analysis of some anatomic-roentgenologic aspects of the brachiocephalic vessels. *AJR* 1964; 91:1222.

2. Williams GD, Edomonds HW. Variations in arrangement of the branches arising from aortic arch in American whites and negroes. *Anat Rec* 1935;62:139.

3. Sutton D, Davies ER. Arch aortography and cerebrovascular insufficiency. *Clin Radiol* 1966;17:330.

4. Parkinson D. Collateral circulation of cavernous carotid artery: Anatomy. *Can J Surg* 1964;7:251.

5. Wallace S, Goldberg HI, Leeds NE, et al. The cavernous branches of the internal carotid artery. *AJR* 1967;101:34.

6. Gabriele OF, Bell D. Ophthalmic origin of the middle meningeal artery. *Radiology* 1967;89:841.

7. Vignaud J, Hasso AN, Lasjaunias P, et al. Orbital vascular anatomy and embryology. *Radiology* 1974;111:617.

8. Taveras JM, Wood EW. *Diagnostic Neuroradiology.* Baltimore, Williams & Wilkins, 1964.

9. Riggs HE, Rupp C. Variation in forms of circle of Willis. The relation of the variations to collateral circulation: Anatomic analysis. *Arch Neurol* 1963;8:8.

10. LeMay M, Gooding CA. The clinical significance of the azygous anterior cerebral artery (A.C.A.). *AJR* 1966;98:602.

11. Gabrielsen TO, Greitz T. Normal size of the internal carotid middle cerebral and anterior cerebral arteries. *Acta Radiol [Diagn] (Stockh)* 1970;10:1.

12. Greitz T, Lauren T. Anterior meningeal branch of the vertebral artery. *Acta Radiol [Diagn] (Stockh)* 1968;7:219.

13. Stopford JSB. The arteries of the pons and medulla oblongata. *J Anat* 1916;50:131.

14. Takahashi M, Wilson G, Hanafee W. The anterior inferior cerebellar artery: Its radiographic anatomy and significance in the diagnosis of extra-axial tumors of the posterior fossa. *Radiology* 1968;90:281.

15. Kaplan HA, Browder AA, Browder J. Atresia of the rostral superior sagittal sinus: Associated cerebral venous patterns. *Neuroradiology* 1972;4:208.

16. Krayenbuhl HA, Yasargil MG. *Cerebral Angiography,* ed 2. London, Butterworth, 1968.

17. Leeds NE, Taveras JM. *Dynamic Factors in Diagnosis of Supratentorial Brain Tumors by Cerebral Angiography.* Philadelphia, WB Saunders, 1969.

18. Bub B, Ferris EJ, Levy PS, et al. The cerebral venogram: A statistical analysis of the sequence of venous filling in cerebral angiograms. *Radiology* 1968;91:111.

3

Cerebral Blood Flow

John Gilroy, M.D.

AUTOREGULATION

Autoregulation may be defined as the capacity of a circulation that maintains a constant blood flow over a wide range of perfusion pressure in any organ. Autoregulation of cerebral circulation was suggested for the first time in 1890 by Roy and Sherrington,[1] who postulated an intrinsic local chemical control of cerebral blood flow within the brain and stated: "The chemical products of cerebral metabolism contained in the lymph which bathes the walls of the arterioles of the brain can cause variations of the caliber of the cerebral vessels; . . . in this reaction the brain possesses an intrinsic mechanism by which its vascular supply can be varied locally in correspondence with local variations of functional activity." However, Roy and Sherrington were referring to local autoregulation by chemical change within the brain, a factor which may be imposed on general autoregulation of cerebral blood flow. This mechanism is a product of the Bayliss effect[2] described in 1902 by Bayliss, who stated that "the muscular coats of the arteries react like smooth muscle in other situations, to a stretching force by contraction. It also reacts to a diminution of tension by relaxation.[11] While Bayliss was not referring specifically to the cerebral circulation, this principle can be applied to the cerebral vessels and was confirmed in 1933 by Fog,[3] who demonstrated the Bayliss effect on the pial vessels viewed through a skull window. The concept of autoregulation of the cerebral circulation in response to changes in intraluminal pressure was established.

However, the cerebral circulation differs from circulation through other organs in that the circulation is occurring within a rigid structure which has an intrinsic pressure. Intracranial pressure, which is equivalent to extravascular pressure, can influence cerebral blood flow by acting on the walls of cerebral arteries, influencing perfusion pressure. A rise in intracranial pressure can increase pressure in cerebral veins so that perfusion pressure—the difference between intra-arterial pressure in arteries entering the subarachnoid space and the pressure in veins entering the dural sinuses—may be affected by a rise in intracranial pressure. However, pressure in the cerebral veins is maintained at a slightly higher level than intracranial pressure over a wide range of intracranial pressures as high as 100 mmHg,[4] and cerebral perfusion pressure can be defined as the difference between intra-arterial pressure and intracranial pressure over a wide range of intracranial pressure changes. A cerebral perfusion pressure between 50 and 130 mmHg is associated with a constant flow due to a reduction in the caliber of smaller cerebral arteries 0.5–1.0 mm in diameter.[5] A reduction in cerebral perfusion pressure within the same limits of 130 mmHg to 50 mmHg will result in dilatation of cerebral arteries maintaining a constant blood flow. However, observation of pial vessels has shown a differential response to mean arterial pressure changes. Larger vessels (200 μm or more in diameter) begin to dilate when the mean arterial pressure falls to 90 mmHg, while smaller vessels (less than 70 μm in diameter) dilate when the pressure falls below 60 mmHg.[6]

While the intrinsic myogenic mechanism in response to stretching of the arterial muscle is generally accepted as the basis for autoregulation,[7] as proposed by Bayliss, it is possible that changes in transmural pressure may be the key factor. The short latency of the response in autoregulation supports this concept since alterations in transmural pressure can produce changes in arteriolar responses within seconds.[6]

However, an attractive alternative hypothesis suggests that autoregulation is a metabolically mediated mechanism since adenosine concentrations in rat brain probably generated by perivascular astrocytes increase very rapidly in hypotension.[8] Adenosine is a patent cerebral vasodilator found in increasing concentrations in the brain as systemic arterial pressure falls; it may play a role in autoregulation in hypotensive states. This could be accomplished by reducing calcium influx through calcium channels in the cell membrane[9] or preventing calcium release from intracellular sites. The lower calcium iron concentration would reduce free calcium interaction with actinomycin complexes in the muscle cells in the arteriolar wall.[10]

Autonomic innervation does not appear to influence autoregulation under physiological conditions. Sympathic activity has no role in the control of cerebral blood flow during hypotension,[11] hypoxia,[12] or hypercapnia,[13] but it may promote vasoconstriction of large proximal cerebral arteries during acute severe hypertension, protecting smaller arterioles from damage.[14] Nevertheless, sympathetic stimulation is believed to elevate the limits of autoregulation toward higher pressures,[15] while acute sympathetic paralysis of denervation reduces the limits toward lower pressures.[16]

Parasympathetic activity may influence cerebral blood flow, and stimulation of parasympathetic projections to the cerebral vasculature increases cerebral blood flow.[17] It is possible that parasympathetic activity influences the development of collateral circulation during cerebral ischemia. In one study, the volume of cerebral infarction in rat brain increased by 30–50% following middle cerebral artery occlusion after chronic parasympathetic ablation.[18]

HYPERTENSION

The absolute level of cerebral blood flow is the same in healthy, normotensive individuals and in patients with essential hypertension.[19] Nevertheless, there is an increased risk of stroke in hypertension,[20] and treatment of hypertension is one of the major recommendations in prevention of stroke.[21] The fact that resting cerebral blood flow is the same in normotensive and hypertensive individuals indicates that vascular resistance must be higher in the hypertensive patient. This is in part due to morphological changes in cerebral arteries, with thickening of the media due to muscle cell hypertrophy and hyperplasia,[22] followed by degeneration of muscle cells and by deposition of hyaline material and fibrin.[23] Thus, while hypertension may lead to morphological changes in cerebral arteries, it is not the primary factor in the increased risk of stroke, whether the stroke is a result of cerebral infarction or cerebral hemorrhage. Cerebral blood flow is maintained in the hypertensive individual; it is the morphological changes in the cerebral arteries that result in the increased risk of both thrombosis and hemorrhage.

Changes in the larger vessels in hypertension, by increasing vascular resistance, impair tolerance to acute hypotension but improve tolerance to hypertension. Consequently, the upper and lower limits of autoregulation are shifted to higher levels of arterial blood pressure in the hypertensive individual.[24]

Adequate treatment of hypertension reverses the shift in autoregulation, and the lower limit of autoregulation moves to lower levels of arterial blood pressure.[25,26] This may be the result of a reversal of morphological changes in cerebral arteries, although they have been reported to be persistent,[27] suggesting that other mechanisms are responsible.

The upward shift in the limits of autoregulation is important in clinical practice since the rapid reduction of arterial blood pressure in the hypertensive patient to normotensive levels may induce cerebral ischemia. The risk is higher in acute stroke since autoregulation may be further impaired by several factors in this condition. Consequently, blood pressure should be controlled at high normal or low hypertensive levels in such cases. Similarly, chronic cerebrovascular disease and hypertension require gradual reduction of blood pressure, using mild antihypertensive agents to avoid a sudden reduction in arterial blood pressure to levels which may abolish autoregulation.[27,28]

The viscosity of blood alters blood flow in the cerebral circulation, with an increase in cerebral blood flow in anemia despite the arteriolar constriction which occurs following reduction of the baseline hematocrit.[29] Conversely, a rise in hematocrit in polycythemia vera is associated with a decrease in cerebral blood flow, which is partially compensated for by the increased oxygen-carrying capacity of the blood. However, reduced blood flow increases viscosity and may lead to temporary stasis in arterioles and capillaries.[30] On the other hand, the secondary polycythemia of emphysema is usually associated with normal cerebral blood flow since vasodilation occurs in response to increased cerebrovascular resistance resulting from increased viscosity.[31]

MODIFICATIONS OF AUTOREGULATION

Carbon dioxide reactivity is an important factor in the regulation of cerebral blood flow. A high arterial CO_2 tension ($PaCO_2$) causes vasodilatation; a low $PaCO_2$ tension results in vasoconstriction. $PaCO_2$ has an important role in the regulation of cerebral blood flow and cerebral blood volume. Carbon dioxide rapidly crosses the blood–brain barrier, inducing pH changes in the cerebrospinal fluid, which results in changes in cerebrovascular diameter.[32] The flow response induced by changes in arterial pCO_2 begins with 2 min and normal CO_2 reactivity in humans at approximately 3%/mmHg. However, prolonged changes in pCO_2 are countered by effective buffering systems which keep the pH in the cerebrospinal fluid (CSF) within narrow limits.[33] In sustained hyperventilation, the pH in the CSF returns to baseline within 24 hr, with return of vessel diameter to slightly above baseline.[34]

Changes in arterial oxygen tension (pO_2) have a much smaller effect on cerebral blood flow than alterations in pCO_2. This is due in part to the shape of the oxygen dissociation curve, and cerebral blood flow does not begin to increase until pO_2 has fallen below 50 mmHg. The increase does not occur in severe hypoglycemia, suggesting that lactic acid produced by anaerobic glycolysis causes a rise in extracellular H^+ concentration and an increase in cerebral blood flow in hypoxia.[35]

AGING

There has been no general agreement on changes in cerebral blood flow in normal aging. While autoregulation remains intact, several authors have reported a decline in cerebral blood flow; however, studies by others have not confirmed this finding. The results have varied when either the nitrous oxide technique,[36,37] 133XE inhalation,[38] or positron emission tomography (PET) scanning[23,39,40] has been utilized. It is possible that the discrepancies are the result of several factors, including the state of arousal, partial volume averaging, cerebral atrophy, or the presence of mild cerebrovascular disease.[41]

The significance of areas of increased signal intensity

in the deep cerebral white matter and the periventricular region seen on magnetic resonance imaging (MRI) studies in the elderly remains controversial. Many patients are neurologically intact,[42,43] but pathology studies have revealed arterial ectasia with enlargement of perivascular spaces or lacunar infarction in some cases.[44,45] The common factor is probably ischemia secondary to fibrinoid necrosis and lipohyalinosis of small, penetrating arteries supplying the deep cerebral white matter in the boundary zone of the arterial supply, which is more susceptible to ischemia.[42] Minor changes are unlikely to affect autoregulation and cerebral flow, whereas the diffuse changes in the cerebral white matter due to diffuse arteriolar involvement are likely to reduce in cerebral blood flow. Perhaps this accounts for some of the discrepancies among different studies of cerebral blood flow in older individuals.

DEMENTIA

Reduction in cerebral blood flow has been demonstrated in most cases of established dementia,[46] although cerebral blood flow may be normal in the early stages of Alzheimer's disease. Moderate or severe cases of Alzheimer's disease show global reduction of circulation blood flow, which is especially pronounced in the temporal and parietal lobes measured by single photon emission computed tomography (SPECT)[47] or PET.[48] In contrast, relative hypoperfusion occurs in the frontal and temporal lobes in Pick's disease.[49] Multiinfarct dementia is characterized by asymmetry of cerebral blood flow, with focal abnormalities.[35] Primary progressive aphasia shows hypoperfusion in the left inferior frontal, left temporal, and left parietal regions.[50]

THE EFFECT OF COLLATERAL CIRCULATION

The brain has an efficient system of collateral circulation which may affect both cerebral blood flow and autoregulation. The system occurs primarily at two levels. The circle of Willis has long been recognized as the ultimate example of collateral circulation at the base of the brain, allowing final distribution of blood in an even volume before the blood is circulated over and through the brain. While the circle of Willis is often incomplete and has many anatomical variants, it still provides a unique and vital collateral circulation in all of its many forms.

The intracerebral vasculature does not consist of rigid

anatomical compartments supplied by major vessels. The carotid artery system and the vertebral basilar system are not isolated vascular territories but communicate through a rich system of collateral vessels.

Since the circle of Willis forms the first major anatomical channel on the inflow pathway, an occlusion of significant (greater than 70%) stenosis of an internal carotid artery leads to increased perfusion of the ipsilateral hemisphere as blood from the opposite internal carotid artery is shunted through the anterior circle of Willis to the ischemic side. Retrograde flow from the external carotid system through the ophthalmic artery to the terminal internal carotid artery is another route of potential collateral flow when there is a reduction flow in the internal carotid artery. Another example of collateral flow in carotid insufficiency is the shunting of blood from the vertebral basilar system to the carotid system through the posterior communicating arteries.[51] Similarly, it is possible to demonstrate collateral flow from the carotid system through the posterior communicating arteries to the posterior cerebral arteries in the presence of vertebral-basilar insufficiency.

Areas supplied by the smaller intracerebral arteries such as the middle cerebral artery, anterior cerebral artery, or posterior cerebral arteries possess overlapping boundaries through a system of interdigitating arteries, arterioles, and capillaries. However, the boundaries or boundary zones (sometimes called *watershed zones*—a completely inaccurate use of the term) are not fixed in location but can vary, depending on functional needs. If, for example, there is a reduction in blood flow through the middle cerebral artery because of atherosclerosis and stenosis, the boundary zone between the posterior cerebral artery and the middle cerebral arteries will change and move toward the origin of the middle cerebral artery. There will be a similar adjustment to the boundary zone between the anterior cerebral artery and the middle cerebral artery. Thus the area of brain supplied by the diseased middle cerebral artery will contract. Consequently, an occlusion of the stenosed middle cerebral artery will result in an infarction which is situated closer to the origin of the middle cerebral artery and smaller than an unexpected occlusion of the middle cerebral artery by an embolism in a healthy individual. Consequently, a young patient with a previously healthy cerebral circulation tends to suffer a large cerebral infarction owing to cerebral embolism in the middle cerebral distribution. An elderly patient with multiple areas of narrowing in the carotid and middle cerebral arteries may have a smaller area of infarction at the time of occlusion because of a well-developed collateral supply. The relocation of the boundary zones and the decrease in size of relatively ischemic areas in the brain are gradual processes occurring over a period of months or years. Ultimately, a collateral circulation may provide the principal blood supply to an ischemic area, and loss of the primary arterial blood supply by thrombosis may be asymptomatic.

If this principle is accepted, cerebral infarction should be regarded as an infarction occurring in a recognized anatomical area of brain rather than in the territory of an arterial supply. It would be more accurate to describe a constellation of symptoms and signs as a stroke in an anatomical location rather than as occurring in a vascular territory. A good example of this principle is the *lateral medullary infarction,* the correct term for an infarction which is often called *posterior inferior cerebellar artery thrombosis.* In fact, this condition is associated with occlusion of the terminal portion of the ipsilateral vertebral artery in at least 50% of cases.[52]

The symptoms and signs of the most frequently encountered strokes are listed in Chapter 1. The appreciation of these findings should draw the attention of the neuroradiologist to a restricted area of the brain identified as the area of concern where an abnormality is likely to be located.

THE INFLUENCE OF PERIVASCULAR INNERVATION ON CEREBRAL BLOOD FLOW

Sympathetic innervation of cerebral vasculature originates in the superior cervical ganglion and is widely distributed to the internal carotid, external carotid, and vertebral basilar systems. The innervation seems to be richer in the carotid than in the vertebral basilar system. A second system originating in the locus coeruleus, which innervates the cerebral microvasculature, is also recognized. This system may be under the control of the paraventricular nucleus of the hypothalamus and may play a key role in migraine. The nerve fibers in both systems contain norepinephrine and neuropeptide Y as neurotransmitters, both of which produce potent constriction of cerebral vessels.

Parasympathetic innervation probably originates in the brain stem, with connections through the facial nerve to the sphenopalatine ganglion. Certainly there is a widespread distribution of parasympathetic fibers from the sphenopalatine ganglion to the cerebral vasculature. These fibers contain acetylcholine, which interacts with muscarinic receptors which subserve relaxation of cerebral vessels.

Another important system of serotinergic innervation also supplies cerebral vessels. This system originates in the median and dorsal raphe nuclei in the brain stem and is distributed in part through the superior cervical ganglion. There is also a more direct distribution from the brain stem to the pial vessels of the cerebral cortex. The 5-hydroxytryptamine released by stimulation of these fibers is an extremely potent vasoconstrictor and may have a more important role than norepinephrine in modifying the cerebral circulation.

The cerebral vasculature has a network of sensory fibers which contain substance P, calcitonin gene-related peptide (CGRP), vasoactive intestinal peptide, and neurokinin A, all of which have vasodilator properties but which are also concerned with afferent transmission of pain impulses from the blood vessels and the pia. This system is probably involved in the pathogenesis of headache.

FAILURE OF AUTOREGULATION

Acute Ischemic Cerebral Infarction

Acute cerebral infarction resulting from thromboembolism is associated with an immediate disturbance of autoregulation.[53] The occlusion of a major vessel by thrombosis in situ or embolism from the heart or major vessels results in a sudden reduction of blood flow distally and death of tissue. The infarcted area may be surrounded by a peripheral zone of reduced blood flow supplied by collateral vessels where the viability of the neurons depends upon the increased extraction of oxygen from the blood. This peripheral zone, or *penumbra*, is potentially salvageable if blood flow can be maintained or increased. Should this be the case, the neurons will survive and function will return in the penumbra once lysis of the occluded thrombus with migration of fragments has occurred and blood flow increases—often to a state of hyperemia[54] which can last for several days. Ultimately, the blood flow decreases again in response to the lower level of metabolism in the infarcted area.

It is apparent that the changes in cerebral blood flow which occur in acute cerebral infarction are essentially passive and that autoregulation is lost. Consequently, it is questionable whether hypertension should be treated in the patient with an acute stroke. In any case, hypertension often shows spontaneous reduction or resolution within a few days after a stroke, and vigorous treatment of hypertension in the early stages may lead to a decrease in perfusion in the penumbra and extension of the area of infarction.[55] The risk of accepting untreated hypertension is the theoretical transformation of an ischemic infarct into a hemorrhagic infarct, once lysis of the clot has occurred and the in-

farcted area is hyperemic, or the acceleration of edema in the surrounding tissue by the same mechanism.[56] One suggestion would be to leave the hypertension to decline spontaneously unless the diastolic pressure exceeds 120 mmHg[57] and to use a serial computed tomography (CT) scan[58] to monitor the infarcted area for the development of edema.

ACUTE HYPERTENSIVE ENCEPHALOPATHY

Hypertensive encephalopathy may be defined as a condition of severe headache and impaired intellectual functioning associated with a reduced level of consciousness or focal or generalized seizures in an individual with a sudden severe rise in blood pressure or malignant hypertension.[57] This usually implies the presence of grade 3 or grade 4 retinopathy, but papilledema (grade 4 retinopathy) is not a necessary requirement for the diagnosis of hypertensive encephalopathy.

The condition is associated with loss of autoregulation,[59] forced vasodilatation of arteries and arterioles, disruption of the blood–brain barrier, and brain edema.[60,61,62]

This is a medical emergency requiring immediate measures to lower the blood pressure to low hypertensive levels. This process allows the reestablishment of autoregulation and avoids relative hypotension and cerebral ischemia.[63]

MIGRAINE

The early phase of migraine is associated with a phase of spreading depression—a wave of abnormal electrical activity beginning in the occipital region and spreading anteriorly at a steady velocity of 2–3 mm/min. This condition, first described by Leao,[58] is accompanied by local hypoperfusion. Some studies have indicated impaired autoregulation in the affected cortex,[64] but spreading depression is now believed to be a primary neuronal phenomenon, with secondary reactive hypoperfusion and intact autoregulation.[56]

SUBARACHNOID HEMORRHAGE

Impaired autoregulation is a frequent accompaniment of subarachnoid hemorrhage.[65] This condition, which is caused by a rupture of a berry aneurysm in the majority of nontraumatic cases of subarachnoid hemorrhage, carries an overall mortality of 50%, with some degree of disability in 50% of the survivors.[53] Furthermore, 50% of cases of subarachnoid hemorrhage develop localized or generalized vasospasm with ischemic damage to the brain in the presence of a global impairment of autoregulation.[66] This may occur early and, while most severe during the first 7 days,[67] may persist for 3 weeks[68] or more in patients with a poor prognosis.

The current therapy of subarachnoid hemorrhage by hyperventilation, calcium channel blocking agents, and induced hypertension in the postoperative period remains a controversial issue at this time.

HYPERPERFUSION

Hyperperfusion, which can be a focal phenomenon or a generalized complication of brain dysfunction, has been described in a number of pathological conditions. Hyperperfusion is a feature of recovery from systemic hypotension and hypocapnia[69] and may follow even brief episodes of cerebral ischemia.[70] Hyperperfusion has been recognized during or following carotid endarterectomy[71] in cases of stenosis greater than 70%, with an associated reduction in cerebral blood flow.[72] The complication may occur during the surgical procedure, or there may be a delay of several days[73] before hyperperfusion is established. The risk is highest in patients with bilateral stenosis of the internal carotid arteries, unilateral occlusion with contralateral high-grade stenosis, or unilateral stenosis with poor cross-filling from the opposite carotid system.[75,76,77,78] Some 40% of patients develop intracerebral hemorrhage.[74]

The clinical features include unilateral headache in the frontal area involving the orbit and face, seizures, and cerebral edema with increased focal neurological deficits in cases complicated by intracerebral hemorrhage.[79,80]

In cerebral infarction, lysis of a thrombus or fragmentation and migration of embolic fragments leads to reperfusion of the ischemic area and results in hyperperfusion or intraparenchymal hemorrhage in some cases.[81] It is probable that most cases of circulation infarction exhibit hyperemia and hyperperfusion of variable degree at some time after onset.[82]

Increased cerebral blood flow begins within seconds during a generalized seizure.[32] Hyperperfusion is a feature of status epilepticus [83] and far exceeds the metabolic needs of the involved neurons.[84]

Other conditions associated with hyperperfusion include head injury where hyperemia has been associated with a poor prognosis.[85] Surgical obliteration of an arteriovenous malformation may be followed by severe hyperperfusion of the previously ischemic brain surrounding the area of the malformation secondary to an abrupt closure of a shunting mechanism.[86,87] Severe cerebral edema and hemorrhage can occur in such cases.[88]

Occasionally, removal of a large mass lesion such as a meningioma or subdural hematoma can result in focal hyperperfusion. The condition can also occur in a more generalized form during recovery from cardiac arrest[89] and bacterial meningitis.[90]

Ischemia is associated with the release of vasoactive metabolites including lactic acid, adenosine, and free oxygen radicals, all of which can contribute to hyperperfusion.[91,92,93,94] However, the common factor in the rather diverse conditions associated with hyperperfusion seems to lie in the periventricular sensory neurons, which may have the capacity to influence the regulation of cerebral blood flow.[95,96,97] These sensory nerve fibers contain several polypeptides, including substance P, CGRP, vasoactive intestinal peptide, and neurokinin A. The most potent vasodilator in this group is CGRP, which may act by producing vasodilatation through an axonal reflex mechanism, although other vasoactive substances such as adenosine triphosphate[10,98] or adenosine[99] could mediate a similar response.[54]

HEAD INJURY

Head trauma is associated with cerebral arterial vasospasm in 61–85% of cases.[100,101,102] The changes are similar to those observed in subarachnoid hemorrhage but also have been seen in head trauma patients without hemorrhage.[100] Vasospasm can occur within 24 hr of the traumatic event but may be delayed for several days in some cases. Delayed onset of arterial spasm tends to be associated with a milder clinical course. However, vasospasm and loss of autoregulation after head injury[103] is not a uniform finding and may be a response to more than one mechanism.

Hyperemia and loss of autoregulation may occur within the first few days following severe head injury, or may follow a period of vasospasm and the development of increased intracranial pressure, which is closely associated with the development of hyperemia.[85] However, the relationship is not a uniform feature of all cases of head injury, and further studies are needed to clarify the changes following head trauma and to develop a rational approach to therapy.[104]

REFERENCES

1. Roy CS, Sherrington CS. On the regulation of the blood supply of the brain. *J Physiol* 1890;11:85–108.

2. Bayliss WM. On the local reactions of the arterial wall to changes of internal pressure. *J Physiol (Lond)* 1902; 28:220–231.

3. Fog M. Influence of intracranial hypertension upon the cerebral circulation. *Act Psychiatr Neurol* 1933;8: 191–198.

4. Meyer JS, Gilroy J. Regulation and adjustment of the cerebral circulation. *Diseases of the Chest* 1968;53:30–37.

5. Johnston IH, Rowan JO. Raised intracranial pressure and cerebral blood flow. 3. Venous outflow tract pressures and vascular resistance in experimental intracranial hypertension. *J Neurol Neurosurg Psychiatry* 1974; 37:392–402.

6. Kontos HA, Wei EP. Responses of cerebral arteries and arterioles to acute hypotension and hypertension. *Am J Physiol* 1978;234:H371–H383.

7. Bevan JA, Hiva JJ. Myogenic tone and cerebrovascular autoregulation: The role of a stretch dependent mechanism. *J Biomed Eng* 1985;13:281–286.

8. Winn HR, Welsh JE, Rubio R, et al. Brain adenosine production in rat during sustained alteration in systemic blood pressure. *Am J Physiol* 1980;239:H636–H641.

9. Fenton RA, Bruttig SP, Rubio R, et al. Effect of adenosine on calcium uptake by intact and cultured vascular smooth muscle. *Am J Physiol* 1982;242:H797–H804.

10. Kovach AGB, Dora E, Szedlacsek S, et al. Effect of the calcium antagonist D-600 on cerebrovascular, cortical vascular and redox responses evoked by adenosine, anoxia and epilepsy. *J Cereb Blood Flow Metab* 1983;3: 51–61.

11. Edvinsson L, Mackenzie ET, Robert JP, et al. Cerebrovascular responses to hemorrhagic hypotension in anesthetized cats. Effects of alpha adrenoceptor antagonists. *Acta Physiol Scand* 1985;123:317–323.

12. Edvinsson L. Innervation of cerebral circulation. *Ann NY Acad Sci* 1987;519:334–348.

13. Mueller SM, Heistad DD, Marcus ML. Total and regional cerebral blood flow during hypotension, hypertension and hypocapnia. Effect of sympathetic denervation in dogs. *Circ Res* 1977;41:350–356.

14. Bill A, Linder J. Sympathetic control of cerebral blood flow in acute arterial hypertension. *Acta Physiol Scand* 1976;13:259–265.

15. Faraci FM, Heistad DD. Regulation of large cerebral arteries and cerebral microvascular pressure. *Circ Res* 1990;66:8–17.

16. Fitch W, MacKenzie ET, Harper AM. Effects of decreasing arterial blood pressure on cerebral blood flow in the baboon. Influence of the sympathetic nervous system. *Circ Res* 1975;37:550–557.

17. Pinard E, Purves MJ, Sezlag J, et al. The cholinergic pathway to cerebral blood vessels. II. Physiological studies. *Pflugers Arch* 1979;379:165–172.

18. Kano M, Moskowitz MA, Yokota A. Parasympathetic denervation of pial vessels significantly increases infarction volume following middle cerebral artery occlusion. *J Cereb Blood Flow Metab* 1991;11:628–637.

19. Kety SS, Hafkenscheil JH, Jeffries WA, et al. The blood flow, vascular resistance and oxygen consumption of the brain in essential hypertension. *J Clin Invest* 1948; 27:511–514.

20. Wolf PA, Kannel WB, Verter J. Current status of risk factors for stroke. *Neurol Clin* 1983;1:317–343.

21. Medical Research Council Working Party. MCR trial of treatment of mild hypertension: Principal results. *Br Med J* 1985;291:97–104.

22. Hart MN, Heistad DD, Brody MS. Effect of chronic hypertension and sympathetic denervation on wall/lumin ratio of cerebral vessels. *Hypertension* 1980;2:419–423.

23. DeLeoni MJ, George AE, Ferris SH, et al. Positron emission tomography and computed tomography assessments of the aging human brain. *J Comput Assist Tomogr* 1984;8:88–94.

24. Strandgaard S, Jones JV, Mackenzie ET, et al. Upper limit of cerebral blood flow autoregulation in the baboon with experimental renovascular hypotension. *Circ Res* 1975;37:164–167.

25. Hoffman JE, Miletich DJ, Albracht RF. The influence of antihypertensive therapy on cerebral autoregulation in aged hypertensive rats. *Stroke* 1982;13:701–704.

26. Strandgaard S. Autoregulation of cerebral blood flow in hypertensive patients. The modifying influence of prolonged antihypertensive treatment on the tolerance to acute drug induced hypotension. *Circulation* 1976; 53:720–727.

27. Barry DI, Lassen NA. Cerebral blood flow autoregulation in hypertension and effects of antihypertensive drugs. *J Hypertens* 1984;Suppl 3:519–526.

28. Barry DI. Influence of antihypertensive drugs on cerebral blood flow. *Am J Cardiol* 1989;63:14C–18C.

29. Hudak ML, Jones MD, Popiel AS, et al. Hemodilution causes size dependent constriction of peal arterioles in the cat. *Am J Physiol* 1989;257:H912–H917.

30. Thomas DJ. Whole blood viscosity and cerebral blood flow. *Stroke* 1982;13:285–287.

31. Wade JPH. Transport of oxygen in the brain in patients with elevated hematocrit values before and after venessection. *Brain* 1983;106:513–523.

32. Lassen NA. Control of cerebral circulation in health and disease. *Circ Res* 1974;34:749–760.

33. Siesjo BK. The regulation of cerebrospinal fluid pH. *Kidney Int* 1972;1:360–374.

34. Muizelaar JP, Van Dar Pool H, Li Z, et al. Pial arteriolar vessel diameter and CO_2 reactivity during prolonged

hyperventilation in the rabbit. *J Neurosurg* 1988;69:923–927.

35. Robertson CS, Goodman JC, Grossman RG. Blood flow and metabolic therapy in CNS injury. *J Neurotrauma* 1992;9(Suppl 2):5579–5594.

36. Kety SS. Human cerebral blood flow and oxygen consumption as related to aging. *J Chronic Dis* 1956;3:478–486.

37. Kety SS, Schmidt CF. The nitrous oxide method for the quantitative determination of cerebral blood flow in man: Theory, procedure and normal values. *J Clin Invest* 1948;27:476–483.

38. Yamamoto M, Meyer JS, Sakai F, et al. Aging and cerebral vasodilator response to hypercarbia. *Arch Neurol* 1980;38:488–496.

39. Kuhl DE, Metter EJ, Reige WH, et al. Effects of human aging on patterns of local cerebral glucose utilization determined by the (18 F) fluorodeoxyglucose method. *J Cereb Blood Flow Metab* 1982;2:163–171.

40. Yamaguchi T, Kanno I, Uemura K, et al. Reduction in the regional cerebral metabolic rate of oxygen during human aging. *Stroke* 1986;17:1220–1228.

41. Goldstein S, Reivich M. Cerebral blood flow and metabolism in aging and dementia. *Clin Neuropharmacol* 1991;14(Suppl):S34–S44.

42. Dreyer BP. Imaging of the aging brain, Part 1. Normal findings. *Radiology* 1988;166:785–796.

43. Gerard G, Weisberg LA. MRI periventricular lesions in adults. *Neurology* 1986;36:998–1001.

44. Awad IA, Johnson PC, Spetzler RF, et al. Incidental subcortical lesions identified on magnetic resonance imaging in the elderly II. Postmortem pathological correlations. *Stroke* 1986;17:1090–1097.

45. Awad IA, Spetzler RF, Hodok JA, et al. Incidental subcortical lesions identified on magnetic resonance imaging in the elderly I. Correlation with age and cerebrovascular risk factors. *Stroke* 1986;17:1084–1089.

46. Prohovnik I, Mayeux R, Sackeim HA, et al. Cerebral perfusion as a diagnostic marker of early Alzheimer's disease. *Neurology* 1988;38:931–937.

47. Smith FW, Besson JAO, Gemmell HG, et al. The use of Technetium-99m-HM-PAO in the assessment of patients with dementia and other neuropsychiatric conditions. *J Cereb Blood Flow Metab* 1988;8:S116–S122.

48. Jaimieson DG, Chawluk B, Alawi A, et al. The effect of disease severity on local glucose metabolism in Alzheimer's disease. *J Cereb Blood Flow Metab* 1987;7:S410.

49. Kamo H, McGreer PL, Harrop R, et al. Positron emission tomography and histopathology in Pick's disease. *Neurology* 1987;37:439–445.

50. Chawluk JB, Mesulam M-M, Hurtig H, et al. Slowly progressive aphasia without generalized dementia: Studies with positron emission tomography. *Ann Neurol* 1986;19:68–74.

51. Petty GW, Wiebers DO, Meissner I. Transcranial Doppler ultrasonography: Clinical applications in cerebrovascular disease. *Mayo Clin Proc* 1990;65:1350–1364.

52. Gilroy J. *Basic Neurology* New York, McGraw-Hill 1990, p 144.

53. Philips LH, Whemant JP, O'Fallon WM. Unchanged patterns of subarachnoid hemorrhage in a community. *Neurology* 1980;3:1034–1040.

54. MacFarlane R, Moskowitz MA, Sales DE, et al. The role of neuroeffector mechanisms in cerebral hyperfusion syndromes. *J Neurosurg* 1991;75:845–855.

55. Yatsu FM, Zivin J. Hypertension in acute stroke. Not to treat. *Arch Neurol* 1985;42:999–1000.

56. Spence JD, del Maestro RF. Hypertension in acute ischemic stroke. Treat. *Arch Neurol* 1985;42:1000–1002.

57. Strandgaard S, Paulson OB. Regulation of cerebral blood flow in health and disease. *J Cardiovasc Dis* 1992;19(Suppl 6):S89–S93.

58. Symon L. Pathological regulation in cerebral ischemia in cerebral blood flow: Pathologic and clinical aspects, in JH Wood (ed), New York, McGraw-Hill, 1987.

59. Strandgaard S, Oleson J, Skinhoj E, et al. Autoregulation of brain circulation in severe arterial hypertension. *Br Med J* 1973;1:507–510.

60. Baumbach GL, Heistad DD. Heterogeneity of brain blood flow and permeability during acute hypertension. *Am J Physiol* 1985;249:H629–637.

61. Lassen NA, Agnoli A. The upper limit of autoregulation of cerebral blood flow—on the pathogenesis of hypertensive encephalopathy. *Scand J Clin Invest* 1973;30:113–116.

62. Strandgaard S, MacKenzie ET, Sengupta D, et al. Upper limit for autoregulation of cerebral blood flow in the baboon with experimental renovascular hypertension. *Circ Res* 1974;34:435–440.

63. Jensen H, Ring-Larsen H, Garsdal P, et al. Carotid artery stenosis exposed by an adverse effect of captopril. *Br Med J* 1986;293:1073–1074.

64. Paulson OB. Cerebral apoplexy (stroke) pathogenesis, pathophysiology and therapy as illustrated by regional blood flow measurements in the brain. *Stroke* 1971;2:327–360.

65. Grubb RL, Raichle ME, Eichling JO. Effects of subarachnoid hemorrhage on cerebral blood flow volume, blood flow and oxygen utilization in humans. *J Neurosurg* 1977;46:446—453.

66. Heros RC, Zervas NT, Varsos V. Cerebral vasospasm after subarachnoid hemorrhage. An update. *Ann Neurol* 1983;14:599–608.

67. Weir B, Grace M, Hansen J, et al. Time course of vasospasm in man. *J Neurosurg* 1978;48:173–178.

68. Meyer CA, Lowe D, Meyer M, et al. Progressive changes in cerebral blood flow during the first three weeks after subarachnoid hemorrhage. *Neurosurgery* 1983; 12:58–76.

69. Symon L, Ganz JC, Dorsch NWC. Experimental studies of hyperaemic phenomena in the cerebral circulation of primates. *Brain* 1972;95:265–278.

70. Gourley JK, Heistad DD. Characteristics of reactive hyperemia in the cerebral circulation. *Am J Physiol* 1984; 146:H52—H58.

71. Sundt TM Jr, Sharbrough FW, Piepgrass DG, et al. Correlation of cerebral blood flow and electroencephalic changes during carotid endarterectomy. With results of surgery and hemodynamics of cerebral ischemia. *Mayo Clin Proc* 1981;56:533–543.

72. Russel D, Dybevold S, Kjartansson O, et al. Cerebral vasoactivity and blood flow before and three months after carotid endarterectomy. *Stroke* 1990;21:1029–1032.

73. Bernstein M, Fleming JFR, Deck JHN. Cerebral hyperperfusion after endarterectomy: A cause of cerebral hemorrhage. *Neurosurgery* 1984;15:50–56.

74. Pomposelli FB, Lamparello PJ, Riles TS, et al. Intracranial hemorrhage after carotid endarterectomy. *J Vasc Surg* 1988;7:248–255.

75. Reigel MM, Holker LH, Sundt TM Jr, et al. Cerebral hyperperfusion syndrome: A cause of neurologic dysfunction after endarterectomy. *J Vasc Surg* 1987;5: 628–634.

76. Solomon RA, Loftus CM, Quest DO, et al. Incidence and etiology of intracerebral hemorrhage following carotid endarterectomy. *J Neurosurg* 1986;64:29–34.

77. Sundt TM Jr. The ischemic tolerance of neural tissue and the need for monitoring and selective shunting during carotid endarterectomy. *Stroke* 1983;14:93–98.

78. Sundt TM Jr, Sandok BA, Whissant JP. Carotid endarterectomy. Complications and pre-operative assessment of risk. *Mayo Clin Proc* 1975;50:301–306.

79. Dolan JG, Mushlin AI. Hypertensive vascular headaches and seizures after carotid endarterectomy. Case report and therapeutic considerations. *Arch Intern Med* 1984;144:1489–1491.

80. Messert B, Black JA. Cluster headaches, hemicrania and other head pains. Morbidity of carotid endarterectomy. *Stroke* 1978;9:559–562.

81. Olson TS, Lassen NA. A dynamic concept of middle cerebral artery occlusion and cerebral infarction in the acute state based on interpreting severe hyperemia as a sign of embolic migration. *Stroke* 1984;15:458–468.

82. Olson TS, Larsen B, Skriver EB, et al. Focal cerebral hyperemia in acute stroke. Incidence, pathophysiology and clinical significance. *Stroke* 1981;12:598–607.

83. Franck G, Sadzot B, Salmon E, et al. Regional cerebral blood flow and metabolic rates in human focal epilepsy and status epilepticus. *Adv Neurol* 1986;44:935–948.

84. Ingvar M. Cerebral blood flow and metabolic rate during seizures. Relationship to epileptic brain damage. *Ann NY Acad Sci* 1986;462:194–206.

85. Obrist WD, Gennorelli TA, Segawa H, et al. Relation of cerebral blood flow to neurological status and outcome in head-injured patients. *J Neurosurg* 1979;51: 292–300.

86. Batzer HH, Devous MD Sr, Seibert JB, et al. Intracranial arteriovenous malformation: Relationship between clinical and radiographic factors and ipsilateral steal severity. *Neurosurgery* 1988;23:322–328.

87. Mullan S, Brown FD, Patrones NJ. Hyperemic and ischemic problems of surgical treatment of arteriovenous malformations. *J Neurosurg* 1979;51:757–764.

88. Spetzer RF, Wilson CB, Weinstein, et al. Normal perfusion pressure breakthrough theory. *Clin Neurosurg* 1978;25:651–672.

89. Beckstead JE, Tweed WA, Lee J, et al. Cerebral blood flow and metabolism in man following cardiac arrest. *Stroke* 1978;9:569–573.

90. Tauber MG. Brain edema, intracranial pressure and cerebral blood flow in bacterial meningitis. *Pediatr Infect Dis* 1989;8:915–917.

91. Berne RM, Rubio R, Curnish RR. Release of adenosine from ischemic brain. Effect on cerebral vascular resistance and incorporation into cerebral adenine nucleotides. *Cir Res* 1974;35:262–271.

92. Kontos HA. Oxygen radicals in cerebral vascular injury. *Circ Res* 1985;57:508–516.

93. Wei EP, Ellison MD, Kontos HA, et al. O_2 radicals in arachidonate-induced increased blood-brain barrier permeability to proteins. *Am J Physiol* 1986;251: H693–H699.

94. Wei EP, Kontos HA. Oxygen radicals in cerebral ischemia (abstract). *Physiologist* 1987;30:122.

95. MacFarlane R, Tasdemeroghe E, Moskowitz MA, et al. Chronic trigeminal ganglionectomy or topical copsiacin application to pial vessels attenuates postocclusive hyperemia but does not influence postischemic hypoperfusion. *J Cereb Blood Flow Metab* 1991;11:261–271.

96. Moskowitz MA, Sakos DE, Wei EP, et al. Postocclusive cerebral hyperemia is markedly attenuated by chronic trigeminal ganglionectomy. *Am J Physiol* 1989;257: H1736–H1739.

97. Sakes DE, Moskowitz MA, Wei EP, et al. Trigeminovascular fibers increase blood flow in cortical gray matter by axon reflex-like mechanisms during acute severe hypertension or seizures. *Proc Natl Acad Sci USA* 1989;86: 1401–1405.

98. Berne RM, Rubio R, Curnish RR. Release of adenosine from ischemic brain. Effect on cerebral vascular resistance and incorporation into cerebral adenine nucleotides. *Neurosurgery* 1984;15:50–56.

99. Fredholm BB, Henquist P. Modulation of neurotrans-

mission by purine nucleotides and nucleosides. *Biochem Pharmacol* 1980;29:1635–1643.

100. Goraj B, Rifkinson-Mann S, Leslie DR, et al. Cerebral blood flow velocity after head injury: Transcranial Doppler evaluation. *Radiology* 1993;188:137–141.

101. Sanker P, Richard KE, Weigl HC, et al. Transcranial Doppler sonography and intracranial pressure monitoring in children and juveniles with acute brain injuries of hydrocephalus. *Child Nerv Syst* 1991;7:391–393.

102. Weber M, Grolemund P, Seiler RW. Evaluation of posttraumatic cerebral blood flow velocities in trans-cranial Doppler ultrasonography. *Neurosurgery* 1990; 27:106–112.

103. Kwan-Hon Chan, Miller JD, Deardon NM, et al. The effect of changes in cerebral perfusion pressure upon middle cerebral artery blood flow velocity and jugular venous oxygen saturation after severe brain injury. *J Neurosurg* 1992;77:55–61.

104. Bouma GJ, Muizelaar JP. Cerebral blood flow, cerebral blood volume, and cerebrovascular reactivity after severe head injury. *J Neurotrauma* 1992;9(Suppl 1): S333–S348.

4

Cerebrovascular Pathology

T. Edgar Huang, M.D.

Diseases of the cerebral blood vessels, i.e. cerebrovascular diseases, encompass a wide variety of lesions that often have an abrupt disease onset and cause considerable morbidity and mortality.[1-3] During the acute stages, the initiating disease process often elicits a strong reaction in the surrounding brain, resulting in a space-occupying lesion. This may lead to shifting and displacement of the brain and blood vessels in the rigid intracranial cavity, causing further tissue damage and even death. When a patient survives the acute episode, a variable and often unpredictable degree of recovery ensues, with residual morbidity. Cerebrovascular diseases have now become the third leading cause of death in the United States after heart diseases and cancers. The cost of continuing care for the disabled survivors is also escalating at an astronomical pace.

Of particular interest to diagnostic angiographers are the occlusive vascular diseases and intracranial hemorrhage, with lesions including aneurysms and vascular malformations. The resulting infarct or hemorrhage in the brain shows a territorial or diffuse distribution. Structural shifting and secondary brain changes are common. With the advent of selective interventional angiography, the natural progression of some of these diseases may sometimes be ameliorated or even averted early.

OCCLUSIVE VASCULAR DISEASES
(Table 4-1)

Arterial Occlusion

Atherosclerosis and arteriosclerosis are among the common causes of arterial occlusion in the central nervous system.[4] Intracranial arteries and extracranial neck arteries are often involved in atherosclerosis. The severity does not always parallel that seen in the systemic blood vessels such as the aorta and the limb arteries. Certain anatomical sites of predilection are usually more severely affected. The end results of arterial occlusions are infarcts that are often definable by the arteries involved (Table 4-2).

Carotid Artery and Vertebral Artery[4-6]
Atherosclerosis of the carotid artery is most severe at the bifurcation and carotid sinus, a consequence of the special hemodynamic status in the area. As the atherosclerotic plaque grows, there is gradual narrowing of the lumen. Ulceration with thrombus formation, sometimes associated with hemorrhage in the plaque, and dissection of the arterial wall may cause sudden exacerbation of the stenosis.[7] Before the artery is completely occluded, the patient may experience episodic transient ischemic attacks, without demonstrable structural changes in the brain. Small infarcts can result from distal migration of dislodged emboli. Large hemispheric infarcts eventually develop as the occlusion of the internal carotid artery becomes complete. The inferior surface of the temporal lobe and the occipital pole may be spared, for these areas derive their blood supply mainly from the posterior circulation.

Atherosclerosis of the vertebral artery is less common, and complete occlusion is rare.[8] Unilateral occlusion of the vertebral artery may be asymptomatic if the collateral circulation is adequate. When the contralateral vertebral artery is hypoplastic, large infarcts in the brain supplied by the posterior circulation may result.

TABLE 4-1   Occlusive Cerebrovascular Diseases

Arterial occlusion
  Atherosclerosis with thrombosis
    Carotid and vertebral arteries
    Circle of Willis
  Embolism and thromboembolism
    Left atrium
    Vulvular vegetation
    Mural thrombus
    Paradoxical embolus
    Fat
    Cholesterol crystal
    Air
    Infected embolus
    Tumor
  Inflammatory disease of the cerebral artery
    Infection
    Collagen vascular disease
    Hypersensitivity
    Drug induced
    Idiopathic
      Primary central nervous system vasculitis
      Moyamoya disease
      Giant cell arteritis
  External compression
    Cerebral herniation
      Subfalcian—anterior cerebral artery
      Uncal and parahippocampal—posterior cerebral
        artery
      Cerebellar tonsillar—posterior inferior cerebellar
        artery
      Axial and caudal—basilar artery
    Osteoarthritic bony spur
    Strangulation
  Arterial dissection
    Thoracic aortic dissection
    Ulceration of atherosclerotic plaque
    Marfan's syndrome
  Vasospasm
    Subarachnoid hemorrhage
    Infection
    Drug abuse
    Trauma
    Idiopathic
Venous occlusion
  Thrombosis of the cerebral vein and sinus
    Cachexia in infants
    Hypercoagulative state
    Polycythemia
    Infection
    Idiopathic
  Compression or invasion by tumor

TABLE 4-2   Effects of Occlusive Cerebrovascular Disease

Hypoxic-ischemic encephalopathy
  Selective vulnerability
    Cerebral cortex—pseudolamilar necrosis
    Ammon's horn—Sommer's sector
    Cerebellum—Purkinje cell
  Boundary zone necrosis—watershed
Infarction
  Arterial
  Venous
Respirator brain necrosis

Intracranial Arteries in the Circle of Willis[9]
Symptomatic intracranial atherosclerosis is almost always limited to the basilar artery. Hardening and thickening of the arterial wall, atheromatous plaque deposits, vascular ectasia, and accentuated tortuosity occur. At times, these conditions may lead to the formation of a fusiform atherosclerotic aneurysm. When occlusion of the blood vessels becomes severe, infarction of the areas they supply may result.[10–17] Atheromatous plaques in the arterial branches distal to the Circle of Willis may occasionally be seen.

Embolism and thromboembolism are important causes of cerebral infarcts.[18] Bland emboli may arise from the atrium in atrial fibrillation. Valvular vegetation from bacterial infection or rheumatic valvulitis may be carried to the brain.[19] Acute myocardial infarction with mural thrombi may give rise to fibrin emboli[20] (Fig. 4-1). Paradoxical emboli arising in the pulmonary circulation may reach the brain through an atrial or ventricular septal defect. Open fracture and decompression sickness can cause fat, cholesterol, or air embolism.[21–25] Infection of the face around the nose may pass infective material intracranially through the venous plexus. Intravascular or intracardiac tumors such as myxoma rarely may lead to embolization.[26]

Despite elaborate anastomoses in the cerebral arteries, when an artery is occluded, the collateral circulation may not be sufficient to keep up with the metabolic requirement. A definable territorial distribution of arterial infarction follows. Anatomical variation in the arterial trees may modify the actual outcome.

Complete occlusion of the internal carotid artery causes ipsilateral cerebral hemispheric infarction, sparing the basal temporal lobe and the occipital pole. Anterior cerebral artery occlusion causes cingulate gyrus and frontal pole infarcts (Fig. 4-2). Middle cerebral artery occlusion causes infarction of most of the lateral

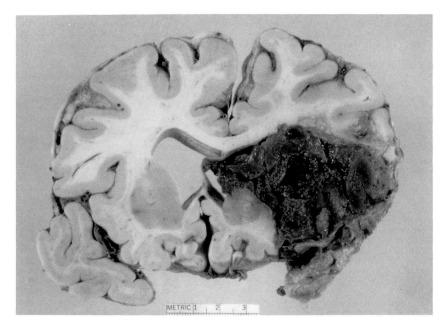

Fig. 4-1 Massive hemorrhagic infarct secondary to acute myocardial infarction with mural thrombosis and complete embolic occlusion of the right middle cerebral artery.

surface of the cerebral hemisphere and the deep gray matter, including the thalamus and the basal ganglia (Figs. 4-3, 4-4). Posterior cerebral artery occlusion causes temporo-occipital infarcts. Vertebrobasilar occlusion leads to pontine infarcts (Fig. 4-5). Occlusion of more distal branches of the cerebral arteries causes smaller, limited foci of infarction. Posterior inferior cerebellar artery occlusion is responsible for lateral medullary and cerebellar infarcts with a characteristic clinical presentation (Wallenberg syndrome).

Inflammatory diseases of the intracranial arteries may cause damage to the vessel, with thickening of the wall and thrombotic occlusion of the lumen. Infections, collagen vascular diseases, hypersensitivity, and drug-induced vasculitis may be responsible.[27–30] Idiopathic disorders such as primary central nervous system vas-

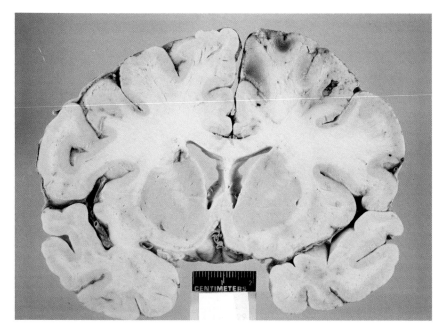

Fig. 4-2 Acute cerebral infarct due to complete thrombotic occlusion of the right anterior cerebral artery.

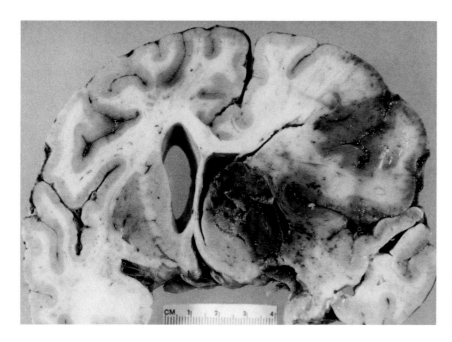

Fig. 4-3 Complete right middle cerebral artery occlusion with massive acute infarct, midline shift, and subfalcian and transtentorial herniation.

culitis,[31–35] moyamoya disease,[36–39] and giant cell arteritis[40,41] often cause arterial occlusion and infarction in addition to their characteristic clinical presentation.

Direct extrinsic compression of the cerebral arteries, if prolonged, may compromise the blood supply sufficiently to cause infarction.[42–44] Direct compression by a tumor or herniated brain tissue is often responsible for arterial compression. Thus, an ipsilateral cingulate gyrus infarct may result from subfalcian herniation and

compression of the anterior cerebral artery. Uncal and parahippocampal herniations may compress the posterior cerebral artery, leading to infarction of the temporal and occipital lobes (Figs. 4-6, 4-7A). Acoustic neuroma may compress the anterior inferior cerebellar artery directly. Cerebellar tonsillar herniation may compress the posterior inferior cerebellar artery, with cerebellar and medullary infarcts (Fig. 4-7B). Axial and caudal herniation of the thalamus and the midbrain

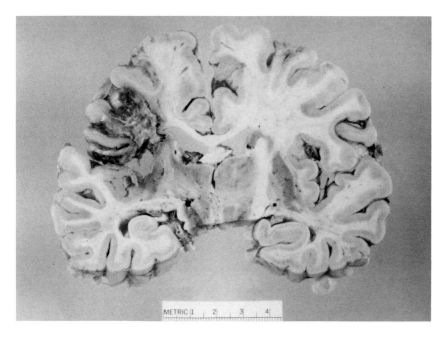

Fig. 4-4 Chronic cerebral infarct with a cystic cavity due to severe atherosclerosis of the left middle cerebral artery.

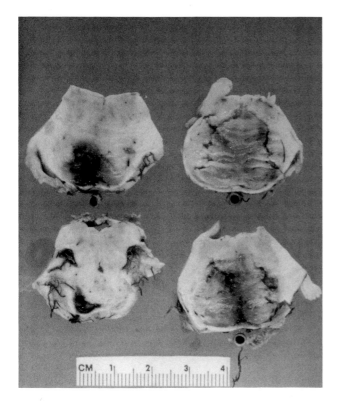

Fig. 4-5 Basilar artery thrombosis with extensive pontine infarct.

may stretch and compress the basilar artery, with resultant central brain stem infarcts (Duret's hemorrhage). Osteoarthritic spurs in cervical spines may impinge on the vertebral artery and compromise the blood flow. Strangulation is the extreme form of extrinsic compression; it may lead to extensive brain damage if the victim survives.

Arterial dissection caused by extension of thoracic aortic dissection, ulceration of atheromatous plaques, or Marfan's syndrome may compress and occlude the arterial lumens significantly.[45–47] Persistent arterial vasospasm, whether secondary to subarachnoid hemorrhage, infection, drug abuse, trauma, or idiopathic, also may be sufficient to cause infarction of the brain.[48]

Venous Occlusion

The blood circulation in the cerebral veins and the venous sinuses is a low-pressure, slow-flow system. Alteration in the hemodynamic pattern or constitutional components of the blood may cause thrombus formation and gradual or sudden occlusion of the venous channels. Severe dehydration in cachexia, the hypercoagulative state in the postpartum period, and polycythemia are the major causes.[49–54] Intracranial extension of fungal sinus-orbital infection in diabetics may cause infectious thrombi[55] (Fig. 4-8). Tumors may occasion-

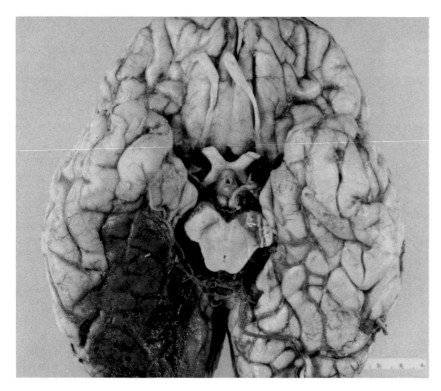

Fig. 4-6 Acute hemorrhagic infarct in the right occipital and medial temporal region due to compression of the right posterior cerebral artery.

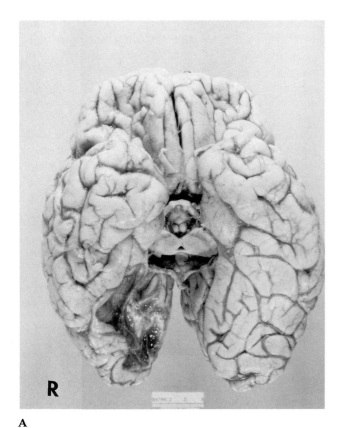

A

ally compress and invade the venous sinuses, with secondary tumorous or fibrinous thrombosis.[56] When venous sinuses are occluded, the cortical veins are often markedly congested and engorged, and extensive cortical hemorrhagic infarction follows (Fig. 4-9).

HEMORRHAGE

Intracranial hemorrhage may be spontaneous (Table 4-3) or secondary to recognizable events (Table 4-4).[57] Spontaneous intracranial hemorrhage may be mainly intracerebral or subarachnoid. Magnetic resonance imaging (MRI) is very sensitive to early intracerebral hemorrhage. Computed tomography (CT) scanning appears to locate intracerebral hematomas better. Intracerebral hemorrhage with rupture into the ventricles and cerebral herniations with brain stem compression remain the two major causes of death in spontaneous intracerebral hemorrhage. Subarachnoid hemorrhage may cause early death when widespread ischemic brain damage or concomitant intracerebral hemorrhage occurs.

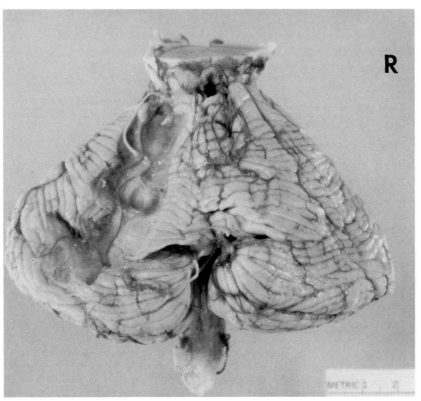

B

Fig. 4-7 Chronic infarcts due to atherosclerotic occlusion of (*A*) the right posterior cerebral artery and (*B*) the left anterior cerebellar artery.

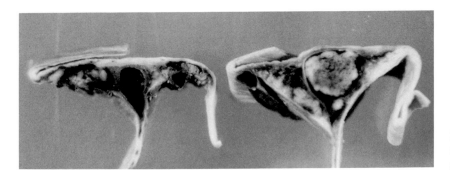

Fig. 4-8 Superior sagittal sinus thrombosis in a diabetic patient with oculocerebral aspergillosis.

Hypertensive Cerebrovascular Disease

Hypertension is the presumed cause of intracerebral hemorrhage in 70–90% of cases. The majority of massive intracerebral hemorrhages occur in hypertensive patients.[56–61] There is a relatively high incidence of hypertensive hemorrhage into the basal ganglia and the thalamus (Figs. 4-10, 4-11 and 4-12), but the cerebellum and brain stem may also be involved. The areas

supplied by the penetrating branches of the middle cerebral and basilar arteries are most susceptible to hypertensive hemorrhage.

In patients with hypertension, widespread changes in blood vessels are found throughout the body. The carotid and intracranial arteries may also show increased atherosclerosis. The smaller arteries and arteri-

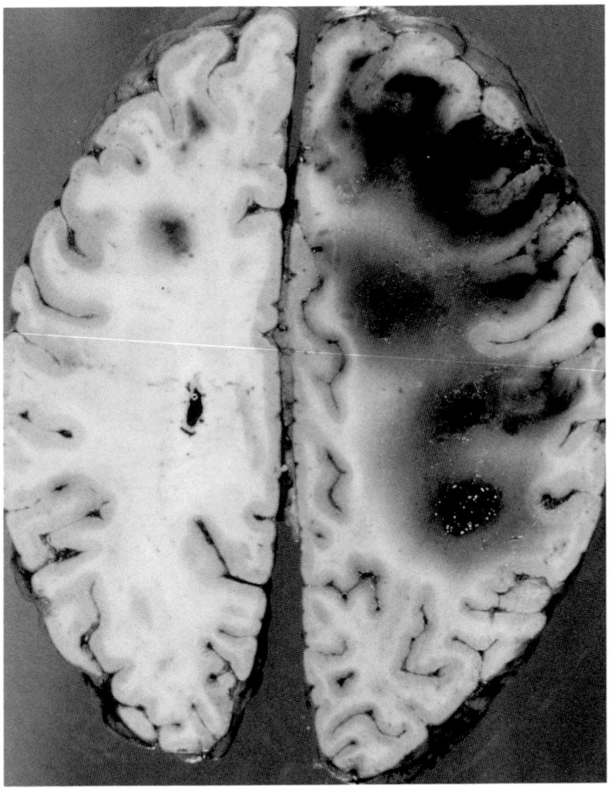

Fig. 4-9 Hemorrhagic infarcts due to complete occlusion of the right transverse sinus and partial occlusion of the superior sagittal sinus.

TABLE 4-3 Spontaneous Intracranial Hemorrhage

Hypertensive cerebrovascular disease
  Basal ganalia
    Lateral ganglionic type
    Medial ganglionic type
  Thalamus
  Pons
  Cerebellum
  Cerebral white matter
  Malignant hypertension
Nonhypertensive intracranial hemorrhage
  Primary and metastatic tumor
  Congophilic angiopathy
  Complication of anticoagulation
  Clotting disorder
  Moyamoya disease
  Drug abuse
  Acquired immunodeficiency syndrome
Aneurysm
  Saccular
  Fusiform
  Traumatic
  Mycotic
  Carotid cavernous fistula
Vascular malformation
  Capillary telangiectasia
  Cavernous/venous malformation
  Arteriovenous malformation
  Vein of Galen aneurysm
  Dural arteriovenous shunt

TABLE 4-4 Secondary Intracranial Hemorrhage

Cerebral herniation
  Duret's hemorrhage
  Kernohan's notch
  Contusion infarct
Trauma
  Extradural—middle meningeal artery
  Subdural—bridging vein
  Subarachnoid
  Intracerebral
    Contusion
    Contrecoup
    Penetrating
Perinatal hypoxia
  Subependymal germinal matrix
  Choroid plexus
  Intraventricular
  Subarachnoid
Tumors
  Glioblastoma multiforme
  Oligodendroglioma
  Metastatic tumors
Small blood vessel disease
  Disseminated intravascular coagulation
  Drug hypersensitivity
  Hemorrhagic leukoencephalopathy
  Fat embolism
  Thrombotic thrombocytopenic purpura

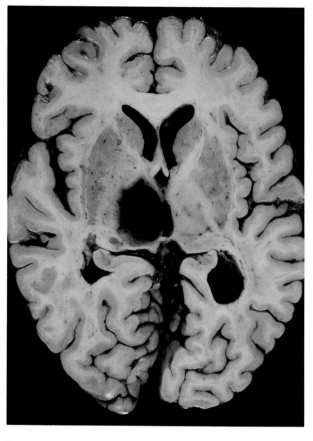

Fig. 4-10 Hypertensive intracerebral hemorrhage in the left thalamic region.

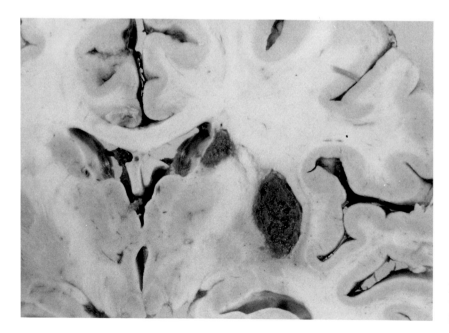

Fig. 4-11 Acute hemorrhagic infarct involving the right caudate nucleus and the right putamen.

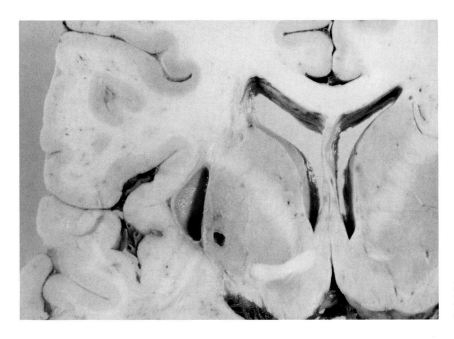

Fig. 4-12 Chronic cavitary infarct in the left basal ganglia with a hemosiderin-stained capsule.

oles show accentuated thickening and hyalinization of vessel walls, which occur with normal aging. These vascular changes are most pronounced in older hypertensive patients. Segments of a blood vessel or only part of its circumference may be affected. There may be necrosis of the vessel wall with aneurysmal dilatation, perivascular hemorrhage, or thrombotic occlusion of the lumen. Usually little or no lipid deposition is found.

The role of miliary aneurysms (Charcot-Bouchard microaneurysms) in hypertensive intracerebral hemorrhage has been much debated and remains unsettled.[62,63] These aneurysms are identified in a high percentage of hypertensive patients, often in the regions of the brain where small and massive cerebral hemorrhages occur. These areas include the central gray matter, the subcortical area, and the internal capsule. Miliary aneurysms may also be found in a small number of normotensive individuals. Histological evidence of asymptomatic hemorrhage may sometimes be found.

In malignant hypertension, endothelial cell damage, fibrinoid necrosis of arteriolar walls, and thrombotic occlusion have been seen in the acute states.[64]

Nonhypertensive Cause of Cerebral Hemorrhage[65–68]

Aside from vascular diseases, a variety of nonhypertensive disorders may cause intracranial hemorrhage. Primary and metastatic tumors in the brain account for about 10% of spontaneous intracranial hemorrhage.[69,70] Primary brain tumors such as glioblastoma multiforme, oligodendroglioma, and astrocytoma frequently bleed. Metastases from choriocarcinoma, malignant melanoma, and bronchial carcinoma are also prone to bleed. In 5–10% of primary nonhypertensive cerebral hemorrhage, amyloid accumulation in and around small arteries and arterioles in the brain and meninges results in cerebral amyloid angiopathy (congophilic angiopathy)[71–75] (Fig. 4-13). Complications of anticoagulation and clotting disorders may present as intracerebral or subarachnoid hemorrhages.[76–78] Recurrent intracerebral hemorrhages have been reported in moyamoya disease, cocaine abuse,[79,80] and acquired immunodeficiency syndrome.[28]

Aneurysm and Vascular Malformation

Aneurysms[81–84]
Aneurysms are defined as focal distensions and outpouchings of the arterial wall. They are a common cause of intracranial hemorrhage and are of great clinical and radiographic interest (Fig. 4-14). The common types include saccular, fusiform, dissecting, and mycotic aneurysms. Most aneurysms are formed secondary to a congenital or acquired structural defect in the vessel wall giving way to the tremendous pressure in the lumen.

Saccular Aneurysm[85] Saccular intracranial aneurysms occur in 1–2% of the population. Sixty percent are

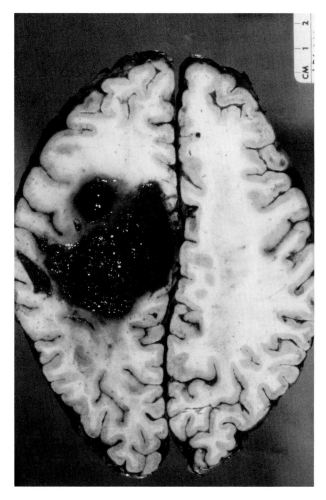

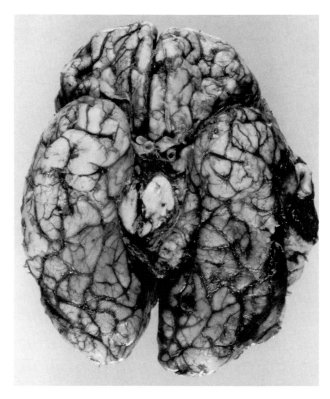

Fig. 4-14 Hypertensive intracerebral hemorrhage with rupture of the cerebral cortex, uncal and parahippocampal herniation, Kernohan's notch, and Duret's hemorrhage.

Fig. 4-13 Lobar intracerebral hemorrhage secondary to congophilic angiopathy in a normotensive patient.

diagnosed in patients 40 to 60 years of age. They may be found in any part of a cerebral artery but tend to occur more often at the bifurcations of arteries[86,87] (Fig. 4-15). Multiple aneurysms may occur, more frequently on the middle cerebral artery. Approximately 95% of aneurysms are visible in the circle of Willis and its main branches. A small number of aneurysms are located at the basilar and vertebral arteries or at more distal arterial branches.[88,89] Saccular aneurysms may rupture and give rise to subarachnoid or intracerebral hemorrhage (Figs. 4-16, 4-17), and may do so in the absence of arterial hypertension. Their locations may be defined by cerebral angiography and CT scanning. Rupture of a saccular aneurysm on the internal carotid artery projecting into the cavernous sinus may be the cause of some carotid-cavernous sinus fistulas.

Grossly, saccular aneurysms present as thin-walled but rigid, berry-like lesions at the arterial bifurcations.

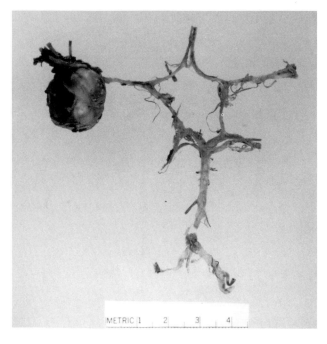

Fig. 4-15 A previously ruptured and thrombosed saccular aneurysm located at the right middle cerebral artery.

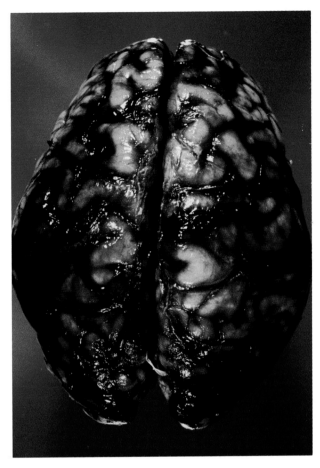

Fig. 4-16 Diffuse subarachnoid hemorrhage due to rupture of a saccular aneurysm located at the anterior communicating artery.

A blood clot attached to the distal tip and orange discoloration of the arachnoid and adjacent brain are evidence of previous hemorrhage. These aneurysms may occasionally be buried in the brain substance and may not be externally visible. The lumen may be completely occluded by lamellated blood clots or fibrotic tissue. Giant aneurysms, defined as those larger than 2.5 cm in diameter, rarely rupture due to frequent spontaneous thromobosis. They are sometimes not visualized by cerebral angiography for the similar reason. Variable amounts of recent or organizing blood clots may surround the frayed edges of ruptured aneurysms.

Microscopically, the wall of the aneurysm consists of thickened, fibrotic intima and adventitia. The muscular media and elastic lamina are missing or attenuated at the opening into the aneurysmal sac. Calcification may be seen in the walls of larger aneurysms. A thrombus is often present, partially or completely occupying the aneurysmal sac.[90] Hemosiderin-laden macrophages may be seen in the adjacent tissue even without gross rupture of the aneurysmal sac.

Atherosclerotic Fusiform Aneurysm In patients with severe atherosclerosis, fusiform dilatations of the basilar or the internal carotid arteries are common.[91,92] The arterial wall may stretch due to fibrous replacement of the smooth muscle media. When the dilatation is severe, a fusiform aneurysm (Fig. 4-18) is formed. Compression of adjacent structures, intraluminal thrombosis, atherosclerotic obstruction, and embolism may cause transient ischemic attacks and even infarcts of

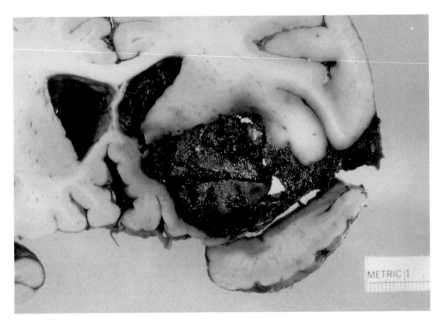

Fig. 4-17 Right middle cerebral artery saccular aneurysm rupture with intracerebral and subarachnoid hemorrhage.

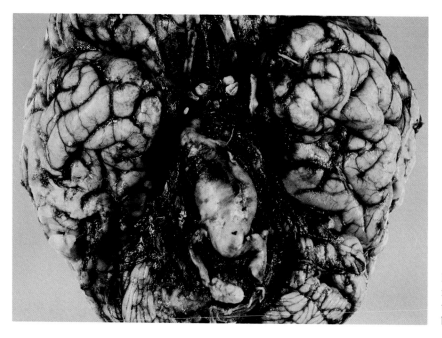

Fig. 4-18 A massive fuisform atherosclerotic aneurysm of the basilar artery ruptured at the superior surface, with massive brain stem and subarachnoid hemorrhage.

the brain stem and cerebellum.[93] Although rare, these aneurysms may occasionally lead to massive hemorrhage.

Dissecting Aneurysm Dissecting aneurysms may be found in association with blunt injury to the neck, open or closed head injury, or fibromuscular dysplasia of the artery.[47,94] The basilar, vertebral, middle cerebral, and intracranial parts of the internal carotid arteries may be affected. Infarcts may result from occlusion of the involved blood vessels, while hemorrhage occurs when these vessels rupture.

Bacterial/Fungal Aneurysm[95–98] Bacterial or fungal infection of the intracranial arteries may occasionally give rise to observable small aneurysms at the distal cerebral arteries. *Staphylococcus aureus* and *Streptococcus viridans* in infective endocarditis and *Aspergillus* from nasal sinus infection or endocarditis may be responsible. The lesions are often found at the gray–white junctions; they are multiple, and frequently rupture and bleed.

Vascular Malformations
Vascular malformations in the cerebral blood vessels can be classified into three major categories.

Capillary Telangiectasia Often an incidental finding, capillary telangiectasias (Fig. 4-19A) occur commonly in the cerebral hemispheres and the pons. Grossly, they may present as an ill-defined area of darker discolor-

ation. Microscopically, they are formed by clusters of dilated channels of vessels with thin capillary walls and a simple endothelial lining. The intervening brain tissue is often unremarkable, without evidence of gliosis or hemorrhage. Bleeding from a capillary telangiectasia is rare.

Cavernous/Venous Malformations[99–106] Cavernous/venous malformations (Fig. 4-19B) are often an incidental finding but may occasionally give rise to major hemorrhage (Fig. 4-20). They can be found in the hemispheric white matter and brain stem and may be multiple. They are not usually visualized angiographically. MRI is more sensitive than CT and angiography in detecting these lesions. Grossly, aggregates of prominent blood vessels may be visible, but they are often obscured by a large blood clot. Microscopically, they consist of dilated venous channels in loosely or tightly arranged clusters enclosing gliotic brain tissue that often shows evidence of previous hemorrhage. Cavernous channels with shared vascular walls are often found.

Arteriovenous Malformations[107–116] Arteriovenous malformations (Fig. 4-21A,B) are the major vascular malformations that most often lead to recurrent subarachnoid or intracerebral bleeds. In situ, they are often grossly visible at the cortical surface as tight tangles of angry-looking, engorged blood vessels. They can also be found deep in the hemisphere (Fig. 4-22). In a sec-

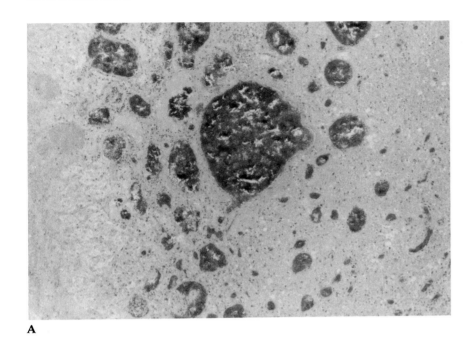

A

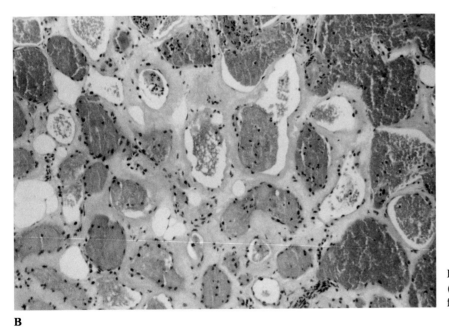

B

Fig. 4-19 (*A*) Capillary telangiectasia (H&E stain). (*B*) Cavernous/venous malformation (H&E stain).

tion through the long axis, they are often conical, with the apex pointing toward the ventricles. Microscopically, they consist of collections of dilated, poorly formed blood vessels of variable types, including arterial, venous, and hybrid forms. Focal thickening of the smooth muscle layers, so-called pseudomyomatous hyperplasia, is commonly seen. There is often evidence of previous hemorrhage and gliosis in the adjacent or entrapped brain tissue. An association with saccular an-

eurysms has been noted occasionally. Special forms of arteriovenous malformation may include great vein of Galen aneurysm[117] (Fig. 4-23) and dural arteriovenous shunt.[118–120]

Secondary Intracranial Hemorrhage

Specific intracranial events may give rise to various forms of hemorrhage. Cerebral herniations with com-

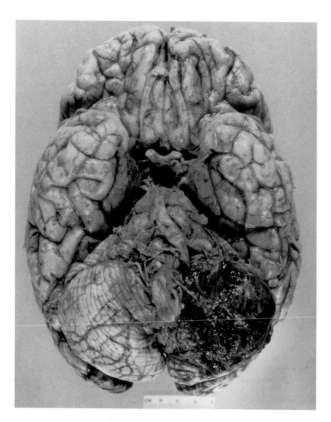

Fig. 4-20 Cerebellar hemispheric hemorrhage after rupture of a venous malformation located at the cerebellopontine angle.

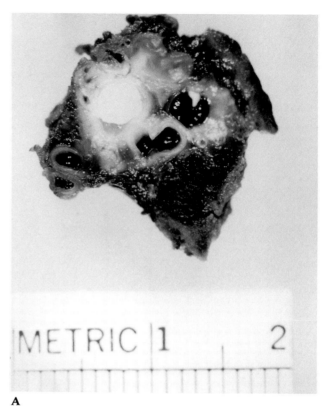

A

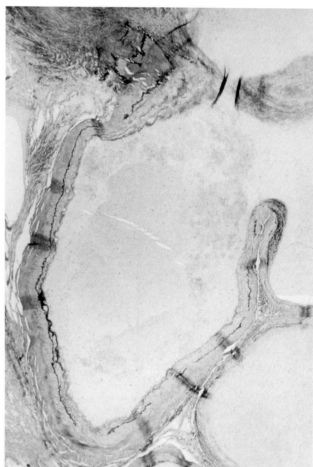

B

Fig. 4-21 (*A*) Arteriovenous malformation. (*B*) Arteriovenous malformation (elastic stain) showing interrupted elastic lamina in the hybrid arteriovenous vessel wall.

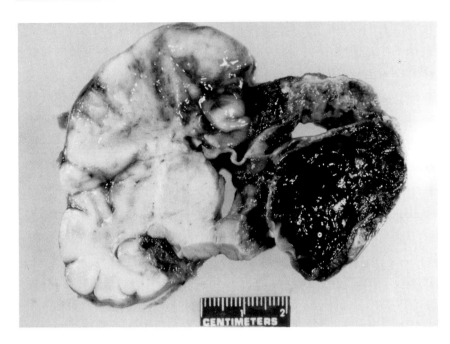

Fig. 4-22 Massive arteriovenous malformation with nearly complete replacement of the right cerebral hemisphere.

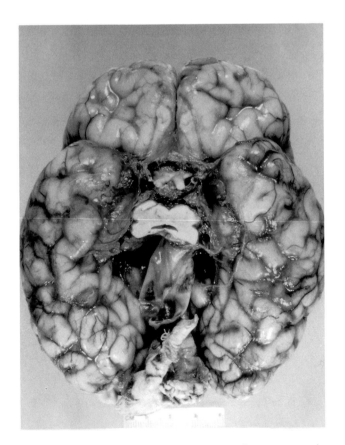

Fig. 4-23 Vein of Galen aneurysm presenting as a posterior fossa mass and heart failure.

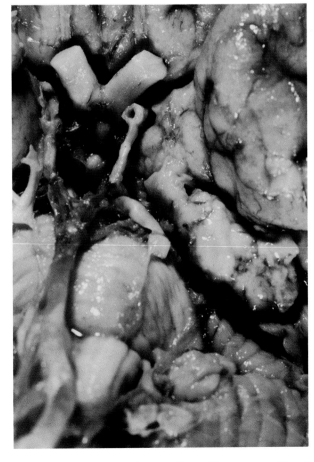

Fig. 4-24 Supratentorial mass effect with acute uncal herniation and necrosis.

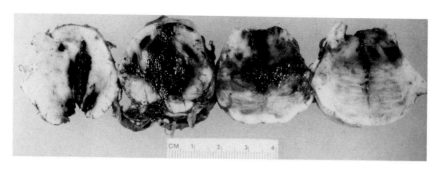

Fig. 4-25 Increased supratentorial intracranial pressure with axial brain herniation and brain stem hemorrhage (Duret's hemorrhage).

pression of brain tissue against rigid intracranial structures may lead to contusion, necrosis, and hemorrhage such as Kernohan's notch and contusion infarction of the hippocampus (Fig. 4-24). Stretching and occlusion of the basilar artery due to axial herniation lead to Duret's hemorrhage (Fig. 4-25). Open or closed head injuries may cause localized or extensive extracranial and intracranial hemorrhage. Perinatal hypoxia with hemorrhage in the subependymal germinal matrix or choroid plexus may result in intraventricular and subarachnoid hemorrhage[121] (Fig. 4-26). Hemorrhage in tumors may extend to the adjacent brain tissue. Small blood vessel occlusion due to various disease processes may give rise to petechial or massive hemorrhage.

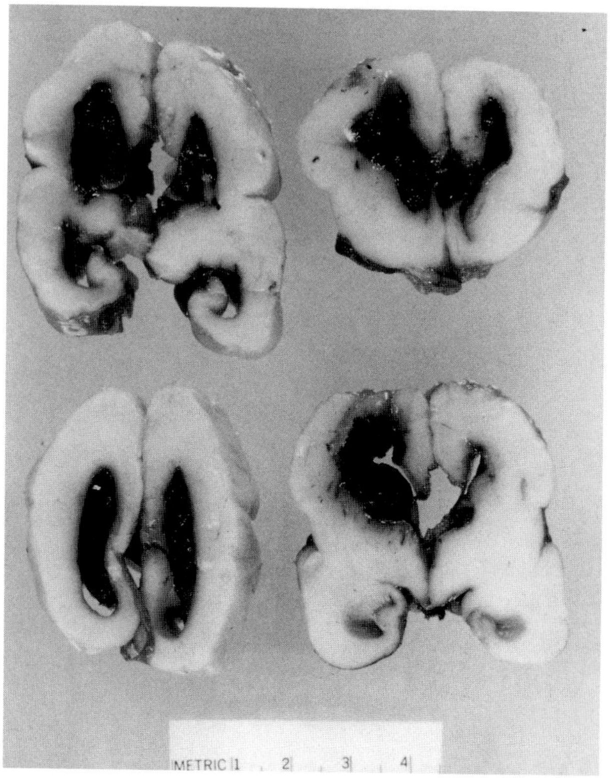

REFERENCES

1. Garcia JH, Anderson ML. Circulatory disorders and their effects on the brain, in Davis RL, Robertson DM (eds): *Textbook of Neuropathology*. Baltimore, Williams & Wilkins, 1991, pp 621–718.
2. Graham DI. Hypoxia and vascular disorders, in Adams JH, Duchen LW (eds), *Greenfield's Neuropathology*. New York, Wiley, 1992, pp 153–268.
3. Socco RL, Ellenberg JH, Mohr JP, et al. Infarcts of undetermined cause: The NINCD stroke data bank. *Ann Neurol* 1989;25:382–390.
4. Fisher CM, Gore I, Okabe N, et al. Atherosclerosis of the carotid and vertebral arteries—extracranial and intracranial. *J Neuropathol Exp Neurol* 1965;24:455–476.
5. Levine S, Welch KMA. Common carotid artery occlusion. *Neurology* 1989;39:178–186.
6. Fisher CM. Occlusion of internal carotid artery. *Arch Neurol Psychiatr* 1951;65:346–377.
7. Bornstein NM, Krajewski A, Lewis AJ, et al. Clinical significance of carotid plaque hemorrhage. *Arch Neurol* 1990;47:958–959.
8. Castaigne P, Lhermitte F, Gautier J, et al. Arterial occlusions in the vertebral-basilar system. A study of 44 patients with postmortem data. *Brain* 1973;96:133–154.
9. Hosoda Y. Pathology of so-called "spontaneous occlusion of the circle of Willis." *Path Annu* 1984;19(2):221–244.
10. Levine RL, Lagreze HL, Dobkin JA, et al. Large subcortical hemispheric infarctions. Presentation and prognosis. *Arch Neurol* 1988;45:1074–1077.
11. Caplan LR, Schmahmann JD, Kase CS, et al. Caudate infarcts. *Arch Neurol* 1990;47:133–143.
12. Donnan GA, Baldin PF, Berkovic SF, et al. The stroke

Fig. 4-26 Perinatal hypoxia in a premature baby with supependymal germinal matrix, intraventricular hemorrhage, and subarachnoid hemorrhage.

syndome of striatocapsular infarction. *Brain* 1991;114: 51–70.

13. Phillips S, Sangalan V, Sterns G. Basal forebrain infarction. A clinicopathologic correlation. *Arch Neurol* 1987;44:1134–1138.

14. Degos JD, Gary F, Louarn F, et al. Posterior callosal infarction. Clinicopathological correlations. *Brain* 1987; 110:1155–1171.

15. Jagiella WM, Sung JH. Bilateral infarction of the medullary pyramids in humans. *Neurology* 1989;39:21–24.

16. Amarenco P, Hauw J-J. Cerebellar infarction of the territory of the anterior and inferior cerebellar artery. A clinicopathological study of 20 cases. *Brain* 1990;113: 139–155.

17. Anderson NE, Willoughby EW. Infarction of conus medullaris. *Ann Neurol* 1987;21:470–474.

18. Jeynes BJ, Warren BA. Cerebral atheroembolism. An animal model. *Stroke* 1982;13:312–318.

19. Calandre L, Ortega JF, Bermejo F. Autoregulation and hemorrhagic infarction in cerebral embolism secondary to rheumatic heart disease. *Arch Neurol* 1984;41: 1152–1154.

20. Cerebral Embolism Task Force: Cardiogenic brain embolism. *Arch Neurol* 1986;43:71–84.

21. Haymaker W, Johnston AD. Pathology of decompression sickness. A comparison of the lesions in airman with those in caisson workers and divers. *Mil Med* 1955; 117:285–306.

22. von Hochstetter AR, Friede RL. Residual lesions of cerebral fat embolism. *J Neurol* 1977;216:227–233.

23. McCarthy M, Norenberg MD. Pontine hemorrhagic infarction in nontraumatic fat embolism. *Neurology* 1988; 38:1645–1647.

24. McDonald WI. Recurrent cholesterol embolism as a cause of fluctuating cerebral symptoms. *J Neurol Neurosurg Psychiatry* 1967;30:489–496.

25. Brierly JB, Meldrum BS. The nature and distribution of brain damage due to air embolism, in Arfel G, Naquet R (eds), *L'Embolie Gazeuse due Systemie Carotidien.* Paris, Doin, 1974;180–183.

26. O'Neill BP, Dinapoli RP, Okazaki H. Cerebral infarction as a result of tumor emboli. *Cancer* 1987;60:90–95.

27. Koeppen AM, Lansing LS. Peng SK, et al. Central nervous system vaculitis in cytomegalovirus infection. *J Neurol Sci* 1981;51:395–410.

28. Mizusawa H, Hirano A, Llena JF, et al. Cerebrovascular lesions in acquired immunodeficiency syndrome (AIDS). *Acta Neuropathol* 1988;76:451–457.

29. Del Brutto OH. Cysticercosis and cerebrovascular disease: A review. *J Neurol Neurosurg Psychiatry* 1992;55: 252–254.

30. Moore PM, Cupps TR. Neurological complications of vasculitis. *Ann Neurol* 1983;14:155–167.

31. Burger PC, Burch JG, Vogel FS. Granulomatous angiitis: An unusual etiology of stroke. *Stroke* 1977;8: 29–35.

32. Koo EH, Massey EW. Granulomatous angiitis of the central nervous system: Protean manifestations and response to treatment. *J Neurol Neurosurg Psychiatry* 1988; 51:1126–1133.

33. Sabharwal UK, Keogh LH, Weisman MH, et al. Granulomatous angiitis of the nervous system: Case report and review of the literature. *Arthritis Rheum* 1982; 25(3):342–345.

34. Caccamo DV, Garcia JH, Ho KL: Isolated granulomatous angiitis of the spinal cord. *Ann Neurol* 1992;32: 580–582.

35. Matsell DG, Keene DL, Jimenez C, et al. Isolated angiitis of the central nervous system in childhood. *Can J Neurol Sci* 1990;17:151–154.

36. Maki Y, Enomoto T. Moyamoya disease. *Child's Nerv Syst* 1988;4:204–212.

37. Rolak LA, Rokey R. Magnetic resonance imaging in Moyamoya disease. *J Child Neurol* 1986;1:67–70.

38. Kaufman M, Little BW, Berkowitz BW: Recurrent intracranial hemorrhage in an adult with Moyamoya disease: Case report, radiographic studies and Pathology. *Can J Neurol Sci* 1988;15:430–434.

39. Enomoto H, Goto H. Moyamoya disease presenting as intracranial hemorrhage during pregnancy: Case report and review of the literature. *Neurosurgery* 1986;20: 33–35.

40. Gibb WGR, Urry PA, Lees AJ. Giant cell arteritis with spinal cord infarction and basilar artery thrombosis. *J Neurol Neurosurg Psychiatry* 1985;48:945–948.

41. McDonell PJ, Moore GW, Miller NR, et al. Temporal arteritis: A clinicopathologic study. *Ophthalmology* 1986;93:518–530.

42. Lindenberg R. Compression of the brain arteries as a pathogenic factor for tissue necrosis and their areas of predilection. *J Neuropathol Exp Neurol* 1955;14: 223–243.

43. Sheehan S, Bauer RD, Meyer JS. Vertebral artery compression in cervical spondylosis. *Neurology* 1960;10: 968–986.

44. Lynch DR, Dawson TM, Raps EC, et al. Risk factors for the neurologic complications associated with aortic aneurysms. *Arch Neurol* 1992;49:284–285.

45. Josien C. Extracranial vertebral artery dissection: Nine cases. *J Neurol* 1992;239:327–330.

46. Linden MD, Chou SM, Furlan AJ, et al. Cerebral arterial dissection. A case report with histologic and ultrastructural findings. *Cleve Clin J Med* 1987;54:105–114.

47. Luscher TF, Lie JT, Stanson AW, et al. Arterial fibromuscular dysplasia. *Mayo Clin Proc* 1987;62:931–952.

48. Macdonald RL, Weir BKA, Grace MGA, et al. Mecha-

nism of cerebral vasospasm following subarachnoid hemorrhage in monkeys. *Can J Neurol Sci* 1992;19: 419–427.

49. Martin JP. Thrombosis in superior longitudinal sinus following childbirth. *Br Med J* 1941;2:537–540.

50. Srinivasan K. Puerperal cerebral venous and arterial thrombosis. *Semin Neurol* 1988;8(3):222–225.

51. Thron A, Wessel K, Linden D, et al. Superior sagittal sinus thrombosis: Neuroradiological evaluation and clinical findings. *Neurology* 1986;36:283–288.

52. Imai WK, Everhart FR, Sanders JM. Cerebral venous sinus thrombosis: Report of a case and review of the literature. *Pediatrics* 1982;70:965–970.

53. Cross JN, Castro PO, Jennette WB: Cerebral strokes associated with pregnancy and the puerperum. *Br Med J* 1968;2:214–218.

54. Chievitz E, Thiede T. Complications and causes of death in polycythemia vera. *Acta Med Scand* 1962;172: 513–523.

55. Southwick FS, Richardson EP Jr, Swartz MN. Septic thrombosis of the dural venous sinuses. *Medicine* 1986; 65(2):82–106.

56. Hickey WF, Garnick MB, Henderson IC, et al. Primary cerebral venous thrombosis in patients with cancer—a rarely diagnosed paraneoplastic syndrome. Report of three cases and review of the literature. *Am J Med* 1982; 73:740–750.

57. Ojemann RG, Heros RS. Spontaneous brain hemorrhage. *Stroke* 1983;14:458–475.

58. Baker ABA, Resch JA, Loewenson RB. Hypertension and cerebral atherosclerosis. *Circulation* 1969;39: 701–710.

59. Byrom FB. The evolution of acute hypertensive arterial diseases. *Prog Cardiovasc Dis* 1974;17:31–37.

60. Chester EM, Agamanolis DP, Banker BQ, et al. Hypertensive encephalopathy: A clinicopathologic study of 20 cases. *Neurology* 1978;28:928–939.

61. Disdale HB. Hypertensive encephalopathy. *Stroke* 1982; 13:717–719.

62. Fisher CM. Cerebral miliary aneurysm in hypertension. *Am J Pathol* 1972;66:313–330.

63. Challa VR, Moody DM, Bell MA. The Charcot-Bouchard aneurysm controversy: Impact of a new histologic technique. *J Neuropathol Exp Neurol* 1992;51(3): 264–271.

64. Rosenblum WI. The importance of fibrinoid necrosis as the cause of cerebral hemorrhage in hypertension, commentary. *J Neuropathol Exp Neurol* 1993;52(1): 11–13.

65. Mendelow AD. Spontaneous intracerebral hemorrhage. *J Neurol Neurosurg Psychiatry* 1991;54:193–195.

66. Mehler MF, Ragone PS. Primary spontaneous mesencephalic hemorrhage. *Can J Neurol Sci* 1988;15:435–438.

67. Cole FM, Yates PO. Comparative incidence of cerebrovasular lesions in normotensive and hypertensive patients. *Neurology* 1968;18:255–259.

68. Kase CS. Intracerebral hemorrhage: Non-hypertensive causes. *Stroke* 1986;17(4):590–595.

69. Minette SE, Kimmel DW. Subdural hematoma in patients with systemic cancer. *Mayo Clin Proc* 1989;64: 637–642.

70. Nutt SH, Patchell RA. Intracranial hemorrhage associated with primary and secondary tumors. *Neurosurg Clin North Am* 1992;3(3):591–599.

71. Kalyan-Raman UP, Kalyan-Raman K. Cerebral amyloid angiopathy causing intracranial hemorrhage. *Ann Neurol* 1984;16:321–329.

72. Ishii N, Nishihara Y, Horii A. Amyloid angiopathy and lobar cerebral hemorrhage. *J Neurol Neurosurg Psychiatry* 1984;47:1203–1210.

73. Okazaki H, Regan TJ, Campbell RJ. Clinicopathologic studies of primary cerebral amyloid angiography. *Mayo Clin Proc* 1979;54:22–31.

74. Mandybur TI. Cerebral amyloid angiopathy: The vascular pathology and complications. *J Neuropathol Exp Neurol* 1986;45(1):77–90.

75. Roosen N, Martin J-J, De La Porte C, et al. Intracerebral hemorrhage due to cerebral amyloid angiopathy. Case report. *J Neurosurg* 1985;63:965–969.

76. Greaves M. Coagulation abnormalities and cerebral infarction. *J Neurol Neurosurg Psychiatry* 1993;56: 433–439.

77. Carlson SE, Aldrich MS, Greenberg HS, et al. Intracerbral hemorrhage complicating intravenous tissue plasminogen activator treatment. *Arch Neurol* 1988;45: 1070–1073.

78. Ramsay DA, Penswick JL, Robertson DM. Fatal streptokinase-induced intracerebral hemorrhage in cerebral amyloid angiopathy. *Can J Neurol Sci* 1990;17: 336–341.

79. Shibata S, Mori K, Sekine I, et al. Subarachnoid and intracerebral hemorrhage associated with necrotizing angiitis due to metamphetamine abuse—an autopsy case. *Neurol Med* 1991;31(1):49–52.

80. Nolte KB, Gelman BB. Intracerebral hemorrhage associated with cocaine abuse. *Arch Pathol Lab Med* 1989; 113:812–813.

81. Ljunggren B, Saveland H, Brandt L. Aneurysmal subarachnoid hemorrhage—historical background from a Scandinavian horizon. *Surg Neurol* 1984;22:605–616.

82. Meyer FB, Sundt TM, Fode NC, et al. Cerebral aneurysms in childhood and adolescence. *J Neurosurg* 1989; 70:420–425.

83. Reynolds AF, Shaw C-M. Bleeding patterns from ruptured intracranial aneurysms: An autopsy series of 205 patients. *Surg Neurol* 1981;15(3):232–235.

84. Inagawa T, Hirano A. Autopsy study of unruptured incidental intracranial aneurysms. *Surg Neurol* 1990;34: 361–365.

85. Rhoton AC. Anatomy of saccular aneurysms. *Surg Neurol* 1980;14:59–66.

86. Sindou M, Pellisou-Guyotat I, Mertens P, et al. Pericallosal aneurysms. *Surg Neurol* 1988;30:434–440.

87. Gerber CJ, Neil-Dwyer G. A review of the management of 15 cases of aneurysms of the posterior cerebral artery. *Br J Neurosurg* 1992;6:521–527.

88. Maiuri F, Corriero G, D'Amico L, et al. Giant aneurysm of the pericallosal artery. *Neurosurgery* 1990;26: 703–706.

89. Pia HW. Classification of vertebro-basilar aneurysms. *Acta Neurochir* 1979;47:3–30.

90. Batjer HH, Purdy PD. Enlarging thrombosed aneurysm of the basilar artery. *Neurosurgery* 1990;26:695–700.

91. Tommasi-Davanas C, Demiaux B, Kzaiz M, et al. Giant and thrombosed aneurysm of the left vertebral artery developed in the fourth ventricle. *Rev Neurol (Paris)* 1989;145(11):799–801.

92. Little JR, St Louis P, Weinstein M, et al. Giant fusiform aneurysm of the cerebral arteries. *Stroke* 1982;12: 183–188.

93. Cohen AR, Aleksic S, Budzilovich GM, et al. Giant intracranial aneurysm presenting as a posterior fossa mass. *Surg Neurol* 1983;20:160–164.

94. Arabi B. Traumatic aneurysms of brain due to high velocity missile head wounds. *Neurosurgery* 1988;22: 1056–1063.

95. Clare CE, Barrow DL: Infectious intracranial aneurysms. *Neurol Clin North Am* 1992;3(3):551–556.

96. Frazee JG, Cahan LD, Goldstein MN, et al. Pathogenesis of cerebral mycotic aneurysms. *Neurology* 1973;23: 325–332.

97. Frazee JG, Cahan LD, Winter J. Bacterial intracranial aneurysms. *J Neurosurg* 1980;53:633–641.

98. Horten BC, Abbott GF, Porro RS. Fungal aneurysms of intracranial vessels. *Arch Neurol* 1976;33:577–579.

99. Rigamonti D, Spetzler RF, Medina M, et al. Cerebral venous malformations. *J Neurosurg* 1990;73:560–564.

100. Rigamonti D, Hadley MN, Drayer BP, et al. Cerebral cavernous malformations. Incidence and familial occurence. *N Engl J Med* 1988;319:343–347.

101. Ferrante L, Palma L, d'Addetta R, et al. Intracranial cavernous angioma. *Neurosurg Rev* 1992;15:125–133.

102. Farmer J-P, Cosgrove GR, Villemure J-G, et al. Intracerebral cavernous angiomas. *Neurology* 1988;38: 1699–1704.

103. Zimmerman RS, Spetzler RF, Lee KS, et al. Cavernous malformations of the brain stem. *J Neurosurg* 1991;75: 32–39.

104. Pozzati E, Giuliani G, Nuzzo G, et al. The growth of cerebral cavernous angiomas. *Neurosurgery* 1989;25: 92–97.

105. Matias-Guiu X, Alejo M, Sole T, et al. Cavernous angiomas of the cranial nerves. *J Neurosurg* 1990;73: 620–622.

106. Kubota T, Kuroda E, Fujii T, et al. Orbital varix with a pearly phlebolith. *J Neurosurg* 1990;73:291–295.

107. Miyasaka K, Wolpert SM, Prager RJ. The association of cerebral aneurysms, infundibula, and intracranial arteriovenous malformation. *Stroke* 1982;13:196–203.

108. Suzuki J, Omuna T. Intracranial aneurysms associated with arteriovenous malformation. *J Neurosurg* 1979;50: 742–746.

109. Deruty R, Pelissou-Guyotat I, Mottolese C, et al. Ruptured occult arteriovenous malformation associated with an unruptured intracranial aneurysm: Report of three cases. *Neurosurgery* 1992;30:603–607.

110. Ondra SL, Troupp H, George ED, et al. The natural history of symptomatic arteriovenous malformations of the brain: A 24-year follow-up assessment. *J Neurosurg* 1990;73:387–391.

111. Spetzler RF, Martin NA. A proposed grading system for arteriovenous malformations. *J Neurosurg* 1986;65: 476–483.

112. Suarez JC, Viano JC. Intracranial arteriovenous malformations in infancy and adolescence. *Child's Nerv Syst* 1989;5:15–18.

113. Fong D, Chan S: Arteriovenous malformation in children. *Child's Nerv Syst* 1988;4:199–203.

114. Yokoyama K, Asano Y, Murakawa T, et al. Familial occurrence of arteriovenous malformation of the brain. *J Neurosurg* 1991;74:585–589.

115. Itakura T, Takifuji K, Ozaki F, et al. Cystic arteriovenous malformation. A case report. *Acta Neurochir (Wien)* 1989;96:154–158.

116. Willinsky R, TerBrugge K, Lasjaunias P, et al. The variable presentations of craniocervical and cervical dural arteriovenous malformation. *Surg Neurol* 1990;34: 118–123.

117. Lasjaunias P, Rodesch G, Pruvost P, et al. Treatment of vein of Galen aneurysmal malformation. *J Neurosurg* 1989;70:746–750

118. Tomlinson FH, Rufenacht DA, Sundt TM, et al. Arteriovenous fistulas of the brain and the spinal cord. *J Neurosurg* 1993;79:16–27.

119. Izuka Y, Rodesch G, Garcia-Monaco R, et al. Multiple cerebral arteriovenous shunts in children: Report of 13 cases. *Child's Nerv Syst* 1992;8:437–444.

120. Volpe JJ. Intraventricular hemorrhage in the premature infant—current concepts. Part I. *Ann Neurol* 1989; 25:3–11.

121. Perlman JM, Volpe JJ. Intraventricular hemorrhage in extremely small premature infants. *AJDC* 1986;140: 1122–1124.

Section 2

Imaging Modalities

5

Ocular Imaging with Fluorescein Angiography

Edward M. Cohn, M.D., John L. Johnson, CRP,
Tarek Hassan, M.D., Jane Werner, M.D.

INTRODUCTION

The eye is said to be the window of the body, and it provides a direct view of blood vessels. As an extension of the brain, the optic nerve is often viewed without difficulty. Moreover, the eye is a neurologic organ, with layers and characteristics similar to those of the brain, and is ideal for neuroimaging. Neuroimaging of the eye is obtained with direct visualization and photography, which can be accomplished with or without intravascular injection of materials such as sodium fluorescein or, more recently, indocyanine green, which allow contrasting images. This chapter is meant to make the reader aware of the eye and an important, but very specialized, form of neuro-imaging. We can not be exhaustive in the subject with so little space and refer those interested to some other sources.

The eye has three basic layers. The outer layer, or sclera, is an extension of the dura mater. The inner layer is the retina, which, in turn, is made up of 10 layers of first-, second-, and third-order neuron cell bodies, their axons, and neural support cells. The middle, or choroidal, layer of the eye is very vascular and is similar to the pia-arachnoid of the central nervous system.

Since the first successful fundus photograph of a human, taken by Jackman in 1886, color fundus photography has been considered one of the most impor-

tant methods of documenting retinal disease. It was not until the early 1960s that another photographic procedure, fluorescein angiography, became available to further assist contrast imaging.

Fluorescein angiography is a diagnostic procedure which permits documentation and demonstration of choroidal and retinal circulation. Venous injection of sodium fluorescein allows photographing of dye as it circulates in the retinal vasculature. In 1961, Novotny and Alvis discovered this photographic technique during their research as medical students. Since 1961, the standard fundus camera has been modified and redesigned to provide ophthalmologists with detailed microcirculatory findings using sodium fluorescein, special filters, and black-and-white film.

The methodology of photographing fluorescence is based upon the quantum theory, which states when certain substances are exposed to a form of short-wave electromagnetic radiation, energy will be absorbed and its electrons will be raised to a higher level of energy. As the molecules return to their original state, the substance will emit radiation of a longer wavelength. This phenomenon is known as *luminescence,* of which there are two types: phosphorescence and fluorescence. Phosphorescence occurs after the stimulating source is removed, while fluorescence occurs only in the presence of a stimulating source.

Two filters are required to photograph fluorescence:

(1) the exciter and (2) the barrier. The exciter filter converts the illumination flash from the fundus camera to the correct wavelength of light necessary to excite sodium fluorescein dye molecules and create fluorescence. The barrier filter blocks out unwanted reflected blue light from the camera flash and allows only yellow-green fluorescence to pass through the filter onto the film plane.

These same two filters are used to document autofluorescence when giant drusen of the optic nerve is suspected and pseudopapilloedema is present. Autofluorescence does not require the injection of fluorescein.

Sodium fluorescein dye is excited by light energy at 465–490 nm and emits fluorescence at 520–530 nm. The dye normally leaks from all vessels in the body except those in the retina and central nervous system because of firmly connected endothelial cells. Sodium fluorescein dye is eliminated from the liver and kidneys within 24–48 hr, although traces have been found more than a week postinjection. Fluorescein dye also stains skin and mucous membranes for a period of 2–4 hr postinjection. The standard dose for angiography is 5 cc of a 10% solution. Chemically, fluorescein is a compound which binds with serum protein in the blood. It is an orange-red crystalline hydrocarbon in powdered form that becomes bright yellow with green fluorescence when mixed in a diluted alkaline solution. Fluorescein dye is artificially made from coal tar and should not be referred to as a vegetable dye.

FLUORESCEIN ANGIOGRAPHY OF THE NORMAL FUNDUS

Prior to fluorescein angiography, a few color fundus photographs are obtained to provide documentation and assist the angiographic interpretation. Once color fundus photos are taken, the camera body is exchanged with another and loaded with black-and-white 400 ASA film for the angiogram. Red-free (green filter) identification photos (Fig. 5-1A) of the central or posterior pole of the retina are taken, and the filter is replaced with the barrier filter. A control photograph tests the integrity of the exciter and barrier filters and determines possible autofluorescent pathology in the eye (see Figure 5-6B). A flash setting of 150–200 watt-seconds is needed to excite the sodium fluorescein, which is injected at a rate of approximately 1 cc/sec or more. At injection, a timer is started.

Normally, within 8–12 sec of the injection, background fluorescence occurs, and the choroid is seen and often visualized as patchy or mottled. Dye then enters the central retinal artery as the early arterial phase. Complete arterial filling occurs after approximately 1.0–1.5 sec (Fig. 5-1B).

The next phase of fluorescence is seen at the posterior pole and the peripapillary region, with increasing fluorescence in the choroidal vessels. Following this, the venous phase (Fig. 5-1C) is marked by an outflow of dye via the venous system. Fluorescence can be observed when the dye enters the macular venules and laminar flow occurs in the large veins. It can take 4–5 sec for the fluorescein dye and the venous blood to mix totally for complete filling of the venules (Fig. 5-1D).

One frame every other second for the first 25–30 sec is usually adequate to capture the initial early phases. Stereoangiography further demonstrates circulation patterns, abnormal fluorescence, and elevations.

The mid-phase (Fig. 5-1E) occurs after 20–30 sec. The late phase (Fig. 5-1F) is considered to occur 5–10 min postinjection and is recognized when fluorescein dye almost disappears from the retinal vessels; the residual diffuse choroidal fluorescence gradually disappears. Fluorescence can normally be seen at the optic disc margin because of collagen staining. Hyperfluorescence of the disc itself is abnormal and indicates vessel leakage, as in edema. An angiogram can be completed in 36 frames or less.

CHOROIDAL CIRCULATION

The choroidal circulation is first visualized in the fluorescein angiogram by a background choroidal flush. This is seen several seconds prior to filling of the retinal arterioles because of the rapid flow to the choroid through the posterior ciliary arteries. The blood is distributed in lobules with generous collateral circulation.

The aqueous phase containing the fluorescein dye almost immediately diffuses from the choriocapillaries because of the lack of tight junctions. The result is a diffuse, generalized hypofluorescence, not visualization of the individual arteries, veins, and capillaries of the choroid itself. This is unlike the retinal circulation, in which the individual vessels can be well visualized.

In cases of choroidal pathology, as in malignant melanoma of the choroid (Fig. 5-2A–D), this background choroidal fluorescence can be quite altered. In metastatic tumors, the choroidal circulation is also altered.

Choroidal inflammation may be found with meningeal inflammation in a poorly understood and rarely documented association. Choroidal inflammation (Fig. 5-3A) is seen on fluorescein as large or small, isolated

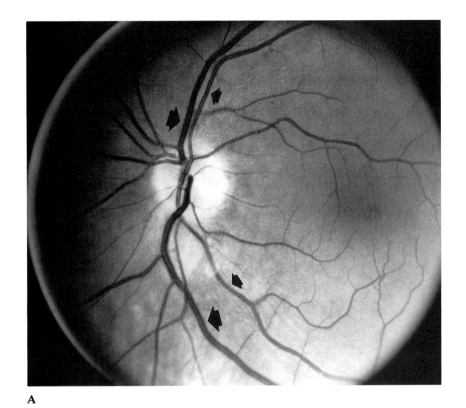

A

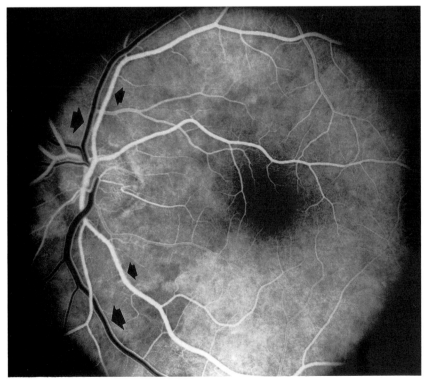

B

Fig. 5-1 (*A*) Red-free photograph of a normal posterior pole. The pale appearance of the optic nerve is due to overexposure from a very bright flash and from the green filter blocking out the healthy red/pink color (arterioles are pointed out with small arrows and venules with larger arrows). (*B*) at 13.9 sec, we see the normal background choroidal filling blush. The arteriole (small arrows) circulation is normally filled, and the early venous (large arrows) filling is seen as a lamellar flow.

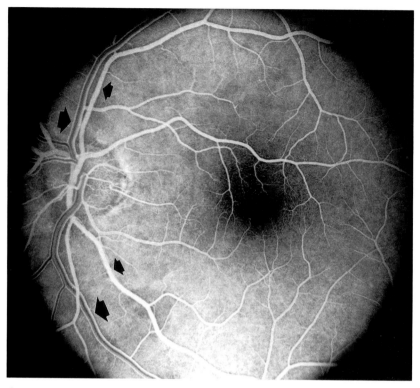

C

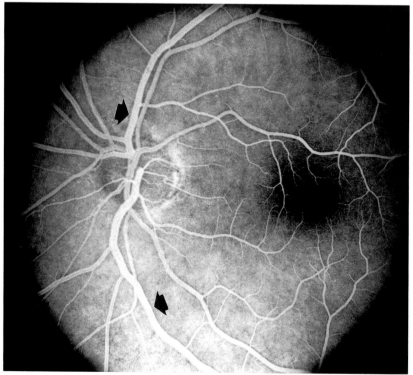

D

Fig. 5-1 (*C*) At 16.1 sec, fluorescein transit is in the midvenous phase (small arrows to the arteriole and large arrows to the venules). (*D*) At 21.6 sec, the venous phase is normally completed, as evidenced by complete filling of both arterioles (small arrow) and venules (large arrow).

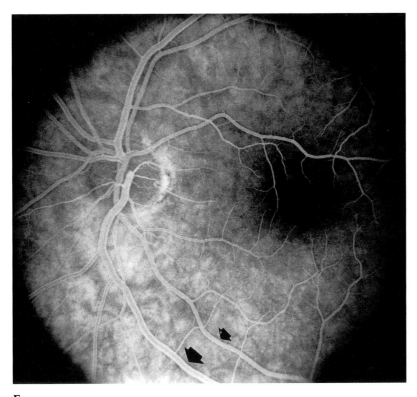

E

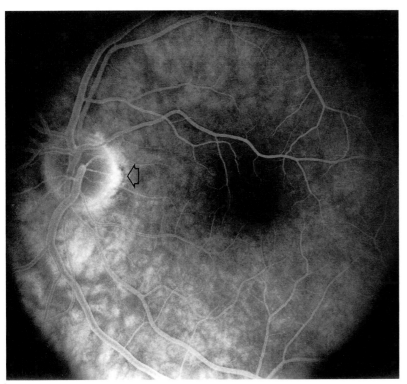

F

Fig. 5-1 (*E*) By 40.8 sec, the dye is gradually fading from the retinal circulation as it is removed by the body (small arrow pointing to the arteriole and large arrow pointing to the venule). (*F*) In the late phase (363.9 sec or 6 min), the retinal fluorescein angiogram shows some normal staining of the disc margin (open arrow) but no abnormal staining of the body of the disc.

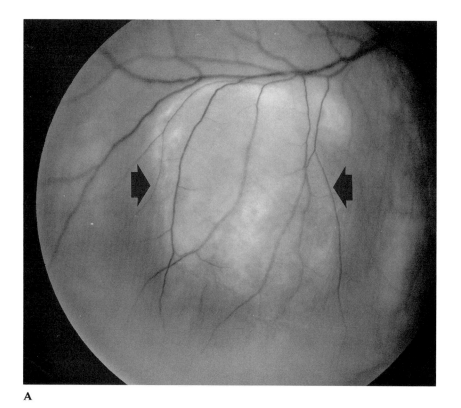

A

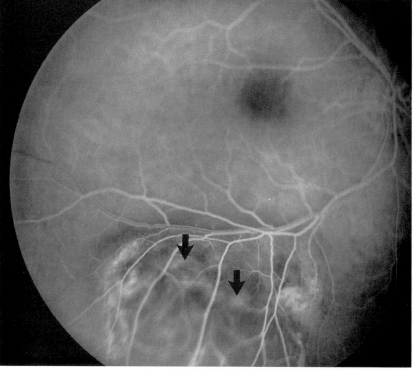

B

Fig. 5-2 (*A*) Malignant melanoma of the choroid (arrows in a red-free photo) of a 60-year-old male. (*B*) The same tumor is elevated, and fluorescein dye is seen at 25 sec in tumor vessels (arrows).

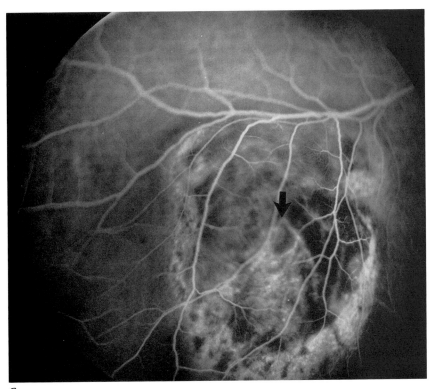

C

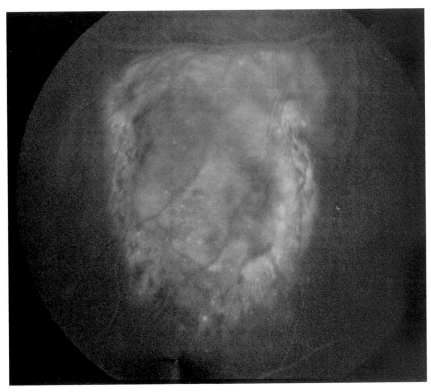

Fig. 5-2 (*C*) Dye in tumor vessels (arrow) is more apparent in the midvenous (31.6 sec) phase in the same eye. (*D*) Dye fades with recirculation in the late phase (10 min or 612 sec).

D

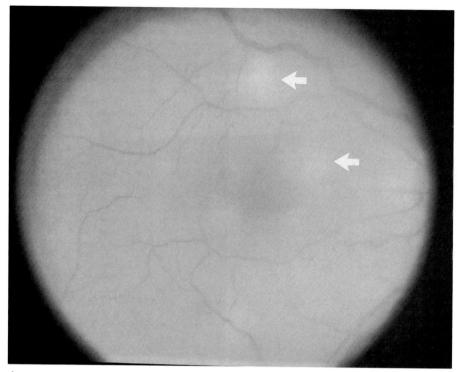

A

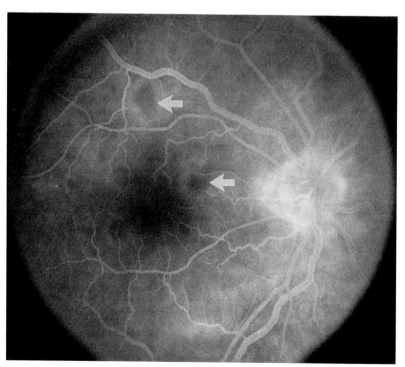

B

Fig. 5-3 (*A*) Creamy yellow lesions (arrows) in the retina of a patient with multifocal choroiditis. (*B*) Midphase (80.6 sec) fluorescein dye finds the choroidal blush hypointense (arrows) in choroiditis.

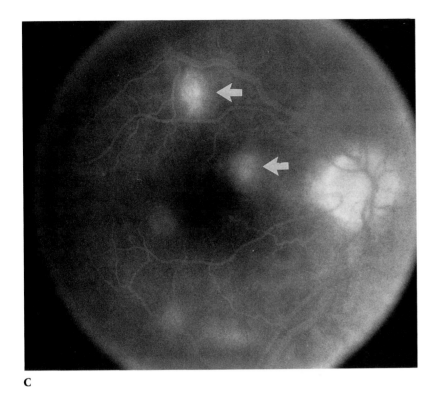

C

Fig. 5-3 (*C*) The same eye in the late phase (10 min or 602 sec) finds the same areas with persistent staining of the choroidal inflammatory lesions and hyperintense staining of the optic nerve (open arrow) from dye leakage.

areas that initially hypofluoresce (Fig. 5-3B); these areas later become hyperintense (Fig. 5-3C) due to vessel leakage of dye. Persistent fluorescein staining is observed in late-phase photos. Inflammatory conditions of the orbit, such as orbital pseudotumor or dysthyroid orbitopathy, can cause swelling or apparent indentation of the globe. This can then be seen as altering the background choroidal fluorescence, and folds in the choroid may appear. In systemic diseases that cause vasculitis, such as systemic lupus erythematosus, choroidal vessels can be markedly affected and cause fluid to accumulate under the retina.

RETINAL ARTERIAL AND VENOUS CIRCULATION

The two main circulations are to the inner (retinal) and middle (choroidal) layers of the eye. The outer (scleral) layer has minimal circulation and is basically a dense collagenous tunic of fibrous tissue similar to dura mater. The retina is supplied by the central retinal artery and vein, which enter and exit the eye through the central portion of the nerve to supply the inner layer of the eye. The choroid and optic nerve are mainly supplied by the posterior ciliary arteries, which

arise from the circle of Zinn vessels surrounding the optic nerve. These vessels typically enter the choroid to the middle layer of the retina, but may occasionally enter the inner layer of the retina to supply a small portion through anomalous cilioretinal arteries.

As a result of this separation of circulations to the ocular layers, vascular disorders of the retina may occur with sparing of the choroidal circulation, and vice versa. For example, the two most common disorders are carotid occlusive disease and vasculitis.

OCCLUSIVE DISEASE

In retinal occlusive disease, the posterior pole of the eye may be seen to contain a continuous or intermittent flow of emboli. This may be documented in the acute phase by the characteristic appearance in color fundus photographs (Fig. 5-4A). The retina supplied by this circulation is ischemic, pale, and edematous. A typical cause of retinal artery emboli is a cholesterol plaque from occlusive atheromatous carotid artery disease.

Some retinal areas may remain healthy and well perfused when other branches of the central retinal artery are spared or there is anomalous circulation to the ret-

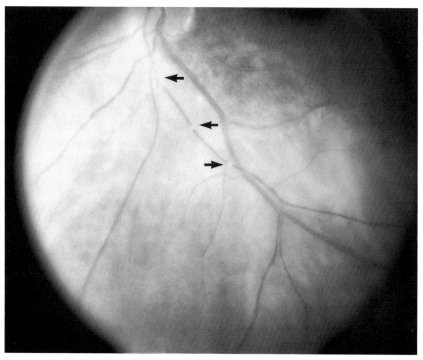

A

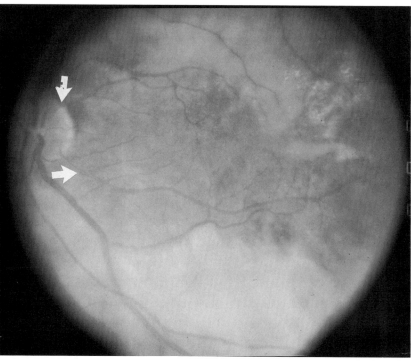

B

Fig. 5-4 (*A*) The posterior pole of the left eye demonstrates central retinal artery emboli (black arrows) in a patient with acute total left carotid occlusion. The retina supplied by this circulation is ischemic, pale, and edematous. (*B*) The healthy central retina is perfused by two fortuitous, but normally anomalous, cilioretinal arterioles (large white arrows) coming from the posterior ciliary circulation to the retina. These vessels are found to enter the retina from the 4 o'clock and 2 o'clock positions of the optic nerve head; their origins can be traced in subsequent fluorescein photos.

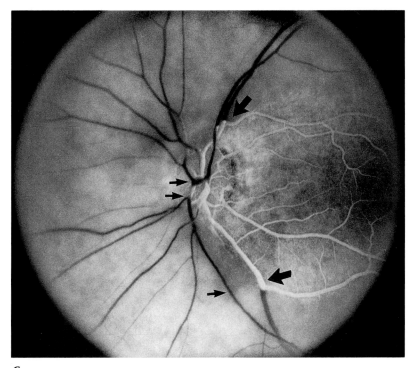

 C

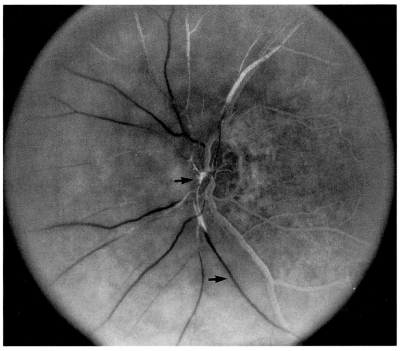

D

Fig. 5-4 (*C*) Cilioretinal perfusion is seen returning in branches of the central retinal vein (large black arrows) at 28.9 sec. There is no filling of central retinal artery branches (smaller arrows) because of carotid emboli. (*D*) Fluorescein photos at 1 min (63.3 sec) show minimal dye in the central retinal artery circulation and minimal filling in some but not all branches of the central retinal artery.

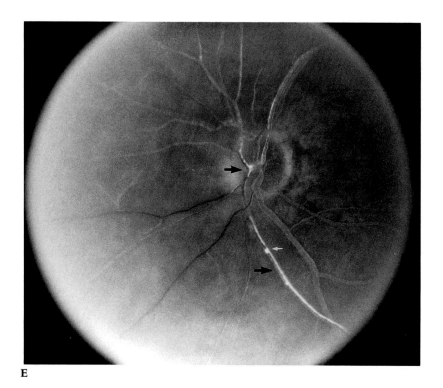

E

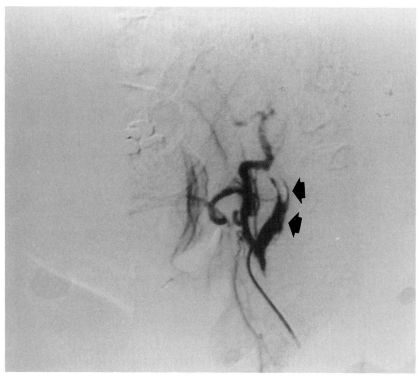

F

Fig. 5-4 (*E*) Late-phase photos at 5 min (314.4 sec), show only partial filling of the inferior temporal branch of the central retinal artery. An occluding Hollenhorst or cholesterol plaque may be seen to "light up" as a small, hyperfluorescent rectangle (small white arrow) between the black arrows. (*F*) Carotid angiogram of the same patient demonstrating acute total left internal carotid occlusion.

ina from the posterior ciliary arteries in the form of fortuitous cilioretinal vessels (Fig. 5-4B). In these cases the occluded branches of the central retinal artery do not fill the fluorescein, although branches of the central retinal vein may partially fill with fluorescein from returning blood of the perfused retina (Fig. 5-4C).

Normally, the midphase (after 20–30 sec after dye injection) is characterized by fading fluorescence in the retinal circulation. With delayed filling caused by vascular occlusive disease, it is not uncommon to see delayed and incomplete filling in central retinal artery branches (Fig. 5-4D), even into the late phase (Fig. 5-4E) 5–10 min postinjection. Retinal emboli are often caused by showers of atheromatous plaque material in acute carotid occlusion (Fig. 5-4F).

DIABETIC RETINOPATHY AND NEOVASCULARIZATION

Diabetes mellitus causes widespread multiorgan system morbidity in many of the 14 million Americans it afflicts. The progressive retinopathy it produces is the leading cause of new cases of legal blindness in working-age Americans, affecting 8,000 people per year. Though both types I and II diabetes lead to retinopathy, type I is associated with more frequent and more severe retinopathy, though it affects fewer patients than type II. After 5 years, 25% of type I diabetics have some retinopathy; after 10 and 15 years, approximately 60% and 80%, respectively, have some retinopathic change. Though they are less likely to develop retinopathy, type II diabetics make up a greater percentage of the diabetic population. Thus there are more legally blind type II than type I diabetics in the United States.

The progressive fundus changes that occur in diabetic retinopathy fall into two major categories: (1) background (or nonproliferative) diabetic retinopathy (BDR), in which the anatomical abnormalities occur within the retina, and (2) proliferative diabetic retinopathy (PDR), in which the anatomical abnormalities are anterior to the retina, including those in the vitreous cavity. This categorization describes changes occurring in a spectrum, with BDR associated with earlier and milder visual effects and PDR associated with a significantly increased risk of visual loss. Though BDR does not invariably progress to PDR, it always precedes its development.

Diabetic retinopathy (Fig. 5-5A) of both types results from numerous pathophysiological changes occurring in the retinal blood vessels. These include capillary basement membrane thickening, loss of microvascular

intramural pericytes, microaneurysm formation, and capillary acellularity, all of which contribute to both abnormal retinal vessel permeability and retinal vessel closure. Retinal vessel closure leads to retinal ischemia, which, through the production of a still unknown angiogenic factor by the retina, in turn stimulates the development of abnormal neovascularization on the iris, optic nerve, and retinal surface and into the vitreous cavity.

There are numerous characteristic ophthalmoscopic manifestations of BDR. Microaneurysm formation is generally the initial detectable fundus change, occurring first on the venous side of the capillaries and then on the arterial side. When capillary or microaneurysm walls become significantly weakened, intraretinal dot, blot, or splinter hemorrhages develop. Diffuse capillary or microaneurysm leakage of intracellular fluid and protein leads to macular edema formation, which is the leading cause of legal blindness in diabetics, and to lipid deposition in the macular and paramacular retina known as *hard exudation.*

Dilated collateral capillary networks known as *intraretinal microvascular abnormalities* are also seen. A subclassification of diabetic retinopathy termed *preproliferative diabetic retinopathy (PPDR)* is used for advanced BDR. It is characterized by increasing retinal hypoxia that manifests as large areas of capillary nonperfusion, cotton wool spots (nerve fiber layer infarctions), and increased intraretinal hemorrhages. Venous beading and loop formation (Fig. 5-5A) occur suggesting slowed retinal circulation.

The primary ophthalmoscopic manifestation of PDR is the development of newly formed blood vessels and associated fibrous tissue arising from the iris, retina, and optic nerve. This neovascularization extends along the inner retinal surface and/or into the vitreous cavity and stains brightly with fluorescein. Because of the great tendency to bleed, neovascularization often leads to vision-threatening vitreous or retinal hemorrhage. A fibrovascular frond (Fig. 5-5B) growing over the retinal surface leads to tissue contraction, with visual distortion or loss from traction detachment of the retina.

Fundus fluorescein angiography (FFA) is necessary in the diagnostic evaluation and therapeutic management of diabetic retinopathy. Patients with BDR lose vision largely from macular edema and capillary nonperfusion, both of which are well defined on FFA. During the transit phase of FFA, microaneurysms appear as small, punctate areas (Fig. 5-5C) of hyperfluorescence in cases of macular edema. Dot/blot hemorrhages, which are often confused with microaneurysms on clinical exam and do not have the same potential for

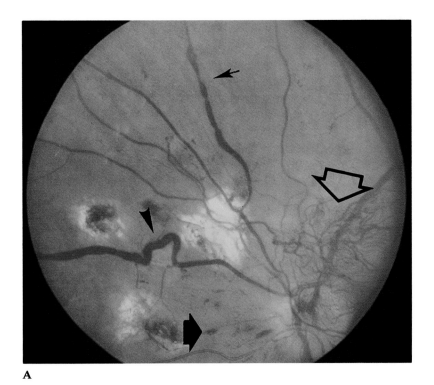

A

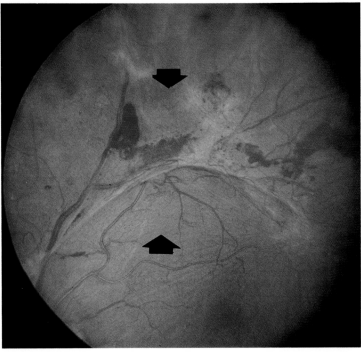

B

Fig. 5-5 (*A*) Venous beading (small arrow) and venous loop formation (arrowhead) in diabetic retinopathy are suggestive of sluggish circulation. Neovascularization (open arrow) and splinter hemorrhages (large arrow) occur. (*B*) Large frond of fibrovascular tissue (between the arrows) creates visible macular traction, leading to the final PDR stage of retinal detachment.

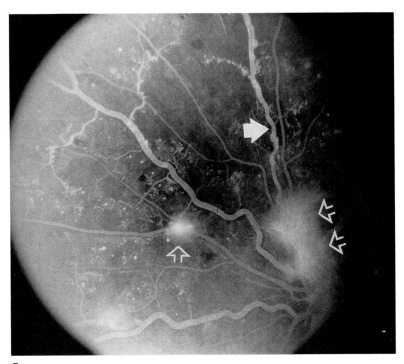

C

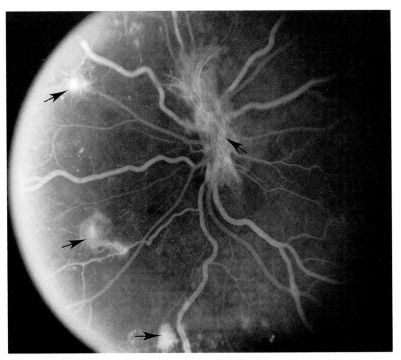

D

Fig. 5-5 (*C*) Diabetic retinopathy showing venous beading (arrow), hypofluorescent patchy capillary nonperfusion (arrow with stem), hyperfluorescent leaking neovascular tufts (open arrows), and multiple tiny, punctate hyperfluorescent microaneurysms (not marked but clearly visible). (*D*) Neovascular tufts of fragile vessels likely to rupture and bleed are found to hyperfluoresce as they continue to leak fluorescein during the angiogram.

leading to macular edema, appear as areas that remain hypofluorescent throughout FFA.

The early Treatment Diabetic Retinopathy Study demonstrated the therapeutic efficacy of, and established guidelines for, laser photocoagulation of patients with clinically significant macular edema. By clearly defining the location of the leaking microaneurysms, FFA determines the areas requiring laser treatment. Patients with poor macular function who lack visible fundus changes to explain their poor visual acuity often suffer from macular capillary nonperfusion, in which there is significant retinal ischemia that can only be seen with FFA. These areas and cotton wool spots of ischemia appear as large patches of consistent hypofluorescence.

Numerous studies have demonstrated the beneficial effect of panretinal laser photocoagulation in the treatment of eyes with active PDR. The abnormal neovascularization emanating from the optic disc and retinal surface hyperfluoresces (Fig. 5-5D) early during the arterial phase of FFA and continues to increase in brightness, with extensive leakage of fluorescein by the late phases. Clinically obvious areas of neovascularization are easily seen on FFA, but subtle or occult areas not seen clinically are also revealed. Thus, eyes that otherwise would not be treated with laser photocoagulation early in the course of PDR come to the attention of the physician with the use of FFA.

HAMARTOMAS, ANOMALIES, AND VARIATIONS

Phakomatoses are of great interest to ophthalmologists because these tumors cause complex symptoms affecting many organs, including the central nervous system. Neurofibromatosis (von Recklinghausen), tuberous sclerosis (Bournville), and angiomatosis retinae (von Hippel) and cerebellae (Lindau), and encephalotrigeminal angiomatosis (Sturge-Weber) are the most well known to neuroradiologists and neuro-ophthalmologists alike. Ataxia-telangiectasia may also be included in this group.

These diseases are so characteristic as to be well recognized. Less well understood and occasionally confused are anomalies and variations such as pseudopapilledema caused by drusen of the optic nerve. Drusen of the optic nerve are elevated optic nerve head anomalies. The impression of papilledema rather than pseudopapilledema leads to neurological and neuroradiological evaluation in otherwise asymptomatic, normal, and healthy patients with no symptoms of an expanding

intracranial mass. The drusen may be on the surface of the nerve (Fig. 5-6A) or buried below the surface. These drusen bodies fluoresce without dye injection and demonstrate autofluorescence (Fig. 5-6B) and occasional visualization on computed tomography (CT) scans (Fig. 5-6C). Drusen of the disc may be associated with hemorrhages at the margin of the disc (Fig. 5-6D) that further suggest papilledema if not recognized; fluorescein angiography demonstrates the lack of hyperintensity of the optic nerve head commonly associated with papilledema (Fig. 5-6E).

EFFECTS OF DEMYELINATING DISORDERS

Central nervous system demyelination may be associated with intraocular inflammation; uveitis and iritis are infrequently encountered. These inflammatory changes are incompletely understood and inadequately studied. Nonetheless, this rare association should be searched for and recognized. Vasculitis that is manifest as staining or sheathing or retinal vessels (Fig. 5-7), both arterial and venous, may occasionally be found on careful examination.

CAROTID CAVERNOUS AND DURAL ARTERIOVENOUS FISTULAS

Common ophthalmic findings of carotid cavernous fistulas are proptosis, bruit, diplopia, and a red eye from arterialization of conjunctival veins. More subtle findings are often found in dural sinus or low-flow shunts. Venous dilation from arterialization is not limited to the conjunctival vessels but may involve the retinal venules as well.

The normal arteriole:venule caliber ratio in the retina is 2:3 (Fig. 5-8A). Dilated, tortuous retinal venules can be documented with fluorescein dye. The dilation of arterialized veins can result in a 1:3 arteriolar venule (AV) ratio (Fig. 5-8B), and this can be followed by serial fluorescein angiography (Fig. 5-8C–G). A cerebral vessel neuroimaging study (Fig. 5-8H) demonstrates the extent of arterial shunting.

INFLAMMATIONS AND VASCULITIS

By far the most common vasculitis to affect the visual system is giant cell arteritis (known also as *temporal arteritis* or *arteritis of the elderly*). The characteristic clini-

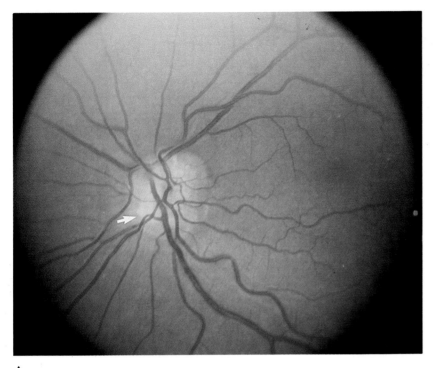

A

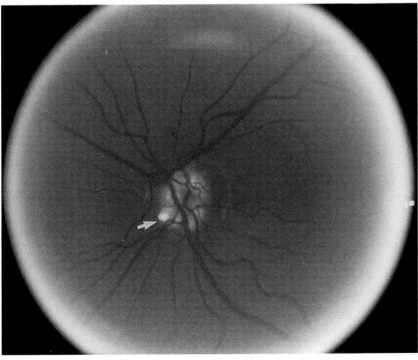

B

Fig. 5-6 (*A*) Drusen of the optic nerve head (arrow). (*B*) Drusen of the optic nerve head demonstrating autofluorescense (arrow pointing to the same area as part A).

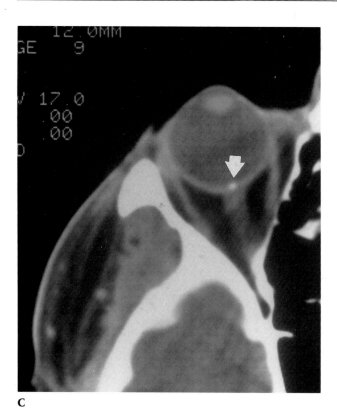

C

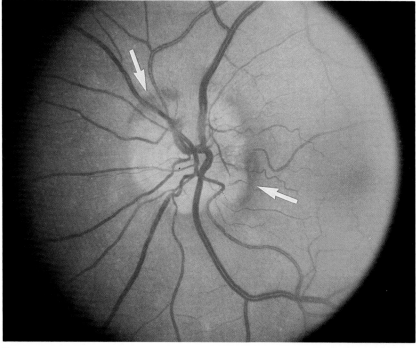

Fig. 5-6 (*C*) CT scan of the orbit demonstrating drusen of the optic nerve. (*D*) The opposite eye of the same patient shows hemorrhage (arrows) at the disc margin and an appearance suggestive of papilledema from buried disc drusen.

D

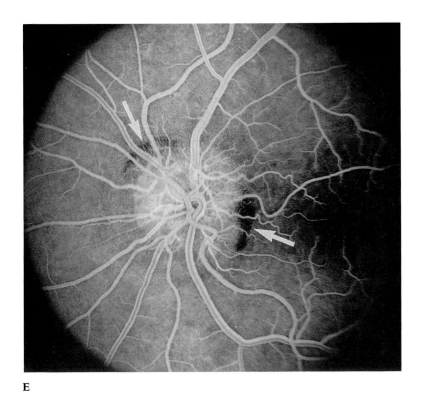

E

Fig. 5-6 (*E*) Fluorescein photo of the same eye demonstrates no hyperfluorescence of the disc itself and hypofluorescence of areas covered by hemorrhage (arrows).

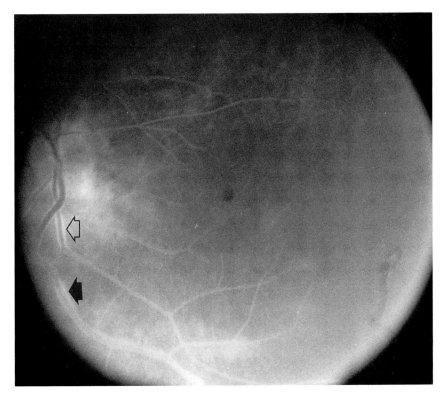

Fig. 5-7 Focal staining of the walls of both arteries (open arrows) and veins (closed arrows) in a 36-year-old female with multiple sclerosis. Histologically, inflammatory cells infiltrate the perivascular tissues. Vascular walls are partially incompetent and allow hyperfluorescence from leaking dye.

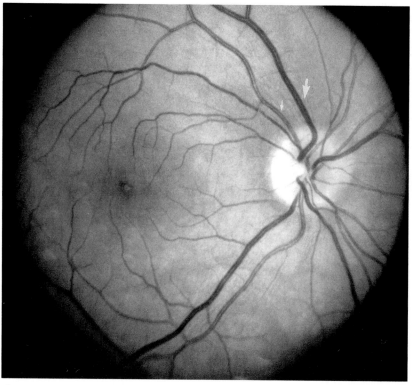

A

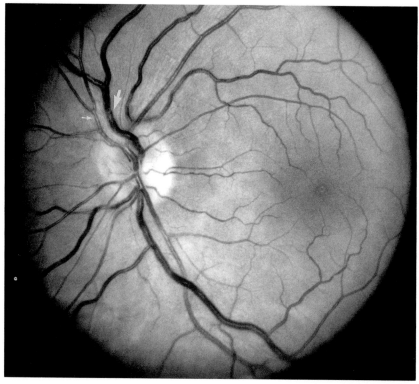

B

Fig. 5-8 (*A*) Red-free photo of the normal right eye in a 37-year-old female with a low-flow arterial to cavernous sinus fistula. The normal arteriole (small arrow) to venuole (large arrow) ratio is 2:3. (*B*) Red-free photo of the affected left eye of the patient in part (*A*). Arteriovenous shunting has expanded the vein caliber, so that the arteriole (small arrow) to venule (large arrow) ratio is 1:3.

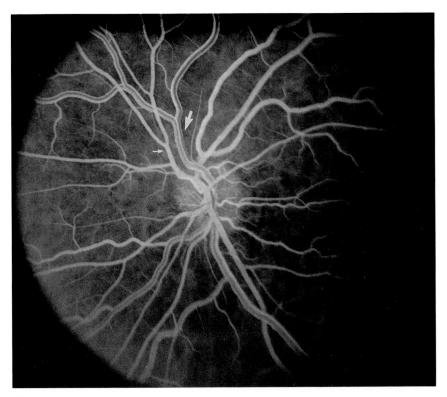

C

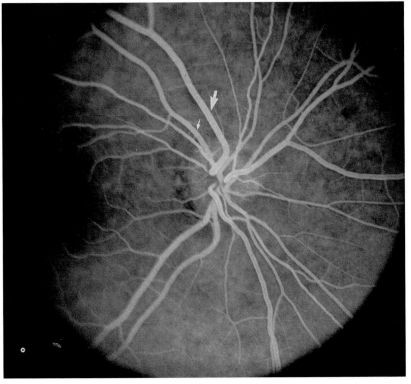

D

Fig. 5-8 (*C*) At 31.4 sec, lamellar flow is occurring in the dilated venules of the affected left eye. (*D*) Midphase (48 sec) fluorescein photo of the unaffected right eye shows a normal AV ratio of 2:3.

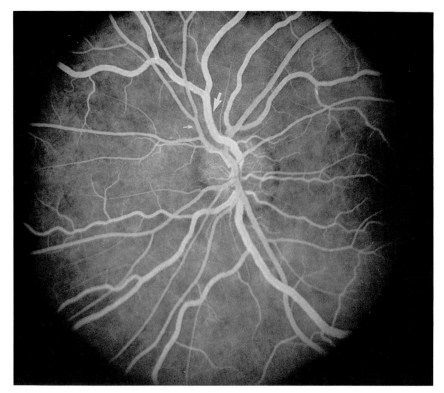

E

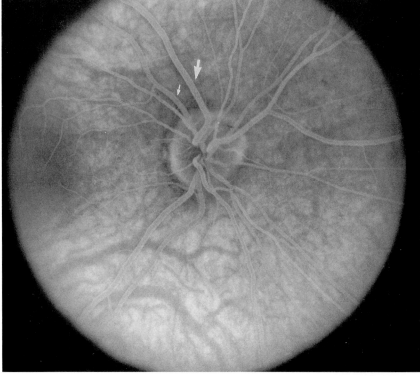

Fig. 5-8 (*E*) Midphase (69.7 sec) fluorescein photo of the affected left eye demonstrates the 1:3 AV ratio. (*F*) Late-phase
(5 min or 327.8 sec) right eye.

F

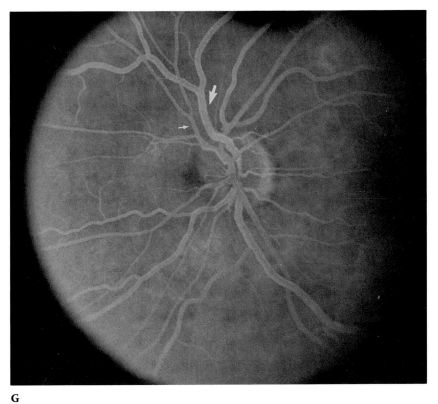

G

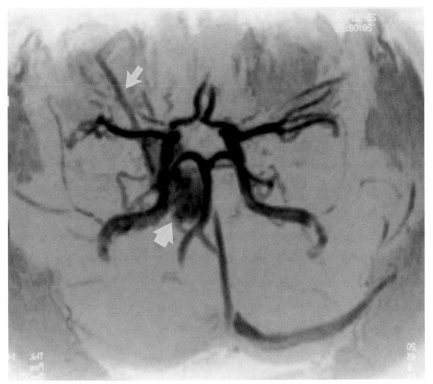

H

Fig. 5-8 (*G*) Late-phase (5 min or 341.2 sec) left eye. (*H*) Magnetic Resonance Angiography study of the same patient showing an enlarged left superior ophthalmic vein (arrow) and prominent asymmetry of cavernous sinus filling on the left side (larger arrow).

cal symptom complex in an individual over the age of 60 consists of some combination of the following: headaches, jaw claudication, polymyalgia, weight loss, anemia, or acute visual loss.

In giant cell arteritis, the posterior ciliary circulation of the eye is typically involved. The dozen or so short posterior ciliary arteries form a ring around the optic nerve adjacent to the globe. When the posterior ciliary circulation makes an anomalous contribution to the retinal circulation with cilioretinal arteries, retinal ischemia may be the initial result (Fig. 5-9A). In arteritis and the resultant occlusion of these posterior ciliary end arteries, the optic nerve becomes ischemic. Within a short time, there is resulting optic nerve swelling and varying, irreversible visual loss from this extreme ischemia (Fig. 5-9B), which often leaves the patient legally blind.

Fluorescein filling of vessels undergoing progressive occlusion from arteritis can be expected to be delayed or absent (Fig. 5-9C). While symptoms of amaurosis fugax are typically described as loss of monocular vision for several minutes at most and associated with carotid occlusive disease, these same symptoms may herald the onset of arteritis. Occlusion of posterior ciliary arteries causing ischemic optic neuropathy is the hallmark of giant cell arteritis. Temporal artery biopsy

documents the presence of arteritis (Fig. 5-9D), as opposed to the atherosclerotic vessel changes (Fig. 5-9E).

While temporal arteritis is rarely associated with cranial arteritis and cerebral infarction, the above case may be illustrative. Most neuroimaging studies suggestive of a diagnosis of arteritis do not have confirmatory pathology. Central nervous system involvement in cases of arteritis from polyarteritis nodosa is usually secondary to damage from hypertensive changes. Wegener's granulomatosis principally affects the peripheral nervous system and cranial nerves. Lymphomatoid granulomatosis involves the central nervous system in 20% of cases, as well as inflammation of the arterial wall with destruction, lymphocytes, plasma cells, histiocytes, and atypical lymphoreticular cells.

Takayasu's arteritis is characterized by intimal proliferation and luminal occlusion; early granulomatous inflammation is associated with patchy destruction of the media and elastica of the vessel wall. In these cases, intimal proliferation and late adventitial fibrosis may or may not be associated with vessel thrombosis. In systemic lupus erythematosus (SLE), brain artery disease is nonspecific and probably that of hypertension rather than SLE changes in the choroid plexus.

Isolated arteritis of the central nervous system is not always granulomatous, and disseminated or focal artery

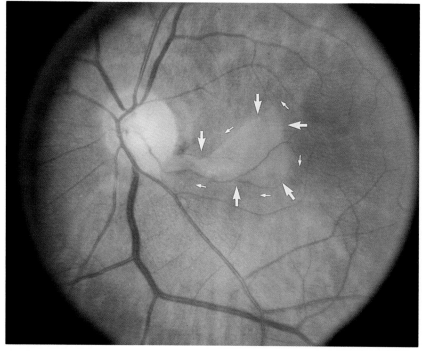

Fig. 5-9 (*A*) Occlusion of the cilioretinal artery causing very localized retinal edema (arrows surround the ischemic retina supplied by this normally anomalous vessel). The patient was found to have minimal carotid occlusive disease after carotid angiography 1 week earlier when evaluated for amaurosis fugax in the right eye. Put on aspirin and dipyridamole, she returned 1 week later with visual loss in the left eye, as documented here.

A

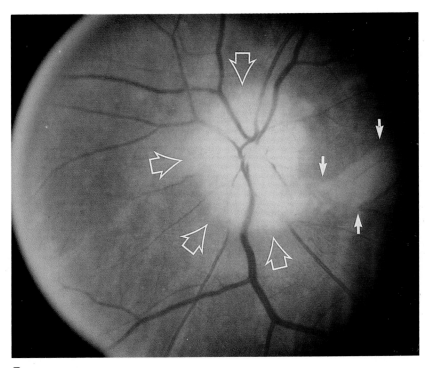

B

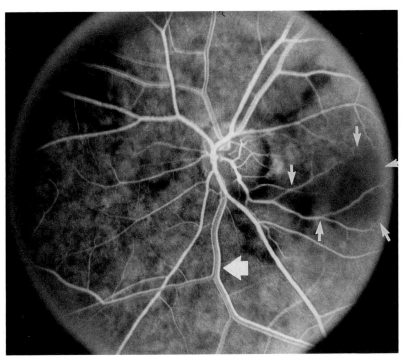

C

Fig. 5-9 (*B*) Same patient 3 days later demonstrating progressive occlusion of short posterior ciliary arteries with ischemic infarction of the optic nerve (surrounded by large open arrows) in addition to an initially ischemic retina (surrounded by small solid arrows). (*C*) Midphase fluorescein photo (53.6 sec) documents laminar venous flow (large arrows) due to sluggish retinal circulation. Normally, fluorescein is fading in this phase. Background choroidal circulation is absent in the region of ischemic retinal edema (surrounded by small arrows).

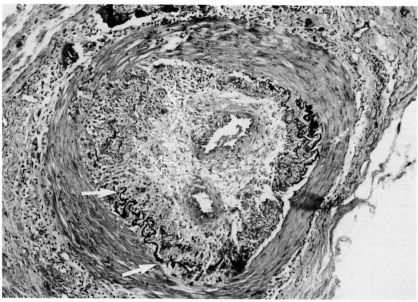

D

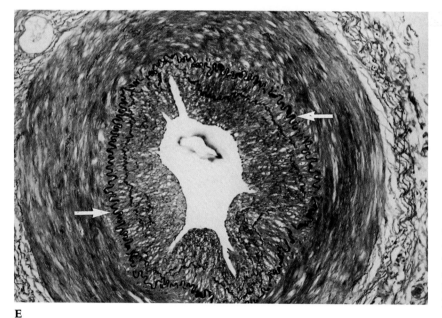

E

Fig. 5-9 (*D*) With posterior ciliary circulation occlusion in this 63-year-old female, a temporal artery biopsy was performed in spite of a normal sedimentation rate. Giant cells (open arrows), massive intimal fibrous proliferation, diffuse chronic inflammatory infiltration with fragmentation, and loss of the ribbon of elastic lamina (solid arrows) are present. (*E*) Atherosclerotic vessel for comparison demonstrates an open lumen, lack of inflammatory cell infiltration, and intact (though duplicated) elastic lamina (arrows) at the border between vessel intima and muscularis layers.

involvement occurs with luminal narrowing. Moyamoya disease involves arteries of the circle of Willis, with intimal fibrous thickening, and the elastic lamina is duplicated or triplicated, along with thinning of the media. Large collaterals may develop. Thrombotic thrombocytopenic purpura exhibits thrombosis in small vessels and capillaries from fibrin and platelet thrombi. Finally, endarteritis obliterans is found with vessel wall inflammation associated with syphilis, tuberculosis, bacteria, and fungal infections.

HYPERTENSIVE RETINOPATHY

Hypertension, which affects over 50 million adults in the United States, is associated with vascular lesions in the brain, heart, kidney and eyes. Its ocular effects are primarily manifested as hypertensive retinopathy resulting from both vasospastic and arteriosclerotic changes in the retinal arterioles. Most patients with mild to moderate hypertension have no visual symptoms and only minimal funduscopic changes, while those with longer-standing or more severe hypertension develop prominent characteristic changes in the retina with associated potential visual loss. However, it is important to note that there is significant variability in the types of hypertensive changes, and that there is no direct correlation between the changes and the particular level of systemic blood pressure.

Early or mild, non-vision-threatening retinopathic changes include arteriolar narrowing, increased arteritis reflexes, and arteriovenous crossing changes. Focal and diffuse narrowing of the retinal arterioles is the hallmark of hypertensive retinopathy. It is most commonly seen in chronic hypertension, though it can be seen as an acute vasospastic response during episodes of acute elevated blood pressure. Diffuse narrowing is manifest as a reduction in arteriole caliber; thus, the normal AV ratio of 2:3 is decreased. Hypertension induces progressive increases in the amounts of elastic and muscular tissue in the arteriole walls, which, in turn, induce changes in the light reflexes coming from the wall of the vessel. These reflexes range from simple broadening of the light reflex on the vessel surface to "copper wire" and "silver wire" appearances. Atherosclerotic changes in the intima of the larger vessels such as lipid deposition, calcification, and fibrosis can compromise the lumen and predispose the vessel to occlusion. Thickening of the vessel wall alters the appearance of the arteriovenous crossing. The arteriole and venule share a common adventitial sheath, with the venule lying in the anterior position. Glial cell proliferation around the vessels and sclerosis of the vessel walls lead to compression of the venule and the appearance of arteriovenous "nicking," venous banking, deviation of the vein, and right-angled crossings.

Severe hypertension (Fig. 5-10A) leads to more prominent and visually significant fundus changes. There is marked arterial and arteriolar constriction with areas of vessel wall damage, particularly at the origins of the first- and second-order retinal arterioles. Narrowing or closure of arterioles occurs, with leakage of blood elements into the vessel wall. As a result, cotton-wool spots and areas of capillary nonperfusion develop in the retina (Fig. 5-10B). There is remodeling of the capillary bed in the areas of ischemia. Microaneurysm and telangiectatic formation is seen and there is breakdown of the inner blood–retina barrier, with extravasation of plasma and red blood cells, producing dot/blot intraretinal hemorrhages and lipid deposition. There may be marked ischemic arteriolar and capillary permeability changes in the optic nerve head as well, especially in cases of accelerated acute hypertension,

and the optic nerve head will leak fluorescein, appearing hyperintense

Complications of severe hypertension include marked abnormalities in venous flow, evidenced by tortuous, dilated retinal veins (Fig. 5-10C) among the aforementioned arterial abnormalities. Medical treatment of severe hypertension can significantly improve the pathological fundus changes and associated venous statis retinopathy. With subsequent successful blood pressure control, significant resolution of funduscopic abnormalities (Fig. 5-10D–F), including disappearance of cotton-wool spots, decreased venous dilation and tortuosity, increased arterial caliber, and resolution of retinal hemorrhage are seen.

FFA is of significant benefit in delineating areas of breakdown of the blood–retina barrier. Most microvascular angiographic changes in hypertensives occur outside the central macular area. Microaneurysms, capillary telangiectasias, capillary nonperfusion, and retinal edema from leaking capillaries are all identified on FFA. Microaneurysms appear as small, punctate areas of hyperfluorescence scattered in areas of blood–retina breakdown. Microaneurysmal leakage from these areas results in retinal edema, though somewhat less commonly than in diabetic patients, and appears as diffuse increased hyperfluorescence in the regions with prior punctate hyperfluorescence (Fig. 5-10E). In areas of vascular occlusion, capillary nonperfusion is seen as patches of hypofluorescence which maintain their appearance throughout the late phases of the angiogram. Remodeling of the capillary network occurs in areas of prior ischemia, and capillary telangiectasias and collateral vessels may develop. Cotton-wool spots appear as hypofluorescent areas of retinal ischemia. Optic nerve swelling appears as both early and late hyperfluorescence of the neural rim.

Hypertension causes specific retinal, choroidal, and optic nerve abnormalities. The associated arteriolar sclerosis of the retina and optic nerve, however, is pathogenetically important in the causes of other posterior segment conditions as well, including arterial macroaneurysm, ischemic optic neuropathy, branch retinal vein occlusion, central retinal vein occlusion, and venous stasis retinopathy. Patients with venous stasis retinopathy are generally asymptomatic or complain of mild, sometimes transient decreased vision. Their fundi demonstrate mild to moderate venous dilation, scattered retinal hemorrhages, and many of the aforementioned funduscopic and angiographic signs associated with hypertensive retinopathy.

FFA is a useful diagnostic tool in the evaluation of many of the microvascular retinal, choroidal, and optic

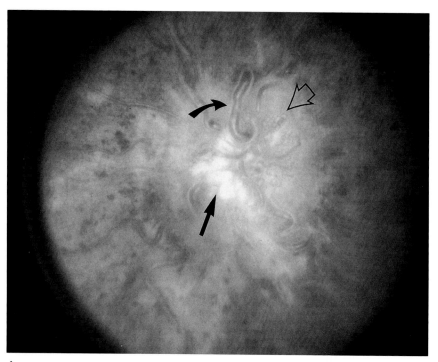

A

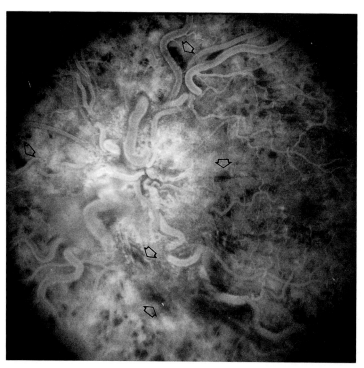

B

Fig. 5-10 (*A*) Severe hypertensive retinopathy with optic disc edema, cotton-
wool spots with capillary nonperfusion
(solid arrow), microaneurysm and telangiectatic vessel formation (open arrow), and
dilated, tortuous veins of abnormal venous
flow (curved arrow). (*B*) During the fluorescein midvenous phase (58.1 sec), hemorrhages are seen as hypointense areas
(open arrows).

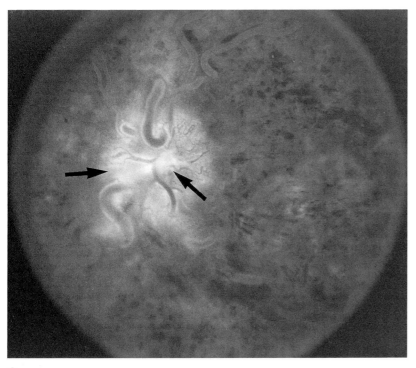

C

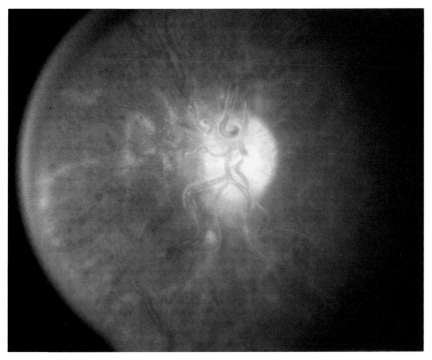

D

Fig. 5-10 (*C*) The late phase (207.4 sec) reveals optic disc edema hyperfluorescence (arrows) from leaking fluorescein. (*D*) Two months later, disease in the same eye has resolved significantly as control of the patient's blood pressure is achieved.

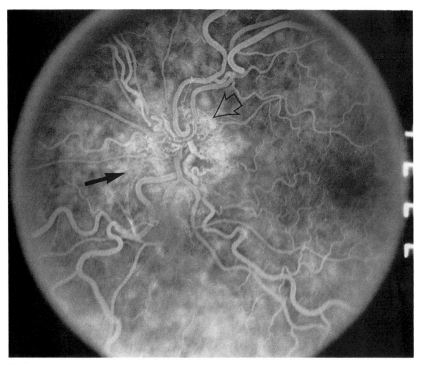

E

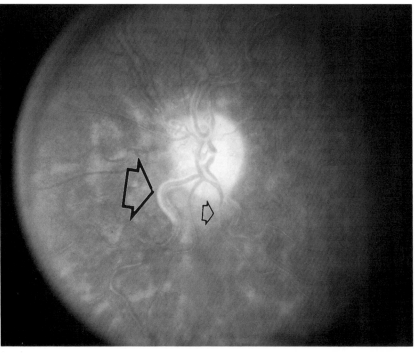

F

Fig. 5-10 (*E*) Corresponding fluorescein of 2-month photo in part (*D*) demonstrates remodeling of the capillary network in areas of prior ischemia (arrow), capillary telangiectasias, and collateral vessels (open arrow). (*F*) Same retina at 2.5 years. Vessel sheathing (large open arrow) and both focal (small open arrow) and diffuse arteriolar attenuation are seen.

nerve abnormalities seen in patients with hypertension. It is vital in the management of these patients and is most important in defining and following the extent of disease.

SUGGESTED READINGS

Daniel AM, Frederick JA (ed). Principles and Practice of Ophthalmology. W.B. Saunders, 1994.

Feman SS (ed). *Ocular Problems in Diabetes Mellitus.* Boston, Blackwell Scientific, 1991.

Gass JDM. *Stereoscopic Atlas of Macular Diseases,* vol 1. St Louis, CV Mosby, 1987.

Ryan SJ (ed). *Retina,* vol 2. St Louis, CV Mosby, 1989.

Schatz H, Burton TC, Yannuzzi LA, et al. *Interpretation of Fundus Fluorescein Angiography.* St Louis, CV Mosby, 1978.

Yannuzzi LA, Slakter JS, Sorenson JA, et al. *Digital Indocyanine Green Videoangiography and Choroidal Neovascularization,* Retina, vol 12. St Louis, CV Mosby, 1992, pp 191–192.

Early Treatment Diabetic Retinopathy Study Group: Early photocoagulation for diabetic retinopathy. ETDRS No. 9. *Ophthalmology* 98:766, 1991.

The Diabetic Retinopathy Study Research Group: Photocoagulation treatment of proliferative diabetic retinopathy. Clinical applications of DRS findings. DRS Report No. 8. *Ophthalmology* 88:583, 1981.

6

Conventional Cerebral Angiography

Richard A. Baker, M.D., Daniel K. Kido, M.D., Calvin L. Rumbaugh, M.D.

HISTORY AND INDICATIONS

Carotid angiography was first described by Egas Moniz[1] in 1927. Since then, there have been progressive improvements in techniques for needle and catheter introduction and contrast injection, in contrast agents, and in imaging techniques. Today most carotid angiography is carried out via the Seldinger[2] catheter technique, usually through the femoral artery, although the brachial or carotid artery occasionally is still used for catheter introduction, especially for interventional procedures.

Although rapid film changers are still in use for imaging, digital subtraction equipment is replacing them.[3–5] In addition, substantial improvements in computed tomography (CT) and magnetic resonance imaging (MRI) have resulted in techniques with excellent, rapid visualization of much of the vaculature of the head and neck with noninvasive or minimally invasive techniques.

At one time, conventional film cerebral angiography was not only the primary diagnostic tool for confirming cerebrovascular disease, it was the only method available. Now, high-resolution digital subtraction angiography is excellent for confirming occlusive vascular diseases, arteriovenous malformations, and aneurysms.[6,7] Small vessel diseases such as vasculitis or occlusive changes may be more optimally imaged on conventional 2 × magnification film because of the better resolution. Because of the high resolution obtained with some digital subtraction units, and with the promise of further improvements in the resolution of small structures, conventional cut-and-roll film changers are becoming obsolete. Furthermore, conventional angiography and digital subtraction angiography are both being replaced, to some degree, by color flow Doppler, high-resolution CT and MRI vascular imaging. However, aneurysm clips still present a serious problem both for CT and MRI, and these special situations may continue to necessitate the use of angiography.

PRELIMINARY PATIENT ORIENTATION AND PREPARATION

The neuroradiologist should always, when feasible, discuss with the patient and family the nature of angiography, the reasons for this study, alternative diagnostic and therapeutic algorithms which may be available, and the risks. Optimally, this discussion will occur before the patient is given any premedications. The patient's clinical chart, including laboratory findings, must be reviewed, with special vigilance for possible complicating factors such as heart failure, renal or hepatic disease, diabetes, and bleeding tendencies. In children, homocystinuria is an added contraindication.

This clinical review should clearly establish the critical questions to be answered by angiography.

The patient needs to be adequately hydrated before arriving for the examination. Preliminary angiographic orders should ensure the avoidance of solid food for the preceding 8–12 hr. Except when the study is performed immediately preoperatively, the patient is encouraged to maintain the oral intake of fluids until arrival in the angiography suite. If the patient's condition does not allow oral intake, intravenous hydration may be provided.

Many neuroradiologists prefer that the patient be premedicated for this study. An intravenous line may be positioned at or before angiography to ensure access if intravenous medication or volume expanders are required during this study. Low-flow oxygen by nasal cannula is becoming more routine and is especially important if intravenous sedation is used. Pulse oximetry, frequent blood pressure monitoring, and electrocardiographic monitoring are the standard of care when intravenous sedation is employed.[8] Frequent verbal interchange with the patient, however, remains the most sensitive means of detecting subtle neurologic compromise.

TECHNIQUE

The Seldinger method for catheter introduction by the femoral arteries is preferred for most angiographies.[2] Many excellent references describing catheter techniques for this method, as well as axillary, brachial, subclavian, and carotid approaches, along with catheter selection, positioning of the patient's head, filming sequence, and contrast agents, are available.[9,10]

Nonionic contrast agents have been shown to be less neurotoxic and produce significantly fewer side effects than ionic agents.[11,12] These positive features are responsible for ionic agents becoming more routine for cerebral angiography. Most angiographers agree that nonionic agents are especially desirable for spinal angiography.

Vital signs are generally checked every 15 min for the first hour and every 30 min for the next 2 hr following angiography. The puncture site should be inspected for bleeding and/or hematoma formation, and the pulses and temperature of the extremity must be checked, with vital sign monitoring. The patient should be kept on bed rest for at least 5–6 hr postangiography, and physical activity should be modestly restricted for 24 hr. The patient must be encouraged to maintain good hydration. When possible, the neuroradiologist or his assistant should check the patient for any evidence of complications and document this in the hospital record.

COMPLICATIONS

Complications of cerebral angiography generally are classified into three groups: general systemic or allergic reactions, local complications related to the vessel puncture, and neurologic deficits.

General Systemic Reactions to Contrast Agents or Medications

Patients should be screened before the procedure for a history of allergies or sensitivity reactions to drugs or iodine exposure such as contrast agents used in radiology procedures, severe renal disease, and multiple myeloma. A positive history for contrast sensitivity should cause reconsideration of magnetic resonance angiography (MRA) and/or noninvasive ultrasound imaging as possible substitutes for angiography. When no substitute is acceptable, steroid preparation (13-hr preparation: 50 mg prednisone PO 13, 7, and 1 hr prior to angiography, with 50 mg Benadryl IM 1 hr before) or, in rare instances, anesthesia stand-by will make angiography feasible and reasonably safe.

Local Complications Related to the Puncture Site

Hematoma formation at the puncture site is one of the more common complications. This is usually a minor problem which can be minimized by careful compression at the puncture site. Compression of the puncture site after removal of the catheter from the vessel for at least 15 min is important. Patients with hypertension or clotting problems or those taking antiplatelet agents or heparin may require longer compression periods. In addition to visible bleeding or hematoma formation, when the puncture site is unusually high, bleeding may occur within the pelvic region and go undetected. A kidney, ureter, bladder study or CT scan should be considered if a patient becomes hypotensive following angiography to exclude the uncommon but life-threatening consequence of pelvic hematoma. Thrombosis of the femoral artery, pseudoaneurysm formation, and dissection at the puncture site are rare but occasionally occur in a badly diseased artery or in cases where the initial puncture has been difficult and hence more traumatic than usual. The puncture needle, guidewire, and cathether should all be handled and manipulated gently to minimize possible damage to vessel walls. Smaller catheters (5 French and smaller) appear to produce less vessel injury.[13] At one time, treatment usually required surgical intervention, but now other techniques, including clot lysis methods, may be considered.[14] Pseudoaneurysm compression with ultrasound monitoring is successful as well as noninvasive.

Neurologic Deficits or Stroke

These conditions are occasionally seen with cerebral angiography. They occur rarely, and fortunately are usually transitory. Sometimes the problem may be due to contrast sensitivity; at other times, small iatrogenic blood clots are thought to be the cause. Frequently, the cause is unclear.[14,15] This is especially true of the rare cortical blindness and the more common postangiography confusion. Personal experience suggests that fever or vasculitis is a more likely precursor of these generalized toxic reactions to contrast agents.

A number of precautions may minimize neurological complications. Some angiographers recommend that each patient be given an initial small dose of heparin before initiation of the angiographic procedure.[16] Others recommend continuous, slow irrigation of the catheter with a heparinized solution via an infusion pump during the entire procedure. Still others recommend that with the nonionic contrast agents, heparin be added to the contrast solution. Some workers believe that all of the above measures should be used.[17,18]

Mani et al.,[13,19,20] reviewing 5,000 cerebral angiograms, reported higher complication rates in older patients (over 40 years of age), in those with cerebrovascular occlusive disease, and in those whose angiographic procedures lasted for more than 80 min. Angiographer expertise and contrast volumes are also related to morbidity.[19]

There is a fourth type of angiographic complication, often not considered, at the time of the event. This is the "pseudocomplication," which is a relatively common problem, frequent, and not always appreciated by the neuroradiologist.[21] Pseudocomplication is an untoward event which is actually not related to the procedure but is coincidental. It may consist of progression of the patient's disease process or may be a totally unrelated occurrence such as a coronary occlusion in a patient not known, prior to the event, to have heart disease. These occurrences pose a diagnostic problem when they occur during or shortly after the procedure.

Their true nature may not be recognized; therefore, appropriate treatment may be delayed. The importance of having the clinician requesting the study readily available for consultation in the event of any untoward event cannot be overstated.

REFERENCES

1. Moniz E. L'encephalographie arterielle, son importance dans la localisation des tumeurs cerebrales. *Rev Neurol (Paris)* 1927;2:72.

2. Seldinger SI. Catheter replacement of the needle in percutaneous arteriography. A new technique. *Acta Radiol (Stockh)* 1953;39:368.

3. Amplatz K. Rapid film changes, in H.L. Heram (ed), *Abrams Angiography*, Vol 1, ed 3. Boston, Little, Brown, 1983, p 105.

4. Levin DC. Noncardiac angiographic facilities, in H.L. Heram (ed), *Abrams Angiography*, Vol 1, ed 3. Boston, Little, Brown, 1983, p 175.

5. Ouitt TW. Digital subtraction angiography, in H.L. Heram (ed), *Abrams Angiography*, Vol 1, ed 3. Boston, Little, Brown, 1983, p 180.

6. Kruger RA, Riederer SJ. *Digital Subtraction Angiography.* Boston, G.K. Hall, 19.

7. Foley WD, Milde MW. Intra-arterial digital subtraction angiography. *Radiol Clin North Am* 1985;23:293–320.

8. Young WL, Pile-Spellman J. Anesthetic considerations for interventional neuroradiology. *Anesthesiology* 1994; 80:427.

9. Taveras JM, Wood EH. *Diagnostic Neuroradiology.* Baltimore, Williams & Wilkins, 1976.

10. Amundsen P, Dugstad G, Slettebo M. Clinical testing of amipaque for cerebral angiography. *Neuroradiology* 1978; 15:89.

11. McIvor J, Steiner TJ, Perkin GD, et al. Neurological morbidity of arch and carotid arteriography in cerebrovascular disease. The influence of contrast medium and radiologist. *Br J Radiol* 60:117.

12. Mani RL, Eisenberg RL, McDonald EJ, et al. Complications of catheter cerebral arteriography: Analysis of 5,000 procedures: I. Criteria and incidence. *AJR* 1978; 131:861.

13. Davis DO, Rumbaugh CL, Gilson JM. Angiographic diagnosis of small vessel cerebral emboli. *Acta Radiol (Diagn) (Stockh)* 1969;9:264.

14. Zatz LM, Iannone AM. Cerebral emboli complicating cerebral angiography. *Acta Radiol (Diagn) (Stockh)* 1966; 5:621.

15. Wallace S, Medellin H, DeJongh D, et al. Systemic heparinization for angiography. *AJR* 1972;116:204.

16. Rasuli P. Blood clot formation in angiographic syringes containing nonionic contrast media. Letter to the editor.

17. Dawson P, Strickland NH. Thromboembolic phenomena in clinical angiography: Role of materials and technique. *JVIR* 1991;2:125.

18. Mani RL, Eisenberg RL. Complications of catheter cerebral arteriography: Analysis of 5,000 procedures: II. Relation of complication rates to clinical and arteriographic diagnoses. *AJR* 1978;131:867.

19. Mani RL, Eisenberg RL. Complications of catheter cerebral arteriography: Analysis of 5,000 procedures: III. Assessment of arteries injected, contrast medium used, duration of procedure, and age of patient. *AJR* 1978;131:871.

20. Pelz DM. Complication rates of DSA and conventional film cerebral angiography. Letter to the editor.

21. Baum S, Stein GN, Kuroda KK. Complications of "no arteriography." *Radiology* 1996;86:835.

7

Digital Subtraction Angiography: Introduction, Equipment, Techniques

Robert A. Ellwood, M.D., Matthias J. Kirsch, M.D.

INTRODUCTION, EQUIPMENT, TECHNIQUES

Introduction

The fascination with digitization of images, first introduced experimentally by Meyers et al. in 1963,[1] continued to grow with the development of computed tomographic scanners during the 1970s. Later in that decade and in the early 1980s, adaptation of those methods to traditional imaging techniques such as angiography came to the fore. Researchers at the University of Wisconsin described computed fluoroscopy, in which images from an image intensifier were collected, amplified allegorically, and digitized before being integrated, processed, and redisplayed on a monitor.[2] Similar research was being done at the University of Arizona.[3] Workers at the Cleveland Clinic were the first to use the term *digital subtraction angiography* (*DSA*).[4]

While these techniques were being developed, there was some apprehension in both the radiographic professional and manufacturing communities about the future of this modality. Some of this apprehension was due to two factors. Professionally, there was a feeling that digital imaging—proposed, as it was, initially for intravenous administration—perhaps represented a retreat in quality from the sophisticated level of vascular imaging that had already been developed. This was coupled with the fact of new jargon and the variety of adaptations utilized by manufacturers as they entered the marketplace.

Today, digital imaging is common in most vascular laboratories, to the point where digital radiography has totally replaced film screen angiography in some laboratories.

This chapter attempts to review the components of the digital angiography system, the technical performance of the examination, and, in particular, the role of DSA in evaluation of the cervicocephalic vasculature.

DSA, like conventional subtraction angiography, attempts to increase the contrast between the temporally transient (contrast-enhanced vasculature) and the temporally permanent (bones and soft tissue).[5] This requires the generation of a series of images and a postprocessing function. For digital subtraction, the latter function is performed by the use of computer technology and generally requires a high-quality imaging chain for the generation of images.

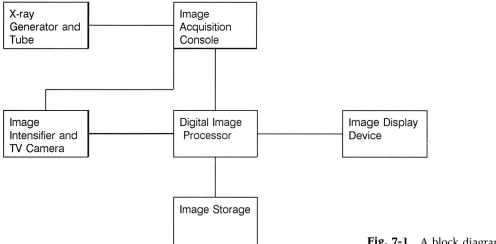

Fig. 7-1 A block diagram of a digital subtraction unit.

Equipment

Two basic DSA systems exist: integrated and add-on.[6] The integrated systems are produced by major x-ray equipment manufacturers and are fully dedicated DSA units with complex interfacing between the x-ray and image acquisition systems. The components have been designed to produce the best images possible. Integrated systems are more expensive than add-on systems. Add-on systems take the television signal from a fluoroscopic system and digitize it. Because of the high signal-to-noise ratio, several frames are often integrated to improve the image. Add-on systems are cheaper and can be mobile. Mixing of equipment has potential problems due to the complicated synchronization required and the need to optimize all links in the imaging chain. After some initial success, add-on systems became less popular.[7]

Understanding and evaluating DSA equipment requires a component-by-component evaluation of the entire imaging chain. Figure 7-1 delineates the basic requirements of DSA. To achieve low-contrast visualization, all the links of the imaging chain must be optimal.

Standard angiographic x-ray tubes and generators are generally adequate for DSA.[8] The x-ray generator must be capable of producing high-flux, short-exposure images to reduce motion artifacts and constant x-ray output for each exposure. A high-heat-capacity tube is needed to allow multiple high-intensity exposures.[9]

The modern cesium-iodide image intensifier is one of the strongest links in the DSA image chain.[7] The image intensifier absorbs a certain fraction of incident x-ray photons and produces a quantity of light proportional to the number of incident x-ray photons. A light diaphragm is used to control the amount of light from the image intensifier that reaches the television camera tube, as in the case of changing photographic F-stops. The size of the image intensifier is an important factor in determining the size of the area imaged. Large image intensifiers offer greater imaging areas and superior contrast resolution capabilities but have the disadvantages of decreased spatial resolution due to the fixed matrix size of the image processor and increased cost.[8] The image intensifier should be mounted on a C-arm apparatus to allow angulated views while the patient remains supine, decreasing patient motion artifact.

The television system produces an electronic video signal from the light emitted from the image intensifier. Many believe that this limits the overall resolution of the system.[8] Noise is anything that obscures the signal being measured. Signal-to-noise ratio (SNR) is the ratio of the signal voltage to the noise voltage. Several methods are utilized by various manufacturers to perform DSA imaging and optimize the SNR.

One method is sequential or progressive video scanning after a short-pulsed radiation exposure. In this method the x-ray tube is pulsed, causing an x-ray exposure for a fixed period, and one television frame is digitized for each image after the pulse has terminated. The sequential scanning method scans the lines of the television target in consecutive order. This method results in significant shortening of exposure time, thus decreasing motion artifacts.[10] Frames are not wasted while waiting for video signal stabilization, allowing optimum dose efficiency to be achieved.[11] If biplane DSA is installed, it allows alternating pulses of the two tubes to prevent scatter.[12] However, this method places stringent requirements on the noise level of both the television camera and the analog-to-digital converters. Higher SNR cameras (1,000:1) are needed to reduce video noise.[10] The shorter exposure times necessitate the use of significantly higher amperage levels,[10,13,14] which requires higher-power generators and x-ray tubes.

Another technique used in earlier systems is the continuous-during-readout method. Here x-ray exposure is continuous, and one or more television frames are digitized and averaged to form an image. The target of the television is read out in an interlaced pattern, resulting in scanning of only the even-numbered lines in the first half of the frame, followed by scanning of the odd-numbered lines in the second half of the frame. Extending x-ray exposure periods can improve the SNR by using the simple technique of frame averaging. By digitally adding multiple frames, improvements in the effective SNR of the camera and the effective precision of the analog-to-digital converter can be achieved.[15] This allows utilization of a system with a television camera having a lower SNR. A major drawback of frame integration is that it lengthens the effective exposure time.[10] Therefore, motion artifacts are likely to degrade the image. Another disadvantage is that the first few television fields are wasted to allow the video signal to stabilize, thus adding to patient exposure and x-ray tube load.[10]

Some have suggested that it is difficult to obtain high-quality DSA images with older video cameras operating with an SNR in the 100:1 or 200:1 range.[10] Newer Plumbicons (lead oxide cameras) with SNRs well in excess of 1,000:1 at a 5-MHz bandwidth are available, which have improved dynamic ranges and reduced lag. Stein and Swift[15] have concluded that lower SNR cameras can be used in DSA without performance degradation and that conventional vidicons have better performance than newer Plumbicons. The dynamic range of the vidicon far exceeds that of the Plumbicon, making it easier to achieve good image quality when examining parts of the body exhibiting a wide range of x-ray transmissions. The use of a vidicon in a pulsed DSA system is difficult due to its properties of "lag," but it may be incorporated into a continuous DSA system.[16]

The digital image processor is where subtraction and image enhancement take place. The major functions are to digitize television frames, store the digital images,

MATRIX SIZE

Field Size of Image Intensifier (inches)	128²	256²	512²	1024²
4.5	.56	1.1	2.2	4.4
6.0	.42	.84	1.7	3.4
9.0	.28	.56	1.1	2.2
14.0	.18	.36	.72	1.4
16.0	.15	.31	.63	1.26

Fig. 7-2 Table demonstrates that spatial resolution (lp/mm) decreases as larger field intensifiers are used for a fixed matrix size.

display them on a monitor or allow photographing, and allow manipulation of the digital images.

The matrix of the image processor is a rectangular array of picture elements, or pixels, the size of which is defined by the number of pixels on a side. Typically, the acquisition matrix is 512 × 512, with new systems having a 1,024 × 1,024 matrix. The spatial resolution of the system is limited by the pixel size. With a fixed matrix, spatial resolution decreases as larger field intensifiers are used (Fig. 7-2). Some users of large-field image intensifiers have found that the loss of spatial resolution is outweighed by the increased field size and contrast sensitivity of such advanced intensifiers.[8] If matrix size were increased to 1,024 × 1,024, in theory the spatial resolution should be increased; but in practice, the gain is less than expected.[17]

Methods utilized for digital subtraction include temporal, energy, and hybrid subtraction. Temporal subtraction uses a mask (a single image or integrated series of images) which is subtracted from images containing contrast acquired later in the run. Energy subtraction has been used experimentally in DSA and utilizes pulses of high- and low-energy x-rays. Following digitization and subtraction of images, residual images display bone and vessels. This is not particularly helpful in displaying vessels without overlying bone.[6] Hybrid

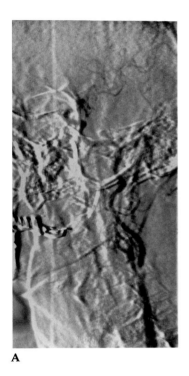

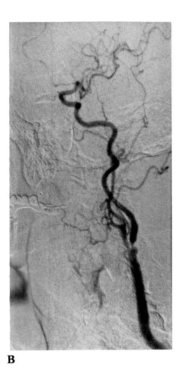

A   B

Fig. 7-3   The role of pixel shift. (*A*) Distorted image using mask 4 and image 18 without pixel shift. (*B*) Improved image quality following pixel shift, using the same images.

subtraction uses energy-subtracted images as a sequence for temporal subtraction, and eliminates bone and motion artifacts.

Misregistration artifacts are caused by voluntary and involuntary patient motion during the time interval between the mask and contrast images. Artifacts caused by slight motion may be reduced by reregistration or pixel shifting.[10] This allows shifting of pixel information horizontally, vertically, or even obliquely to improve the match of the mask and contrast images (Fig. 7-3).

Technique

It was felt that because of the increased conspicuousness of the contrast material utilizing computerized enhancement of digital imaging, utilization of the intravenous route would provide sufficient signal to perform digital angiography. Accordingly, the initial studies in this field were done with intravenous boluses injected at the antecubital area.[18] It soon became apparent, however, that utilization of the peripheral venous site for injection involved the loss of cohesive dispersion of the contrast bolus; therefore, the placement of central catheters became the preferred method. Despite the more central placement, there was felt to be a loss of the cohesive contrast bolus secondary to cardiac effects. Some authors recommended an increased rate of injec-

tion of the contrast agent, but with a reduction in overall volume.[19]

The intravenous digital subtraction method, while it is valid and remains valid in patients in whom intra-arterial access may be difficult or contraindicated, provides less detail than standard angiography.[20] Consequently, there was a shift from the intravenous method to the intra-arterial method as small-bore catheters became more readily available. The intra-arterial method allowed delivery of the contrast agent with less fear of cohesive dispersion. It also provided a greater contrast signal, with reduction in both contrast volume and concentration. The reduction in the contrast volume and concentration is particularly great in imaging larger vascular structures. As one attempts to image smaller and smaller vessels in the cervicocephalic region, however, the degree of contrast reduction becomes more modest. This finding is similar to the experiments proposed by Rose,[21] in which the diameter of the test spot and the contrast level are seemingly inversely proportional. For practical purposes, most authors[22] reduce the volume of contrast injections by one-quarter to one-third of that used in conventional angiography. There is usually a concomitant reduction in the iodine concentration. The catheter selected for digital studies should have the smallest caliber capable of delivering the desired contrast rate and volume.

Conclusion

Introduction of the digital subtraction technique has provided the diagnostic radiologist with a modality to enhance his or her current angiographic techniques. Injection rates, volumes, and concentrations of contrast material require modest alterations with this technology. Familiarization with the basic concepts of digital imaging is imperative when utilizing the digital method or in contemplating the purchase of new equipment.

EVALUATION OF CERVICOCEPHALIC VASCULATURE

Transvenous Evaluation

As digital angiography made its debut, the hope was that the enhanced digitized clarity of the vasculature would allow screening of major patient population groups with hypertension or extracranial occlusive disease using the intravenous approach. However, despite the proven safety of this method,[23] upon comparison of the intravenous method with standard film screen angiography,[18,20,24–27] the intravenous method fell into disfavor.

Transbrachial Evaluation

The inability to adequately evaluate the extracranial circulation by the intravenous method in 20% of cases and to exquisitely provide quality and correlative exams in but 60%, led to a shift to the second phase of digital subtraction angiography, in which evaluation of the cervicocephalic system was performed by intra-arterial digital angiography. Concomitant with this development was the development of thin-wall, small-bore catheters which were capable of delivering the smaller volumes of contrast material required for intra-arterial digital angiography but which also, by virtue of their size, allowed intra-arterial access with fewer puncture site complications. To maintain an acceptable procedure for outpatients, the transbrachial method became popular.[28] In our experience[29] with 404 patients evaluated by transbrachial arch studies for extracranial occlusive disease, the incidence of puncture site complications requiring surgical intervention was 0.5%; of these patients, 66% were female. In cases where multiple catheter exchanges were utilized or manipulative studies were performed by the transbrachial route, the complication rate increased. In our experience, this resulted in a 3.2% rate of brachial injuries requiring sur-

TABLE 7-1 Surgically Correlated Brachial Injuries

Institution	No. of Patients	Surgery
Blodgett Memorial[32]	660	2 (0.3%)
University of Indiana[30]	361	2 (0.6%)
William Beaumont[29]	404	2 (0.5%)
Presbyterian University[31]	355	2 (0.6%)

gical intervention. Because of this apparent complication, when required to use the brachial approach for the evaluation of extracranial disease, we limit that study to midstream thoracic injections and employ systemic heparinization at the time of the study, as well as a beta-blocking agent, in an attempt to reduce catheter-induced vasospasm at the puncture site. Our experience, as well as that of others[29–32] (Table 7-1), demonstrates a relatively low incidence of complications at the puncture site. In correlative examinations of intra-arterial DSA studies with standard angiography, there appeared to be nearly 100% correlation with clinically useful information.[33,34]

Transfemoral Evaluation

Although the transbrachial route seemed to provide fewer suboptimal exams than standard arch studies[35] (17%) and intravenous DSA (20%), there continued to be suboptimal exams (3%), primarily due to overlap and motion. Furthermore, although the rate of puncture site surgical complications was usually below 1%, that rate was 10 times greater than the rate of surgical repair of the puncture site when we used the femoral route (0.04% vs. 0.5%). In addition, the intracranial portions of the examination were of poorer quality than the cervical portions.[35] Accordingly, with the introduction of high-flow, small-bore catheters, we and others[36,37] have returned to evaluating the cervicocephalic vasculature by the transfemoral route, when feasible, utilizing the digital method for the majority of

Fig. 7-4 Arch anomalies. (*A*) Common anomaly of the left common carotid (arrow) arising from the innominate. (*B*) Unusual common trunk (arrow) giving rise to both common carotids. (*C*) Low-lying carotid bifurcations (arrows). (*D*) Multiple brachiocephalic anomalies: aberrant right vertebral from the common carotid (open arrow); left vertebral from the arch (double arrow) and anomalous right subclavian (solid arrows).

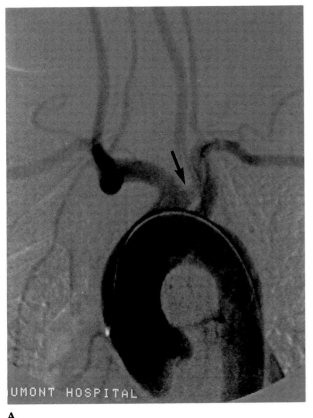

A

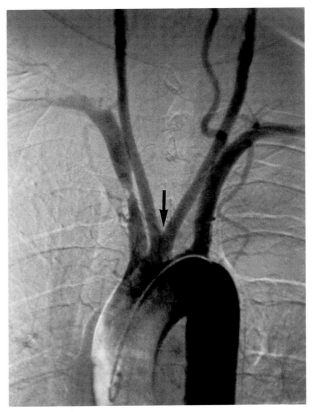

B

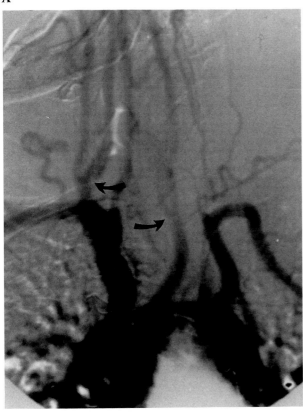

C

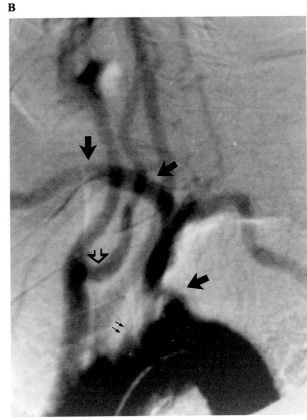

D

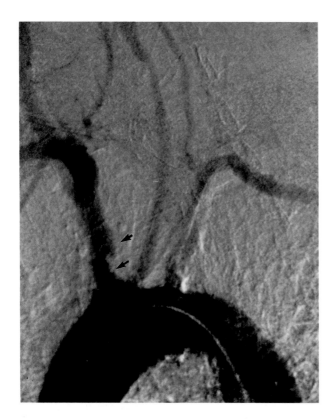

Fig. 7-5 Irregular atheromatous plaque in the innominate artery (arrows).

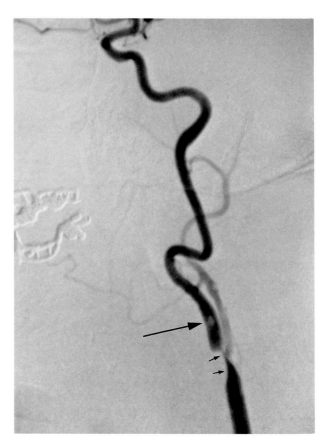

Fig. 7-6 Critical distal common carotid artery stenosis with extension into the proximal internal carotid (small arrows). Note also the intraluminal thrombus (long arrow) in the internal carotid.

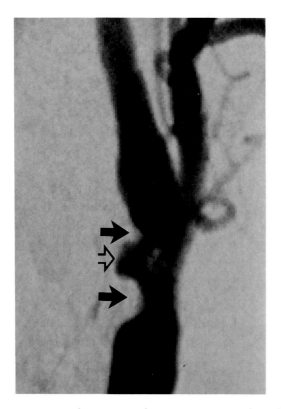

Fig. 7-7 Large atheromatous ulcer (open arrows) within a distal common/proximal internal carotid plaque (solid arrows).

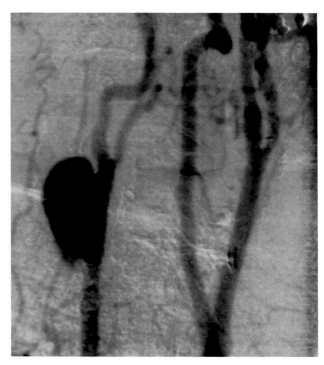

Fig. 7-8 Aneurysmal development at a previous atherectomy site.

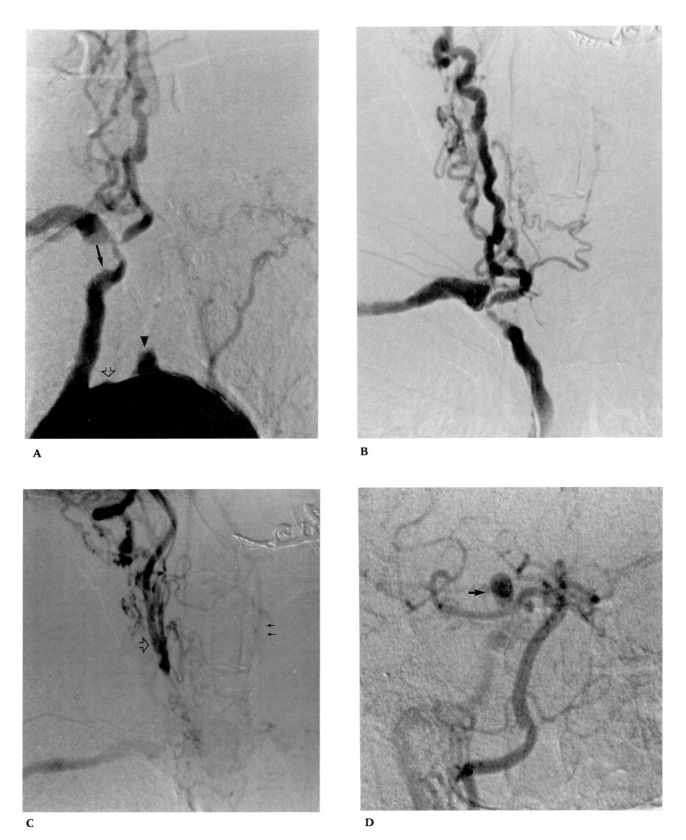

Fig. 7-9 Severe cervicocephalic occlusive disease. (*A*) Arch injection demonstrates occlusion of the right common carotid (long arrow), left common carotid (open arrow), and left subclavian (arrow head). (*B*) Early innominate injection reveals a perivertebral plaque and stenosis. (*C*)Delayed innominate injection reveals reconstitution of the right carotid bifurcation (open arrow) and faint opacification of the left carotid bifurcation (arrows). (*D*) Intracranial imaging after an innominate injection reveals an incidental posterior communicating aneurysm (arrow).

the examination. By using this procedure since 1987, our intraprocedural transischemic attack rate has been reduced approximately 70%: from 1.5% when the majority of the film sequences were done by conventional angiography to 0.4% when the majority were obtained utilizing digital imaging.

It is presumed that digital angiography facilitates the cervicocephalic examination in two ways. First, because the digital method requires little contrast volume, one can perform an initial arch survey examination, which provides a baseline directing the angiographer to further selective catheter requirements in patients with anomalous (Fig. 7-4) or subtle pathological processes (Fig. 7-5). Further, the digital method reduces the image acquisition time compared to standard imaging. Both of these factors reduce the intraprocedural catheterization time, which had been suggested as one cause of intraprocedural neurological complications.[38]

The synergy of the transfemoral and digital methods allows examination of the patient with cervicocephalic disease in the most expeditious and comfortable way, with the lowest puncture site complication rate. In our experience and that of others, it also reduces the rate of intraprocedural neurological deficits (from 1.7% to 0.55%).[34]

We believe that delineation of cervicocephalic pathology (Figs. 7-6, 7-7, and 7-8) is achieved as well as, if not more easily than (Fig. 7-9) the standard film-screen method.

Conclusion

DSA is the mainstay of most angiographic laboratories today. The efficiency and increased safety provided by digital techniques in terms of contrast volume and patient tolerance, along with the rapidity of image acquisition, make DSA most effective.

REFERENCES

1. Meyers PH, Becker HC, Sweeney JW, et al. Evaluation of a computer-retrieved radiographic image. *Radiology* 1963;81:201–206.
2. Kruger RA, Mistrcha CA, Houk TL, et al. Computerized fluoroscopy in real time for noninvasive visualization of the cardiovascular system. *Radiology* 1979;130:49–57.
3. Ovitt TW, Christenson PC, Fisher HD, et al. Intravenous angiography using digital video subtraction: X-ray imaging system. *Am J Roentgenol* 1980;135:1141–1144.
4. Meaney TF, Weinstein MA, Buonocore E, et al. Digital subtraction angiography of the human cardiovascular system. *Am J Roentgenol* 1980;135:1153–1160.
5. Boxt LM, Taus RH. Imaging processing technique for digital subtraction arteriography in Harvard Medical School CME syllabus, 1985, pp 66–70.
6. Jeans WD. The development and use of digital subtraction angiography. *Br J Radiol* 1990;63:161–168.
7. McLean ID, Collins LT. Some DSA testing methods and an evaluation of eight available units. *Australas Radiol* 1989;33:259–265.
8. Harrington DP, Boxt LM, Murray PD. Digital subtraction angiography: Overview of technical principles. *Am J Roentgenol* 1982;139:781–786.
9. Ovitt TW, Newell JD. Digital subtraction angiography: Technology, equipment, and techniques. *Radiol Clin North Am* 1985;23:177–184.
10. Levin DC, Schapiro RM, Toxt LM, et al. Digital subtraction angiography: Principles and pitfalls of image improvement techniques. *Am J Roentgenol* 1984;143:447–454.
11. Strother CM, Sackett JF, Crummy AB, et al. Clinical applications of computerized fluoroscopy: The extracranial carotid arteries. *Radiology* 1980;136:781–783.
12. Crummy AB, Strother CM, Lieberman RP, et al. Digital video subtraction angiography for evaluation of peripheral vascular disease. *Radiology* 1981;141:33–37.
13. Enzmann DR, Djang WT, Riederer SJ, et al. Low-dose, high-frame rate versus regular-dose, low-frame digital subtraction angiography. *Radiology* 1983;146:669–676.
14. Buonocore E, Pavlicek WA, Modic MT, et al. Anatomic and functional imaging of congenital heart disease with digital subtraction angiography. *Radiology* 1983;147:647–654.
15. Stein JA, Swift RD. Digital subtraction angiography: A new perspective. Advanced Technology Laboratories, Bedford, Massachusetts 1982.
16. Riederer SJ. Digital radiography: General Electric's approach to digital fluoroscopy and scanned projection imaging. In Mistretta CA, Crummy AB, Strother CM, et al (eds): *Digital Subtraction Arteriography: An Application of Computerized Fluoroscopy.* Chicago, Year Book Medical, 1982, pp 142–150.
17. Gomes AS, Papin PJ, Mankovich NJ, et al. Digital subtraction angiography: A comparison of 512^2 and 1024^2 imaging. *Am J Roentgenol* 1986;146:835–838.
18. Chilcote WA, Modic MT, Pavlicek WA, et al. Digital subtraction angiography of the carotid arteries: A comparative study in 100 patients. *Radiology* 1981;139:287–295.
19. Saddekni S, Sos T, Sniderman KW, et al. Optimal injection technique or intravenous digital angiography. Animal and clinical studies of right arterial injection using small volumes (25 ml) at a high rate (35 ml/sec). *Radiology* 1984;150:655–659.
20. Earnest F IV, Houser OW, Forbes GS, et al. The accuracy

and limitations of intravenous digital subtraction angiography in the evaluation of atherosclerotic cerebrovascular disease: Angiographic and surgical correlation. *Mayo Clin Proc* 1983;58:735–746.

21. Rose A. *Vision—Human and Electronic.* Plenum, pp 1–28.

22. *Digital subtraction angiography (DSA)* in Kadir S (ed): *Diagnostic Angiography.* Philadelphia, WB Saunders, 1986, pp 101–122.

23. Pinto RS, Manuell M, Kricheff II. Complications of digital intravenous angiography: Experience in 2,488 cervicocranial examinations. *Am J Roentgenol* 1984;143:1295–1299.

24. Glover JL, Bendick PJ, Jackson VP, et al. Duplex ultrasonography, digital subtraction angiography, and conventional angiography in assessing carotid atherosclerosis. *Arch Surg* 1984;119:664–669.

25. Russell JB, Watson RM, Modi JR, et al. Digital subtraction angiography for evaluation of extracranial carotid occlusive disease: Comparison with conventional arteriography. *Surgery* 1983;94(4):604–611.

26. Foley WD, Smith DF, Milde MW, et al. Intravenous DSA examination of patients with suspected cerebral ischemia. *Radiology* 1984;151:651–659.

27. Connolly JE, Brownell DA, Lenine EF, et al. Accuracy and indication of diagnostic studies for extracranial carotid disease. *Arch Surg* 1985;120:1229–1232.

28. McCreary JA, Schellhas KP, Brant-Zawadzki M, et al. Outpatient DSA in cerebrovascular disease using transbrachial arch injections. *Am J Neuroradiol* 1985;6:795–801.

29. Ellwood RA. Personal communication. Excerpts from quality care reviews: 1986–1992, William Beaumont Hospital. Unpublished.

30. Hicks ME, Kreipke DL, Becker GJ, et al. Cerebrovascular disease: Evaluation with transbrachial intraarterial digital subtraction angiography using a 4F catheter. *Radiology* 1986;161:545–546.

31. Barnett FJ, Lecky DM, Freiman DB, et al. Cerebrovascular disease: Outpatient evaluation with selective carotid DSA performed via a transbrachial approach. *Radiology* 1989;170:535–539.

32. Gritter KJ, Laidlaw WW, Peterson NT. Complication of outpatient transbrachial intraarterial digital subtraction angiography. *Radiology* 1987;162:125–127.

33. Lipchik EO, Mewissen MW. A comparison of normal intraarterial digital subtraction angiography with standard angiography in patients with symptomatic cerebrovascular ischemia. *Am J Neuroradiol* 1990;11:837–838.

34. Brant-Zawadzki M, Gould R, Normal D, et al. Digital subtraction cerebral angiography by intraarterial injection: Comparison with conventional angiography. *Am J Roentgenol* 1983;140:347–353.

35. Zimmerman RD, Goldman MJ, Auster M, et al. Aortic arch digital arteriography: An alternative technique to digital venous angiography and routine arteriography in the evaluation of cerebrovascular insufficiency. *Am J Neuroradiol* 1983;4:266–270.

36. Waugh JR, Sacharias N. Arteriographic complications in the DSA era. *Radiology* 1992;182:243–246.

37. Forbes GS, Earnest F IV, Kispert DB, et al. Digital angiography—introducing digital techniques to clinical cerebral angiography practice. *Mayo Clin Proc* 1982;57:683–693.

38. Mani RL, Eisenberg RL. Complications of catheter cerebral arteriography: Analysis of 5,000 procedures. III. Assessment of arteries injected, contrast medium used, duration of procedure and age of patient. *Am J Roentgenol* 1978;131:871–874.

8

Intra-arterial Digital Subtraction Angiography: Clinical Application

Yukunori Korogi, M.D., Mutsumasa Takahashi, M.D.

CLINICAL APPLICATION

Basic Principles

It is generally accepted that conventional cerebral angiography or intra-arterial digital subtraction angiography (IADSA) is essential to confirm the presence of extracranial and intracranial vascular lesions.[1] Noninvasive studies of the cerebral vasculature, such as duplex ultrasonography and magnetic resonance angiography (MRA), can identify the disease of the extracranial carotid bifurcation in a high percentage of cases. As a screening procedure of the carotid bifurcation, MRA may replace cerebral angiography.[2–6] However, there are some limitations that prevent full reliance on its use as a diagnostic modality for surgical intervention.[7]

Conventional cerebral angiography with suitable subtraction imaging is the most accurate and most widely used modality at present, but IADSA is gaining wider acceptance. In the last several years the general conditions for cerebral angiography have changed significantly.[8] Modern digital equipment has a 1024 × 1024 matrix, which approaches the resolution of a standard radiographic film screen combination on an angiographic changer. Film costs are significantly reduced with digital subtraction equipment. Concomitantly with the introduction of digital subtraction angiography (DSA) into the neuroradiological routine, new nonionic contrast media have been developed. There are potential advantages of IADSA over conventional cerebral angiography; they include a shorter procedure time and the use of lower volumes of contrast medium and smaller catheters.[1] This may lead to lower complication rates.

For patients with mild ischemic cerebrovascular diseases undergoing cerebral angiography, the risk of suffering a neurological complication (transient ischemic attack or stroke) is about 4%, and the deficit may be permanent in 1%.[1] The mortality rate is <0.1%. It is generally accepted that patients suffering from arteriosclerotic cerebral vascular disease have a higher risk with angiography than other patients. One major series recorded the remarkably low neurological deficit complication rate of 0.09% in a series of 1,095 patients undergoing cerebral IADSA.[8] Warnock et al.[9] reported that the permanent neurological complication rate of cerebral IADSA was 0.5% in the high-risk group, which is the lower range of the rates recorded in previous studies of conventional cerebral angiography.

Stereoscopic DSA

The value of stereoscopic DSA has been emphasized for obtaining detailed information on tumorous and vascular lesions and their relationship to the normal vascular structure. With the recent development of x-ray tube technology, twin focal x-ray tubes are widely available for angiographic uses.[10] Stereoscopic DSA is considered an important tool in IADSA.[11] In vascular tumors and arteriovenous malformations (AVMs), feeding arteries and draining veins can be visualized stereoscopically, and the relation of the lesion to the normal vasculature is clearly shown (Fig. 8-1). The neck and direction of the aneurysm are also well shown. In less vascular tumors, displacement and stretching of the vessels can be evaluated. The superimposition of the normal vascular structures can often be separated, and invaluable information can be obtained for evaluation of the lesions.[11]

Intraoperative DSA

The value of intraoperative cerebral DSA as a diagnostic and therapeutic tool has been stressed by both radiologists and neurosurgeons.[12,13] If the neurosurgeon can visualize the cerebral vasculature intraoperatively after clipping an aneurysm or resecting an AVM, the decision to modify the operative procedure may be made immediately, thereby improving the surgical outcome and obviating a repeat surgical procedure.[14] Furthermore, intraoperative DSA may facilitate an other-wise impossible therapeutic procedure such as the selective embolization of AVMs, by direct catheterization of intracranial feeding arteries that are otherwise inaccessible by angiographic technique.[14]

In intraoperative cerebral angiography, the development of portable DSA equipment allows the rapid acquisition of multiple angiographic series in various projections, without the delay inherent in the processing and subtraction of standard radiographic film.[14] The relatively small field size is thought to be a disadvantage of portable DSA equipment compared with fixed equipment.[15]

EXTRACRANIAL CAROTID-VERTEBRAL DISEASE

Occlusive Vascular Disease

Atherosclerotic Disease
The aortic arches are not routinely studied since detection of clinically significant lesions is extremely low and an added systemic risk exists with arch opacification.[16] However, the proximal subclavian, innominate artery, and vertebral artery origins may be affected[17] (Figs. 8-2, 8-3). In the presence of hemodynamically

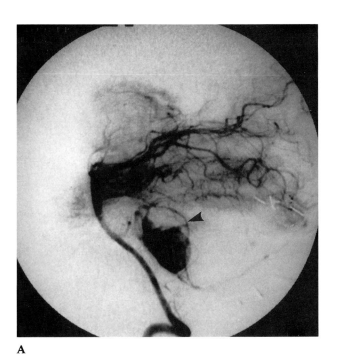

A

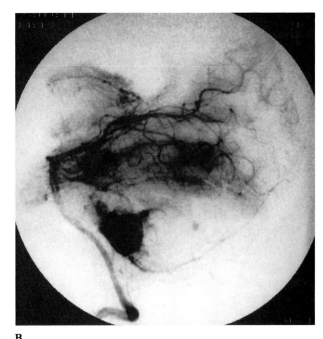

B

Fig. 8-1 Vertebral angiogram of hemangioblastoma. (*A,B*) Stereoscopic IADSA (lateral view) shows a markedly hypervascular tumor. The relation of the lesion to the posterior inferior cerebellar artery (arrowhead) is well demonstrated.

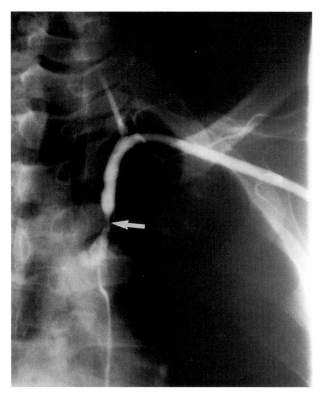

Fig. 8-2 Conventional arteriogram shows stenosis of the prevertebral part of the left subclavian artery (arrow).

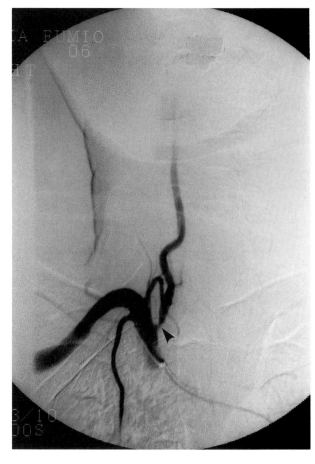

Fig. 8-3 Right subclavian arteriogram shows stenosis at the origin of the right vertebral artery (arrowhead).

significant occlusive vascular disease, collateral blood flow from other vessels may develop. For example, when a vertebral artery is occluded or stenotic, collateral blood flow may develop via the muscular branches of the external carotid artery, the contralateral vertebral artery, or thyrocervical and intercostal collaterals[18] (see Fig. 8-8).

At the common carotid bifurcation, atheromas are often found on the posterior wall (Figs. 8-4, 8-5). The flow reversal that is normally seen in the posterior carotid bulb may be a contributing factor to platelet adhesion and initial plaque formation.[17] Intimal fatty streaks are the earliest macroscopically visible lesions in atherosclerosis. As the disease progresses, a fibrotic cap is formed that covers a core of foam cells, necrotic debris, and cholesterol crystals. Eventually, intraplaque subintimal hemorrhage and necrosis occur.[17] Most ulcerated atheromas are located on the posterior carotid wall, no more than 2.5 cm from the bifurcation.[19] True plaque ulceration frequently results in the formation of platelet fibrin clots on their surface from the exposed collagen; these clots can embolize to the intracranial circulation, giving rise to transient ischemic attacks and strokes.[20,21] Characteristically, the ulceration presents as an elon-

gated, irregular cavity within the atheroma, the ostium of the crater being directed downstream.

The three most important goals of carotid angiography in atherosclerotic vascular disease are as follows[16,17]: (1) determine the degree of carotid stenosis, (2) identify "tandem" lesions in the carotid siphon or intracranial circulation (see Fig. 8-10), and (3) evaluate the existing and potential collateral circulation. The degree of stenosis may be divided into one of three groups[16]: (1) complete vascular occlusion, presumably caused by thrombotic formation, (2) severe flow-reducing stenosis (Fig. 8-5), and (3) normal or minor stenosis of a vessel that does not impede flow. Atherosclerotic ulceration can accompany any of these groups.

Atherosclerotic disease in the carotid artery contributes to cerebral ischemia or infarction by either hemodynamic effects or emboli from atherosclerotic plaques. Accurate determination of the degree of stenosis in the carotid bifurcation is critical since a recent joint study

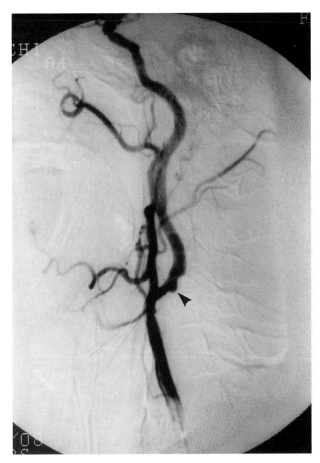

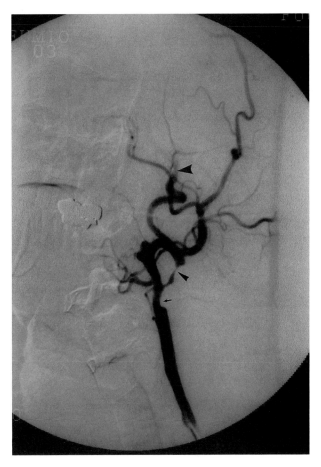

Fig. 8-4 Left common carotid angiogram (lateral view) shows an ulcerated plaque (arrowhead) on the posterior wall of the carotid bifurcation.

Fig. 8-5 Left common carotid angiogram (lateral view) shows a severe stenosis at the origin of the internal carotid artery (ICA) (arrowhead). A smooth plaque is also present on the posterior wall of the terminal common carotid artery (arrow). Note the slow opacification of the distal ICA (large arrowhead).

has indicated that a 75% or greater stenosis has the best prognosis with surgical endarterectomy.[22] The degree of stenosis is determined by relating the minimum residual luminal diameter at the stenosis to the luminal diameter of the distal internal carotid artery beyond the carotid bulb in an area where no atherosclerotic disease is present[22] (Figs. 8-4, 8-5). It is imperative to obtain additional oblique anteroposterior and lateral views of the carotid bifurcation whenever no significant stenosis is identified on the standard views or when the proximal internal carotid cannot be fully delineated on both the anteroposterior and lateral routine projections.[20] Although angiography can accurately show stenosis or occlusion, it may not be as accurate in showing ulceration. In one series, ulcers were detected angiographically in only 60% of carotid bifurcations that showed ulceration at surgery.[23]

In the event of cervical or intracranial vascular occlusion or hemodynamically significant stenosis, the adequacy of the collateral circulation becomes critical.[17] The most important potential collateral pathway is through the circle of Willis, the large, anastomotic vascular ring at the base of the brain (see Fig. 8-8). Extra-to intracranial pathways from external carotid branches to the ophthalmic artery or cavernous internal carotid artery (ICA) are also important. Intracranial pial and leptomeningeal collaterals may develop, but they are often inadequate to prevent a neurological deficit.[17]

MRA offers a sensitive and specific evaluation of atherosclerotic narrowing of the carotid artery bifurcation and may supplant cerebral angiography.[2–6]

Fibromuscular Dysplasia
Fibromuscular dysplasia (FMD) is a nonatheromatous, noninflammatory vascular disease that involves pri-

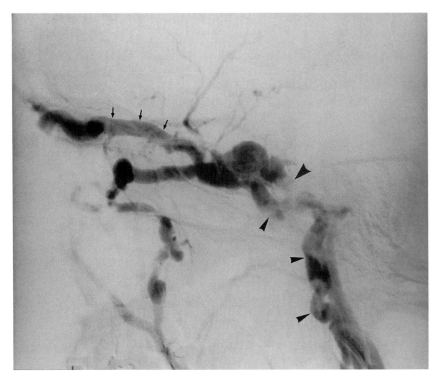

Fig. 8-6 Conventional ICA angiogram (lateral view) of the carotid-cavernous fistula due to FMD. The ICA (arrowheads) is elongated and irregularly dilated. The carotid-cavernous fistula is demonstrated. (arrows = superior ophthalmic vein; large arrowhead = inferior petrosal sinus).

marily the renal and internal carotid arteries, and, less often, the vertebral, iliac, subclavian, and visceral arteries. Although its pathogenesis is not completely understood, humoral, mechanical, and genetic factors as well as mural ischemia may play a role.[24] Histopathological classification of FMD is based on the predominant site of dysplasia in the arterial wall: the intima, media, or adventitia. Three main types of FMD have been identified: intimal fibroplasia, medial FMD, and periadventitial fibroplasia.

The natural history of FMD is relatively benign, with progression occurring in only a minority of patients. FMD is a histological diagnosis; however, the diagnosis can be made with a degree of accuracy on the basis of the angiographic appearance.[24] Classic string-of-beads stenoses are consistent with the presence of FMD. However, both intimal and medial hyperplasia may sometimes be confused with atherosclerotic plaques on the angiogram.

In patients undergoing carotid angiography, FMD is present in 0.25–1%. Cerebrovascular FMD constitutes 25 to 30% of the published cases.[25,26] Cervical FMD is bilateral in approximately 65% of all cases.[18] It occurs in the middle and upper cervical segments of the ICA adjacent to the first and second cervical vertebrae. Characteristically, changes of FMD extend from the C1 or C2 level to the entrance of the ICA into the petrous carotid canal.[18] The common carotid bifurcation and

proximal ICA are spared in nearly all cases. The symptoms are usually those of transient ischemic attacks, cerebral infarction, or subarachnoid hemorrhage from a coexisting aneurysm. Rarely, spontaneous dissection of the arterial wall of the ICA causes carotid-cavernous fistulas (Fig. 8-6).

Arteritis
Arteritis of the cerebral vessels can result from a variety of causes: viral, mycotic, and bacterial agents; necrotizing angiitis; and autoimmune disorders.[18] Arteritis affecting the aortic arch vessels classically produces either long-segment stenosis or proximal occlusion of its major branches. In either instance, the distal portions of the vessels are usually spared.

Takayasu's arteritis, one of the most common vascular diseases in Japan, as well as in China and some other parts of Asia, is a nonspecific inflammatory process of unknown cause segmentally affecting the aorta and its branches.[27] According to recent studies, the pathology of this entity is rather complicated; it not only leads to stenosis and obstruction but also causes dilatation and aneurysm formation[28] (Fig. 8-7). The disease is a form of panarteritis involving mainly the media. The wall of the artery is diffusely or irregularly thickened and fibrotic. Microscopically, extensive fragmentation, destruction, and fibrosis of the elastic and smooth muscle fibers are found in the media, in combi-

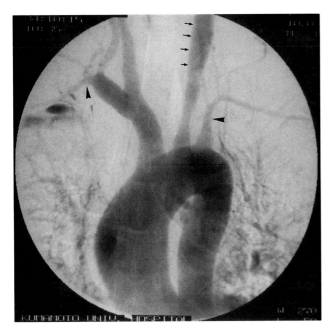

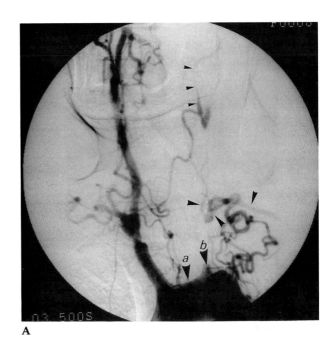

A

Fig. 8-7 Aortic arch angiogram (IVDSA) of Takayasu's arteritis. Smooth stenoses of both subclavian arteries (arrowheads) are shown. Dilatation of the left common carotid (arrows) and proximal left subclavian arteries is also demonstrated.

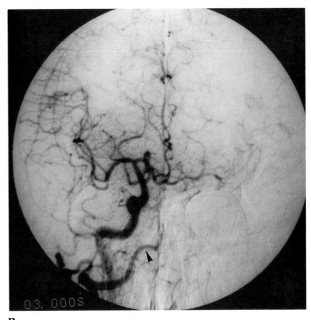

B

nation with inflammatory cell infiltration, predominantly of lymphocytes and monocytes, and granulation tissue proliferation.[28] Aneurysm formation in this disease results from extensive destruction of the elastic fibers in the media of the arterial wall.[29]

In about 30–47% of patients, the brachiocephalic arteries are involved, with the common carotid and subclavian arteries, particularly on the left side, being the sites of predilection[28,30] (Fig. 8-8). The luminal stenosis of the brachiocephalic arteries varies from mild to total occlusion, but localized or segmental severe stenosis and occlusion constitute the most common angiographic patterns and usually involve the proximal portion or midportion of the artery. Dilatations and aneurysms in the left carotid and left subclavian arteries are rare, whereas 31% of the lesions in the right-sided brachiocephalic vessels are either aneurysms or dilatations.[30] The ischemic phenomenon of the brain is uncommon.

Aneurysms

Dissecting Aneurysm

Dissecting aneurysms are usually identified in the middle and upper cervical segments of the ICAs or in the intraforaminal segment of the vertebral artery.[31] In the

Fig. 8-8 Severe occlusive disease of the aortic arch. This patient has presumed Takayasu's arteritis affecting the aortic arch and its major branches. Aortic arch angiogram (A: right posterior oblique view) demonstrates total occlusion of the left common carotid (arrow a), left subclavian (arrow b), and right vertebral arteries. An extensive network of collateral vessels has developed. The left subclavian and left vertebral arteries are faintly visible (arrowheads). The left ICA (small arrowheads) is also demonstrated via the collateral of the neck. The AP view (B) from a right innominate artery injection demonstrates opacification of the left middle cerebral artery as well as the right vertebral artery (arrowhead) from the occipital branch of the right external carotid artery.

ICA, they may occasionally extend down to the origin of the artery and may extend distally into the petrous segment. They may develop as a result of penetrating or blunt trauma to the neck; spontaneously; or from a rapid force of spontaneous, vigorous head and neck rotation, flexion, or extension.[7] They may also occur as a result of chiropractic neck-adjusting maneuvers. These head and neck rotation/flexion-extension maneuvers may cause impingement of the ICA on the C1 transverse process and trauma to the vertebral arteries as they pass through the C1 and C2 transverse bony foramina. Spontaneously occurring dissections may be seen in association with fibromuscular dysplasia, cystic medial necrosis, atherosclerotic disease with subintimal ulceration, and idiopathic causes.[7]

Dissecting aneurysms in the internal carotid and vertebral arteries are usually not of the double-lumen variety, as seen with dissection aneurysms of the aorta, but represent dissecting hematomas within the wall of the artery. They may produce a characteristic appearance referred to as the *string sign*, which results in a tapered narrowing of the vessel proximally and distally.[32] The dissection may result in complete occlusion of the lumen. In most instances, cerebral symptoms are the result of embolization from a site on the dissection to the brain.[33] Occasionally cerebral ischemic symptoms are the result of vascular stenosis caused by the dissection.

Aneurysms of the Cavernous Segment of the ICA
The most frequent site of extradural ICA aneurysms is the cavernous segment (Fig. 8-9). Most of these aneurysms have been considered to be of atherosclerotic origin. However, many studies indicate that these are true developmental or congenital lesions.[34,35] Atherosclerotic changes, which occur commonly in the cavernous portion of the ICA, may further weaken the

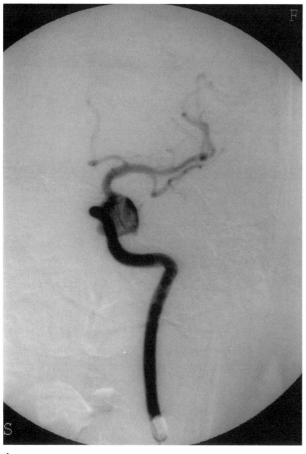

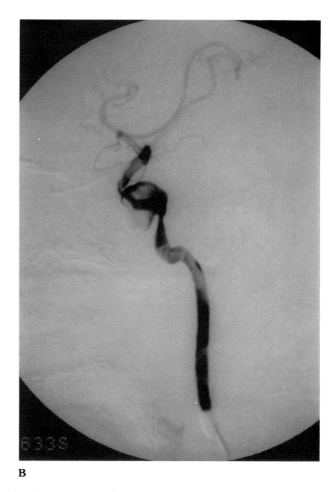

A   **B**

Fig. 8-9 AP (*A*) and lateral (*B*) views from an ICA angiogram. Under balloon occlusion, a lumen of a large, cavernous ICA aneurysm is gradually opacified.

arterial wall and may be an aggravating factor in the evolution of aneurysms.[36] Mirror-image, asymptomatic aneurysms and asymptomatic cavernous aneurysms were found in 11% and 3% of patients respectively.

Typically, patients harboring these lesions present with ophthalmoplegia or with symptoms referable to another cerebral aneurysms and, less commonly, with retro-orbital pain or signs of a spontaneous carotid-cavernous fistula.[37] Both cerebral ischemic episodes and subarachnoid hemorrhage are rare. In a review of 70 cases of aneurysm of the cavernous carotid artery, Kupersmith et al.[37] concluded that this aneurysm is rarely associated with life-threatening complications, and treatment should be considered principally for patients with intolerable pain or problems related to vision.

INTRACRANIAL VASCULAR DISEASE

Occlusive Vascular Disease

Atherosclerotic Disease
In the evaluation of patients with cerebral ischemic symptoms, it is critical that the intracranial circulation be adequately studied along with the extracranial vessels. In a small percentage of cases (approximately 5%), a significant intracranial stenosis exists in association with a significant extracranial vascular lesion.[20] The intracavernous and supraclinoid segments of the ICA are frequently involved in hypertensive individuals. These vessels generally demonstrate an irregular circumferential or eccentric stenosis over a short to moderate-length segment of the artery.[20]

The most frequent and severe atheromatous changes in the cerebral vascular system itself are localized to the circle of Willis and the large arteries at the base of the brain. The upper basilar artery, the ICA bifurcation, the proximal aspect of the MI segment of the middle cerebral artery (MCA), and the P1 segment of the posterior cerebral artery are most commonly involved[18] (Figs. 8-10, 8-11, 8-12). The clinical sequelae of actual vascular occlusions involving the circle of Willis and its small branches vary, depending on the level of the occlusion, the branches implicated, and the available collateral flow.[18] Sudden occlusion of the ICA is often accompanied by severe contralateral hemiplegia and hemianesthesia.[18] If occlusion occurs gradually and collateral blood flow through the circle of Willis is adequate, there may be few or no symptoms.

Wolpert et al.[16] have proposed seven rules for proper

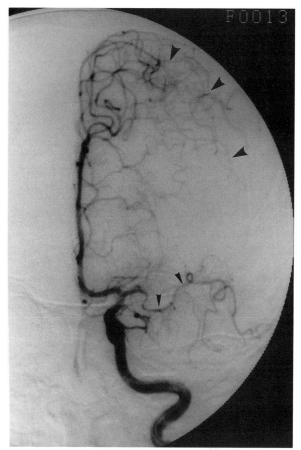

A

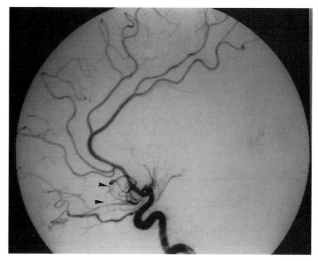

B

Fig. 8-10 Left ICA angiogram depicting complete occlusion at the M1 segment of the left MCA. AP (*A*) and lateral (*B*) views. The anterior temporal arteries (arrowheads) are visible. Note the leptomeningeal collateral pathway from the ACA to the MCA territory (large arrowhead).

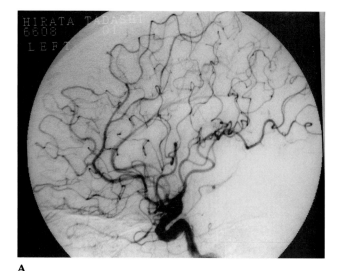

A

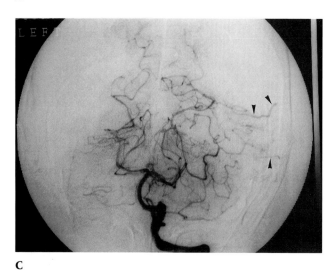

C

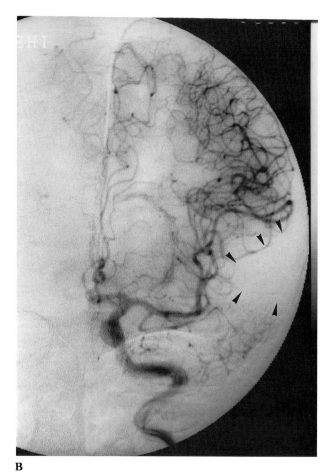

B

Fig. 8-11 Left ICA angiogram depicting posterior temporal artery branches. Lateral (*A:* arterial phase) and AP (*B:* late arterial phase) views demonstrate lack of opacification (note the "bare area" = arrowheads) of the posterior temporal branches. Left vertebral angiogram (*C*) shows filling of these vessels via pial and leptomeningeal collaterals (arrowheads).

study of cerebral angiography in patients with atherosclerotic cerebrovascular diseases:

1. Angiography is indicated only when it is likely to answer clinically relevant questions.
2. Neuroimaging (computed tomography [CT] and/or MRI) and noninvasive sonography should be performed first.
3. During angiography, the vessel supplying the ischemic zone should be studied first.
4. The decision on imaging of opacifying a vessel should be made sequentially.
5. The amount of contrast material injected during angiography and the length of the procedure should be minimized.

6. Studies that provide optimal and clinically useful data require close cooperation between the clinician and the angiographer.
7. The patient should be examined frequently between injections in order to detect problems or complications as soon as possible.

Moyamoya Disease
Moyamoya disease is a rare cerebrovascular occlusive disease the cause of which is unknown.[38] Diagnosis of moyamoya disease primarily depends on the angiographic demonstration of stenosis and occlusion of the carotid fork and extensive parenchymal, leptomeningeal, and transdural collaterals[39] (Fig. 8-13). Its paren-

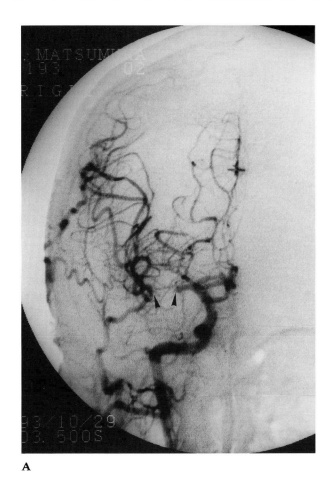
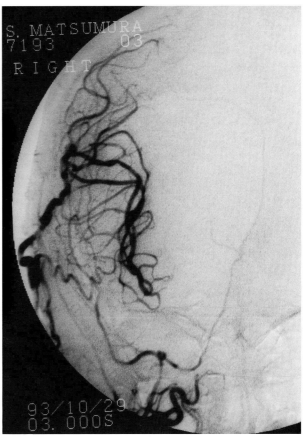

A   B

Fig 8-12   Right common carotid angiogram (*A:* AP view) showing occlusion of the M1 segment (arrowheads). Right external carotid angiogram (*B:* AP view) shows excellent retrograde filling of the left MCA branches via the superficial temporal artery (STA)–MCA anastomosis.

chymal collateral vessels from the suprasellar cistern to the basal ganglia are known as *moyamoya vessels.* The diagnostic criteria set by the Research Committee on Spontaneous Occlusion of the Circle of Willis include (1) stenosis or occlusion at the terminal portion of the ICA and/or at the proximal portion of the anterior cerebral artery (ACA) and/or the MCA, (2) abnormal vascular moyamoya networks in the vicinity of the areas mentioned above, and (3) bilateral involvement.[40] In children, its clinical manifestations are due to brain ischemia and consist of hemiplegia, paresthesia, headaches, and convulsions. In adults, the most common symptom is intracranial hemorrhage, sometimes occurring suddenly as intraventricular, subarachnoid, or intracerebral bleeding.[39] Small aneurysms arising from the moyamoya vessels and their feeding arteries may be a source of hemorrhage, in addition to the generally accepted rupture from the moyamoya vessels.[41]

Arteritis (Vasculitis)

Cerebral vasculitis is a rare disorder with numerous causes. Infectious causes include predominantly bacterial and viral diseases (Fig. 8-14). Purulent bacterial arteritis is most often a complication of severe bacterial meningitis. The arteritis associated with tuberculous meningitis has a marked tendency to involve arteries at the base of the brain. The noninfectious vasculitides include granulomatous angiitis, the systemic necrotizing vasculitides, vasculitis associated with collagen vascular disease, neurosarcoid vasculitis, and drug-abuse vasculitis.[42]

One such entity, noninfectious granulomatous angiitis of the nervous system, is an extremely rare disease with a predilection for leptomeningeal and parenchymal arteries and veins.[42,43] Histological findings include necrosis of the vessel wall, which is infiltrated by lymphocytes, plasma cells, large mononuclear cells, and giant cells. Characteristically, these vasculitic lesions re-

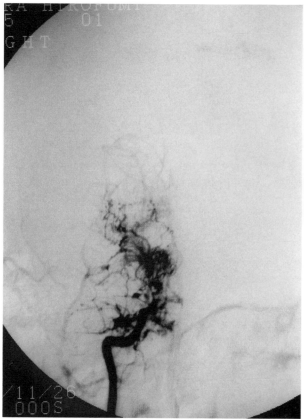

A

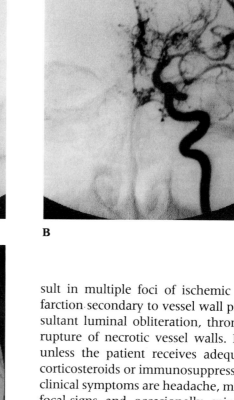

B

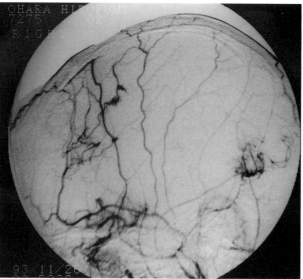

C

Fig. 8-13 Moyamoya disease. Right ICA angiogram (*A:* AP view) shows complete occlusion of the terminal ICA and a moyamoya blush. Left ICA angiogram (*B:* AP view) shows severe stenosis of the proximal ACA and MCA and a moyamoya blush. Right external carotid angiogram (*C:* lateral view) shows development of a transdural anastomosis.

sult in multiple foci of ischemic or hemorrhagic infarction secondary to vessel wall proliferation, with resultant luminal obliteration, thrombotic occlusion, or rupture of necrotic vessel walls. It is frequently fatal unless the patient receives adequate treatment with corticosteroids or immunosuppressives.[44–47] The typical clinical symptoms are headache, mental status changes, focal signs, and, occasionally, spinal cord involvement and seizure activity. Patients are usually middle-aged, and there is no sex-related predominance.[43] Granulomatous angiitis has also been referred to in the literature as "isolated angiitis of the central nervous system"[45] and, more recently, as "primary angiitis of the central nervous system."[47]

Definitive diagnosis of cerebral vasculitis can be made only on the basis of positive brain biopsy results; a highly presumptive diagnosis of cerebral vasculitis may be made on the basis of a positive cerebral angiogram. Characteristic angiography features include segmental narrowing or "beading" of the affected arteries, although angiography was found to be negative in 29% of 48 cases, presumably because very small vessels are

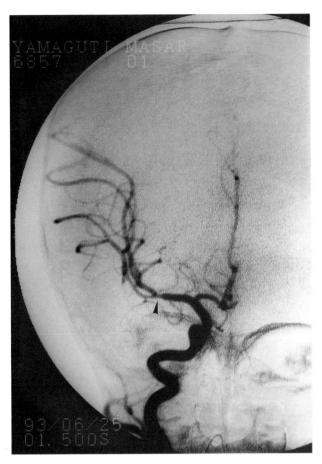

Fig. 8-14 Right ICA angiogram (AP view) of presumed vasculitis due to viral infection in a 1-year-old boy. Moderate stenosis is present at the distal M1 segment (arrowhead).

primarily involved.[47] Other causes, such as systemic inflammation or infection, must be excluded.

Venous Occlusive Disease

Dural venous sinus thrombosis has a variable clinical presentation including headache, behavioral changes, paraparesis, and seizures. Before the discovery of antibiotics, venous sinus thrombosis was often associated with mastoid sinusitis and facial infections, and the transverse sinus was most frequently involved. It is now seen more commonly with altered coagulation states in pregnancy, the puerperium, systemic infection, oral contraceptive use, polycythemia, hypercoagulability related to malignancy, thrombotic purpura, neurovascular diffuse intravascular coagulation, severe malnutrition, and dehydration.[48]

Patients with cerebral venous thrombosis typically present with nonspecific symptoms and signs of in-

creased intracranial pressure, with or without the subsequent development of focal neurological abnormalities. Hemorrhagic infarction, brain edema, and ventricular compression often occur with dural venous sinus thrombosis. Cerebral venous thrombosis is a dynamic process of progressive occlusion, attempted collateralization, and subsequent recanalization. Therefore, the disease may present as a slowly progressive process lasting for weeks to months, with or without a period of rapid deterioration, or as an acute neurological syndrome.[49]

The superior sagittal sinus is the most commonly occluded dural sinus, followed by the transverse, sigmoid, and cavernous sinuses.[17] Internal cerebral vein thrombosis is a less common but clinically devastating event. Radiographic features can be roughly divided into two types[50]: (1) direct evidence of thrombosis and collateral venous drainage and (2) evidence of the complications of cerebral venous thrombosis. At angiography, a thrombosed sinus appears as an empty channel devoid of contrast and surrounded by dilated collateral venous channels in the dural leaves (Fig. 8-15).[17]

Aneurysms

Saccular Aneurysms

Congenital saccular or berry aneurysms commonly affect the circle of Willis and arise predominantly at the bifurcation between two arterial branches. They probably occur because of a congenital arterial wall defect

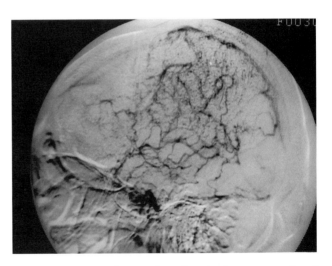

Fig. 8-15 ICA angiogram (lateral projection, venous phase) of dural venous sinus thrombosis. IADSA shows only partial opacification of the superior sagittal sinus and prominent, irregular cortical veins acting as collateral drainage pathways to the cavernous and transverse sinuses.

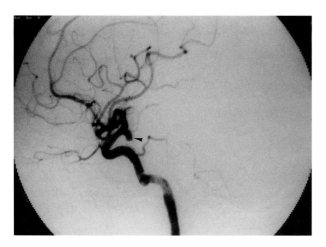

Fig. 8-16 Right ICA angiogram (lateral view) shows a small aneurysm at the origin of the PCA (arrowhead).

and subsequent degenerative changes associated with aging. Most aneurysms are less than 1 cm in diameter. Aneurysms measuring 2.5 cm in diameter or more are called *giant aneurysms*. The most common locations are the anterior and posterior communicating arteries and the MCA trifurcation. Approximately 20% of all intracranial aneurysms arise from the MCA bifurcation. About 30% arise from the anterior communicating artery, and 20–30% arise from the ICA at the origin of the posterior communicating artery (PCA)[18] (Fig. 8-16). Less common sites include the ophthalmic and anterior choroidal artery origins, the ICA bifurcation, the distal basilar artery, the anterior and posterior inferior cerebellar arteries (Fig. 8-17), and the pericallosal artery. From 15% to 20% of intracranial aneurysms are multiple. According to Locksley,[51] location of aneurysms with subarachnoid hemorrhage is as follows:

Anterior communicating artery	30%
Origin of PCA	25%
MCA bifurcation	13%
ICA (proximal or distal to PCA)	9%
ICA bifurcation	5%
Proximal MCA	4%
Distal basilar artery	3%

Aneurysms usually present clinically with rupture and subarachnoid hemorrhage. Occasionally, they produce sufficient mass effect to cause neurological symptoms such as PCA aneurysms, causing third nerve palsy. Vasospasm is most common 5–12 days after the aneurysm's rupture. Patients with a large amount of subarachnoid hemorrhage tend to develop more severe spasm.

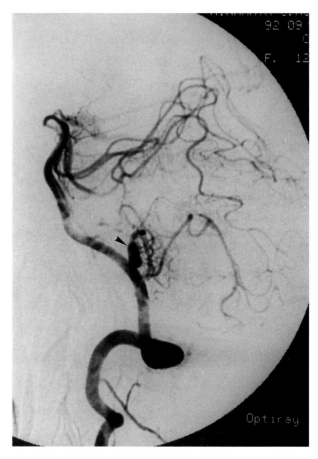

Fig. 8-17 Vertebral angiogram of a posterior inferior cerebellar artery aneurysm (arrowhead).

Despite the dramatic improvement in surgical results for ruptured intracranial aneurysms, the overall management mortality for this disorder remains high. The annual incidence of subarachnoid hemorrhage due to rupture of aneurysm ranges from 6 to 21 per 100,000 population, and 50% of these patients die within the first 30 days after rupture.[52–57] If a subarachnoid hemorrhage is present, and as long as the patient is not comatose, immediate cerebral angiography is usually advised.[16] If the results of initial angiography are normal, angiography should be repeated 2 weeks later, as a small percentage of aneurysms will be found on the second angiography. Aneurysm may not be seen for several reasons[16]: (1) arterial spasm, which temporarily seals off the neck; (2) inadequate technique; (3) thrombosis of the aneurysm, providing a spontaneous cure; and (4) observer error, particularly with multiple lesions or tortuous vessels.

The prevalence of incidental aneurysms in autopsy series is extremely variable and inconsistent, ranging from 0.8% to 7.9%.[52–56] Atkinson et al.[58] reported that the angiographic frequency of unruptured aneurysms was 1%. The natural history of unruptured aneurysms, and especially the risk of rupture, is not precisely known. Studies using current subarachnoid hemorrhage statistics, quoting a small number of autopsy series with a high incidence of aneurysms, suggest that aneurysms are plentiful in the general population and that only a small percentage of aneurysms ever rupture.[58]

Fusiform Aneurysms

Fusiform aneurysms are exaggerated arterial ectasias due to a severe and unusual form of atherosclerosis, and usually occur in older patients. The vertebrobasilar system is commonly affected (Fig. 8-18). Intraluminal clots are common, and perforating branches often arise from the entire length of the involved parent vessel. Intraluminal flow is often very slow and turbulent.

Dissecting Aneurysms

Intracranial dissecting aneurysms have been reported with increasing frequency and are recognized as a common cause of stroke.[59] The true frequency of dissecting aneurysms is not known. The difficulty of diagnosing these lesions may have obscured their true incidence. Yamaura[60] has reported that dissecting aneurysms account for 28% of vertebral artery aneurysms.

Dissecting aneurysms of the carotid arterial system occur in young individuals and are often associated with cerebral infarction resulting from arterial stenosis or occlusion.[61] However, dissecting aneurysms of the intracranial vertebrobasilar system, especially the vertebral artery, have been noted to produce subarachnoid hemorrhage.[62] Patients with dissecting aneurysms of the carotid arterial system are rarely hypertensive, and a few have a history of atherosclerosis. In contrast, most patients with dissecting aneurysms of the posterior circulation are hypertensive.[62] It is noteworthy that almost all patients with dissecting aneurysms of the intracranial vertebral artery complain of sudden, severe headache.[63] Headache may precede neurological deficits by days or weeks, and occasionally the stroke is not complete at its onset.

Histologically, the dissection initially occurs between the intima and media, resulting from diversion of the arterial stream.[62] Subsequently, all arterial layers are destroyed and subarachnoid hemorrhage develops. In younger patients, the dissection tends to be confined within the arterial wall, and brain stem ischemia develops as a result of luminal occlusion.[62]

Many authors have reported the angiographic find-

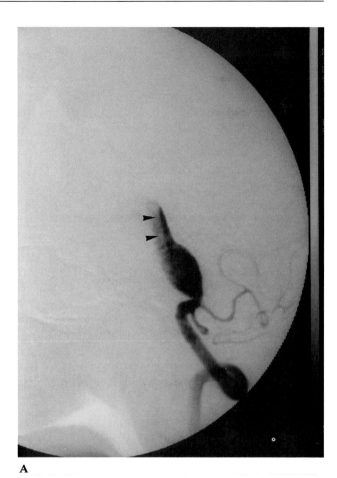

A

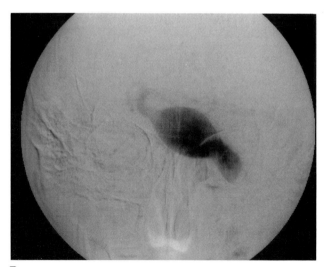

B

Fig. 8-18 Fusiform aneurysm of the vertebrobasilar artery. Lateral view of a vertebral angiogram (*A:* early arterial phase) shows fusiform dilatation from distal vertebral to basilar arteries. Because of markedly slow flow in the aneurysm, the fluid-fluid level consisted of contrast medium, and blood (arrowheads) is demonstrated (*B:* AP view, later phase).

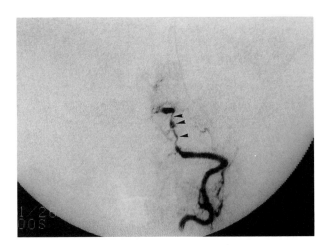

Fig. 8-19 Dissecting aneurysm of the vertebral artery. Left veterbral angiogram (AP view) shows the typical string sign (arrowheads). The distal vertebral artery is almost completely occluded.

ings of intracranial dissecting aneurysms, such as the string sign, occlusion, rosette, intimal flap, proximal and/or distal dilatation, double lumen, retention of contrast medium, and intramural pooling (Fig. 8-19).

Vascular Malformations

Intracranial vascular malformations may fall into one of five categories identified by McCormick[64]: (1) arteriovenous malformations (AVMs), (2) venous malformations, (3) cavernous malformations, (4) capillary telangiectasias, and (5) varices.

Arteriovenous Malformation
Brain AVMs are the most common symptomatic type of vascular malformation and the second most common cause of spontaneous subarachnoid hermorrhage in the adult population.[65] About half of all AVMs hemorrhage, and 25% have seizures as the presenting symptom. Sixty-four percent of these lesions are diagnosed in patients before the age of 40. The majority (90%) of brain AVMs are found in the cerebral hemispheres, and 10% are depicted in the posterior fossa.[66] AVMs are usually solitary lesions, although approximately 2% are multiple. Multiple AVMs are usually associated with extracerebral cutaneous or vascular anomalies, such as Rendu-Osler-Weber and Wyburn-Mason syndromes.[67,68]

The cumulative risk of hemorrhage from a parenchymal AVM is estimated at 2–4% per year.[69] An initial hemorrhage from an AVM carries a 10–17% risk of mortality and about a 30% risk of significant long-term

morbidity.[69–71] Rebleed rates are higher in the first year after an initial hemorrhage from an AVM (up to 6%).

Within the cerebral hemispheres, an AVM is usually a wedge-shaped lesion based at the cortical surface, with its apex pointing toward the lateral ventricle. Macroscopically, AVMs appear as tightly packed masses of abnormal vascular channels without intervening normal brain parenchyma. There is no intervening capillary bed between the arteries and veins. Four anatomical components of AVMs are significant in understanding the anatomy and treatment of these lesions: (1) arterial feeders, (2) arterial collaterals, (3) nidus, and (4) venous outflow (Fig. 8-20). Microscopic studies of AVMs showed the vessel walls to be similar to those of aneurysms. Endothelial gaps were identified; the subendothelial basement membrane was thick, reticulated, or multilaminated.[65] Degenerative changes were often noted within the muscle cells. The surrounding brain also showed important pathological changes associated with the AVM (recent or old hemorrhage, extensive gliosis, dysplastic brain tissue, foci of chronic inflammation, and parenchymal calcification.)[72] Flow-related aneurysms on feeding vessels or within the AVM nidus itself are seen in 8–12% of all cases.[73]

The anatomical relations of the arterial feeders, draining veins, and associated aneurysms are most reliably shown by angiography (Fig. 8-21). Uncomplicated AVMs have minimal or no mass effect unless a hematoma or venous varix is present. Arteriovenous shunting with abnormally early filling of veins that drain the lesions is characteristic of, but not pathognomonic for, AVM.[74] The angiographic differential diagnosis of a patent AVM is limited. Occasionally, highly vascular, anaplastic astrocytomas of glioblastoma multiforme can mimic an AVM.[74]

Venous Malformations (Venous Angioma)
Venous angioma is an incidental finding of little clinical relevance; rarely, it is associated with complications such as hemorrhage.[75] Several authors have reported the association of cavernous hemangioma and venous angiomas; the former are responsible for hemorrhage.[76]

Venous angioma of the brain consists of multiple, radially oriented, dilated medullary veins that drain into a transparenchymal venous system. Intervening brain tissue is present between the veins comprising the lesion. Although the precise etiology of venous angioma is unknown, these lesions are probably not true vascular malformations but instead represent extreme anatomical variants or developmental venous anomalies.[74,77] Arrested venous development after the brain

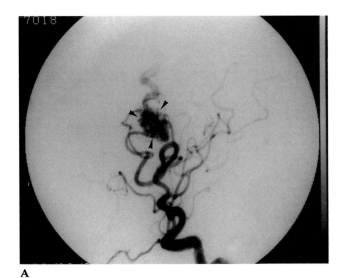

A

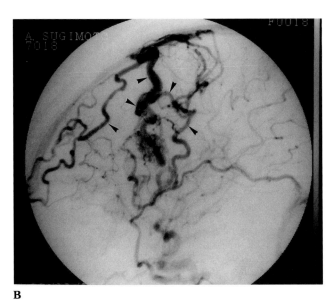

B

Fig. 8-20 Left ICA angiogram (early arterial phase, lateral view) illustrating a frontal lobe AVM (*A:* arrowheads). Late arterial phase film shows multiple tortuous, early draining veins (*B:* arrowheads).

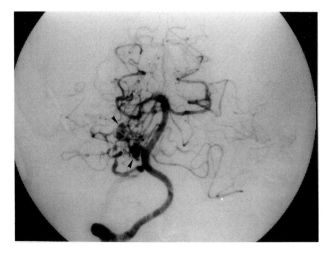

Fig. 8-21 Right vertebral angiogram (arterial phase, AP view) demonstrating a cerebellar AVM. Multiple associated aneurysms (arrowheads) are shown in the nidus.

arterial system has been formed could result in retention of primitive embryological medullary veins that drain into a single, large draining vein and form a venous angioma.[77]

Venous angiomas of the brain have many appearances, ranging from a small, single draining vein, involving at most one small portion of the brain, to a large, hemispheric venous anomaly draining an entire hemisphere.[75] Venous angiomas are located in the deep cerebral or cerebellar white matter, most often near the margin of the adjacent ventricle. The most common

site is adjacent to the frontal horn of the lateral ventricle; the next most frequent location is the cerebellum.[74,78]

The most common angiographic descriptions of venous angioma include a caput medusae appearance of deep, medullary veins during the early to middle venous phase, accompanied by a single large draining vein, most often extending transhemispherically to a superficial cortical vein or dural sinus[75] (Fig. 8-22). Angiographic characteristics also include normal arterial and capillary phases.

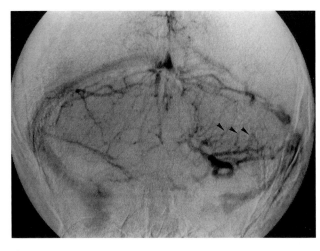

Fig. 8-22 Left vertebral angiogram (venous phase, AP view) of venous angioma of the cerebellum. Note the tuft of enlarged medullary veins (arrowheads). The arterial phase was normal. No arteriovenous shunting was present.

Cavernous Hemangioma

A cavernous hemangioma is a distinct pathological subtype of vascular malformation, appearing as a honeycomb of endothelium-lined sinusoidal vascular spaces, which contain essentially stagnant blood. Thrombosis, calcification, and hemorrhage are frequent occurrences. No brain parenchyma is found within the vascular spaces comprising the malformation. Although these lesions can be asymptomatic, seizures are the most common presenting symptom.

Because most cavernous angiomas are angiographically occult, the common finding is a normal study.[74] If the lesion has hemorrhaged, an avascular area with moderate mass effect can sometimes be identified. Occasionally a faint blush in the late capillary or early venous phase of high-quality cerebral angiograms can be seen.[74]

Posttraumatic Carotid Cavernous Fistulas (CCFs)

Arteriovenous fistulas represent an abnormal communication between an artery and a vein secondary to vessel laceration. Some fistulas may be part of other vascular abnormalities such as preexisting developmental aneurysms or angiodysplasias (see Fig. 8-6). In the craniofacial area, the most frequent type of arteriovenous fistulas are the traumatic CCFs (Fig. 8-23). Between the distal petrosal canal and the anterior clinoid process, the ICA is fixed by a dural attachment; at the time of severe head trauma, with or without skull base fracture, the ICA may be torn between these points of attachment, either by shearing forces or by bony spicules.[79] The tear in the ICA is usually single and large (2–5mm). Posttraumatic CCFs are usually classified as high flow. The ipsilateral ICA angiogram confirms the diagnosis of a single-hole fistula; however, it is often difficult to localize the exact point of shunting. The site of shunting can be localized by injecting the vertebral artery or the contralateral ICA while compressing or balloon-occluding the ICA ipsilateral to the fistula (see Fig. 8-23).

Careful analysis of the venous drainage of CCFs is important. The venous drainage from the cavernous sinus can be multidirectional, and can manifest variable symptoms and signs. Venous drainage is divided into five types[80]:

1. *Anterior:* Drainage to the ophthalmic venous system produces proptosis, chemosis, dilated conjunctiva, lid engorgement, venous retinopathy, disc edema, increased intraocular pressure with secondary glaucoma, and visual loss. The reversed blood flow in

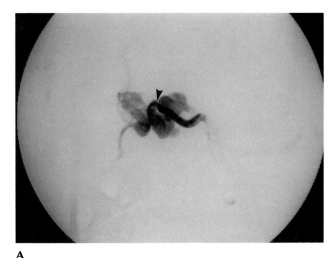

A

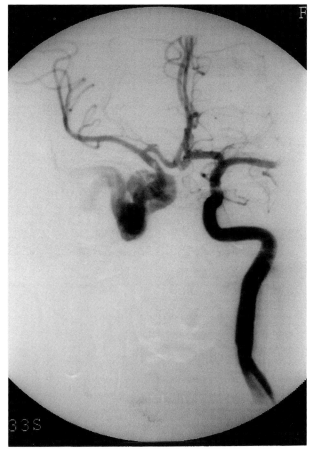

B

Fig. 8-23 Right ICA angiogram (*A*: lateral view) under balloon occlusion of a traumatic CCF. The site of the fistula is well demonstrated (arrowhead). The cavernous sinus is markedly dilated, and superior and posterior drainages are present. AP view from the left ICA angiogram (*B*) under balloon occlusion of the right ICA.

the ophthalmic vein drains toward the facial venous system and external jugular vein.

2. *Posterior:* The fistula often drains directly into the inferior petrosal sinus, the superior petrosal sinus, or the occipital transverse sinus. Only with this drainage, patients are usually asymptomatic, except for the complaint of noise.

3. *Superior:* Drainage to the sphenoparietal sinus or deep sylvian veins involves cortical venous routes.

4. *Contralateral:* Both cavernous sinus plexuses anastomose anteriorly and posteriorly. In general, the more severe symptoms are on the side of the fistula; however, if ipsilateral ophthalmic venous thrombosis is present, the opposite eye will be the more symptomatic one.[80]

5. *Inferior:* This is usually of minor importance; flow can be to the vein of the foramen rotundum or laterally through the vein of the foramen ovale.[80] This inferior drainage then drains into the pterygoid plexus.

Dural Arteriovenous Fistula

Dural arteriovenous fistula (AVF) represent 10–15% of all intracranial arteriovenous shunts.[81] The malformation is probably polyfactorial in origin, with same cases acquired and others congenital. The lesions typically consist of a nidus of numerous small fistulas within the wall of the dura, most typically a dural sinus. Many dural AVFs involve the venous sinuses along the base of the brain; the transverse sinus is most commonly affected.[82] Symptoms may range from mild to very severe, depending on the anatomy and location of the shunt. The clinical symptoms of dural AVFs involving the sagittal, lateral, sigmoid, and straight sinuses are often related to the route of venous drainage.[82] The initial complaints are frequently nonspecific. The pre-angiographic diagnosis of dural AVFs involving the sagittal, lateral, sigmoid, and straight sinuses is difficult and requires a high degree of clinical suspicion. This differs from diagnosis in patients with dural AVFs involving the cavernous sinus, who often present with classic symptoms such as proptosis, chemosis, and bruit.[83] The treatment of these lesions is primarily endovascular, although in selected instances, a surgical or combined surgical and endovascular approach is necessary.

Several authors have postulated that the development of dural AVFs may begin with thrombosis or occlusion of the involved sinus.[82] The rich dural arterial network in the walls of the major sinus may attempt to recanalize the sinus by developing direct artery-to-

sinus communications. This may lead to the angiomatous network of multiple feeding arteries and numerous AV shunts within a partially recanalized sinus that is frequently seen at angiography.[83] The involved dural sinus receives arterialized blood flow that can lead to mechanical obstruction of the sinus and result in retrograde drainage of blood away from the sinus and into cortical veins.[83]

Dural AVFs located in the transverse sigmoid sinus are the most common (Fig. 8-24). The major arterial feeder in these lesions is the occipital artery, which primarily serves the malformation via transosseous

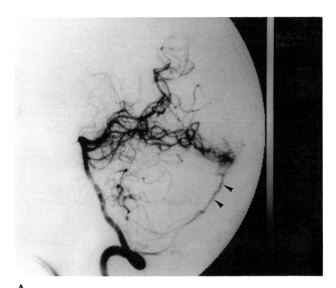

A

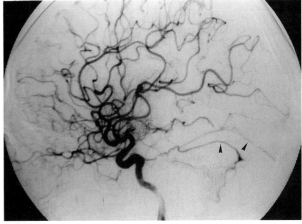

B

Fig. 8-24 Transverse sinus dural AVF. Vertebral angiogram (*A:* lateral view) shows the feeding artery (arrowheads) of a dural AVF as well as opacification of the transverse sinus. The ICA (*B:* lateral view) also supplies the dural AVF via tentorial branches (arrowheads) from the meningohypophyseal trunk.

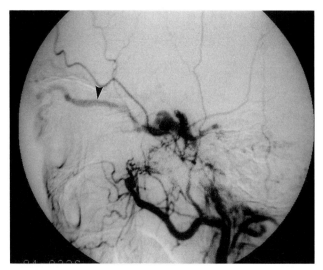

A

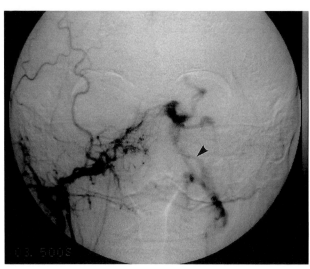

B

Fig. 8-25 Cavernous sinus dural AVF. Left external carotid angiogram (*A:* lateral view) shows the early opacification of the cavernous sinus and the superior ophthalmic vein (arrowhead). Multiple penetrating branches communicate with the cavernous sinus. AP view from the right external carotid angiogram (*B*) shows filling of the contralateral cavernous sinus (arrowhead = inferior petrosal sinuses).

branches.[84] A posterior meningeal artery may also supply the fistula. The meningeal trunk of the ascending pharyngeal artery is usually a significant source of supply to dural AVFs. The ICA can also supply dural AVFs through the meningohypophyseal trunk and its lateral clival or petrous branches.[84]

The major arterial feeders to the cavernous sinus include the middle meningeal artery, the accessory me-

ningeal artery, and the meningohypophseal trunk from the ICA (Fig. 8-25). Additional feeding from the carotid branch of the ascending pharyngeal artery and the recurrent meningeal branch of the ophthalmic artery may also occur.[84] From the distal internal maxillary artery, the artery of the foramen rotundum may also supply the lesion.

REFERENCES

1. Hankey G, Warlow CP, Sellar RJ. Cerebral angiographic risk in mild cerebrovascular disease. *Stroke* 1990;21: 209–222.

2. Masaryk AM, Ross JS, Dicello MC, et al. 3DFT MR angiography of the carotid bifurcation: Potential and limitations as a screening examination. *Radiology* 1991;179: 797–804.

3. Litt AW, Eidelman EM, Pinto RS, et al. Diagnosis of carotid artery stenosis: Comparison of 2DFT time-of-flight MR angiography with contrast angiography in 50 patients. *AJNR* 1991;12:149–154.

4. Polak JF, Bajakian RL, O'Leary DH, et al. Detection of internal carotid artery stenosis: Comparison of MR angiography, color doppler sonography, and arteriography. *Radiology* 1992;182:35–40.

5. Heiserman JE, Drayer BP, Fram EK, et al. Carotid artery stenosis: Clinical efficacy of two-dimensional time-of-flight MR angiography. *Radiology* 1992;182:761–768.

6. Huston J, III, Lewis BD, Wiebes DO, et al. Carotid artery: Prospective blinded comparison of two-dimensional time-of-flight MR angiography with conventional angiography and duplex US. *Radiology* 1993;186:339–344.

7. Goldberg HI. Angiography of extracranial and intracranial occlusive cerebrovascular disease. *Neuroimaging Clin North Am* 1992;2:487–507.

8. Grzyska U, Freitag J, Zeumer H. Selective cerebral intraarterial DSA. *Neuroradiology* 1990;32:296–299.

9. Warnock NG, Gandhi MR, Bergvall U, et al. Complications of intraarterial digital subtraction angiography in patients investigated for cerebral vascular disease. *Br J Radiol* 1993;66:855–858.

10. Takahashi M, Bussaka H, Miyawaki M, et al. Application of stereoscopic technique in digital subtraction angiography. *Radiology* 1985;157:546.

11. Takahashi M, Bussaka H, Miyawaki M. Stereoscopic DSA of the central nervous system. *Neuroradiology* 1986; 28:105–108.

12. Loop JW, Foltz EL. Applications of angiography during intracranial operation. *Acta Radiol [Stockh]* 1966;5: 363–367.

13. Bauer BL. Intraoperative angiography in cerebral aneurysms and AV malformation. *Neurosurgery* 1984;7: 209–217.

14. Hieshima GB, Reicher MA, Higashida RT, et al. Intraoperative digital subtraction neuroangiography: A diagnostic and therapeutic tool. *AJNR* 1987;8:759–767.

15. King JN, Orrison WW, Keck GM, et al. Arteriography with portable DSA equipment. *Radiology* 1989;172:1023–1025.

16. Wolpert SM, Caplan LR. Current role of cerebral angiography in the diagnosis of cerebrovascular diseases. *AJR* 1992;159:191–197.

17. Osborn AG. Stroke, *Diagnostic Neuroradiology.* St Louis, CV Mosby, 1994, pp 330–400.

18. Osborn AG. *Introduction to Cerebral Angiography.* Philadelphia, Harper & Row, 1980.

19. Maddison FE, Moore WS. Ulcerated atheroma of the carotid artery: Arteriographic appearance. *Am J Roentgenol* 1969;107:530–534.

20. Goldberg HI. Angiography of extracranial and intracranial occlusive cerebrovascular disease. *Neuroimaging Clin North Am* 1992;2:487–507.

21. Imparato AM, Riles TS, Gorstein F. The carotid bifurcation plaque: Findings associated with cerebral ischemia. *Stroke* 1979;10:238.

22. North American Symptomatic Carotid Endarterectomy Trial Collaborators. Beneficial effect of carotid endarterectomy in symptomatic patients with high-grade carotid stenosis. *N Engl J Med* 1991;325:445–453.

23. Edwards JH, Kricheff II, Riles T, et al. Angiographically undetected ulceration of the carotid bifurcation as a cause of embolic stroke. *Radiology* 1979;132:369–373.

24. Lüscher TF, Lie JT, Stanson AW, et al. Arterial fibromuscular dysplasia. *Mayo Clin Proc* 1987;62:931–952.

25. Mettinger KL, Ericson K. Fibromuscular dysplasia and the brain: Observations on angiographic, clinical and genetic characteristics. *Stroke* 1982;13:46–52.

26. Houser OW, Baker HL Jr, Sandok BA, et al. Cephalic arterial fibromuscular dysplasia. *Radiology* 1971;101:605–611.

27. Hachiya J. Current concepts of Takayasu's arteritis. *Semin Roentgenol* 1970;5:245–259.

28. Liu YQ. Radiology of aorto-arteritis. *Radiol Clin North Am* 1985;23:671–688.

29. Kozuka T, Nosaki T, Sato K, et al. Aneurysms associated with aortitis syndrome. *Acta Radiol (Diagn)* 1968;7:314–320.

30. Yamato M, Lecky JW, Hiramatsu K, et al. Takayasu's arteritis: Radiographic and angiographic findings in 59 patients. *Radiology* 1986;161:329–334.

31. Simeone FA, Goldberg HI. Thrombosis of the vertebral artery from hyperextension injury to the neck. *J Neurosurg* 1968;29:540.

32. Ojemann RG, Fisher CM, Rich JE. Spontaneous dissection aneurysm of the internal carotid artery. *Stroke* 1972;4:434.

33. McNeil DH, Dreisbach J, Marsden RJ. Spontaneous dissection of the internal carotid artery. Its conservative management with heparin sodium. *Arch Neurol* 1980;37:54.

34. Barr HWK, Blackwood W, Meadows SZ. Intracavernous carotid aneurysm: A clinical pathological report. *Brain* 1971;94:607–622.

35. Drake CG. Giant intracranial aneurysms: Experience with surgical treatment in 174 patients. *Clin Neurosurg* 1979;26:12–95.

36. Rob RC. Arterial aneurysms. *Ann R Coll Surg Eng* 1954;14:35–49.

37. Kupersmith MJ, Hurst R, Berenstein A, et al. The benign course of cavernous carotid artery aneurysms. *J Neurosurg* 1992;77:690–693.

38. Suzuki J, Takau A. Cerebrovascular "moyamoya" disease: Disease showing abnormal net-like vessels in base of brain. *Arch Neurol* 1969;20:288–290.

39. Takahashi M. Magnification angiography in moyamoya disease: New observations on collateral vessels. *Radiology* 1980;136:379–386.

40. Gotoh F. Guidelines to the diagnosis of occlusion of the circle of Willis, in Gotoh F (ed): *Annual Report of 1987 on the Cooperative Study of Occlusion of the Circle of Willis to the Ministry of Health and Welfare.* Tokyo, 1979, p 132.

41. Takahashi M. Magnification angiography of aneurysms associated with moyamoya disease. *AJNR* 1980;1:547–550.

42. Greenan TJ, Grossman RI, Goldberg HI. Cerebral vasculitis: MR imaging and angiographic correlation. *Radiology* 1992;182:65–72.

43. Cravioto H, Feigin I. Noninfectious granulomatous angiitis with a predilection for the nervous system. *Neurology* 1959;9:599–609.

44. Younger DS, Hays AP, Brust CM, et al. Granulomatous angiitis of the brain: An inflammatory reaction of diverse etiology. *Arch Neurol* 1988;45:514–518.

45. Cupps TR, Moore PM, Fauci AS. Isolated angiitis of the central nervous system: Prospective diagnostic and therapeutic experience. *Medicine* 1983;74:97–105.

46. Kolodny EH, Rebeiz JJ, Caviness CVS Jr, et al. Granulomatous angiitis of the central nervous system. *Arch Neurol* 1988;19:510–524.

47. Calabrese LH, Mallek JA. Primary angiitis of the central nervous system: Report of 8 new cases, review of the literature, and proposal for diagnostic criteria. *Medicine* 1987;67:20–39.

48. Grossman CB. Cerebrovascular disorders, in *Magnetic Resonance Imaging and Computed Tomography of the Head and Spine.* Baltimore, Williams & Wilkins, 1990, pp 145–183.

49. Zimmerman RD, Ernst RJ. Neuroimaging of cerebral venous thrombosis. *Neuroimaging Clin North Am* 1992;2:463–485.

50. Buonanno FS, Moody DM, Ball MR, et al. Computed cranial tomographic findings in cerebral sinovenous occlusion. *J Comput Assist Tomogr* 1978;2:281–290.

51. Locksley HB. Report on the cooperative study of intracranial aneurysms and subarachnoid hemorrhage. Section V, Parts I and II. Natural history of subarachnoid hemorrhage, intracranial aneurysms and arteriovenous malformations based on 6368 cases in the cooperative study. *J Neurosurg* 1966;25:219–239, 321–369.

52. Inagawa T, Hirano A. Autopsy study of unruptured incidental aneurysms. *Surg Neurol* 1990;34:361–365.

53. Ross JS, Masaryk TJ, Modic MT, et al. Intracranial aneurysms: Evaluation by MR angiography. *AJNR* 1990;11:449–456.

54. Housepian EM, Pool JL. Systematic analysis of intracranial aneurysms from the autopsy file of the Presbyterian Hospital. *J Neuropathol Exp Neurol* 1958;17:409–423.

55. McCormick WF, Nofzinger JD. Saccular intracranial aneurysms. An autopsy study. *J Neurosurg* 1965;22:155–159.

56. Stehbens WE. Aneurysms and anatomical variation of cerebral arteries. *Arch Pathol* 1963;75:57–76.

57. Kassell NF, Drake CG. Timing of aneurysm surgery. Neurosurgery 1982;10:514–519.

58. Atkinson JLD, Sundt TMJ, Hoser OW, et al. Angiographic frequency of anterior circulation intracranial aneurysms. J Neurosurg 1989;70:551–555.

59. Yonas H, Agamanolis D, Takaoka Y, et al. Dissecting intracranial aneurysms. *Surg Neurol* 1977;8:407–415.

60. Yamaura A. Diagnosis and treatment of vertebral aneurysms. J Neurosurg 1988;69:345–349.

61. Grosman H, Fornasier VL, Bonder D, et al. Dissecting aneurysm of the cerebral arteries. Case report. J Neurosurg 1980;53:693–697.

62. Sasaki O, Ogawa H, Koiek T, et al. A clinicopathological study of dissecting aneurysms of the intracranial vertebral artery. J Neurosurg 1991;75:874–882.

63. Yamaura A, Watanabe Y, Saeki N. Dissecting aneurysms of the intracranial vertebral artery. J Neurosurg 1990;72:183–188.

64. McCormick WF. The pathology of vascular ("arteriovenous") malformations. J Neurosurg 1966;24:807–816.

65. Jellinger K. Vascular malformations of the central nervous system: A morphological overview. *Neurosurg Rev* 1986;9:177–216.

66. Viñuela F. Update on intravascular functional evaluation and therapy of intracranial arteriovenous malformations. *Neuroimaging Clin North Am* 1992;2:279–289.

67. Iizuka Y, Lasjaunias P, Garcia-Monaco R, et al. Multiple cerebral arteriovenous malformations in children (15 patients). *Neuroradiology* 1991;33:538.

68. Salcman M, Scholtz H, Numaguchi Y. Multiple intracerebral arteriovenous malformations: Report of three cases and review of the literature. *Surg Neurol* 1992;38:121–128.

69. Brown RD Jr, Wiebers DO, Forbes G, et al. The natural history of unruptured intracranial arteriovenous malformations. J Neurosurg 1988;68:352–357.

70. Fults D, Kelly DL. Natural history of arteriovenous malformations of the brain: A clinical study. *Neurosurgery* 1984;15:658–662.

71. Graf CJ, Perret GE, Torner JC. Bleeding from cerebral arteriovenous malformations as a part of their natural history. J Neurosurg 1983;58:331–337.

72. Bailey OT. The vascular component of congenital malformations in the central nervous system. *J Neuropathol Exp Neurol* 1961;20:170–187.

73. Marks MP, Lane B, Steinberg GK, et al. Intracranial aneurysms in cerebral arteriovenous malformations: Evaluation and endovascular treatment. *Radiology* 1992;183:355–360.

74. Osborn AG. Intracranial vascular malformations, in *Diagnostic Neuroradiology.* St Louis, CV Mosby, 1994, pp 284–329.

75. Truwit CL. Venous angioma of the brain: History, significance and imaging findings. *AJR* 1992;159:1299–1307.

76. Rigamonti D, Spetzler D. The association of venous and cavernous malformations: Report of four cases and discussion of the pathophysiological, diagnostic and therapeutic implications. *Acta Neurochir (Wien)* 1988;92:100–105.

77. Lasjaunias P, Burrows P, Planet C. Developmental venous anomalies (DVA): The so-called venous angioma. *Neurosurg Rev* 1986;9:233–244.

78. Wims G, Demaerel P, Marchi G, et al. Gadolinium-enhanced MR imaging of cerebral venous angiomas with emphasis on their drainage. *J Comput Assist Tomogr* 1991;15:199–206.

79. Dion J. Acquired cervicocranial arteriovenous fistulas. *Neuroimaging Clin North Am* 1992;2:319–336.

80. Lasjainias P, Berenstein A. Arteriovenous fistulas, in Lasjainias P, Berenstein A (eds): *Surgical Neuroangiography.* Berlin, Springer-Verlag, 1987, pp 175–233.

81. Newton TH, Cronqvist S. Involvement of dural arteries in intracranial arteriovenous malformations. *Radiology* 1969;93:1071–1078.

82. Houser O, Campbell J, Campbell R, et al. Arteriovenous malformation affecting the transverse dural venous sinus: An acquired lesion. *Mayo Clin Proc* 1979;54:651–661.

83. Dural arteriovenous fistulas: Evaluation with MR imaging. *Radiology* 1990;175:193–199.

84. Duckwiler G. Dural arteriovenous fistula. *Neuroimaging Clin North Am* 1992;2:291–307.

9

Color Flow and Duplex Imaging of the Carotid Arteries

Joseph F. Polak, M.D.

THE PHYSICAL PRINCIPLES OF ULTRASOUND

Evaluation of the cerebrovascular system with ultrasound requires that a beam of ultrasound energy or sound waves sent by an imaging device reach the level of the target vessel. Whereas it is possible to clearly image the carotid bifurcation in most patients with a 5-MHz sound wave, evaluation of the intracranial circulation is hampered by the surrounding cranium. This problem can, in part, be overcome by the selection of lower transducer frequencies (2 MHz) and the use of imaging windows where the bone is thinner. Unfortunately, this leads to a trade-off since the resolution and the ability to carefully interrogate the smaller-diameter intracranial vessel are decreased.

There are two aspects to the use of ultrasound in the diagnostic evaluation of the cerebral vessels. The first is the depiction of the arterial structures and changes that occur in the arterial wall secondary to various pathological states. For the second, ultrasound is used to determine the flow dynamics of the cerebral vessels. It is the combination of both, or duplex sonography, that is typically used for diagnostic imaging.

Gray Scale Image: B-Mode Ultrasound

In most imaging applications, the B-mode ultrasound device, consisting of an electronic array of piezoelectric crystals, is used to create a real-time display of the echoes generated by the interaction of sound with the soft tissues of the body.[1]

Sound waves are generated from piezoelectric crystals that translate small electric impulses into a mechanical displacement. This displacement of the crystal creates small pressure waves that are then transmitted as sound waves within the soft tissues of the body. The image is created by the interaction of the sound waves with the soft tissues. The returning echoes are detected by the piezoelectric crystals, which create small electric signals that are amplified, processed, and displayed as a two-dimensional image. Although other forms of imaging such as A-mode and M-mode imaging are in use, most ultrasound imaging of the cerebrovascular system is made with a so-called B-mode display (Fig. 9-1A,B).

Interaction of Sound with Soft Tissues
The ultrasound beam, as it penetrates through the soft tissues of the body, will interact according to three im-

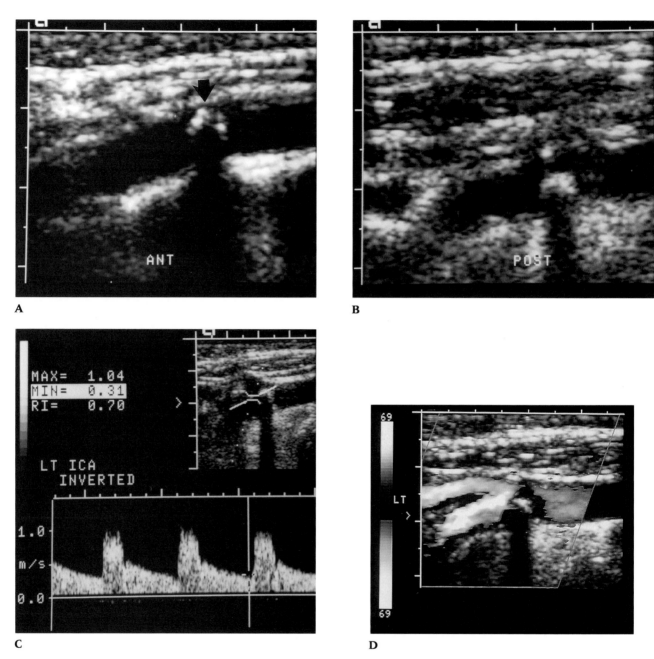

Fig. 9-1 (*A*) This gray scale image taken from the anterior projection shows a plaque in the proximal internal carotid artery (arrow). In this projection, the plaque lies along the anterior wall of the artery. (*B*) This gray scale image is taken from the posterior projection. The plaque previously seen on the anterior wall (*A*) now projects on the posterior wall. This is typical of the eccentric location of plaque in the internal carotid artery. (*C*) This Doppler spectrum is sampled in the proximal internal carotid artery at the plaque shown in parts (*A*), (*B*), and (*D*). There is no significant increase in velocities (above 1.25 m/sec), suggesting that the lesion is not hemodynamically significant. There is, however, some filling in of the Doppler envelope. This is better appreciated when compared to the spectrum shown in part (*A*) and suggests that the focal plaque is large enough to disturb the normal flow patterns expected in the internal carotid artery. (*D*) This color flow image is taken from an anterolateral projection. The plaque seen in parts (*A*) and (*B*) now projects in the middle of the lumen and appears not to be anchored. This "floating" plaque is caused by the limited sampling volume of the ultrasound transducer when it images parallel to the long axis of the artery.

portant physical principles: scattering, attenuation, and reflection. These three interactions occur concurrently and are responsible for the formation of the final image. The relative importance of these interactions is dependent on the tissue, the relative orientation of specific elements within this tissue, and the frequency of the ultrasound beam used for imaging.

Scattering
The basic interaction between the ultrasound beam and the soft tissues of the body is that of scattering. Ultrasound waves interact with the small constituent elements of either muscle, ground substance, or blood in such a way that a portion of the energy is reflected back. Larger target structures such as the myofibrils within muscle reflect the energy from the incoming ultrasound beam as a function of the direction of the beam. The amount of energy reflected and the direction depend on the relative orientation of the structure of interest, its density, and its relative size.

In the case of blood, the plasma does not cause any significant scattering. Most of the ultrasound energy is transmitted through. The smaller elements within the blood, specifically the red cells and, to a lesser extent, the white cells and platelets, are responsible for returning echoes. Because these elements are much smaller than the wavelength of the ultrasound beam, this type of scattering interaction is different from what is seen in the soft tissues. Raleigh scattering has no specific spatial orientation, and the ultrasound energy is scattered in an almost symmetrical fashion. This results in much weaker echoes returning to be detected by the ultrasound transducer. In magnitude, this effect accounts for one ten-thousandth of the strength of signals normally seen in the surrounding soft tissues. This corresponds roughly to a signal 30 to 40 dB lower than the surrounding soft tissues and accounts for the blackness of the vessel lumen on the B-mode image (Fig. 9-1A).

Attenuation
The strength of the transmitted ultrasound beam in soft tissues, even for an ideal homogeneous one, is attenuated. The energy is dissipated as depth increases. This dissipation is in part due to scattering, as well as to direct absorption of the ultrasound energy by the molecules within the soft tissue constituents.

Attenuation tends to be more pronounced at higher frequencies. The ultrasound beam is less capable of penetrating as the carrier frequency increases. Attenuation is greater as frequency increases but is also dependent on the type of tissue. It is more pronounced in muscle than it is in the soft tissues of the brain, for example. It is the lowest in structures containing a clear fluid.

Reflection
Reflection of the ultrasound beam causes a sharp increase in signal strength when the scatterers are aligned in such a fashion that the ultrasound wavefront can be reflected almost perfectly at the interface between tissues of different acoustic characteristics (acoustic impedance). The structure of interest must be oriented perpendicular to the direction of travel of the ultrasound beam. This is more likely to occur at the interface between tissues of high impedance difference such as the transition between the lumen and the intima of the arterial wall. This is pronounced at a transition from low to high acoustic impedance. When the transition is from a zone with high acoustic impedance to one with low acoustic impedance, the nonreflected wavefront can still propagate due to the poor attenuation of the ultrasound beam and create a ringdown artifact, blurring the edge of the interface.

Spatial Resolution
Spatial resolution can be described according to the three spatial coordinates used for imaging. The ability to distinguish two structures lying side by side is normally referred to as *lateral resolution* of the ultrasound beam. This is heavily dependent on focusing of the ultrasound beam and can be adjusted.

The axial resolution of the ultrasound device is critical since it enhances structural detail. This depends on the length and shape of the ultrasound pulse being applied. It is not as greatly affected by the focusing characteristics of the transducer as is lateral resolution. Selection of the transducer frequency or even shaping of the frequency pulse can modify it and dramatically affect imaging quality.

A final type of spatial resolution needs special mention. This deals with the z-axis resolution, or slice thickness definition, of the transducer. Details in the image plane are affected by the thickness of the transducer. The relative shape of the crystal surface affects this type of resolution.

Flow Information: Doppler Ultrasound

The major indication for the use of duplex sonography in patients remains the ability to detect functional stenosis or abnormalities in the flow dynamics within vessels. For this, Doppler ultrasound plays a critical role.[2]

Effect of Motion on Sound

The basic principle underlying the use of Doppler ultrasound is as follows: A sound beam interacts with a moving object in such a way as to cause a net frequency shift in the returning echoes. The magnitude of this frequency shift carries information on the relative motion between the object and the ultrasound beam. Motion toward the transducer tends to increase the frequency of the returning sounds, whereas motion away from the transducer tends to decrease the frequency. The amount of frequency shift is affected by the velocity of blood, as well as by the relative angle between the direction of motion and the direction of propagation of the ultrasound beam. Accurate estimation of the velocity of moving blood requires that the angle between the ultrasound beam and the direction of motion be known (see the section "Steps and Frequency Shift Estimation").

Continuous-wave (C-W) Doppler Ultrasound

A nonimaging probe can be used to continuously transmit and receive sound waves. Motion of blood in the beam of the C-W Doppler ultrasound will cause frequency shifts that can be continuously monitored. The problem with this device is that any moving structure will cause a Doppler signal shift, which can then be detected. Since the actual depth of the returning echoes cannot be determined, there is ambiguity as to the location and orientation of the vessel being imaged.

Pulsed Doppler Ultrasound

This technique is used to send a pulse of finite duration into the soft tissues. The ultrasound device then waits for a finite amount of time. The relative delay between transmission and return of the echoes measures the depth of the returning echoes. By selecting a time delay with respect to the transmission of the ultrasound pulse, signals from a specific depth can be listened to. Within this window, the returning frequency shift information can be used to determine the velocity and direction of the motion of blood. This can be done without the aid of an image, as is the case with traditional transcranial Doppler sonography. If both pulsed Doppler and real-time imaging are done simultaneously, the direction of the sound beam can be depicted on a two-dimensional image. This is known as duplex sonography (Fig. 9-1C). This imaging approach is very useful in evaluation of the extracranial carotid vessels but may be less important for the intracranial circulation since the vessels of interest tend to be located a fixed depth from the temporal bone. Duplex sonography remains the only way to achieve appro-

priate angle correction and subsequent accurate velocity estimation.

Color Flow Imaging

Color flow imaging is a modification of the pulsed Doppler ultrasound principle. With this method, the equivalent of multiple Doppler gates are positioned throughout the imaging field and are used to sample the relative magnitude and direction of moving blood. This information is then processed in a specialized fashion referred to as *autocorrelation*. This method calculates a value related to frequency shift information. Display of pulsed Doppler sonography is traditionally done as a spectrum. The color flow image does not have this level of discrimination and reflects an average velocity value. Such a display is useful in identifying structures that have flowing blood within them, whether arteries or veins. It is more often used as a guide for imaging and selective pulsed Doppler sonography and waveform analysis (Fig. 9-1D).

Conclusion

All of these Doppler techniques rely on the extraction of frequency information from returning echoes. Although the way the information is used varies, the basic principle of the Doppler technique is the detection of the frequency shift generated by moving blood.

INSTRUMENTATION

Gray Scale Imaging

This is a critical component of the sonographic evaluation of the cerebrovascular vessels. The image is a representation of the strength of echoes returning to the ultrasound probe following the interaction of sound beams within the underlying soft tissues.

The quality of the image is dependent on many factors, including the intrinsic resolution of the ultrasound device linked to the frequency used for imaging. Additional factors are beam focusing, as well as the selection of specific frequency components used in the sound beam. In addition, this information must be displayed in real time.

Steps in Image Formation

The creation of the gray scale image proceeds according to the following steps:

1. An appropriate sound pulse is emitted by the ultrasound transducer. For gray scale imaging, the length

of this pulse tends to be one to two cycles of the chosen frequency. Special electronic circuits are used to guarantee that this pulse is of short duration and free of artifacts.

2. The transducer is coupled to the underlying soft tissues by a gel-like substance applied to the skin.

3. The sound waves are then transmitted through the tissues of the skin, muscle, and various facial compartments, where they interact according to the three physical principals we discussed in the section "Gray Scale Imaging: B-Mode Ultrasounds."

4. The returning echoes are captured, and their depth is determined by the time interval between the emission of the ultrasound pulse and reception of the returning echoes. Since the velocity of sound waves in soft tissues is approximately 1,540 m/sec, the delay between emission of the ultrasound pulse and reception of the signal corresponds to the depth of the returning echoes. For example, at a depth of 2 cm, a sound wave must travel a total of 4 cm. This corresponds to a delay of 26 μsec. The time delay is twice this amount at a depth of 4 cm.

The image is created by sequential excitation of smaller crystals within the transducer probe. The linear array transducer has a variable number of crystals, typically between 96 and 128. These are excited in a preselected order. Reception is also encoded as a function of this order by adjusting to the delay between excitation pulses to the crystals. This encoding is responsible for the lateral resolution of the system. Once received, the returning echoes are decoded with respect to their x and y coordinates from knowledge of the delay and relative location of the returning echoes. The intensity of the returning echoes is translated as the intensity of signals displayed on a television monitor. Transformation of the spatial information into an image that can be displayed on a television monitor is accomplished with the help of a scan converter. The final image depicts the real-time distribution of the returning echoes. In general, for evaluation of the carotid vessels, a linear array transducer is used. This transducer has a flat surface and a rectangular shape. For special applications such as transcranial Doppler sonography, the array of crystals is more compact and has a divergent beam. This adapts to the small, accessible window on the skull. The image is displayed as a sector (Fig. 9-2A,B).

Focusing
Focusing is normally accomplished by slight adjustments in the delay between reception and transmission of signals by adjacent crystals in the transducer. Pre-

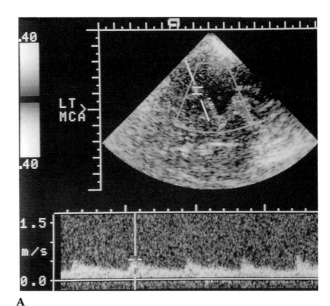

A

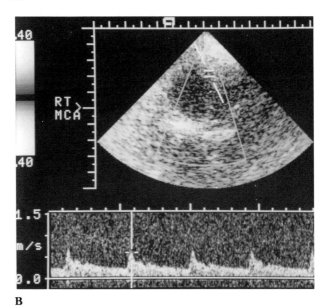

B

Fig. 9-2 (*A*) Transcranial Doppler ultrasound scan through the temporal bone window shows a Doppler spectrum sampled in the left middle cerebral artery on the side contralateral to an internal carotid artery occlusion. It shows a typical low-resistance waveform. (*B*) This Doppler waveform is sampled in the proximal middle cerebral artery on the same side as a total occlusion of the internal carotid artery. Flow is well compensated for due to the presence of collateral flow through the circle of Willis.

selected delays can result in an increase in the signal strength or apparent focusing at a selected depth. This depth is a function of the delay between the exciting pulses delivered to the crystal array. The intrinsic characteristics of the crystal material and width of the emitted sound beam cause difficulty in the near field of the ultrasound device, and focusing is more difficult to accomplish. Newer ultrasound devices now offer advanced digital signal processing and new types of transducers made of epoxy compounds. These have improved coupling between transducer material and skin and decrease imaging difficulties in the near field.

Bandwidth
Bandwidth refers to the actual frequency components emitted by the ultrasound probe. In general, traditional ultrasound devices have used wide bandwidth. The major component of the ultrasound beam has a main frequency component, but a large amount of the ultrasound energy is distributed throughout the spectrum. For example, a 5-MHz imaging probe would transmit some energy at 2.5 MHz. This bandwidth is affected by the interaction with the underlying soft tissues. The bandwidth of returning echoes is different from the emitted bandwidth. The lower-frequency components are less attenuated by the soft tissues and predominate in the image. This accounts for a loss of resolution. Newer transducer materials can increase the imaging bandwidth. Greater emphasis can therefore be given to the high-frequency components in the near-field echoes, while the lower-frequency components are used to characterize the deeper tissues. This, is fact, compensates for some of the effects of attenuation. Another strategy is to limit the bandwidth to a small frequency range and thereby optimize the image. For example, limiting the frequency range to higher values may be useful for the evaluation of a superficially located carotid artery.

Real-time Imaging
The process of creating and displaying the image requires a minimum amount of time, typically 20 to 100 msec. Real-time imaging consists of the transmission and reception of these images in such a way that the information is continuously refreshed and displayed on a monitor screen. This assumes that the ultrasound beam has sufficient time to reach and return from the deeper soft tissues. Therefore, the rate at which the image can be acquired and displayed is dependent on the depth at which imaging is performed. For example, imaging at a depth of 4 cm requires twice the delay needed for a depth of 2 cm.

Although earlier ultrasound devices were capable of static imaging, this approach has been replaced completely by real-time imaging, also referred to as *B-mode imaging*.

Doppler Sonography

Steps and Frequency Shift Estimation
The Doppler principle states that if waves, such as sound or light waves, interact with a moving body, the returning waves acquire a frequency shift which is dependent on the relative motion, direction, and velocity of the body. For example, ultrasound echoes from a body moving toward the source of the sound waves will have a higher frequency when detected. Echoes returning from an object moving away from the detector will have a lower frequency or negative frequency shift. The principle can be summarized by the Doppler equation. This equation basically states that the frequency shift is dependent on the relative motion between the two objects, the carrier frequency, and the angle created between the moving body and the direction of the ultrasound beam. If the ultrasound beam and motion are in the same direction, the frequency shift is maximal. This frequency shift is affected by the angle between the motion and the ultrasound beam. The Doppler equation is given by

$$\Delta v = 2v_0 \left[\frac{V \times \cos \theta}{c} \right]$$

where Δv is the frequency change, v_0 is the original frequency, c is the velocity of sound in the body, V is the blood velocity, and θ is the angle between the direction of blood flow and the direction of the sound beam. This equation makes the Doppler angle crucial in relating a frequency shift to the velocity of flowing blood.

Doppler sonography and the measurement of frequency shifts assume that the length of the packet of ultrasound frequency being emitted is sufficient to permit accurate detection of the frequency shift. For gray scale imaging, pulse lengths of one to two cycles are normally used. For frequency shift detection, pulse lengths of more than 10 cycles are often required to ensure that there is no ambiguity in estimating the frequency shift.

Fourier Transformation: Doppler Waveform Generation
The frequency shift information returning from moving blood tends to be within the audio range when the carrier frequency is between 3 and 7 MHz. This fre-

quency information is extracted from the returning echoes by a process called *Fourier transformation*. In essence, a mathematical representation is made of the different frequency components of the returning echoes. This information is then displayed in a format that contains information on the relative number, distribution, and different velocities of moving red cells. This representation is called the *Doppler spectral waveform* (Fig. 9-1C). The Fourier transformation is applied to echo packets as they return at selected time intervals, varying with the ultrasound device, at increments of 1 to 10 msec. Fourier transformation of the returning echoes is therefore performed for each of these finite blocks of time. The information is displayed in a coordinate system where the amplitude or number of red cells are encoded as intensity. The actual frequency is displayed on the *y*-axis. The *x*-axis is used to encode time information, identifying the specific time when the information is being extracted from the returning echoes. The size of the bins used to create this spectrum varies from 1 to 10 msec. The increase in this spectrum is the peak repetition frequency (PRF).

Color Flow Imaging

Doppler Imaging   The color Doppler approach can be described as the use of a multitude of pulsed Doppler sample gates positioned in the imaging field. The direction of the ultrasound beam is selected by focusing the different crystals within the transducer matrix. The actual distance corresponds to the time interval between emission of the pulse and its reception. The duration of the pulse is selected to be of sufficient length to permit processing and extraction of Doppler shift information with the help of the Fourier transformation process. Hybrid approaches measure the phase shift of the returning pulse wave and accelerate the mathematical extraction of the frequency shift spectrum. This process occurs concurrently with real-time imaging. It therefore reduces the frame rate of real-time gray scale imaging. It is also possible to freeze the real-time image and to focus more attention on Doppler spectral waveform analysis. This gives more detail to the Doppler spectral waveform.

Time-of-flight Imaging   A new approach uses emission of two pulses of ultrasound energy to detect the relative intensity of the returning signals. This intensity is roughly proportional to the number of red blood cells that have moved. This time-of-flight imaging approach offers the advantage that the relative distribution and components of moving blood can be more accurately

displayed. It does, however, suffer from the same restriction as Doppler imaging in regard to absolute velocity measurements: accurate angle correction must be obtained for velocity estimation.[3]

Velocity Estimation

Angle Correction   The Doppler shift information assumes a fixed relationship between the sound wave and the direction of motion of the target of interest. In the case of red blood cells, this angle must be accurately known for the velocity to be estimated. The problem with this angle correction is that it must be performed by the human operator. The operator determines the relative angle between the ultrasound beam and the assumed motion of red blood cells by aligning a digital cursor parallel to the direction of flow in a vessel. This process has an associated error since the operator estimates the actual angle with an accuracy of 1° to 5°. The effect of this inherent error increases as the angle between the direction of motion and the sound beam increases. For example, at angles of close to 70°, a 1° error translates into a 5% error; at 80° this corresponds to a 15% error. The angle should, in general, be kept below 60°.

Aliasing   A finite time delay occurs between transmission and reception of the ultrasound beam. The length of this delay determines the amount of information that can be decoded without ambiguity. This is dependent on a well-known principle for sampling digital signals. This principle states that the upper limit of sampling occurs at twice the rate of the highest frequency component that can be displayed. For example, if sampling can take place only at a maximum of one sample per 10 msec, then information dealing with a wavelength of 20 msec or an absolute frequency of 50 cycles/sec can be displayed. If the sampling interval is increased to a longer value, then the peak-frequency information that can be displayed decreases. This sets an upper limit to the velocities that can be displayed by the ultrasound device. The problem can be partially alleviated by decreasing the size of the wave packet that is being transmitted. This will increase the rate of sampling. The setting on the device that controls this is normally referred to as the *peak repetition frequency (PFR)* of the device and, in essence, limits the maximal velocity information that can be displayed. For most imaging purposes, carrier frequencies are close to 3 MHz and tend not to alias. Higher frequencies are more likely to result in aliasing of the Doppler spectrum.

Since the color flow image is created by processing

information from the full field of view, the time interval between images is longer. This decreases the aliasing frequencies, and color flow imaging will alias at lower velocities than for pulsed Doppler analysis.

HEMODYNAMICS: EVALUATION WITH DOPPLER AND COLOR FLOW SONOGRAPHY

Laminar Flow: Waveform Analysis

Evaluation of the carotid system includes analysis of the flow patterns within the carotid branches. The classic depiction of flow within a straight tube such as the common carotid is that of laminar flow. In the center of the vessel blood moves quickly, while the more peripherally located red cells move more slowly. A depiction of the velocity distribution shows a parabolic contour. This pattern can be seen within the midportion of the common carotid artery. It is lost with irregularities in the walls of the carotid, with angles or curves, and with relative proximity to a bifurcation.

In addition, laminar flow typically applies to constant flow situations. Velocities during peak systole may lose their laminar flow characteristics. These can return during diastole. A narrow sample gate must be used in order to sample a specific portion of the vessel and not artificially broaden the distribution of velocities shown on the velocity spectra.[4]

Effect of Peripheral Impedance

Peripheral arterial impedance has an effect on the shape of the Doppler waveform (Fig. 9-3). For example, high peripheral resistance will decrease diastolic flow. This situation is seen in the external carotid branches (Fig. 9-3A,D). In the internal carotid, flow must continue throughout the cardiac cycle, and the overall resistance of the arterial bed is low (Fig. 9-3B). The waveform therefore shows continuous flow throughout the cardiac cycle, with a strong component during diastole. Changes in distal impedance, such as occlusion of the vessel by an embolus, tend to abolish this low-resistance pattern. However, with time, collaterals partly compensate and tend to reestablish a low-impedance pattern. Conversely, a proximal occlusion tends to reduce the distal impedance (Fig. 9-4A,B). Sampling within the arterial bed distal to a high-grade stenosis (>80% diameter narrowing) may show a rela-

tive increase in the importance of the diastolic component with respect to the systolic component and a delay in the systolic rise time.[5]

Flow at Bends and Bifurcations

Flow Separation
Boundary layer separation is seen at the site of vessel branching. The origin of the internal and external carotid arteries will typically show an area where laminar flow can no longer be maintained. The flow stream separates from the artery wall and is associated with small vortices and reversed flow at the origin of the internal carotid artery. This zone of relative stagnation and low shear stress is thought to promote the formation of early atherosclerotic lesions.[6–9]

Nonlaminar Flow
Loss of the laminar flow pattern can occur whenever a major arterial branch ceases to be straight. In fact, nonlaminar flow is more likely than the more typical laminar flow pattern shown in textbooks. Boundary layer separation and flow separation are examples of nonlaminar flow. The pattern of more homogeneous flow, in which the same velocity affects blood irrespective of its location in the vessel, is termed *plug flow*. Plug flow is present at the level of the smaller capillary bed or at the narrowest portion of a stenosis. The presence of vortices or areas of flow reversal at bifurcations, at stenoses, or at the transition from a small- to a large-diameter vessel are other examples of nonlaminar flow. These situations affect the appearance of the Doppler spectrum and lead to spectral broadening.[10]

Turbulence

Turbulent flow is not equivalent to nonlaminar flow; instead, it is one form of nonlaminar flow. Because of the loss of coherence of this flow pattern, the location of blood cells cannot be tracked in time. In other forms of nonlaminar flow, the location of these cells can be predicted. With turbulent flow, there is loss of coherence and lack of predictability. Turbulence is more likely to occur at a threshold where flow velocity and density and the diameter of the artery cause a large Reynolds coefficient. Typically, turbulence can be seen in larger-diameter arteries such as the aorta at the level of the ascending and aortic roots. Another site for the development of turbulent flow is distal to a stenosis in a small-diameter artery.[11]

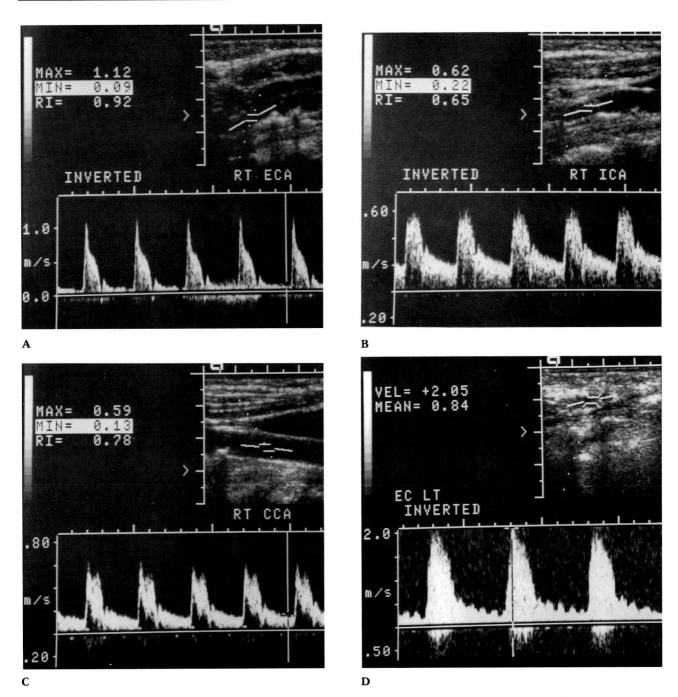

Fig. 9-3 (*A*) This figure shows the typical high-resistance waveform of the external carotid artery, with almost no blood flow seen during diastole. (*B*) This figure shows the typical low-resistance waveform of the internal carotid artery, with preserved blood flow seen during diastole. (*C*) This figure shows the common carotid artery waveform proximal to the corresponding external and internal carotid branches shown in parts (*A*) and (*B*). The waveform shares the appearance of both downstream branches, showing flow during diastole (internal carotid artery) and pulsatility during systole (external carotid artery). (*D*) This Doppler spectrum is taken in the proximal external carotid artery. This waveform shows diastolic flow more typical of an internal carotid artery. The nature of the artery is confirmed by the oscillations in the Doppler spectrum induced by applying pulsations over the preauricular branch of the temporal artery. This maneuver is called the *temporal tap*.

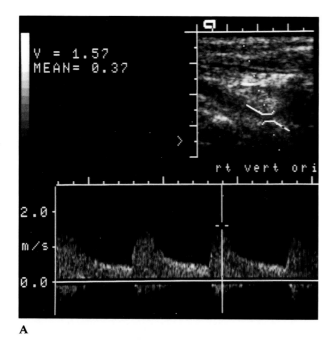

A

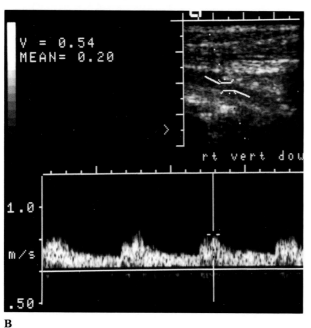

B

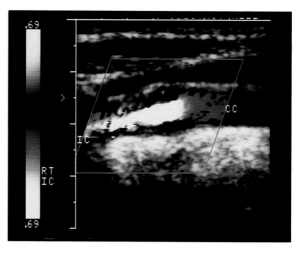

Fig. 9-5 This color Doppler image shows a stenotic jet (in white) with a zone of flow reversal (blue, arrows) beyond an atherosclerotic plaque (curved arrow).

Flow of Stenotic Lesions

Flow Patterns

The development of a typical jet of increased velocity is normally associated with the presence of a hemodynamically significant stenosis (Fig. 9-5). Such stenoses cause a pressure drop across the lesion and therefore are associated with a loss of energy as the blood moves across the stenosis.

Lower-grade stenoses that are not associated with a pressure drop will show an alteration in the normal laminar pattern of flow and the development of spectral broadening.[10,12] In general, however, the more typical stenotic lesion must cause at least a 50% diameter stenotic narrowing before it causes a flow jet and associated areas typical of flow separation distal to the lesion. It is in this transition zone that turbulent flow is present.[11,13]

Flow Separation

A zone of flow separation will develop distal to the stenosis proper as the jet of increased-velocity blood now blends in with more slowly moving blood in a larger-diameter channel. This area of flow reversal is similar to what is seen at a bifurcation. It tends to surround the stenotic jet as it emerges from the stenotic narrowing (Fig. 9-4). This zone of flow separation is variable in length, although it rarely reaches more than 2 cm with simple lesions of the carotid artery.[11]

Fig. 9-4 (*A*) This first of two duplex sonograms shows a high-grade stenosis in the proximal vertebral artery. The peak-systolic velocities are elevated beyond the 0.4- to 0.7-m/sec range that is typical for this artery. (*B*) This duplex ultrasound scan was obtained in the midvertebral artery. It shows a typical pattern for the vertebral artery. Diastolic flow is increased relative to systolic flow when this waveform is compared to that shown in part (*A*).

Stenotic Jet

The stenotic jet proper is the continuation of the zone of increased velocity established at the point of narrowest diameter. This point, or stenosis throat, defines the maximal velocity within the stenotic jet. The jet will typically extend 1 to 2 cm distal to the stenosis in the carotid system. The end and side boundaries of the jet delineate the areas where blood decelerates quickly, thereby generating turbulence.

Turbulence

Alterations in the laminar flow pattern at sites of early atherosclerotic plaque formation have been termed *turbulent flow*. More precisely, however, these alterations are examples of vorticeal flow. True turbulence is more likely to occur at the distal aspect or the boundary of stenotic jets. This is where energy is being rapidly dissipated and generates turbulence. Turbulence is manifested on the Doppler spectrum as a rapid alteration in the amplitude of the velocity envelope or as broadening of the Doppler spectrum (compare Figs. 9-3B and 9-1C).

NORMAL EXAMINATION

Standard protocols are normally followed for the evaluation of the carotid, vertebral, and transcranial vessels. The examination is performed with the aid of gray scale imaging, duplex sonography with Doppler waveform analysis, and finally, color flow imaging. An examination should combine all three types of sonography.

It is possible to conduct a simple survey of the carotid arteries and to detect the presence of atherosclerotic lesions using gray scale imaging alone. However, this has been shown to be unreliable when higher-grade lesions are present.[14–17] Duplex sonography is sufficient for accurate detection and grading of carotid stenoses.[18–22] The addition of color flow imaging facilitates the examination and makes it more time effective.[23]

Carotids

A typical examination of the carotid branches starts with a survey performed in the transverse plane. The course of the common carotid from the base of the neck is followed to the level of the bifurcation and then to the external and internal carotid arteries, typically above the midneck level. The internal carotid artery lies in a posterolateral location, while the external carotid is located anteromedial in most patients. The internal

carotid artery can be distinguished in most cases from the external carotid artery by its greater diameter and the absence of arterial branches. However, in some cases, there may be difficulties in distinguishing between these two branches. The position of the external and internal carotid branches can be reversed in up to 10% of cases.

Following this survey, the carotid artery is imaged in the longitudinal plane. Gray scale imaging is used to evaluate wall thickness and plaque deposits in the carotid branches. The location of these atherosclerotic deposits or wall thickness changes is then clearly documented (Fig. 9-1B).

Duplex sonography is typically performed in the longitudinal plane. This permits accurate placement of the Doppler gate and proper angle correction for subsequent velocity estimations. On occasion, pulsed Doppler sonography is performed in the transverse plane to help distinguish the internal from the external carotid. The internal carotid artery feeds a low-resistance vascular bed, the brain, and has antegrade flow throughout the cardiac cycle (Fig. 9-3B). The lack of major branches accounts for the lack of reflected waves in the systolic portion of the waveform. A dicrotic notch is often seen in early diastole. The external carotid artery waveform has a lower diastolic flow component than that of the internal carotid artery. In addition, since multiple waves are reflected from the branches of the external carotid, the systolic component of the waveform has a pronounced peak (Fig. 9-3A). The Doppler waveform detected in the common carotid artery shares characteristics of both the internal and external carotids.[12] It shows more pulsatility in the systolic component (external carotid) and a significant amount of antegrade flow during diastole (internal carotid) (Fig. 9-3C).

Color flow imaging is used to interrogate the flow patterns within the common, internal, and external carotid artery branches. In the normal patient, flow reversal can be seen at the bifurcation along the lateral wall of the internal carotid.[8] Hemodynamically significant stenoses are normally identified as sites causing aliasing of the color flow image (Fig. 9-6A). These sites should be interrogated and undergo pulsed Doppler waveform analysis (Fig. 9-6B) even when the gray scale image is unremarkable (Fig. 9-6C).

Vertebral

The vertebral arteries lie in the neural foramina. They are difficult to evaluate along their full length.[24] Major

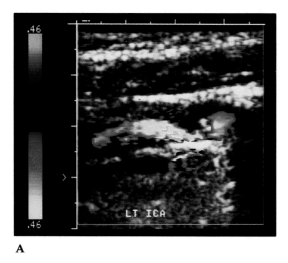

A

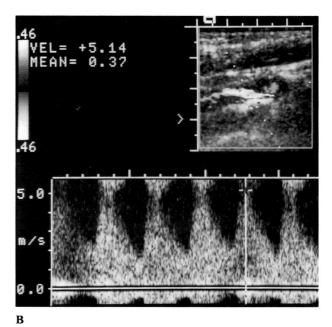

B

Fig. 9-6 This color flow image shows a very eccentric internal carotid artery stenosis. The plaque causing the narrowing is heterogeneous and mostly isoechoic (arrows). (*B*) The Doppler spectrum is sampled in the proximal internal carotid artery, with the Doppler gate directed toward the jet of blood caused by the stenosis. This minimizes the angle between the direction of the sound beam used for Doppler analysis and the direction of blood flow. (*C*) This gray scale image shows a mainly iso- to hypoechoic plaque (arrows) that is also heterogeneous since it has a component with strong echoes. The plaque is barely perceived on the gray scale image. It is more clearly outlined on the color flow image (part *A*), and its significance is confirmed by Doppler analysis (part *B*).

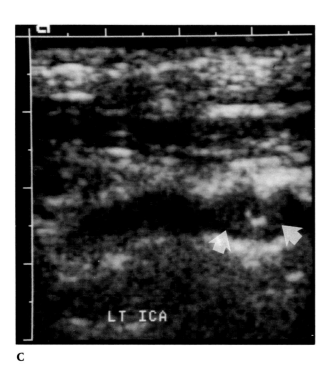

C

portions are obscured by ultrasound shadowing and signal loss due to bone in the transverse processes of the cervical bodies.[25] In general, longitudinal imaging is used (Fig. 9-7). The origin from the subclavian artery is often identified by combined imaging in the oblique and transverse planes.

The flow pattern of the vertebral artery is similar to that of the internal carotid artery (Fig. 9-4A,B). Both feed the intracranial structures. Flow is in the antegrade direction. It can be reversed in the subclavian steal syndrome.[26]

Transcranial Sonography

In general, transcranial sonography is performed with a nonimaging pulsed Doppler probe. The depth of insonation is normally set at 55 mm from contact on the skin over the temporal bone window. The waveforms from the intracerebral vessels are similar to those seen in the internal carotid artery. The systolic component may show slight pulsatility.

The true velocity is difficult to obtain due to the lack of angle correction. Major emphasis is given to analyzing the shape of the waveform, and the pulsatility index is used. This is calculated by taking the difference between systolic and diastolic flow amplitudes and dividing by the average velocity. The relative direction of blood flow in various branches is recorded. This helps to determine the pattern of collateral flow.

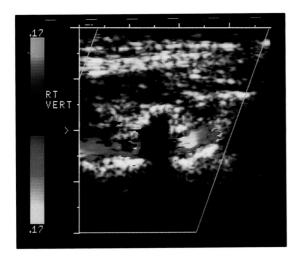

Fig. 9-7 This color flow image shows a stenosis in the mid-right vertebral artery. As with a lesion hidden in the midst of a calcified plaque, the zone of flow abnormality—yellow on the right of the transverse process—extends over a distances of at least 1 cm and shows up as a zone of blue on the left side of the transverse process.

Low-frequency color flow imaging complements duplex sonography[27] and permits the acquisition of angle-corrected velocity profiles. Significant focal lesions,[28] significant spasm,[29] or the intracranial arteries can increase velocities which normally show minimal alterations in flow dynamics (Fig. 9-2A,B). This is mainly due to the significant autoregulation process of the brain vasculature and the presence of collateral pathways through the circle of Willis.[30]

Effect of Age

Doppler waveforms in young patients show increased heart rates and more pronounced pulsatility. This appearance is due to the increased compliance of the vessels, which is reduced with aging.

IMAGING AND WAVEFORM ANALYSIS OF EXTRACRANIAL CAROTID ARTERIES: CLINICAL APPLICATIONS

The major use of sonographic imaging and Doppler waveform analysis of the extracranial carotid arteries is for the detection and grading of atherosclerotic disease. Its major role is as a screening tool for detecting patients with significant stenosis who can potentially benefit from carotid endarterectomy.[31,32] A better understanding of this role is gained by a short review of the pathophysiology of carotid atherosclerotic plaque.

Evaluation of Atherosclerotic Lesions

Atherosclerotic Plaque: Distribution of Disease
Atherosclerotic plaque typically forms in the proximal internal carotid artery at the level of flow bifurcation. The early lesion develops in the wall adjacent to this zone of flow reversal.[7] Another site of preferred plaque growth is the origin of the common carotid artery, but lesions are less common than at the carotid bifurcation. The more distal internal carotid artery at the level of the carotid siphon can also develop focal atherosclerotic lesions. These, as well as middle cerebral artery lesions, are less common than those developing at the bifurcation.[33]

Atherosclerotic plaque consists of an enlarging lipid core that slowly expands the intima into the vessel lumen. When plaque reaches a certain critical size, the shearing forces of flowing blood are believed to pull on the plaque. Since the mechanical integrity of plaque is somewhat less than that of the surrounding artery wall, an intraplaque hemorrhage is likely to develop. This hemorrhage, and possible fissuring of the plaque, may account for rapid plaque growth. These episodes are mostly asymptomatic.[34] Resorption of the hemorrhage and fibrotic deposits likely occur, in addition to continued lipid deposition, and account for the continued increase in the size of the plaque. The plaque contour also becomes more irregular. The plaque content becomes more heterogeneous as fibroatheromatous deposits form.[35,36]

On occasion, the plaque continues to expose its internal elements to flowing blood (i.e., in an ulcer). Platelet thrombi can then form and embolize more distally into the intracranial circulation, thereby causing transient ischemic attacks. Portions of the plaque material can also embolize.

Atherosclerotic Plaque, Relationship to Stroke
Embolic phenomena are often responsible for the development of stroke and transient ischemic attacks. A significant proportion of embolic phenomena (20%) can arise from the cardiac chambers. In addition, stroke may be due to simple ischemia or the development of small vessel disease associated with hypertension. In essence, 50% of episodes of stroke may be linked somehow to atheroembolic phenomena originating from the internal carotid bifurcation lesion. Although it is possible for smaller lesions in the carotid to cause emboli, the risk of embolization increases with the severity of

the stenosis or the narrowing of the lumen diameter. This relationship has recently been documented by the NASCET study,[37] where the relative risk of stroke increased dramatically with the severity of stenosis. Total occlusion of the internal carotid artery is a less likely mechanism for strokes or transient ischemic attacks since collateral circulation can often compensate for occlusion and thrombosis of the extracranial carotid.[38] The presence of embolic phenomena can also be linked to severe carotid stenoses in studies that use transcranial Doppler sonography to detect cerebral embolic events.[39]

Sonographic Classification of Plaque
The sonographic classification of plaque emphasizes detection of zones of intraplaque hemorrhage. Plaques having zones of hemorrhage within them are thought to be more active or unstable. While it is true that most carotid endarterectomy samples show evidence of recent intraplaque hemorrhage, not all episodes of intraplaque hemorrhage are necessarily associated with symptoms.[40,41] As discussed above, many episodes of intraplaque hemorrhage probably occur, and only a few cause significant symptoms.[34]

The sonographic classification of atherosclerotic plaque emphasizes the ability to detect intraplaque hemorrhage. It is thought that this may identify plaques prone to repeated rupture, causing subsequent embolic phenomena culminating in a stroke.

Plaque *density* refers to the type of plaque constituent. Material within the plaque that is relatively iso- or hypoechoic may represent either smooth muscle cells, hematoma, or lipid.[42] Fibrous tissue will cause areas of increased echogenic signals on the B-mode image.

The actual structure of the plaque is typically described as homogeneous or heterogeneous. *Homogeneous* plaque refers to plaque containing material of similar echogenic characteristics. Homogeneous plaque can be isoechoic, hypoechoic, or hyperechoic. Dense plaques do, however, tend to have areas of strong echogenic signals mixed with areas of weak echogenic signals. These heterogeneous plaques probably have previously hemorrhaged. The likelihood of heterogeneous plaque increases with the severity of the stenosis.[43,44]

The surface characteristics of plaque are normally described as the relative smoothness or irregularity of its contour. At one extreme is the excavation 2 mm in size that corresponds to an ulceration. Detecting and documenting the presence of ulceration is, however, difficult by sonography. Accuracy is often quoted to be above 80–85%,[45] while other data suggest that it is

much lower.[46,47] A major problem in determining the accuracy of sonography for lesions not removed at surgery is the variable accuracy of arteriography as a "gold standard." This may be as low as 60–70%.[48,49] Potential sonographic pitfalls include difficulty in fully visualizing a plaque and two separate plaques sitting side by side, thereby mimicking an excavation. Irregularities in the plaque contour by arteriography are known to relate to prevalent transient ischemic attacks and stroke.[50,51] This has to do with the increased likelihood of exposing internal portions of the plaque to blood, and to an increased likelihood of platelet thrombi formation and the release of emboli.

Finally, calcification is treated as a separate category. Calcification hinders penetration of the ultrasound beam and undermines its ability to characterize the underlying lesion. This may mask the flow signals needed to detect significant stenosis. Lesions of 1 cm or more that are likely to obscure these signals can be seen in up to 10% of cases.[23,52]

Hemodynamically Significant Stenoses

A major purpose of the carotid sonographic examination is the detection of hemodynamically significant stenoses. These lesions are defined as having a diameter narrowing of 50% or more. More recently, stenoses of 70% diameter narrowing or more have been considered to be clinically significant.[37]

Although measurement of the cross-sectional area of the stenosis may appear to be a more accurate or more scientific approach to grading stenosis severity, emphasis is now given to grading the lesion by diameter stenosis. This is the strategy adopted by most major studies that have looked at the outcome of carotid endarterectomy. Severity of the stenosis in the internal carotid artery is also determined with respect to the segment of the internal carotid artery above the stenotic lesion.[37]

Diagnostic Criteria
The major diagnostic criterion for the presence of a diameter narrowing of 50% or above is elevation of the peak systolic velocity above 125 cm/sec. This is the threshold above which a lesion is considered hemodynamically significant. This definition assumes a cardiac output within the normal range and common carotid artery velocity values of 60 to 80 cm/sec. In one series, 130 cm/sec was used at the cutoff for a 60% diameter stenosis.[53] This is near the 125 cm/sec cutoff currently recognized for the 50% diameter stenosis.[23]

Besides peak systole, other portions of the Doppler

waveform can be used to grade stenosis severity. A carotid stenosis will also increase the velocity of blood during diastole,[54] but this effect may be more variable.[11] The presence of a high-grade lesion in the internal carotid artery may also affect the waveform in the common carotid artery and decrease the peak systolic and diastolic velocities.[55] This fact can be used to create additional criteria useful for the detection of carotid artery stenosis. The following velocity ratios have been proposed at various times as parameters for grading the severity of internal carotid artery stenosis: (1) the ratio of the peak systolic velocity in the internal divided by that in the common carotid;[21] (2) the ratio of internal carotid peak end-diastolic velocity to common carotid peak end-diastolic velocity;[47,54] (3) and the ratio of peak systolic velocity in the internal carotid divided by peak end-diastolic velocity in the common carotid artery.[56] These different ways of grading the severity of carotid artery stenosis make it difficult to determine which parameter may be useful in the evaluation of the stenosis severity. Few studies have addressed this issue. One of the largest was published in 1988. The authors concluded that end-diastolic velocity was a better parameter for grading stenoses of 60% or more.[47] Other studies have suggested that peak systolic velocity is a more robust parameter[22,57,58] and that other velocity parameters do not appear to contribute significantly to this accuracy.[58]

The peak systolic velocity is obtained at the site of highest velocity within the internal carotid artery. Early studies used pulsed Doppler sonography and duplex devices with early aliasing of the frequency shifts. The end-diastolic velocity frequency shift was then used as a parameter for grading higher-grade stenosis.[59] This circumvents the problem of aliasing (Fig. 9-8). However, subsequent data have suggested that end-diastolic velocity may identify a subset of asymptomatic patients at high risk for subsequent stroke.[60]

Underlying the use of a velocity ratio is the increased likelihood that progression of the internal carotid artery stenosis will depress flow velocity within the common carotid artery.[20,55] Specifically, a high-grade internal carotid artery stenosis can cause a decrease in common carotid velocity or frequency shift.[61] A mean peak systolic velocity below 25 cm/sec in the common carotid has been proposed as a method for detecting significant downstream internal carotid artery stenosis.[55] Unfortunately, this parameter has low sensitivity. Many high-grade internal carotid stenoses may not significantly affect common carotid artery velocity. Presumably, this is due to the development of collateral flow either through the circle of Willis or through the

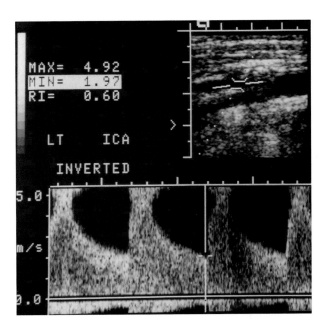

Fig. 9-8 This duplex ultrasound scan shows a high-grade stenosis at the origin of the internal carotid artery. An elevated systolic velocity of 4.92 m/sec is accompanied by an increase in diastolic velocity (1.97 m/sec). Parallel increases in systolic and diastolic velocities are typical of high-grade internal carotid artery stenoses.

ipsilateral external carotid. The ratio of the peak systolic velocity offers a simple means of correcting for changes in cardiac output in patients with concurrent heart disease. Although there are no specific advantages to using the ratio of the end-diastolic velocities, this ratio may be more useful for higher-grade stenosis (80% or more diameter narrowing).[47] Finally, a relatively robust parameter, the ratio of peak systolic velocity within the internal carotid divided by common carotid end-diastolic velocity, appears to distinguish 75% diameter stenosis with high accuracy.[56]

Although velocity ratios may be of use, they add variability to the measurements since more than one parameter has to be measured. A recent review has evaluated the comparative accuracy of these different parameters and suggests that overall, peak systolic velocity is a more robust parameter that offers sensitivity and specificity of about 90%.[58] In addition, it seems to be less affected by selection bias. This is a bias introduced in the population which is specifically looked at in the noninvasive lab since subsequent arteriography is likely to be obtained in patients who have significant stenosis. This selection bias may affect the overall performance of the diagnostic test.[62]

Threshold for Clinical Significance

The cutoff for hemodynamically significant internal carotid artery stenosis has been established to be 125 cm/sec. The problem, however, remains the identification of patients who have clinically significant stenoses. Data from both the NASCET[37] and ECST[63] studies suggest that carotid endarterectomy must be performed in symptomatic individuals who have more than a 70% diameter stenosis. Moneta et al. observe that the threshold of 250 cm/sec or a peak systolic velocity ratio of 4 can identify individuals with a 70% diameter stenosis with high accuracy.[64] Hunink et al. suggest that a threshold of 230 cm/sec peak systolic velocity is sufficient to identify these patients. A regression equation that permits the actual measurement of stenosis from peak systolic velocity and adjusts for common carotid artery velocity can also be used.[58]

The 70% cutoff value applies to individuals with symptoms. Clinically significant lesions needing treatment by carotid endarterectomy may ultimately have a value of 50%, 55%, or 60%. The NASCET and ECST studies are continuing to accumulate data. The 70% threshold is set for institutions that have low morbidity rates with carotid endarterectomy. This obviously affects overall performance and ultimate morbidity of the patient.

Calcification

Calcification obscures the full evaluation of the lumen in the carotid artery in up to 10% of patients presenting for diagnostic sonography and subsequently undergoing carotid angiography. Erickson et al. noted that the presence of calcifications larger than 1.0 cm causes a decrease in the overall sensitivity and specificity of carotid sonography in detecting significant stenosis of the internal carotid.[52] Polak et al. noted a similar phenomenon, but the effect was on the reproducibility of the measurement.[23] Therefore, it appears that calcifications greater than 1 cm compromise the accuracy of Doppler sonography. It is, however, possible to ascertain the presence of a hemodynamically significant stenosis since evidence of a significant flow disturbance or of a jet can be used to infer its presence. This jet will typically extend for 1 cm distal to the throat, or narrowest part, of the stenosis (Fig. 9-9). Although accurate grading of the stenosis may not be possible, the presence of a hemodynamically significant stenosis is very likely.

Subtotal vs. Total Occlusion

Determining the presence of a subtotal occlusion of the internal carotid artery remains the main limitation of the noninvasive sonographic examination.[15,65] There

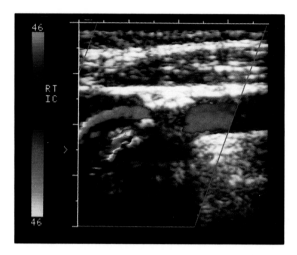

Fig. 9-9 This color flow image shows the internal carotid (zone of blue and yellow on the left) and external carotid (zone of red on the left) arteries beyond a region occupied by a calcified plaque. The color flow signals are aliased in the proximal internal carotid artery, indicating a high-grade stenosis. The zone of flow abnormality associated with a significant carotid artery stenosis often extends over a distance of at least 1 cm. Potential lesions may be missed when the zone of calcification extends over a distance greater than 1 cm.

are two reasons for this. First, the normal relationship between peak systolic velocity and severity of stenosis is one of increasing velocity as the severity of the stenosis increases. However, past a certain threshold at approximately 80–90% diameter stenosis, flow velocities may actually start to decrease.[66] It is therefore possible to have a very-high-grade lesion and depressed flow velocities. Under these circumstances, however, velocity profiles tend to be distorted and may show a tardus-parvus appearance.[5] The rise time during systole is blunted, and the amplitude of the waveform is decreased (Fig. 9-10).

The second reason is the fact that Doppler signals may not be sampled. This occurs in so-called subtotal occlusions, referred to as *pseudo-occlusions* or the *string sign* on arteriograms. The detection of a subtotal occlusion requires accurate placement of the Doppler sample gate, a difficult task since the lumen of the affected vessel may be quite small and the velocity within it significantly depressed. The sensitivity of the Doppler analyzer must therefore be set at lower velocity scales or lower PRF values so that the lower velocity signals can be detected. Color Doppler flow imaging may offer an advantage in detecting these subtotal occlusions (Fig. 9-11). There are no large series addressing the

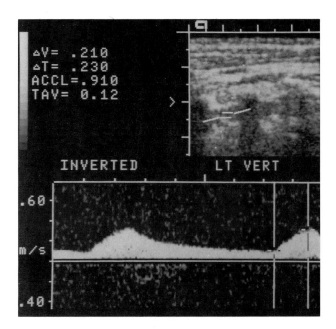

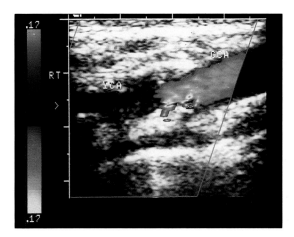

Fig. 9-12 This color flow image shows evidence of total occlusion of the proximal internal carotid artery. The velocity settings have been set to emphasize lower flow velocities in order not to miss a subtotal occlusion. Despite these precautions, classification errors—subtotal versus total occlusions—are still a major limitation of Doppler sonography of the carotid arteries.

Fig. 9-10 This Doppler spectrum sampled in the vertebral artery shows a typical pattern indicating a proximal high-grade lesion. Such a tardus waveform is caused by the delay in the arrival time of blood due to a proximal obstruction. The relative amplitude of diastolic flow also tends to be increased with respect to peak systolic flow. Such a pattern can also be seen in cases of severe aortic stenosis.

issue of sensitivity and specificity of color flow imaging in reaching this diagnosis (Fig. 9-12).

Tandem Lesions
There are three types of tandem lesions. The first lies at the origin of the common carotid or innominate artery, the second within the intracranial portion of the internal carotid, and the third within the common carotid artery. The first two cannot be visualized; the third is accessible to sonographic evaluation.

The first is a relatively rare entity. It was noted in 0.6% of arch aortograms reported in a large series.[67] Direct sonographic evaluation of the origin of the common carotid is not possible in most individuals. For this reason, one must rely on indirect signs to detect the presence of a high-grade stenosis. The presence of a waveform with delayed upstroke and reduced amplitude—tardus-parvus—indicates the presence of hemodynamically significant stenoses. Patients with recurrent symptoms and without significant pathology at the carotid bifurcation may need further evaluation with arch aortography in order to detect this lesion.

The second type of tandem lesion is an intracranial high-grade lesion. An operation performed at the carotid bifurcation will obviously not affect the pathology present within the intracranial portion of the carotid.[33] The issue here is whether the carotid bifurcation lesion should be repaired. Only a few studies have addressed this issue.[68] Recently, a large study looked at the impact

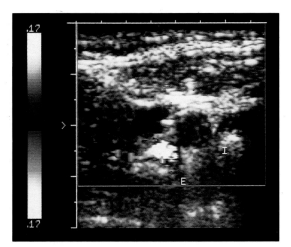

Fig. 9-11 This patient has a subtotal occlusion of the internal carotid artery. The color flow image shows a transverse scan of the proximal internal (I) and external (E) carotid arteries. A full flow lumen is seen in the external carotid (red), whereas the internal carotid has only a trickle of flow (blue). Transverse imaging of the proximal internal carotid with low PRF (velocity scale) settings can be used to help differentiate total from subtotal carotid artery occlusions.

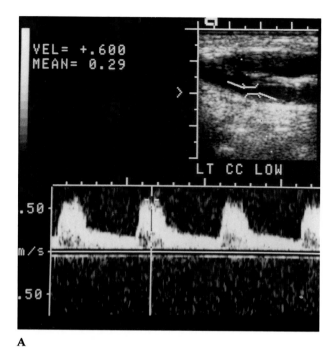

A

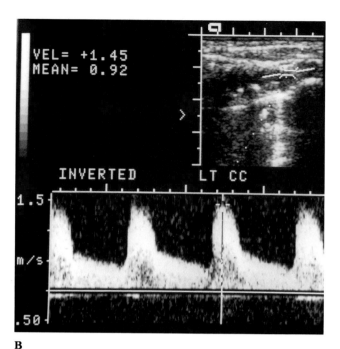

B

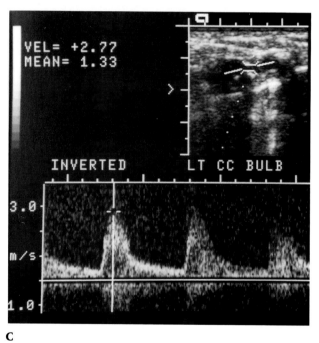

C

Fig. 9-13 (*A*) This Doppler spectrum is sampled in the proximal common carotid artery. Flow velocities are normal in amplitude and do not suggest the presence of a downstream obstruction. (*B*) This Doppler spectrum is sampled downstream to the site shown in part (*A*). The velocity has more than doubled, indicating a common carotid stenosis with more than 50% diameter narrowing. (*C*) This Doppler spectrum is sampled at the level of the carotid bulb, just proximal (upstream) to the bifurcation into the internal and external carotid branches. The severity of this type of stenosis is difficult to grade. Proximal peak systolic velocity in the common carotid artery of this patient was 0.6 m/sec. The current increase in peak systolic velocity results in a velocity ratio of more than 4, which is consistent with a 70% diameter stenosis.

on morbidity following carotid endarterectomy for patients with and without an additional lesion in the intracranial portion of the internal carotid.[69] This study showed, at the outset, greater morbidity for patients with tandem lesions. However, with time, morbid events were almost equivalent in both groups. It there-

fore appears that the presence of a tandem lesion in the intracranial circulation does not affect overall morbidity following carotid endarterectomy. Even if velocity profiles detected in the proximal internal carotid artery point to a high-grade lesion in the head, it is unlikely that this would preclude surgical repair of the lesion.

The third type of lesion lies in a visualized segment of the common carotid. Grading the severity of these lesions relies on a different strategy than using an absolute velocity value. The severity of tandem lesions in the common carotid artery can be graded with the help of the ratio of peak systolic velocities (Fig. 9-13).[21] This ratio is different from the systolic velocity ratio used for the internal carotid artery. A doubling of the common carotid peak systolic velocity corresponds to a 50% common carotid diameter stenosis, while a ratio of 1.5 of the internal to common carotid peak systolic velocities corresponds to a 50% internal carotid diameter stenosis.

Contralateral Lesions

The presence of a contralateral lesion may artifactually elevate the measured velocities in the internal carotid arteries, specifically in cases of total occlusion of the internal carotid.[70] This effect is difficult to document when looking at a large series of cases and, in fact, appears not to cause a significant problem.[22,58]

This effect, if present, is likely to occur with very-high-grade lesions. The contralataral velocity measurements should then be corrected accordingly.[71]

Various Pathologies

Vasculitis

A vasculitis such as Takayasu's arteritis manifests itself by a diffuse inflammatory process of the media and the adventitia. Such a process causes diffuse thickening of the carotid wall, with preferential involvement of the common carotid. This may mimic the appearance of atherosclerosis in a young patient with hypercholesterolemia or hyperlipidemia. Additional involvement of the subclavian artery and axillary arteries is often seen. Carotid sonography can distinguish between atherosclerosis and diffuse vasculitis. The latter tends to spare the region of the carotid bifurcation, and focal lesions are less common. Diffuse thickening of the arterial wall is common.[72]

Radiation

Accelerated atherosclerosis can occur following irradiation. Patients who have had head and neck surgery and subsequent irradiation manifest a diffuse thickening of the common carotid artery wall, with relative spearing of the internal carotid artery bifurcation. Pathologically, this process resembles atherosclerosis. Typically, it manifests itself within 10 years following radiation treatment.[73]

Dissection

Two types of dissection can be detected by carotid sonography. The first is an extension of a dissection arising within the root of the aorta. Such dissections extend into the common carotid artery and to variable levels within the internal carotid artery. The flap or dissected wall can best be visualized on longitudinal imaging, with the interface being perfectly perpendicular to the ultrasound beam.[74,75] The implications of such dissections that persist following graft placement are not clear. A large study that looked at the presence of this entity suggested that conservative management is warranted.[76]

The other type of dissection is a localized internal carotid artery dissection. This is associated with trauma or is idiopathic. Younger patients tend to be affected. Permanent stroke can be seen in up to 20% of cases. Various appearances have been seen, including total occlusion, significant stenosis, and even an almost normal appearance.[77] The lesion typically manifests itself in the high portion of the internal carotid artery as it enters the bony canal. For this reason, the lesion is often not visualized directly. However, flow profiles in the more proximal internal carotid artery show the effect of more distal outflow obstruction. The waveform tends to be blunted—with signals above and below baseline[78]—or almost absent in most cases. Treatment consists of heparinization and observation since recanalization is quite common.[78]

Pseudoaneurysms and Aneurysms

Aneurysms or pseudoaneurysms of the vertebral and extracranial carotid arteries are rare. Possible mechanisms include previous trauma due to penetrating injuries. In addition, aneurysms can arise spontaneously within the bifurcation.

The major role of carotid sonography is to identify the pathology and the level of involvement. Patients typically present with a pulsatile mass.[79] Most of these masses are due to relatively ectatic carotid arteries or slightly asymmetrical enlargement of different segments of the carotid artery. True aneurysms of the carotid artery are quite rare.[80]

Neoplasms

Neoplastic lesions involving the carotid bifurcation are relatively rare. The primary lesion consists of carotid body tumors. These are hypervascular masses that evolve in the carotid bifurcation.[81] They normally cause palpable enlargement in the region.

Other neoplastic masses, such as enlarged lymph nodes, may involve the contiguous region or may extend into the region of the carotid artery. The presence of neoplastic involvement in the wall of the carotid has been described as an obliteration of the interface normally seen between the adventitia and periadventitia of the artery wall.[82]

VERTEBRAL ARTERIES

Evaluation of the vertebral arteries is considered an adjunct to the sonographic evaluation of the extracranial arteries. Because of its location, surrounded by the transverse processes of the cervical vertebra, large portions of the vertebral artery cannot be directly visualized.[24,25] This, however, does not interfere with evaluation of the vertebrolbasilar system for the presence of subclavian steal syndrome.[26]

Normal Waveforms and Extent of Evaluation

The appearance of the Doppler waveform of the vertebral artery is similar to that of the internal carotid artery. It is a low-resistance waveform. The peak systolic velocities range between 0.4 and 0.7 msec, lower than those measured within the internal carotid artery. The diameter of the vertebral artery is quite variable, often showing an asymmetry of 20–25% between the right and left sides.

The normal evaluation includes sampling of the waveforms in the accessible portions of the vertebral artery. This confirms the presence of antegrade flow and is used to characterize the overall appearance of the spectral waveform. More recently, with the aid of color flow imaging, the course of the vertebral artery has been followed. High-grade stenosis can cause zones of flow disturbance projected beyond the areas obscured by the bony processes (Fig. 9-7). Although less severe lesions may be missed, higher-grade lesions with a marked systolic jet of increased flow velocity can project these elevated flow signals beyond the blind spots created by the bone. The accuracy of sonography for stenosis detection varies between 38–67%[25,83] and 83%,[25] the latter when the origin of the vertebral artery is visualized.

Increased peak systolic velocity suggests the use of the vertebral artery as a collateral pathway. For example, in the presence of bilateral internal carotid artery lesions, the vertebral arteries serve as important collateral pathways to the circle of Willis.

Vertebrobasilar Disease

At one end of the spectrum of vertebrobasilar disorders of the circulation is the subclavian steal syndrome. This syndrome is due to the presence of a high-grade stenosis in the proximal subclavian artery, with the vertebral artery ipsilateral to the stenosis then supplying blood to the arm.[26] This situation arises because the vertebral artery normally originates from the subclavian artery,

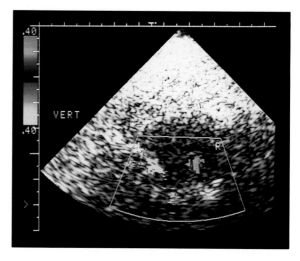

Fig. 9-14 This color flow image is taken from the occipital window. It shows the confluence of the two vertebral arteries into the basilar artery (arrow). Flow in the right vertebral artery is in the normal direction (orange). Flow in the left vertebral artery (blue) shows reversal consistent with a subclavian steal syndrome.

with only a few exceptions when the left vertebral originates directly from the aortic arch in up to 5% of patients.

Since blood normally destined for the brain is shunted to supply the upper extremity, flow within the verterbral artery is reversed. There is a transition where flow within the vertebral artery may be partly reversed. The application of a blood pressure cuff or other method of inducing vasodilatation of the upper extremity in question can increase flow and lead to reveral in flow direction.[84]

Patients with vague symptoms of gait disturbance or unsteadiness may be manifesting vertebrobasilar arterial insufficiency. Compromise of flow may be due to the concomitant presence of a subclavian steal syndrome or of high-grade stenosis or occlusion of the vertebral arteries, since these arteries supply the cerebellum and portions of the occipital lobes. These patients are generally difficult to evaluate. Evaluation of the flow patterns in the vertebral artery may suggest that a vertebral artery lesion is responsible for the problem. Increasingly, this evaluatin is complemented by transcranial sonography (Fig. 9-14).

TRANSCRANIAL SONOGRAPHY

The cranium acts as an obstacle to the penetration of ultrasound energy. Evaluation of the intracerebral vessels is still possible if specific locations or acoustic windows are used in combination with low-frequency ultrasound. The ultrasound signals can then penetrate the thin layer of bone at these locations and interrogate the intracranial vessels.

Most transcranial sonography has been performed using nonimaging probes equipped with range-gated, pulsed Doppler.[29,85] Evaluation of the presence and direction of blood flow is achieved with knowledge of the relative location and depth of the different arteries. This examination can be quite time-consuming. The recent addition of pulsed Doppler sonography[27] and color flow imaging[86,87] may make this evaluation cost effective.

Imaging Windows

There are three windows that permit sonographic evaluation of the intracranial circulation. The posterior window is used when the vertebrobasilar system is evaluated. This is, in essence, imaging through the foramen magnum, with the transducer placed posteriorly. The second window is through the temporal bone in a preauricular region. The transducer can be placed in one of three sites—one more anterior and close to the orbital ridge, the other more posterior and close to the acoustic hiatus. The final window is more posterior just superior to the ear and may actually be inferior to the zygomatic arch. These are the traditional windows for evaluating the intracranial branches of the internal carotid: specifically, the middle cerebral artery and the anterior and posterior cerebral branches, as well as the communicating branches. The third window is direct insonation through the orbit. The window is used to evaluate the direction of flow through the ophthalmic artery. The power output of the ultrasound scanner is reduced to the lowest level possible in order to prevent heating in the ocular globe.

Traditional Criteria

The traditional velocity parameter used in the evaluation of the intracranial branches is mean velocity. The mean velocity values reported in the literature are obtained with the traditional nonimaging approach and lack appropriate angle correction factors. They should be used with caution when duplex sonography is done. The shallow angle of the middle cerebral arteries with respect to the imaging window suggests that the absolute velocity measurements are probably accurate. The pulsatility index and the resistive index can be used since they are not angle dependent. Angle-corrected

peak velocities can be evaluated with duplex sonography.[27]

Pulsatility indices range from 0.6 to 0.8 in the middle cerebral artery. They can be reduced on the side of a high-grade internal carotid lesion.[88] Reversal of the direction of flow within the different branches of the circle of Willis in the presence of total or subtotal occlusions is normally evaluated subjectively.[88]

More subtle changes in intracranial velocities are difficult to measure since brain vasculature has strong autoregulation.[89] For this reason, there are no consistent findings that can be used to predict the presence of significant stenosis within the internal carotid artery.[30]

Color Flow and Pulsed Doppler Sonography

The current generations of color flow and pulsed Doppler sonographic devices rely on transducers with frequencies of 2–2.5 MHz. On gray scale images, the outer table of the contralateral cranium serves as a landmark confirming penetration of the ultrasound beam through the temporal bone. The color flow device can then be used to localize the middle cerebral artery branches of the circle of Willis.

Applications

Most transcranial Doppler sonography has been used to monitor the flow pattern following subarachnoid hemorrhage.[29] It can also be used to evaluate flow dynamics during operations such as carotid endarterectomy.[90] The evaluation of collateral pathways is highly dependent on the technical skill of the operator. The use of this information in clinical decision making has been poorly documented in the literature.

Spasm

Cerebral artery spasm tends to develop approximately 2–7 days following subarachnoid hemorrhage. These spasms may be spontaneous following rupture of an aneurysm, with trauma, or following craniotomy. Symptoms suggesting the presence of spasms can be quite vague. Mean velocities above 200 cm/sec in the middle cerebral artery are consistent with arterial spasm. Increased peak velocities correlate with arteriographic findings of narrowed arteries.[29]

Intracerebral Lesions

There are no large studies giving the overall accuracy of transcranial Doppler sonography in detecting the presence of a tandem lesion in the high internal carotid artery or isolated focal lesions in the middle cerebral branches. The presence of a high-velocity signal within the middle cerebral branches in patients with sickle cell disease is indicative of arterial stenosis.[28] The findings for focal atherosclerotic lesions of the intracranial arteries are variable and include increases in velocity as well as decreases.[91] Decreased pulsatility in major branches may, by inference, suggest the presence of a proximal obstruction. The clinical reliability of this technology to confirm brain death has yet to be systematically studied, but a high-resistance pattern suggests this diagnosis.[92] Accuracy is heavily dependent on the operator, as well as on the adjustment of velocity scales and the sensitivity of the imaging device.

Collateral Pathway Assessment
This is often recognized as the major strength of transcranial Doppler sonography. The presence of a high-grade lesion in arteries can be associated with the development of marked collateralization.[93] Absence of significant collaterals may affect the surgical approach before carotid endarterectomy and lead to the use of a shunt. Conversely, well-developed collaterals despite the presence of an occlusion in an asymptomatic patient who is a high-risk surgical candidate may suggest that repair of this lesion is likely not warranted. In general, however, a provocative test such as a common carotid artery compression can be performed to see if the intracranial flow patterns are affected.[94]

Altered Flow with High-grade Carotid Stenosis
A potential use of transcranial Doppler sonography is for the study of the effect of extracranial stenosis on intracranial flow dynamics. In asymptomatic patients, a high-grade lesion (80% or 90% diameter stenosis) may affect flow dynamics within the intracerebral vasculature.[93] Ultimately, such an evaluation may help identify patients who might benefit from surgical revision. There are as yet no large studies evaluating this hypothesis.

For the asymptomatic patient, a routine evaluation with transcranial Doppler sonography of the collateral pathways is likely unnecessary.

INTRAOPERATIVE SONOGRAPHY

Intraoperative sonography of the carotid system can be utilized in three ways. The first is monitoring the results of carotid surgery following endarterectomy. The second is monitoring vascular flow dynamics in the intracranial circulation during various operations. The final application is direct guidance for intracranial surgery.

Carotid Endarterectomy

High-resolution carotid sonography is increasingly used to monitor the site of previous carotid endarterectomy. This is done to detect significant defects following endarterectomy or the development of platelet clumps that can obstruct flow early or embolize. These lesions may ultimately lead to higher-grade lesions and to complete occlusions.[95] Their early detection and immediate repair reduce subsequent morbidity.[96]

The important issue is the establishment of an appropriate threshold for intervention. Flow perturbations with peak systolic velocity of greater than 1.5 m/sec are arbitrary taken as this threshold. The detection of surgical defects on gray scale imaging is quite common. It is likely that these smaller defects or lesions within the common and internal carotid arteries at the site of carotid endarterectomy will not affect the ultimate prognosis.[97]

Flow abnormalities are commonly seen following carotid endarterectomy and can persist for 6 months to 1 year following surgery. The reason these lesions disappear is not clear. Presumably, they are an adaptive response to the arterial wall that distends with the presence of fibrointimal hyperplasia and reendothelialization of the new wall surfaces created during surgery.[98]

Transcranial Monitoring

Use of transcranial Doppler in intraoperative monitoring may have specific applications in the field of carotid endarterectomy. In those institutions where electroencephalographic monitoring is not available, monitoring of flow dynamics within the cerebral vasculature can indicate changes in cerebral blood flow during surgery[90] or confirm the incidence of microemboli.[99] If occlusion of the ipsilateral collateral causes significant depression and reduced blood flow, the need for a shunt becomes obvious. Development of embolic phenomena, most likely due to air, have also been noted with transcranial monitoring during cardiac bypass surgery.[100] This had led to a change in the technical approaches to placement on and removal of the patient from cardiac pulmonary bypass. This type of monitoring is normally performed with a nonimaging probe.

Therapeutic Guidance of Intracranial Surgery

Ultrasound can be used to identify the quickest path in the placement of needles through burr holes. With full craniotomies, compact ultrasound probes can be used to identify lesions and help guide access to them. More importantly, they can help the neurosurgeon identify structures that need to be circumvented.

PEDIATRIC APPLICATIONS

Evaluation of the extracranial circulation in younger patients is of limited interest. Atherosclerotic lesions do not affect this segment of the population. For this reason, the applications of ultrasound remain limited. They include evaluation for traumatic lesions and possibly vasculitis. Evaluation of the intracranial circulation in the neonatal head can be done through the patent fontanelles.[101] The use of extracorporeal oxygenation devices has been shown to alter intracerebral flow dynamics in the newborn.[102] Color flow imaging and Doppler sonography have been used in these patients to identify possible hemodynamic compromise during these procedures.

Traumatic Lesion

The development of local dissection or penetrating injuries, causing thrombosis and/or pseudoaneurysm formation, is the principal indication for noninvasive evaluation of the neck arteries. Traumatic lesions often present as pulsatile masses. Because of the benign, noninvasive nature of the test, this type of screening can easily be performed.

Appropriate consideration must, however, be given to the fact that heart rates are faster and the overall pulsatility of the Doppler waveform is more pronounced than in older patients. The increase in pulsatility may be due to the more compliant nature of the artery.

Extracorporeal Membrane Oxygenation

Extracorporeal membrane oxygenation is often used in neonates in whom pulmonary oxygenation is compromised. The arterial catheter is normally placed in the right carotid artery because of its ease of access. This traumatic ligation of the carotid artery can diverts flow and can theoretically be the source of a stroke. Preliminary evaluation of the color flow image can be used to ascertain the status of the collateral circulation early and late following the start of therapy.[103,104] Whether the examination has predictive value and can detect the presence of fetal origin of the posterior cerebral artery, a possible compromise in the collateral pathways remains to be seen.

Vasculitis

The principal type of vasculitis seen in this segment of the population is Takayasu's arteritis. During the acute phase, the diffuse inflammatory process affects the media and adventitia of the arterial wall. This causes overall thickening of the arterial wall. The involvement of the adventitia proper is difficult to ascertain by sonography.

Potentially, measurement of wall thickness[105] may be used to monitor the patient's response to therapy with steroids or methotrexate. There are no studies addressing this issue.

CONCLUSION

Carotid Doppler sonography has become an important modality in the evaluation of cerebrovascular diseases. It is no longer limited to evaluation of the extracranial circulation in the neck. It now includes the vertebral artery and the intracranial arteries are now accessible to a more complete examination.

One controversial issue that will be addressed in the next few years is the cost-effective use of this technology. There is also the question of whether carotid sonography, as a noninvasive test, should remain the first step in the evaluation of a specific pathology. Is carotid arteriography still indicated when high-grade stenosis is confirmed by carotid sonography?[106] It has also been suggested that sonography is prone to observer-variability. Conversely, since the presence of tandem lesions often does not affect the nature of surgery, additional arteriography is probably not needed when a high-grade lesion is detected in a symptomatic patient.[69] When contrast administration is contraindicated, carotid sonography is often the only test performed before surgery.[107] Increasingly, carotid Doppler sonography is complemented by magnetic resonance angiography. It appears that arteriography will ultimately be replaced in the large segment of the population for preoperative monitoring detection and therapeutic application of carotid endarterectomy.

REFERENCES

1. Kremkau FW. *Diagnostic Ultrasound Principles, Instrumentation, and Exercises.* Grune & Stratton, 1984.
2. Burns PN, Jaffe CC. Quantitative flow measurements with Doppler ultrasound: Techniques, accuracy, and limitations. *Radiol Clin North Am* 1985;23:641–657.

3. Bonnefous O, Pesque P. Time domain formulation of pulse-Doppler ultrasound and blood velocity estimation by cross-correlation. *Ultrasonic Imaging* 1986;8:73–85.

4. Kassam M, Johnston KW, Cobbold RSC. Quantitative estimation of spectral broadening for the diagnosis of carotid artery disease: Method and in vitro results. *Ultrasound Med Biol* 1985;11:425–433.

5. Kotval PS. Doppler waveform parvus and tardus. A sign of proximal flow obstruction. *J Ultrasound Med* 1989;8:435–440.

6. Phillips DJ, Greene FMJ, Langlois Y, et al. Flow velocity patterns in the carotid bifurcation of young, presumed normal subjects. *Ultrasound Med Biol* 1983;9:39–49.

7. Glagov S, Zarins C, Giddens DP, et al. Hemodynamics and atherosclerosis—insights and perspectives gained from studies of human arteries. *Arch Pathol Lab Med* 1988;112:1018–1031.

8. Middleton WD, Foley WD, Lawson TL. Flow reversal in the normal carotid bifurcation: Color Doppler flow imaging analysis. *Radiology* 1988;167:207–210.

9. Polak JF, O'Leary DH, Quist WC, et al. Pulse and color Doppler analysis of normal carotid artery bifurcation flow dynamics using an-invitro model. *Angiology* 1990;41:241–247.

10. Douville Y, Johnston KW, Kassam M. Determination of the hemodynamic factors which influence the carotid Doppler spectral broadening. *Ultrasound Med Biol* 1985;11:417–420.

11. Hutchison KJ, Karpinski E. Stability of flow patterns in the in vivo poststenotic velocity field. *Ultrasound Med Biol* 1988;14:269–275.

12. Taylor DC, Strandness DEJ. Carotid artery duplex scanning. *JCU* 1987;15:635–644.

13. Rittgers SE, Shu MCS. Doppler color-flow images from a stenosed arterial model: Interpretation of flow patterns. *J Vasc Surg* 1990;12:511–522.

14. Ricotta JJ, Bryan FA, Bond MG, et al. Multicenter validation study of real-time (B-mode) ultrasound, arteriography, and pathologic examination. *J Vasc Surg* 1987;6:512–520.

15. Zwiebel WJ, Crummy AB. Sources of error in Doppler diagnosis of carotid occlusive disease. *AJR* 1981;137:1–12.

16. James EM, Earnest FI, Forbes GS, et al. High resolution dynamic ultrasound imaging of the carotid bifurcation: A prospective study. *Radiology* 1982;144:853–858.

17. Zwiebel W, Austin CW, Sackett JF, et al. Correlation of high-resolution B-mode and continuous-wave Doppler sonography with arteriography in the diagnosis of carotid stenosis. *Radiology* 1983;149:523–532.

18. Jackson VP, Kuehn DS, Bendick PJ, et al. Duplex carotid sonography: Correlation with digital subtraction angiography and conventional angiography. *J Ultrasound Med* 1985;4:239–249.

19. Jacobs NM, Grant EG, Schellinger D, et al. Duplex carotid sonography: Criteria for stenosis, accuracy, and pitfalls. *Radiology* 1985;154:385–391.

20. Garth KE, Carroll BA, Sommer FG, et al. Duplex ultrasound scanning of the carotid arteries with velocity spectrum analysis. *Radiology* 1983;147:823–827.

21. Keagy BA, Pharr WF, Thomas D, et al. Evaluation of the peak frequency ratio (PFR) measurement in the detection of internal carotid artery stenosis. *JCU* 1982;10:109–112.

22. Robinson ML, Sacks D, Perlmutter GS, et al. Diagnostic criteria for carotid duplex sonography. *AJR* 1988;151:1045–1049.

23. Polak JF, Dobkin GR, O'Leary DH, et al. Internal carotid artery stenosis: Accuracy and reproducibility of color-Doppler-assisted duplex imaging. *Radiology* 1989;173:793–798.

24. Bluth EI, Merritt CRB, Sullivan MA, et al. Usefulness of duplex ultrasound in evaluating vertebral arteries. *J Ultrasound Med* 1989;8:229–235.

25. Visona A, Lusiana L, Castellani V, et al. The echo-Doppler (duplex) system for the detection of vertebral artery occlusive disease: Comparison with angiography. *J Ultrasound Med* 1986;5:247–250.

26. Walker DW, Acker JD, Cole CA. Subclavian steal syndrome detected with duplex pulsed Doppler sonography. *AJNR* 1982;3:615–618.

27. Hashimoto BE, Hattrick CW. New method of adult transcranial Doppler. *J Ultrasound Med* 1991;10:349–353.

28. Adams R, McKie V, Nichols F, et al. The use of ultrasonography to predict stroke in sickle cell disease. *N Engl J Med* 1992;326:605–610.

29. Aaslid R, Huber P, Nornes H. Evaluation of cerebrovascular spasm with transcranial Doppler ultrasound. *J Neurosurg* 1984;60:37–41.

30. Kelley RE, Namon RA, Juang S-H, et al. Transcranial Doppler ultrasonography of the middle cerebral artery in the hemodynamic assessment of internal carotid artery stenosis. *Arch Neurol* 1990;47:960–964.

31. O'Leary DH, Clouse ME, Potter JE, et al. The influence of non-invasive tests on the selection of patients for carotid angiography. *Stroke* 1985;16:264–267.

32. Flanigan DP, Schuler JJ, Vogel M, et al. The role of carotid duplex scanning in surgical decision making. *J Vasc Surg* 1985;2:15–25.

33. Rodda RA. The arterial patterns associated with internal carotid disease and cerebral infarcts. *Stroke* 1986;17:69–75.

34. Svindland A, Torvik A. Atherosclerotic carotid disease in asymptomatic individuals: A histological study of 53 cases. *Acta Neurol Scand* 1988;78:506–517.

35. Dixon S, Pais SO, Raviola C, et al. Natural history of nonstenotic, asymptomatic ulcerative lesions of the ca-

rotid artery: A further analysis. *Arch Surg* 1982;117: 1493–1498.

36. Weinberger J, Marks SJ, Gaul JJ, et al. Atherosclerotic plaque at the carotid artery bifurcation: Correlation of ultrasonographic imaging with morphology. *J Ultrasound Med* 1987;6:363–366.

37. North American Carotid Endarterectomy Trial Collaborators. Beneficial effect of carotid endarterectomy in symptomatic patients with high-grade stenosis. *N Engl J Med* 1991;325:445–453.

38. Eklof B, Schwartz SI. Effects of critical stenosis of the carotid artery and compromised cephalic blood flow. *Arch Surg* 1969;99:695–701.

39. Grosset DG, Georgiadis D, Abdullah I, et al. Doppler emboli signals vary according to stroke subtype. *Stroke* 1994;25:382–384.

40. Lusby RJ, Ferrell LD, Ehrenfeld WK, et al. Carotid plaque hemorrhage:Its role in production of cerebral ischemia. *Arch Surg* 1982;117:1479–1488.

41. Imparato AM, Riles TS, Mintzer R, et al. The importance of hemorrhage in the relationship between gross morphologic characteristics and cerebral symptoms in 376 carotid artery plaques. *Ann Surg* 1983;197: 195–203.

42. Widder B, Paulat K, Hackspacher J, et al. Morphological characterization of carotid artery stenoses by ultrasound duplex scanning. *Ultrasound Med Biol* 1990;16: 349–354.

43. Bassiouny HS, Davis H, Massawa N, et al. Critical carotid stenoses: Morphologic and chemical similarity between symptomatic and asymptomatic plaques. *J Vasc Surg* 1989;9:202–212.

44. Lennihan L, Kupsky WJ, Mohr JP, et al. Lack of association between carotid plaque hematoma and ischemic cerebral symptoms. *Stroke* 1987;18:879–881.

45. O'Donnell TF, Erdoes L, Mackey WC, et al. Correlation of B-mode ultrasound imaging and arteriography with pathologic findings at carotid endarterectomy. *Arch Surg* 1985;120:443–449.

46. O'Leary DH, Holen J, Ricotta JJ, et al. Carotid bifurcation disease: Predilection of ulceration with B-mode US. *Radiology* 1987;162:523–525.

47. Bluth EI, McVay LV, Merritt CRB, et al. The identification of ulcerative plaque with high-resolution duplex carotid scanning. *J Ultrasound Med* 1988;7:73–76.

48. Edwards JH, Kricheff II, Riles T, et al. Angiographically undetected ulceration of the carotid bifurcation as a cause of embolic stroke. *Radiology* 1979;132:369–373.

49. Eikelboom BC, Riles TR, Mintzer R, et al. Inaccuracy of angiography in the diagnosis of carotid ulceration. *Stroke* 1983;14:882–885.

50. Thiele BL, Young JV, Chikos PM, et al. Correlation of arteriographic findings and symptoms in cerebrovascular disease. *Neurology* 1980;30:1041–1046.

51. Lo LY, Ford CS, McKinney WM, et al. Asymptomatic bruit, carotid and vertebrobasilar transient ischemic attacks: A clinical and ultrasonic correlation. *Stroke* 1986; 17:65–68.

52. Erickson SJ, Mewissen MW, Foley WD, et al. Stenosis of the internal carotid artery: Assessment using color Doppler imaging compared with angiography. *AJR* 1989;152:1299–1305.

53. Bluth EI, Stavros AT, Marich KW, et al. Carotid duplex sonography: A multicenter recommendation for standardized imaging and Doppler criteria. *RadioGraphics* 1988;8:487–506.

54. Friedman SG, Hainline B, Feinberg AW, et al. Use of diastolic velocity ratios to predict significant carotid artery stenosis. *Stroke* 1988;19:910–912.

55. Vaisman U, Wojciechowski M. Carotid artery disease: New criteria for evaluation by sonographic duplex scanning. *Radiology* 1986;158:253–255.

56. Knox RA, Breslau PJ, Strandness DEJ. A simple paramater for accurate detection of severe carotid disease. *Br J Surg* 1982;69:230–233.

57. Withers CE, Gosink BB, Keightley AM, et al. Duplex carotid sonography. Peak systolic velocity in quantifying internal carotid artery stenosis. *J Ultrasound Med* 1990;9:345–349.

58. Hunink MGM, Polak JF, Barlan MM, et al. Detection and quantification of carotid artery stenosis: Efficacy of various Doppler velocity parameters. *AJR* 1993;160: 619–625.

59. Roederer GO, Langlois YE, Jager KA, et al. A simple spectral parameter for accurate classification of severe carotid disease. *Bruit* 1984;8:174–178.

60. Moneta GL, Taylor DC, Zierler RE, et al. Asymptomatic high-grade internal carotid artery stenosis: Is stratification according to risk favors or duplex spectral analysis possible? *J Vasc Surg* 1989;10:475–483.

61. Blackshear WMJ, Phillips DJ, Chikos PM, et al. Carotid artery velocity patterns in normal and stenotic vessels. *Stroke* 1980;11:67–71.

62. Rozanski A, Diamond GA, Berman D, et al. The declining specificity of exercise radionuclide ventriculography. *N Engl J Med* 1983;309:518–522.

63. European Carotid Surgery Trialists' Collaborative Group. MRC European Carotid Surgery Trial: Interim results for symptomatic patients with severe (70–99%) or with mild (0–29%) carotid stenosis. *Lancet* 1991; 337:1235–1243.

64. Moneta GL, Edwards JM, Chitwood RW, et al. Correlation of North American Symptomatic Carotid Endarterectomy Trial (NASCET) angiographic definition of 70% to 99% internal carotid stenosis with duplex scanning. *J Vasc Surg* 1993;17:152–159.

65. Fell G, Phillips DJ, Chikos PM, et al. Ultrasonic duplex

scanning for disease of the carotid artery. *Circulation* 1981;64:1191–1195.

66. Spencer MP, Reid JM. Quantitation of carotid stenosis with continuous-wave (C-W) Doppler ultrasound. *Stroke* 1979;10:326–330.

67. Akers DL, Markowitz IA, Kerstein MD. The value of aortic arch study in the evolution of cerebrovascular insufficiency. *Am J Surg* 1987;154:230–232.

68. Schuler JJ, Flanigan DP, Lim LT, et al. The effect of carotid siphon stenosis on stroke rate, death, and relief of symptoms following elective carotid endarterectomy. *Surgery* 1982;92:1058–1067.

69. Mattos MA, van Bremmelen PS, Hodgson KJ, et al. The influence of carotid artery siphon stenosis on short- and long-term outcome after carotid endarterectomy. *J Vasc Surg* 1993;17:902–911.

70. Hayes AC, Johnston W, Baker WH, et al. The effect of contralateral disease on carotid Doppler frequency. *Surgery* 1988;103:19–23.

71. Spadone DP, Barkmeier LD, Hodgson KJ, et al. Contralateral internal carotid artery stenosis or occlusion: Pitfall of correct ipsilateral classification—A study performed wtih color-flow imaging. *J Vasc Surg* 1990;11:642–649.

72. Buckley A, Southwood T, Culham G, et al. The role of ultrasound in evaluation of Takayasu's arteritis. *J Rheumatol* 1991;18:1073–1080.

73. Chuang VP. Radiation-induced arteritis. *Semin Roentgenol* 1994;29:64–69.

74. Bluth EI, Shyn PB, Sullivan MA, et al. Doppler color flow imaging of carotid artery dissection. *J Ultrasound Med* 1989;8:149–153.

75. Kotval PS, Babu SC, Fakhry J, et al. Role of the intimal flap in arterial dissection: Sonographic demonstration. *AJR* 1988;150:1181–1182.

76. Zurbrugg HR, Leupi F, Schupbach P, et al. Duplex scanner study of carotid artery dissection following surgical treatment of aortic dissection type A. *Stroke* 1988;19:970–976.

77. Gardner DJ, Gosink BB, Kallman CE. Internal carotid artery dissections: Duplex ultrasound imaging. *J Ultrasound Med* 1991;10:607–614.

78. Steinke W, Rautenberg W, Schwartz A, et al. Noninvasive monitoring of internal carotid artery dissection. *Stroke* 1994;25:998–1005.

79. Wilkinson DL, Polak JF, Grassi CJ, et al. Pseudoaneurysm of the vertebral artery: Appearance on color-flow Doppler sonography. *AJR* 1988;151:1051–1052.

80. Wang A-M, O'Leary DH. Common carotid aneurysm: Ultrasonic diagnosis. *JCU* 1988;16:262–264.

81. Steinke W, Hennerici M, Anlick A. Doppler color flow imaging of carotid body tumors. *Stroke* 1989;20:1574–1577.

82. Gooding GAW, Langman AW, Dillon WP, et al. Malignant carotid artery invasion: Sonographic detection. *Radiology* 1989;171:435–438.

83. Davis PC, Nilsen B, Braun IF, et al. A prospective comparison of duplex sonography vs angiography of the vertebral arteries. *AJNR* 1986;7:1059–1064.

84. Kotval PS, Babu SC, Shah PM. Doppler diagnosis of partial vertebral/subclavian steals convertible to full steals with physiologic maneuvers. *J Ultrasound Med* 1990;9:207–213.

85. Niederkorn K, Myers LG, Nunn CL, et al. Three-dimensional transcranial Doppler blood flow mapping in patients with cerebrovascular disorders. *Stroke* 1988;19:1335–1344.

86. Bogdahn U, Becker G, Winkler J, et al. Transcranial color-coded real-time sonography in adults. *Stroke* 1990;21:1680–1688.

87. Becker G, Lindner A, Bigdahn U. Imaging of the vertebrobasilar system by transcranial color-coded real-time sonography. *J Ultrasound Med* 1993;12:395–401.

88. Lindegaard K-F, Bakke SJ, Grolimund P, et al. Assessment of intracranial hemodynamics in carotid artery disease by transcranial Doppler ultrasound. *J Neurosurg* 1985;63:890–898.

89. Schneider PA, Rossman ME, Bernstein EF, et al. Effect of internal carotid artery occlusion on intracranial hemodynamics. Transcranial Doppler evaluation and clinical correlation. *Stroke* 1985;19:589–593.

90. Bergeron P, Benichou H, Rudondy P, et al. Stroke prevention during carotid surgery in high risk patients (value of transcranial Doppler and local anesthesia). *J Cardiovasc Surg* 1991;32:713–719.

91. deBray J-M, Joseph P-A, Jeanvoine H, et al. Transcranial Doppler evaluation of middle cerebral artery stenosis. *J Ultrasound Med* 1988;7:611–616.

92. Glasier CM, Seibert JJ, Chadduck WM, et al. Brain death in infants: Evaluation with Doppler US. *Radiology* 1989;172:377–380.

93. Rosenkranz K, Langer R, Felix R. Transcranial Doppler sonography: Collateral pathways in internal carotid artery obstructions. *Angiology* 1991;42:819–826.

94. Padayachee TS, Kirkham FJ, Lewis RR, et al. Transcranial measurement of blood velocities in the basal cerebral arteries using pulsed Doppler ultrasound: A method of assessing the circle of Willis. *Ultrasound Med Biol* 1986;12:5–14.

95. Sigel B, Flanigan DP, Schuler JJ, et al. Imaging ultrasound in the intraoperative diagnosis of vascular defects. *J Ultrasound Med* 1983;2:337–343.

96. Schwartz RA, Peterson GJ, Noland KA, et al. Intraoperative duplex scanning after carotid artery reconstruction: A valuable tool. *J Vasc Surg* 1988;7:620–624.

97. Reilly LM, Okuhn SP, Rapp JH, et al. Recurrent carotid stenosis: A consequence of local or systemic factors?

The influence of unrepaired technical defects. *J Vasc Surg* 1990;11:448–460.

98. Cook JM, Thompson BW, Barnes RW. Is routine duplex examination after carotid endarterectomy justified? *J Vasc Surg* 1990;12:334–340.

99. Jansen C, Ramos LMP, van Heesewijk JPM, et al. Impact of microembolism and hemodynamic changes in the brain during carotid endarterectomy. *Stroke* 1994; 25:992–997.

100. van der Linden J, Casimir-Ahn H. When do cerebral emboli appear during open heart operations? A transcranial Doppler study. *Ann Thorac Surg* 1991;51: 237–241.

101. Grant EG, White EM, Schellinger D, et al. Cranial duplex sonography of the infant. *Radiology* 1987;163– 177–185.

102. Taylor GA, Catena LM, Garin DB, et al. Intracranial flow patterns in infants undergoing extracorporeal membrane oxygenation: Preliminary observations with Doppler US. *Radiology* 1987;165:671–674.

103. Mitchell DG, Merton D, Desai H, et al. Neonatal brain: Color Doppler imaging. II. Altered flow patterns from extracorporeal membrane oxygenation. *Radiology* 1988; 167:307–310.

104. Mitchell DG, Merton DA, Graziani LJ, et al. Right carotid artery ligation in neonates: Classification of collateral flow with color Doppler imaging. *Radiology* 1990; 175:117–123.

105. Maeda H, Handa N, Matsumoto M, et al. Carotid lesions detected by B-mode ultrasonography in Takayasu's arteritis: "Macaroni sign" as an indicator of the disease. *Ultrasound Med Biol* 1991;17:695–701.

106. Dawson DL, Zierler RE, Kohler TR. Role of arteriography in the preoperative evaluation of carotid artery disease. *Am J Surg* 1991;161:619–624.

107. Crew JR, Dean M, Johnson JM, et al. Carotid surgery without angiography. *Am J Surg* 1984;148:217–220.

10

Technical Considerations in Computed Tomographic Evaluation of Cerebrovascular Disease

Kenneth Dalen, M.D.

COMPUTED TOMOGRAPHY DESIGN AND GENERATION

Since its introduction to the medical community in the 1970s, computed tomography (CT) has had a dramatic impact on the evaluation of patients with cerebrovascular disease. Over the past two decades, there has been continuous improvement in its hardware and software, resulting in better images with shorter scan times.

A CT image is a computer-generated, mathematically produced pictorial display of a thin slice of anatomy.[1-5] A finely collimated x-ray beam is projected toward an object, and the radiation that penetrates the object is then measured by a series of detectors placed opposite the beam. As the beam is rotated around the patient, data on each view are collected. Following computer manipulation, the data are reconstructed into a CT image.

The initial design of the CT scanner, the *first-generation* scanner, utilized a single detector element that was moved, along with the x-ray tube, in a straight line across the area of interest (Fig. 10-1A). The entire tube-detector system was then rotated by 1°, and a second set of measurements was made. This *translate-rotate* motion was continued until a 180° arc was covered and a sufficient number of measurements had been made to form the image. First-generation scanners required several minutes to complete each slice and several more minutes to reconstruct the image. Although they were a technological marvel at the time, first-generation scanners soon became obsolete due to the length of time for image acquisition and reconstruction, as well as the poor resolution of the resultant image.

Second-generation scanners also utilized a translate-rotate motion. However, they differed from first-generation machines in two respects (Fig. 10-1B). Whereas first-generation units used a highly collimated (2 × 13 mm) x-ray beam, a fan-shaped beam with a diverging angle of 3°–10° was utilized in second-generation scanners. In addition, multiple detectors were used to intercept the beam, thereby increasing the angle of rotation to 10°. The overall construction greatly reduced the number of translations required for image production, with a subsequent decrease in scan time (20–60 sec per slice). Nonetheless, this long scan

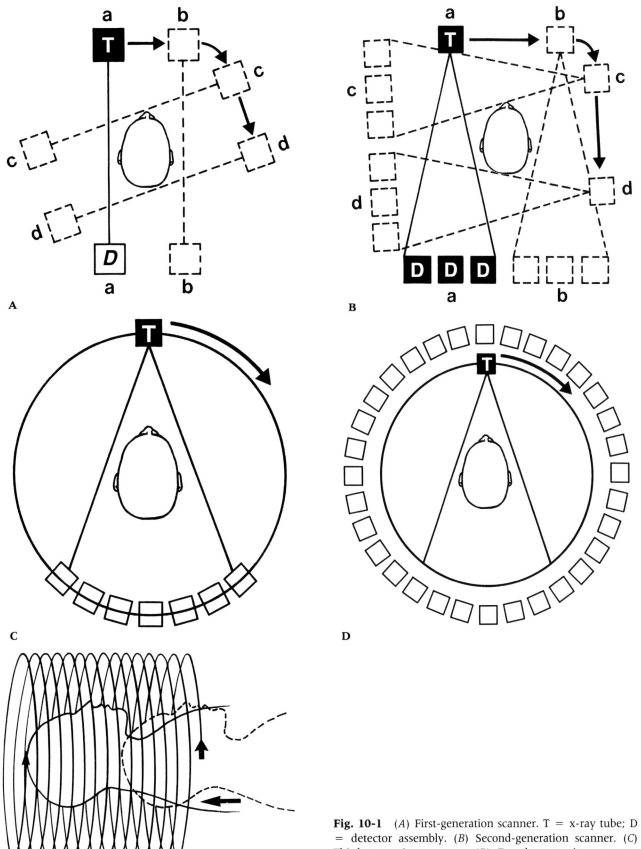

Fig. 10-1 (*A*) First-generation scanner. T = x-ray tube; D = detector assembly. (*B*) Second-generation scanner. (*C*) Third-generation scanner. (*D*) Fourth-generation scanner. (*E*) Spiral CT scanning.

149

time, together with the poor resolution of the final image, spurred further advances, and second-generation scanners also became obsolete.

Third-generation technology represented a significant improvement over its predecessors (Fig. 10-1C). The x-ray diverging beam angle was increased up to 30°–90° so that it could entirely encompass the object without having to perform any type of translate motion. In addition, the number of detectors was increased from approximately 10 to several hundred, and instead of being placed in a straight line perpendicular to the central ray (as in first- and second-generation machines), these detectors were aligned along the arc of a circle whose center was the x-ray focal spot. The detector array was mounted on the gantry along with the x-ray tube, and they rotated simultaneously in a circle (*rotate-rotate*) during the exposure. As the translate motion was eliminated, scan time decreased to 2–3 sec per image. Reconstruction time also decreased from minutes to seconds. Through further refinements in computer components, third-generation units produced a higher-quality image in a shorter period of time.

With the advent of *fourth-generation* machines, the detectors were removed from the rotating gantry and mounted in stationary positions outside the x-ray tube (Fig. 10-1D). While the x-ray tube rotated in a circle inside the stationary ring of detectors (*rotate only*), a fan of detectors was always exposed. As the number of detectors increased to thousands, scan time was reduced to about 1 sec or less and image quality improved. As state-of-the-art technology, most of the scanners in use today are fourth-generation machines.

Dynamic CT scanning is a technique whereby rapid scans with a short interscan delay are performed so that a true picture of the degree of vascularity and the dynamics of blood flow can be obtained.[6] A bolus of intravenous contrast material is delivered over a short span of time (before recirculation occurs), and rapid-sequence CT images are then obtained. By demonstrating the initial passage of contrast material through the area of interest, a measurement of blood flow through vessels as well as an assessment of relative tissue perfusion can be made.

One recent advance whose utility in evaluation of cerebrovascular disease is currently being investigated is *spiral CT angiography*[7–11] (Fig. 10-1E). Spiral scanning involves continuous longitudinal table motion through the gantry, with simultaneous 360° tube rotations during the exposure. This results in continuous data acquisition and avoids omission of levels during scanning as numerous thin, overlapping sections are rapidly acquired during peak intravascular contrast enhance-

ment. Spiral scanners operate on the order of one rotation per second, with scan times of up to 40 sec, permitting data acquisition entirely within the arterial or venous phase of a peripheral intravenous contrast injection. With table speeds of 3 to 5 mm/sec, longitudinal scan volumes of 20 cm can be covered. Following rata data accumulation, three-dimensional reconstruction of the vascular anatomy, with background suppression, provides excellent morphologic detail without visualization of overlapping structures.

IMAGE RECONSTRUCTION

The radiation collected by the detector assembly has many different intensities based on the attenuation coefficients of the structures in its path. The data that reach the detectors are stored in computer memory, awaiting reconstruction. Image reconstruction is a mathematical process whereby scan data for each view are converted to a numerical (*digital*) image, which, in turn, is structured into an array of individual dots or picture elements of varying intensity, called *pixels*. Each pixel in the image corresponds to a volume element, or *voxel*, of tissue in the section being imaged. The numerical value of each pixel, the CT number expressed in *Hounsfield units*, is related to the attenuation coefficient (μ) in the corresponding voxel. In mathematic terms, the equation describing their relationship is:

$$\text{CT number} = \frac{(\mu \text{ tissue} - \mu \, H_2O)}{\mu \, H_2O} \times 1000$$

Water, serving as a reference standard, has a CT number of zero. Materials with positive CT numbers have attenuation coefficients greater than that of water, and those with negative CT numbers have coefficients less than that of water (Table 10-1). At the high kilovolt levels used (approximately 120 kV), CT numbers are closely related to tissue density. Therefore, tissues with a density greater than that of water (specific gravity > 1) have positive CT numbers, whereas those with a density less than that of water have negative CT numbers.[12]

IMAGE RESOLUTION

There are two components to image resolution—spatial resolution and contrast resolution. Spatial resolution in CT is one-tenth that of film screen radiography (five line pairs per centimeter vs. five line pairs per

TABLE 10.1   CT Numbers of Various Materials

Object	CT Number (Hounsfield Units)
Air	−1,000
Fat	−15 to −100
Water	0
Cerebrospinal fluid	5 to 15
White matter	30 to 40
Gray matter	40 to 50
Hemorrhage/hematoma	40 to 90
Vascular structures after enhancement	50 to 100
Calcification	100 to 300
Bone	1,000

millimeter, respectively), but this limitation is largely overcome by CT's superiority in contrast resolution.[1]

The *spatial resolution* of the system denotes its ability to display, as separate images, two objects that are positioned very close to each other. This is determined by three factors: (1) scanner design, (2) motion, and (3) display matrix. First, scanner design affects resolution in CT, just as tube/intensifying screen design affects resolution in conventional radiography. In both systems, resolution increases as the focal spot size decreases. Likewise, resolution in CT is increased by decreasing the size of the detectors, just as it is increased in film screen radiography by decreasing the thickness of the fluorescent intensifying screen. Second, patient motion has a dramatic effect on spatial resolution. Efforts to decrease motion by encouraging patient cooperation and utilizing shorter scan times have resulted in images of improved resolution. Spiral CT yields images of high resolution as large volumes of tissue are imaged over a relatively short period of time, with little or no patient motion. Third, spatial resolution is intimately related to the matrix size used to display the image. By decreasing the size of the pixels so that more pixels are required to cover a specific area, spatial resolution is improved. First-generation scanners had a matrix size of 80 × 80 (6,400 pixels), resulting in a coarse, grainy image with poor resolution. Most fourth-generation machines have a matrix of 512 × 512 (262,144 pixels), yielding an image of high spatial resolution because information that was averaged together in larger adjacent pixels (in early scanners) has become more visible as it is dispersed over more pixels of smaller size.

Contrast resolution refers to the ability of the system to display an image of an object that is only slightly different in density from its surroundings. With standard radiographic technique, even large objects cannot be visualized unless they present a contrast difference of 10–15% with respect to their surroundings. In CT, the contrast resolution is better than 0.25%.[1] The high sensitivity of the CT scanner to small differences in x-ray attenuation is due to three factors: (1) lack of superimposition of adjacent structures, (2) use of a narrow, highly collimated beam, resulting in decreased scatter radiation, and (3) the ability to window the image. The CT window functions as the contrast control and limits viewing to a narrow portion of the total information available. Once the *window center* and *window width* are selected by the operator, tissues can be divided into three categories according to the window setting. The *window center* is the value (in Hounsfield units) of the center of the range of CT values to be displayed. The *window width* is the total range of CT values to be displayed. Tissues with a CT number less than the lower window setting are black, while those with a CT number greater than the upper window setting are white. Tissues with CT numbers between the upper and lower window levels are displayed as varying shades of gray. Most modern scanners have up to 256 shades of gray; therefore, a large number of tissues with varying densities may be displayed. The computer alters CT image contrast by allowing adjustment of the window setting. A large window setting produces an image with relatively low contrast but a wide range of CT numbers, that is, many tissues with varying densities becomes visible. A small window produces high image contrast because small differences in tissue CT numbers are imaged with large differences in shades of gray. Therefore, by manipulating CT window settings, subtle differences can be isolated between tissue densities that are virtually similar.

REFERENCES

1. Thompson TT. *A Practical Approach to Modern Imaging Equipment,* ed 2. Boston and Toronto, Little, Brown, 1985, pp 169–190.

2. Coulam CM, Erickson JJ, Rollo RD, et al. *The Physical Basis of Medical Imaging.* New York, Appleton-Century-Crofts, 1981, pp 189–229.

3. Berland LL. *Practical CT—Technology and Techniques.* New York, Raven Press, 1987, pp 3–131.

4. Sprawls P. *Physical Principles of Medical Imaging.* Rockville, Md, Aspen, 1987, pp 327–353.

5. Tumeh SS, Seltzer SE, Wang AM. Computed tomography in vascular disorders, in Loscalzo J, Creager MA,

Dzau VJ (eds): *Vascular Medicine—A Textbook of Vascular Biology and Diseases.* Boston, Toronto, and London, Little, Brown, 1992, pp 509–513.

6. Michael AS, Mafee MF, Valvassori GE, et al. Dynamic computed tomography of the head and neck: Differential diagnostic value. *Radiology* 1985;154:413–419.

7. Dillon EH, van Leeuwen MS, Fernandez MA, et al. Spiral CT angiography. *AJR* 1993;160:1273–1278.

8. Kallender WA, Seissler W, Klotz E, et al. Spiral volumetric CT with single-breath-hold technique and continuous transport and scanner rotation. *Radiology* 1990;176: 181–183.

9. Suojanen JN, Mukherji SK, Dupuy DE, et al. Spiral CT in evaluation of head and neck lesions: Work in progress. *Radiology* 1992;183:281–283.

10. Marks MP, Napel S, Jordan JE, et al. Diagnosis of carotid artery disease: Preliminary experience wtih maximum-intensity-projection spiral CT angiography. *AJR* 1993; 160:1267–1271.

11. Castillo M. Diagnosis of disease of the common carotid artery bifurcation: CT angiography vs. catheter angiography. *AJR* 1993;161:395–398.

12. Williams AL, Haughton VM. *Cranial Computed Tomography—A Comprehensive Text.* St Louis, CV Mosby, 1985, pp 12–38, 214.

11

Computed Tomography of Cerebrovascular Disease

Ay-Ming Wang, M.D., John H. Bisese, M.D., Jackson C.T. Lin, M.D.

INTRODUCTION

For evaluation of cerebrovascular disease, the noncontrast head computed tomography (CT) scan can delineate the regions or territories supplied by major cerebral arteries (Figs. 11-1, 11-2) and detect intracranial hemorrhage, brain edema, mass effect, hydrocephalus, blood clots in the cerebral vessels, and calcifications. In addition, the contrast-enhanced head CT scans can depict normal and pathological vessels, as well as abnormal enhancement of the areas of the injured brain, with breakdown of the blood–brain barrier. The key role of CT in evaluation of cerebrovascular disease is to exclude the presence of intracranial hemorrhage.[1]

STROKE

Cerebral ischemia (transient ischemic attack, TIA) is a temporary nutritional deprivation of the brain resulting in reversible neurological dysfunction; it does not cause any permanent damage. The head CT scan usually shows no brain changes referable to TIA.[2]

Cerebral infarction (stroke) is the result of prolonged nutritional deprivation that injures the affected neurons, and brain necrosis occurs.[2] Cerebral infarctions can be bland (ischemic) and hemorrhagic (vessels wall ruptured due to necrosis), focal, or global. Focal cerebral infarction can be due to arterial or venous vascular disorders, connective tissue disorder, embolism, or hematological disorders; global cerebral infarction (Fig. 11-3) can result from decreased cardiac output, decreased peripheral vascular resistance, increased intracranial pressure, metabolic disorders, anemia, or respiratory failure causing diffuse brain edema and bilateral basal ganglia infarction.[3] Temporary generalized cerebral hypoperfusion can result in watershed (arterial border zone or distal perfusion zone) infarction (Fig. 11-4) in the border zone between the anterior, middle, and posterior cerebral artery territories; watershed infarction is often associated with preexisting cerebral vascular (usually atherosclerotic and/or hypertensive) disease, and there is usually bilateral involvement.[4] Lacunar infarcts (Fig. 11-5) are small (less than 15 mm) infarcts, most often located in the basal ganglia, periventricular regions, and brain stem; they result from occlusive vascular disease of the small arteries which is commonly associated with hypertension and diabetes.[5] In patients with cerebral venous and/or dural sinus thrombosis, obstruction of venous outflow causes increased intracranial venous pressure, resulting in decreased perfusion pressure and cerebral infarctions. The

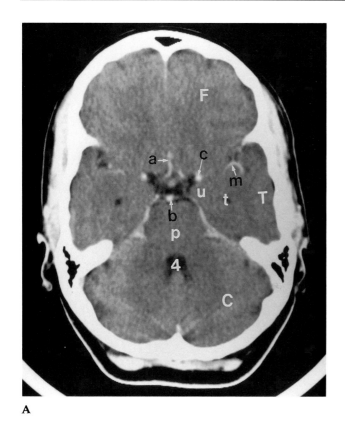

A

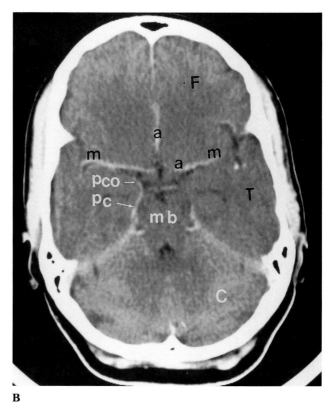

B

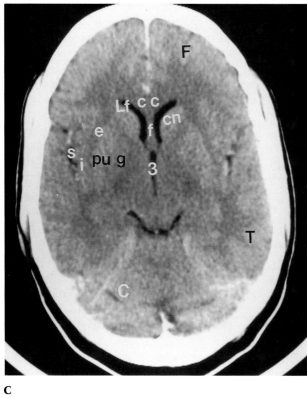

C

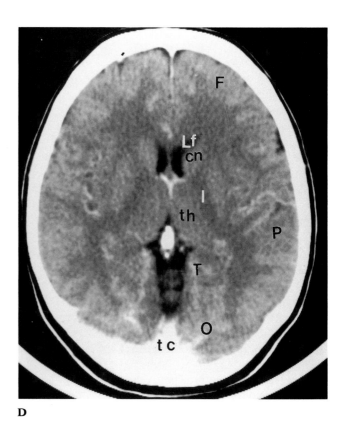

D

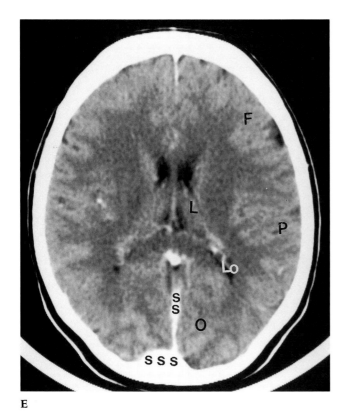

E

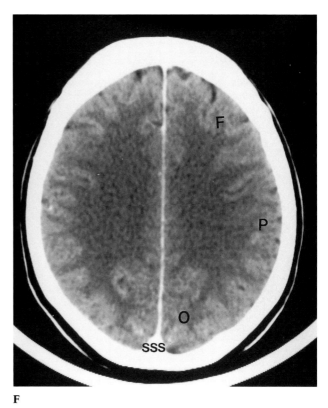

F

Fig. 11-1 Normal axial contrast-enhanced cranial CT scans at the levels of the fourth ventricle (*A*), midbrain (*B*), third ventricle (*C*), occipital horn of the lateral ventricles (*D*), body of the lateral ventricles (*E*), and high cerebral convexity (*F*). a = anterior cerebral artery; b = basilar artery; c = internal carotid artery; C = cerebellum; cc = corpus callosum; cn = head of the caudate nucleus; e = external capsule; F = frontal lobe; f = fornix; g = globus pallidus; I = internal capsule; i = insula; L = body of the lateral ventricle; Lf = frontal horn of the lateral ventricle; Lo = occipital horn of the lateral ventricle; m = middle cerebral artery; mb = midbrain; O = occipital lobe; P = parietal lobe; p = pons; pc = posterior cerebral artery; pco = posterior communicating artery; pu = putamen; s = sylvian fissure; ss = straight sinus; sss = superior sagittal sinus; T = temporal lobe; t = temporal horn of the lateral ventricle; tc = Torcular Herophili; th = thalamus; u = uncus; 3 = third ventricle; 4 = fourth ventricle.

goals of head CT in evaluating stroke are to exclude the presence of hemorrhage within the infarct or intracranial hemorrhage due to a ruptured aneurysm or other etiologies; to demonstrate the location and extent of the insult; and to exclude other pathologies mimicking stroke clinically, such as brain tumors. On the noncontrast head CT study, the intracranial hemorrhage appears as a focus of increased density (usually 50–70 Hounsfield units), while ischemic infarction appears as either an isodense area or an area of decreased density in the brain parenchyma. In the early stage of infarction, cytotoxic brain edema is the first abnormality demonstrated on CT scan; it appears as an area of decreased density in the cerebral gray matter. By contrast, vasogenic brain edema is the predominant abnormality in brain tumor, which appears as decreased density in

the cerebral white matter. On the contrast-enhanced head CT study, the early infarction does not show pathological enhancement, in contrast to the usually observed pathological enhancement in brain tumor.

HEMORRHAGIC INFARCTION

Hemorrhagic infarction is a hemorrhage originating within and secondary to infarction appearing within 24 hr, whereas hemorrhagic transformation is a delayed appearance of hemorrhage 24 hr after the ictus.[6,7] Hemorrhagic infarction is most common in embolic stroke and large infarcts. Acute hemorrhagic infarction may be seen as small, slightly hyperdense bands within a larger, hypodense infarct. These hemorrhages are

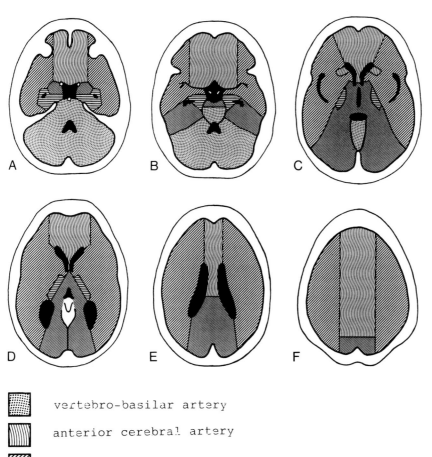

vertebro-basilar artery

anterior cerebral artery

middle cerebral artery

posterior cerebral artery

anterior choroid artery

Fig. 11-2 Axial views of the major cerebral arterial territories corresponding to Fig. 11-1 at the levels of the fourth ventricle (*A*), midbrain (*B*), third ventricle (*C*), occipital horn of the lateral ventricles (*D*), body of the lateral ventricles (*E*), and high cerebral convexity (*F*).

most commonly seen in the cerebral cortex or at the margin of the infarct, but they can also be seen centrally in the deep cerebral gray matter. The hemorrhages can become confluent, resulting in more striking hyperdensity (Fig. 11-6). Such predominant hyperdensity, combined with extension into the cerebral white matter, can mimic nontraumatic primary intracerebral hematoma. However, the nontraumatic primary intracerebral hematoma (Fig. 11-7) tends to be more homogeneous in density, round or oval in shape, and more sharply defined than the hemorrhagic infarct. The noncontrast head CT study can define an acute cerebral hemorrhage as a hyperdense lesion, but it cannot differentiate a subacute (isodense) or chronic (low-density) cerebral hemorrhage from a nonhemorrhagic infarction. Hemorrhagic transformation may be due to embolic migration and a collateral supply to a distal arterial throm-

botic occlusion; it appears as a petechial hemorrhage and may have been underdiagnosed on CT.[8] Magnetic resonance imaging (MRI) has been reported to be better than CT in differentiating the subacute and chronic, nonhemoorhagic infarction from the hemorrhagic infarction and in identifying hemorrhagic transformation because it can detect the presence of methemoglobin and hemosiderin by their characteristic signal intensity changes on T_1- and T_2-weighted images.[9,10] The contrast head CT study may demonstrate rim enhancement along the hemorrhage[11] (Fig. 11-8).

ISCHEMIC INFARCTION

The CT findings of stroke are related to the time of scanning from the ictus; there are four stages: su-

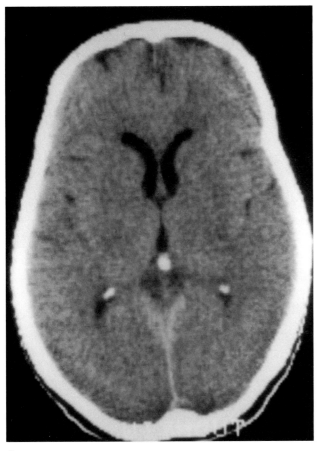 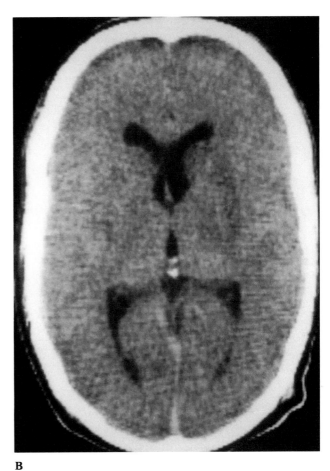

A   B

Fig. 11-3 Noncontrast head CT scans of two patients with global cerebral infarctions. (*A*) A 32-year-old male with cardiopulmonary arrest secondary to IV drug overdose. The CT scan obtained 6 hr after the arrest shows diffuse, decreased density in the bilateral basal ganglia. (*B*) A 46-year-old female with carbon monoxide poisoning and deep coma. The CT scan obtained 12 hr after the event shows a marked decrease in density of the head of the caudate nucleus bilaterally, as well as of the left putamen. There is diffuse brain edema and decreased density in the bilateral occipital lobes.

peracute (to 24 hr), acute (24 hr to 7 days), subacute (8 to 21 days), and chronic (more than 21 days).[8,12]

Superacute Stage Infarction

The major roles of CT in this stage are (1) to exclude the presence of hemorrhage (noncontrast CT study) and (2) to exclude disease entities such as brain tumors that could clinically mimic stroke (contrast CT study). With improvement in spatial and contrast resolution, the ability of the state-of-the-art CT scanner to directly identify infarcted brain tissue has markedly improved. However, the sensitivity of CT in early detection of ischemic infarction remains limited, and only about half of all strokes are visualized within the first 48 hr.[13] The detectable noncontrast CT changes associated with

superacute stage stroke are the subtle mass effect with effacement of the surface sulci in cerebral cortical infarction (Fig. 11-9), ventricular compression in deep cerebral infarction (Fig. 11-10), and loss of the distinction between the densities of cerebral gray matter and white matter (Fig. 11-11) due to the presence of a slightly decreased density in the cerebral gray matter from cytotoxic brain edema,[14-17] as well as visualization of a hyperdense cerebral artery.[21,22] The larger the area of infarction in the presence of cytotoxic brain edema, as well as of mass effect, the more likely the ischemic infarction will be seen on a high-quality CT study 6 to 12 hr after the ictus.

Gray matter hypodensity reflects the presence of cytotoxic brain edema, which usually begins immediately after the onset of cerebral hyperperfusion. Cytotoxic

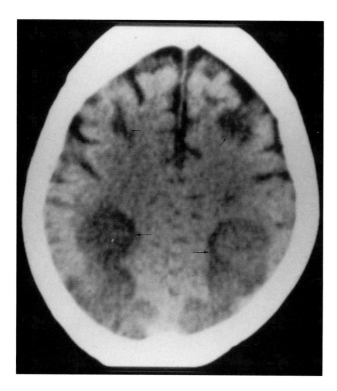

Fig. 11-4 Noncontrast head CT scan of a 70-year-old male with mental status changes shows acute watershed infarctions (arrows) involving the bilateral parietal lobes at the arterial border zone of the anterior and middle cerebral arteries bilaterally.

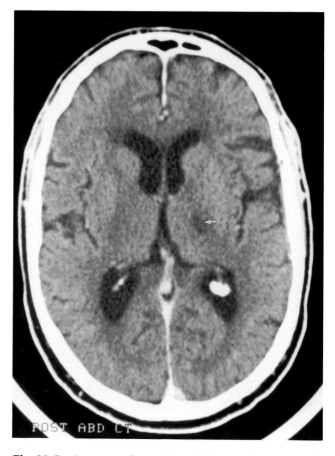

Fig. 11-5 Contrast-enhanced head CT scan of a 77-year-old male with right hemiparesis shows a lacunar infarction (arrow) involving the posterior limb of the left internal capsule.

brain edema is caused by a redistribution of sodium and water from the extracellular to the intracellular compartment, with minimal change in the overall water content of the brain.[18,19] It is not associated with changes in the blood–brain barrier and is reversible if perfusion is restored. Because of the lack of changes in the blood–brain barrier in cytotoxic brain edema, there is usually no pathological enhancement on a contrast-enhanced CT study in the superacute stage of stroke.[20] Visualization of pathological enhancement requires at least 24 hr after the ictus, when blood–brain barrier damage is sufficient to allow leakage of the contrast material on the contrast-enhanced CT study. Increased density in a cerebral artery, most commonly in the horizontal (M1) segment of the middle cerebral artery (Fig. 11-12) and also commonly in the basilar artery (Fig. 11-13), can be seen in the superacute stage of stroke on the noncontrast CT study.[21,22] It represents an intraluminal thrombus or embolus.

The use of intravenous iodinated contrast agents in the superacute or acute stage of stroke is controversial. Some authors[13,23] have found contrast-enhanced CT to

be of great value for the diagnosis and characterization of infarcts; others[24,25] have stated that recovery from stroke is better among those who had not received intravenous iodinated contrast. These latter authors also stated that the prognosis was poorer for stroke patients with enhanced lesions than for those with nonenhanced lesions, indicating neurotoxicity of the iodinated contrast medium, which might cause ischemic but not yet infarcted brain tissue to undergo irreversible damage. These authors gave only a few indications of a contrast-enhanced CT scan for a suspected infarction.

Contrast head CT may show enhancement of the normal cortical gray matter[26] and may occasionally show curvilinear enhancement of the cortical arterial vessels in the region of the superacute ischemic infarction but no enhancement in the zone of the infarction.[20] In the superacute stage of stroke, we recommend that head CT be performed without contrast to

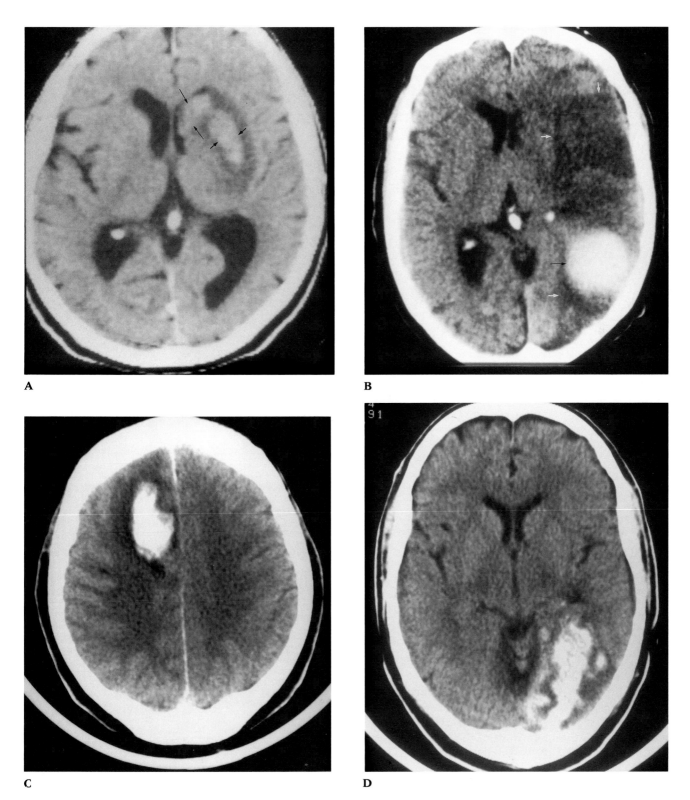

Fig. 11-6 Noncontrast head CT scans of four patients with hemorrhagic infarctions. (*A*) Acute hemorrhagic infarctions (arrows) involving the head of the caudate nucleus and putamen on the left in the left lenticulate striate artery territory associated with mass effect and edema. (*B*) Extensive low-density infarction (white arrows) in the left middle cerebral artery territory; in the posterior aspect of this infarction, a large area of hemorrhage (black arrows) is seen. (*C*) Large hemorrhagic infarction in the right frontal lobe in the right anterior cerebral artery territory. (*D*) Large hemorrhagic infarction in the left occipital lobe in the left posterior cerebral artery territory.

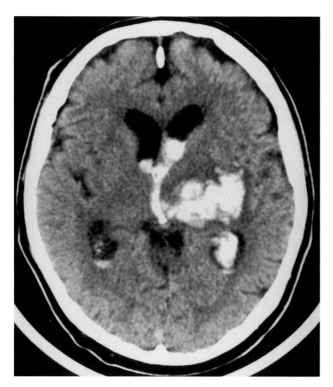

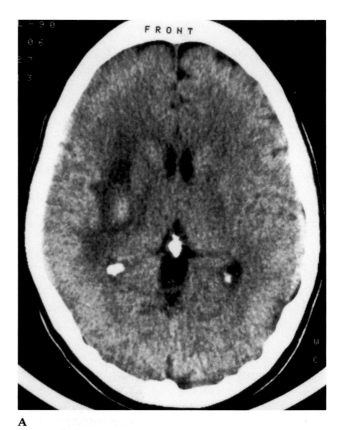

A

Fig. 11-7 Noncontrast head CT scan of a 71-year-old male with a history of hypertension with acute headache and right hemiparesis. The scan shows left thalamic hemorrhage dissecting to the third ventricle and extending to the left basal ganglia. Intraventricular hemorrhage is also seen involving the frontal and occipital horns of both lateral ventricles. The third ventricle is displaced to the right.

exclude the presence of hemorrhage. If a noncontrast head CT study suggests the presence of a focal mass and/or vasogenic edema; then a contrast-enhanced head CT scan is recommended to exclude a brain tumor.

Acute Stage Infarction

During the first week of the stroke, the visibility of a sharply delineated hypodensity involving both the cerebral gray and white matter of the infarcted brain, conforming to a vascular distribution on a head CT study (Fig. 11-14), increases beyond 24 hr after the

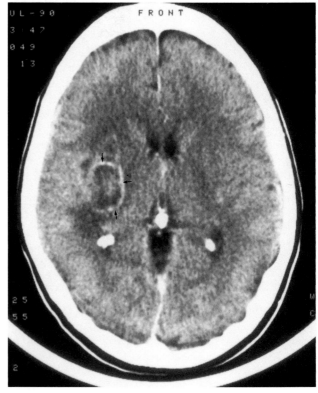

Fig. 11-8 A 44-year-old female with headache for 1 week. (*A*) Noncontrast head CT scan shows subacute parenchymal hemorrhage with edema in the right lateral basal ganglia. (*B*) Contrast-enhanced head CT scan shows rim enhancement (arrows) along the periphery of the hemorrhage.

B

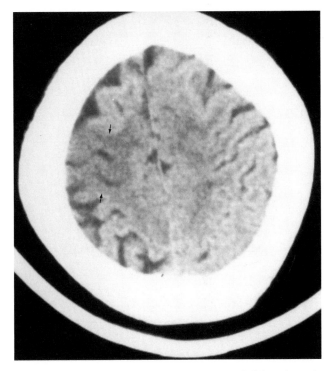

Fig. 11-9 An 85-year-old female with acute left hemiparesis for 8 hr. A noncontrast head CT scan shows an ill-defined, low-density, hyperacute infarction (arrows) with effacement of the surrounding sulci.

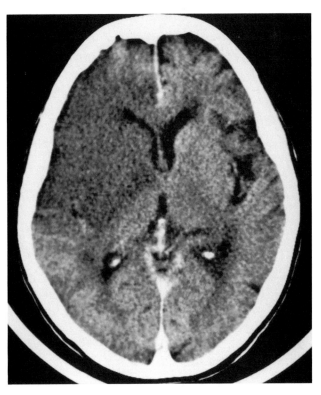

Fig. 11-10 A 78-year-old female with acute mental confusion and left hemiparesis for 22 hr. The noncontrast head CT scan shows diffuse, decreased density areas of hyperacute infarction involving the right frontoparietal opercula, right insular cortex, and right basal ganglia, with mass effect on the frontal horn of the right lateral ventricle and effacement of the surrounding sulci and cisterns.

ictus. Cerebral cortical infarcts are usually triangular or wedge-shaped, while deep cerebral infarcts are usually round or oval. Brain edema and mass effect usually reach their maximum during the third to fifth days.

Subacute Stage Infarction

On a contrast head CT study, enhancement within the infarction usually appears during the second week after the ictus. The enhancement may be gyral in configuration, involving the cortex (Fig. 11-15), or a homogeneous (Fig. 11-16) ring enhancement in deep gray matter. The patterns of enhancement are nonspecific and reflective of several pathophysiological mechanisms, including disruption of the blood–brain barrier, enhanced capillary filling of the affected gyri (luxury perfusion), reactive hyperemia, and neovascularity. Brain edema and mass effect decrease during the subacute stage and usually resolve completely by 2–3 weeks. The attenuation values of the infarcted brain increase as brain edema subsides. Some infarcts can become temporarily normal in density on noncontrast as well as contrast head CT studies (foggy effect)[27] (Fig. 11-17) during the subacute stage and then revert to hypoden-

sity. Fogging can occur in all or part of an infarct and represents the phase of phagocytization of necrotic brain after resolution of edema. Areas of fogging may enhance intensely (Fig. 11-18). Ischemic infarcts may develop secondary to hemorrhagic transformation, which is most likely to be seen with embolic infarcts. Due to lack of autoregulation in the capillary beds of embolic infarcts once exposed to systemic arterial pressure following fragmentation and lysis of the clot and reestablishment of normal antegrade flow it may produce hemorrhagic transformation.[25] These reperfusion hemorrhages are usually petechial and clinically silent. They are difficult to see on noncontrast head CT studies but are easily visualized on MRI studies (Fig. 11-19).

Chronic Stage Infarction

The areas of infarction are replaced by a well-defined, sharply marginated focal zone of cystic encephalomala-

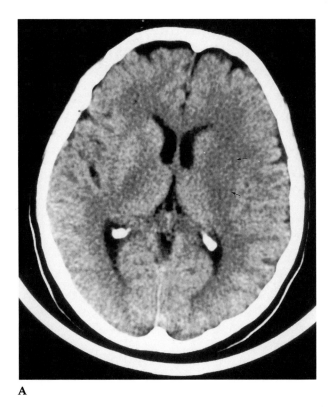 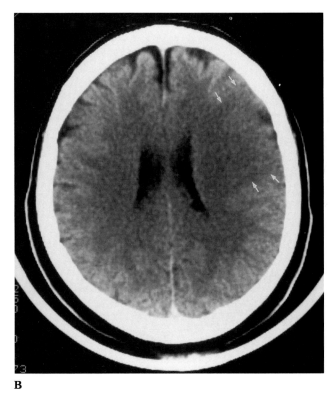

A   **B**

Fig. 11-11   Noncontrast head CT scans of two patients with hyperacute infarction, with loss of distinction between the densities of the cerebral gray matter and white matter. (*A*) A 65-year-old female with acute right hemiparesis for 6 hr. The noncontrast head CT scan shows decreased density in the left putamen (arrows). (*B*) A 53-year-old male with acute mental status changes and right hemiparesis for 8 hr. The noncontrast head CT scan shows decreased density in the left frontal and left anterior parietal lobes (arrows).

cia and gliosis involving both cerebral gray and white matter. On noncontrast head CT studies, cystic encephalomalacia is isodense to cerebrospinal fluid, and the gliotic rim is slightly hyperdense to cerebrospinal fluid (Fig. 11-20). Dilatation of the ipsilateral ventricle and sulci and retraction of the midline structure toward the infarcted brain are often seen. Contrast enhancement begins to decrease during the third week after the ictus and is unusual after the second month.[26] A ribbon of preserved cortex may be seen overlying a zone of infarction since the outer layers of the cerebral cortex are more resistant to ischemic infarction than the deep structures. Once the large, old infarcts affect the motor cortex or internal capsule, an ipsilateral cerebral peduncle and pontine atrophy can be demonstrated on CT. However, these can be better seen on MRI from antegrade degeneration of an axon and its myelin sheath following injury to the proximal portion of the axon or the neuronal cell body (Wallerian degeneration).[28] Calcification may also occasionally be seen in the old infarct (Fig. 11-21).

CEREBRAL VENOUS AND DURAL SINUS THROMBOSIS

A large number of disease processes[29] can cause cerebral venous and dural sinus thrombosis. They can be divided into three groups: (1) local diseases such as infection, trauma, neoplasm, and arterial infarction, as well as subarachnoid hemorrhage; (2) systemic conditions such as pregnancy, puerperium, collagen vascular disease, migratory thrombophlebitis, inflammatory bowel disease, cardiac disease, and hematological disorders; and (3) idiopathic conditions. Direct involvement of a dural sinus, venous stasis, hypercoagulable state, and increased blood viscosity resulting from polycythemia or dehydration are the most common causes of cerebral venous and dural sinus thrombosis. The clinical findings depend upon the location and extent of the thrombosis, the rate and degree of propagation into the cerebral veins and dural sinuses, the presence of collateral venous drainage, and the degree of recanalization. The role of CT in evaluation of cerebral

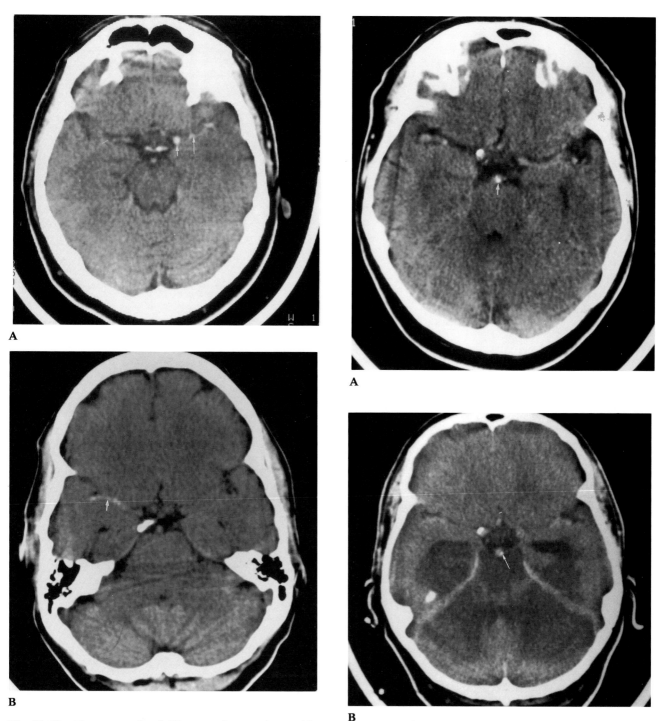

A

B

A

B

Fig. 11-12 Noncontrast head CT scans of two patients with a hyperdense middle cerebral artery sign of hyperacute infarction. (*A*) A 53-year-old male with acute onset of aphasia and right hemiparesis for 8 hr. The head CT scan shows a hyperdense blood clot in the supraclinoid portion of the left internal carotid artery and M1 segment of the left middle cerebral artery. There is diffuse, decreased density in the gray matter of the left anterior temporal lobe. (*B*) A 43-year-old female with acute onset of left hemiparesis for 4 hr. The head CT scan shows a linear, hyperdense blood clot (arrow) in the M1 segment of the right middle cerebral artery.

Fig. 11-13 A 41-year-old male with acoute coma for 8 hr. (*A*) The noncontrast head CT scan shows a hyperdense blood clot in the basilar artery (arrow). (*B*) The noncontrast head CT scan 6 days later demonstrates interval diminution of the hyperdense blood clot in the basilar artery (arrow), with diffuse, low-density infarction in the brain stem, bilateral posterior temporal lobes, and cerebellum, and mass effect and effacement of the fourth ventricle. There is dilatation of the temporal horns of both lateral ventricles, suggesting hydrocephalus.

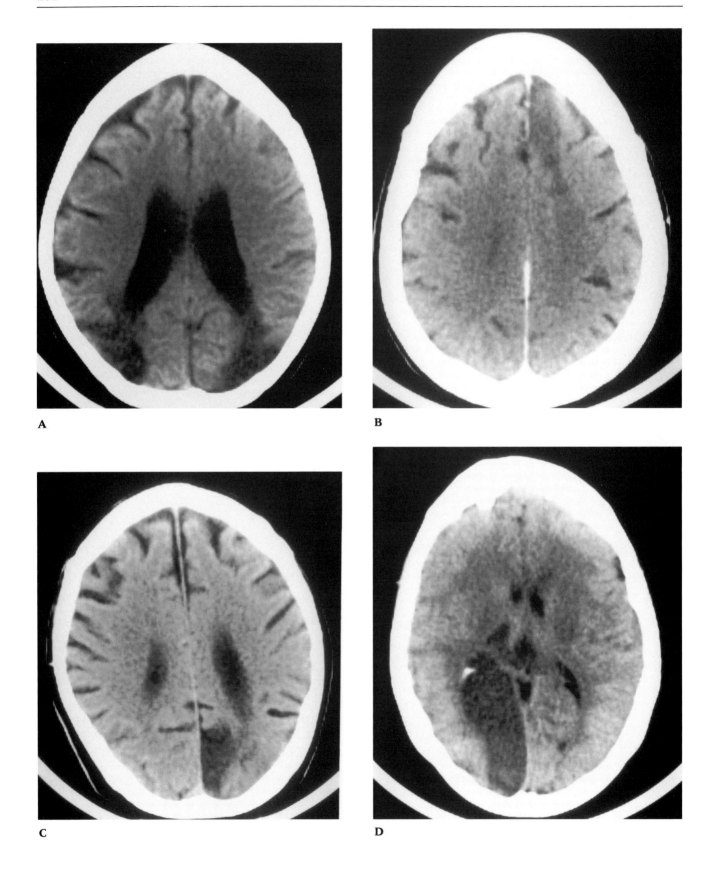

A

B

C

D

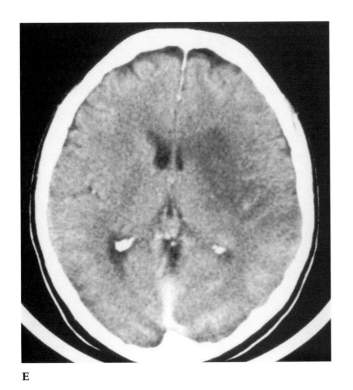

E

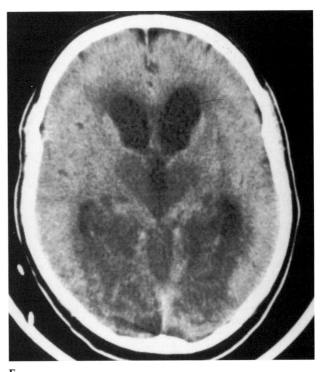

F

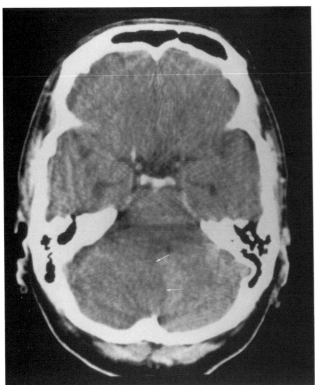

G

Fig. 11-14 Noncontrast head CT scan of seven patients with acute ischemic infarction. (*A*) Bilateral occipital lobe infarctions in the bilateral middle and posterior cerebral arterial border zones. (*B*) Left frontal lobe infarction in the left anterior cerebral artery territory. (*C*) Left parieto-occipital infarction in the left posterior pericallosal artery territory. (*D*) Right thalamic, posterior temporal lobe, and occipital lobe infarctions in the right posterior communicating artery and right posterior cerebral artery territory. (*E*) Left basal ganglia and frontoparietal lobe infarctions with mass effect in the left middle cerebral artery territory. (*F*) Bilateral thalamic, occipital lobe, and posterior temporal lobe infarctions with mass effect and hydrocephalus in the bilateral posterior communicating artery and bilateral posterior cerebral artery territories due to occlusion of the basilar artery (same patient as Fig. 11-13B). (*G*) Ischemic infarction involving the right cerebellar hemisphere (arrows), with mass effect and effacement of the fourth ventricle in the right posterior inferior cerebellar artery territory.

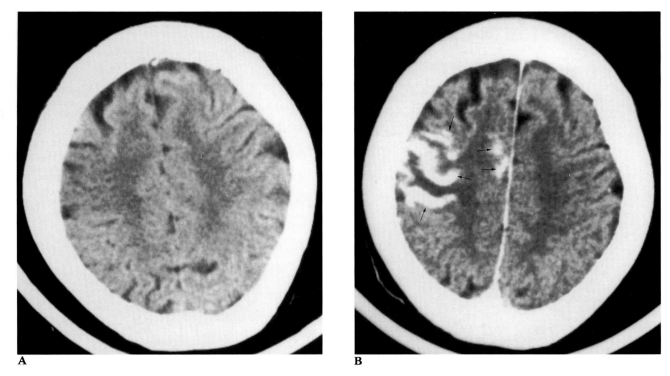

A   B

Fig. 11-15 Precontrast (*A*) and postcontrast (*B*) head CT scans of a 61-year-old male with left hemiparesis for 8 days show a low-density infarction involving the gray and white matter of the right frontoparietal lobe with enhancement of the gyri (arrows).

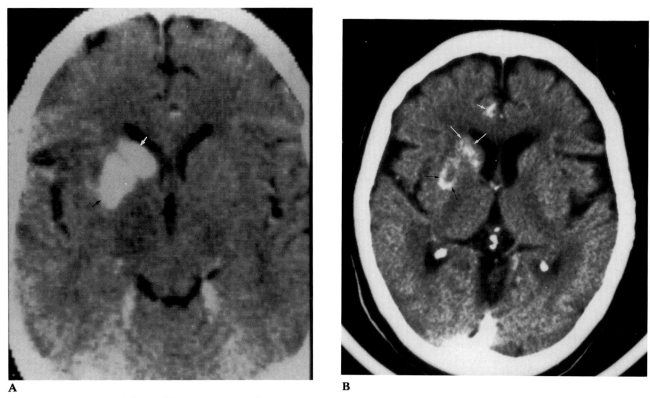

A   B

Fig. 11-16 Contrast-enhanced head CT scans of two patients with subacute infarction involving the right basal ganglia with enhancement. (*A*) Homogeneous enhancement of the head of the caudate nucleus (white arrow) and the putamen (black arrow). (*B*) Slight, inhomogeneous enhancement of the head of the caudate nucleus (white arrow) and rim enhancement of the putamen (black arrow). Enhancement of the gyri is also seen involving the cingulate gyrus (small arrow).

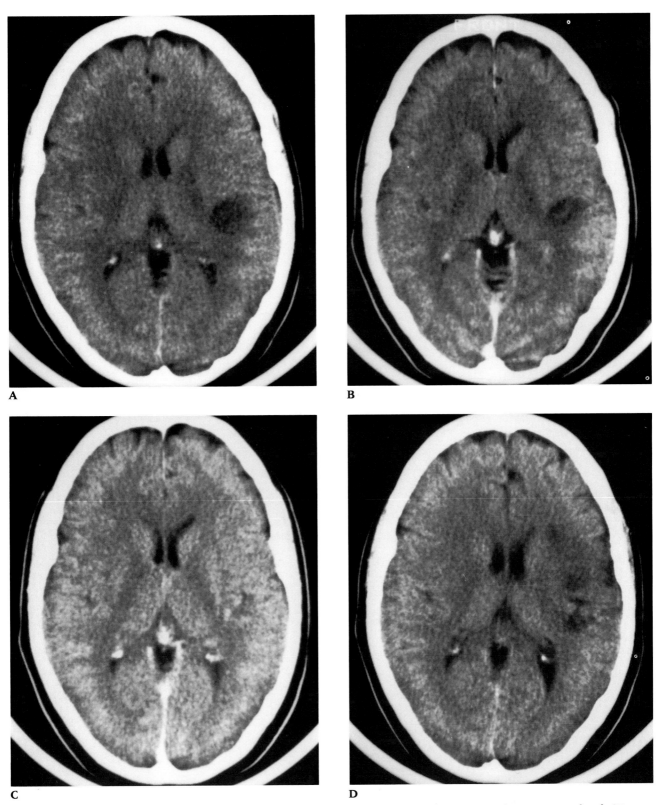

Fig. 11-17 A 30-year-old female with acute onset of right hemiparesis. (*A*) Noncontrast and (*B*) contrast head CT scans obtained 3 days postictus demonstrate a low-density, acute ischemic infarction in the region of the left parietal operculum, with absence of pathological enhancement. (*C*) Contrast-enhanced head CT scan 2 weeks after the ictus shows the foggy effect. (*D*) Noncontrast head CT scan 4 months later shows that the infarction has reverted to hypodensity, with dilatation of the ipsilateral lateral ventricle.

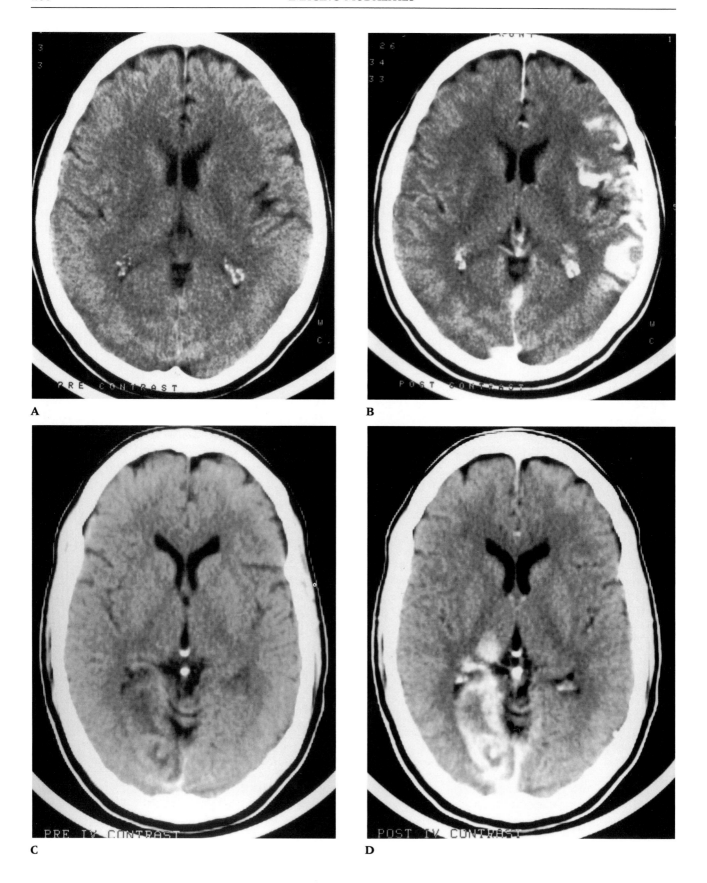

A

B

C

D

venous and dural sinus thrombosis[30-36] is to detect complications (Fig. 11-22) such as hemorrhage, infarctions, brain edema, and hydrocephalus, as well as to visualize thrombosed veins. On noncontrast head CT studies, thrombosed veins and dural sinuses can be directly visualized as foci of significantly increased density (measured as 50–70 Hounsfield units), the so-called cord sign (Fig. 11-23), for the first week after the thrombosis forms. The cord sign has been reported[29,35] in fewer than 20% of cases of cerebral venous thrombosis. However, mild hyperdensity can be seen in patent veins because the state-of-the-art CT scanner can visualize routinely the intrinsic mild hyperdensity (relative to cerebral gray matter) of unclotted intraluminal blood in the cerebral veins and dural sinuses. On the contrast-enhanced head CT study, there is enhancement of the surrounding collateral venous channels and normal enhancement of the dura. The hypodense central portion, relative to the enhanced peripheral portion, produces the empty delta sign[29,30,31,34,35] (Fig. 11-24), which is best seen in patients with superior sagittal sinus thrombosis. The empty delta sign was reported as a pathognomonic sign for superior sagittal sinus thrombosis; however, its incidence varies from 25%[29,35] to 70%.[31]

ANEURYSMS

Intracranial aneurysms are classified[37] as saccular or berry (most common), atherosclerotic, mycotic (Fig. 11-25), tumor-induced, traumatic, or dissecting. Most common intracranial aneurysms are saccular or berry aneurysms which result from a congenital defect in the arterial wall. Two percent of the normal population may harbor saccular aneurysms (range, 0.2–9%).[38,39] Most berry aneurysms form at branch points of intra-

cranial vessels, probably related to the intrinsic structural weakness in the walls of cerebral arteries,[37,40,41] with an increase in the number of fenestrations in the internal elastic membrane and media at the apex of branching cerebral arteries and in hemodynamic stresses by axial impingement of the bloodstream on branch points of cerebral arteries to reduce tensile strength. The most common locations of berry aneurysms are at the junction of the anterior cerebral artery and the anterior communicating artery (30%), the junction of the internal carotid artery and the posterior communicating artery (25%), the middle cerebral artery bi/trifurcation (13%), the supraclinoid carotid ophthalmic artery junction and bi/trifurcation of the supraclinoid segments (15%), and the vertebrobasilar artery system (5%).[42] Ninety-five percent of aneurysms are supratentorial. The incidence of mutiple aneurysms is 20–25%.[43]

The CT findings are as following: direct visualization of the aneurysms, and evaluation of findings and complications related to the rupture of the aneurysms.

Direct Visualization of Aneurysms

The role of CT in aneurysm screening is somewhat undefined at the present time. Contrast head CT can be used to screen for intracranial aneurysms that are 5 mm or larger if thin slices (1.5 mm) are used through the region of the circle of Willis.[44] An aneurysm (Fig. 11-26) is usually a rounded area of hyperdensity on a noncontrast head CT scan and is often enhanced homogeneously on a contrast-enhanced head CT scan close to the circle of Willis. Enhancement of a thrombosed aneurysm can be seen centrally, due to enhancement of the patent lumen with peripheral thrombus formation (Fig. 11-27), or peripherally due to enhancement of a centrifugally organizing thrombus via the peripheral vasa vasorum, or a combination of both. Areas of calcification are occasionally seen.

CT Findings of the Ruptured Aneurysm and Related Complications

Noncontrast head CT is of great value in detecting acute subarachnoid and parenchymal hemorrhage, as well as ventricular hemorrhage complicated by a ruptured aneurysm. Noncontrast head CT offers high diagnostic accuracy in predicting the site of hemorrhage when an intracerebral hematoma is present.[45,46] The pattern of cisternal blood also helps to suggest the bleeding site if an intracerebral hematoma is absent.[47] Although lumbar puncture yields the diagnosis of subarachnoid hem-

Fig. 11-18 Contrast-enhanced head CT scans of two patients with foggy effect in a subacute ischemic infarction with pathological enhancement. (A) Noncontrast and (B) contrast head CT scans of a 63-year-old male 15 days after acute onset of right hemiparesis show gyral enhancement of an isodense, ischemic infarction of the left frontal and parietal opercula, as well as of the left insular cortex. (C) Noncontrast and (D) contrast head CT scans of a 43-year-old male 2 weeks after acute onset of right homonymous hemianopsia show isodense, ischemic infarction with homogeneous enhancement involving the right posterior thalamus and inhomogeneous enhancement involving the right occipital lobe. The low-density infarction involving the right occipital lobe does not show pathological enhancement.

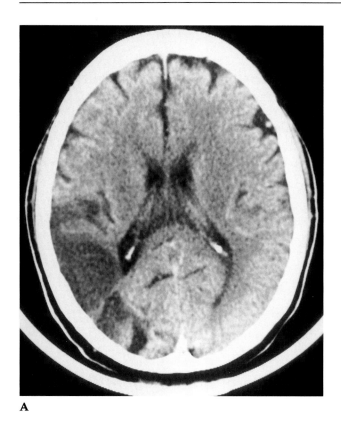

A

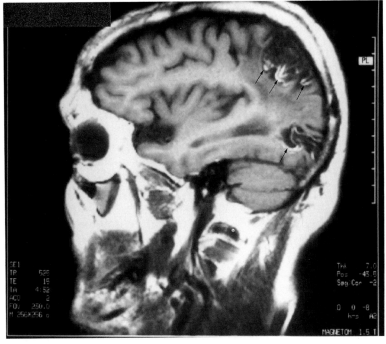

B

Fig. 11-19 (*A*) A noncontrast head CT scan obtained 3 weeks postictus shows a low-density, ischemic infarction involving the right parietal and occipital lobes. (*B*) T$_1$-weighted sagittal image of the brain shows patechial hemorrhages (arrows) representing reperfusion and hemorrhagic transformation.

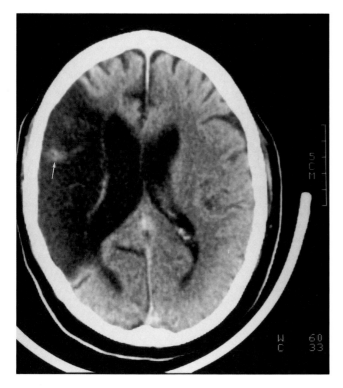

Fig. 11-20 Noncontrast head CT scan of chronic ischemic infarction. A 60-year-old male 6 months after right middle cerebral artery territory stroke. The CT scan shows a large area of well-defined low density of the right frontal and parietal lobes, with dilatation of the right lateral ventricle. A gliotic band (arrow) is seen within the infarction.

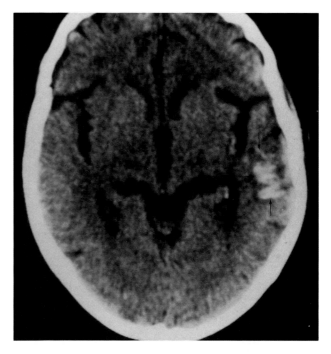

Fig. 11-21 Noncontrast head CT scan obtained 2 years after ictus shows gyral calcifications (arrows) in the left parietal opercular region.

orrhage, acute subarachnoid hemorrhage can be visualized as increased density in the cisterns, sulci, and fissures of the brain on the plain head CT scan. The increase in density is related to the hematocrit and the amount of blood released into the subarachnoid space. Within the first 24 hr after the development of subarachnoid hemorrhage, noncontrast head CT can detect more than 90% of these cases.[48–50] After the first week, subarachnoid hemorrhage is usually not detected on noncontrast head CT; if subarachnoid hemorrhage is obvious on CT more than 1 week following the initial event, rebleeding has probably happened. When a CT scan shows a subarachnoid hemorrhage with more blood in the interhemispheric fissure and/or in the septum pellucidum, with or without the presence of hemorrhage in the deep frontal lobe, suggesting rupture of an anterior communicating artery aneurysm (Fig. 11-28); with more blood in the unilateral sylvian fissure cistern, with or without the presence of temporal lobe hemorrhage suggesting rupture of a middle cerebral artery aneurysm (Fig. 11-29A); with more

blood in the suprasellar cistern, with or without the presence of hemorrhage in the medial temporal lobe, suggesting rupture of a posterior communicating artery aneurysm (Fig. 11-29B); with more blood in the posterior fossa cistern, suggesting rupture of an infratentorial aneurysm; and diffuse, symmetrical cistern blood, suggesting rupture of an aneurysm of unknown origin. If subarachnoid hemorrhage is seen only in the prepontine cistern, this indicates a venous or capillary rupture rather than an aneurysm rupture[51] (Fig. 11-30).

Cerebral arteriogram is the best diagnostic procedure to evaluate the cerebral aneurysm; given the prediction of the site of a ruptured aneurysm by CT, the cerebral arteriogram can be shortening by limiting the study to the appropriate projection to define the aneurysm in a critical and unstable patient. In the literature,[46] contrast head CT has been found to identify the ruptured aneurysm in 30% of patients with subarachnoid hemorrhage related to a ruptured aneurysm (Fig. 11-31). Subarachnoid hemorrhage enhancement was also reported to be demonstrated in these patients by contrast CT even with a normal precontrast CT study.[52] Subarachnoid hemorrhage enhancement may be related to the leakage of contrast into the cisterns or related to leptomeningeal changes due to meningeal hyperemia from chemical irritation of the meninges related to sub-

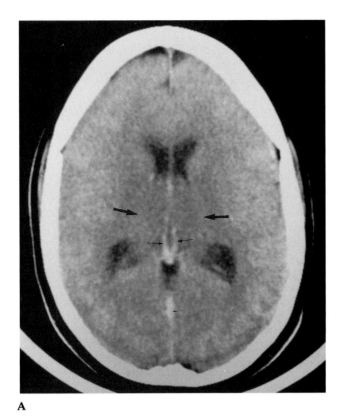

A

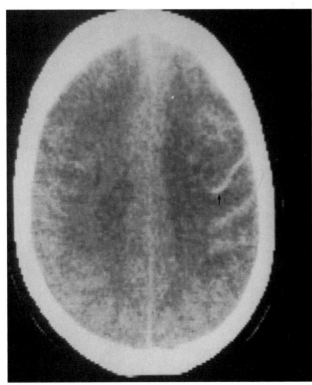

C

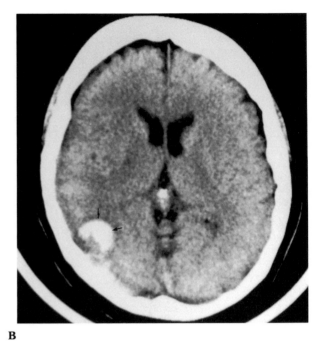

B

Fig. 11-22 Noncontrast head CT scans related to complications of cerebral venous and dural sinus thrombosis. (*A*) Diffuse, decreased density in the bilateral thalami representing interstitial edema (long arrows). Hyperdense blood clots are seen in the internal cerebral veins (arrows) and straight sinus (small arrow). (*B*) Right occipital lobe hemorrhage (arrows) related to right sigmoid sinus thrombosis. (*C*) Cortical vein thrombosis (arrow) is seen in the left frontal region, with infarction of the left frontoparietal lobe and mass effect.

arachnoid hemorrhage. Other complications, such as hydrocephalus (Fig. 11-32) and infarction (Fig. 11-33) related to vascular spasm, can also be adequately evaluated by noncontrast head CT.

VASCULAR MALFORMATIONS

Vascular malformations are commonly classified into four categories: arteriovenous malformation (AVM), venous angioma, cavernous angioma, and capillary hemangioma/telangiectasia.[53] The most common vascular malformation is AVM. The goal of CT in evaluation of the vascular malformations are to detect their complications, such as subarachnoid hemorrhage, intraventricular hemorrhage, parenchymal hemorrhage, venous infarction, calcifications, mass effect, and hydrocephalus, and to identify the vascular malformation.

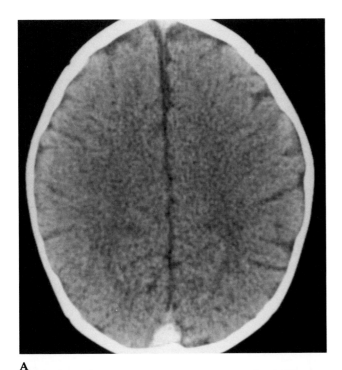

A

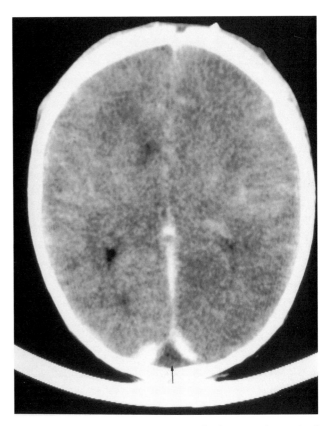

Fig. 11-24 Contrast-enhanced head of a superior sagittal sinus thrombosis shows the empty delta sign in the superior sagittal sinus (arrow) and diffuse infarction in the left cerebral hemisphere with mass effect.

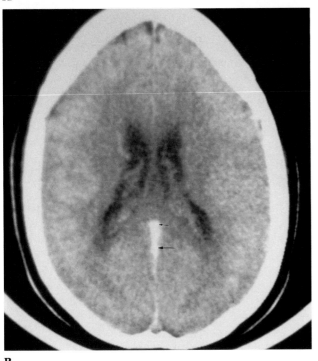

B

Fig. 11-23 (*A*) Noncontrast head CT scan of a superior sagittal sinus thrombosis shows a cord sign in the superior sagittal sinus (arrow). (*B*) Noncontrast head CT scan of a straight sinus thrombosis shows a cord sign in the straight sinus (arrow), as well as in the great cerebral vein of Galen (small arrow).

Arteriovenous Malformations

Dural AVMs are sometimes considered acquired and may be traumatic, atherosclerotic, or spontaneous. Parenchymal and ependymal AVMs are congenital. At normal 3 weeks' gestation, the primitive intracranial arteries, capillaries, and veins form; however, localized arrest results in a direct arteriovenous communication. Failure to form an intervening capillary bed between essentially normal feeding arteries and draining veins results in an AVM. The subsequent dilatation of the feeding and draining vessels is the result of increased flow through a low-pressure system. AVMs are named according to their anatomical location and their blood supply. They most commonly occur in the supratentorial region, usually involve the cerebral hemispheres, particularly the parietal lobe, and are generally 2 cm or more in diameter. Twenty percent of AVMs are infratentorial in location. Approximately 6% are multi-

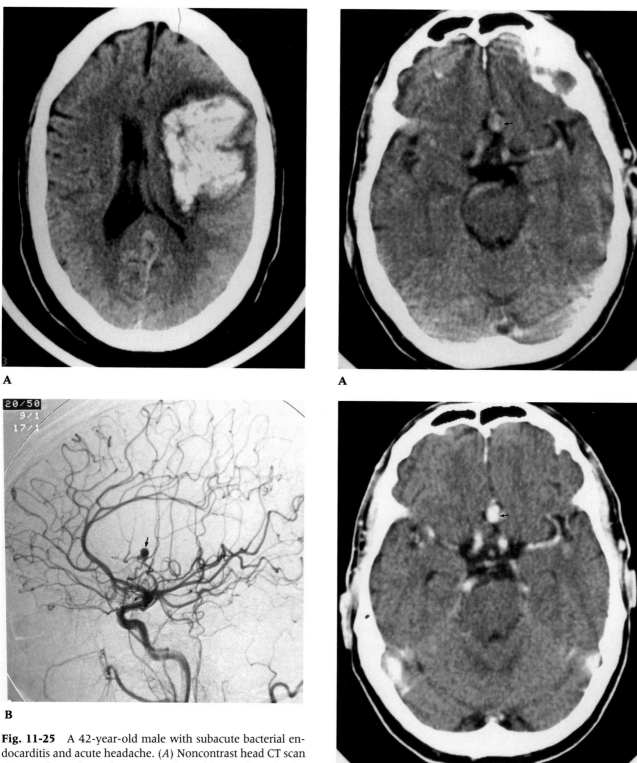

A

B

Fig. 11-25 A 42-year-old male with subacute bacterial endocarditis and acute headache. (*A*) Noncontrast head CT scan shows a large, hyperdense parenchymal hemorrhage in the left frontoparietal region. (*B*) Left carotid arterial digital subtraction angiography shows a 5-mm-diameter aneurysm in the ascending frontal branch of the left middle cerebral artery (arrow). Mycotic aneurysms tend to be peripherally located.

A

B

Fig. 11-26 CT demonstration of cerebral aneurysms.

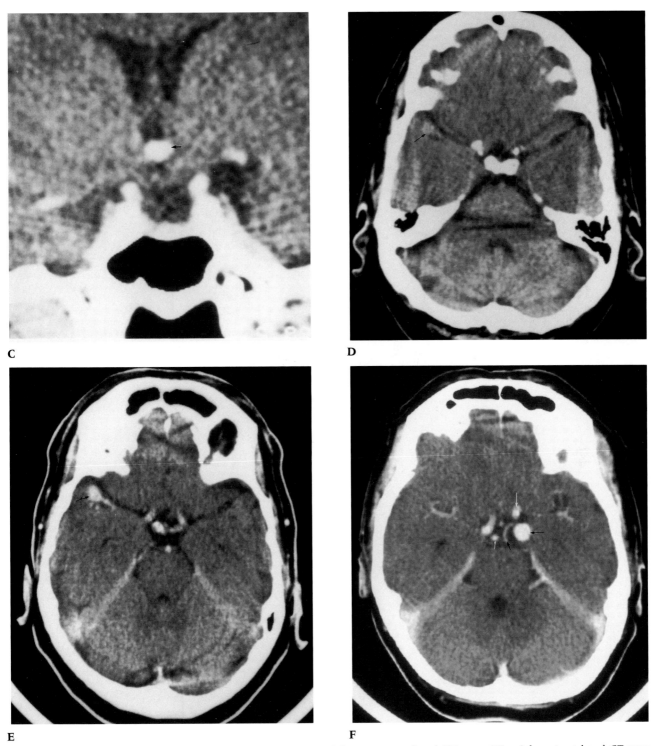

Fig. 11-26A–F *Anterior communicating artery aneurysm:* (*A*) axial noncontrast head CT scan, (*B*) axial contrast head CT scan, and (*C*) coronal contrast head CT scan demonstrate a 7-mm-diameter, hyperdense aneurysm (arrow) with homogeneous enhancement at the anterior communicating artery. *Middle cerebral artery aneurysm:* (*D*) axial noncontrast head CT scan and (*E*) axial contrast head CT scan demonstrate a 6-mm-diameter, hyperdense aneurysm (arrow) with homogeneous enhancement at the trifurcation of the right middle cerebral artery. *Posterior communicating artery aneurysm:* (*F*) axial contrast head CT scan shows a 1-cm-diameter, homogeneously enhanced aneurysm at the junction of the left internal carotid artery and the left posterior communicating artery (black arrow = aneurysm, short black arrow = left posterior communicating artery, white arrow = left internal carotid artery, short white arrow = basilar artery). *Anterior cerebral artery aneurysm:*

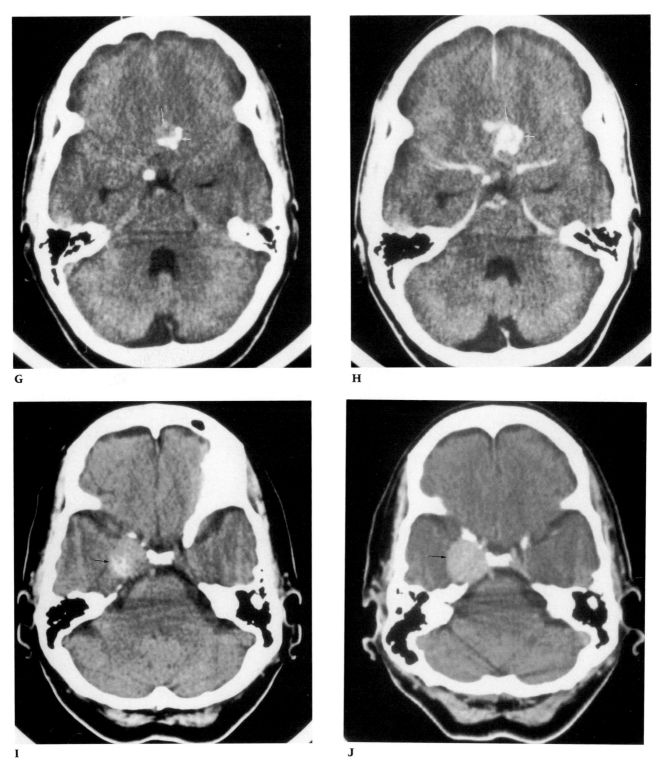

G

H

I

J

Fig. 11-26G–J (*G*) noncontrast axial head CT scan and (*H*) axial contrast head CT scan demonstrate a 12-mm, hyperdense aneurysm with homogeneous enhancement (white arrow) with a calcified wall (small white arrow) at the A2 segment of the left anterior cerebral artery. *Giant cavernous carotid aneurysm:* (*I*) axial noncontrast head CT scan and (*J*) axial contrast head CT scan show a 3-cm-diameter, hyperdense aneurysm (arrow) with homogeneous enhancement at the cavernous segment of the right internal carotid artery.

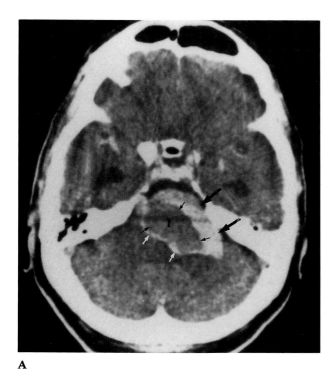

A

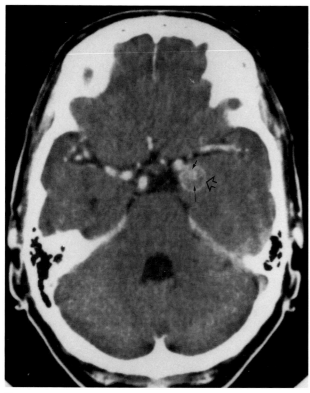

B

ple.[53] A superficial AVM can be pial, dural, or mixed. A pial AVM derives its blood supply from branches of the internal carotid or vertebrobasilar system. A dural AVM is supplied by the meningeal system, the external carotid artery, and muscular branches of the vertebral artery. A mixed AVM has a combination of the two types of blood supply. An ependymal AVM occurs on the ventricular surface and may penetrate the brain for a variable distance. Anatomical specimens show a nidus of vascular channels supplied by a variable number of dilated arteries and drained by multiple dilated veins. The interstitial neural tissue within the AVM usually shows gliosis and is largely nonfunctional. The patient's symptoms may be related to hemorrhage,[54] stealing of blood from normal brain structures,[55] and mass effect as well as resistance of drainage of the normal cerebral veins to the arterialization of drainage veins of the AVM.

A noncontrast head CT scan can detect the common pattern of a poorly defined area with both increased and decreased densities (Fig. 11-34), as well as mass effect in the areas of the AVM; it can also detect the acute hemorrhage. The low-density areas within the brain parenchyma observed in the mixed CT pattern most commonly represent atrophy, which is usually due to ischemia resulting from vascular steal by the AVM. The areas of increased density in and around the site of an AVM that has not recently hemorrhaged may be due to vascular and/or parenchymal calcifications or to blood in the dilated vessels. An AVM that has never bled has approximately a 25% chance of bleeding within 15 years. If an AVM has bled once, the risk of rebleeding rises to 25% in 5 years, and if it has bled more than once, the risk of rebleeding is 25% each year.[54]

Since approximately 20–25% of AVMs cannot be identified on noncontrast head CT, contrast-enhanced head CT is recommended to complete the CT evalua-

Fig. 11-27 Head CT scans of two patients with thrombosed aneurysms. (*A*) Contrast head CT scan shows a basilar artery aneurysm with thrombosis (large black arrow = patent basilar artery with enhancement, small black arrows = thrombosed aneurysm without enhancement, white arrows = enhanced wall of the thrombosed aneurysm). (*B*) Contrast head CT scan shows a partially thrombosed aneurysm of the left posterior communicating artery (small black arrow = patent lumen with enhancement, larger black arrow = thrombosed portion of the aneurysm without enhancement, open black arrow = enhanced wall of the aneurysm).

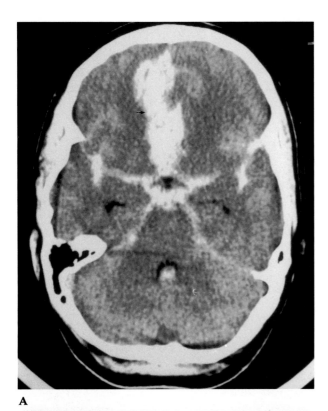

A

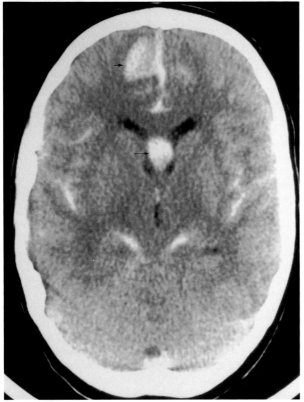

B

tion of AVMs. Most AVMs are heterogeneous, with a serpiginous, tubular, or linear pattern of enhancement, occasionally associated with diffuse or nodular enhancement on the contrast-enhanced head CT study (Fig. 11-35). The patterns of contrast enhancement are more likely to represent the central vascular nidus and adjacent draining veins (larger vessels), as well as the feeding arteries (smaller vessels). Although approximately 25% of AVMs have aneurysms on feeding arteries,[56] it is difficult to determine with CT alone whether aneurysms to be present with AVMs because the feeding arteries tend to be tortuous. Contrast-enhanced head CT may fail to demonstrate enhancement of the AVMs when they are thrombosed or are in a dural location.

Venous Angioma

Venous angioma[57] consists of a cluster of radially oriented, dilated medullary veins of the normal brain that drain into a single dilated, transparenchymal vein which empties into a cortical vein, dural sinus, or deep venous system. No abnormal arterial component is present. There is no nidus. The venous angioma probably represents pathways of collateral or alternate venous drainage resulting from fetal venous occlusions or underdevelopment of the medullary venous structures in the sixth to ninth week of fetal life. With the advent of CT and MRI, venous angioma has been found to be probably the most common anomaly of the intracranial vasculature demonstrated on neuroimaging studies and is usually an incidental finding of little clinical relevance.[57–59] Some reports[60–62] have suggested that patients with venous angioma are at considerable risk for parenchymal intracranial hemorrhage. Several authors[63–65] have reported the association of cryptic vascular malformations and venous angiomas; the former are responsible for hemorrhage.

Fig. 11-28 Noncontrast head CT scan of a 32-year-old female with acute rupture of an anterior communicating artery aneurysm. (*A*) At the suprasellar cistern level, there is diffuse subarachnoid hemorrhage in the suprasellar cistern, sylvian fissure cistern, basal cistern, fourth ventricle, interhemispheric fissure cistern, and right frontal lobe (arrow). (*B*) At the level of the frontal horns of the lateral ventricle, there is diffuse subarachnoid hemorrhage in the anterior interhemispheric fissure cistern, bilateral sylvian fissure cistern, and quadrigeminal plate cistern. Hemorrhage is also seen in the right frontal lobe (small arrow) and in the fornix (arrow).

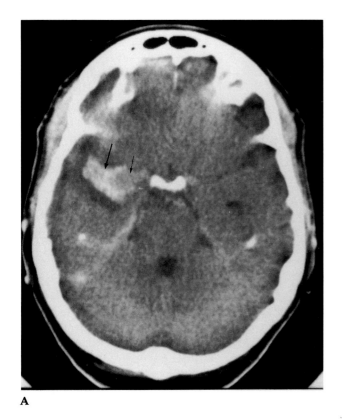

A

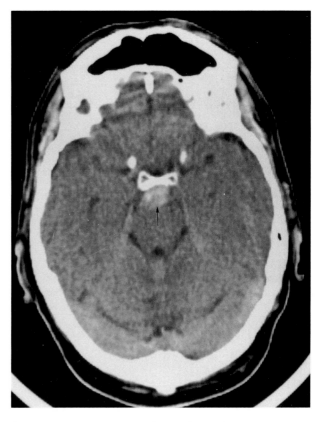

Fig. 11-30 Nonaneurysmal prepontine cistern subarachnoid hemorrhage. Noncontrast head CT scan of a 59-year-old male with acute onset of severe headache shows a large focal area of subarachnoid hemorrhage in the prepontine cistern (arrow). Cerebral arteriogram fails to demonstrate an aneurysm.

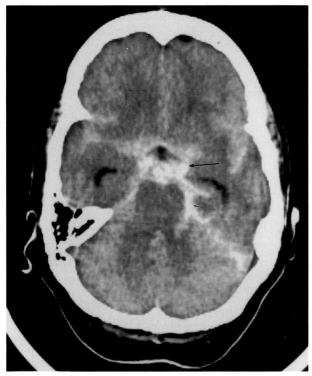

B

Fig. 11-29 (*A*) Noncontrast head CT scan of a 62-year-old female with rupture of the right middle cerebral artery shows a right temporal lobe hemorrhage (arrow) which is denser than the aneurysm (small arrow). (*B*) Noncontrast head CT scan of a 62-year-old female with rupture of a left posterior communicating artery aneurysm. There is more subarachnoid hemorrhage in the suprasellar cistern (arrow) and Ambien's cistern (small arrow) on the left side. There is faint subarachnoid hemorrhage in the bilateral sylvian fissure cisterns, as well as blood clots in the fourth ventricle. There is dilatation of the temporal horns of the lateral ventricle suggesting early obstructive hydrocephalus.

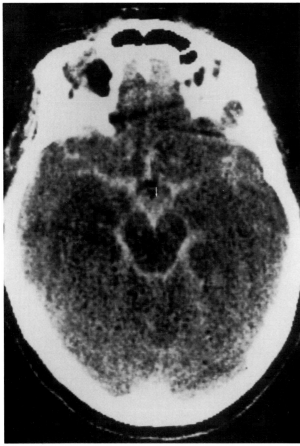

A

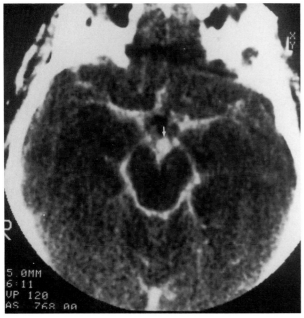

B

Venous angiomas are most frequently solitary but can be multiple. They can occur anywhere on the brain; favored sites include the frontal lobes and the posterior fossa. They are typically unilateral, although bilateral ones have been reported, particularly in the posterior fossa.[66] Noncontrast head CT may show a linear or punctate, faint, hyperdense lesion in the brain (Fig. 11-36). The contrast head CT scan shows a linear or curvilinear focus of enhancement with a "Medusa's head" appearance (Fig. 11-36), typically coursing from the deep white matter to a cortical or deep vein or to a dural sinus.[67] Occasionally, a nodular area of hyperdensity is seen on the noncontrast head CT study, with faint enhancement or an area of nodular enhancement following contrast administration.[68]

Sturge-Weber syndrome is a phakomatosis characterized by a facial vascular nevus in the territory of the trigeminal nerve. Intracranially, patients with Sturge-Weber syndrome consistently have venous angiomatosis of the leptomeninges. The meningeal abnormality is found most commonly in the anterior occipital lobe, with variable extension to the posterior parietal and temporal lobes.[69] The intracranial lesion is usually ipsilateral to the nevus, but contralateral and bilateral lesions have also been described.[70] Calcifications are frequently noted in the brain parenchyma adjacent to the leptomeningeal abnormality; they can be demonstrated on a noncontrast head CT study (Fig. 11-37). Pathologically, these calcifications occur in a pericapillary distribution, usually in the fourth layer of the atrophied cerebral cortex (which can be seen on a noncontrast head CT scan) and are thought to be related to chronic tissue hypoxia.[69] Contrast head CT may show postictal cortical enhancement or abnormal venous drainage and an enlarged choroid plexus. Direct visualization of venous angiomas is seldom possible on a contrast head CT scan but can be seen clearly on Gadopentetate dimeglumine-enhanced T_1-weight MRI images.[71]

Fig. 11-31 Rupture of a basilar artery aneurysm. (*A*) Noncontrast head CT scan and (*B*) contrast head CT scan show diffuse subarachnoid hemorrhage. A 9-mm aneurysm at the tip of the basilar artery (arrow) is well identified on the contrast head CT scan as a rounded, homogeneously enhanced area in the interpeduncular cistern. The aneurysm is less dense than the subarachnoid hemorrhage on the noncontrast head CT scan.

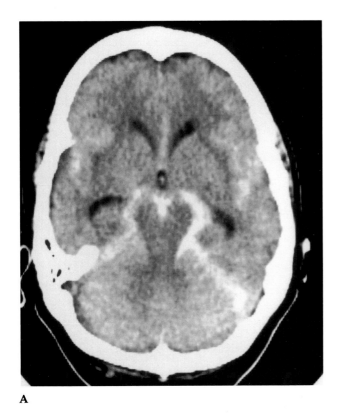

A

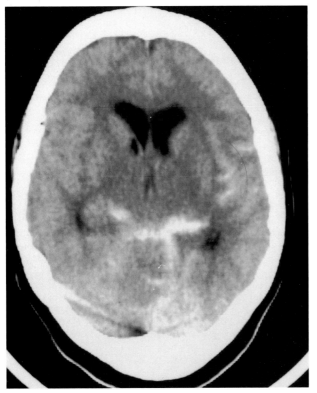

B

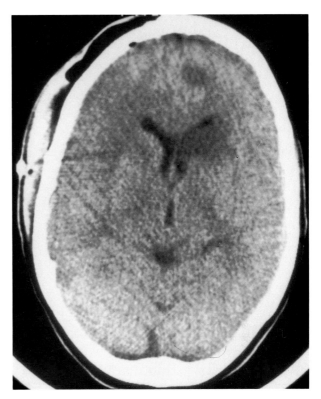

Fig. 11-33 Noncontrast head CT scan of a 20-year-old female in coma after surgical clipping of an acutely ruptured anterior communicating artery aneurysm shows diffuse, decreased density in the right frontal and parietal opercula, as well as in the left basal ganglia and left frontal lobe, consistent with acute ischemic infarction.

Fig. 11-32 A noncontrast head CT scan of a 62-year-old female with acute rupture of a left posterior communicating artery aneurysm. Noncontrast head CT scan at the levels of the midbrain (A) and of the lateral ventricles (B) shows diffuse subarachnoid hemorrhage in the perimesencephalic cisterns and faint subarachnoid hemorrhage in the bilateral sylvian fissure cistern. There is moderate dilatation of the temporal and frontal horns of both lateral ventricles, as well as in the third ventricle, suggesting early obstructive hydrocephalus. Blood clot is also seen in the third ventricle. Lacunar infarction is seen involving the head of the caudate nucleus on the right.

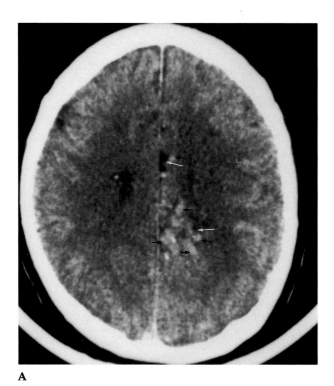

A

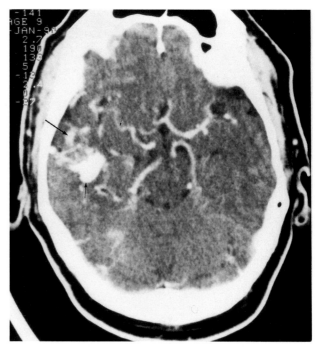

Fig. 11-35 Contrast head CT scan of a 40-year-old female with AVM of the right temporal lobe shows a large nodular enhancement (arrow) representing a nidus, a larger tubular enhancement representing the draining veins (larger arrow), and a small tubular enhancement representing the arterial feeder (small arrow).

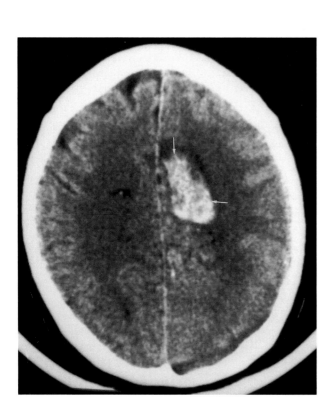

B

Fig. 11-34 A 63-year-old male with seizure. (*A*) Noncontrast head CT scan shows a poorly defined area of mixed increased (black arrows) and decreased (white arrows) densities in the left frontoparietal region representing a parenchymal AVM. (*B*) Noncontrast head CT scan 4 days later, on acute onset of severe headache, shows parenchymal hemorrhage (white arrows) in the left frontal lobe at the anterior aspect of the AVM.

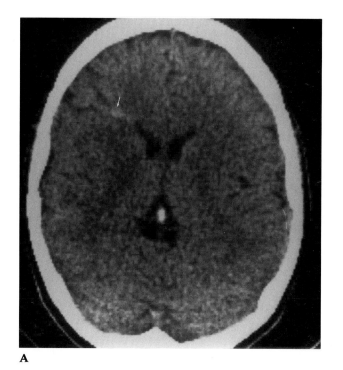

A

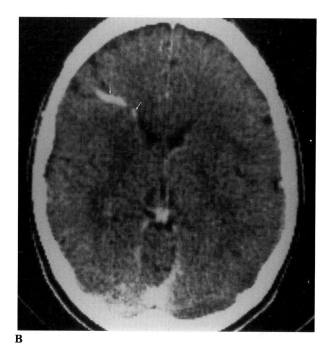

B

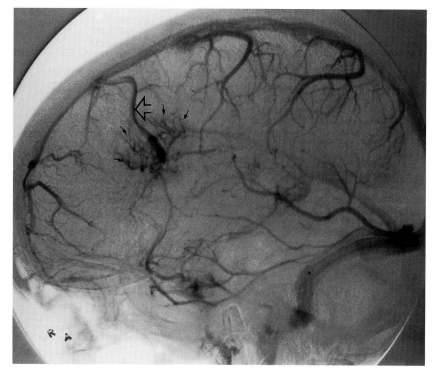

C

Fig. 11-36 *Case 1: Right frontal venous angioma.* (*A*) Noncontrast and (*B*) contrast head CT scans show a hyperdense, densely enhanced venous angioma (arrow) with the appearance of Medusa's head in the right frontal lobe. (*C*) Lateral view of the venous phase of the right internal carotid arteriogram shows dilated medullary veins (small arrows) drained to a large cortical vein (open arrow) and then drained to the superior sagittal sinus.

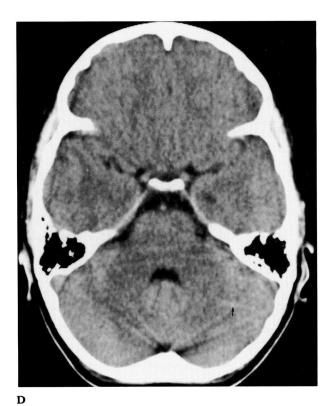

D

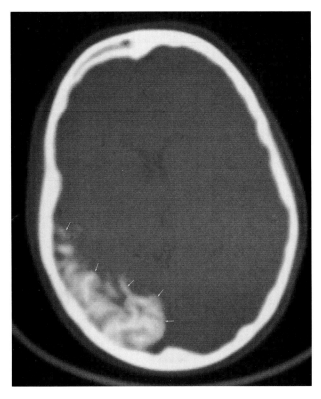

Fig. 11-37 Noncontrast head CT scan of a patient with Sturge-Weber syndrome shows dense calcifications of the right parieto-occipito-temporal region (arrows).

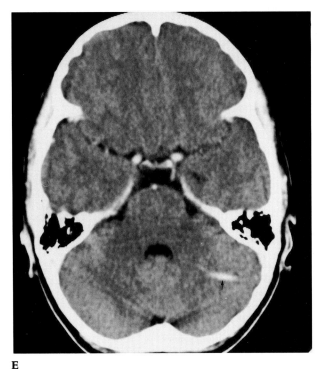

E

Fig. 11-36 *Case 2: Left cerebellar venous angioma.* (*D*) Noncontrast and (*E*) contrast head CT scans show a linear, faint, hyperdense, densely enhanced venous angioma (arrow) in the left cerebellum which appears to drain to the left sigmoid sinus.

Cavernous Angioma

Cavernous angiomas of the brain consist of endothelium-lined sinusoidal spaces without intervening neural tissue. Their walls have no muscular or elastic tissue. They may be familial[72] and can be multiple as well as solitary. Hemorrhages in different stages of evolution are commonly present. Noncontrast head CT shows a dense parenchymal lesion (Fig. 11-38A) that produces no mass effect and enhances with intravenous administration of contrast (Fig. 11-38B).[73] Granular calcifications radiating from the center of the lesion can be seen on the noncontrast head CT scan.

Capillary Hemangiomas/Telangiectasias

Capillary hemangiomas/telangiectasias are small vascular spaces lined by a single layer of endothelium. Normal neural tissue can be found interspersed between the small vascular spaces. The feeding arteries and draining veins are typically normal in size. The pons is the most common location. Multiple lesions are

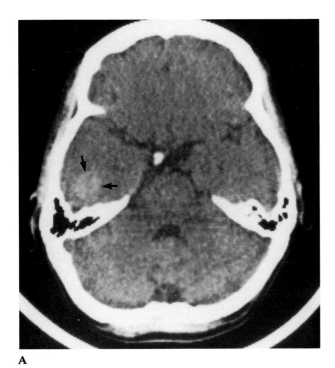

A

B

Fig. 11-38 CT scan of a patient with surgically proven cavernous angioma in the right temporal lobe. (*A*) Noncontrast and (*B*) contrast head CT scans show a parenchymal calcified lesion in the right temporal lobe (arrows) with dense enhancement (arrows). There is no associated mass effect or edema.

relatively common. They are usually clinically silent but may produce symptoms when they bleed. Noncontrast head CT usually cannot detect the lesions; however, contrast head CT may show minimal to moderate enhancement of them. The lesions are almost always undetectable on cerebral angiography. MRI is usually more useful for detecting capillary hemangiomas/telangiectasias because it is very sensitive to hemosiderin from a prior hemorrhage.

REFERENCES

1. Wang AM, Lin JCT, Rumbaugh CL. What is expected of CT in the evaluation of stroke? *Neuroradiology* 1988;30: 54–58.

2. Hecht ST, Eelkema EA, Latchaw RE. Cerebral ischemia and infarction in Latchaw RE (ed): MR and CT Imaging of the head, neck, and spine. St. Louis, Mosby Year Book, 1991, pp. 145–169.

3. Wodarz R. Watershed infarctions and computed tomography: A topographical study in cases with stenosis or occlusion of the carotid artery. *Neuroradiology* 1980; 19(5):245–248.

4. Brown JJ, Hesselink JR, Rothrock JF. MR and CT of lacunar infarcts. *AJNR* 1988;9:477–482.

5. Hart RG, Easton JD. Hemorrhagic infarcts. *Stroke* 1986; 17:586–589.

6. Hornig CR, Dorndorf W, Agnoli AL. Hemorrhagic infarction—a prospective study. *Stroke* 1986;17:179–185.

7. Bozzao L, Angeloni U, Bastianello S, et al. Early angiographic and CT findings in patients with hemorrhagic infarction in the distribution of the middle cerebral artery. *AJNR* 1991;12:1115–1121.

8. Gomori JM, Grossman RI, Goldberg HI, et al. Intracranial hematoma: Imaging by high field MR. *Radiology* 1985; 157:87–93.

9. Hecht-Leavitt C, Gomori J, Grossman RI. High field MRI of hemorrhagic cortical infarction. *AJNR* 1986;7: 581–585.

10. Lee Y, Mosei R, Bruner JM, et al. Organized intracerebral hematoma with acute hemorrhage: CT, patients and pathological correlations. *AJR* 1986;147:111–118.

11. Weingarten K. Computed tomography of cerebral infarction. *Neuroimag Clin North Am* 1992;2(3):409–419.

12. Houser OW, Campbell JK, Baker HL, et al. Radiologic evaluation of ischemic cerebrovascular syndromes with emphasis on computed tomography. *Radiol Clin North Am* 1982;20:123–142.

13. Inoue Y, Takemoto K, Miyamoto T. Sequential computed tomography scans in acute cerebral infarction. *Radiology* 1980;135:655–662.

14. Wall SD, Brant-Zawadzki M, Jeffrey RB, et al. High fre-

quency CT findings within 24 hours after cerebral infarction. *AJNR* 1981;2:553–557.

15. Truwit CL, Barkovich AJ, Gean-Marton A, et al. Loss of the insular ribbon: Another early CT sign of acute middle cerebral artery infarction. *Radiology* 1990;176:801–806.

16. Bryan RN, Levy LM, Whitlow WS, et al. Diagnosis of acute cerebral infarction: Comparison of CT and MR imaging. *AJNR* 1991;12:611–620.

17. Katzman R, Casen R, Klatzo I, et al. 1V. Brain edema in stroke. *Stroke* 1977;8:512–540.

18. Millikan CH, McDowell F, Easton JD. General pathology and neuropathology of stroke, in Millikan CH, McDowell F, Easton JD (eds): *Stroke*. Philadelphia, Lea & Febiger, 1987, pp 33–44.

19. Kuroiwa T, Seida M, Tomida S, et al. Discrepancies among CT, histological and blood–brain barrier findings in early cerebral ischemia. *J Neurosurg* 1986;65:517–524.

20. Pressman BD, Tourje EJ, Thompson JR. An early CT sign of ischemic infarction: Increased density in a cerebral artery. *AJNR* 1987;8:645–648.

21. Tomsick TA, Brott TG, Chambers AA, et al. Hyperdense middle cerebral artery sign on CT: Efficacy in detecting middle cerebral artery thrombosis. *AJNR* 1990;11:473–477.

22. Goldberg HI, Lee SH. Stroke, in Lee SH, Rao KCVG (eds): *Cranial Computed Tomography and MRI*, ed 2. New York, McGraw-Hill, 1987, pp 643–716.

23. Kendall BE, Pullicino P. Intravascular contrast injection in ischemic lesions. 11. Effect on prognosis. *Neuroradiology* 1980;19:241–243.

24. Pullicino P, Kendall BE. Contrast enhancement in ischemic lesion. 1. Relationship to prognosis. *Neuroradiology* 1980;19:235–239.

25. Grossman CB. Cerebrovascular disorders, in Grossman CB (ed): *Magnetic Resonance Imaging and Computed Tomography of the Head and Spine*. Baltimore, Williams & Wilkins, 1991, pp 145–183.

26. Becker H, Desch H, Hacker H, et al. CT fogging effect with ischemic cerebral infarcts. *Neuroradiology* 1979;18:185–192.

27. Kuhn MJ, Hohnson KA, Davis KR: Wallerian degeneration: Evaluation with MR imaging. *Radiology* 1988;168:199–202.

28. Bousser MG, Chiras J, Bories J, et al. Cerebral venous thrombosis—a review of 38 cases. *Stroke* 1985;16:199–213.

29. Buonanno FS, Moody DM, Ball MR, et al. Computed cranial tomographic findings in cerebral sinovenous occlusion. *J Comput Assist Tomogr* 1978;2:281–290.

30. Rao KC, Knipp HC, Wagner EJ. Computed tomographic findings in cerebral sinus and venous thrombosis. *Radiology* 1981;140:391–398.

31. Eick JJ, Miller KD, Bell KA, et al. Computed tomography of deep cerebral venous thrombosis in children. *Radiology* 1981;140:399–402.

32. Gabrielson TO, Seeger JF, Knake JE, et al. Radiology of cerebral vein occlusion without dural sinus occlusion. *Radiology* 1981;140:403–408.

33. Zilkha A, Stenzler SA, Lin JH. Computed tomography of the normal and abnormal superior sagittal sinus. *Clin Radiol* 1982;33:415–425.

34. Virapongse C, Cazenave C, Quisling R, et al. The empty delta sign: Frequency and significance in 76 cases of dural sinus thrombosis. *Radiology* 1987;162:779–785.

35. Goldberg AL, Rosenbaum AE, Wang H, et al. Computed tomography of dural sinus thrombosis. *J Comput Assist Tomogr* 1989;10:16–20.

36. Sekhar LN, Hervas RC. Origin, growth and rupture of saccular aneurysms (a review). *Neurosurgery* 1981;8:248–260.

37. Chason JL, Hindman WM. Berry aneurysms of the circle of Willis: Results of a planned autopsy study. *Neurology* 1958;8:41–44.

38. Jellinger K. Pathology and aetiology of intracranial aneurysms, in Pia HW, Langmaid L, Zierski J (eds): *Advances in Diagnosis and Therapy*. New York, Springer, 1979, pp 5–19.

39. Ferguson GG. Physical factors in the initiation, growth, and rupture of human intracranial saccular aneurysms. *J Neurosurg* 1972;37:666–677.

40. Campbell GJ, Roach MR. Fenestrations in the internal elastic lamina at bifurcations of human cerebral arteries. *Stroke* 1981;12:489–496.

41. McCormick WF, Acosta-Rua GJ. The size of intracranial saccular aneurysm: An autopsy study. *J Neurosurg* 1970;33:422–427.

42. McKissock W, Richardson A, Walsh L, et al. Multiple intracranial aneurysms. *Lancet* 1964;1:623–631.

43. Schmid U, Steiger HJ, Huber P. Accuracy of high resolution computed tomography in direct diagnosis of cerebral aneurysms. *Neuroradiology* 1987;29:152–159.

44. Kendall BE, Lee BCP, Claveria E. Computerized tomography and angiography in subarachnoid hemorrhage. *Br J Radiol* 1976;49:483–501.

45. Hayward RD, O'Reilly GVA. Intracerebral hemorrhage: Accuracy of computerized transverse axial scanning in predicting the underlying etiology. *Lancet* 1976;1:1–4.

46. Yuichi I, Saiwai S, Miyamoto T, et al. Postcontrast computed tomography in subarachnoid hemorrhage from ruptured aneurysms. *J Comput Assist Tomogr* 1981;5:341–344.

47. Ghoshhajra K, Scotti L, Marasco J, et al. CT detection of intracranial aneurysm in subarachnoid hemorrhage. *AJR* 1979;132:613–616.

48. Liliequist B, Lindquist M, Valdimarsson E. Computed to-

mography and subarachnoid hemorrhage. *Neuroradiology* 1977;14:21–26.

49. Lim ST, Sage DJ. Detection of subarachnoid blood clot and other thin, flat structures by computed tomography. *Radiology* 1977;123:79–84.

50. Rinkel GJE, Wijdicks EFM, Vermenlen M, et al. Nonaneurysmal perimesencephalic subarachnoid hemorrhage: CT and MR patterns that differ from aneurysmal rupture. *AJNR* 1991;12:829–834.

51. Yuichi I, Shigeo S, Takeshi M, et al. Postcontrast computed tomography in subarachnoid hemorrhage from ruptured aneurysms. *J Comput Assist Tomogr* 1981;5(3): 341–344.

52. McCormick WF. The pathology of vascular "arteriovenous" malformations. *J Neurosurg* 1966;24:807–816.

53. Forster DMC, Steiner L, Hakanson S. Arteriovenous malformation of the brain. A long term clinical study. *J Neurosurg* 1972;37:562–568.

54. Marks MP, O'Donahue J, Fabricant JI, et al. Cerebral blood flow evaluation of arteriovenous malformations with stable xenon CT. *AJNR* 1988;9:1167–1175.

55. Newton TH, Troost BT. Arteriovenous malformations and fistulae, in Newton TH, Potts DG (eds): *Radiology of the Skull and Brain*. St Louis, CV Mosby, 1974, p 2512.

56. Saito Y, Kobayashi N. Cerebral venous angiomas. Clinical evaluation and possible etiology. *Radiology* 1981;139: 87–94.

57. Rothfus WE, Albright AL, Casey KF, et al. Cerebellar venous angioma: Benign entity. *AJNR* 1984;5:61–66.

58. Garner TB, Curling OD Jr, Laster DW. The natural history of intracranial venous angiomas. *J Neurosurg* 1991; 75:715–722.

59. Maehara T, Tasaka A. Cerebral venous angioma: Computerized tomography and angiographic diagnosis. *Neuroradiology* 1978;16:296–298.

60. Wendling LR, Moore JS, Kieffer SA, et al. Intracerebral venous angioma. *Radiology* 1976;119:141–147.

61. Malik GM, Morgan JK, Boulos RS, et al. Venous angio-

mas: An underestimated cause of intracranial hemorrhage. *Surg Neurol* 1988;30:350–358.

62. Sasaki O, Tanaka R, Koike T, et al. Excision of cavernous angioma with preservation of coexisting venous angioma. *J Neurosurg* 1991;75:461–464.

63. Goulao A, Alvarez H, Garcia Monarco R, et al. Venous anomalies and abnormalities of the posterior fossa. *Neuroradiology* 1990;31:476–482.

64. Rigamonti D, Spetzier D. The association of venous and cavernous malformations: Report of four cases and discussion of pathophysiological, diagnostic and therapeutic implications. *Acta Neurochir (Wien)* 1988;92:100–105.

65. Hacker DA, Latchaw RE, Chou SN, et al. Bilateral cerebellar venous angioma. *J Comput Assist Tomogr* 1981;5: 424–426.

66. Olson E, Gilmor RL, Richmond B. Cerebral venous angiomas. *Radiology* 1984;151:97–104.

67. Sordet D, Beroud P, Pharaboz C, et al. Angioma veineux cerebral aspects angiographique et tomo denis tometrique. *J Radiol* 1986;67:285–287.

68. Coulam CM, Brown LR, Reese DF. Sturge-Weber syndrome. *Semin Roentgenol* 1976;11:55–60.

69. Boltshauser E, Wilson J, Hoare RD. Sturge-Weber syndrome with bilateral intracranial calcification. *J Neurol Neurosurg Psychiatry* 1976;39:429–435.

70. Elster AD, Chen MYM. MR Imaging of Sturge-Weber syndrome: Role of gadopentetate dimeglumine and gradient-echo techniques. *AJNR* 1990;11:685–689.

71. Rigamonti D, Hadley MN, Drayer BP, et al. Cerebral cavernous angiomas: Incidence and familial occurrence. *N Engl J Med* 1988;319:343–347.

72. Soviardo M, Strata L, Passerini A. Intracranial cavernous hemangiomas: Neuroradiologic review of 36 operated cases. *AJNR* 1983;4:945–950.

73. Baker DH, Townsend JJ, Kramer RA, et al. Occult cerebrovascular malformations: A series of 18 histologically verified cases with negative angiography. *Brain* 1979; 102:279–287.

12

Neurodiagnostic Applications of Spiral Computed Tomography

Richard B. Schwartz, M.D.

INTRODUCTION

Intrinsic pathology of the cervical and intracranial vasculature, such as carotid stenosis or intracerebral aneurysms, constitutes an important risk factor for the development of intracerebral infarcts or hemorrhage. Such abnormalities are most reliably evaluated using conventional angiography, but that technique is associated with a complication rate of approximately 3% in the general population.[1] Consequently, radiologists have pursued the development of noninvasive methods for evaluating neurovascular anatomy. Duplex sonography provides accurate flow-related information of the carotid bifurcation, but provides limited spatial information and is presently of little value for the intracranial vasculature. Magnetic resonance angiography (MRA) provides accurate imaging of the cervical and intracranial vessels, but a significant number of patients cannot undergo successful MRA examinations owing to anxiety or obesity or, more important, because of the presence of indwelling electromechanical or metallic devices.

Spiral computed tomography (CT) is a recently developed imaging technique in which a patient is scanned while being drawn through the gantry of the CT scanner, resulting in an uninterrupted volume of data which can be reconstructed to produce a three-dimensional representation of CT information (Fig. 12-1). If imaged at an appropriate time after the intravenous injection of contrast material, the cervical or intracranial vasculature may be selectively studied. In this chapter, the technique of spiral CT will be discussed, followed by the consideration of specific neuroradiological applications.

GENERAL METHODS

Spiral CT requires installation of new CT equipment or upgrading of existing hardware and software. We are using the Siemens Somatom Plus or Plus-S CT scanner system (Siemens Medical Systems, Iselin, NJ), but the majority of CT manufacturers now offer spiral capability. For a typical spiral protocol, an intravenous catheter is placed in an antecubital vein, and the patient is placed supine on the CT table. A lateral topogram is obtained through the area of interest, and the starting point of the spiral acquisition is chosen. A nonenhanced baseline scan may be obtained by scanning while the patient is withdrawn through the scanner. These data are stored, and then another scan is performed at a standard time (we use 20 sec) after intravenous injection of a bolus of contrast material; we use 75 cc of Hypaque 60 or Omnipaque 240 (Sanofi Winthrop, New York) at a rate of 2.5 cc/sec. The velocity of the table feed determines the effective slice thickness.

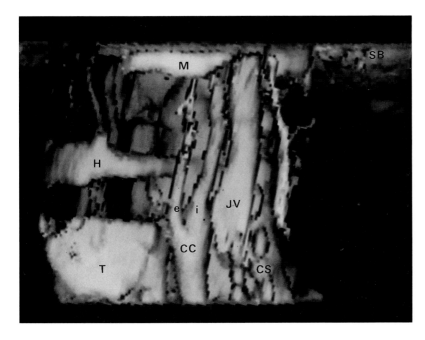

Fig. 12-1 Three-dimensional reconstruction of cervical region. Lateral projection from the three-dimensional reconstruction of an enhanced spiral CT scan prior to postprocessing shows the left common carotid artery bifurcation (CC); the internal (i) and external (e) carotid arteries are demonstrated. The left jugular vein (JV) is partially opacified from above. Various bony and cartilaginous structures such as the mandible (M), hyoid bone (H), thyroid cartilage (T), cervical spine (CS), and skull base (SB) are also shown.

Slower table speeds give a tighter spiral with greater resolution in the z-axis but a smaller volume covered relative to faster table speeds. The duration of the scan determines the total volume of the data set, but this is limited by the amount of heat produced by the x-ray tube during the continuous exposure necessary during the spiral acquisition. With available machinery, scan durations of up to 40 sec are now possible.

The spiral data acquired must then be reconstructed to provide three-dimensional representations of the vasculature. First, the surrounding bony structures must be removed from each image by manual subtraction techniques. The remaining information is then reconstructed using either of two software algorithms; the shaded-surface rendering (SSR) or the maximum-intensity projection (MIP) technique. SSR provides a high-resolution rendition of the vasculature, but with this technique, calcification has the same appearance on the SSR as does the intraluminal contrast; this may require additional data manipulation using a workstation with customized segmentation software to separate calcification from the enhancement within the vessel. In MIP reconstructions, attenuation values in the final reconstructed image more accurately reflect those in the axial images; thus, calcium is easily distinguished from intraluminal contrast, but the image is somewhat less sharp than with SSR. For purposes of display, reconstructions are filmed in 15° intervals of rotation in all three planes.

Carotid Stenosis

For spiral CT of the carotid bifurcation, a topogram of the cervical spine is obtained and the C6 vertebral body is localized. A gantry tilt parallel to the disc space is used routinely unless artifact from dental hardware requires the gantry to be angled several degrees. The CT table is then withdrawn through the gantry, using a table speed of 4 mm/sec; scanning is performed beginning at the mid-C6 level (165 mA, 125 kVp, 24 sec continuous exposure, depending on the equipment, 4 mm collimation), resulting in a three-dimensional volume acquisition of approximately 9.6 cm. This nonenhanced scan serves two purposes: it provides a means to identify calcium within the vessel wall prior to contrast injection, and it gives the exact localization of the bifurcations (a point located midway between the two bifurcations is assigned as the center for the contrast-enhanced scan). For the enhanced scan, the patient is withdrawn through the scanner 20 sec after the onset of an intravenous injection using a power injector (75 cc of Hypaque 60% or Omnipaque 180, 2.5 cc/sec); it is imperative that patients remain motionless and not swallow during the scans. In most cases, spiral CT is performed using a 2-mm/sec table feed velocity starting at a table position 2.4 cm below the predetermined center and using 2-mm collimation. This covers a distance of 4.8 cm if a scan duration of 24 sec is used to 9.6 cm if a scan duration of 40 sec is used. If a larger

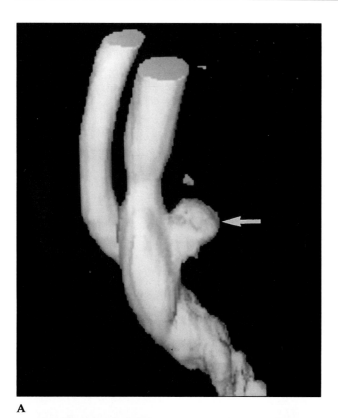

A

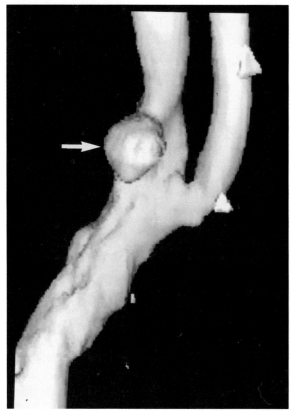

B

volume of data is needed, a 4 mm/sec table velocity will cover twice the distance. The 2-mm sections are reconstructed at 1-mm increments. In both the SSR and MIP algorithms, each axial image must be edited prior to the three-dimensional reconstruction. Regions of interest are drawn around the adjacent bony structures and jugular veins, and these are erased. In the SSR technique, the attenuation value of the intraluminal contrast at the vessel's narrowest point is used to determine the lower threshold for data exclusion. All pixels less than this value (usually 90–100 HU) are automatically removed, leaving only the enhanced carotid bifurcation in the image. This information is then automatically reconstructed to produce a three-dimensional SSR. This process requires approximately 30 min for both carotid arteries and results in a highly accurate representation of the carotid bifurcation (Fig. 12-2).

Because of the inability to distinguish easily calcium from the intravascular contrast column using SSR, however, the MIP protocol is now the technique of choice to reconstruct the carotid vessels. Since calcification within plaques can be differentiated from the contrast-filled lumen, rotating the vessel in various planes usually allows the stenosis to be judged accurately, without the need for additional reconstruction in most cases (Fig. 12-3). If calcium completely surrounds an arterial structure and impedes visualization of the underlying vessel contour, additional postprocessing using a workstation and segmentation software may be required (Fig. 12-4). We have used a Sun workstation (Sun Microsystems, Mountain View, CA) with customized segmentation software[2] to allow automatic differentiation of calcification from enhancing arterial structures on the basis of attenuation differences. This requires approximately an additional 30 min of postprocessing time for each carotid artery if performed by a technologist familiar with the Sun workstation. Reference to cross-sectional images may be helpful in evaluating the true lumen diameter in the presence of calcium.

In our study of 40 carotid bifurcations using SSR

Fig. 12-2 Carotid bifurcation using SSR reconstruction; demonstration of ulcer arising from the internal carotid artery. Later (*A*) and anteroposterior (*B*) views from spiral CT reconstruction obtained using the SSR program show a large ulcer of the left internal carotid artery (arrow). Note the irregularity of the distal common carotid artery caused by calcium of attenuation similar to that of the contrast column surrounding the vessel.

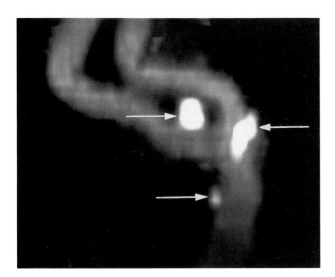

Fig. 12-3 Carotid bifurcation using MIP reconstruction. Lateral view from spiral CT reconstruction obtained by using the MIP reconstruction protocol shows small flecks of calcium (arrows) discernible from the intraluminal contrast.

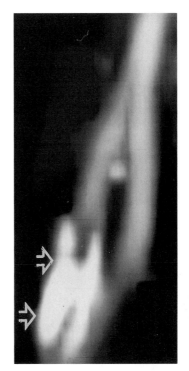

A

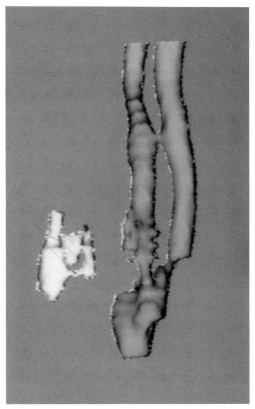

B

presented previously,[3] we estimated the severity of stenosis and compared these rankings to those determined using intra-arterial digital subtraction angiograms, duplex ultrasound examinations, and MRA images. We found that the results of spiral CT correlated with those of contrast angiography in 93% of cases, with ultrasound in 97% of carotids, and with MRA in 100%. Indeed, spiral CT performs better than MRA in patients with tortuous vessels; on MRA, in-plane flow can result in loss of signal and overestimation of stenoses; however, since there are no flow-related artifacts on CT, these vessels can be imaged accurately with the spiral technique (Fig. 12-5). Other advantages of spiral CT over MRA include its rapidity, as well as its safety in patients with indwelling MRA-incompatible devices. On the other hand, the presence of calcium may result in inaccurate depictions of stenosis severity using spiral

Fig. 12-4 Differentiation of calcification from the carotid bifurcation using MIP and the Sun workstation. (A) Lateral projection of a spiral CT MIP reconstruction using the Siemens protocol shows a large, irregular mass of calcium surrounding the distal common carotid artery and proximal internal carotid artery (arrows). The intraluminal contrast column is concealed by the calcification. (B) Lateral projection of a spiral CT reconstruction obtained using the Sun workstation segmentation program separates calcium (white) from the enhancing lumen of the internal carotid artery (red).

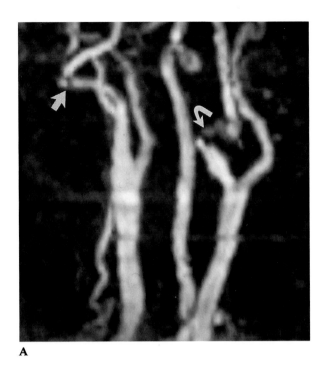

A

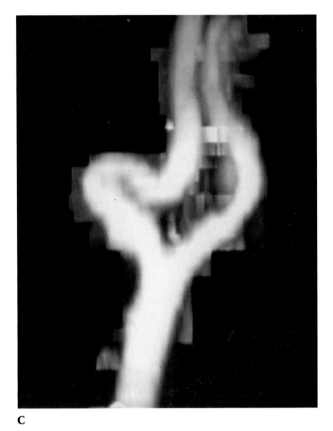

C

Fig. 12-5 Carotid bifurcations demonstrated more accurately by spiral CT than by MRA. (A) Two-dimensional time-of-flight angiogram obtained in the right anterior oblique (RAO) projection shows tortuous internal carotid arteries bilaterally, with loss of signal in the proximal portion of the right (straight arrow) and left (curved arrow) internal carotid arteries. On this study, it is unclear whether this is due to stenosis or an in-plane flow phenomenon. Spiral CT of the right (B) and left (C) carotid bifurcations in the lateral projection shows the internal carotid arteries to be tortuous but completely patent.

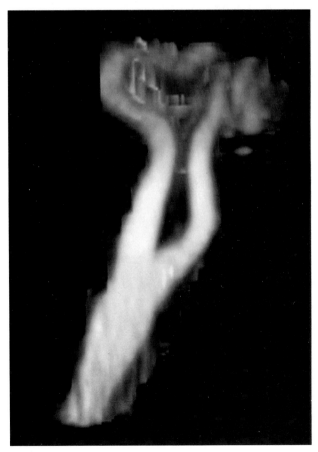

B

CT. There is a tendency for small flecks of calcium to blend in with the contrast column, resulting in slight underestimation of stenosis; conversely, removal of calcium from the image may remove neighboring pixels, which may result in overestimation of stenosis. Thus, as with MRA, correlation with another noninvasive test is always suggested if surgery is considered. We consider MRA or spiral CT to be adequate to provide anatomical detail of the bifurcation, although Doppler ultrasound is essential to determine the flow dynamics at the stenosis. These tests, used in conjunction, can provide the surgeon with the necessary information required to operate.

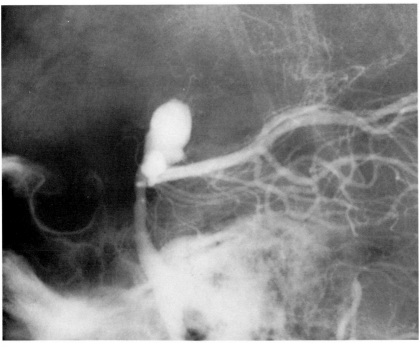

A

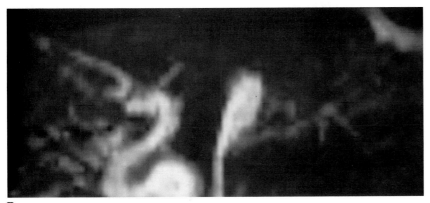

B

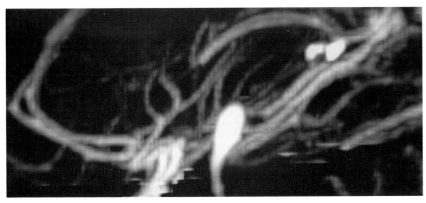

C

Fig. 12-6 Conventional angiography, MRA, and spiral CT in aneurysm assessment. Lateral views of a conventional angiogram (vertebral injection, *A*), MRA (*B*), and spiral CT using the MIP reconstruction algorithm (*C*) show a basilar tip aneurysm 9 mm in the greatest dimension.

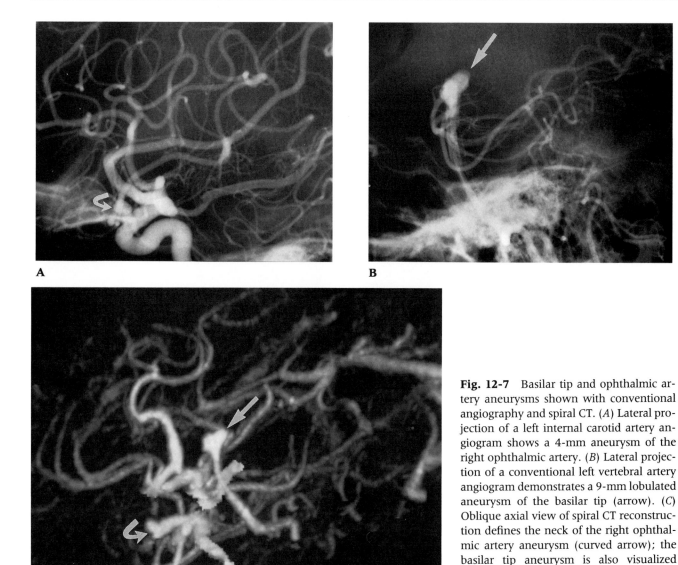

A

B

C

Fig. 12-7 Basilar tip and ophthalmic artery aneurysms shown with conventional angiography and spiral CT. (*A*) Lateral projection of a left internal carotid artery angiogram shows a 4-mm aneurysm of the right ophthalmic artery. (*B*) Lateral projection of a conventional left vertebral artery angiogram demonstrates a 9-mm lobulated aneurysm of the basilar tip (arrow). (*C*) Oblique axial view of spiral CT reconstruction defines the neck of the right ophthalmic artery aneurysm (curved arrow); the basilar tip aneurysm is also visualized (straight arrow).

It is very important that the operator follow the prescribed protocol in acquisition of the spiral data and reconstruction of the images. Appropriate timing of the scan relative to the contrast bolus is essential so that the carotid bifurcation is maximally opacified at the time of scanning; the table speed must be slow enough to provide sufficient anatomical detail; the jugular vein must be edited from the axial images prior to reconstruction so that the carotid vessels can be viewed without obstruction; a workstation should be employed, if possible, to extract calcium from the bifurcation; and axial images should be used in the interpretation of the scan, especially if calcium obscures the bifurcation.

Failure to follow these guidelines may result in unsatisfactory studies.[4]

Intracranial Aneurysms

The protocol for spiral CT of the intracerebral vessels is similar to that for the carotid bifurcation. Following placement of an intravenous catheter, a topogram of the head is obtained. A gantry tilt along the orbitomeatal line is used, and a starting point is selected at the base of the sella turcica. Imaging is started 20 sec after the intravenous injection of 75 cc of contrast using a power injector at a rate of 2.5 cc/sec. The CT table is

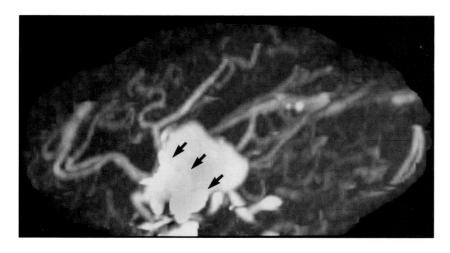

Fig. 12-8 Lateral projection of a spiral CT shows a giant (3 × 3 × 2 cm) aneurysm of the left internal carotid artery bifurcation; note the calcium within the walls of this aneurysm (small black arrows).

withdrawn through the gantry at a velocity of 2 mm/sec while scanning is performed (165 mA, 125 kVp, 32- or 40-sec continuous exposure, 2-mm collimation). This results in a three-dimensional volume acquisition of approximately 6.4 or 8.0 cm. The 2-mm sections are reconstructed at 1-mm increments. The bony structures at the skull base are excluded from the axial images, and the resulting data are reformatted using MIP. Images are displayed as a series of projections rotated at 15° intervals in three planes.

We have studied 24 aneurysms in 16 patients with conventional angiography, MRA, and spiral CT. We found that spiral CT and MRA were equivalent in their ability to delineate the location, contour, and neck of intracranial aneurysms (Fig. 12-6). With both techniques, all of the aneurysms larger than 3 mm were seen, whereas none of the aneurysms measuring less than 3 mm were demonstrated on either the three-dimensional reformatted images or the axial source images.[5] Rotating the reconstructed images in space allows the information to be viewed from virtually any perspective in order to display vascular anatomy to maximal advantage (Fig. 12-7). Saccular (Figs. 12-6, 12-7), giant (Fig. 12-8), and fusiform (Fig. 12-9) aneurysms are well demonstrated with this technique.

Spiral CT offers several advantages over MRA in the evaluation of aneurysms. Most important, the conspicuity of aneurysms on CT is dependent on the volume, not the flow rate, of contrast; hence, there are no flow-related artifacts to interfere with visualization of aneurysms, as may occur with MRA (Fig. 12-10). Calcification within the walls of aneurysms is clearly delineated with CT (Figs. 12-11, 12-12); this may be of surgical importance since the presence of calcium in

the aneurysm neck can increase the difficulty of clipping the aneurysm. Also, thrombus within aneurysms may be appreciated on spiral CT (Fig. 12-13). The relationship of the aneurysm to surrounding bony structures also is well defined on CT, and this can influence the surgeon's approach.

Spiral CT has some disadvantages relative to MRA

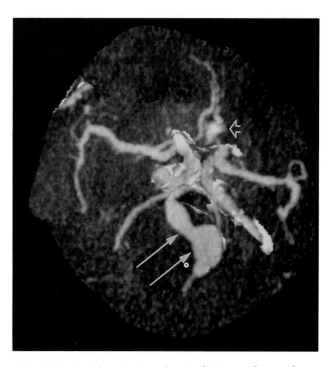

Fig. 12-9 Axial projection of a spiral CT scan shows a large, fusiform aneurysm of the right vertebrobasilar confluence (arrows). A smaller aneurysm of the anterior cerebral artery is also seen (arrowhead).

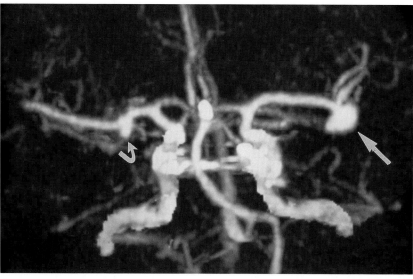

A

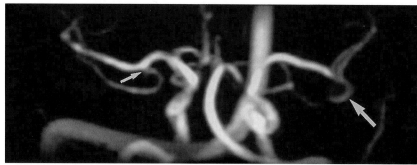

B

Fig. 12-10 Bilateral middle cerebral artery aneurysms studied with spiral CT and three-dimensional phase contrast (PC) MRA. (*A*) AP view of a spiral CT reconstruction demonstrates a lobulated aneurysm of the left middle cerebral artery (MCA) bifurcation, 12 mm in the largest dimension (large arrow), and a 3-mm aneurysm of the right MCA bifurcation (small arrow). (*B*) AP view of a three-dimensional PC MRA does not clearly identify the lumen of either the left MCA (large arrow) or the right MCA (small arrow) aneurysm.

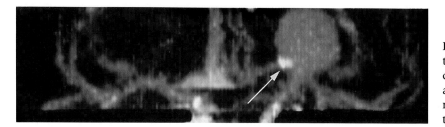

Fig. 12-11 Demonstration of calcium in the wall of an internal carotid artery bifurcation aneurysm by spiral CT. AP view of a spiral CT scan shows a large MCA aneurysm and a small focus of calcium within the aneurysm wall (arrow).

in the evaluation of intracranial aneurysms. Postprocessing is necessary, generally taking 40–60 min in the hands of an experienced technologist. However, since there are no venous structures of any significance to obscure the circle of Willis, and since vascular calcifications are generally sparse distal to the intracavernous carotids, it is only necessary to delete the anterior and posterior clinoids and the lesser sphenoid wing from the axial images; a workstation generally is not neces-

sary. However, small aneurysms at the skull base also may be more difficult to define with spiral CT than with MRA due to bony artifact. Similarly, evaluation of intracavernous internal carotid artery aneurysms may be limited by partial volume effects from surrounding bony structures and calcifications in the vessel wall or from venous opacification of the cavernous sinuses; however, aneurysms in this location are not usually considered amenable to resection.

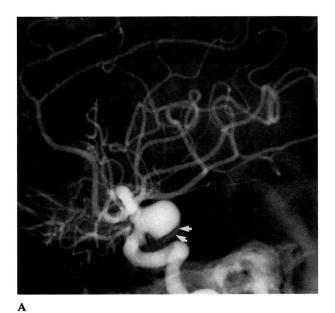

A

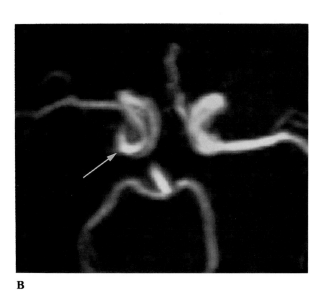

B

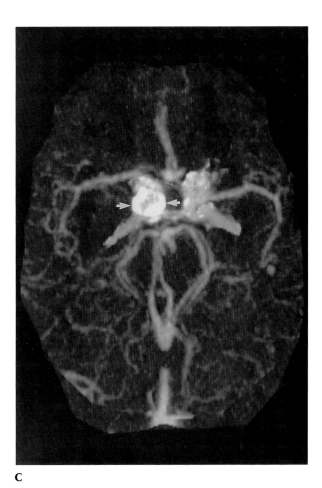

C

Fig. 12-12 Calcified aneurysm shown by spiral CT. (*A*) Lateral view of a conventional angiogram shows calcium in the margin of a left posterior communicating artery aneurysm. (*B*) Axial view of a three-dimensional time-of-flight MRA shows high signal in the periphery of the aneurysm (arrow) but does not demonstrate either the aneurysm lumen or calcification in its walls. (*C*) An axial view of a spiral CT reconstruction shows the dense calcium surrounding the internal carotid artery aneurysm (arrows), as well as its contrast-filled lumen.

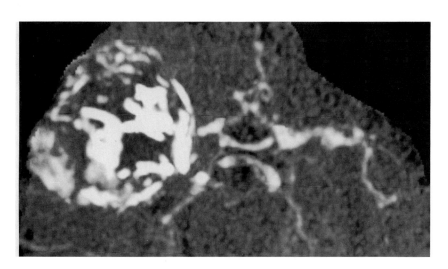

Fig. 12-13 Thrombosed, calcified giant right MCA aneurysm imaged on three-dimensional PC MRA and spiral CT. (*A*) Axial projection of a reconstructed spiral CT shows a 5-cm thrombosed aneurysm of the right MCA, with dense collections of calcium in the wall of the aneurysm.

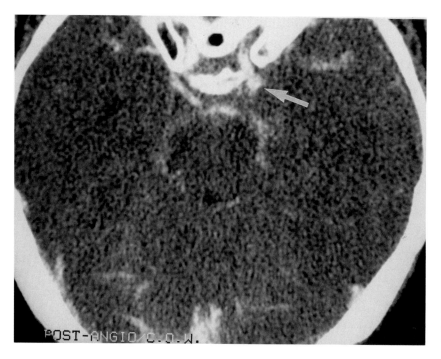

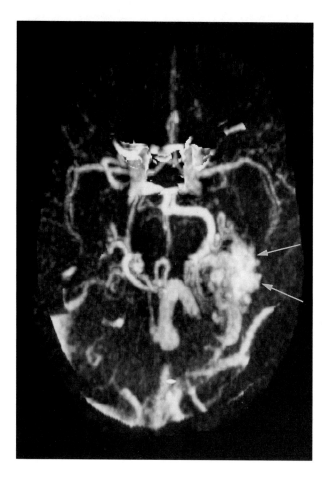

Fig. 12-14 Subarachnoid hemorrhage obscuring an aneurysm on CT. An axial CT image shows a small aneurysm of the left posterior cerebral artery (arrow) partially obscured by subarachnoid blood after rupture.

Another relative disadvantage of spiral CT is the possibility that subarachnoid blood may obscure an aneurysm owing to the similarity in attenuation of blood and contrast material (Fig. 12-14). Thus, spiral CT may be of limited usefulness soon after aneurysm rupture; however, the short T1 of hemorrhage also may obscure an aneurysm on three-dimensional time-of-flight MRA, and a patient with a subarachnoid hemorrhage may be too unstable to cooperate for the time required to obtain an MRA. Thus, conventional angiography is likely to remain the procedure of choice in the setting of subarachnoid hemorrhage.

The postoperative patient presents a special challenge. Although neither spiral CT nor MRA is likely to be useful in the evaluation of clip placement due to metallic artifact, these techniques may be used to determine the presence of other aneurysms. Spiral CT and MRA may both be limited due to artifact, depending on the location of the clip to the other arterial structures; however, CT can be performed in all postoperative patients without risk, whereas recent guidelines militate against using MRA in any patient after aneurysm clip-

Fig. 12-15 AVM shown by spiral CT. Axial projection of a spiral CT scan shows a 3-cm AVM of the posteromedial left temporal lobe (arrows) supplied by the left posterior cerebral artery. Drainage is via the straight sinus.

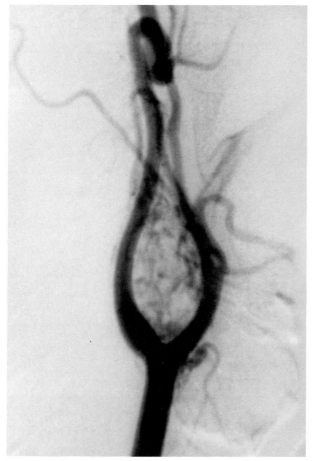

A

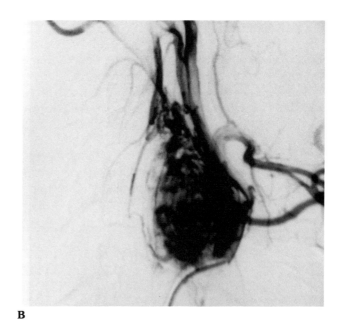

B

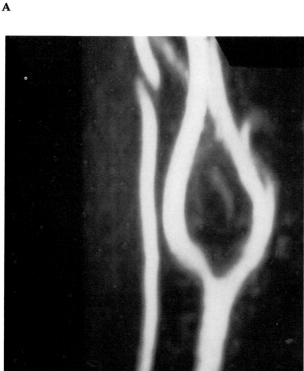

C

D

Fig. 12-16 Carotid body tumor demonstrated by angiography, MRA, and spiral CT. (*A*) Lateral view of a right common carotid conventional angiogram shows an enhancing mass within the carotid bifurcation splaying the internal and external carotid arteries. (*B*) Lateral view of a right external carotid angiogram shows the vascular nature of this carotid body tumor supplied by branches of the external carotid artery. (*C*) Lateral view of a two-dimensional time-of-flight MRA shows the right carotid bifurcation to be splayed by a mass, but the nature of the lesion is not apparent. (*D*) Lateral view of a spiral CT scan shows the carotid body tumor nestled within the carotid bifurcation.

ping without absolute assurance of the composition of the clip.

Spiral CT provides information similar to that of MRA with respect to aneurysm location and structure, and in some ways is superior to MRA. However, as with the evaluation of the carotid vessels, spiral CT of aneurysms should be treated as an adjunct to other noninvasive imaging techniques and should not be considered a replacement for conventional angiography at present.

Miscellaneous Applications

Spiral CT may prove useful in a variety of other intracranial applications. Arteriovenous malformations (AVMs) are usually well seen on spiral CT (Fig. 12-15), although several issues limit the utility of this technique in the primary evaluation of all AVMs. The complete evaluation of large AVMs and their venous drainage would require that the entire cranial vault be studied; this, in turn, would necessitate the use of a rapid table velocity, with resultant decreased resolution in the z-axis. Also, due to rapid shunting into the venous system, both arterial and venous components are visualized essentially simultaneously. We feel that the main usefulness of spiral CT in the evaluation of AVMs is in the follow-up of treated malformations; in this scenario, the location and maximum size of the lesion would be known already, so that spiral CT could be performed through the area of interest and the volume of the nidus measured over successive scans obtained at intervals before and after therapy.

Carotid body tumors (chemodectomas) also are well visualized on spiral CT, and this technique appears to be better suited for evaluating these lesions than does MRA. Flow through these vascular tumors is too slow to be visualized on two-dimensional time-of-flight angiography; however, these carotid body tumors are well seen on spiral CT as an enhancing mass nestled within the splayed carotid bifurcation (Fig. 12-16).

Intracranial thrombosis or stenosis can also be evaluated using spiral CT (Fig. 12-17); moreover, since flow rate is not as important an issue in CT as it is in MRA, spiral CT may prove to be more sensitive than MRA in distinguishing between slow flow and total thrombosis. Spiral CT also may prove useful in evaluating arterial encasement by tumor (Fig. 12-18). In all of these applications, spiral CT should not be considered a replacement for conventional angiography, but it is well suited as an alternative to MRA for initial screening and follow-up.

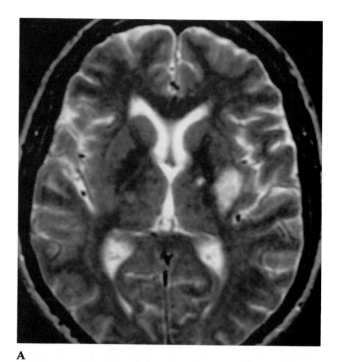

A

B

Fig. 12-17 Focal stenosis of MCA shown by spiral CT. (*A*) Axial T$_2$-weighted MRA image shows an infarct of the left posterior putamen and a smaller infarct of the left internal capsule. (*B*) An axial view of a three-dimensional reconstruction shows focal narrowing of the proximal left MCA at the origin of the lenticulostriate vessels (arrow).

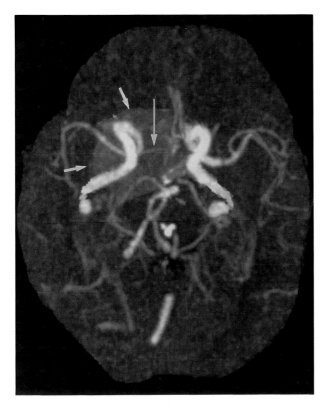

Fig. 12-18 Encasement of the right MCA shown by spiral CT. An axial view of a spiral CT reconstruction shows circumferential narrowing of the A1 segment of the right anterior cerebral artery (long arrow) due to encasement by a large pituitary adenoma (small arrows).

CONCLUSIONS

Spiral CT is a reliable, reproducible, and easily performed examination which is virtually equivalent to MRA in accuracy and provides additional information which complements angiography. This technique is well suited as a screening test for carotid stenosis or intracranial aneurysms, particularly in patients who cannot tolerate an MRA examination due to anxiety, body size, or the presence of MRA-incompatible implanted devices. In addition, spiral CT takes less time and is less expensive than MRA.

Disadvantages of spiral CT over other noninvasive imaging techniques include the requirement of an intravenous contrast injection and ionizing radiation, as for any enhanced CT, although it requires less contrast and a small radiation dose per scan than does a standard head CT. The conspicuity of calcium and bone in the CT image is both an advantage and a disadvantage; demonstration of these densities may be of benefit to the surgeon, but anatomical details may be obscured. Software advances which will allow the automatic exclusion of structures with very high attenuation (i.e., calcium and bone) from the images are in development. With continued refinements in spiral CT equipment, more accurate images will become possible. We envision an important role for spiral CT in the noninvasive evaluation of the cervical and intracranial vasculature.

REFERENCES

1. Earnest F, Forbes G, Sandok BA, et al. Complications of cerebral angiography: Prospective assessment of risk. *AJR* 1984;142:247–253.
2. Kikinis R, Jolesz FA, Gerig G, et al. 3D morphometric and morphologic information derived from clinical brain MR images. NATO ASI Series, Vol F60, 1990;441–454.
3. Schwartz RB, Jones KM, Chernoff DC, et al. Evaluation of the common carotid artery bifurcation using spiral CT. *Radiology* 1992;185:513–519.
4. Castillo M. Diagnosis of disease of the common carotid artery bifurcation: CT angiography vs. catheter angiography. *AJR* 1993;161:395–398.
5. Schwartz RB, Tice HM, Hooten SM, et al. Evaluation of cerebral aneurysms with helical CT: correlation with conventional angiography and magnetic resonance angiography. *Radiology* 1994;192:717–722.

13

Principles of Magnetic Resonance Imaging

Anil N. Shetty, Ph.D., John E. Kirsch, Ph.D.

INTRODUCTION

The introduction of magnetic resonance imaging (MRI) in medicine has opened a new era in diagnostic interpretation of various disease processes in the human body. Over the years, MRI has steadily increased its ability to provide superior image quality in terms of tissue contrast. Compared to other modalities such as x-ray and computed tomography (CT), MRI has the obvious advantages of being noninvasive and eliminating the use of ionizing radiation. Because of its high tissue contrast, lack of side effects, multiplanar imaging capability, and high patient acceptability, it has become the modality of choice.

MRI uses a hydrogen nucleus or proton as a probe to image tissue characteristics. The superior sensitivity and natural abundance of hydrogen make it the nucleus of choice. The signal characteristic of a tissue is based on the concentration of hydrogen and its intrinsic properties under the action of magnetic and gradient fields.

The development of MRI dates back to the early work in nuclear magnetism in solids by Gorter in 1936.[1] The existence of magnetic moment, which is a key to obtaining the magnetic resonance signal, was first demonstrated by Rabi and colleagues at Columbia University in 1938.[2] The first successful demonstrations of the magnetic resonance signal were done independently by Purcell and coworkers at Harvard[3] and by Bloch and coworkers at Stanford.[4] Much of the early work by the above investigators determined nuclear induction by subjecting the spin system to an intense, short radiofrequency power. Subsequent theoretical treatment by Torreys[5] and practical applications by Hahn[6] formed the beginning of pulsed nuclear magnetic resonance (NMR).

The early NMR experiments were performed in solids and polymers to determine the structural details of molecular arrangement in various samples. The chemical shift was key to obtaining spectral information on individual species. The idea of using a Fourier transform to obtaining the multiline spectra by Ernst and Anderson[7] revolutionized the way NMR spectroscopy was done, and a new form of high-resolution spectroscopy was created. The transition from spectroscopy to imaging was based on ideas by Lauterber,[8] who showed that by intentionally varying the magnetic field, spatial encoding can be achieved. This formed the basis for MRI. Since then, several different approaches to MRI have been proposed. The vast majority of scanners currently use the spin-warp imaging technique to perform MRI.

This chapter introduces the reader to MRI, beginning with the fundamental concepts of NMR experiments.

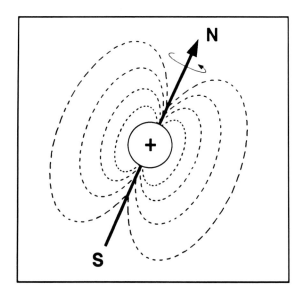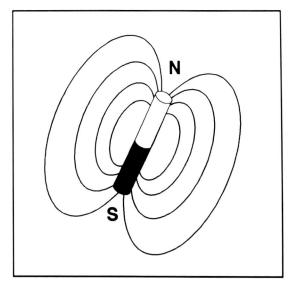

Fig. 13-1 The presence of magnetic moment in a proton results in a magnetic field surrounding the proton in a way similar to a simple bar magnet. However, there is a major difference between the two situations: the angular momentum possessed by the proton moment resulting in a precessional motion when placed in an external magnetic field.

MACROSCOPIC PROPERTIES OF NUCLEAR MAGNETISM

Nuclear Magnetic Moment

Protons and neutrons constitute the nucleus of an atom. The proton is a positively charged particle, whereas the neutron is a neutral particle. The electric charge of the proton is distributed and rotates around a central axis. In some nuclei, electric charges are distributed asymmetrically, causing these nuclei to behave as magnetic dipoles.[9-11] It is known from classical mechanics that a mass undergoing circular motion about a fixed point in a plane has a classical angular momentum.

In addition, these charges spin around their own axes, and the total angular momentum is a result of the orbital and spinning motion of the charges. The combined motion provides a total angular momentum, which, in turn, produces a magnetic dipole moment that is proportional to the net angular momentum.[12,13] As shown in Fig. 13-1, a single proton acts like a tiny magnet with a magnetic dipole moment; this key concept is fundamental to an understanding of the magnetic resonance phenomenon.

The strength of the magnetic moment is a property of the type of nucleus and determines the detection sensitivity of the magnetic resonance experiment. Not all nuclei have a magnetic moment. Each nuclear species (isotope), being composed of different numbers of protons and neutrons, has its own total angular momentum. Furthermore, depending on these values and on the nuclear charge, there may be a strong magnetic moment or no moment whatsoever. Also, nuclei with a net spin produce a resonance signal, and those without a net spin do not produce any resonance signal. Nuclei with an even number of protons and an even number of neutrons have no intrinsic spin. For example, ^{12}C, with six protons and six neutrons, does not possess spin and therefore produces no NMR signal, whereas ^{13}C does produce NMR signal. Hydrogen (^{1}H) generates one of the strongest magnetic moments and is abundant biologically; it is therefore the nucleus of choice for MRI.

Nuclei in a Static Magnetic Field

Basic physical properties of the nuclear magnetic moment in the presence of a magnetic field are best understood using a vector description. A vector in space describes both direction and magnitude. A spatial coordinate system is established to specify the orientation and magnitude of a vector. Thus, a vector in a two-dimensional $(x:y)$ or three-dimensional $(x:y:z)$ coordinate system can be broken down into component vectors in the direction of the x-, y-, and z-axes by projecting the respective components of the vector along those axes. Thus, a system (such as a nucleus, consisting of many protons and neutrons which are directly or indirectly coupled together as a state of the nucleus) is defined collectively by its total angular momentum J and a magnetic moment μ.[13] These are vector quantities possessing both magnitude and direction, and they are parallel to each other. One can define a total magnetic moment in terms of total angular momentum:

$$\mu = \gamma J \qquad (13\text{-}1)$$

where γ is called the *gyromagnetic ratio,* which is a unique property of the nucleus and is used in comparing different species. For example, γ for ^{1}H is 2.67 $\times$ 10^8 radians/sec-Tesla or 42.58 MHz/Tesla.[11]

Motion of the Nuclear Magnetic Moment: Semiclassical Approach

Based on simple vector interpretation, the ^{1}H (or proton) magnetic moment may be described as behaving like a tiny bar magnet with north and south poles. However, the protons have an additional property that bar magnets do not have: angular momentum because of their spin. It is this property that causes magnetic moments to precess around in the direction of an externally applied magnetic field. This is analogous to a precessing top in a gravitational field. Classically, precessional motion can be explained as follows: a spinning top experiences torque due to the gravitational force which tends to make the top rotate, or precess, around the axis of the force. Similarly, when a nucleus possessing nonzero magnetic moment is placed in an external magnetic field B, the total angular momentum experiences torque due to an applied magnetic field and is given by[13–15]

$$\tau = \frac{dJ}{dt} = \mu \times B. \qquad (13\text{-}2)$$

The symbol "$\times$" in eq. 13-2 signifies the vector cross-product between μ and B. When a magnetic field is applied, the axis of the magnetic moment μ precesses around the applied magnetic field in such a way that the torque due to force from the applied magnetic field is counterbalanced by the spinning proton. This will form a conical region of rotation around the axis of the applied magnetic field. Equation 13-2 suggests that the change in angular momentum dJ is always perpendicular to $\mu(J)$ and B. The only way to describe this is if the magnetic moment precesses around the magnetic field B, forming a cone, as shown in Fig. 13-2. Thus,

when a nucleus with a nonzero magnetic moment μ is placed in an external magnetic field B, the magnetic moment vector precesses around the direction of the magnetic field with an angular frequency based on the angle between μ and B. This type of precession is called the *Larmor precession,* and the precessional rate (frequency) is given by[10,15]

$$\omega = \gamma B \qquad (13\text{-}3)$$

where γ and B have their usual meaning. Alternatively, one can explain precessional motion using a purely classical mechanical description. The change in energy resulting from the rotation due to torque in the presence of a magnetic field can be determined using the classical expression for the change in potential energy. The assumption here is that the change in energy is zero when the magnetic moment is experiencing maximum torque (oriented perpendicular to the field). This energy is due to the rotation and is a completely rotational potential energy. One can calculate the energy required to rotate from its zero energy position to any angle. The change in energy is written as

$$\Delta E = \int_{90}^{\theta} \tau d\theta = \int_{90}^{\theta} \mu B \sin\theta \, d\theta$$
$$= -\mu \cdot B. \qquad (13\text{-}4)$$

For $\theta = 90°$, $\Delta E = 0$; for $\theta = 0°$, $\Delta E = -\mu B$; and for $\theta = 180°$, $\Delta E = \mu B$. The position of minimum energy occurs when the angle between the magnetic moment and the field is 0, while $\theta = 180°$ corresponds to a position of maximum energy.

Thus, when a nucleus with a nonzero magnetic moment is placed in a magnetic field, the magnetic moment tries to align with the field, putting the system into a state of minimum energy. Less than exact alignment results from a change in the rotational energy from its original value. In doing so, the system (nuclei) tries to dissipate the additional energy.[15] But since there is no process by which it can effectively do so, the tendency to dissipate energy results in a precessional motion around the magnetic field, keeping the angle θ and the change in energy fixed at some equilibrium.

The characteristic precessional frequency from the application of a given external magnetic field is different for different nuclei and is dependent on the gyromagnetic ratio γ. The γ factor for hydrogen nucleus is 42.58 MHz/Tesla. From eq. 13-3, for a hydrogen nucleus placed in a 1-Tesla magnetic field the frequency of precession is 42.58 MHz. Table 13-1 describes the

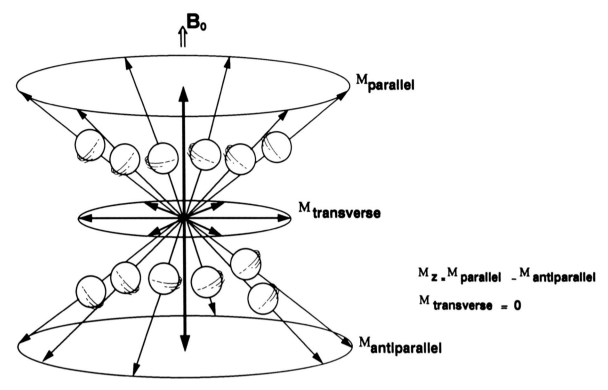

Fig. 13-2 A classic picture of proton moments when placed in a magnetic field. The difference between parallel and antiparallel components in the direction of magnetic field gives rise to the net magnetic moment or magnetization. However, due to random orientation of moments, the transverse component has no net effect due to cancellation among components in opposite directions.

TABLE 13-1 Magnetic Resonance Properties of Some Nuclei of Interest in the Human Body

Isotope	Spin	Natural Abundance (%)	Sensitivity Relative*	Sensitivity Absolute†	MR Frequency (MHz at a field of 1.5 Tesla)	Gyro-magnetic Ratio (MHz/Tesla)
^{1}H	$\frac{1}{2}$	99.980	1.00	1.00	63.87	42.58
^{13}C	$\frac{1}{2}$	1.108	1.59×10^{-2}	1.76×10^{-4}	16.07	10.71
^{19}F	$\frac{1}{2}$	100	0.83	0.83	60.075	40.05
^{23}Na	$\frac{3}{2}$	100	9.25×10^{-2}	9.25×10^{-2}	16.89	11.26
^{31}P	$\frac{1}{2}$	100	6.62×10^{-2}	6.62×10^{-2}	25.845	17.23
^{39}K	$\frac{3}{2}$	93.1	5.08×10^{-4}	4.73×10^{-4}	2.985	1.99

*At a constant field for an equal number of nuclei.
†Product of relative sensitivity and natural abundance. It is clear that hydrogen is the most abundant and also has the maximum sensitivity for a magnetic resonance study. Other nuclei with nonzero spins, however, will also contribute to the signal. Isotopes like ^{12}C and ^{16}O have zero net spin and therefore do not contribute to a resonance signal.

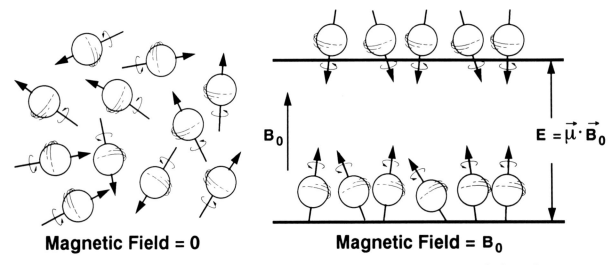

Fig. 13-3 A quantum mechanical view of spin moments when an external magnetic field is switched on. The excess moments are in a low-energy ground state. The difference between energy levels of occupation is given by μB_0.

γ factor for various nuclei and associated precessional frequencies at a constant magnetic field strength of 1.5 Tesla.[11]

Macroscopic Magnetization

Net magnetization is a vector sum of all individual proton magnetic moments that align in the direction of the external magnetic field. Thus, the state in which the proton magnetic moments exist becomes crucial in defining net magnetization. When describing the motion of an isolated nucleus at the atomic level, classical theory is inadequate in explaining the possible states in which spins exist. The net signal is based on the statistical distribution of precessing spins with their collective net vector in a specific orientation with the magnetic field. Classically, the magnetic moment can exist in any orientation with respect to the magnetic field. However, according to atomic and nuclear theory, and the quantum nature of the nucleus of a spinning moment, one assigns (based on transition selection rules) restricted and discrete orientations to the magnetic moment. This results in only certain states that a given nucleus can achieve during the precessional motion. For a nucleus with spin 1/2, such as hydrogen, there are only two possible states associated with two distinct levels of energy. For a nucleus with spin 3/2, there are four possible states in which spins can exist. In a classical description, the orientations for a nucleus with spin 1/2 may be thought to be restricted to parallel and antiparallel to the magnetic field's direction.[12]

In the absence of the external magnetic field, there is

no difference between spin states and all are randomly oriented in space. When these spins are placed in a magnetic field, they distribute themselves between the two states (in the case of proton spin magnetic moments) after a period of time. If spin magnetization vectors were distributed in equal amounts, there would be no net magnetization because all the vectors pointing in one direction (parallel) would cancel the effect of all the vectors pointing in the opposing direction (antiparallel). In reality, spins are distributed unequally, obeying Boltzmann's law of thermal distribution, as described in eq. 13-5a. Here the population of the two states will reach some equilibrium distribution such that spins in a state that is parallel to the magnetic field are slightly in excess of the remaining spins in a state that is anti-parallel. Figure 13-3 shows the distribution of spin moments when a magnetic field is applied.

$$\frac{N_{\text{antiparallel to the field}}}{N_{\text{parallel to the field}}} = e^{-\mu B/kT}. \qquad (13\text{-}5a)$$

The excess population defined as $n = (N_{\text{parallel}} - N_{\text{antiparallel}})$ is given by

$$n = N \frac{(e^{+\mu B/kT} - 1)}{(e^{+\mu B/kT} + 1)} \qquad (13\text{-}5b)$$

where $N = (N_{\text{parallel}} + N_{\text{antiparallel}})$, the total number of spin moments. The spins that are parallel to the magnetic field are at a lower energy state, whereas the spins that are antiparallel to the magnetic field are at a higher energy state. The Boltzmann distribution of these states increases with magnetic field strength. It is this excess of spins in the energy states which contributes to the net magnetization and the eventual magnetic resonance signal intensity. Thus, working at a higher field strength gives the advantage of having more protons contributing to the overall net magnetization, increasing the amount of potential signal.

For a sample at room temperature, from eq. 13-5b the excess population is only a small fraction and is about 3×10^{-6}. For a sample with a mass of 1 g, the total number of nuclei is on the order of 10^{23}, so the excess population is actually substantial. The population difference depends on the thermal temperature of the environment. Also, in the absence of any external field ($B = 0$), these spinning moments are randomly oriented, so the net magnetization is very small because the Earth's magnetic field is too weak to overcome the random motion caused by the thermal effects.

The net magnetic moment, or magnetization, per unit volume is

$$M_z = \mu \cdot n \qquad (13\text{-}6)$$

where n is the population difference (excess population) between the two allowed states of nuclei with spin $= 1/2$ and μ is the magnetic dipole moment. The z-direction given by convention to the applied field is arbitrary and can be associated with any physical direction. We will describe the magnetic resonance signal in terms of this magnetization that is present in a sample when placed in a magnetic field.

MAGNETIC RESONANCE PHENOMENON

Response of a Magnetization Vector to a Radiofrequency (RF) Field

In an externally applied magnetic field B, the collective magnetization from all proton moments at equilibrium will be aligned along the direction of the magnetic field, which we define as the z direction. Because the net magnetization of a system of spins in human tissue is aligned with the powerful external magnetic field along z, it is not possible to detect it as long as both are parallel to each other. The only measurable component will be a transverse, or xy, component of $M(M_{xy})$. Therefore, to produce a measurable NMR signal, the equilibrium magnetization must be tilted away from main magnetic

field's z direction. This is the principle behind NMR signal measurement.

Using quantum mechanical theory, it is possible to show that the signal emission is actually due to the transition of spins from an excited state to the ground state. The occurrence of such a transition is probable when the external stimulus is transverse or perpendicular to the direction of the main magnetic field. By applying a small, oscillating magnetic field B_1, in the transverse xy plane at a frequency that is exactly equal to the Larmor frequency of precession, one can stimulate spins from one orientation state to the other. This is called *resonance absorption*. The phenomenon is called *magnetic resonance*.[9-12]

Free Induction Decay and Resonance Signal

The transition of spins from a state of higher energy to one of lower energy is associated with the release of excess energy. The excess energy released is exactly the difference of the two spin energy states (ΔE) and is a specific line of finite frequency. To induce such a transition, an external energy source is first applied to cause resonance absorption. To observe an absorption/emission line, external energy in the form of a B_1 field has to be applied. One way to ensure proper coupling and energy exchange between a B_1 field and the precessing moments is to apply the B_1 field transverse to the equilibrium magnetization direction of the main external field B_0. In addition, maximum efficiency of energy transfer occurs when the B_1 field rotates at the same frequency as the Larmor precessional frequency. This ensures maximum torque on the precessing moments so that the orientation of moment is changed during the time the external energy source is applied. The effect of rotation depends on the frequency difference between B_1 frequency and the Larmor frequency. The larger this difference, the smaller the torque effect of B_1 on the magnetic moments. As shown in Fig. 13-4, the angle through which the magnetization rotates from its equilibrium position is called the *flip angle* and is given by

$$\alpha = \gamma B_1 \tau_p \qquad (13\text{-}7)$$

where γ is the gyromagnetic ratio, B_1 is the strength of the applied field, and τ_p is the duration of the B_1 field.[16]

Equation 13-7 shows that the flip angle is a function of the B_1 amplitude. How does this affect the transition between two spin states? As the energy is increased beyond the difference between energy states, does the transition still take place? This may appear to be con-

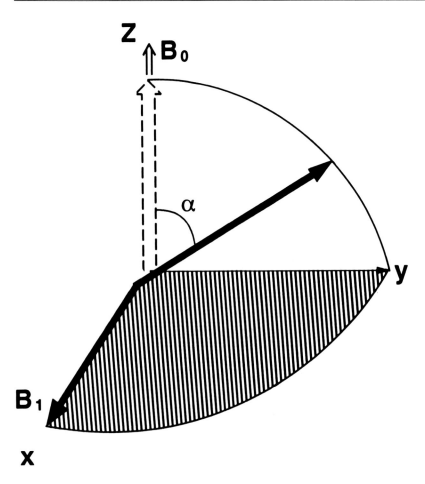

Fig. 13-4 The collection of excess moments that produce magnetization M in the direction of the main magnetic field B_0 is tipped away from the z-direction onto the x-y plane by an angle a due to the presence of a transverse B_1 field applied along the x-direction.

tradictory when we talk strictly in terms of the energy due to the B_1 field, which should be exactly the difference between the energies of the two allowed spin states. In actuality, it is the power of the B_1 field, or the rate of energy absorption by the spin moments in the low energy states, that determines the transition of the moments. It should be noted that the probability of transition is proportional to the square of the B_1 field. Therefore, the rate at which the energy is absorbed depends on the power due to the applied B_1 field. The probability of transition, however, increases as the B_1 amplitude is increased (more spins absorb the energy from the low-energy state and jump to the high-energy state) and will continue to do so as long as the probability is much less than the rate of transition back to their original state (a mode of energy relaxation). However, once the probability is large enough to equal the rate of relaxation, the absorbed energy levels off even though the probability increases. This effect on magnetic resonance is called *saturation*.[10]

Concept of the Rotating Frame

The concept of the rotating frame of reference simplifies our understanding of complex spin motion under the action of both a main field B_0 and the transverse oscillating field B_1.[17] The motion of spin moments under the action of two simultaneously applied fields is complicated. The spin moment vectors tend to spiral along the direction representing the resultant collective orientation of the two applied field directions. The precession is a result of torque exerted by a static B_0 field and an oscillating B_1 field. Due to the rapid precession of spin moments about the resultant field, any change in energy or frequency associated with the transition is very small compared with the total energy of the system E and the Larmor frequency. In fact, in NMR we are dealing with small changes which, in terms of frequency, are in the kilohertz range compared to the Larmor frequency, which is in the megahertz range. In order to simplify our understanding of the complex

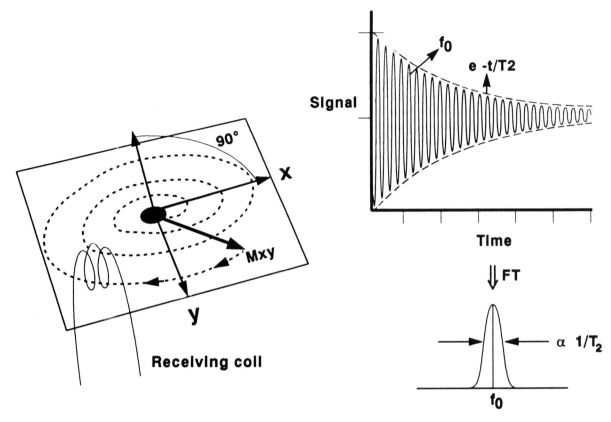

Fig. 13-5 The free induction decay of magnetization is shown in the form of an exponentially decaying signal. The decay is due to spin-spin interaction that causes random dephasing with an exponential modulation. The Fourier transform of such a monoexponentially decaying signal is centered on the resonance frequency, and the width of the line is determined by the relaxation time constant. Placing a suitably tuned and matched receiver coil in a plane where magnetization is maximum will pick up the signal based on a simple Faraday effect.

motion of spin moments, a simple coordinate transform of the measuring device to a reference frame that precesses at the Larmor frequency is made in which the effect of the main field B_0 is eliminated.

The oscillating field may be treated as a combination of two rotating component fields in which one rotates clockwise and the other counterclockwise. The resulting motion is a precession about both stationary and rotating field directions. A convenient way to observe this is to view the motion of magnetization vectors in a reference coordinate frame that is rotating at the Larmor frequency along the direction of one of the rotating components. In this frame, the magnetization vector would appear stationary to the observer. The other component of the oscillating field is at twice the Larmor frequency and will have no effect on the magnetization. By setting the coordinate frame of the detecting system at the Larmor frequency, any change above or below it may be detected easily as a spectral line in the audio frequency range (hertz to kilohertz).

When the applied B_1 field ceases, the resulting spin state transition process is called the *free induction decay,* or *FID* ("free" from any further external induction). The FID is received by placing an antenna (receive coil) at an angle to the magnetization where it will detect a maximum amplitude. Figure 13-5 shows the FID signal and its Fourier transform. It turns out that by placing the receiver coil in the transverse plane and rotating the magnetization to this plane (at an angle of 90° from the longitudinal), the maximum amplitude of the FID will be detected. The FID is a continuous and decaying signal damped by relaxation effects when the B_1 field is applied exactly on-resonance.

The relaxation effects influence the signal to behave exponentially during the FID. On the other hand, if B_1 is slightly off-resonance, the resulting FID will be an alternating sine or cosine wave with an exponential damping factor due to relaxation. The offset frequency is the rate at which the FID oscillates. In fact, when considering off-resonance magnetization in a rotating frame, the resulting magnetic field seen by this magnetization is not simply B_1 but a combination of a residual static B_0 field (due to off-resonance) and the B_1 field. The residual field exists because the effect of B_0 is not completely canceled. The proton magnetic moments then see an effective field which in a coordinate system rotating at $-\omega$ about the z-axis is given by

$$B_{\text{eff}} = z\left(B_0 - \frac{\omega}{\gamma}\right) + xB_1 \qquad (13\text{-}8)$$

where the effective field along the z direction is $[B_0 - (\omega/\gamma)]$ and is zero when the rotational frequency ω of the rotating coordinate system exactly equals γB_0. The flip angle of rotation is $\gamma B_{\text{eff}}\tau_p$, which is same as eq. 13-7 when ω equals γB_0. An easy way to view this is to take the Fourier transform of the FID. If B_1 was on-resonance, the Fourier transform of the FID yields a signal line centered on the Larmor frequency. If there was an off-resonance between B_1 and the Larmor frequency, the Fourier transform will yield a line shifted from the Larmor frequency by an amount equal to the offset value.

As seen above, the transformation to a rotating frame is equivalent to eliminating terms related to main magnetic field effects. A similar feature employed in communication electronics is called *demodulation*, which in principle has the same result. Therefore, the rotating frame concept is utilized the same way the detection system is used. The detection system frame of reference is matched with the Larmor frequency of the nuclei of interest. This is achieved by producing a carrier frequency for detection that is at the Larmor frequency. Any change in resonance frequency that occurs due to transition of spin moments will be small. Thus, the received signal will be a modulation of the carrier frequency by the offset frequency. The resulting offset frequency is detected as a difference between the received signal and that of the carrier frequency. Such a detecting system is called a *phase-sensitive detector*. By working exactly at resonance frequency, any deviation from the Larmor frequency is directly related to the frequency offset generated by the configuration of magnetization in the sample. For a sample containing nuclei in different molecular configurations, this technique of observing differences in offset frequency is used in NMR spectroscopy to identify the conformation of chemical shift frequencies. Because of the broad range of chemical shift frequencies, the B_1 field RF pulse must be quite broad in its frequency bandwidth to excite all chemical shift frequencies simultaneously.

In the time domain, such a pulse is very narrow and intense. On the other hand, in imaging, one should be able to excite a narrow band of frequencies for the excitation of a slice section. Here, a broader RF pulse is used in a time domain.

Nevertheless, it is important to note that although it is desirable to have all the protons in the human body resonate at the same frequency, it is not possible in reality and a broader rather than a narrower frequency band may be necessary. This could result from inhomogeneous frequency distributions within the system or from external effects such as field inhomogeneity. In both cases, the Larmor frequency at different parts of the human body could be either greater or less than the frequency of the B_1 field (detecting system) and must be kept broad enough to ensure proper excitation.

Relaxation Phenomenon

Relaxation is a process by which the excited proton spins return to their original state; it influences the signal intensity. The interest here is in observing the signal difference that exists between proton spin moments originating from different local molecular surroundings. The spins (nuclei) make a transition from a state of higher energy to one of lower energy by emitting excess energy in the form of RF electromagnetic radiation. In general, a spin can spontaneously make a transition (relaxation) or can be stimulated (excitation) to make a transition. Unlike optical transitions, the probability of spontaneous transitions is too small to be detected.

However, spins may be stimulated by an external B_1 field, causing first absorption of energy and then dissipation of this excess energy following a transition. The process of absorption is almost instantaneous due to very efficient coupling between the external B_1 source and the spins. When a single proton is placed in the magnetic field and is stimulated by a B_1 field to jump into an anti-parallel state, it may remain in that state for a long time (years) when the external stimulus is removed. The only way the excited proton spin would return to the original state (parallel to the static field) is by contact with a field at the same frequency. In the case of a bulk sample, such an external field is provided by several means, such as molecular motion or internal interactions among the protons themselves. Dissipation of the excess energy is most efficient when there is a local field fluctuating at the same frequency as that of the precessing nuclei. Due to efficient coupling with such fields, relaxation or energy transitions of the nuclei occur. The processes by which excess energy is dissipated are described by spin-lattice (T_1) and spin-spin (T_2) relaxation, and the mechanism is assumed to be in the form of a simple exponential. These mechanisms also describe how the components of magnetization behave after the B_1 field is turned off.

Detailed phenomenological equations of the motion and relaxation of magnetization based on experimental observation were first provided by Bloch and coworkers at Stanford and by Purcell and colleagues at Harvard. They were first described mathematically by Bloch in 1947.[4,18] The basic idea was to express the interaction of the magnetization with the external static (B_0) and alternating (B_1) fields, using a simple model in which signal growth and decay were then expressed as a result of interaction of the spins with the surrounding lattice (T_1 relaxation) and the interaction between neighbors (T_2 relaxation).

Spin-Lattice Relaxation (T_1)
Consider a sample containing proton spins (magnetic moments) in the absence of an external magnetic field. The magnetic moments will occupy two allowed states with spin at $+1/2$ or $-1/2$. The population difference n decays exponentially, and the rate of change in n is given by

$$\frac{dn}{dt} = -\frac{n}{T_1} \qquad (13\text{-}9)$$

where T_1 is a constant and is called *spin-lattice relaxation time*. Since magnetization is proportional to n, one can further show that

$$\frac{dM_z}{dt} = -\frac{M_z}{T_1}. \qquad (13\text{-}10)$$

By introducing an external magnetic field, B, M_z no longer vanishes at thermal equilibrium but has the value M_0. The relaxation of M_z now obeys the equation

$$\frac{dM_z}{dt} = -\frac{(M_z - M_0)}{T_1}. \qquad (13\text{-}11)$$

Solving for M_z,

$$M_z = M_0[1 - e^{(-t/T_1)}]. \qquad (13\text{-}12)$$

This equation describes the exponential growth of magnetization M_z as a function of elapsed time t. As shown in Fig. 13-6A, when $t = T_1$, the magnetization would grow to 63% of its full value of M_0. When $t = 2T_1$, it would grow to 87% of M_0.

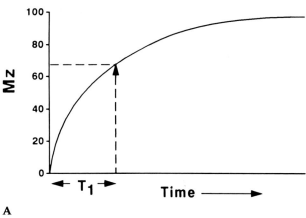

A

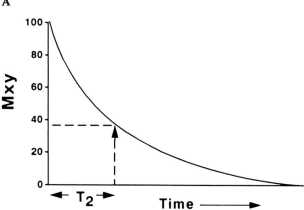

B

Fig. 13-6 The signal growth and decay curves following a 90° RF pulse. (*A*) Signal growth along the longitudinal (parallel to the main magnetic field) direction. The signal immediately following a 90° RF pulse is zero and grows exponentially according to eq. 13-12. The time T_1 is the longitudinal relaxation time at which the signal is 63% of the full signal amplitude. (B) Decay of a transverse signal following a 90° RF pulse. The signal immediately following the pulse is at its maximum. It decays exponentially according to eq. 13-14. The time T_2 is the spin-spin relaxation time at which the signal is 37% of its maximum amplitude.

Spin-Spin Relaxation (T_2)

Similarly, the transverse (*xy*) components of magnetization decay exponentially, but at a different rate, given by

$$\frac{dM_{xy}}{dt} = -\frac{M_{xy}}{T_2}. \qquad (13\text{-}13)$$

Solving for M_{xy},

$$M_{xy} = M_0 e^{(-t/T_2)}. \qquad (13\text{-}14)$$

TABLE 13-2 Summary of MRI Tissue Characteristics at a Field Strength of 1.5 Tesla

| | Relaxation Time (msec) | | Image Contrast | | |
	T_1	T_2	Spin Density	T_1w	T_2w
Skeletal muscle	863 ± 155	47 ± 6	Isointense	Isointense	Dark/gray
CSF	3000 ± 600	1400 ± 250	Gray	Dark	Bright
White matter	783 ± 133	92 ± 20	Gray/dark	Bright/gray	Dark
Gray matter	917 ± 156	101 ± 13	Isointense	Gray	Gray
Heart muscle	862 ± 138	57 ± 9	Gray	Gray	Dark
Liver	490 ± 108	43 ± 6	Gray	Gray	Dark
Kidneys	650 ± 175	58 ± 8	Gray	Dark/gray	Bright
Spleen	778 ± 148	62 ± 17	Gray	Dark	Bright

Source: Partain CL, Price RR, James AE, et al. *Magnetic Resonance Imaging.* Philadelphia, WB Saunders, 1988, p 1082.

The spin-spin relaxation process, unlike the spin-lattice relaxation process, involves the phase of individual spins. The net signal in the transverse plane immediately following a 90° RF pulse is maximum because all spins are coherent and in phase with each other. However, as time progresses, the relative phase between spins evolves from zero to a value that depends on the nature of the microscopic surroundings. This environment constitutes neighboring moments that act like tiny magnetic field centers. Thus, the degree of order or organization among spins is important in defining the signal variation. The process can be described as a non-energy-related process or an entropy process in which the relative phase between individual spins determines the actual signal strength. The time T_2 determines the decay time such that at $t = T_2$, the signal would be 37% of its maximum M_0. Figure 13-6B shows the magnetization decay as a function of time. For pure liquids, $T_1 = T_2$, while $T_1 \gg T_2$ for solids. Table 13-2 depicts T_1 and T_2 values for various tissue components at $1.5T$ field strength.[19]

Origin of Spin Interaction

The term *lattice* refers to the surrounding nuclei. Coupling of spin motions to the thermal motions of the lattice provides a means of energy exchange between the spin system and the surrounding lattice structure.[20,21] In order for the two relaxation processes (T_1, T_2) to exist, the system of spins must experience a direct interaction, and it should be time dependent. Finally, only a certain time scale of interaction is responsible for facilitating the relaxation process.

Just as energy absorption is facilitated by applying a B_1 field at the Larmor frequency, the dissipation of en-

ergy is facilitated at the Larmor frequency. However, the source of this energy is available not from the B_1 field originating from the RF coil, but from various molecular interactions taking place in the spin system. Interactions occurring at a rate much faster than the magnetic resonance frequency (Larmor frequency) will have little or no effect on the exchange of energy. Therefore, molecular movement that possesses a fluctuating field with a frequency close to the resonance frequency is very important for spin-lattice relaxation. The precession of the spin moments away from the z-axis is caused by the transverse fields that are static in the rotating frame. Therefore, the components of the local field that are transverse to the z-axis in rotating frames with frequencies at the Larmor frequency determine the spin-lattice T_1 relaxation. This is the basis on which the tissue T_1 is characterized. The actual value of T_1 will be based on the surrounding molecular structure forming the lattice environment. Figure 13-7 shows the spectral characteristics of rapidly fluctuating motion for various types of molecules. For example, freely moving water, which has a rapidly fluctuating magnetic field at a rate much larger than the resonance frequency does not constitute an efficient scenario for exchange. On the other hand, carbon bonds at the ends of fatty acids fluctuate with a frequency near the Larmor frequency, thus resulting in an effective energy transfer. This is why the protons of fat have shorter T_1 values.

Similarly, local fields that are static or that have a frequency close to zero are primarily responsible for spin-spin relaxation. The change in the z component of the local field adds or subtracts with the main magnetic field, causing spins to precess faster or slower than the Larmor frequency about the z-axis. The degree of

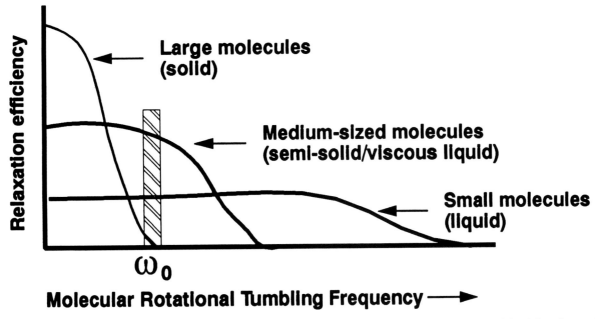

Fig. 13-7 The relaxation efficiency of molecules of various sizes influences the signal line and the width of the observed line. This is due to tumbling of molecules in the presence of neighboring molecules. For example, large molecules which are immobile (in solids) tend to dephase magnetization quickly due to a large, inhomogeneous field created by local fixed sites. This is in contrast to pure liquid, in which the random motion of molecules (due to their small size) produces a smaller dephasing field which results in slow decay of the magnetization in the transverse plane. The intermediate-size molecules are represented between these extremes.

dephasing depends on the frequency broadening around the Larmor frequency. On the basis of this, free water has a long T_2 compared to long chain molecules in fat. Water molecules move about rapidly and have motions that average out, resulting in no field change and therefore little spin dephasing. Large molecules with slow motion create comparatively large differences in magnetic field, resulting in a strong dephase of spins and therefore smaller T_2 values.

In a system composed of complex tissues, there are several types of motion, such as rotational, translational, and vibrational motion, which occur on different time scales. The frequency range for these motions is not always in the vicinity of the Larmor frequency. The local fields are also time dependent and random, depending mostly on the size of the nuclei. One collective representation of the various types of motion is the motional correlation time, which is a measure of the molecular resident time in a particular state of orientation. Thus, it can be said that spin-lattice T_1 relaxation is most efficient when the molecular correlation frequency is near the resonance frequency. On the other hand, spin-spin T_2 relaxation is most efficient for static field changes at slow correlation times or molecular correlation frequencies far from the resonance fre-

quency. The spin-lattice relaxation time T_1 determines the degree of saturation, and the spin-spin relaxation time T_2 determines the unsaturated spectral line width.

Bloch Equations

The seminal paper in 1946 by Felix Bloch describes the behavior of magnetic moments in a system of minimally interacting spins in the presence of an externally applied magnetic field.[18] In what are described as *phenomenological equations*, Bloch incorporated both relaxation terms, T_1 and T_2, to describe magnetization behavior. Using previously described equations, the time dependence of longitudinal (M_z) and transverse (M_x, M_y) magnetization is described by the vector equation

$$\frac{dM}{dt} = \gamma M \times B - \frac{(M_x i + M_y j)}{T_2}$$
$$- \frac{(M_z - M_0) k}{T_1}$$

(13-15a)

where i, j, and k are unit vectors of direction in the laboratory frame of reference. Although there is no analytical solution to this differential equation, it can be solved under certain boundary conditions. However, a much easier set of solutions can be found by transforming it into a rotating frame coordinate system. The rotating coordinate system coincides with the rotational frequency of the magnetization vector so that the magnetization vector appears stationary in that frame of reference.

$$\frac{dM}{dt} = \gamma M \times B_{\text{eff}} - \frac{(M_{x'}i' + M_y j')}{T_2}$$
$$- \frac{(M_{z'} - M_0)k'}{T_1} \qquad (13\text{-}15b)$$

where i', j', and $k' = k$ are unit vectors in the rotating frame and B_{eff} is given by eq. 13-8. Equation 13-15a can be rewritten to provide the solution to the problem of magnetization M in each of the three orthogonal directions. An additional condition, $\omega = \gamma B_0$, is imposed.

The solution of the coupled differential equation has a simple form. The transverse signal components M_x and M_y can be written as

$$M_{x'}(t) = M_0 \sin(\omega t) \exp(-t/T_2)$$
$$M_{y'}(t) = M_0 \cos(\omega t) \exp(-t/T_2). \qquad (13\text{-}16)$$

Thus, in a rotating coordinate frame, the transverse components become a sine or cosine function with an exponential decay factor based on T_2 relaxation. The signal, which is an FID in the transverse plane, describes the time evolution of transverse magnetization. The signal in the frequency domain may be obtained by a straightforward Fourier transformation. The resulting signals after Fourier transformation are known as the *absorption* and *dispersion signals*.

Echo Formation

The transverse magnetization M_{xy} and its associated signal after the application of a 90° RF pulse decay due to intrinsic spin dephasing caused by spin-spin T_2 relaxation. The exponential form of decay modulated by magnetic field inhomogeneities also dephases the transverse components. Thus, the resulting decay is a combination of spin-spin interaction and magnet inhomogeneity. However, the component arising from the magnetic field inhomogeneity can be reversed because the spins possess phase memory due to the fact that the inhomogeneities do not change over time.

The gain or loss in phase due to extrinsic variables can be reversed by applying a second RF pulse of 180°.

The first demonstration of such a method was by Hahn in 1950, and the term *echo* was used.[6] By applying a 180° RF pulse at an echo time, TE, of TE/2, a signal echo of the magnetization is formed at exactly TE/2 after the 180° pulse. The pulsing sequence is of the form 90 − TE/2 − 180° − TE/2 − echo. A simplified evolution of magnetization subjected to 90° and 180° RF pulses is presented in a rotating frame in Fig. 13-8. To explain the behavior of net magnetization, a simplified approach is used in which net magnetization is considered to be an assembly of packets of spins called *isochromats*. At the end of the 90° RF pulse, all of the isochromats are in the transverse plane, with the relative phases between all isochromats being zero. Thus, the signal is maximum immediately after the 90° RF pulse. As time elapses, the isochromats fan out or disperse in the transverse plane, where some rotate faster than others due to variable magnetic field inhomogeneities across the sample. Therefore, the signal in the transverse plane is effectively reduced due to the intrinsic spin-spin relaxation process and extrinsic field inhomogeneities.

An application of a 180° RF pulse at time TE/2 will reverse the vector position in the transverse plane. Under this condition, faster-moving isochromats are reversed and are now behind slowly rotating isochromats. At time TE/2 after the 180° RF pulse, all isochromats will meet, forming an echo of maximum phase coherence which has an amplitude affected only by the T_2 relaxation process. This amplitude is given by

$$M_{y'} = M_0 \exp(-\text{TE}/T_2). \qquad (13\text{-}17)$$

This pulse sequence is called a *spin-echo pulse sequence*, where the effects of magnetic field inhomogeneities are removed. An additional advantage of using a 180° RF pulse is that the echo peak position is detected, which can be rather difficult to observe in a FID at the end of a 90° RF pulse by itself due to systematic receiver dead time. The finite delay between the receiver on-time and the RF off-time will result in information loss at the beginning of the FID signal.

FUNDAMENTALS OF IMAGE FORMATION

The previously discussed treatment is based strictly on information about the net signal obtained from a sample in a relatively uniform magnetic field. It provides no spatial information about the sample. This is due to the fact that under a uniform magnetic field, all nuclei

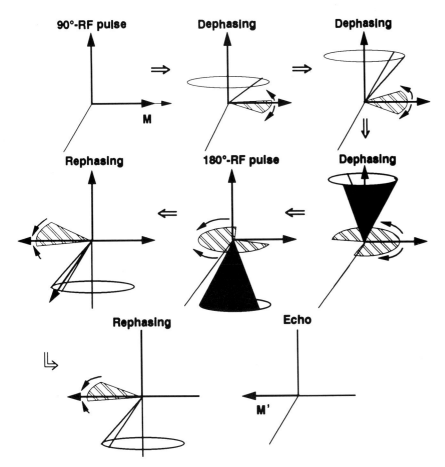

Fig. 13-8 The behavior of magnetization in the presence of 90° and 180° pulses is shown. At the end of a 90° RF pulse, the magnetization starts to spread out in either direction in the transverse plane. This is due to the fact that the internal magnetic field is never perfectly homogeneous. As dephasing takes effect, transverse magnetization amplitude decreases exponentially; at the same time, longitudinal magnetization begins to grow exponentially. When a 180° RF pulse is applied, motional behavior is completely reversed. The moments moving faster will be slower, and vice versa. Thus, at exactly the time that is twice the time between the 90° and 180° RF pulses, magnetization refocuses, producing a signal. This signal is never equal to the signal it started with. This is because the T_2 decay is inherently random and cannot be reversed by a 180° RF pulse.

belonging to the same chemical environment will resonate at the same Larmor frequency. Thus, any variation in the detection frequency will only cause a spread in linewidth at the center frequency. A technique by which magnetic fields are intentionally varied to alter resonance conditions is used to encode different spatial locations. Such a technique was first demonstrated by Lauterbur in 1973.[8] In this technique, use of magnetic field gradients in three orthogonal directions provided spatially dependent resonance frequencies, which were then used to obtain spatial information using projection reconstruction in each direction. A modified technique using pulse Fourier transformation was first demonstrated in imaging by Kumar et al. in 1975.[22]

Behavior of Magnetization in the Presence of Magnetic Field Gradients

The exact precessional frequency is determined by the magnitude of the magnetic field that is experienced by the spins. The static magnetic field B_0 may be changed slightly in any direction by simply adding a field in that same direction or in the opposing direction. A small time-dependent field is superimposed on the static field for a short period and alters the net field seen by precessing protons. During the time the field is altered, the precessional frequency of the spins is changed by an amount determined from eq. 13-18. Such a variation in static field is achieved by producing fields using an additional set of coils called *gradient coils*. These coils produce spatially varying magnetic fields in three orthogonal directions, thus altering precessional frequencies in those directions. The coil windings are such that the field produced varies linearly with the distance from the center of the coil. The precessional frequency in the presence of a gradient field is written as[23,24]

$$\omega(r) = \gamma\left(B_0 + \frac{dB}{dr}\,dr\right)$$
$$= \gamma B_0 + \gamma \vec{G}_r \cdot \vec{r} \tag{13-18}$$

where r is a vector which assumes the x-, y-, or z-direction and G_r is the strength of the gradient magnetic field along r. The basic principle underlying the spatial encoding is as follows. The presence of a gradient alters the frequency of the magnetization as described by

$$M_{xy} = M_{xy} \exp(-i\gamma \vec{G} \cdot \vec{r}t). \qquad (13\text{-}19)$$

The signal intensity following a gradient is determined by taking the integral over the entire x and y direction and is given by

$$S = \int \int M_{xy} \exp(-i\gamma \vec{G} \cdot \vec{r}t)\, dx\, dy. \qquad (13\text{-}20)$$

When magnetic field gradients are present, the resulting precessional frequency assumes a complex motion when viewed from a laboratory frame. However, when viewed from a rotating frame that is also precessing at the Larmor rate, the effect of gradient is simply to make spins precess at a rate given by $\gamma G_r r$. When the gradients are switched off, the spins return to the Larmor precessional frequency, however, with an additional phase shift introduced by the former presence of the gradient. Depending on their physical location, the set of spins, or isochromats, may advance or lag in phase when the gradient field is switched off. This is the principle behind spatial encoding of spins. The degree of spatial encoding that is achieved through position vector r is described in eq. 13–18. Thus, when a gradient in the x-direction is applied, the corresponding precessional frequency increases or decreases with the distance x from the center of the gradient, depending on the gradient's direction. Commercial scanners have gradient coils capable of providing a maximum gradient strength of typically 1 Gauss/cm. For example, using a gradient of 1 Gauss/cm, the precessional frequency, as viewed from a rotating frame at a distance of 100 cm from the center, would be around 420 kHz.

To demonstrate the effect of gradients on spatial encoding, consider three test tubes containing water placed in a static magnetic field, as shown in Fig. 13-9. The test tubes are equidistant from each other and are also within the magnetic field gradient coils. When no gradient is applied, an FID obtained from these tubes will display only one component of frequency when the collective FID signal is Fourier transformed into the frequency domain. Now consider the application of a

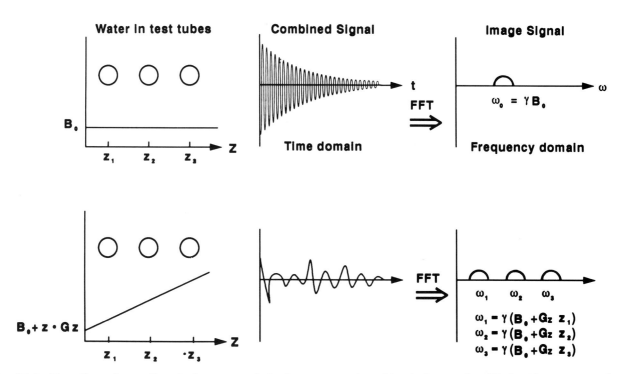

Fig. 13-9 The effect of a gradient is demonstrated. In the top row, three identical test tubes filled with water are placed equidistant in a fixed external magnetic field and the gradient field is zero. The combined signal, which is the sum of exponentially decaying signals from each test tube, provides a single peak signal when Fourier transformed. The bottom row has a similar situation, except that the gradient field is turned on. The linear gradient field provides a linear change in the static magnetic field, thus providing resonance at three different frequencies. The combined signal when Fourier transformed provides peaks at three distinct frequencies based on static field and the superposing gradient field at that location.

gradient along the direction of the test tubes. The net signal after excitation of all the spins in the sample is a combination of the signals derived from each of the test tubes, which individually resonate at different Larmor frequencies. This signal is then Fourier transformed to locate the signal amplitude as a function of position. Thus, each test tube is at a unique magnetic field (frequency), as described by eq. 13-18. The Fourier transformation enables us to decode the RF signal to produce a map in the z-direction of the applied gradient field. This process yields three distinct frequencies, with a separation proportional to their actual spatial separation. The process is then repeated in the x- and y-directions to provide a full map in all directions in three-dimensional space.

In mathematical terms, the action of applying a magnetic field gradient in the presence of a static magnetic field produces a signal that is given by

$$S(t) = \int_{z1}^{z2} D(z)\, e^{i(\gamma/2\pi)(B + zG_z)t}\, dz. \qquad (13\text{-}21)$$

This equation represents the signal in one dimension which is the signal at the Larmor frequency modulated by the integral of the signal generated by the gradient applied between distances $z1$ and $z2$. Thus, the distribution of signal between $z1$ and $z2$ of a sample is contained in the above integral. The product $\gamma G_z t$ is defined as k_z (for reasons that will be discussed in the next section), and in general, k has the dimension of 1/distance and is called the *spatial frequency*.

The distribution of $D(z)$ is determined by simply applying a Fourier transform to the above signal $S(t)$. On simplification

$$S(k_z) = \int_{z1}^{z2} D(z)\, e^{-izk_z}\, dz \qquad (13\text{-}22)$$

where the effect of the static field is ignored. This will be the case when the high-frequency term is eliminated by demodulating the function at the Larmor frequency. Using standard Fourier transformation, the quantity $D(z)$ can be written as

$$D(z) = \int_{-\infty}^{\infty} S(k_z)\, e^{izk_z}\, dk_z \qquad (13\text{-}23)$$

In an imaging setup, five events take place: RF pulsing, x-gradient pulsing, y-gradient pulsing, z-gradient pulsing, and receiver signal collection. Individual events in a given physical direction are active for only a brief time, and sometimes the intervals during which

a certain event is active may overlap with the activity of other events along any other direction.

Spatial Localization in MRI

The effect of an RF pulse is to excite spins and change the orientation of their magnetization relative to the main field. However, when such a pulse is applied, all of the spins in the body that are within the magnetic field will become excited. Such pulses are called *nonselective RF pulses*. The use of selective excitation forms a basis for two- or three-dimensional MRI.[8,26] In doing so, protons in a selected section of the human body are excited and the signal emitted only from that section is recorded, while protons from outside this section remain unaffected. The process of selecting sections in a three-dimensional object is achieved by the use of magnetic field gradients. The presence of a magnetic field gradient introduces spatial encoding along the direction in which it is applied.

Slice Encoding (Plane Selection)
For selective excitation, a shaped RF pulse is used in the time domain such that its shape in the frequency domain is fairly uniform across the slice. It is desirable to have all spins within a slice experience the same excitation when the RF pulse is applied. A pulse containing a single frequency has a zero bandwidth and is very simple to generate. In the time domain, this is a sine wave of infinite duration which will excite an infinitesimally thin slice. By contrast, a pulse containing all possible frequencies has an infinite bandwidth. Such a pulse is a spike of infinitesimally short duration in the time domain and has infinite thickness.

In MRI, we use pulse shapes that provide a pulse of finite duration and bandwidth between these two extremes. The flip angle across the slice should be the same when excited by such an RF pulse. The rectangular slice profile in the frequency domain is ideally suited to achieve uniform excitation. To obtain a rectangular profile, a mathematical sinc-shaped pulse is usually applied in the time domain. In most commercial scanners, pulses such as SINC ($[\sin x]/x$) and GAUSSIAN (e^{-ax^2}) are commonly used. The pulse duration is adjusted so that the RF power deposition is equal for all frequencies within the desired pulse frequency bandwidth. Figure 13-10 shows the excitation of a finite section within the human body placed in a magnetic field. As can be seen, the amplitude or strength of the gradient can be varied for a fixed-bandwidth RF pulse in such a way that it changes the slice thickness. The specific location x of the slice is calculated by offsetting

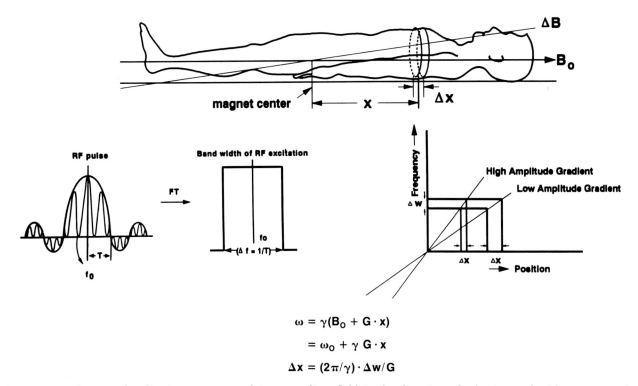

$$\omega = \gamma(B_0 + G \cdot x)$$
$$= \omega_0 + \gamma\, G \cdot x$$
$$\Delta x = (2\pi/\gamma) \cdot \Delta w / G$$

Fig. 13-10   Selection of a slice in MRI. By applying a gradient field in the direction of selection and with an appropriate bandwidth RF pulse, a slice of desired thickness is selected for excitation. In most scanners, the bandwidth of the RF pulse is fixed and the gradient amplitude is varied. The slice offset is provided by the modulation of the RF carrier wave used in creating the pulse.

the RF pulse using pulse modulation of the carrier, or reference wave.

A simple relationship between the excited slice thickness, the RF pulse bandwidth, and the applied gradient strength is given by eq. 13-24 and illustrated in Fig. 13-10:

$$\text{Slice thickness} = \frac{2\pi\ \text{RF pulse bandwidth}}{\gamma\ \text{gradient strength}}. \quad (13\text{-}24)$$

It is clear from eq. 13-24 that for a constant gradient strength, the slice thickness will depend on the RF bandwidth of excitation. Conversely, keeping the pulse bandwidth constant (most RF pulses are designed with a predetermined frequency bandwidth), the desired slice thickness is achieved via gradient amplitude adjustment. Thus, by using the proper gradient amplitude, one can excite a slice of a desired thickness. An off-center slice can be excited either by moving the slice-selection gradient to the center position with respect to the isocenter of the magnet or, more simply, by creating an RF pulse that is shifted from the center

frequency by an amount related to the off-center physical location. In most scanners, the offset in slice location is obtained by modulating the carrier frequency by an amount equal to the offset frequency calculated from the magnitude of the magnetic field gradient along that direction.

For a fixed-bandwidth RF pulse, the minimum slice thickness that is achievable depends on the maximum available gradient strength. In most commercial scanners, the limiting value for the gradient strength is about 1 Gauss/cm (10 mT/m). Once this limit is reached, reducing the slice thickness further necessitates the use of smaller-bandwidth RF pulses. This is achieved simply by extending the RF duration, however, at the expense of increasing the TE. For example, the magnetic field variation over one slice caused by the gradient is $\Delta B = G * SL$. The bandwidth of the RF pulse is $\Delta f = (\gamma/2\pi)\Delta B$ or $(\gamma/2\pi)\,G * SL$. Thus, for a 10-mm slice and using a 0.1 Gauss/cm (1 mT/m) gradient strength, the required bandwidth of the RF pulse is 420 Hz. For a 5-mm cut using the same gradient strength, the RF bandwidth is 210 Hz. On the other hand, using the same bandwidth of 420 Hz, the gradient must be doubled to 0.2 Gauss/cm (2 mT/m) to provide a 5-mm cut.

Frequency Encoding
After selecting a slice encoding direction, another gradient is applied along one of the two remaining orthogonal directions. This time, however, the gradient is applied while the data are being collected to frequency-encode the information. Since a computer is used for processing the data, the data must be sampled discretely while the gradient is present. Remember that the presence of a gradient moment provides only the phase information based on the position. There are two ways one can achieve variation in gradient moment: either by changing the amplitude and holding the duration constant or by changing the duration while keeping the same amplitude throughout the data acquisition period. In this case, the latter method is used. For example, in order to sample m points in a given direction, the gradient time duration axis is divided into m equal parts. The interval over which the signal is sampled is called the *sampling window* or *readout period*. The corresponding gradient that is active during this period is called the *readout gradient*.

The term *bandwidth* is also used here, but it does not refer to the RF bandwidth described in the slice selection process. Rather, it refers to a range of frequencies involved during data sampling. However, discrete sampling should satisfy the Nyquist criterion. This states that the sampling rate must be at least twice the maximum frequency to be uniquely sampled. The upper and lower limits of maximum frequency are dictated by the extent of the field of view (FOV). For example, if the object dimension along the frequency encoding direction is $(FOV)_x$, the bandwidth of sampled frequency is given by $\Delta f = (\gamma/2\pi) G_x FOV_x$. Thus, the maximum frequency to sample is f_{max}, which is half of the bandwidth. The Nyquist criterion dictates that the sampling frequency should be at least twice the f_{max}; $f_s = 2f_{max}$. Thus, the sampling rate is $1/f_s = 2\pi/(\gamma G_x FOV_x)$. The relationship between receiver sampling frequency bandwidth, the FOV, and the readout gradient strength can be expressed as

$$FOV = \frac{2\pi \text{ receiver bandwidth}}{\gamma \text{ gradient strength}}. \quad (13\text{-}25)$$

Phase Encoding
Phase encoding is applied in one of the last remaining orthogonal directions. In this direction, the gradient is incremented in amplitude, keeping its duration constant. As seen in eq. 13-23, the inverse Fourier transform of $S(t)$ projects the density information of the object along the direction in which the Fourier transform is directed. Thus, one can provide a distribution of frequencies for an object to create an array of density projections. To achieve this, a gradient is applied and incremented stepwise each time the data are recorded. For each gradient step, there is a projection defined by eq. 13-21. Note that each time the gradient is switched off, the spins precess with the same Larmor frequency but with different phase. Each time the gradient is activated, the spin phase along that direction is linearly changed. Mathematically, the phase at each gradient value is given by

$$\phi(t) = \phi(0) + \gamma y \int_0^t G_y(t)\, dt. \quad (13\text{-}26)$$

The shift in phase depends on the gradient's strength and on its location in the y direction. However, due to the cyclic nature of phase, the maximum allowable unique phase shift is 2π. Any increment $\partial\phi$ beyond 2π [i.e., $(2\pi + \partial\phi)$] will form an aliasing based on phase ambiguity with $\partial\phi$. The increment in amplitude is also in accordance with the Nyquist criterion. According to the Nyquist criterion, the maximum phase shift along one end of FOV_y for n steps in gradient is given by

$$\phi_{max} = 2\pi \quad (13\text{-}27)$$
$$\times \frac{n}{2} = \frac{\gamma}{2\pi} \frac{FOV_y}{2} n \int_0^t \Delta G(t')\, dt' = n\pi.$$

To distinguish each of the steps along the phase encode direction, it is necessary to divide the phase encode direction into N steps. In the above case, n takes on values from $-N/2, -N/2 + 1 \ldots -1, 0, 1, \ldots N/2 - 1$. Thus, repeating a single loop through n different gradient steps in G_y produces data with N points along the y direction. To create 256 encoding steps, the gradient is equally divided into 256 steps to provide 256 distinct phase values for the spins.

Spatial Frequency Domain (K-Space)
An important aspect of Fourier imaging is the ability to transform information from one domain to its reciprocal domain.[27] In MRI, we deal with two such domains: temporal and spatial. The MRI signal is represented in a spatial domain which is the Fourier transform of the magnetization distribution within the

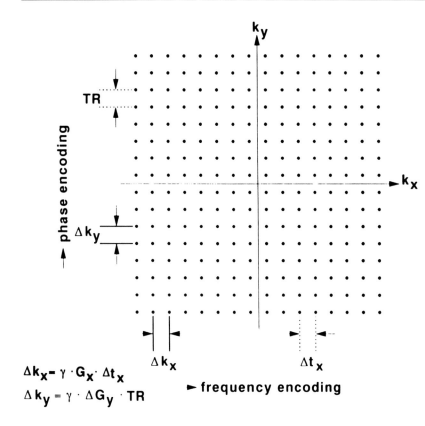

$$\Delta k_x = \gamma \cdot G_x \cdot \Delta t_x$$

$$\Delta k_y = \gamma \cdot \Delta G_y \cdot TR$$

► **frequency encoding**

Fig. 13-11 The matrix of discrete spatial frequency points. The separation between points along the frequency direction is determined by the sampling interval, whereas the separation along the phase direction is determined by the gradient amplitude. The higher (outer) spatial frequency components determine resolution, whereas the lower (near-zero) spatial frequency components determine the signal content.

object that is being imaged. In a spatial domain which is called the *k-space domain,* the spatial frequency information at one point is a function of all the other points. Thus, to generate an image, the entire *k*-space must be mapped.

The knowledge of *k*-space provides a basis for understanding the resolution and signal/noise in the final image. The size of the object dictates the extent of *k*-space coverage to obtain an image of proper resolution. The entire *k*-space is mapped simply by changing the gradient moment (amplitude and duration) along each direction in a stepwise manner. *K*-space is formed as a matrix of k_x and k_y points, as shown in Fig. 13-11. The spacing between points along the frequency and phase-encoding directions are determined by Eq. 13-28. The variable along the phase direction is the gradient amplitude, and the variable along the frequency direction is the sampling interval. The outer regions of *k*-space lines are obtained using high-gradient amplitudes, while the inner regions are acquired with low-gradient amplitudes. The central region of *k*-space, which is at or near zero gradient strength, contains most of the signal information. This is due to the fact that these lines in *k*-space have minimal spin dephasing caused by the gradient and conse-

quently contain most of the signal information. The more cycles per unit length of the object that are used, the greater the accuracy of the spatial map. Thus, higher *k*-space values are required to improve the spatial resolution. The data are then subjected to a two- or three-dimensional Fourier transform to form an image in a spatial domain.

In fact, the application of a gradient transforms the data to the spatial domain, which can be explained as follows. The spatial frequency *k* along any direction where the gradient is applied is defined as

$$K_x = \frac{\gamma}{2\pi} \int G_x(t)\, dt$$

$$K_y = \frac{\gamma}{2\pi} \int G_y(t)\, dt. \tag{13-28}$$

When $G(t) = G$, $k_x = (\gamma/2\pi) G_x t$ and $k_y = (\gamma/2\pi) G_y t$. Thus, one can map *k*-space simply by changing either *t* or *G*. As described previously, this is achieved in two spatial encoding directions. Along the phase-encoding direction, the gradient amplitude is varied, keeping the duration constant, along the frequency-encoding direction, the gradient amplitude is kept constant and the duration is varied. The result is a matrix of k_x by k_y points (or pixels) in a k-space data matrix. The signal in each of these pixels may be written under the action of three orthogonal gradients as

$$S(t) = \int\int \rho(x,y; z = z0) e^{i(\gamma/2\pi)\int_0^t [xGx(t') + yGy(t')]\,dt'}\,dx\,dy. \quad (13\text{-}29)$$

Upon substitution for k,

$$S(k_x, k_y) = \int\int \rho(x,y; z = z0) e(ik_x x) e(ik_y y)\,dx\,dy. \quad (13\text{-}30)$$

In the most general case where relaxation effects are also included, the net signal is obtained by multiplying $S(t)$ by $\exp(-t/T_2)$ and $[1 - \exp(-TR/T_1)]$.

The above type of k-space sampling along the two orthogonal directions is discrete, and each sampling point satisfies the Nyquist criterion. The spatial resolution, Δx and Δy, along the x- and y-directions, respectively, is defined by

$$\frac{1}{2k_x} = \Delta x = \frac{2\pi}{2\gamma G_x T_x}$$
$$\frac{1}{2k_y} = \Delta y = \frac{2\pi}{2\gamma G_y T_y}. \quad (13\text{-}31)$$

The FOV, in terms of spatial resolution, is then written as

$$(\Delta x)_{min} = \frac{(FOV)_{min}}{n_x} = \frac{2\pi}{2\gamma G_x T_x}. \quad (13\text{-}32)$$

Upon substituting the receiver bandwidth,

$$(FOV)_{min} = \frac{2\pi \text{ receiver bandwidth}}{\gamma \text{ gradient strength}} \quad (13\text{-}33)$$

which is exactly eq. 13-25.

As can be seen from eq. 13-33, the allowed unique frequency range determined by the Nyquist criterion is also related to the desired FOV. This relationship among FOV, pixel size, and the receiver bandwidth allows one to determine the smallest possible size of a pixel based on the bandwidth. The bandwidth is chosen so that the frequency spread per pixel is usually greater than the frequency difference between fat and water signals. For example, on a 1.5-Tesla system, the fat/water frequency separation is approximately 220 Hz. This corresponds to a receiver bandwidth of 28.16 kHz for a 256 × 256 matrix. However, using a pixel

spread of 125 Hz, the maximum frequency at the edge of the FOV is 16 kHz and the receiver sampling bandwidth is ± 16 kHz. The receiver bandwidth is kept high enough to produce less chemical shift misregistration artifact. In the above case, for fat/water separation of 220 Hz, the pixel misregistration is only 1.8. In actuality, MRI applications are sometimes employed, so that one can use a lower bandwidth to improve the signal/noise ratio when the imaging area is devoid of fat. However, it should be clear that the lowest bandwidth possible is dictated only by the Nyquist criterion. Under the approximation where the finite sampling effect on pixel broadening is ignored, the smallest pixel size is useful in defining the spatial resolution in an image.

Note that the time interval between sampling points along the frequency-encoding direction is on the order of microseconds, whereas along the phase-encoding direction it is approximately the repetition time when a single acquisition is used. Thus, any motion-related artifacts will be more prominent along the phase-encoding direction due to gross phase-to-phase variability during the repetition time, caused mainly by the motion of the object. Along the frequency-encoding direction, the variation is negligible due to very short time sampling intervals.

Spin-Warp Pulse Sequence

The simplest form of spin-echo pulse sequence utilizes two RF pulses to provide a 90° and 180° rotation of magnetization. In addition, there are gradient activities that take place at different time intervals in the three orthogonal directions. Figure 13-12 shows activities of various gradients and RF pulses on a time scale. In a single cycle, RF, gradient, and receiver activities take place. Such a cycle is then repeated, each time modifying the phase-encode gradient amplitude. The purpose of the 90° pulse, as described earlier, is to rotate the magnetization that exists along the longitudinal direction into the transverse plane. The purpose of the 180° pulse is to refocus the magnetization once it is in the transverse plane to form a spin echo, which is collected during its formation. The available magnetization that initially resides along the longitudinal direction depends on its history from the previous pulsing cycle.

In a standard spin-echo pulse sequence, the signal intensity in a tissue, including the combined effects of T_1 and T_2, can be written as

$$S = N(H)[1 - e^{-(TR/T_1)}]e^{-(TE/T_2)}. \quad (13\text{-}34)$$

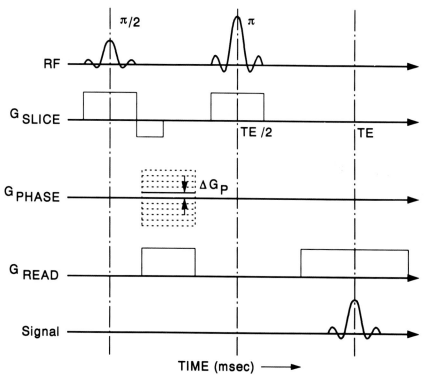

Fig. 13-12 RF pulse and gradient pulse activities in a simple spin-echo pulse sequence. The RF pulse shape is SINC to provide a fairly uniform excitation profile in a frequency domain. A slice is selected by applying gradients G_{slice} along with RF pulses. This provides encoding along one of the three orthogonal directions. The other two directions are encoded using two other orthogonal gradients indicated by G_{phase} and G_{read}.

Inversion-Recovery Pulse Sequence

This pulse sequence incorporates an additional 180° RF pulse applied at the beginning of each TR cycle. It is apparent from the name of this sequence that the longitudinal magnetization M_z is first inverted to lie along the negative z direction. If the 180° pulse is precise, there will be no magnetization along the xy transverse plane. To acquire signal, this is followed by a 90° RF pulse to bring the $-M_z$ component along the transverse plane, as shown in Fig. 13-13. It is the time delay after the inversion from the application of the first 180° pulse that determines the amount of signal available in the transverse plane after the 90° RF pulse. Thus, the contrast can be manipulated simply by adjusting the delay between the first 180° and 90° RF pulses. The magnetization takes longer to recover, as it must first pass through zero and then continue to grow along $+z$ until it reaches M_z. It takes longer to establish thermal equilibrium, and thus a longer TR is needed to complete a cycle of full recovery. The signal based on T_1, T_2 in this type of pulse sequence may be written as

$$S = N(H)[1 - 2e^{-(TI/T_1)} + e^{-(TR/T_1)}]e^{-(TE/T_2)}. \quad (13\text{-}35)$$

An interesting consequence of eq. 13-35 is the null signal originating from either water or fat obtained by

adjusting the delay time, TI. To null a tissue of known T_1, substituting T_1 and setting the bracketed quantity to zero,

$$TI_{null} = T_1 \ln\left[\frac{2}{1 + e^{-(TR/T_1)}}\right]. \quad (13\text{-}36)$$

For example, if TR = 1000 msec and T_1 of fat is about 250 msec at 1.5 Tesla, the TI null point for fat is approximately 168 msec. This sequence is sometimes used to suppress the fat signal by setting TI = 168 msec.

Contrast Phenomenon

The signal intensity within each pixel in an image is a function of the concentration of protons (proton density, $N(H)$) and their relaxation behavior. In imaging, just prior to each cycle (90° − delay − 180° − delay − echo), all tissue signals are zero. At the end of the first cycle, tissues begin to regain their longitudinal magnetization. Depending on where during the growth of longitudinal magnetization the signal is collected, the signal in a pixel can be made to vary according to T_1, T_2 or the $N(H)$ of protons within that pixel. Thus,

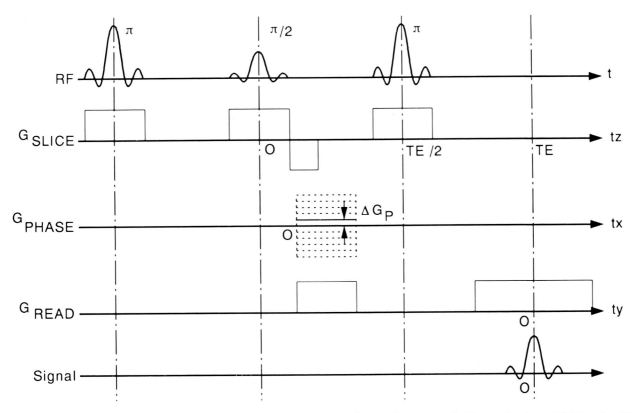

Fig. 13-13 In an inversion recovery pulse sequence, the selective 90° RF pulse is preceded by a selective 180° RF pulse. The first RF pulse provides 180° inversion to all spins. During the delay between 180° and 90° RF pulses, there will be growth of the longitudinal magnetization of fat and water spins. In fact, by carefully controlling the delay between these pulses, one can selectively image a desired signal originating from either fat or water.

the contrast between tissues is based on the collective pixel information based on T_1, T_2, and $N(H)$. Figure 13-14 shows the growth curve for tissues A and B and the time at which the magnetization is acquired.

Spin density–based tissue contrast may be observed by extending TR sufficiently so that the recovered longitudinal magnetization is near 100% before the onset of the next 90° RF pulse. At this point, the magnetization has reached a maximum level of growth due to T_1 relaxation. Generally, TR is selected to be quite long (2000–2500 msec). TR must be such that TR $\gg$ T_1 for nearly full longitudinal recovery of the magnetization. TE is adjusted to a very small value (TE $\ll$ T_2), so that there is no significant dephasing between spins within each of the tissues due to T_2 relaxation. Thus, the longitudinal magnetization from a previous cycle becomes independent of T_1 and T_2 and is strictly a result of the concentration $N(H)$ of protons within each pixel (voxel). The signal difference, therefore, between adjacent tissues will be simply a difference between $N(H)$. Figure 13-15 describes the process of a spin-echo train with TE and TR along the longitudinal growth and

transverse decay curves for two adjacent tissues. A typical spin-echo pulse sequence uses a TE of 10–15 and a TR of 2000–2500 msec in order to obtain density-weighted images.

T_1-weighted contrast, on the other hand, is obtained by acquiring magnetization during its recovery. As shown in Fig. 13-16 the signal behavior during the early part of the recovery cycle is greatly influenced by the T_1 of the tissue. Therefore, the selection of TR should be such that the T_1 contrast is significant between adjacent tissues. Although T_1 contrast is increased at low TR, the overall signal may be reduced due to only partial recovery of the longitudinal magnetization. If TR is increased, the overall signal may increase but the T_1 contrast is reduced. A good compromise is to use TR nearly equal to the T_1 of the tissues. This provides good contrast and reasonable signal intensity. Therefore, using a short TE (10–15 msec) and short TR (500–700 msec), one can generate images based on T_1 weighting between tissues.

Images based on T_2 weighting is obtained by allowing T_2 relaxation to occur. From the magnetiza-

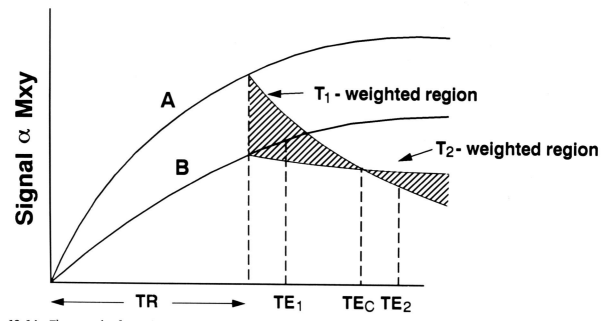

Fig. 13-14 The growth of two tissue magnetizations (*A*, *B*) is shown. The relative contrast between these two tissues depends on when the growth cycle is interrogated. As can be seen, during short TR, the T_1 difference is quite large, providing an image based on T_1 differences when sufficiently short TE (TE_1) is chosen. On the other hand, by increasing TE (TE_2), one allows for T_2 decay to take place, thus introducing T_2-based contrast. At an intermediate TE (TE_c), the signal difference between tissues is zero and therefore does not produce any contrast. In imaging, one is either in a short or very long TE range, never in an intermediate range.

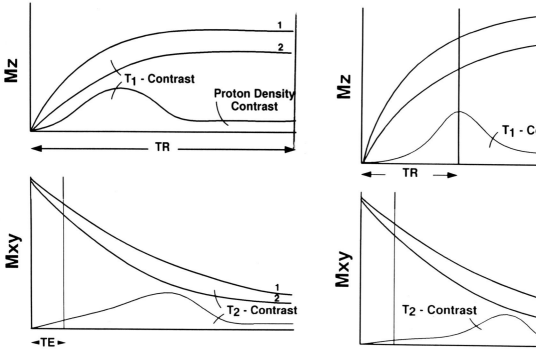

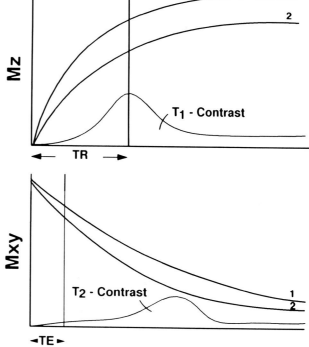

Fig. 13-15 Contrast in a spin-density-weighted image. Using a long TR, the signal growth is interrogated where the difference between tissue signals is based strictly on their density. At the same time, shortening TE, the signal dephasing due to T_2 is minimized. Thus, the overall contrast is based on the density difference between tissue protons.

Fig. 13-16 Contrast in a T_1-weighted image. In this case the signal growth is interrogated at a short TR where the growth is primarily influenced by the T_1 of protons in a tissue. Again, using short TE, T_2 dephasing is reduced, so that the influence of T_2 is minimized.

224

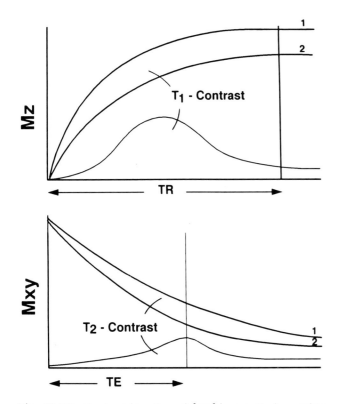

Fig. 13-17 Contrast in a T_2-weighted image. By increasing TE, the signal is allowed to dephase due to the T_2 mechanism. Using long TR again avoids changes influenced by T_1 growth.

tion evolution cycle, it is clear that when TE is sufficiently large, there will be sufficient dephasing among spins in the transverse plane caused by T_2 relaxation. Thus, the T_2 relaxation process begins at a TE of zero and develops as TE is increased. Figure 13-17 shows the magnetization curve for TE and TR to generate T_2-based contrast. With longer TE the net signal will be reduced due to losses from dephasing, even though the T_2 contrast is increased. In a clinical setup, a long TR is used when the signal does not suffer from T_1 relaxation; at the same time, TE is kept long so that T_2 relaxation is dominant. In a clinical situation, TE = 90 msec and TR is approximately 2000–2500 msec, which provides images with heavily T_2-weighted contrast.

Paramagnetic contrast agents such as gadopentetate dimeglumine (GD-DTPA) can be used to enhance the contrast between tissues. It is well known that the presence of gadolinium quickens the relaxation processes, thereby shortening T_1 and T_2 relaxation times.[28,29] The paramagnetic characteristic of gadolinium forms the basis of this MRI contrast enhancement. The rapid rotation and tumbling of the gadolinium molecule result in fluctuation of the magnetic field surrounding the

proton. Thus, protons close to gadolinium rapidly relax due to severe dephasing of the transverse magnetization. Although the tumbling motion of gadolinium change T_1 and T_2 relaxation rates equally, the change in T_1 is more pronounced than the change in T_2. For example, the net change in the relaxation rate can be written as

$$\frac{1}{(T_1)_{eff}} = \frac{1}{T_1} + \frac{1}{(T_1)_{Gd}} \qquad (13\text{-}37a)$$

$$\frac{1}{(T_2)_{eff}} = \frac{1}{T_2} + \frac{1}{(T_2)_{Gd}}. \qquad (13\text{-}37b)$$

Consider an unenhanced T_1 changing from 600 msec to 200 msec due to the presence of gadolinium. On substitution in eq. 13-27a, the relaxation rate change from Gd ($1/T_1$ Gd) is 0.3030×10^{-3} msec^{-1}. Since the rate of change is the same in T_1 and T_2, substituting in eq. 13-27b using an unenhanced T_2 of 60 msec, the change in T_2 is only 10 msec, to 50 msec. Therefore, it is clear that the change in relaxation time is more dramatic in T_1 than in T_2. Contrast-enhanced studies, therefore, are usually performed using T_1-weighted sequences. Once the contrast agent is injected, there will be perfusion of the contrast medium where there is blood–brain barrier (BBB) breakdown, such as in areas of tumors. Normal tissue with an intact BBB will not contain a significant amount of contrast. Therefore, only the T_1 of the tissue or tumor where the contrast is present is greatly reduced making its magnetization recovery curve more rapid, as shown in Fig. 13-18. The change in signal is increased manyfold and is used as a contrast enhancement mechanism between tissues.

FAST IMAGING PRINCIPLES

Standard spin-echo pulse sequences show that the flip angles are 90° and 180° for the excitation and refocusing RF pulses, respectively. The 90° degree excitation pulse is most useful when the repetition time TR is infinitely long compared with T_1 of the tissue. This, however, may not be an optimal flip angle for obtaining maximum signal, especially when TR is finite and much less than T_1, such as in fast imaging applications. Instead, if a variable flip angle for the excitation RF pulse is applied, then the specific flip angle can be optimized based on the Ernst angle relationship.[16] By solving the Bloch steady-state equations for the simple spin-echo type pulse sequence: $\alpha^0 - 180° - SE$, one can write the signal behavior as a function of RF flip

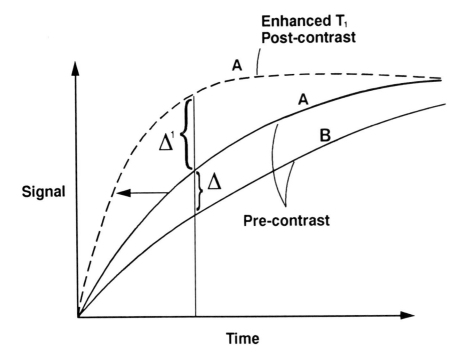

Fig. 13-18 The use of gadolinium chelate enhances the relaxation of spins in which the contrast agent is present. As shown, tissue (A) after the administration of the contrast agent recovers much faster than tissue (B). The signal difference increases tremendously (from Δ to $\Delta + \Delta^1$), and the contrast between (A) and (B) is greatly improved.

angle (as TR $\gg$ TE) as

$$S(\cong M_{xy}) = N(H) \frac{\sin \alpha (1 - e^{-(TR/T_1)})}{(1 + \cos \alpha e^{-(TR/T_1)})} e^{-(TE/T_2)} \quad (13\text{-}38)$$

which reduces to eq. 13-34 when $\alpha = 90$. The optimum flip angle is given by

$$\alpha_E = \cos^{-1}(-e^{-(TR/T_1)}). \qquad (13\text{-}39)$$

The dependence of signal on the flip angle of the RF pulse is shown in Fig. 13-19. For a given TR, tissues with shorter T_1 will give maximum signal when the RF flip angle is near 90° compared with the tissues of longer T_1. Also, it is clear from eq. 13-38 that the optimal flip angle for maximum signal is in the range between 90° and 180°. This is true when sufficiently long TR is used, which is the case in a spin-echo pulse sequence.

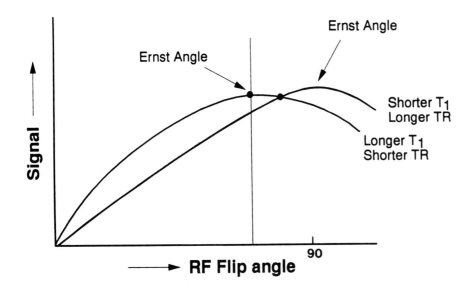

Fig. 13-19 Signal growth as a function of flip angle. The Ernst angle is the flip angle at which transverse magnetization is maximum. At shorter T_1 and longer TR, the flip angle, more nearly 90°, provides a higher signal compared to the same tissue with longer T_1 and shorter TR.

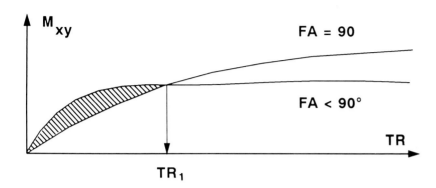

Fig. 13-20 Signal growth as function of TR at various flip angles. It is clear from the figure that at short TR the tissue with a small flip angle has more signal than the tissue with a large flip angle. The short flip angle and short TR form the basis for gradient recalled echoes.

Gradient-Echo Pulse Sequence

In conventional spin-echo imaging, the scan time is dependent on TR, the number of phase-encoding steps, and the number of acquisitions for each of these phase-encoding steps and is given by

$$\text{Scan time} = \text{TR} * (\text{number of phase encodes})$$
$$* (\text{number of acquisitions}).$$

The phase-encoding steps and the number of acquisitions are used to improve resolution and the signal/noise ratio, respectively. TR is the time necessary to establish the desired contrast. In addition, TR is used to reestablish magnetization in the z-direction before the onset of the next RF pulse. The longitudinal magnetization recovers between successive RF pulses to reach a steady-state value that is proportional to $(1 - \exp[-\text{TR}/T_1])$. In a spin-echo pulse sequence, it is assumed that all the magnetization is in the transverse plane following a 90° RF pulse. The TR is set in such a way that all transverse magnetization is decayed before the onset of the next 90° RF pulse. Typically, TR is about four or five times the T_1 of the tissue. When TR is reduced, however, there will be incomplete dephasing of transverse magnetization before the next 90° RF pulse. We begin to saturate the spin system severely and the signal becomes weaker scaling with $(1 - \exp[-\text{TR}/T_1])$. Contrary to spin-echo, under these conditions a flip angle of the RF pulse that is less than 90° becomes more effective. Since low flip angle RF pulses cause only a short excursion of magnetization, a steady state is achieved in which most magnetization remains longitudinal. Thus, by reducing the RF flip angle, one can reduce TR accordingly to provide similar contrast, as observed in a spin-echo pulse sequence. This follows from eq. 13-38, where the flip angle can be optimized as a function of TR. It is interesting to note that the actual transverse magnetization is larger in magnitude than that obtained using a 90° RF pulse at short TR. As shown in Fig. 13-20, as long as TR is sufficiently short, there is more M_{xy}, with a corresponding increase in the overall signal/noise ratio. A net signal advantage can be achieved with short TR times with the use of a reduced flip angle, or alpha pulse.

Due to the large component of magnetization that still remains in the z-direction after an alpha pulse, the effect of a 180° refocusing pulse in a spin-echo sequence would invert this magnetization, thereby requiring a long TR to regain M_z. Instead of a 180° refocusing RF pulse to generate a spin echo, gradients are used to refocus the magnetization in the transverse plane, as shown in Fig. 13-21, hence the name *gradient-recalled echo (GRE)*. The phase of spin isochromats is changed by a fixed amount during the first part of the gradient pulsing. During the next part, the polarity of the gradient is reversed. This results in the phase evolution becoming reversed so that the net phase is zero at the point where the echo is formed.

The formation of the signals associated with gradient-recalled echos in MRI was first analyzed by Carr in 1958.[30] He applied a series of closely spaced RF pulses to obtain a steady-state free precession. When three or more RF pulses were applied successively, they formed stimulated echoes that coincided with spin echos if the RF pulses were spaced equidistant in time. When these RF pulses were applied rapidly, they provided a dynamic equilibrium steady state in which the FID overlapped with the spin echo and stimulated echoes.

Contrast Phenomenon

The optimal contrast in a gradient-echo sequence is dependent on TR, TE, and the flip angle.[31,32] Because of the absence of a 180° RF pulse, gradient-echo pulse sequences are susceptible to extrinsic variables such as magnetic field inhomogeneities, chemical shifts, local

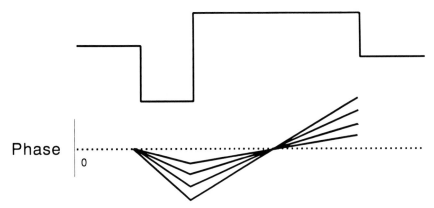

Fig. 13-21 Rephasing of the spins in a transverse plane is done by applying a gradient. At the end of the RF pulse, the phase difference between spins is zero. As time progresses, they experience the first part of the gradient, which introduces phase by a known amount. During the second part of the gradient and due to reversal of polarity of the gradient, the phases are also reversed by the same amount and spins are refocused, forming an echo.

field distortions, and so on. The net spin dephasing, therefore, is a result of spin-spin relaxation (T_2) and field inhomogeneities and is determined collectively by T_{2*} rather than T_2.[33] Another problem is the phase cycling of fat and water spins within a voxel. The frequency separation between water and fat spins is about 220 Hz in 1.5 Tesla. Thus, at every multiple of 2.3 msec, there will be phase change of 180° between fat and water spins. In this case, for TE = 2.3 and 6.8 msec, the fat and water spins will be opposed in their phase, causing signal cancellation within the voxel, whereas at TE = 4.5 and 9.1 msec, the fat and water spins will be in phase.

A generic form of gradient echo pulse sequence is shown in Fig. 13-22. Based on dynamic steady-state equilibrium of the magnetization between rapidly successive repeat cycles, there are two versions of basic gradient echo pulse sequences. In the first type, the residual transverse magnetization is spoiled just after data acquisition. The magnetization that is available for the next cycle is therefore purely longitudinal magnetization, M_z. Thus, only the longitudinal magnetization reaches a steady state. This form of gradient echo pulse sequence is called *Fast Low Angle Shot* (*FLASH*), one of the many acronyms used in the literature.[34,35]

The transverse magnetization in a low flip angle GRE

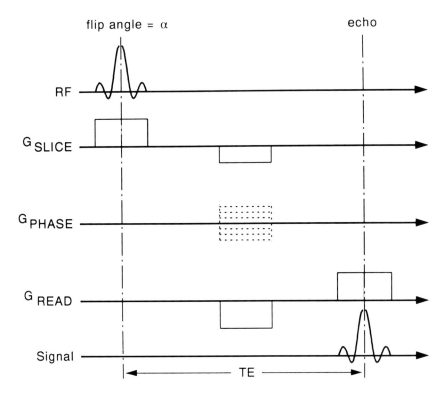

Fig. 13-22 A generic form of GRE pulse sequence. The RF pulse provides a tilt of magnetization by an angle *a*. The gradient activities are shown along three orthogonal directions. The READ gradient is adjusted to refocus the magnetization to form an echo.

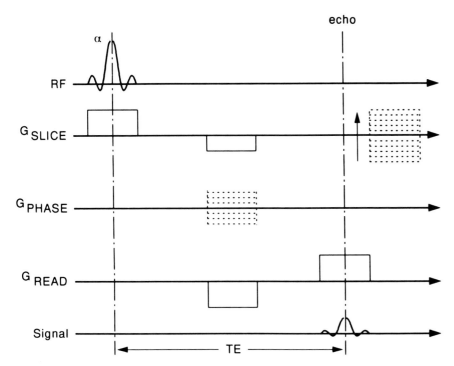

Fig. 13-23 A FLASH pulse sequence. The residual transverse coherence is destroyed after the data are acquired and before the onset of the next RF pulse. The signal amplitude is defined by eq. 13-42.

sequence is given by eq. 13-40, which is similar to eq. 13-38 when TR $\gg$ T$_2$.

$$S \approx N(H) \; \frac{(1 - e^{-(TR/T_1)}) \sin \alpha}{[1 - e^{-TR/T_{1_e} - TR/T_2}} \; e^{-TE/T_{2*}}. \quad (13\text{-}40)$$
$$- \cos \alpha (e^{-TR/T_1} - e^{-TR/T_2})]$$

If TR $\ll$ T$_{2*}$, transverse magnetization coherence is destroyed before the next RF pulse with the use of "spoiler" gradient pulses. Using the Ernst angle (eq. 13-39) for a given TR/T$_1$, eq. 13-40 can be simplified and the signal can be written as

$$S = N(H) \left(\tan \frac{\alpha}{2} \right) e^{-(TE/T_{2*})}. \quad (13\text{-}41)$$

For small flip angles, $\alpha/2 \approx \sqrt{TR/2T_1}$. Upon substituting,

$$S \cong N(H) \sqrt{\frac{TR}{2T_1}} \, e^{-(TE/T_{2*})}. \quad (13\text{-}42)$$

According to eq. 13-42, FLASH signal depends on TR and T$_1$ of the tissue. If TR is sufficiently long to allow T$_1$ recovery, the signal is proportional to the proton density, $N(H)$. For short TR, the signal is T$_1$ weighted. The TE in eq. 13-42 reflects the T$_{2*}$ contribution to the signal. For sufficiently short TE we can ne-

glect effects of the last term involving T$_{2*}$. Figure 13-23 shows a FLASH pulse sequence with various gradient activities necessary for imaging and for gradient echo formation.

There is another variation of the gradient echo pulse sequence in which residual transverse magnetization is maintained instead of being destroyed. This type of pulse sequence is called Gradient-Recalled Acquisition in the Steady State (GRASS) or Fast Imaging with Steady-state Precession (FISP).[35] In this variation, the net effect of the imaging gradient is made to be zero from cycle to cycle to minimize spin dephasing due to the gradients. Therefore, both longitudinal and transverse magnetization achieve a steady state and contribute to the signal. In a sense, FISP is the opposite of FLASH in the gradient echo sequence family. While FLASH specifically destroys transverse magnetization, FISP is designed to sustain it. Once again, the signal behavior may be predicted by solving eq. 13-40 under a different set of conditions. For TR $\ll$ T$_2$, the optimum FISP signal using eq. 13-41 with TR $\ll$ T$_2$ is given by

$$S \approx \frac{N(H)}{2} \sqrt{\frac{T_2}{T_1}} \, e^{-TE/T_{2*}}. \quad (13\text{-}43)$$

As can be seen, the signal is independent of TR as long as TR $\ll$ T$_2$. It depends on the ratio T$_2$/T$_1$ and on

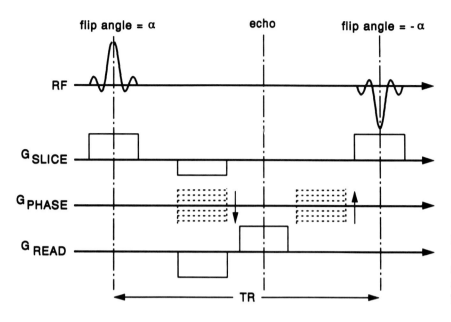

Fig. 13-24 A FISP pulse sequence. In contrast to FLASH, this sequence preserves residual transverse magnetization after data acquisition. The signal amplitude is defined by eq. 13-43.

the proton density, $N(H)$. For fluids with long T_2, the signal appears bright because the steady-state magnetization is large due to persistent transverse magnetization from cycle to cycle. When one looks at soft tissue which has $T_2 < 100$ msec, it will appear dark because of the smaller T_2 effect. Surrounding tissues appear dark while fluids such as cerebrospinal fluid appear bright. The signal from fat appears moderately bright (yet darker than that of fluids) due to a large ratio of T_2/T_1. Figure 13-24 shows a FISP-type GRE with various gradient activities for imaging and echo formation. The phase variation from cycle to cycle is shown in Figure 13-25, indicating that net phase is zero, thus sustaining transverse coherence.

The contrast in FISP is based on T_1 and T_2, and the steady state effect tends to dominate at very short TR or with long T_2 tissues. Thus, to obtain a myelogram-like image of the spine, a short TR sequence will be sufficient. As TR is increased when TR $> T_2$, the transverse relaxation effect will dephase the transverse magnetization sufficiently on its own, so that during the next cycle there is no transverse component left over to induce coherence by adding to the longitudinal component of the signal, thereby approaching FLASH-like contrast. Also, at long TR the effect is predominantly due to longitudinal magnetization. Therefore, at sufficiently long TR, FLASH and FISP have identical contrast behavior.

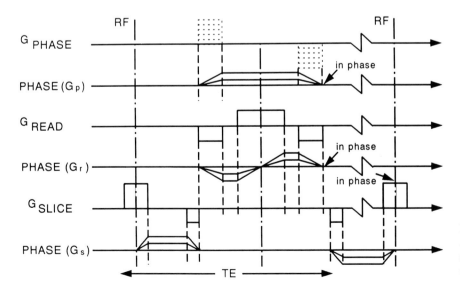

Fig. 13-25 The phase information in a FISP pulse sequence. The net phase shift at the echo is zero along each of the three orthogonal directions.

REFERENCES

1. Gorter CJ. *Physica* 1936;3:995.
2. Rabi II, Zacharias JR, Millman S, et al. *Phys Rev* 1938; 53:318.
3. Purcell EM, Torrey HC, Pound RV. *Phys Rev* 1946;69:37.
4. Bloch F, Hansen WW, Packard M. *Phys Rev* 1946;70:474.
5. Torreys HC. *Phys Rev* 1949;76:1059.
6. Hahn EL. *Phys Rev* 1950;80:580.
7. Ernst RR, Anderson WA. *Rev Sci Instrum* 1966;37:93.
8. Lauterber PC. *Nature* 1973;242:190.
9. Abragam A. *Principles of Nuclear Magnetism.* Oxford, Clarendon Press, 1961.
10. Slichter CP. *Principles of Magnetic Resonance.* New York, Harper & Row, 1963.
11. Gerstein BC, Dybowski CR. *Transient Techniques in NMR of Solids: An Introduction to Theory and Practice.* New York, Academic Press, 1985.
12. Carrington A, McLachlan AD. *Introduction to Magnetic Resonance.* London, Harper & Row, 1980.
13. Rose ME. *Elementary Theory of Angular Momentum.* New York, Wiley, 1957.
14. Shaw D. *Fourier Transform NMR Spectroscopy,* ed 2. Amsterdam, Elsevier, 1984.
15. Arya AP. *Elementary Modern Physics.* Reading, Mass, Addison-Wesley, 1974.
16. Ernst RR, Bodenhausen G, Wokaum A. *Principles of Nuclear Magnetic Resonance in One and Two Dimensions.* Oxford, Clarendon Press, 1987.
17. Rabi II, Ramsey NF, Schwinger J. *Rev Mod Physics* 1954; 26(2):167.
18. Bloch F. *Phys Rev* 1946;70:460.
19. Bottomly PA, Hardy CJ, Argersinger RE, et al. *Med Phys* 1987;14:1.
20. Bloembergen N, Purcell EM, Pound RV. *Phys Rev* 1948; 73:679.
21. Solomen I. *Phys Rev* 1955;99:559.
22. Kumar A, Welti D, Ernst RR. *J Magn Reson* 1975;18:69.
23. Callaghan PT. *Principles of Magnetic Resonance Microscopy.* Oxford, Clarendon Press, 1991.
24. Farrar TC, Becker ED. *Pulse and Fourier Transform NMR.* New York, Academic Press, 1971.
25. Mansfield P, and Morris PG. *NMR Imaging in Biomedicine.* New York, Academic Press, 1982.
26. Mansfield P, Grannell PK. *J Phys* 1973;C6:L422.
27. Stark DD, Bradley WG (eds): *Magnetic Resonance Imaging.* St. Louis, CV Mosby, 1988.
28. Bloembergen N, Morgan LO. *J Chem Phys* 1961;34:842.
29. Lauffer RB. *Chem Rev* 1987;87:901.
30. Carr HY. *Phys Rev* 1958;80:580.
31. Haacke EM, Wielopolski W, Tkach JA. *Rev Magn Reson Med* 1991;3:53.
32. Haacke EM, Tkach JA. *Radiology* 1990;155:951.
33. Carr HY, Purcell EM. *Phys Rev* 1954;94:630.
34. Haase A, Frahm J, Matthaei D, et al. *J Magn Reson* 1986; 67:258.
35. Pub. No. MG/5000-217-121. Iselin, N.J., Siemens Medical System, Inc, 1987.

14

Imaging of Intracranial Hemorrhage

Amir A. Zamani, M.D.

Hemorrhage and hemorrhagic conditions constitute a significant proportion of disease entities a neuroradiologist deals with every day. With the addition of computed tomography (CT) and then magnetic resonance imaging (MRI), the investigation of these entities has improved dramatically during the past two decades. With these two diagnostic tools, the radiologist is not only capable of identifying a hemorrhage (which was not so easy before) but is also able to determine, with some accuracy, the age of the lesion. Frequently, CT and MRI enable the radiologist to determine the cause of the hemorrhage, obviating the need for more invasive procedures.

In this chapter, we will describe the imaging findings of intracerebral hemorrhage in general. A discussion of the causes of intracerebral hemorrhage will follow. Consideration of subarachnoid hemorrhage is followed by a review of the causes of this important entity.

INTRACEREBRAL HEMORRHAGE

MRI and CT Appearance

With newer imaging sequences and higher-strength magnetic fields, MRI is capable of detecting acute intracranial hemorrhage. In addition, in subacute and chronic hemorrhage, MRI is able to determine the approximate age of the lesion better than CT. Emergency imaging of an acute hemorrhage is, however, usually relegated to CT.

The appearance of hematoma on MRI depends on the age of the lesion and the imaging sequence employed.[1,2] According to Bradley,[1] hematomas evolve in five stages: intracellular oxyhemoglobin, intracellular deoxyhemoglobin, intracellular methemoglobin, extracellular methemoglobin, and finally, ferritin and hemosiderin.

On CT, a few hours after formation, a clot is visible as a high-attenuation lesion; by contrast, on MRI, hemorrhage less than 12 hr old may not differ from any other lesion. Therefore, CT should be the imaging modality of choice during the first 12 hr of an ictus. The appearance on MRI of later stages of hematoma depends primarily on two paramagnetic phenomena:

1. Paramagnetic dipole–dipole interaction, seen with methemoglobin, causes T_1 shortening.
2. The magnetic susceptibility effect, seen with *intracellular* deoxyhemoglobulin, methemoglobin, and hemosiderin, causes T_2 shortening.

Hyperacute hematoma (first few hours) appears iso- to hypointense to brain on T_1-weighted images. Because most of a hematoma at this stage is composed of oxyhemoglobin (which has no paramagnetic properties), there is no significant T_2 shortening. CT is more sensitive than MRI at this stage.

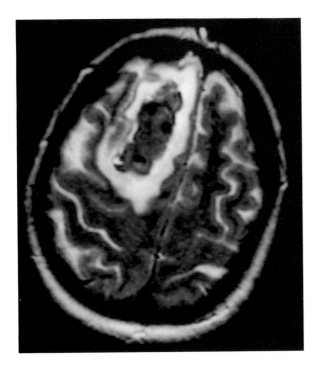

Fig. 14-1   Acute hematoma. Intracellular deoxyhemoglobin causes significant T_2 shortening.

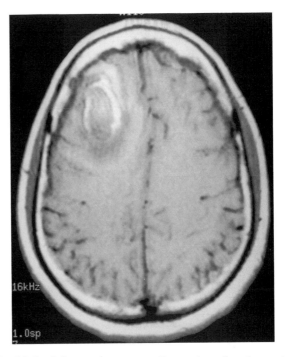

Fig. 14-2   Subacute hematoma. Formation of methemoglobin starts at the periphery and causes T_1 hyperintensity.

Acute Hematoma (1 to 3 Days)
At this stage, deoxyhemoglobin within intact red cells causes T_2 shortening. Hemoconcentration, red cell dehydration, and clot retraction contribute to this situation. The hematoma is very hypointense on long TR/ TE images. It is isointense on T_1-weighted images (deoxyhemoglobin does not cause T_1 shortening) (Fig. 14-1).

Early Subacute Hematoma (3–7 Days)
At this stage, the red cells are still intact and contain methemoglobin. The formation of methemoglobin starts at the periphery of a parenchymal hematoma (where the oxygen level is higher in the adjacent normal brain). It then progresses centrally. Methemoglobin causes significant T_1 shortening. T_2 shortening, seen with deoxyhemoglobin formation, continues with the formation of intracellular methemoglobin. The hematoma has a bright periphery on T_1-weighted images and is very hypointense on T_2-weighted images (Fig. 14-2).

Late Subacute Hematoma (More Than 7 Days)
The hematoma is bright on both T_1 and T_2 images. The T_1 shortening is caused by methemoglobin, which is now extracellular, as lysis of the red blood cells has

occurred. Because of this lysis, the T_2 shortening which had resulted from compartmentalization of methemoglobin is lost (Fig. 14-3).

Chronic Hematoma (More Than 2 Weeks)
At this stage, hemosiderin and ferritin are present within macrophages that ring the hematoma. The intracellular hemosiderin causes significant T_2 shortening and causes a ring of hypointensity at the periphery of a hematoma (Fig. 14-4). Eventually the center of the hematoma becomes filled with nonparamagnetic heme pigments such as hematoidin.

It should be noted that magnetic susceptibility effects (SE) are enhanced with higher magnetic fields and on gradient echo images; and they are reduced with fast SE techniques[3,4] (Fig. 14-5).

The CT appearance of hemorrhage is well known. Increased density, which is seen initially, is dependent on the globin part of the hemoglobin molecule. Clot formation and retraction are important in formation of this high density lesion. If the hemoglobin level is less than 10%, detection of an intracerebral hemorrhage may be difficult. The low-density, vasogenic edema surrounding the hemorrhage becomes maximal around the fifth day and then decreases. The density of the clot starts to decrease, beginning at the periphery, after the third

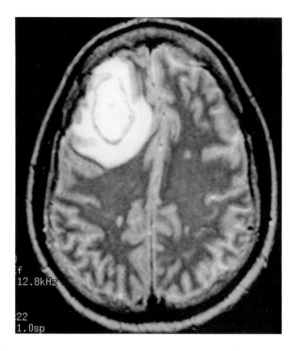

Fig. 14-3 Late subacute hematoma. Extracellular methemoglobin is bright on T_2 images. Surrounding brain edema is evident.

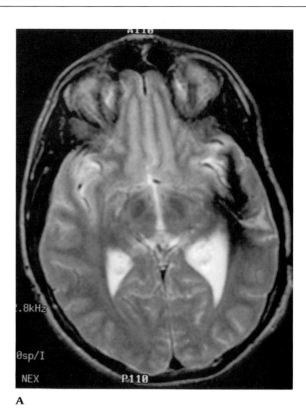

A

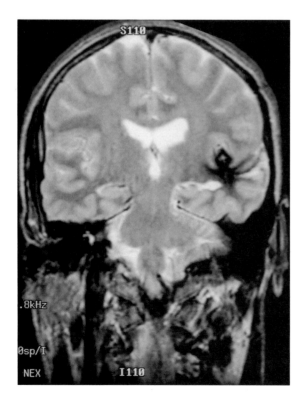

Fig. 14-4 Hemosiderin in an old hematoma site causes significant T_2 shortening.

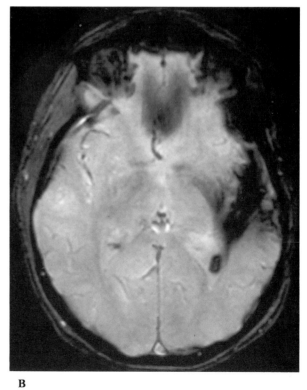

B

Fig. 14-5 A T_2-weighted fast spin echo and B-gradient echo images. T_2 hypointensity of hemosiderin is enhanced on gradient echo images.

day; after 1 or 2 months, there should be no residual hyperdensity. Ring enhancement may be seen after the fifth day and may last for 1 or 2 months.[5] At this late stage, the CT appearance may be confusingly similar to that of an abscess or tumor (Fig. 14-6). Previous studies and an MRI examination may help the differentiation. After 2 months, only a slit-like, low-attenuation cavity remains. There is no surrounding edema and no enhancement. Adjacent cerebrospinal fluid (CSF) spaces may begin to dilate.

Causes of Nontraumatic Intracerebral Hemorrhage

In adult life, the common causes of intracerebral hemorrhage include hypertension, anticoagulant therapy (especially coumadin), aneurysms, and vascular malformations.[6] Amyloid angiopathy, hemorrhage in an infarct, hemorrhage in a tumor, blood dyscrasias, coagulopathies, drug abuse, and vasculitis are other causes.

HYPERTENSIVE INTRACRANIAL HEMORRHAGE

In recent years, there has been a reduction in the incidence of these hemorrhages with better and more widespread therapy for hypertension. Most of these hemorrhages occur in the basal ganglia and thalami; the pons, cerebellum, and frontal lobe are other common sites. These lesions are frequently quite large. Rupture into the ventricular system is common, and hypertension is the most common cause of intraventricular hemorrhage. Lentiform nucleus hemorrhages usually rupture into the frontal horn or temporal horn; thalamic hemorrhages open in the third ventricle. Depending on the site of hemorrhage, the clinical symptoms vary and include hemiparesis, hemianopsia, altered mental status, pupillary findings, and so on. Often there is acute onset of headache, with nausea and vomiting.

Pathology

Eighty percent of hypertensive hemorrhages are supratentorial, with 80% of these occurring in the basal ganglia and thalami. Ten percent of intracranial hypertensive hemorrhages occur in the pons and 10% in the cerebellum.[7] The tendency of these hemorrhages to occur in certain areas of the brain corresponds to the frequency of microaneurysms in small vessels (50–200 μm) in these areas of the brain. These aneurysms,

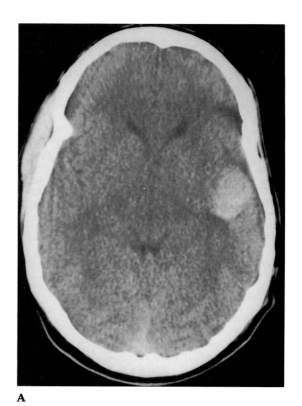

A

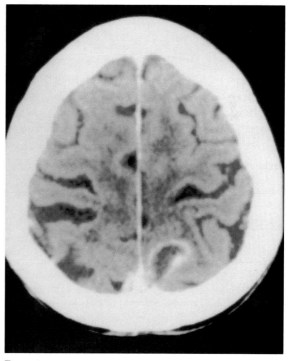

B

Fig. 14-6 (*A*) Classical CT appearance of an acute intracerebral hemorrhage. (*B*) An old hematoma shows peripheral enhancement and can be confused with an abscess or a tumor.

called *Charcot-Bouchard aneurysms,* are associated with total disruption of the endothelial, muscular, and elastic layers, and predispose the weakened arteriole to rupture and hemorrhage. The development of these aneurysms and the role of hypertension in nontraumatic parenchymal hemorrhage is still controversial, however.

In any event, once hemorrhage happens, it dissects along white matter fibers. Soon it stops accumulating, and liquefaction begins. After weeks to months, all that is left is a cyst-like cavity with hemosiderin-filled macrophages in its walls.

Radiological Examination

In the acute stage, the patient is usually not cooperative or able to undergo MRI. In these early hours, CT may be even more sensitive (and clearly easier to perform) than MRI. The changes demonstrated are those of acute hematoma seen with other causes (Fig. 14-7). Hypertension in the etiology of the hemorrhage is suspected primarily because of the location of the hemorrhage and the patient's clinical history. CT or MRI may show evidence of prior hypertensive bleeds (a cystic, shrunken cavity with hemosiderin in its walls) or lacunar infarcts in the basal ganglia.

AMYLOID ANGIOPATHY

This is a disease of the elderly. It may be found incidentally at autopsy. Lobar hemorrhage is the most common presentation. Dementia with acute onset is rare. Leukoencephalopathy has been recently described.[8]

In this entity, amyloid is deposited in the blood vessels of the cerebral cortex and leptomeninges. Secondary changes of double barreling, clefts, fibrinoid changes, vessel ectasia, and occlusion also occur. These changes are rather common in the elderly; their incidence is more than 60% in individuals above the age of 80. As a result of these changes, these vessels are extremely fragile. Hemorrhages which result from this disease are typically superficial. There is a predilection for the temporal and occipital lobes; the brain stem and basal ganglia are usually spared. Subarachnoid hemorrhage may occur. Amyloid angiography accounts for 5–12% of sporadic cerebral hemorrhages.[9-11]

Imaging demonstrates intralobar/subarachnoid hemorrhage (Fig. 14-8). There may be evidence of prior intracerebral hemorrhages, as there is a tendency toward recurrent hemorrhages in this disease. There are no typical angiographic findings.

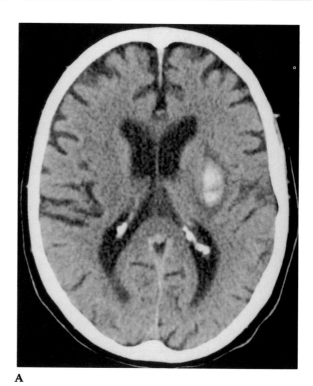

A

B

Fig. 14-7 Hypertensive intracerebral hemorrhage. (*A*) and (*B*) show a putaminal hemorrhage with surrounding edema.

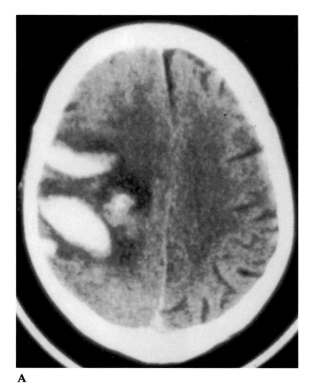

A

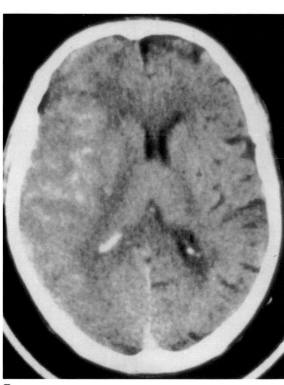

B

Fig. 14-8 Hemorrhage in amyloid angiopathy. (*A*) Superficial intralobar and (*B*) subarachnoid hemorrhage.

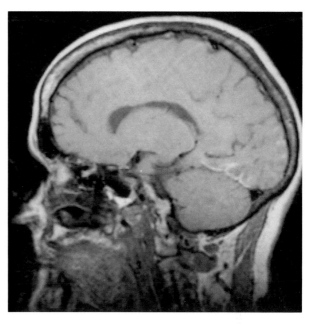

Fig. 14-9 Hemorrhagic conversion of an infarct is a common event. Hemorrhage is usually scant and superficial.

HEMORRHAGE IN AN INFARCT

Petechial gyral hemorrhage in a cerebral infarct is fairly common and is seen in at least 25% of cases. Detection of this infarct by CT is usually difficult. This degree of hemorrhage is usually asymptomatic and is most commonly seen in embolic infarctions.

Visualization of areas of gyral hyperintensity in an infarcted area on T_1-weighted MRI images presumably corresponds to the formation of methemoglobin (Fig. 14-9). It has been reported that methemoglobin forms faster in an infarcted area than in the noninfarcted normal brain because the infarcted area is rich in oxidizing free radicals. Early vascularization and luxury perfusion by increasing the local partial pressure of oxygen (PO_2), may contribute to this condition.[12]

Rarely, a large hemorrhage is observed. It may even rupture into the ventricular system (Fig. 14-10). These larger hemorrhages are more common in larger infarcts, in the hypertensive patient, and during the early days of infarction.[13] The radiological manifestations are those of an infarcted area containing hemorrhage. Rarely, confusing pictures is seen in which differentiation from a hemorrhagic tumor may be difficult.

Venous infarcts, especially those secondary to superior sagittal and lateral sinus thrombosis, tend to be hemorrhagic[14] (Fig. 14-11).

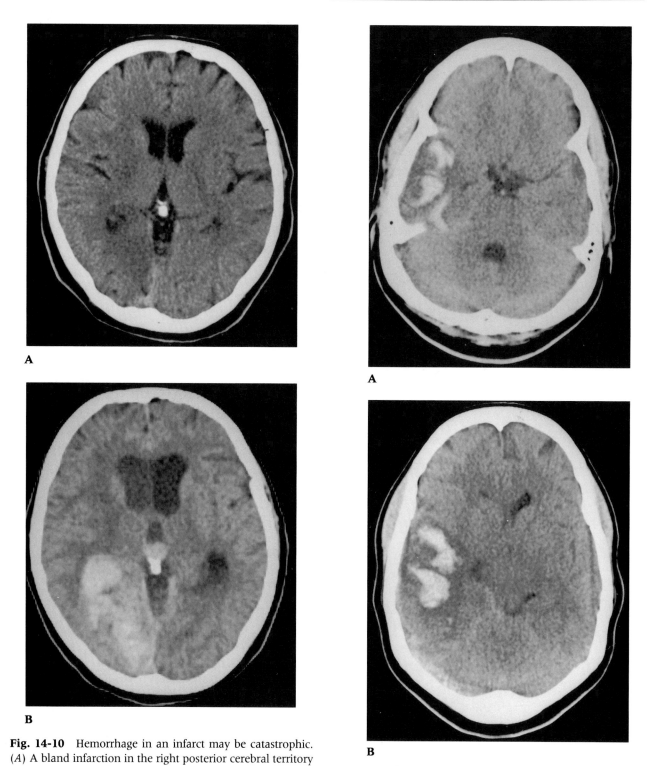

A

B

A

B

Fig. 14-10 Hemorrhage in an infarct may be catastrophic. (*A*) A bland infarction in the right posterior cerebral territory that became hemorrhagic 1 week later, with blood rupturing into the right lateral ventricle (*B*).

Fig. 14-11 Hemorrhagic venous infarction. Severe headache developed 10 days after delivery in this young woman. (*A*) and (*B*) demonstrate temporal lobe hemorrhage surrounded by infarcted brain. On (*B*) a dense, thrombosed lateral sinus is partially seen.

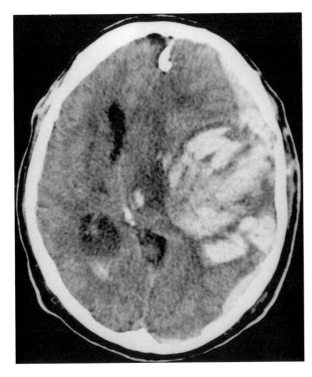

Fig. 14-12 Hemorrhage in a glioblastoma. This was the first clinical presentation in this patient. Note the significant mass effect and midline shift.

HEMORRHAGE IN A TUMOR

Tumors, both benign and malignant, may become hemorrhagic. Hemorrhage is seen in oligodendrogliomas and ependymomas, as well as in glioblastomas and metastatic lesions. Metastatic lesions with a hemorrhagic tendency are those seen with melanomas, choriocarcinomas, and renal and thyroid primaries.[15] These hemorrhages may be multiple. Accurate diagnosis of the disease requires historical data, a positive (for metastasis) chest x-ray, and comparison with previous studies. In the absence of this evidence, there are three helpful radiological signs:

1. There is an inordinate amount of edema around a hemorrhage that, clinically, is 1–2 days old. Edema persists even after 1 to 2 months (Fig. 14-12).

2. There are areas of abnormal enhancement on contrast-enhanced images that cannot be explained on the basis of hemorrhage alone.

3. The evolution of hemorrhage in a tumor is different from that of hemorrhage in the normal brain. Methemoglobin does not form. Formation of hemosiderin is either delayed or does not occur at all. The

ring of hemosiderin, if it forms at all, is incomplete.[16,17]

Hemorrhage in Coagulopathies, in Blood Dyscrasias, and in Patients Receiving Anticoagulants
Intracranial hemorrhage may be seen in patients with hemophilia and von Willebrand's disease, in thrombocytopenic patients (with idiopathic thrombocytopenic purpura, leukemia, aplastic anemia, etc.), and in patients receiving anticoagulants. Anticoagulant therapy carries a risk of 1–2% of intracerebral hemorrhage per year. Coumadin can cause intracranial hemorrhage in different compartments. Spinal epidural hematoma may occur.[18] Intracranial hemorrhage may complicate thrombolytic therapy in patients with myocardial infarction. In one study, the incidence was less than 1%. Of these patients, 62% died during hospitalization. Intracerebral and supratentorial locations were the most common sites.[19]

Drug Abuse and Intracranial Hemorrhage
Cerebral ischemia, subarachnoid hemorrhage, and intracerebral hemorrhage have been reported in cocaine users. The mechanisms of these neurological complications are not clear. Hypertension and abnormal neurovascular control may have a role.[20] There is usually no evidence of vasculitis. In one report, patients who suffered from intracranial hemorrhage frequently had underlying aneurysms or vascular malformations.[21] Amphetamine use may be associated with vasculitis.

SUBARACHNOID HEMORRHAGE

Head trauma is the most common cause of bloody CSF. Hypertension is the second most common cause of subarachnoid hemorrhage (SAH), with intralobar blood gaining access to the CSF via ventricular rupture. Bleeding from a saccular arterial aneurysm is the next most common cause.

In the United States, 26,000 cases of SAH each year cause about 10% of all deaths from stroke. Vascular malformations account for less than 10% of all SAH. Bleeding may occur at any age but is most likely in patients less than 30 years old. Other causes of SAH include blood dyscrasias, primary or secondary brain neoplasms, infections (bacterial endocarditis), arterial or venous hemorrhagic infarctions, and vasculitis. Some cases of SAH remain undiagnosed even at autopsy.[22]

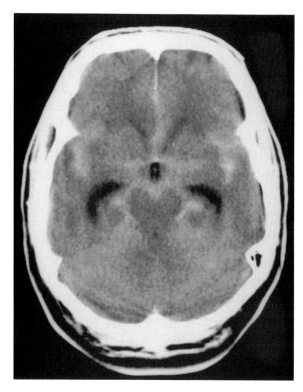

Fig. 14-13 SAH. Blood is seen in the suprasellar cistern, interhemispheric fissure, and sylvian fissures. There is mild hydrocephalus.

Radiological Examination

For a variety of reasons, CT remains the diagnostic tool of choice in the early diagnosis of SAH. CT is sensitive and easily performed. The appearance of high-density blood in the basal cisterns, especially the suprasellar and perimesencephalic cisterns, sylvian fissures, and interhemispheric fissures, is virtually diagnostic (Fig. 14-13). In abut 20% of cases, there is also parenchymal hemorrhage. CT may also demonstrate the causative aneurysm (especially if it is larger than 1.5 cm) or the vascular malformation. Finally, hydrocephalus secondary to SAH may be seen. Sensitivity of CT in detecting SAH varies with time: 95% of average SAHs can be detected early; after 1 week, the yield decreases to 50%. The location of the dominant subarachnoid blood may point to the site of an aneurysm. The amount of subarachnoid blood is directly proportional to the risk of spasm seen later.[23]

MRI is not as sensitive as CT. Blood in the subarachnoid space is mixed with CSF where ambient oxygen levels are high. As a result, significant methemoglobin formation does not occur for several days to 1 week. Due to the increased protein in CSF immediately after SAH, there is a subtle T_1 shortening. This causes the "dirty CSF" sometimes seen.[1] After several days to 1 week, increased signal intensity of CSF is due to methemoglobin formation (Fig. 14-14). The detection rate of SAH, according to Ogawa et al.,[24] is 36% on T_1- and 50% on T_2-weighted images (0.5 T magnet).[24,25]

In chronic, repeated SAH, there may be staining of leptomeninges, subpial tissue, spinal cord, and cranial nerves with hemosiderin, causing the typical decreased signal intensity on T_2-weighted images called *superficial siderosis*. Deafness, other cranial nerve findings, cerebellar dysfunction, and dementia may be associated[26] (Fig. 14-15).

Intracranial aneurysms

The great majority of intracranial aneurysms are berry aneurysms. These account for 70–90% of all aneurysms. Atherosclerotic and mycotic aneurysms also occur. Saccular aneurysms were found in 5–6% of consecutive autopsies performed by Stebbens.[27] They are probably slightly more common in females (3/2 ratio). Aneurysms usually occur at the site of branching of a vessel. The most common sites are the posterior communicating–internal carotid junction, anterior cerebral–anterior communicating junction, middle cerebral artery trifurcation, and internal carotid bifurcation. Ninety-five percent of *single* aneurysms are seen in the anterior circulation. Twenty percent of all aneurysms are multiple. There is an association with polycystic kidney disease and coarctation of the aorta.

Aneurysms may grow. When they reach a certain size, the danger of rupture increases. The size at which aneurysms are prone to rupture is probably between 5 and 10 mm (7 mm on a cooperative study).[28] The risk of rupture of an aneurysm is roughly 2–3% per year. It is much higher in the first 2 months after a SAH.

Despite significant progress in magnetic resonance angiography (MRA) visualization of aneurysms, angiography remains the procedure of choice. It is felt that aneurysms less than 4 mm in size may be missed by current MRA techniques.[29]

In some cases of SAH, angiography will not demonstrate the aneurysms. The usual reason is spasm and thrombosis of the aneurysm. Repeat angiography may demonstrate these aneurysms. Even after a second angiogram, however, a certain percentage of SAH remains unexplained.[30] In this context, a certain number of SAHs occur predominantly in perimesencephalic cisterns. These lesions have a very good prognosis, and

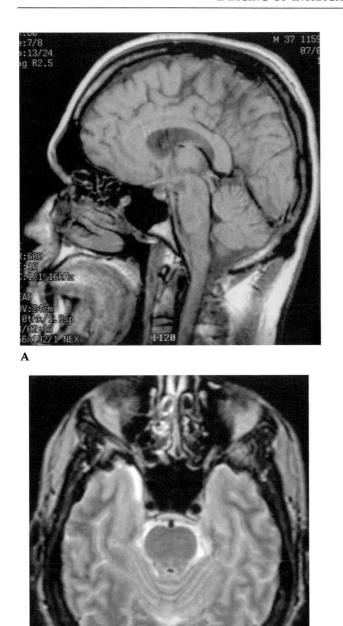

A

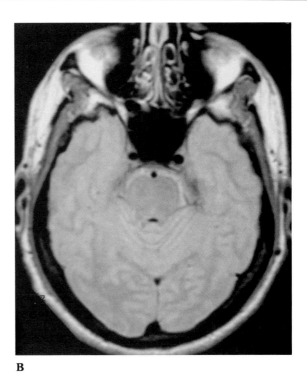

B

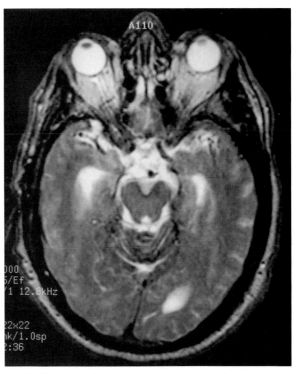

C

Fig. 14-14 SAH seen on MRI. Hemorrhage in (A) the pre-pontine, (B) interpeduncular, and (C) suprasellar cisterns.

Fig. 14-15 Superficial hemosiderosis. The T_2 hypointensity seen around the midbrain and folia of the vermis represents hemosiderin deposited in the meninges and subpial tissue as a result of repeated SAH.

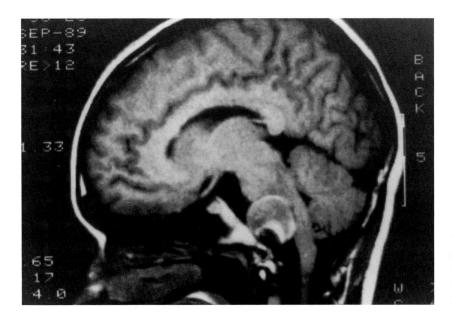

Fig. 14-16 Giant, partially thrombosed aneurysm. The MRI appearance, with an eccentric flow void surrounded by layers of hemorrhagic products of different ages, is virtually diagnostic.

the chance of recurrence is very low. The source of these subarachnoid blood "leaks" is not clear.[31]

An aneurysm larger than 2.5 cm in diameter is designated a *giant aneurysm.* The most common locations of these aneurysms are the cavernous carotid artery and middle cerebral artery. These lesions rarely bleed. They have a tendency to enlarge over time. They present most commonly with symptoms caused by increased intracranial pressure and mass effect. Quite often they become thrombosed. Calcification is frequent.

Atlas et al. described the MRI features of a giant thrombosed aneurysm.[32] There is usually an eccentric area of signal void corresponding to the patent lumen; signal loss is due to blood flow in this lumen. This is usually surrounded by a rim of methemoglobin. A lamellar arrangement of layers of thrombosis at different ages, calcification, and hemosiderin formation surround this complex. The resultant picture is usually diagnostic (Fig. 14-16).

Mycotic aneurysms account for 2% of all aneurysms. These aneurysms are usually small and are seen in more peripheral locations, especially along the middle cerebral artery branches. They are caused by inflammation of the vessel wall triggered by a septic embolus. Therefore, they are usually seen in patients with bacterial endocarditis and septicemia. By conservative estimates, the incidence of these aneurysms in bacterial endocarditis may be as high as 10%.[33] Rupture may be fatal in a high percentage (20–80%) of these patients. Subarachnoid and intracerebral hemorrhage may be

seen (Fig. 14-17). The hematomas may become secondarily infected.

Inflammatory aneurysms may be seen in polyarteritis nodosa, in cerebral arteritis secondary to herpes zoster ophthalmicus,[34] and in fungal and syphilitic infections.

VASCULAR MALFORMATIONS

Arteriovenous Malformations (AVMs)

Ninety-three percent of AVMs are supratentorial; 7% are in the posterior fossa. Eighteen percent are located in the basal ganglion/internal capsule regions. Presenting symptoms are seizures, intracranial (usually intralobar) hemorrhage, and headaches and symptoms referable to the steal phenomenon.

Ten percent of AVMs are associated with aneurysms. The aneurysms may occur on the arterial or venous side of an AVM. Intranidal aneurysms have been implicated in a higher risk of hemorrhage in an AVM.[35] Other factors associated with increased risk include a central location and central venous drainage.[36] The risk of hemorrhage is estimated at 2–4% per year. Lesions smaller than 3 cm have a higher tendency to hemorrhage. After an initial hemorrhage, the risk of hemorrhage is 6% in the first year. A grading system proposed by Spetzler and Martin considers size, the pattern of venous drainage, and the eloquence of the brain areas adjacent to the AVM in assigning grades (I to V) in an

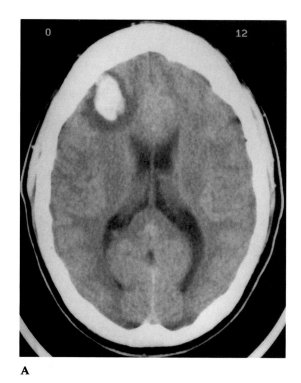

A

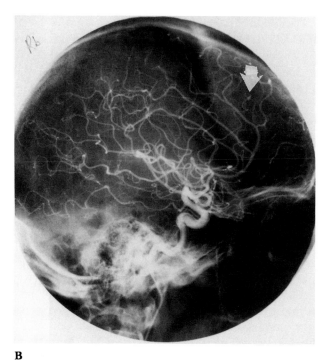

B

Fig. 14-17 Intralobar hemorrhage in subacute bacterial endocarditis. (*A*) A right frontal hematoma is demonstrated. (*B*) There was a small mycotic aneurysm in a branch of the right middle cerebral artery on angiography.

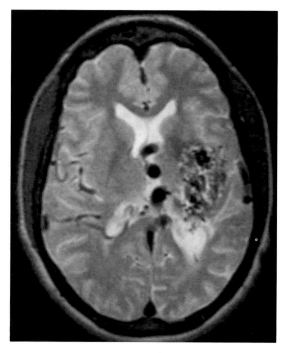

Fig. 14-18 A deep basal ganglionic AVM is demonstrated. Multiple flow voids seen above the third ventricle represent dilated, tortuous central venous drainage.

AVM.[37] The higher the grade, the greater the risk of surgical resection.

CT demonstrates serpiginous areas of increased density, sometimes with calcification. There is intense enhancement of these vessels after IV injection of contrast. There is usually no mass effect; recent hemorrhage and large draining veins may cause mass effect, however.

MRI, with its multiplanar capability, is superior to CT in demonstrating the relations of these lesions. MRI may show hemorrhage, either new or old, the feeding arteries, the nidus, and the draining veins. These capabilities can be further enhanced by judicious use of different MRA techniques. Thus, phase contrast MRA can be utilized to demonstrate the nidus, the draining veins, and the feeding arteries almost separately (Fig. 14-18).

Dural AVM, more commonly found in the posterior cranial fossa, should be considered separately. Here there are feeders from dural vessels; drainage is toward venous sinuses or collateral pial veins. The role of venous occlusive disease in these AVMs is controversial. These AVMs should be suspected whenever there is visualization of large superficial veins draining into a venous sinus in the absence of a parenchymal nidus.[38]

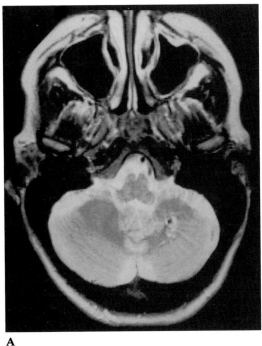

A

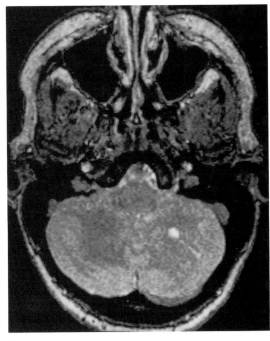

B

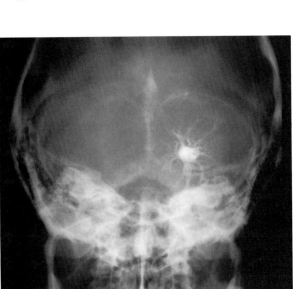

C

Fig. 14-19 Venous angioma. (*A*) (T$_2$-weighted) and (*B*) (flow-sensitive gradient echo) images demonstrate a venous angioma of the left cerebellar hemisphere. (*C*) The corresponding angiogram.

Treatment strategies include embolization, surgery, and radiosurgery, both separately and in combination. Sometimes embolization is used to reduce a large AVM to a size amenable to surgery or radiation therapy. Radiosurgery (treating a lesion with radiation focused on the lesion) is reserved for round lesions less than 2.5 cm in size. For complete obliteration of an AVM with radiosurgery, a period of about 2 years is usually required.[39] In these cases, enhancement on CT at the site of a previous AVM does not prove that the AVM is still patent. This determination can be made only with angiography.

Venous Angioma

Venous angioma is perhaps the most common vascular malformation. In one autopsy series its incidence was 2.6%.[40] Usually these lesions are found incidentally during CT or MRI. These structures, although anomalous, perform a normal function: They are part of the venous system draining that part of the brain. Most supratentorial venous angiomas do not cause hemorrhage (2 out of 30 in the Rigamonti series); posterior fossa venous angiomas may cause hemorrhage. The role of an associated cavernous angioma in hemorrhage is controversial.[41] If a hemorrhage occurs, treatment should focus on evacuation of the hematoma rather than resection of the venous angioma.

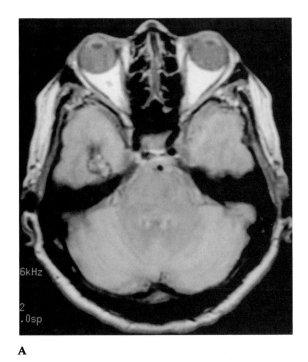

A

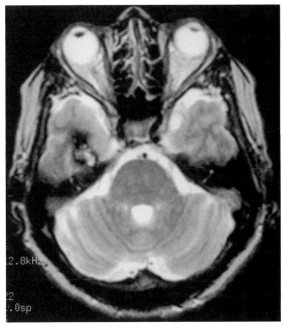

B

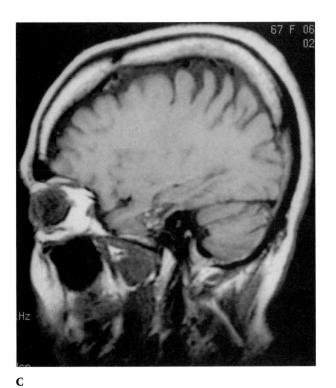

C

Fig. 14-20 Cavernous angioma. (*A*) (intermediate), (*B*) (T$_2$-weighted), and (*C*) (T$_1$-weighted) show a cavernous angioma of the right temporal lobe. Note the typically increased hypointensity of the periphery of the lesion with increasing T$_2$ weighting.

CT or MRI usually show a vein starting deep within the white matter and extending to the surface. This vein usually starts at a point where multiple smaller venous channels oriented in a radial distribution come together. It usually decreases in caliber as it extends to the surface (Fig. 14-19).

Cavernous Angiomas

Cavernous hemangiomas account for 10–15% of all intracranial and intraspinal malformations. These are thin-walled vascular caverns, the walls of which are devoid of smooth muscles. They do not have brain parenchyma in their interstices. Macroscopically, they are seen as distinct, well-defined "mulberry" malformations.[42]

Cavernous hemangiomas can be sporadic or familial. In the familial form, there is a high incidence of multiple lesions.[43]

Seizure is the most common presentation. Hemorrhage is rare: The risk of *symptomatic* hemorrhage is 0.7 per lesion per year in Robinson's series and 0.11 per lesion per year in Curling's series.[42] Hemorrhage did not change the outcome. Treatment is surgical and is indicated in patients with intractable seizures or with hemorrhage. Progressive neurological deficit is another reason for surgery. Brain stem lesions that are close to the outer surface or close to the fourth ventricle can be removed with minimal risk. Radiation therapy cannot be recommended at this time.

Radiologically, these lesions have a distinctive appearance and are usually inhomogeneous on T_1 and T_2 images. The center has a mixed-intensity "popcorn," multilobular appearance. Here the T_1 hyperintensity is attributed to methemoglobin. The periphery, best seen on T_2-weighted images, consists of a ring of hemosiderin (Fig. 14-20). So much of the radiological appearance of these lesions depends on different blood products that it is plausible that their appearance is the result of multiple asymptomatic hemorrhages.

A cavernous hemangioma is not surrounded by edema unless it has bled recently. The peripheral ring of hemosiderin must be complete. These features, along with a lack of any other components and additional soft tissue masses in the vicinity, help to differentiate them from hemorrhagic lesions, such as metastatic tumors which may resemble them.

Capillary telangiectasia, another vascular malformation, is usually small, consisting of dilated, thin capillaries with brain tissue interspersed between them. The pons is the most common site. It cannot be differentiated radiographically from a cavernous angioma.

REFERENCES

1. Bradley WG. MR appearance of hemorrhage in the brain. *Radiology* 1993;189:15–26.

2. Gomori JM, Grossman RI, Goldberg HI, et al. Intracranial hematomas: Imaging by high field MR. *Radiology* 1985; 157:87–92.

3. Zyed AM, Hayman LA, Bryan RN. MR imaging of intracerebral blood: Diversity in the temporal pattern at 0.5 and 1.0 T. *AJNR* 1991;12:469–474.

4. Jones KM, Mulkern RV, Mantello MT, et al. Brain hemorrhage evaluation with fast spin-echo and conventional dual spin-echo images. *Radiology* 1992;182:53–58.

5. Zimmerman RD, Leeds NE, Nadich TP. Ring blush with intracerebral hematoma. *Radiology* 1977;122:707–711.

6. Toole JF. Vascular disease, in *Merritt's Textbook of Neurology*, ed 7. Philadelphia, Lea & Febiger, 1984, p 149.

7. Escourolle R, Poirier J. Vascular pathology 1. Cerebral and/or meningeal hemorrhage, in *Manual of Basic Neuropathology*, ed 2. Philadelphia, WB Saunders, 1978, pp 67–81.

8. Case Records of the Massachusetts General Hospital: Case 27-1991. *N Engl J Med* 1991;325(1):42–54.

9. Loes DJ, Biller J, Yuh WTC, et al. Leukoencephalopathy in cerebral amyloid angiopathy: MR imaging in four cases. *AJNR* 1990;11:485–489.

10. Vinters HV, Gilbert JJ. Cerebral amyloid angiopathy: Incidence and complications in the aging brain II. The distribution of amyloid vascular changes. *Stroke* 1983;14: 924–928.

11. Wagle WA, Smith TW, Weiner M. Intracerebral hemorrhage caused by cerebral amyloid angiopathy: Radiologic–pathologic correlation. *AJNR* 1984;5:171–176.

12. Grotta JC. Can raising cerebral blood flow improve the outcome after acute cerebral infarction? *Stroke* 1987;18: 264–267.

13. Ott BR, Zamani AA, Kleefield J, et al. The clinical spectrum of hemorrhagic infarction. *Stroke* 1986;17: 630–637.

14. Buonamo FS, Moody DM, Ball RM. CT scan findings in cerebral sinovenous occlusion. *J Comput Assist Tomogr* 1978;2:281–290.

15. Zimmerman RA, Bilaniuk LT. Computed tomography of intratumoral hemorrhage. *Radiology* 1980;135:355–359.

16. Atlas SW, Grossman RI, Gomori JM, et al. Hemorrhagic intracranial malignant neoplasms: Spin-echo MR imaging. *Radiology* 1987;164:71–77.

17. Sze G, Krol G, Olsen WL, et al. Hemorrhagic neoplasms: MR mimics of occult vascular malformations. *AJNR* 1987;8:795–802.

18. Snyder M, Renaudin J. Intracranial hemorrhage associated with anticoagulation therapy. *Surg Neurol* 1977;7: 31–34.

19. Uglietta JP, O'Connor C, Boyko OB, et al. CT pattern of intracranial hemorrhage complicating thrombolytic therapy for acute myocardial infarction. *Radiology* 1991;181: 555–559.

20. Jacobs IG, Roszler M, Kelly JK, et al. Cocaine abuse: Neurovascular complications. *Radiology* 1989;170:223–227.

21. Levine ST, Brust JCM, Futrell N, et al. Cerebrovascular complications of the use of the "crack" form of alkaloidal cocaine. *N Engl J Med* 1990;323:699–704.

22. Brust JCM. Subarachnoid hemorrhage, in *Merritt's Textbook of Neurology*, ed 7. Philadelphia, Lea & Febiger, 1984, pp 185–191.

23. Davis JM, Davis KR, Crowell RM. Subarachnoid hemorrhage secondary to rupture in intracranial aneurysm: Prognostic significance of cranial CT. *AJR* 1980;134: 711–715.

24. Ogawa T, Inugami A, Shimosegawa E, et al. Subarachnoid hemorrhage: Evaluation with MR imaging. *Radiology* 1993;186:345–351.

25. Atlas T. MR imaging is highly sensitive for acute subarachnoid hemorrhage . . . NOT! *Radiology* 1993;186: 319–322.

26. Gomori J, Grossman RI, Bilaniuk LT, et al. High field MR imaging of superficial siderosis of the central nervous system. *J Comput Assist Tomogr* 1985;9:972–975.

27. Stebbens WE. *Pathology of Cerebral Blood Vessels.* St Louis, CV Mosby, 1972, p 383.

28. Locksey HB. Report on the cooperative study of intracranial aneurysms and subarachnoid hemorrhage, Section 5, Part 1, Natural history of subarachnoid hemorrhage, intracranial aneurysms and arteriovenous malformations. *J Neurosurg* 1966;25:219–239.

29. Glicklich M, Ross JS. MR angiography: Clinical applications. *Appl Radiol* 1992;77–83.

30. Suzuki S, Kayama T, Sakurai Y, et al. Subarachnoid hemorrhage of unknown cause. *Neurosurgery* 1987;21:310–313.

31. Rinkel GJE, Wijdicks EFM, Vermenden M, et al. Outcome in perimesencephalic (nonaneurysmal) subarachnoid hemorrhage: A follow-up study in 37 patients. *Neurology* 1990;40:1130–1132.

32. Atlas SW, Grossman RI, Goldberg HI, et al. Partially thrombosed giant intracranial aneurysms: Correlation of MR and pathologic findings. *Radiology* 1987;162:111–114.

33. Frazer JG, Cahan LD, Winter J. Bacterial intracranial aneurysms. *J Neurosurg* 1980;53:633–651.

34. O'Donoghue JM, Enzmann DR. Mycotic aneurysm in angiitis associated with herpes zoster ophthalmicus. *AJNR* 1987;8:615–619.

35. Marks MP, Lane B, Steinberg GK, et al. Intranidal aneurysms in cerebral arteriovenous malformations: Evaluation and endovascular treatment. *Radiology* 1992;183:355–360.

36. Chappell PM, Steinberg GK, Marks MP. Clinically documented hemorrhage in cerebral arteriovenous malformations: MR characteristics. *Radiology* 1992;183:719–724.

37. Spetzler RF, Martin NA. A proposed grading system for arteriovenous malformations. *J Neurosurg* 1986;65:476–483.

38. De Marco JK, Dillon WP, Holbach VV, et al. Dural arteriovenous fistulas: Evaluation with MR imaging. *Radiology* 1990;175:193–199.

39. Kjellberg RN, Hanamura T, Davis KR, et al. Bragg-peak proton beam therapy for arteriovenous malformations of the brain. *N Engl J Med* 1983;309:269–274.

40. Sarwar M, McCormick WF. Intracerebral venous angioma. Case report and review. *Arch Neurol* 1978;35:323–325.

41. Rigamonti D, Spetzler RF, Medina M, et al. Cerebral venous malformations. *J Neurosurg* 1990;73:560–564.

42. Golfinos JG, Warcher TM, Zabramski JM, et al. The management of unruptured intracranial vascular malformations. *BNI Q* 1992;8(3):2–11.

43. Rigamonti D, Hadley MN, Drayer BP. Cerebral cavernous malformations incidence and familial occurrence. *N Engl J Med* 1988;319:343–347.

15

Magnetic Resonance Imaging of Acute Ischemic Infarcts

Ay-Ming Wang, M.D., William T.C. Yuh, M.D.

INTRODUCTION

The diagnosis of cerebral ischemia in its very early stages by clinical and radiological methods can be difficult. Magnetic resonance imaging (MRI) has been shown to be more sensitive than computed tomography (CT) in the detection of acute cerebral ischemia within the first 72 hr.[1-9] Vascular flow–related abnormalities, including the absence of normal flow void and the presence of arterial enhancement, are the earliest MRI findings detected within minutes of onset.[9] Morphological changes (brain edema) on T_1-weighted images without signal changes on T_2-weighted images can be detected within the first few hours. Signal changes are not usually found before 8 hr on T_2-weighted images or before 16 hr on T_1-weighted images. Paramagnetic contrast administration often provides valuable information in detecting and characterizing complete cerebral infarction and transient brain ischemia and helps to predict the accuracy of the prognosis in patients with ischemic stroke.

TECHNIQUE

Sagittal and axial T_1-weighted (short repetition time (TR), short echo time (TE)) and axial T_2-weighted (long TR, long TE) spin-echo images of the brain are obtained with a 3-mm to 10-mm slice thickness and a 10–50% slice gap.

Postcontrast T_1-weighted imaging should be performed immediately after IV injection of 0.1 mmol/kg of paramagnetic contrast (e.g., Magnevist, Berlex Laboratories, Inc., Wayne, NJ). Postcontrast pulse parameters and imaging planes should be identical to those of the precontrast T_1-weighted sequences.

MRI FINDINGS

The detection of acute cerebral ischemia by MRI may depend on many pathophysiological factors (Table 15-1) that are often coexistent. Alteration of normal blood flow is a flow-kinetics phenomenon that should be detected immediately. The remaining factors are biophysiological phenomena that may take time to be appreciated by MRI. The use of paramagnetic contrast may increase the sensitivity in detecting acute ischemia, probably due to either accentuation of the underlying flow derangement or accumulation of abnormal amounts of contrast agent in the ischemic tissue. Normal arterial structures are generally devoid of intraluminal MRI signal due to rapid and/or turbulent flow, the so-called flow-void phenomenon, which is best seen on T_2-weighted images.

Absence of normal flow-void phenomenon in major intracranial vessels has been reported to be an indicator of early cerebral ischemia.[9,10] However, the absence of normal flow-void phenomenon in smaller arterial ves-

TABLE 15-1 Pathophysiologic Mechanisms for MRI Findings in Brain Ischemia

Mechanism	MRI Findings	Possible Causes	Estimated Time*
Flow kinetics	Absent flow void	Slow flow; occlusion	Immediately
	Arterial enhancement	Slow flow	Immediately
Biophysiological	T_1 morphologic change (swelling)	Cytotoxic edema (free water)	2–4 hr
	T_2 signal change	Blood–brain barrier (BBB) breakdown; vasogenic edema; macromolecular binding	8 hr
	T_1 signal change	BBB breakdown; vasogenic edema; macromolecular binding	16–24 hr
Combination	Progressive parenchymal enhancement‡	Impaired delivery of significant amount of contrast agent	>120 hr†
	Early exaggerated enhancement§	Intact delivery of contrast agent; focal hyperemia	2–4 hr

*Time at which findings generally may first be detected by available MRI examinations; this does not necessarily imply the exact time of onset.
†Usually not detected before 5–7 days.
‡Typical findings in completed cortical infarctions.
§Found in cases with transient or partial occlusions and in watershed infarctions.
Source: Adapted with permission from Yuh et al.[9]

sels (such as cortical branches of the middle cerebral artery) may not be appreciated on unenhanced MRI studies. The presence of a dense artery sign seen on the CT scan has been reported to be an early sign of ischemic infarction,[11–13] but this finding may be less conspicuous than that of contrast-enhanced MRI studies. Arterial enhancement has been shown in nearly half of the acute ischemic lesions studied,[14] on T_1-weighted images usually in cortical lesions; it can appear immediately after ictus and can persist for 7 days. The abnormal arterial enhancement can be seen in large arteries in both anterior (Fig. 15-1) and posterior circulation lesions, as well as in smaller arteries in distal cortical distributions. However, enhancement of the terminal arteries supplying isolated, deep noncortical lesions cannot be detected, probably due to their small size. Arterial enhancement can be seen both in complete proximal occlusion with retrograde collateral flow and in incomplete occlusion with slow antegrade flow. Although the mechanism of arterial enhancement is unknown, slow flow is the most likely explanation.

Morphological Changes

Morphological changes in the brain caused by brain tissue swelling can be best seen on T_1-weighted MRI studies in the first 24 hr after the onset of symptoms. Brain swelling can be detected either by gross enlargement of structures or, more often, by distortion of the normal adjacent structures. Morphological changes occur frequently in cortical lesions, where swelling is best demonstrated by obliteration of cortical sulci. Morpho-

logical changes in isolated noncortical lesions, including those in the deep white matter, noncortical gray matter, and brain stem, are less obvious. The incidence of morphological changes seen on T_1-weighted images of acute ischemic lesions is identical to that of arterial enhancement. However, arterial enhancement is far more obvious.

Signal Changes

Abnormal increases in signal (T_2 prolongation) on T_2-weighted images usually cannot be detected until 8 hr after the onset of cerebral ischemia. Compared with incomplete ischemia, complete ischemia tends to have earlier and more extensive T_2 prolongation. Compared with T_2-weighted images, signal changes on T_1-weighted images are much less sensitive in detecting early cerebral ischemia.

Brain Parenchymal Enhancement

Enhancement of ischemic brain parenchyma by a paramagnetic contrast agent depends on the availability of the contrast agent in the ischemic zone. Adequate vascular delivery of the contrast agent, as well as abnormal local tissue accumulation of contrast, are the two basic steps to determine this availability. Parenchymal enhancement can occur only when the delivery of contrast material is intact. In contrast to the typically progressive gyriform cortical enhancement seen in the subacute to chronic phases of ischemic infarct,[15,16] early and/or intense enhancement of brain parenchyma may

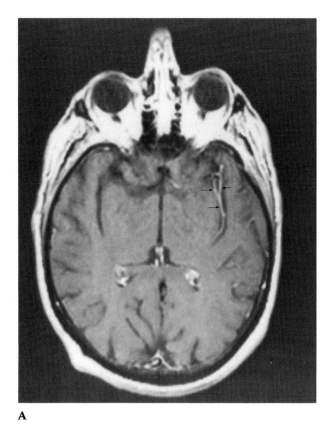 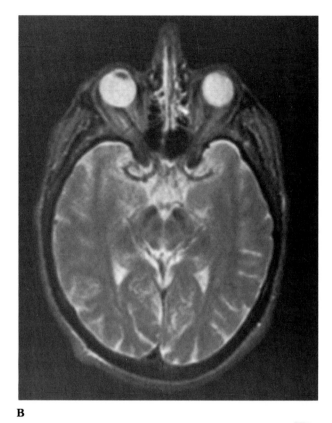

A   B

Fig. 15-1   Complete ischemia in a 62-year-old man with acute left hemispheric stroke symptoms. (*A*) Gadopentetate dimeglum-ine–enhanced axial T$_1$-weighted (TR 700/TE 20) image obtained 3 hr after the onset of symptoms shows abnormal arterial enhancement (arrows) in the distribution of the left middle cerebral artery. No abnormal parenchymal enhancement is seen. (*B*) Axial T$_2$-weighted (TR 2200/TE 90) image at a corresponding level shows no parenchymal T$_2$ signal changes.

also be seen in the first 24 hr after the onset of symptoms.[9,10]

Virapongse et al.[17] divided tissue perfusion during an acute ischemic insult in two categories: complete ischemia (no perfusion) and incomplete ischemia (some perfusion). In the setting of complete proximal vascular occlusion without preexisting collateral flow (complete ischemia, no perfusion) (Fig. 15-1), no early parenchymal enhancement occurs. In incomplete is-chemia (some perfusion), early parenchymal enhance-ment (Fig. 15-2) can be seen due to the delivery of contrast material during the acute stage. This enhance-ment may be maintained with partial vessel occlusion or may be promptly restored after interruption of flow in transient vessel occlusion. Ischemic lesions with early parenchymal enhancement in incomplete ischemia tend to have a better prognosis than ische-mic lesions without early parenchymal enhancement in complete ischemia.

There is an inverse relationship between arterial and parenchymal enhancement, with arterial enhancement occurring in the acute phase of ischemia only when perfusion is absent (complete ischemia). Arterial en-hancement dissipates and parenchymal enhancement develops in the subacute stage (7–30 days) as collateral flow is established. In the acute phase, the area of parenchymal enhancement also appears to be inversely related to the area of signal abnormality on T$_2$-weighted images. Parenchymal enhancement tends to be absent when the area and intensity of signal abnor-mality on T$_2$-weighted are greatest, both indicating a severe ischemic insult.

SUMMARY

1. With an increasing armamentarium of stroke thera-pies, early, precise radiological diagnosis is becom-ing more and more important. MRI with paramag-netic contrast enhancement will play an important

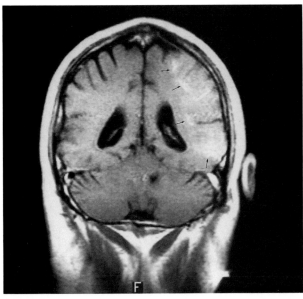

A

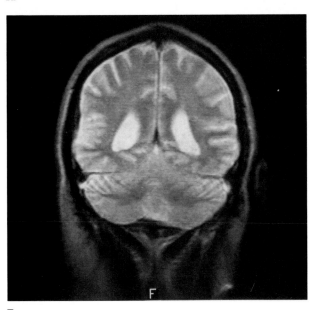

B

Fig. 15-2. Incomplete ischemia in a 67-year-old man who underwent a preoperative balloon occlusion test of left internal carotid artery and developed acute ischemic symptoms after 2 min of carotid occlusion. After balloon deflation, preservation of carotid flow was demonstrated angiographically. (*A*) Gadopentetate dimeglumine–enhanced coronal T_1-weighted image (TR 583/TE 20) obtained 2 hr after the onset of symptoms shows diffuse parenchymal enhancement of the left cerebral hemisphere (arrows). Parenchymal morphological changes (swelling with mass effect) are noted, without evidence of discrete arterial enhancement. (*B*) Axial T_2-weighted coronal image (TR 2000/TE 100) at the corresponding level shows no parenchymal signal changes.

role in early detection of stroke and will improve the prognosis as a result of adequate early treatment.

2. MRI imaging of the brain with paramagnetic contrast enhancement is very useful in detecting and characterizing complete cerebral infarction and transient brain ischemia in their acute stages.

3. In complete ischemia, arterial enhancement appears early and is paralleled by parenchymal T_2-weighted image prolongation, while parenchymal enhancement slowly develops subacutely. Incomplete brain ischemia, by contrast, typically demonstrates early intense parenchymal enhancement, with minimal or no T_2-weighted parenchymal signal abnormalities or arterial enhancement.

REFERENCES

1. Bryan RN, Wilcott MR, Schneiders NJ, et al. Nuclear magnetic resonance evaluation of stroke. *Radiology* 1983; 149:189–192.

2. Sipponen JT, Kastle M, Ketonen L, et al. Serial nuclear magnetic resonance (NMR) imaging in patients with cerebral infarction. *J Comput Assist Tomogr* 1983;7:585–589.

3. Sipponen JT. Visualization of brain infarction with nuclear magnetic resonance imaging. *Neuroradiology* 1984; 26:590–594.

4. Biller J, Adams HP Jr, Dunn V, et al. Dichotomy between clinical findings and MR abnormalities in pontine infarction. *J Comput Assist Tomogr* 1986;10:379–385.

5. Rothrock JF, Lyden PD, Hesselink JR, et al. Brain magnetic resonance imaging in the evaluation of lacunar stroke. *Stroke* 1987;18:781–786.

6. Brown JJ, Hesselink JR, Rothrock JF. MR and CT in lacunar infarcts. *AJNR* 1988;151:367–372.

7. Kinkel PR, Kinkel WR, Jacobs L. Nuclear magnetic resonance imaging in patients with stroke. *Semin Neurol* 1986;6:43–52.

8. Kertesz A, Black SE, Nicholson L, et al. The sensitivity and specificity of MRI in stroke. *Neurology* 1987;37:1580–1585.

9. Yuh WTC, Crain MR, Ioes DJ, et al. MR imaging of cerebral ischemia: Findings in the first 24 hours. *AJR* 1991;157:565–573.

10. Biller J, Yuh WTC, Mitchell GW, et al. Early diagnosis of basilar artery occlusion using magnetic resonance imaging. *Stroke* 1988;19:297–306.

11. Pressman BD, Tourje JF, Thompson JR. An early CT sign of ischemic infarction: Increased density in a cerebral artery. *AJNR* 1987;8:645–648.

12. Tomsick TA, Brott TG, Chamber AA, et al. Hyperdense

middle cerebral artery sign on CT: Efficacy in detecting middle cerebral artery thrombosis. *AJNR* 1990;11: 473–477.

13. Schuknecht B, Rutzka M, Hoffman E. The "dense artery sign"—major cerebral artery thromboembolism demonstrated by computed tomography. *Neuroradiology* 1990; 32:98–103.

14. Crain MR, Yuh WTC, Greene GM, et al. Cerebral ischemia: Evaluation with contrast-enhanced MRI imaging. *AJNR* 1991;12:631–639.

15. Imakita S, Nishimura T, Naito H, et al. Magnetic resonance imaging of human cerebral infarct: Enhancement with Gd-DTPA. *Neuroradiology* 1987;29:422–429.

16. Imakita S, Nishimura T, Yamada N, et al. Magnetic resonance imaging of cerebral infarct: Time course of Gd-DTPA enhancement and CT comparison. *Neuroradiology* 1988;30:372–378.

17. Virapongse C, Mancuso A, Quisling R. Human brain imaging: Gd-DTPA-enhanced MR imaging. *Radiology* 1986; 161:785–794.

16

Computed Tomography and Magnetic Resonance Imaging of Subacute and Chronic Infarcts

Amir A. Zamani, M.D.

PATHOLOGY

Detection of a blind acute infarction with the naked eye is difficult in the first few hours. After 8 hr the damaged zone is usually pale and softer than adjacent brain. The distinction between gray and white matter becomes less distinct. Microscopically and after 6 hr, the neurons and glial cells undergo ischemic changes. The nuclei become pyknotic. There is swelling of neurons and endothelia.

Phagocytic activity occurs rapidly. Between 24 and 48 hr, the predominant cells are polymorphonuclear. After 48 hr, foamy macrophages dominate. Edema remains for 2 to 10 days but gradually decreases, and the boundaries of the infarcted area become more evident. After 10 days liquefaction begins. Cavitation becomes evident after 3 weeks. It takes about 3 months for 1 cm^3 of the infarcted tissue to be removed. After a few months, a cystic cavity is all that remains. This is traversed by vascular–connective tissue septae and surrounded by glial proliferation. There is dilatation of the adjacent ventricles and subarachnoid spaces.[1-3]

IMAGING WITH COMPUTED TOMOGRAPHY (CT) AND MAGNETIC RESONANCE IMAGING (MRI)

Findings on imaging studies reflect the pathological changes described above. A subacute infarct on CT is seen as an area of low absorption in a vascular distribution. The lesion may be slightly inhomogeneous. This inhomogeneity is caused by petechial hemorrhage, the beginning of liquefaction, and vascular proliferation. If there is mass effect, it is usually decreasing.

During the second and third weeks, infarcts appear smaller and occasionally are difficult to detect. This so-called fogging phenomenon was described in 1979 by Becker et al.[4] At this time, active phagocytosis of the dead tissue is taking place. There is also ingrowth of neovascular channels and often petechial hemorrhage (Fig. 16-1). Intense enhancement is usually present at this time.

After the third week infarction reappears, and from then on the density of the lesion gradually decreases, in time approaching that of cerebrospinal fluid (CSF).

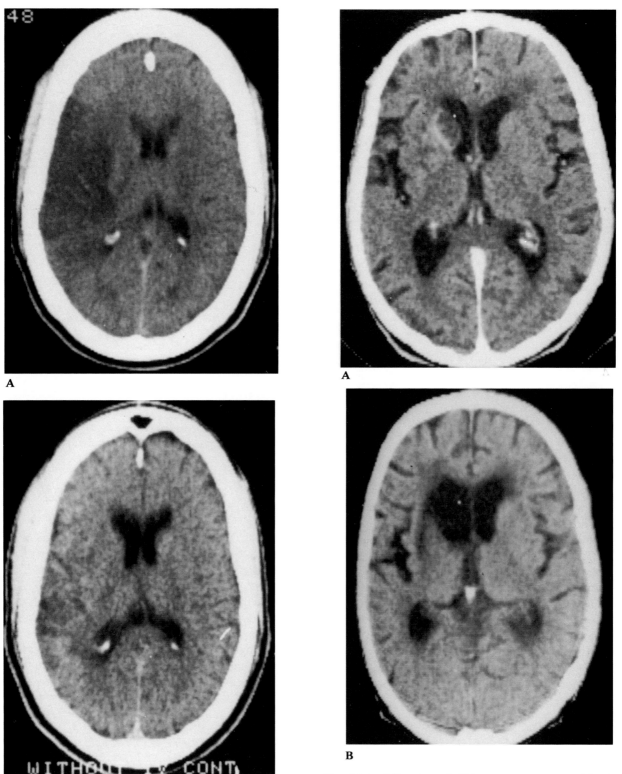

Fig. 16-1 Fogging effect. (*A*) Acute middle cerebral artery territory infarct. (*B*) Two weeks later, the infarct is less visible.

Fig. 16-2 Dilatation of CSF spaces next to an old infarct. (*A*) Acute basal ganglionic infarct with mass effect and enhancement. (*B*) Three months later, there is dilatation of the adjacent right frontal horn.

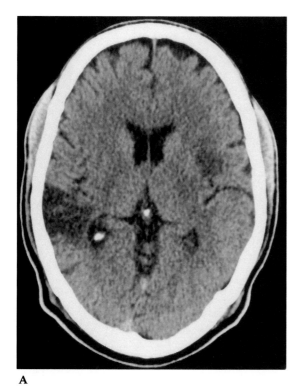

A

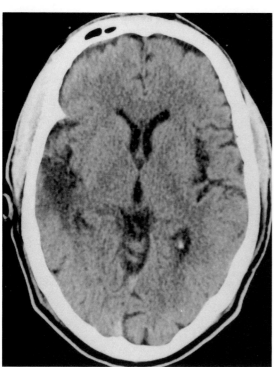

B

Fig. 16-3 (*A*) Acute left insular infarct. (*B*) Eighteen months later, all that is left is mild dilatation of the left sylvian fissure.

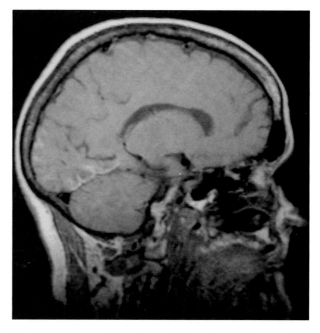

Fig. 16-4 Hemorrhage in an infarct is usually superficial and small.

There is gradual widening of the ventricles and subarachnoid spaces near the lesion.[5] There may be shrinkage of the ipsilateral brain stem (see below) (Fig. 16-2). There is usually no calcification.

Contrast enhancement is usually not employed in the evaluation of a known old infarct; enhancement is a feature of new infarcts. If a lesion considered to be an infarct continues to enhance after 1 or 2 months, the diagnosis should be seriously reconsidered.

If a small cortical infarct is examined months after the ictus occurs, an abnormally widened sulcus may be the only finding (Fig. 16-3). It may be difficult to differentiate this from cortical atrophy.

The MRI appearance of a subacute or chronic infarct is a reflection of the pathological changes described above. Formation of methemoglobin as a result of hemorrhage in an infarct is fairly common. This methemoglobin may last for a long time in an infarcted area (Fig. 16-4).

On T_2-weighted images, an old infarct may look superficially similar to an acute infarct (Fig. 16-5). The differentiation on T_1-weighted images is less problematic, as one notes the associated ex vacuo dilatation of adjacent CSF spaces seen with old infarcts. On intermediate images, a chronic infarct may have a (gliotic) border which is brighter than the center (macrocystic change). This difference is less evident on more heavily T_2-weighted images.[6]

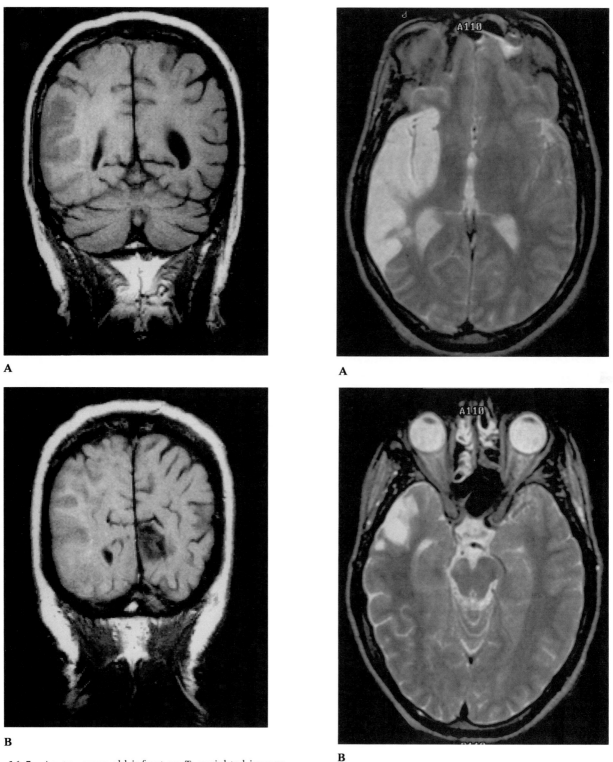

A

B

Fig. 16-5 Acute versus old infarct on T$_1$-weighted images. (A) New right occipitoparietal infarct. (B) Old parasagittal infarct on the left side. The intensity difference is obvious.

A

B

Fig. 16-6 Wallerian degeneration. (A) Old right middle cerebral artery infarct. Dilatation of the right atrium. (B) Shrinkage of the right cerebral peduncle and cord. A focal area of T$_2$ hyperintensity appears in it.

Wallerian degeneration may be visible in the ipsilateral brain stem in a brain harboring a chronic infarct. Following sizable cortical or capsular infarction, this change may take weeks to develop, but it lasts indefinitely. It is seen as punctate areas of increased T_2 intensity along the course of the corticospinal tract in the brain stem. Associated shrinkage of the ipsilateral brain stem is best appreciated on axial T_1-weighted images (Fig. 16-6). Wallerian degeneration may be seen with other pathological entities such as demyelination and tumors.[7]

REFERENCES

1. Escourolle R, Poirier J. Vascular pathology, in *Manual of Brain Neuropathology*. Philadelphia, WB Saunders, 1978, pp 82–104.

2. Schochet SS, McCormick WF. *Neurovascular disease,* in *Essentials of Neuropathology.* New York, Appleton-Century-Crofts, 1979, pp. 87–100.

3. Burger PC, Vogel FS. Cerebrovascular disease, a teaching monograph. Bethesda, MD, American Association of Pathologists, 1978, pp 257–313.

4. Becker H, Desch H, Hocker H, et al. CT effect with ischemic cerebral infarcts. *Neuroradiology* 1979;18:185–192.

5. Hakin IV, Rynder-Cooke A, Melanson D. Sequential computerized tomographic appearance of strokes. *Stroke* 1983; 14:893–897.

6. Wong WS, Tsuruda JS, Kortman DE, et al. in *Practical MRI.* Rockville, MD, Aspen Publishers, 1987, pp 87–89.

7. Kuhn MJ, Johnson KA, Davis KR. Wallerian degeneration evaluated by MR imaging. *Radiology* 1988;168:199–202.

17

Principles of Magnetic Resonance Angiography

John E. Kirsch Ph.D., Anil N. Shetty Ph.D.

INTRODUCTION

Magnetic resonance imaging (MRI) has rapidly become the mode of choice for the diagnosis of numerous diseases and disorders, particularly in the brain. Much of the reason lies in the fact that MRI possesses the ability to achieve a high level of soft tissue contrast owing to its multiparametric dependence on inherent properties of the tissues. Hydrogen proton density, T_1 and T_2 relaxation, magnetic susceptibility, and chemical shift are all intrinsic characteristics that influence the magnetic resonance (MR) signal of a given technique that eventually leads to the image contrast.

Long before MRI became accepted in the clinical setting, however, it was well known that the signal intensity in an in vivo experiment was also extremely sensitive to flow and motion.[1-5] Techniques were developed to quantitate both the macroscopic motion associated with bulk flow and the microscopic motion related to molecular diffusion.[4] Even in the early development of MRI, artifactual effects of bulk motion and blood flow were observed.[6-8] However, soon after MRI was developed as an anatomically based diagnostic tool, imaging methods to visualize blood flow and the vasculature were pursued.[9-11] *Magnetic resonance angiography (MRA)* has rapidly progressed, becoming an accepted adjunct to the routine MRI examination. Aside from the overall inherent advantage of MRI as an imaging modality that does not use ionizing radiation, MRA is noninvasive and can be performed without the use of an injected dye or contrast medium.

The conceptual approach to visualizing vessels with MRA is simple. If static tissue information is minimized and blood flow information is maximized, then in principle a high degree of contrast will result from the vasculature. In general, the MRI "information" lies in the MR radiofrequency signal that is detected. This signal is in actuality no different from any other form of electromagnetic radiation (albeit nonionizing) and therefore possesses two fundamental types of information—a magnitude and a phase. In the vast majority of conventional MRI applications, the signal phase is typically discarded and the magnitude is displayed in the image as tissue intensity or brightness. The diagnostic utility of an MRI application is based on whether the signal magnitudes coming from different tissues can be manipulated in such a way as to maximize the difference between them, leading to high tissue contrast in the image. The image quality depends on whether this can be achieved without too severely compromising the overall magnitude of the signals. In the MRA application, the strategy is very different. In order to highlight the MRI information coming from the signal of blood, the information from stationary tissue must be suppressed, not maximized.

Although numerous MRI methods exist to visualize

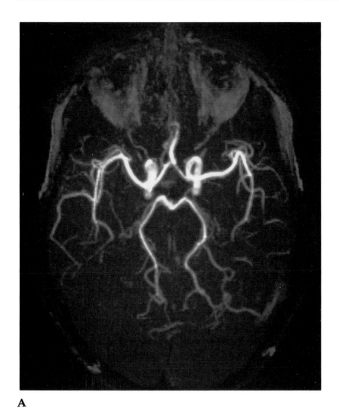

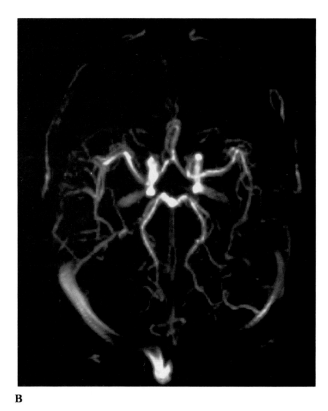

A   B

Fig. 17-1   MRA using (A) TOF, and (B) PC techniques. In TOF, vessel contrast is obtained by maximizing the signal magnitude from blood. In PC, visualization of the vessels results from maximizing the signal phase difference from blood.

blood flow, they fall into two main categories that exploit the effects of motion on the two basic types of information that come from the MR signal. Of these, several techniques have gained the widest acceptance in the clinical setting and are the primary focus of this chapter. *Time-of-flight (TOF) MRA* detects the difference in the *signal magnitude* information between moving blood in the vasculature and that of the surrounding stationary tissue. Vessel contrast comes from the ability to maximize the signal from blood while minimizing it from tissue. *Phase contrast* (PC) *MRA* observes changes in the *signal phase* information between static tissue and flowing blood. Here, contrast and visualization of the vasculature arise from maximizing the phase difference seen in the blood while minimizing this difference in surrounding tissue. Figure 17-1 illustrates the comparative results that can be typically obtained by TOF and PC MRA. In neither case was a contrast medium or dye administered. Vascular contrast was obtained solely on the basis of the differences in the signal information from stationary tissue and moving blood. Although each possesses the ability to portray vessels, subtle differences between the two can clearly be seen.

Whether maximizing the signal magnitude in TOF or the phase difference in PC techniques, knowledge of how both are affected by motion is critical to their successful implementation. In the first part of this chapter, fundamental principles of how motion influences signal magnitude and phase is presented. This is followed by an introduction to the concepts of the TOF and PC MRA techniques, along with their advantages and disadvantages. In the final section, potential pitfalls and artifacts commonly seen with the use of current MRA methods are presented.

THEORETICAL CONCEPTS IN FLOW IMAGING

At any given time during MRI, the bulk magnetization of a tissue, whether it is moving or stationary, is comprised of two vector components. The longitudinal component, M_z, which lies in the z-direction of the main external magnetic field, grows in magnitude toward its thermal equilibrium value M_0 at a rate governed by the T_1 relaxation time. The transverse component, M_{xy}, lying in the x-y plane that is perpendicular to the main external field, decays in magnitude based on its phase evolution at a rate governed by the T_2 relaxation time and by any other mechanism that induces phase changes in the transverse magnetization. In general, the study of flow in MRI is simply the study of how motion directly and independently affects the longitudinal magnetization, M_z, through spin saturation and the transverse magnetization, M_{xy}, through phase changes.

In virtually all MR imaging techniques, it is only the transverse component, M_{xy}, that is ultimately detected. The MR signal related to M_{xy} has a magnitude and phase associated with it at any point in time during imaging acquisition and at any point in space, whether in a blood vessel or in brain tissue. The following sections will demonstrate that both the signal magnitude and signal phase are influenced by motion such as the flow of blood through vessels. Changes in magnitude and phase due to motion constitute the two main categories of methods used to visualize flow in MRI. TOF MRA exploits the differences seen in the magnitude of the signal from flow relative to the surrounding stationary tissue, and PC MRA uses the differences observed in the phase of the signal associated with flow.

Spin Saturation (Magnitude)

In studying how signal magnitude is affected by flow, it is easiest to consider only the magnitude of M_{xy} immediately after radiofrequency (RF) pulsing, where, under this condition, the evolution of the phase is negligible and can be ignored in the treatment.

One RF Pulse and Magnetization
The action of applying an *RF pulse* in an MR experiment consists of rotating the *bulk magnetization* from an initial vector direction to a final direction by the *flip angle* θ_{rf}. The *transverse magnetization, M_{xy}*, immediately following the application of an RF pulse of flip angle θ_{rf} can be expressed as

$$M_{xy}(+) = M_0 \sin \theta_{rf}, \quad (17\text{-}1)$$

where M_0 designates the *thermal equilibrium magnetization* that originally lies longitudinally along the z-axis of the main external magnetic field. In other words, $M_z(-) = M_0$ and $M_{xy}(-) = 0$ in the original thermal equilibrium state. The notations $(-)$ and $(+)$ denote the state of magnetization immediately prior to or following the RF pulse, respectively. The magnitude of $M_{xy}(+)$ clearly depends on the RF flip angle, θ_{rf}, as also depicted in Fig. 17-2. If θ_{rf} is small, then the amount

of magnetization that becomes transverse and available for detection as a signal will also be small by the fractional amount of $\sin\theta_{rf}$. On the other hand, a 90° RF pulse will convert all the longitudinal magnetization into transverse magnetization, where $M_{xy}(+) = M_0$, yielding the maximum possible signal after a single RF pulse.

Longitudinal magnetization immediately following the RF pulse, $M_z(+)$, does not contribute to the immediate signal. Nevertheless, it is important and will be seen to have major consequences in subsequent RF pulsing. It can be expressed as

$$M_z(+) = M_0 \cos\theta_{rf}. \quad (17\text{-}2)$$

It is important to note that for small flip angles, the majority of M_0 remains longitudinal. Conversely, a large flip angle of 90° will convert all of M_0 to $M_{xy}(+)$, leaving $M_z(+) = 0$. An even larger RF flip angle of 180° will invert the longitudinal magnetization so that $M_z(+) = -M_0$.

T_1 Relaxation and Longitudinal Recovery
After rotation by an RF pulse, magnetization evolves by the magnetic resonance processes known as *relaxation*. Transverse magnetization, M_{xy}, relaxes by losing its coherence and exponentially decays in magnitude over time. However, if M_{xy} is examined immediately following the RF pulse, then this aspect of relaxation need not be considered further in this treatment.* Longitudinal magnetization, M_z, relaxes by exponentially growing back to the magnitude, M_0, with a characteristic time constant known as the T_1, *or spin-lattice relaxation time*, a fundamental property of the tissue. This relaxation behavior or, more specifically the *longitudinal magnetization recovery*, is depicted in Fig. 17-3 and can be expressed as

$$M_z(t) = M_z(+) e^{-t/T_1} + M_0(1 - e^{-t/T_1}), \quad (17\text{-}3a)$$

*Note: In the strictest sense, this is accurate only if the coherence of the transverse magnetization (see the section "Spin Magnitude and MRA") is destroyed before each RF pulse that is applied and does not influence the magnetization upon subsequent RF pulsing. This would be the case for Fast Low Angle Shot (FLASH), spoiled Gradient Recalled Acquisition in the Steady State (GRASS), or spoiled Steady State Free Precession (SSFP) gradient echo imaging techniques. In some applications, however, the coherence might be purposely maintained. This would be true for techniques such as Fast Imaging with Steady-State Precession (FISP), rephased GRASS, or SSFP. A substantive review of these specific types of rapid gradient echo imaging techniques is given elsewhere.[12] For the sake of simplicity, it will be assumed that the transverse coherence is deliberately spoiled or destroyed prior to each RF pulse. It should be mentioned that studying this special case in no way deters from the ability to understand the theory, and in actual fact should facilitate this understanding.

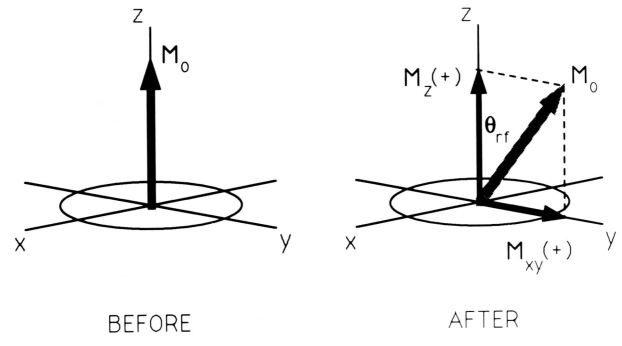

Fig. 17-2   Effect of a single RF pulse of flip angle θ_{rf} on the equilibrium magnetization.

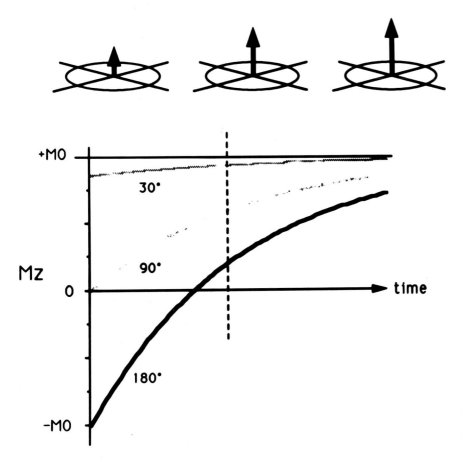

Fig. 17-3 T_1 relaxation and the longitudinal recovery of magnetization after various RF flip angle excitations.

or

$$M_z(t) = M_z(0)\, e^{-t/T_1} + M_0(1 - e^{-t/T_1}),\quad (17\text{-}3b)$$

where 0 now denotes the magnetization at time $t = 0$ immediately after the RF pulse and t denotes the relaxed state of the magnetization at a time t after the RF pulse. Note that $M_z(+)$ from the previous section is identical to $M_z(0)$. From Eq. 17-3 and from Fig. 17-3, it can be seen that the initial magnitude of M_z is simply $M_z(0)$ (or $M_z(+)$) and the final magnitude is M_0. Therefore

Initial state: $M_z(t) = M_z(0)$ for $t = 0$,   (17-4a)

Final state: $M_z(t) = M_0$ for $t = \infty$.   (17-4b)

Recall that according to eq. 17-2, the initial state of $M_z(0)$ depends on the RF flip angle. Figure 17-3 demonstrates the T_1 relaxation and longitudinal recovery of M_z following three different RF pulse flip angles. For $\theta_{rf} = 180°$, M_z becomes inverted and begins its longitudinal recovery from a magnitude of $-M_0$. In this case, growth back to full recovery of the thermal equilibrium value of M_0 requires the longitudinal recovery of $M_0 - (-M_0) = 2M_0$, the difference between the initial and final magnitudes of M_z. Consequently, it takes a long time for this amount of recovery to occur. For $\theta_{rf} = 90°$, M_z begins with a value of zero, which means that full recovery requires only the growth of the amount $M_0 - 0 = M_0$, half of that required with a 180° pulse. Finally, for $\theta_{rf} = 30°$, M_z begins with the majority of its magnetization (0.866 M_0) and requires the growth of only $M_0 - (0.866M_0) = 0.134M_0$, which takes very little time relative to pulsing with larger flip angles.

Although the rate of recovery is entirely dependent on the T_1 relaxation time, which is a property of the tissue, it should be clear that the total time it takes for full recovery will depend on the RF flip angle used. If insufficient time is allowed for complete recovery back to M_0, then the degree of *partial recovery* at some time t will be greatly influenced by the RF flip angle, as shown in Fig. 17-3.

Two RF Pulses and Magnetization
After a single RF pulse is followed by a period of time for relaxation of the magnetization to occur, a second RF pulse can be applied. If it can be assumed that no transverse magnetization exists just prior to the RF pulsing [ensuring that the coherence of the magnetization is destroyed, $M_{xy}(-) = 0$; see the section "Spin

Dispersion (Phase)"], then the only magnetization that contributes to what subsequently occurs is $M_z(-)$, the longitudinal magnetization that exists just prior to the second RF pulse. Therefore, if the RF flip angle is θ_{rf}, then the magnetization immediately following the second RF pulse will be

$$M_{xy}(+) = M_z(-) \sin \theta_{rf},\quad (17\text{-}5a)$$

$$M_z(+) = M_z(-) \cos \theta_{rf}.\quad (17\text{-}5b)$$

Note the similarities of eq. 17-5a and eq. 17-1 with eq. 17-5b and eq. 17-2. The only difference is that M_0 is replaced by $M_z(-)$. In fact, eq. 17-5 is the general expression that can be used to describe the state of the magnetization after the application of an RF pulse, whether it was the first, second, or nth pulse. If this was the first pulsing of RF, then clearly the magnetization would initially be in a state of thermal equilibrium, which means that $M_z(-) = M_0$, and eq. 17-5 would reduce to eqs. 17-1 and 17-2.

The most important aspect of eq. 17-5 is that the magnitude of $M_{xy}(+)$ depends not only on the RF flip angle, θ_{rf} but equally on $M_z(-)$, the amount of longitudinal magnetization that exists just prior to the pulsing. Once again, if this is the first RF pulse, then $M_z(-) = M_0$. However, if this is the second RF pulse, $M_z(-)$ will be some value less than M_0. Recall from the previous section that the magnitude of $M_z(-)$ depends on the amount of time that is allowed for longitudinal recovery to occur at the rate dictated by the characteristic T_1 relaxation time of the tissue, according to eq. 17-3. Furthermore, this will depend on what the flip angle was from the previous RF pulsing.

Consider the following scenarios, as shown in Fig. 17-3. If a small flip angle is used, then the $M_z(-)$ that is available for the second RF pulse will be large and will reach a maximum value of M_0 in a short period of time. Therefore, it is not strongly dependent on the time interval between pulses. However, if a large flip angle is used, then $M_z(-)$ will in general be small and largely dependent on the time between the RF pulses, requiring a long period of time for recovery to occur and make $M_z(-)$ large. Looking at it in another way, if the time between the RF pulses is kept extremely short, then little time is allowed for longitudinal recovery. Hence, $M_z(-)$ will in general be small and primarily dictated by the flip angle. On the other hand, if a large amount of time is allowed between RF pulses, then significant longitudinal relaxation will occur, leading to a large $M_z(-)$ that approaches the value of M_0 and is less dependent on the flip angle.

Multiple RF Pulses and the Steady State

In most conventional methods of MRI, data are progressively acquired through the repetition of multiple RF pulsing. As seen in the previous sections, for a given T_1 of a tissue, the magnitude of M_{xy} immediately following an RF pulse that contributes to the signal intensity of the image is based on θ_{rf} and the magnitude of $M_z(-)$. In turn, $M_z(-)$ depends on θ_{rf}, as well as on the amount of time between RF pulses that allows for longitudinal recovery of the magnetization.

For a given *repetition time (TR)* of successive RF pulsing, θ_{rf} contributes to M_{xy} in two different ways. First, it contributes directly to M_{xy} by RF excitation through the expression given in eq. 17-5a. Large flip angles lead to a larger degree of $M_z(-)$ that is converted to M_{xy}. Second, θ_{rf} contributes indirectly to M_{xy} by T_1 relaxation through the expression given in eq. 17-5a. An important observation in a multiple RF pulse scenario is that $M_z(+)$ in eq. 17-5b is $M_z(-)$ for the next RF pulse. Here, then, large flip angles lead to a lesser amount of $M_z(-)$ that can be converted to M_{xy} on further pulsing.

Therefore, there are two effects that counter each other in the way they influence M_{xy} in a multiple RF pulse situation. As a result, a *dynamic steady-state of spin saturation* of M_{xy} is achieved. The relative contributions of direct excitation effects and indirect relaxation effects of the RF pulsing ultimately depend on the TR of the pulsing as it relates to the T_1 of the tissue. The range of the magnitude of M_{xy} will exist somewhere at a level between zero (TR → 0, independent of direct effects from RF excitation, dependent only on indirect effects

of T_1 relaxation) and $M_0\sin\theta_{rf}$ (TR → ∞, dependent only on direct effects of RF excitation, independent of indirect effects of T_1 relaxation). If the TR is long enough to allow some degree of longitudinal recovery but short enough so that only partial recovery occurs (typically, when $0 < TR < T_1$), then several interesting aspects emerge from the dynamic steady-state behavior of M_{xy}.

First, for a given TR and T_1, there exists a specific RF flip angle, θ_{rf}, that yields a maximum M_{xy}. This is shown graphically in Fig. 17-4. At the lowest flip angles, the direct effect of excitation dominates and yields an M_{xy} that is very small. At the highest flip angles, the indirect effect of relaxation dominates and also results in a very small M_{xy}. Thus, it seems perfectly plausible that there should be some intermediate flip angle for which M_{xy} is a maximum, where neither excitation nor relaxation dominates the magnitude of M_{xy}. It also is logical that this should depend on the TR and T_1 that determine the amount of the contribution made by the relaxation effects. If TR is large enough relative to T_1 (namely, TR/ T_1 is large) then sufficient recovery of the longitudinal magnetization prior to the RF pulse occurs. This yields a larger M_{xy} overall, with a maximum value predominantly dictated by the direct excitation. If TR is too short, then no time is allowed for recovery, resulting in a small M_{xy}, regardless of the flip angle. The RF flip angle θ_{rf} that determines the maximum value of M_{xy} for a given TR and T_1 is known as the *Ernst angle* and is given by

$$\theta_{max} = \cos^{-1}(e^{-TR/T_1}). \qquad (17\text{-}6)$$

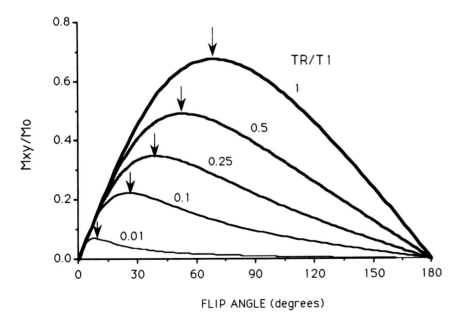

Fig. 17-4 Steady-state transverse magnetization as a function of RF flip angle. For a given TR and T_1, maximum transverse magnetization in the steady-state occurs between 0° and 180° at an RF flip angle defined as the Ernst angle (arrows).

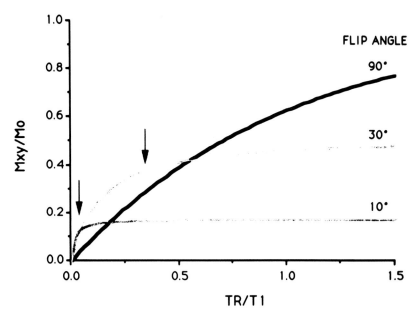

Fig. 17-5 Steady-state transverse magnetization as a function of TR. At an RF flip angle of 90°, maximum magnetization is reached at large TR. At smaller flip angles, maximum magnetization is reached at shorter TR. With smaller flip angles, greater transverse magnetization results if short TR is used (arrows).

Another interesting feature of the dynamic steady-state is that the extent of what TR must be in order to achieve full longitudinal recovery is dependent on the RF flip angle. This is demonstrated in Fig. 17-5. If the flip angle is large, then the amount of longitudinal magnetization for full recovery is large. This was previously shown in Fig. 17-3. Thus, for a given T_1, the TR will necessarily be long for full recovery. However, at a reduced flip angle, two things occur, as shown in Fig. 17-5. First, because some magnetization remains longitudinal, a smaller TR is needed to reach full recovery. Second, smaller flip angles have greater M_{xy} at short TR. In certain rapid imaging applications where very short TR values are required, this signal advantage at smaller flip angles is often exploited.

In-Flow and the Approach to Steady State
It has been seen how the magnitude of M_{xy} behaves in the dynamic steady-state of spin saturation. Under normal circumstances when tissues are stationary, the signal and contrast will be associated with this steady-state behavior. This, however, will not be the case if blood flows into the *volume of excitation*. Whether imaging is performed in a two-dimensional (2D) or three-dimensional (3D) mode, the slice or slab that ultimately becomes spatially encoded must first be regionally excited by the RF. This means that defined boundaries of excitation exist. Vessels carrying flowing blood that originate outside of these boundaries may traverse the slice or slab, setting up a scenario whereby flowing blood continually enters and exits the excitation volume.

Consider the simple situation shown in Fig. 17-6, where a unidirectional vessel passes orthogonally through an imaging slab from left to right. Everywhere within the stationary volume of excitation, the spins experience an infinite number of RF pulses and exhibit a magnitude of M_{xy} equal to the dynamic steady-state value. At the point of immediate entry into the slab on the left, however, the spins associated with the inflowing blood have never experienced a single RF pulse since it came from outside the slab. As the blood flows further into the volume of excitation, it will be hit with more successive RF pulses. If the slab is thick enough or if the flow of the blood is slow enough, then the blood will eventually experience a large enough number of excitations to reach a dynamic steady-state of M_{xy}. Therefore, the *TOF of the in-flowing blood* determines how many RF pulses the blood experiences.

If the blood flow velocity, v_b, is assumed to be constant, then the number of RF pulses, n_{rf}, that a bolus of blood has experienced within the slab after traversing a path length of L is

$$n_{rf} = \frac{L}{v_b TR}, \qquad (17\text{-}7)$$

where TR is the repetition time between successive RF pulses. Note that even if the vessel changes direction within the volume, it is the total path length that determines the number of RF pulses and not necessarily the thickness of the slab.

At the point of entry into the excitation volume by any vessel, L is small and therefore $n_{rf} = 1$. On the other hand, a tortuous vessel that winds in different

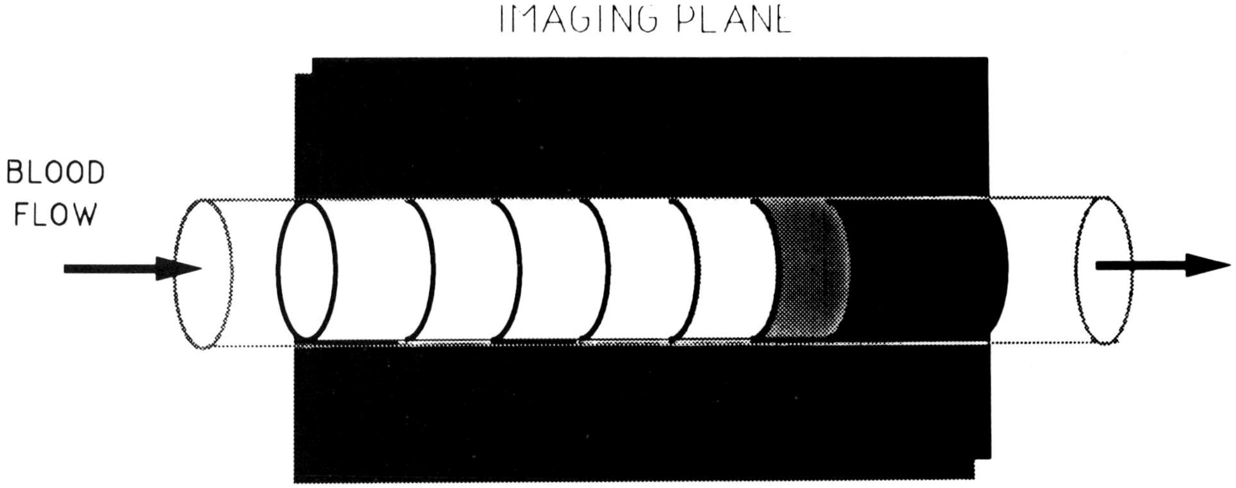

IMAGING PLANE

Fig. 17-6 Schematic depiction of the time-of-flight effects of blood flowing into a region of RF excitation. At the entry (left), fresh unsaturated blood enters the region of excitation. As it penetrates the volume, it experiences an increasing number of RF pulses and the blood magnetization begins to saturate. At the exit to the volume, blood achieves a steady-state of transverse magnetization similar to that of the stationary tissue throughout the region of excitation.

directions within the slab, such as what may be associated with an arteriovenous malformation, will have a large L and n_{rf} will typically be large. Slow flow (small v_b) will reside in the volume longer and will therefore have a larger n_{rf} than faster flow (large v_b), regardless of the path length. Finally, a short TR means that n_{rf} will be large. Conversely, if TR is long enough, then all of the in-flowing blood will experience only a single RF pulse since it will be completely replenished with fresh spins during each TR interval. Thus due to *time-of-flight effects*, in-flowing blood will experience a range of n_{rf}, from one RF pulse at the point of entry, to two RF pulses as it penetrates the slab, to many RF pulses deep within the excitation volume.

Therefore, the magnitude of M_{xy} associated with in-flowing blood is not related to the dynamic steady-state, as it is with stationary tissues that experience close to an infinite number of RF pulses in an imaging application. Rather, it is related to *the approach to the steady-state of M_{xy}*, and will be different, depending on where the blood is located within the volume of excitation and how many RF pulses it has seen.

Recall that for $n_{rf} = 1$, M_{xy} is solely dependent on the RF flip angle of excitation, as shown in eq. 17-1. Since the spins have never experienced any previous RF pulsing, M_{xy} is based on $M_z(-) = M_0$, the thermal equilibrium magnetization. For $n_{rf} > 1$, however, M_{xy} also depends on the degree of longitudinal recovery of $M_z(-)$ from the previous RF pulsing, which will be based on TR and T_1, as described in eq. 17-5. For $n_{rf} \to \infty$ in the steady state, the magnitude of M_{xy} will

be something less than M_{xy} after a single RF pulse. As shown in Fig. 17-7, the approach of M_{xy} to the steady-state is strongly dependent on the RF flip angle and on the TR relative to a given T_1.

There are a number of important features in the behavior of the approach to steady-state of the magnetization. For the sake of clarity, consider a vessel containing blood with a given T_1 relaxation moving at a given velocity, v_b. Then the number of RF pulses, n_{rf}, is directly proportional to the path length, L, that the vessel traverses, according to eq. 17-7. Figure 17-7 can therefore be interpreted in terms of how M_{xy} (and thus the signal magnitude) changes as the moving blood penetrates the excitation volume.

With a small RF flip angle, Fig. 17-7 demonstrates that there is a slow approach to the steady-state. This means that many RF pulses are required to reach the steady-state and that blood will travel quite far before it reaches it. However, there is little difference overall between the magnitude of M_{xy} of the penetrating blood and the steady-state value ($n_{rf} \to \infty$). Even at the point of entry ($n_{rf} = 1$) there is only a small difference. In addition, regardless of the number of RF pulses the blood has experienced, the overall magnitude of M_{xy} is small because of the small flip angle. Conversely, at a large RF flip angle, Fig. 17-7 shows that there is a rapid approach to the steady-state. At the entry, large M_{xy} is observed. However, after only a small number of RF pulses, M_{xy} decreases significantly to a steady-state value which is lower than that for the smaller flip angle situation.

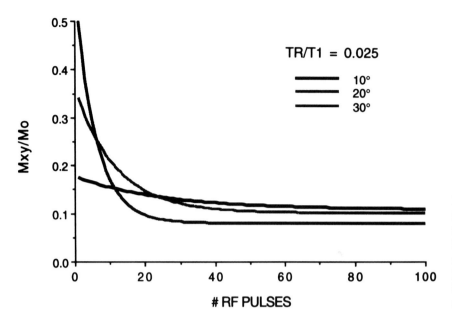

Fig. 17-7 Steady-state approach of transverse magnetization as a function of the number of RF pulses experienced. Higher RF flip angles begin with larger magnetization but rapidly approach a low steady-state value. Lower flip angles begin with smaller magnetization but slowly approach the steady-state.

Spin Magnitude and MRA

In an MRI technique, the signal that is collected possesses a magnitude and a phase. The spin magnitude, or intensity, of this signal is directly related to the magnitude of the transverse magnetization, M_{xy}. Given the intrinsic properties of the tissue, and in particular T_1 relaxation, the magnitude will be determined primarily by the RF flip angle, the number of times the tissue is hit with the RF, and the time allowed between RF pulses for T_1 longitudinal recovery to occur, as defined by the TR. Time-of-flight effects are specifically related to how the spin magnitude approaches the steady-state of M_{xy}.

Vessel contrast in time-of-flight MRA is achieved by maximizing the signal from moving blood and minimizing it from surrounding stationary tissues. By definition, the latter will be governed by the steady-state magnitude of M_{xy}. On the other hand, the signal from blood in a vessel that penetrates the volume of excitation will be dictated by the behavior of the approach to the steady-state of M_{xy} and how many times the blood has been hit with RF as it flows into the volume. Imaging protocols (RF flip angle and TR) and strategies to obtain good visualization of vessels in a particular application depend on numerous factors, such as the blood flow velocities that are characteristic of the vessels; the tortuosity of the vessels, and therefore the path lengths associated with them; the volume of excitation; and the size of the region of interest. This becomes complicated by the fact that large flip angles

provide good contrast at the point of entry into the imaging volume but poor depth penetration, and small flip angles provide poor contrast but good depth penetration.

In PC MRA, vessel contrast is based on the spin phase differences between stationary tissue and moving blood, not on the magnitude of the signal. Therefore, time-of-flight effects are not crucial. Nevertheless, unless precise quantification of the flow velocities is desired, the processed phase information that is ultimately used to visualize the vessels with this technique is weighted by the magnitude of the signal. If M_{xy} is too small, there will be poor vessel depiction even if the contrast due to the phase differences is large. On the other hand, depth penetration is not an issue, since the vasculature will still be well delineated based on the phase differences even when the M_{xy} of the blood reaches approximately the same steady-state value as the surrounding tissue at the greater depths. The only importance is that M_{xy} is large enough so that signal exists from the in-flowing blood.

Spin Dispersion (Phase)

Frequency and Phase
Transverse magnetization, M_{xy}, is the vector component of the total bulk magnetization that lies perpendicular to the external magnetic field that conventionally lies in the z-direction. As shown in Fig. 17-8A, M_{xy} characteristically precesses about the z-axis at the *Larmor frequency* according to the relation

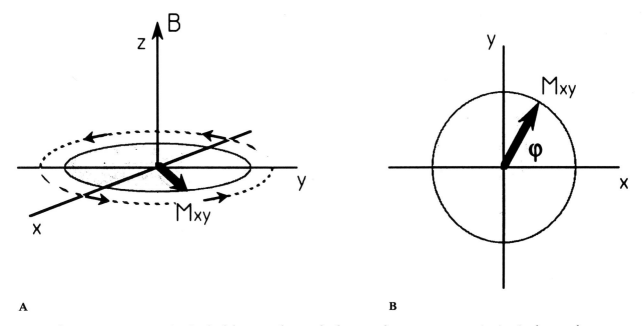

A   **B**

Fig. 17-8 (*A,B*) Rotation in the laboratory frame of reference of transverse magnetization in the *x-y* plane.

$$\omega = \gamma B, \qquad (17\text{-}8)$$

where B is the external magnetic field strength; ω is the precessional frequency; and γ is the gyromagnetic ratio, which is a constant and a unique property of the nuclei (42.5758 MHz/Tesla for hydrogen). Thus, the precessional frequency of M_{xy} is directly dictated by the external magnetic field strength that it experiences. Put another way, M_{xy} is the component of the total bulk magnetization that is sensitive to magnetic field through its precessional frequency.

As M_{xy} precesses, its *phase* at any given time, ϕ, is related to the direction in which it points in the *x-y* plane, as shown in Fig. 17-8B. Over time, M_{xy} will rotate in the *x-y* plane and increase in its phase relative to some initial starting value. At a precessional frequency ω, the phase of M_{xy} at some time t can be described as

$$\phi(t) = \omega t = \gamma B t, \qquad (17\text{-}9)$$

where the initial condition is taken here as $\phi = 0$ at $t = 0$.

Rotating Frame

The evolution of the phase of M_{xy} can be examined more easily by observing how it changes relative to some reference frequency, ω_0. If the *x-y* axes are al-lowed to rotate at this reference frequency, then the phase of M_{xy} in this *rotating frame of reference* becomes

$$\begin{aligned}\Delta\phi(t) &= \phi(t) - \phi_0(t)\\ &= (\omega - \omega_0)t = \gamma(B - B_0)t,\end{aligned} \qquad (17\text{-}10)$$

where $\phi_0(t)$ represents the phase of the rotating frame at some time, t, based on the reference frequency, ω_0, and a reference field, B_0. By defining magnetic field, frequency, and phase in terms of the rotating frame of reference, this simplifies to the expression

$$\phi'(t) = \omega't = \gamma B't, \qquad (17\text{-}11)$$

where $B' = (B - B_0)$, $\omega' = (\omega - \omega_0)$, and $\phi'(t) = \Delta\phi(t) = \phi(t) - \phi_0(t)$ for the magnetic field, frequency, and phase in the rotating frame, respectively.

Note that eq. 17-11 appears identical to eq. 17-9. However, in a real or laboratory frame of reference, there is no such thing as a magnetic field or frequency that is negative and less than zero. Nevertheless, ac-cording to eq. 17-11, in the rotating frame of reference, B' can be negative if the field B is less than the reference field B_0. Therefore, ω' can be negative and the phase evolution over time is negative. As shown in Fig. 17-9, in the rotating frame of reference, the phase of M_{xy} evolves counterclockwise if $B < B_0$ and evolves clock-

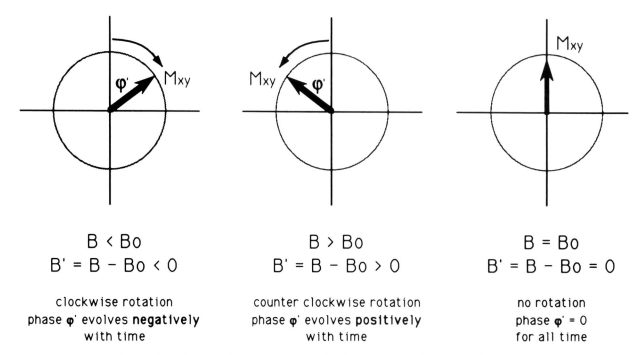

$$B < Bo \qquad\qquad B > Bo \qquad\qquad B = Bo$$
$$B' = B - Bo < 0 \qquad B' = B - Bo > 0 \qquad B' = B - Bo = 0$$

clockwise rotation   counter clockwise rotation   no rotation
phase **φ'** evolves **negatively**   phase **φ'** evolves **positively**   phase **φ'** = 0
with time   with time   for all time

Fig. 17-9   Behavior of transverse magnetization in the rotating frame of reference.

wise if $B > B_0$. In the special case when $B = B_0$, $B' = 0$ and no rotation occurs, with the phase being a constant and equal to zero.

Spin Isochromats

The transverse magnetization, M_{xy}, and the bulk magnetization as a whole are representative of the sum of all of the microscopic nuclear dipole moments from the hydrogen nuclei, or spins. The phase of M_{xy} reflects the average of all of the phases associated with the individual spins. In order to understand more clearly how moving spins affect the overall macroscopic magnetization, it is useful to introduce the concept of *spin isochromats*.[13]

An isochromat is a collection of spins, or nuclei, that precess at exactly the same specified Larmor frequency. This also means that all of the spins that make up an isochromat experience the same external magnetic field. Different isochromats have different precessional frequencies. An isochromat may be comprised of one nucleus or many nuclei, depending on the situation. Nevertheless, the sum total of all the isochromats representing all the nuclei yields M_{xy}. Since phase evolves based on frequency, it is more relevant to study the behavior of isochromats, not just individual spins that may have the same frequency or M_{xy} that may be comprised of a large number of different frequencies.

Coherence and Phase Dispersion

If all the nuclei began with the same phase and precess at the same frequency, then they would remain together in phase over time as one isochromat that described all the spins. In this situation, all the magnetic dipoles of the spins would add up to yield a maximum magnitude for M_{xy} (Fig. 17-10A). The transverse magnetization is said to be *coherent*. Stated another way, if M_{xy} is comprised of only one isochromat, the magnetization will be coherent and its magnitude will be a maximum.

On the other hand, if several isochromats exist, then a certain degree of *phase dispersion* will occur over time, leading to *incoherence* of M_{xy}, as shown in Fig. 17-10B. In the rotating frame of reference, one isochromat may be rotating counterclockwise, with a frequency larger than the reference frequency, whereas another isochromat may be rotating clockwise, with a frequency smaller than the reference frequency. In this case, the magnitude of the transverse magnetization will be reduced due to the collective result of the dispersed isochromats.

In the limit, if many isochromats represent magnetization in the transverse plane, a large degree of phase dispersion occurs over time and M_{xy} approaches zero magnitude, since the contributions to M_{xy} made by isochromats progressing counterclockwise in phase will

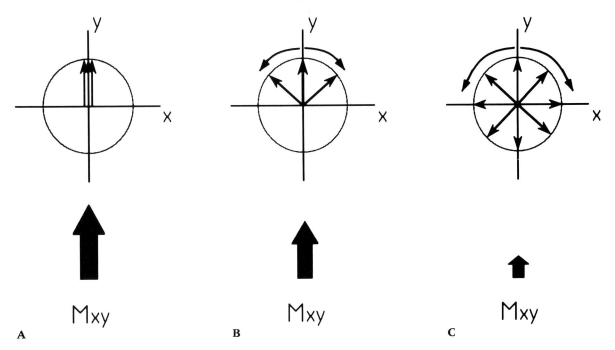

Fig. 17-10   Spin phase dispersion in the rotation frame of reference. Shown is the behavior of spins (*A*) in phase with no dispersion, (*B*) diverging with partial dispersion, and(*C*) out of phase with nearly complete dispersion. The magnitude of the transverse magnetization decreases progressively with increasing phase dispersion.

be canceled out by contributions made by other isochromats rotating clockwise in phase (Fig. 17-10C). Since the detected MR signal is directly proportional to the magnitude of M_{xy}, it can be seen that large phase dispersions in isochromats lead to incoherence and a reduced magnitude of M_{xy}, resulting in signal loss.

Gradients and Phase
The causes of phase evolution, phase dispersion, and changes in the magnitude and phase of M_{xy} are based on differences in the external magnetic field experienced by the spins, as seen in eq. 17-11. The significance of this relationship is that the phase will always be directly proportional to whatever the external magnetic field strength is at the time. Therefore, if a slight change, ΔB, in the magnetic field occurs from B' to $B' + \Delta B$, then ω' will change accordingly to $\omega' + \Delta\omega$, setting up a different isochromat with a phase evolution of

$$\phi'(t) + \Delta\phi'(t) = (\omega' + \Delta\omega)t = \gamma(B' + \Delta B)t. \quad (17\text{-}12)$$

There can be many origins of ΔB. For example, spatially varying external magnetic field inhomogeneities cause spins from a macroscopic sample to sense a different ΔB, depending on where they reside in the sample. As a result, the large number of isochromats that represent the sample leads to a rapid phase dispersion of M_{xy} and a rapid signal decay. Often this dominates the exponential signal loss of a free induction decay (FID) by the characteristic decay time of T_2^*.

However, by far the most dominant magnetic field changes that occur in an MRI experiment are those associated with the spatially varying *linear magnetic field gradients* which are purposely used to encode the signal spatially. The application of a gradient field causes the main external magnetic field to vary linearly in a given direction, as shown in Fig. 17-11. A *gradient coil* within the MRI system is capable of generating these spatially varying fields in all three of the physical, or Cartesian, directions: *x*, *y*, and *z*. Therefore, if a group of spins are located physically in space at a position along the *x* direction, then they will experience a ΔB according to the relation

$$\Delta B = G_x x, \quad (17\text{-}13a)$$

where the applied gradient field is defined as

$$G_x = \frac{\delta B}{\delta x}. \quad (17\text{-}13b)$$

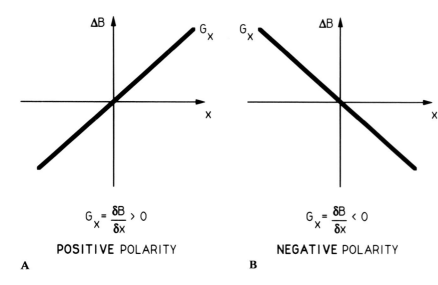

$$G_x = \frac{\delta B}{\delta x} > 0$$

POSITIVE POLARITY

A

$$G_x = \frac{\delta B}{\delta x} < 0$$

NEGATIVE POLARITY

B

Fig. 17-11 Depiction of the polarity of a spatially varying linear magnetic gradient field. Spatial variation of a gradient field with (*A*) positive and (*B*) negative polarity.

Gradient fields can be generated as positive or negative field changes. Normally, if G is positive, the field simply increases with increasing distance (Fig. 17-11A). If the *gradient polarity* is reversed so that G is negative, this means that the field decreases with increasing distance (Fig. 17-11B). The *gradient strength* refers to the amount of field change that is generated at a given distance and is the magnitude of G in eq. 17-13.

When the gradient field, G_x, is applied, it can be seen from eq. 17-13a that the magnetic field change, ΔB, is equal to zero in the center of the magnet where $x = 0$. This is typically referred to as the magnet's *isocenter,* or electronic center, the position along a given axis at which the applied gradient field, either positive or negative, causes no change in the main external field ($\Delta B = 0$). However, if $x > 0$ and $G_x > 0$, then ΔB is positive, and the phase evolution of the spins in the rotating frame is counterclockwise and positive, according to eq. 17-12. With the same applied gradient field ($G_x > 0$), if the spins are now located on the opposite side of the isocenter where $x < 0$, then ΔB is negative, and the phase evolution is clockwise and negative. How the phase evolves for spins located at different positions along a positive gradient field is shown in Fig. 17-12.

In virtually all MRI experiments, spatially selective RF excitation and spatial encoding of the signal are accomplished by pulsing gradient fields at the appropriate time and in the appropriate physical direction. When a gradient field is turned on for a certain duration and then turned off thereafter, this constitutes a *gradient pulse,* as shown in Fig. 17-13. If all other sources of field change ΔB are ignored, then the spin phase will evolve only when a gradient pulse is applied.

The rate at which the phase progresses will depend basically on the strength of ΔB, and according to eq. 17-13a, this means it will depend on the strength of the gradient field and the position of the spins in space relative to the isocenter. As long as the gradient field is on at a constant strength, ΔB will be a constant and the phase will vary linearly with time, as dictated by eq. 17-12. However, as soon as the gradient pulse is turned off, the phase will no longer evolve but will remain at the value it had immediately before the gradient was set to zero.

Figure 17-13 demonstrates that if all other magnetic field differences are ignored, the phase of the spins that make up M_{xy} will be equal and zero as long as a gradient pulse is not applied. M_{xy} will remain maximally coherent, and no phase dispersion will occur. Figure 17-13 also demonstrates that as soon as a gradient pulse is applied, the phase of all the isochromats will evolve linearly in time at different rates, according to their spatial position along the physical direction in which the pulse was applied. Collectively, this causes a phase dispersion, or *dephasing,* that continues as long as the gradient pulse remains on. Finally, once the pulse is turned off, M_{xy} will be incoherent to some degree and the signal will be reduced accordingly.

This may appear to pose a dilemma in imaging. If gradient pulses are required to encode the signal spatially, then it remains to be considered how this can be achieved without simultaneously dephasing the signal so that it becomes vanishingly small. For an isochromat located at a given position, the amount of phase that evolves depends on the gradient pulse's strength, duration, and polarity. This phase can be completely negated, or *rephased,* by applying a second gradient pulse

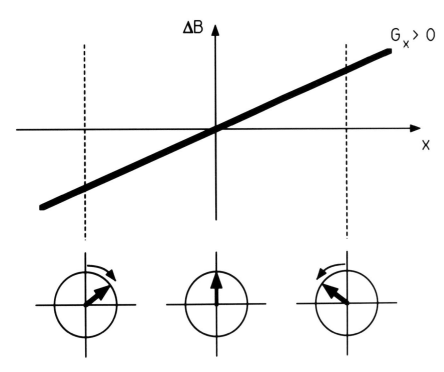

Fig. 17-12 Effect of a spatially varying linear magnetic gradient field in the rotating frame. For a positive polarity gradient field, spins located in the negative direction rotate clockwise, while spins located in the positive direction rotate counterclockwise.

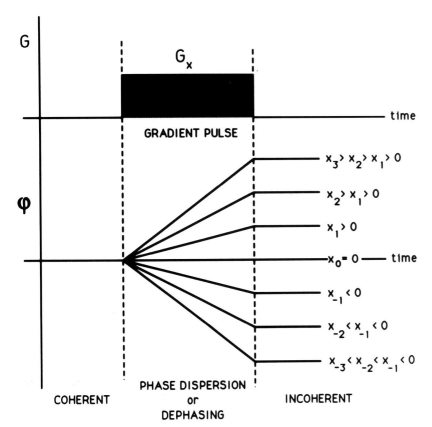

Fig. 17-13 Effect of a pulsed gradient field on time evolution of spin phase and coherence of the transverse magnetization. Spins located farther away from the center evolve in phase faster than spins located closer to the center when a gradient field is applied. The resulting collective effect is a phase dispersion causing a loss of transverse magnetization coherence.

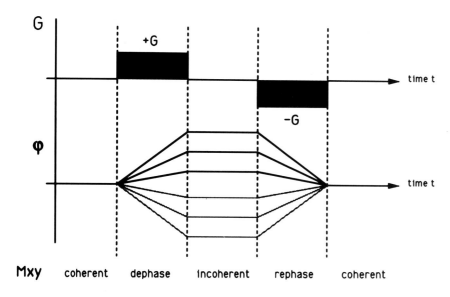

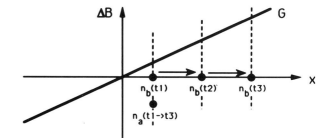

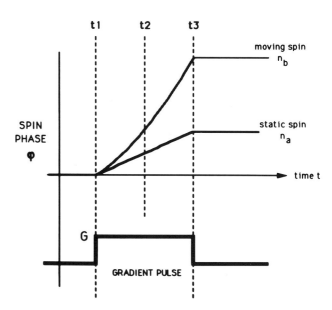

Fig. 17-14 Spin phase evolution with bipolar gradient pulsing. Spins begin in phase, with maximum coherence of the transverse magnetization. Application of the first positive polarity gradient pulse causes phase dispersion and loss of coherence in the magnetization. With the application of a second negative polarity gradient pulse, spins rephase and return to the same phase, resulting in coherence of the magnetization.

of equal strength and duration, but of opposite polarity, as shown in Fig. 17-14. If a negative gradient pulse is applied along with a positive one, for any given position the evolution of the phase will reverse, according to eq. 17-12. Therefore, spatial encoding can be accomplished while maintaining the coherence of M_{xy} by the application of additional gradient pulses in a precise and predictable manner.

Motion, Phase Evolution, and Moments
The study of spin phase evolution in the presence of gradient pulses is straightforward and simple, provided that it can be assumed that the hydrogen nuclei do not move from a fixed position in all space over the course of all time. However, this is certainly not true with respect to blood flow, as well as cerebrospinal fluid (CSF) flow, respiration, heart motion, and all other physiological motions. Therefore, it can be expected that M_{xy} and its associated magnitude and phase may behave differently if it originates from moving tissue. Not necessarily obvious is the fact that relative to the types of physiological motion, ΔB from sources other than gradient pulses causes negligible differences in M_{xy} between static and moving tissues. In other words, motion-induced phase changes can be assumed to occur only when a gradient pulse is applied.

Consider the situation shown in Fig. 17-15, where two nuclei, n_a and n_b, initially begin at the same physical position in space. They possess the same phase of zero immediately preceding the application of a gradient pulse (time, t_1). When the positive gradient pulse is applied, the stationary nucleus, n_a, begins to increase linearly in phase, as expected and described in Fig.

Fig. 17-15 Effect of a gradient pulse on moving spins. As an isochromat of spins (n_b) travels along the physical direction of an applied gradient field, its phase evolves faster than the phase of a static isochromat of spins (n_a) since it senses a progressively larger external magnetic field.

17-13. However, n_b moves in the positive direction of increasing magnetic field. As it travels, it changes its position and experiences a continuously increasing field strength, over and above that experienced by n_a. As a result, the phase of n_b becomes slightly larger than that of n_a at some time t_2 into the duration of the gradient pulse because it is continually sensing a larger magnetic field. As long as n_b continues to move, its phase will progress at a faster rate than the phase of n_a. Finally, when the gradient pulse is turned off at some time t_3, the moving spin, n_b, will have a substantially larger phase than n_a.

The actual phase behavior of a moving isochromat with respect to time depends on the type of motion. Since it will never experience the same ΔB at any two points in time (provided that its motion is continuous), the progression of its phase in the very least will never be linear. It can be shown that the total phase evolution of an isochromat can be represented as the sum of its individual components of motion. In the simplest form, the total phase, ϕ_{tot}, is equal to a static component, ϕ_s, and a motion component, ϕ_m. This can be expressed as

$$\phi_{tot}(t) = \phi_s(t) + \phi_m(t), \qquad (17\text{-}14)$$

where the apostrophe denoting the rotating frame of reference from before has been dropped for simplicity. Therefore, in the situation of Fig. 17-15, if the phase of n_a and n_b could be measured at any given point in time, the difference between the two would be the phase associated with the motion of n_b, that is, $\phi_{m,b}$. This is because the static components of n_a and n_b are equal ($\phi_{s,a} = \phi_{s,b}$) and would cancel upon subtraction. Note that in this case, since n_a is stationary, its total phase equals its static component ($\phi_{m,a} = 0$).

Specifically, the motion component of phase, $\phi_m(t)$, can be separated into more detailed *components*, or *moments, of motion*. It is known in the physics of mechanics that generalized motion can be described in terms of a *position*, a *velocity*, an *acceleration*, and even more complex motions. Position is considered the zeroth *order of motion*. Velocity is the first order of motion. Acceleration is the second, and all others are of successively higher orders. Therefore, eq. 17-14 can be expanded as

$$\phi_{tot}(t) = \phi_s(t) + \phi_v(t)$$
$$+ \phi_a(t) + [\text{higher orders}], \qquad (17\text{-}15)$$

where $\phi_v(t)$ and $\phi_a(t)$ now designate velocity and acceleration *moments* of the total spin phase evolution, respectively.

It can be further shown that each phase component

of increasing order of motion has a time dependence that increases as the power of time. From eq. 17-12, it is known that in the presence of a constant gradient field, stationary spins progress in phase linearly with time. The phase associated with the velocity component of motion can be shown to vary with the square of time. There is a cubic time dependence of phase due to the second order of motion, acceleration. Higher orders of motion have phase terms with higher powers of dependence on time. Thus,

0th order : static phase term : $\phi_s(t) \propto t$,

1st order : velocity phase term : $\phi_v(t) \propto t^2$,

2nd order : acceleration phase term : $\phi_a(t) \propto t^3$,

$\cdots$ $\cdots$ $\cdots$

nth order : nth phase term : $\phi_n(t) \propto t^{n+1}$,

$$(17\text{-}16)$$

where the actual phase contributions of each moment would depend on both the gradient strength, G, and the degree of the motion. For example, it is known that if the position of the spin is far from the isocenter, then the static phase term will be large. In addition, if the velocity of the motion is large, the corresponding velocity phase term will also be large. If pulsatility described the motion accurately, then the acceleration might be large and its associated phase component could be significant.

There are a number of consequences to eq. 17-16 that are worth noting:

• First and most important, if no gradient pulse is applied, then no difference in phase will be seen among spins, regardless of whether they are stationary or moving.

In other words, the deviations in phase between spins that are traveling and spins that remain in one place will begin to occur only when the first gradient pulse is applied and the resulting magnetic field differences are sensed.

• Second, if the motion occurs in a direction other than the direction in which the gradient pulse is applied, then no difference will be observed in the phase between static and moving spins.

If a gradient pulse is applied, for example, in the x-direction and the spins are moving in the z-direction, then no phase component will be associated with motion that will be generated because no velocity or acceleration occurs in the x-direction. Even though the spins move and change position in the z-direction, their position along the x-direction remains constant. Since the only gradient pulse that is applied is along the x-direction, only a static phase term will evolve.

- Third, the more complex the motion, the greater the deviation in phase from stationary spins and the greater the overall phase dispersion.

Complex motion is associated with large contributions from acceleration and higher-order motions. Therefore, as seen in eq. 17-16, if these components are significant, the resulting phase contributions will be extremely large because of their greater power dependence on time.

- Last, the longer the time allowed for spins to move before the signal is collected, the greater the deviation in phase from stationary spins and the greater the overall phase dispersion.

Spin phase evolves with time, and motion is associated with dependencies on time that are greater than for static spins, as seen in eq. 17-16. Provided that a gradient field is present, as time progresses the difference between static and moving spins becomes greater.

Gradient Moment Nulling

All MRI techniques require the pulsing of gradient fields to resolve the signal spatially. As a result, spin dephasing occurs, accompanied by a loss of coherence in the transverse magnetization, M_{xy}, and a subsequent signal reduction. If, however, the spin phase evolves in a precise and predictable manner, then the deleterious effects of the gradient pulsing can be negated while still accomplishing the task of spatial encoding by applying an additional gradient pulse. A simple but useful example of this was shown in Fig. 17-14.

In a situation where motion exists, such as in blood flow, isochromats from the moving spins evolve in their phase quite differently from isochromats of static spins when gradient pulses are applied. If the phase evolution of a moving spin is compared to that of a stationary spin in the pulsing configuration previously shown in Fig. 17-14, the resulting phases at the end of the gradient pulses will be quite different, as seen in Fig. 17-16A. Stationary spins will have a zero net phase ($\phi_{tot} = 0$, since $\phi_s = 0$), maximum coherence of M_{xy}, and therefore high signal. Moving spins, however, will have a nonzero phase ($\phi_{tot} \neq 0$, since $\phi_m \neq 0$), the

value of which will depend on their position and motion. Phase dispersion occurs with a loss of coherence in M_{xy} and a potentially large reduction in signal as a result of the motion.

Figure 17-16A basically demonstrates that in the presence of two gradient pulses, only the *zeroth-order moment* (static phase term, ϕ_s) can be *nulled* ($= 0$). In other words, $\phi_s = 0$ but $\phi_m \neq 0$. This is commonly known as zeroth-order *gradient moment nulling*. It can be shown, however, that by introducing a third gradient pulse, both zeroth- and first-order gradient moment nulling can be accomplished simultaneously, as shown in Fig. 17-16B. In this configuration, the net moments after the third gradient pulse are $\phi_s = 0$ and $\phi_v = 0$. Therefore, static and moving spins will both be maximally coherent, yielding large M_{xy} and large signal, provided that the motion does not contain higher-orders moments such as acceleration. If acceleration does exist, then $\phi_a \neq 0$, and there will be a net phase dispersion resulting from this type of motion. Simultaneous moment nulling that accommodates static (zeroth order), velocity (first order), and acceleration (second order) can be achieved, but it requires the introduction of a fourth gradient pulse.

Gradient moment nulling, *motion compensation*, or *gradient motion rephasing*, is a well-established method of minimizing image artifacts and general signal loss associated with motion in many MRI techniques.[10,14-19] However, because it requires additional gradient pulses to zero the phase contributions by various orders of motion, it places demands on the gradient hardware capabilities and typically lengthens the echo time, TE. If the nulling cannot be achieved within a reasonable time, one reaches a point of diminishing returns. Moment nulling can be achieved only if the motion remains precise, predictable, and unidirectional during the interval of gradient pulsing. With larger time intervals, motion becomes less precise and far less predictable, and very possibly will change direction; thus it becomes more difficult to null their phase contributions effectively. As a result, nulling is rarely performed beyond second-order compensation for acceleration. In the typical TE time frame of an MRI technique, most types of bulk motion can be well approximated as being of constant velocity and unidirectional. Thus, in many cases, gradient moment nulling is performed only to the first order.

Gradient Moment Encoding

If moment nulling can be achieved successfully, then there is every reason to believe that *gradient moment*

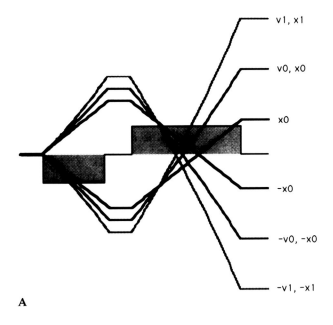

A

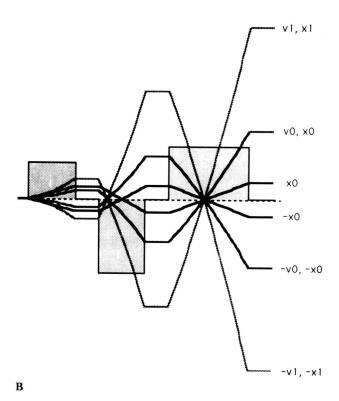

B

Fig. 17-16 Evolution of the phase of moving spins with multiple gradient pulsing. Shown is the phase evolution of both static and moving spins associated with (*A*) bipolar gradient pulsing and (*B*) tripolar gradient pulsing. In (*B*), specific gradient amplitudes and timing result in a situation where moving spins come into phase with static spins. This effect is known as *gradient moment nulling.*

encoding can also be attained. In fact, moment nulling is simply a special case of moment encoding in which the encoded phase is set to zero. The purpose of nulling is to minimize phase dispersion and maximize the coherence of M_{xy}. However, if the motion is well behaved, then it is possible to induce a nonzero net phase that has a direct relationship to the characteristics of the motion.

Consider a vessel containing flowing blood that moves in one direction with a velocity that can be approximated as being constant in a given time interval, TE. In effect, it is then expected only that there will be two phase terms, ϕ_s and ϕ_v. All other components of motion can be considered negligible. Figure 17-16A shows that a pair of equal and opposite gradient pulses will produce a nulling of the static component of the phase, $\phi_s = 0$, but will generate a nonzero velocity moment, $\phi_v \neq 0$, that can be considered an encoding of the motion. The actual phase of the velocity term will depend on the gradient's strengths and durations and on the actual velocity of the flowing blood. From eq. 17-13a, it is clear that the ΔB associated with the phase evolution will be greater with larger gradient strength, G, and/or larger velocity, v, that in a given period of time produces a larger change in position, x. The exact relationship between ϕ_v and the actual velocity, v, for a *bipolar gradient pulse pair*, as shown in Fig. 17-16A, is

$$\phi_v = \gamma v G \tau_1 \tau_2, \qquad (17\text{-}17)$$

where γ is the gyromagnetic ratio, τ_1 is the duration of each gradient pulse, and τ_2 is the time separating the two pulses. Figure 17-17, in conjunction with eq. 17-17, indicates that for a specific pulse timing of a bipolar gradient pair, a given gradient strength, G, will induce a specific ϕ_v that represents a one-to-one linear correspondence to a precise velocity, v. By applying a larger gradient strength, ϕ_v will become larger for a given velocity. Slow flow, for example, can be encoded with a significant phase in ϕ_v by ensuring that a strong enough gradient strength, G, is used.

It might be expected from the previous discussions that by inducing a nonzero phase term, static or motion related, there will be a certain degree of phase dispersion that can lead to incoherence in M_{xy} and signal loss. Since it can be expected that not all stationary spins are located in the same physical position, for $\phi_s \neq 0$ this certainly would be true. However, if it can be assumed that all of the flowing spins have approximately the same velocity in a blood vessel, then there may be no phase dispersion associated with a net effect of

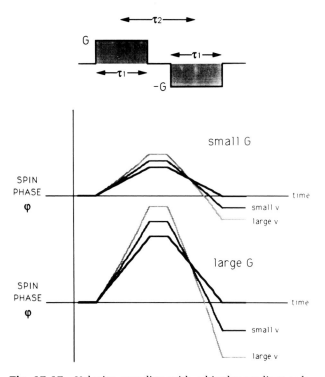

Fig. 17-17 Velocity encoding with a bipolar gradient pulsing scheme. Moving spins from blood can be encoded with a phase after bipolar gradient pulsing that is directly proportional to its velocity. Larger velocities are associated with larger phase shifts. The phase is also linearly proportional to the gradient field strength. Therefore, larger phase shifts are seen with a stronger bipolar gradient pulsing. Note that static spins end with a zero net phase after such a pulsing scheme.

different isochromats on the velocity term, ϕ_v. M_{xy} will maintain coherence, but will possess a phase ϕ_v that is not zero but is directly proportional to the velocity.

Spin Phase and MRA

The transverse magnetization, M_{xy}, is the component of the bulk magnetization that is detected in an MRI experiment. M_{xy}, being perpendicular to the main external magnetic field, will be sensitive to field changes. Gradient pulses are used to encode the signal spatially in order to generate an image and therefore sensitize M_{xy} to large phase changes and phase dispersions. Additional gradient pulses, however, can be used to negate these effects while still ensuring that spatial encoding is achieved. However, if motion is a part of M_{xy}, then the evolution of the phase of moving spins will behave differently from stationary spins that collectively make up M_{xy}. This may still result in phase

changes, phase dispersion, incoherence, and ultimately signal loss.

In TOF MRA, the contrast between vessels and surrounding tissue is produced by maximizing the magnitude of the signal from blood while minimizing it from stationary tissue. Therefore, a primary goal would be to maximize the coherence of M_{xy} by minimizing phase dispersions associated with motion-induced phase changes in the isochromats of the moving blood. This means that gradient moment nulling of the velocity phase term, and possibly even of the acceleration phase term, is a crucial part to the ultimate success of any TOF technique.

Vessel contrast in PC MRA is generated by purposely encoding blood with a nonzero phase shift that is directly proportional to the blood velocity. Stationary tissues with a velocity very close to zero should yield little or no velocity phase term, whereas fast flow should induce large phase shifts in the velocity term. The essence of PC MRA is not to nullify motion-induced phases, as in TOF techniques, but to encode them.

TOF MRA

Theory

TOF MRA is one of the two major methods used to visualize vascular structures. Its primary source of vessel contrast lies in the difference between the signal magnitudes of flowing blood and the surrounding stationary tissues. To achieve this difference, the method relies on the magnetic resonance phenomenon of inflow enhancement that is based on the time-of-flight of moving blood into the volume of RF excitation. Several different TOF techniques will be described here. All of them are based on in-flow enhancement, and all of them attempt to improve vessel contrast and delineation by either maximizing the signal magnitude from blood or minimizing the signal magnitude from stationary tissue. Theoretical details of the fundamental principles of how signal magnitude and phase are affected in flowing blood have been presented in the section "Spin Magnitude and MRA" and will not be discussed here. Rather, based on this foundation, the concepts of how TOF MRA is accomplished and how these principles are applied to this MRA method will be described.

In general, *in-flow enhancement* is based on the fact that a selective volume of RF excitation sets up a situation whereby the transverse magnetization (and thus the MR signal magnitude) from blood experiences a very different history of RF pulsing than for stationary tissue. During acquisition, magnetization from blood lying within the volume will be continuously replenished by fresh, unsaturated magnetization entering the volume from outside the excitation boundaries. Stationary tissue, on the other hand, experiences a continuous pulsing of RF excitation within the volume. In this scenario, the transverse magnetization of the blood will be dictated by the transverse magnetization approach to the steady-state, whereas that of the stationary tissue will be governed by the steady-state.

What gives rise to *flow-related enhancement* by inflow effects is the fact that the signal during the approach to the steady-state of moving blood is larger than the signal associated with the stationary tissue which is in the steady-state. Vessel contrast in TOF MRA will ultimately be determined by the amount of difference in their signal magnitudes. Therefore, the strategy of this angiography technique consists of finding ways to lower the steady-state magnitude while increasing the magnitude during the approach to the steady-state.

As described in detail in the section "Spin Saturation (Magnitude)," the number of RF pulses that a given tissue experiences determines the transverse magnetization and the magnitude of the signal. Stationary tissue that resides within the imaging volume throughout the examination will experience a number of RF pulses that approaches infinity, and its transverse magnetization will be in a steady-state. In-flowing blood immediately at the point of entry at all times during the scan will experience only a single RF pulse. As the blood penetrates the volume of excitation, it will experience more RF pulses as it approaches the steady-state. Eventually, if the volume is large enough, the blood reaches a steady-state, and the magnitude of the signal will approximately equal that of the stationary tissue.

The steady-state will depend on numerous factors related to the imaging technique, as well as on intrinsic properties of the tissue. As shown previously in Figs. 17-4 and 17-5, the steady-state magnitude of the transverse magnetization is based on the repetition time TR, the spin-lattice relaxation time T_1, and the RF flip angle. For a given T_1 of the tissue, rapid pulsing with a short TR does not allow sufficient time for longitudinal magnetization recovery, which leads to small signal magnitude due to saturation effects. In addition, using RF flip angles that are either small (near 0°) or large (near 90°) at a short TR will further reduce the steady-state signal. The maximum steady-state signal will be achieved at some intermediate flip angle that is determined by TR and T_1. Therefore, in order to minimize

the signal from stationary tissue in TOF MRA techniques, a short TR should be used with either a small or large RF flip angle.

To decide what TR and flip angle to use, however, one must also consider how in-flow effects influence the blood signal. The approach to the steady-state of the in-flowing blood is also based on TR, T_1, and the flip angle. However, the rate of the approach depends on an additional factor—the number of RF pulses experienced, as shown in Fig. 17-7. From eq. 17-7, it is also seen that this will be determined by the flow scenario related to the vessel path length and blood velocity. First, for a given blood flow velocity, as the flow penetrates the imaging volume, it is hit with more and more RF pulses. In other words, the number of RF pulses it experiences increases. If TR is small, it will be hit with more RF pulses at some depth within the volume and will approach the steady-state at that depth much more quickly than with a larger TR. Second, if the path of the blood vessel is tortuous, so that it turns and remains within the excitation volume, then the blood will experience a larger number of RF pulses than for a straight vessel at the same depth because its path length is effectively longer. Finally, slower flow velocities will result in a larger number of RF pulses at some depth than faster velocities.

Figure 17-7 shows that for a given TR and T_1, large RF flip angles have a large initial signal (one RF pulse) and a rapid approach to the steady-state, taking only a few RF pulses to reach it. Conversely, small RF flip angles have a small initial signal and a slower approach to the steady-state. In the final analysis, in nearly all TOF MRA protocols, good stationary tissue suppression requires TR to be kept short relative to the T_1 values of the tissues and therefore is typically not a very flexible acquisition parameter. However, determining the use of the proper RF flip angle will greatly depend on the situation and on the types of vessels to be visualized. The appropriate flip angle can vary widely. The incorrect choice of its value for a particular TOF application can lead to major compromises in both vessel contrast and overall diagnostic utility.

Moment Nulling in TOF MRA

Since the primary goal of TOF MRA is to maximize the signal magnitude from moving blood, an additional issue related to the spin phase needs to be addressed. Theoretical details of spin phase and how it is influenced by motion has been described in the section "Spin Dispersion (Phase)." Immediately following excitation, all spins are precessing at the same phase and are in a state of *maximum coherence*. The transverse magnetization and the corresponding signal are also at their maximum. Ideally, in a TOF MRA application, this is the time when the signal should be collected for processing. However, spatial encoding of the signal is necessary in imaging and requires a certain TE interval. This finite time delay can lead to substantial signal loss, particularly in moving blood.

Gradient moment nulling (discussed in the section "Gradient Moment Nulling") is a crucial method used to minimize the signal loss from moving blood and is incorporated in virtually every TOF MRA application. By introducing gradient pulses within the TE interval in addition to that used for spatial encoding, it can be shown that at the time the signal is collected, the phase of moving spins can be nulled, leading to maximal signal coherence and magnitude. Furthermore, moment

nulling can be used to correct for different orders of motion such as velocity and acceleration.

The effect of overall gradient moment nulling on the performance of TOF MRA is shown in Fig. 17-18. A 2D application in the transverse orientation was performed for the purpose of demonstration. Figures 17-18A, C, and E are representative slices at the same anatomical position acquired with static (zeroth-order), velocity (first-order), and acceleration (second-order) moment nulling, respectively, in the slice excitation and frequency encoding directions. All other acquisition parameters were identical. Figures 17-18B, D, and F are the corresponding maximum intensity projections of all the slices in the acquisition, respectively. (A maximum-intensity projection, or MIP, is a postprocessing procedure which allows visualization of complete vascular structures in a projected image based on

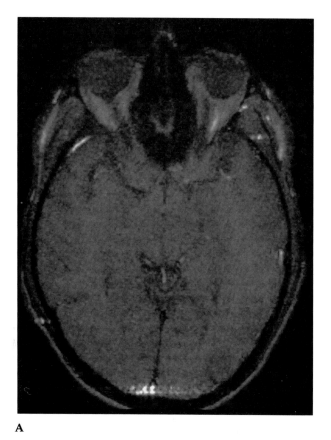 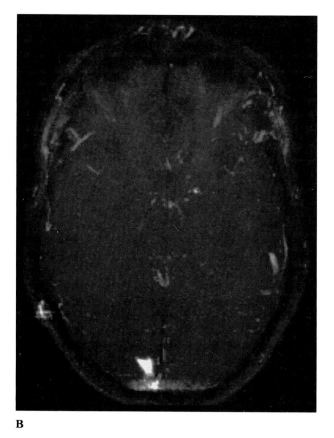

A   **B**

Fig. 17-18 Effects of overall gradient moment nulling in TOF MRA. A 2D acquisition (TR/TE/FA = 25/14/60°, 4-mm thickness, 30 slices, 50% overlap) was acquired in the transverse plane. Moment nulling was performed in the slice excitation and frequency encoding directions with (*A,B*) zeroth/static, (*C,D*) first/velocity, and (*E,F*) second/acceleration order motion correction. Images (*A*), (*C*), and (*E*) show the acquired data at the same anatomical location. Images (*B*), (*D*), and (*F*) are the corresponding maximum-intensity projections through all of the slices in the acquisition. Note the ghosting artifacts from regions of high pulsatility with only velocity correction (arrows).

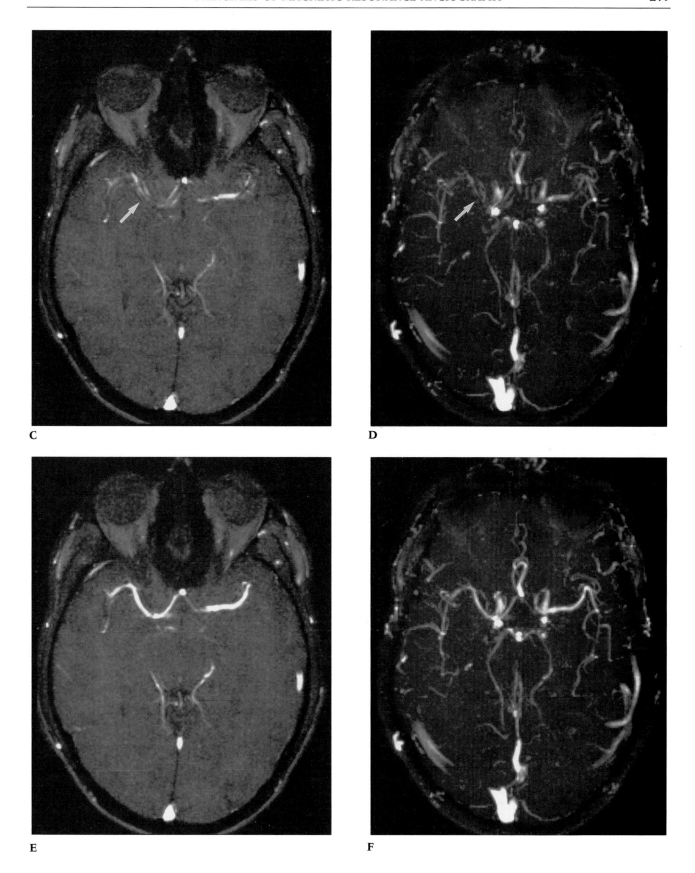

C

D

E

F

ray tracing algorithms that select only the largest signal intensity for display. Further details of postprocessing can be found in the section "Processing and Display.")

With only moment nulling of static tissues (Figs. 17-18A, B), signals from nearly all of the vessels are reduced to the background level due to phase incoherence of the magnetization from flowing blood. Some vessels, such as those near the area of the sagittal sinus, may be relatively insensitive to motion in the phase-encoding direction of the image (anatomically from left to right). When velocity moment nulling is applied, as shown in Figs. 17-18C and D, numerous vessels appear in the acquisition slice as well as in the MIP. However, due to the pulsatility of higher-order motion or faster flow, velocity correction may not be sufficient, as seen in the region of the middle cerebral artery. Ghosting artifacts due to pulsatility and ineffective higher-order moment nulling can lead to poor vessel delineation. With the incorporation of second-order moment nulling that corrects for phase incoherences due to acceleration motion, maximum signal from blood flow is achieved (Figs. 17-18E, F). Most of the improvements in vessel depiction using higher-order correction occur in areas of faster flow, tortuous vessels, and regions that possess a high degree of pulsatility.

Since the effect of the motion on the transverse magnetization of moving spins is also direction dependent, gradient moment nulling is typically performed in at least two of the three spatial directions. The phase-encoding direction of data acquisition usually does not require correction for motion, since little phase incoherence occurs in this direction even though the motion from blood flow exists. However, significant signal loss due to incoherence can result if the flow is in the slice excitation and frequency (readout)-encoding directions. Figure 17-19 demonstrates the effect of moment nulling in the frequency-encoding direction. Figures 17-19A, B, and C are MIP images with static, velocity, and acceleration correction, respectively, in the readout direction (anatomically, anterior to posterior). Second-order (acceleration) moment nulling in the slice excitation direction was performed in all three cases. Figure 17-19A shows clearly that a significant amount of flow occurs in the readout direction, requiring more than zeroth-order (static) correction for successful TOF MRA. Little difference, however, is seen between first (Fig. 17-19B) and second (Fig. 17-19C) order correction, with most vessels being equally visualized. Note, however, that specific areas of faster flow from vessels that traverse in the readout direction can still benefit from higher-order moment nulling, such as in the middle cerebral arteries. In Fig. 17-20, the effect

of moment nulling in the slice excitation direction is shown in similar fashion. Here second-order moment nulling was now performed in the readout direction in all cases.

In TOF MRA, gradient moment nulling is an absolute requirement, at least to the first order, to correct for phase incoherences associated with velocity motion of blood flow. This must also be performed in both the slice excitation and frequency-encoding direction. Second-order acceleration correction may also be warranted in imaging fast or complex flow such as pulsatility. This, however, requires the application of more gradient pulses of stronger amplitude and often is not considered practical. Introducing more pulses to correct for higher-order motion such as acceleration can also lengthen the TE, which may counter the efforts used to correct the motion. At some time, this reaches a point of diminishing returns and may not be considered useful. Note that in order to demonstrate the differences in moment nulling between first and second order, the data obtained for Figs. 17-18 to 17-20 using a relatively long TE (14 msec) are not typical of state-of-the-art techniques that can usually achieve first-order moment nulling with TE values well below 10 msec. In general, most TOF MRA techniques incorporate only first-order moment nulling (velocity correction) in the two directions of slice excitation and frequency encoding, and attempts are made to keep the TE as short as possible.

2D TOF MRA[20–26]

Application
In 2D TOF MRA applications, slices are acquired in a time sequential manner. If the slices are sufficiently thin, then most blood vessels that reside within the volume of excitation have relatively small path lengths. As a result, even with a short TR, most of the blood, including slow flow, will in principle experience only a few RF pulses before it exits the volume and is replenished with fresh unsaturated spins. Therefore, a large RF flip angle can be used to increase the signal from blood. In conjunction with a low steady-state signal from stationary tissue, this can lead to very high vessel contrast.

The effect of using different RF flip angles is depicted in Fig. 17-21. At 20°, the MIP (see the section "Processing and Display" for details) shown in Fig. 17-21A demonstrates poor vessel contrast for several reasons. First, with a low flip angle, only a small difference in signal magnitude will be achieved between blood and stationary tissue, as described in Fig. 17-7. Even at the

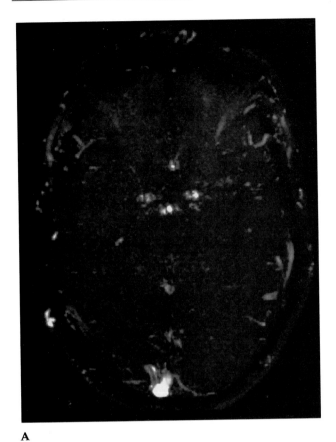

A

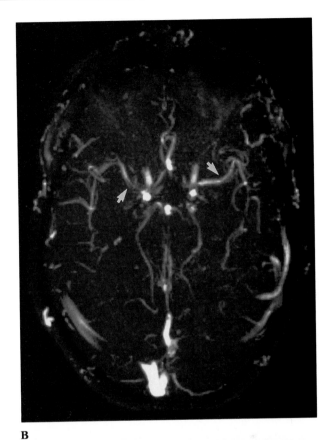

B

Fig. 17-19 Effects of gradient moment nulling in the frequency encoding direction. A 2D acquisition (TR/TE/FA = 25/14/60°, 4-mm thickness, 30 slices, 50% overlap) was acquired in the transverse plane. Second-order moment nulling (acceleration) was performed in the slice excitation direction in all cases, with (*A*) zeroth, (*B*) first-, and (*C*) second-order correction in the frequency encoding direction. Note the increased vessel delineation in regions of fast flow (arrows) with second- compared to first-order correction.

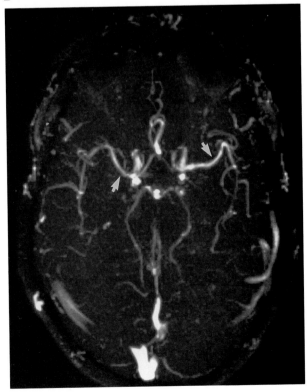

C

entry to the slices when the blood signal is maximal, this difference is small. The good penetration characteristics afforded by using low flip angles is not exploited when thin sections are used in a 2D application. Vessel contrast is also further reduced due to partial voluming effects with stationary tissue within the slice even though they may be thin sections. Relative to the sizes of the intracerebral vessels, 2D slices that may be on the order of 2–5 mm are large and partial voluming can be significant. In Fig. 17-21B, which was acquired with 40°, vessel contrast is substantially improved due to in-flow enhancement. However, the steady-state signal from stationary tissue is also near maximum at 40° for the TR used (25 msec) and the T_1 value of brain

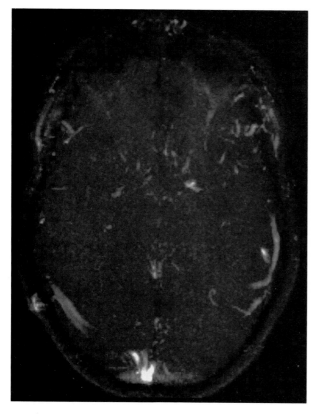

A

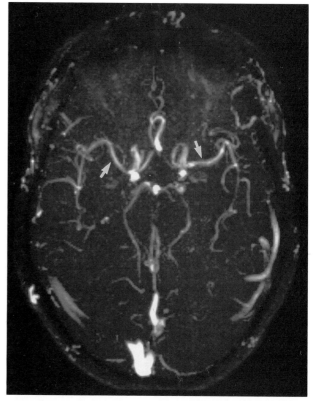

B

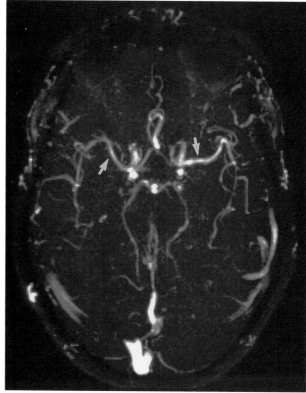

C

Fig. 17-20 Effects of gradient moment nulling in the slice excitation direction. A 2D acquisition (TR/TE/FA = 25/14/60°, 4-mm thickness, 30 slices, 50% overlap) was acquired in the transverse plane. Second-order moment nulling (acceleration) was performed in the frequency encoding direction in all cases, with (A) zeroth, (B) first-, and (C) second-order correction in the slice excitation direction. Note the increased vessel delineation in regions of fast flow (arrows) with second- compared to first-order correction.

matter. Therefore, background can be more conspicuous. At the 60° flip angle shown in Fig. 17-21C, the vessel signal is even higher due to in-flow enhancement from TOF effects; however, due to the steady-state behavior of magnetization at short TR, the background is now further suppressed.

Overall the vessel contrast is superior at the highest flip angle used. The dangers of losing vessel contrast at depth with such large flip angles is negligible if sufficiently thin sections are employed. In Fig. 17-21, 2D slices of 2-mm thickness were obtained with a 50% overlap to ensure vessel continuity on MIP processing. Comparing Figs. 17-21B and 17-21C, no secondary or tertiary vessels are lost at the higher flip angle with 2-mm sections. Only higher vessel contrast and delin-

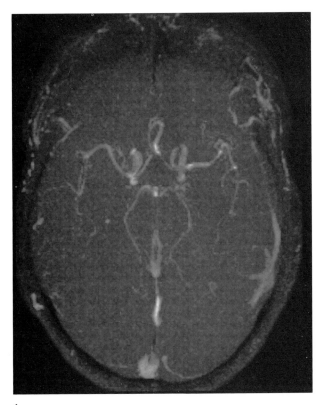

A

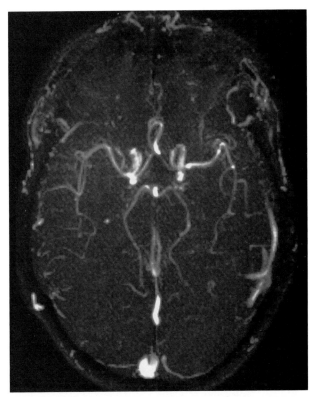

B

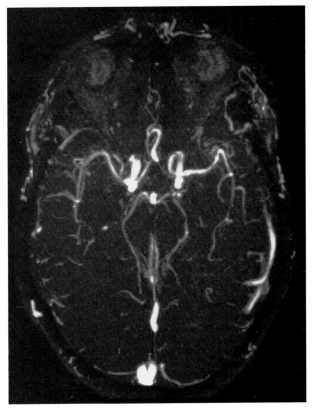

C

Fig. 17-21 Influence of RF flip angle in 2D TOF MRA (TR/TE = 25/10, 2-mm thickness, 64 slices, 50% overlap). Data were acquired in the transverse plane with flip angles of (A) 20°, (B) 40°, and (C) 60°. Postprocessed MIP images of the data are shown. Poor vessel contrast is seen at the lowest flip angle. The intermediate flip angle shows improved vessel contrast but also increased background from stationary tissue. At the highest flip angle, superior vessel contrast is observed, based on good in-flow enhancement and decreased stationary tissue signal.

eation are achieved. The use of thicker slices, however, may result in some loss of vessel branches at the same flip angle due to a combination of poor depth penetration and partial voluming effects. This is demonstrated in Fig. 17-22 when section thickness is varied from 2 mm to 8 mm. Progressive loss, particularly in smaller vessels, is observed. At 8 mm, only the largest vessels remain.

Therefore, the optimal method for 2D TOF MRA applications is to use as thin a section as possible and as large an RF flip angle that will not suffer from signal losses due to poor depth penetration. In some circumstances, however, thin slices may not be practical. For example, since the sections are acquired sequentially in time, the total scan time for an examination may be

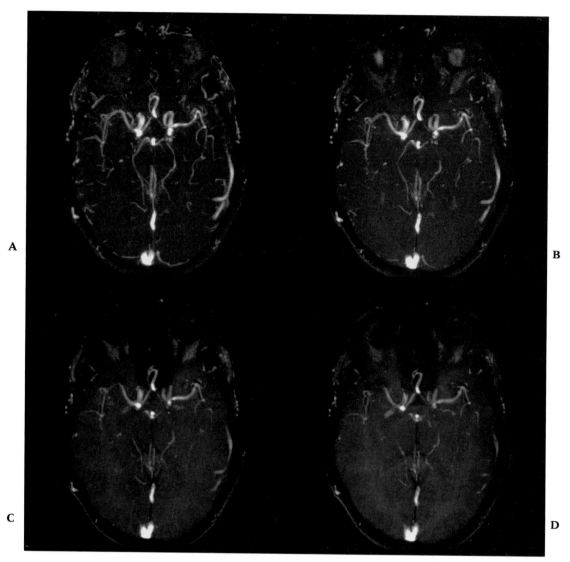

Fig. 17-22 Influence of section thickness in 2D TOF MRA (TR/TE/FA = 25/10/60°, 50% overlap). Data were acquired in the transverse plane with thicknesses of (A) 2 mm, (B) 4 mm, (C) 6 mm, and (D) 8 mm. The number of slices acquired was varied to cover the same anatomical regions. Postprocessed MIP images of the data are shown. Vessel contrast and delineation at larger slice thicknesses are degraded. This is due to a combination of poor depth penetration using a large RF flip angle and partial voluming effects with thick sections.

quite long if a large number of thin slices are required for complete coverage. If the region of interest is relatively localized and does not require large coverage, it may be worth the additional scan time to reduce the slice thickness and increase the number of slices so that a large flip angle can be used.

Although a high degree of vessel contrast can be achieved with 2D TOF MRA applications, there are several limitations due to the fact that these methods are 2D. All 2D MRI techniques suffer in spatial resolution along the direction of slice excitation because of

limits on how thin a slice can be acquired. Whenever high resolution is required in all three directions, a 3D method is usually used, since the third dimension of slice excitation becomes additionally phase encoded and can yield as small a pixel dimension as in the plane of the other two directions. Spatial resolutions of less than 0.8 mm in both the frequency and phase-encoding directions of an image can be achieved. Slice thicknesses in a 2D application are rarely less than 2 mm.

MIP images can be processed in any orientation rela-

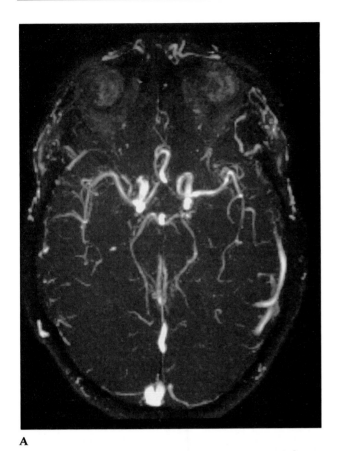

A

B

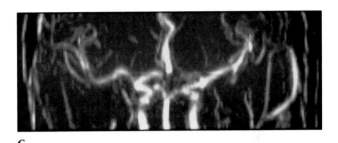

C

Fig. 17-23 Spatial resolution loss with orthogonal MIP images in 2D TOF MRA. Data were acquired axially with TR/TE/FA = 25/10/60°, a slice thickness of 2-mm with 50% overlap, an in-plane FOV of 210 mm, and a 256 × 256 matrix. MIP images were processed in the (A) transverse, (B) sagittal, and (C) coronal orientations. Note the directional spatial losses seen in the sagittal and coronal MIPs in their respective axial directions associated with the slice thickness.

tive to the acquired data. If a 2D TOF MRA technique is processed so that a MIP is projected orthogonally to the direction of slice excitation, the image will exhibit an observable loss of spatial resolution due to the limitations of the slice thickness. This can be seen in Fig. 17-23. If a MIP is processed in the same plane as the acquisition, no spatial resolution loss occurs since it possesses the same in-plane resolution as the acquisition data of 0.82 mm (Fig. 17-23A). However, Figs. 17-23A and 17-23C exhibit sagittal and coronal MIPs that are orthogonal to the data acquired in the axial direction with slice thicknesses of 2 mm. Noticeable loss of spatial resolution and blurring are seen in the

transverse direction of the orthogonal MIPs. Less conspicuous is the fact that this blurring is unidirectional and occurs only in the axial direction of excitation. Overlapping slices during data acquisition is normally done to ensure vessel continuity in the MIP. However, increasing the degree of overlap may also improve spatial resolution in the slice direction if appropriate postprocessing is performed. Yet doing so will also require a greater number of slices for coverage, will increase the overall scan time, and may not be a feasible alternative.

Another consequence of 2D TOF MRA is the *preferential directionality* to the vessels acquired with this

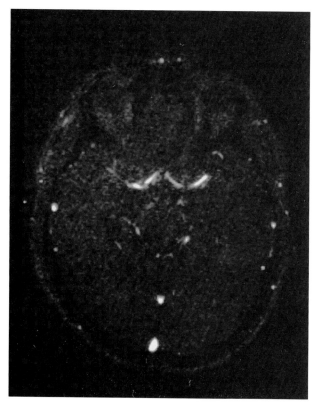

A

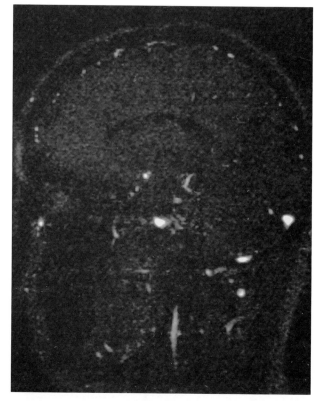

B

Fig. 17-24 Directional dependence of 2D TOF MRA (slices). Acquisition parameters were TR/TE/FA = 19/10/90°, 2-mm slice thickness, a 50% overlap, a 192 × 256 mm FOV, and a 192 × 256 matrix. Three separate datasets were acquired: (A) transverse, (B) sagittal, and (C) coronal planes. Total scan time for each acquisition was 4:18 min (64 slices). Extremely high vessel contrast is seen primarily in vessels that traverse orthogonally through the slices.

technique. Even though thin slices are primarily used, the use of a relatively large RF flip angle tends to generate the largest signal from blood at the immediate entry to the slice. Any vessel that traverses the section at an angle will have a certain degree of compromise to its signal relative to a vessel that travels perfectly orthogonal to the slice orientation. As a result, vessel contrast will ultimately be weighted preferentially in the direction of the slice. This, of course, will be accentuated with larger flip angles that yield inherently less depth penetration, shorter TR, and thicker slices.

Figure 17-24 depicts three representative 2D TOF MRA slices obtained with separate acquisitions in the transverse, sagittal, and coronal planes. Few in-plane vessels are observed. Maximum vessel contrast was achieved by using an extremely short TR of 19 msec

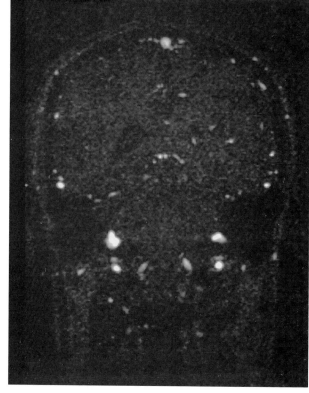

C

that greatly suppresses stationary tissue and a flip angle of 90° that produces the maximum possible signal from blood flow at the immediate entry to the slices. In this scenario, any angulation of the vessel to the slice will rapidly lose signal and the directionality will be accentuated. Figure 17-25 shows the MIP images in all three directions of the transverse acquisition. In the axial MIP (Fig. 17-25A), increased contrast is seen from vessels that primarily run transversely, suggesting directional

preference to the flow enhancement. This becomes obvious on the sagittal and coronal MIPs of the axially acquired data (Figs. 17-25B,C). Few lateral vessels are seen relative to the high contrast from axially oriented vessels. MIP images from the sagittal acquisition (Fig. 17-26A,B) and from the coronal acquisition (Fig. 17-26C,D) clearly show the directional dependence of the 2D TOF MRA application that is preferential to their respective slice directions.

Acquiring three separate datasets in the three orthogonal directions is never used as a 2D TOF MRA application primarily because the examination would take three times as long. However, if the TR is reduced to extremely short times that are even advantageous for vessel contrast, the scan time would not necessarily be unreasonable. For example, using a TR of 19 msec and a 192×256 matrix, 64 slices in all three orientations can be obtained in just over 12 min, with no compromise in spatial resolution or inherent vessel contrast. Although the datasets have clearly been shown to possess vessel directionality, it is possible to postprocess all three datasets together, so that the high vessel contrast contributions from all directions would be combined into one MIP. Such a result is shown in Fig. 17-27. The maximum depiction of all vessels, regardless of their direction, will occur in the region where all three acquisitions intersect and are combined in the MIP processing.

Advantages and Disadvantages
Time sequential slice acquisition of 2D TOF MRA has the ability to attain high vessel contrast based on its

A

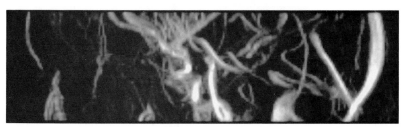

B

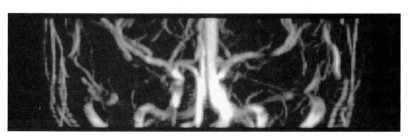

C

Fig. 17-25 Directional dependence of 2D TOF MRA (MIP images of an axial acquisition). (*A*) Axial, (*B*) sagittal, and (*C*) coronal MIP images are displayed from the transverse acquisition shown in Fig. 17-24. Note the preferential depiction of the vessel structures in the transverse direction of the acquisition.

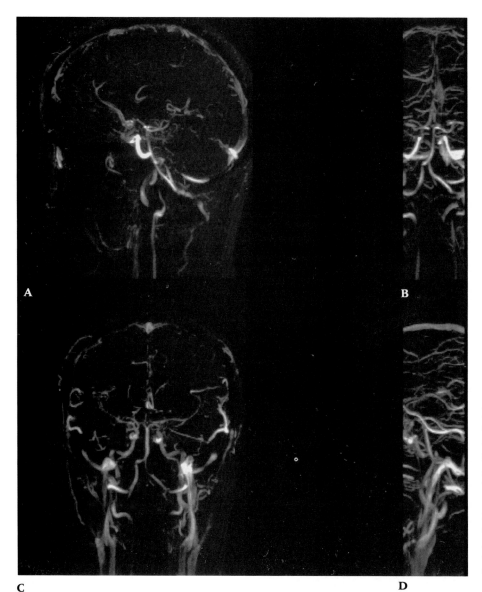

Fig. 17-26 Directional dependence of 2D TOF MRA (MIP images of a sagittal and coronal acquisition). (*A*) Sagittal and (*B*) coronal MIP images of the sagittal acquisition shown in Fig. 17-24 and (*C*) coronal and (*D*) sagittal MIP images of the coronal acquisition shown in Fig. 17-24 are displayed. A clear preferential direction of the vasculature to the plane of acquisition is observed.

use of short TR, thin sections, and high RF flip angle. This offers one of its primary advantages: the ability to image slower flow that may otherwise lose its contrast at depth. Entry in-flow enhancement can be extremely large, but high flip angles provide inherently poor depth penetration. Vessels that enter the slices at an angle may have reduced signal magnitude that can be further aggravated by the use of very small TR values and thicker sections. Partial voluming with larger thicknesses may also decrease contrast of the smaller secondary and tertiary vessels. As a result, 2D TOF MRA tends to be preferential in its direction of vessel depiction based on the orientation of the acquired

slices, losing vessels that traverse laterally in the plane of acquisition. Its 2D nature usually introduces a poor 3D resolution based on the slice thickness that is typically larger than the in-plane pixel resolution of the phase- and frequency-encoding directions of the image. Finally, because 2D TOF MRA data are acquired in a time sequential manner, the total scan time for the examination is directly proportional to the number of sections. Depending on the degree of slice overlap, targeting of smaller regions of interest that require only a small number of them to be collected can lead to attractively short imaging times (i.e., a few minutes). Nevertheless, the possible misalignment of sequentially

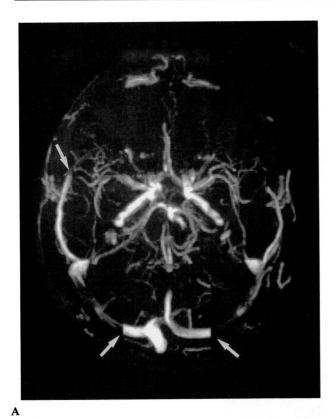

A

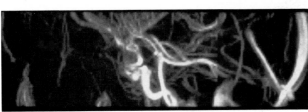

B

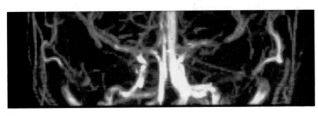

C

Fig. 17-27 Combined MIP display of three orthogonal 2D TOF MRA acquisitions. All three data acquisitions described in Fig. 17-24 were combined in postprocessing to yield (*A*) axial, (*B*) sagittal, and (*C*) coronal MIP images. Although similarities are seen with Fig. 17-25, no preferential vessel direction is seen in the regions of slice intersection where the maximum signal was chosen in the MIP processing coming from the slice that generated the largest in-flow enhancement. Note, however, the abrupt signal changes in vessels that traverse outside of the data acquisition boundaries (arrows).

acquired slices within the stack due to bulk patient motion can cause wholesale displacement artifacts of the vessels in the MIP display of the complete vascular structures.

3D TOF MRA[26–34]

Application

3D imaging techniques offer the ability to attain high spatial resolution in all directions. This is the primary reason to use TOF MRA as a 3D method. Unlike the use of thin slices in 2D TOF MRA, the slab of excitation is quite thick in the third dimension (on the order of 30 to 100 mm), depending on the coverage required. Since this slab becomes spatially encoded during the 3D acquisition, equal dimensions of the encoded partitions through the slab with respect to the in-plane pixels can easily be achieved. *Isotropic resolutions* with equal dimensions on all three sides of a voxel may be as high as 0.7 mm.

With the use of a thick slab of excitation, vessel path lengths can be quite long as the blood travels through it. Therefore, good vessel contrast in 3D TOF MRA can be attained only by ensuring good depth penetration of the flow-related enhancement. Based on the time-of-flight behavior of moving blood and the approach to steady-state of its magnetization as it traverses the volume of excitation, it was shown in Fig. 17-7 that maintaining the signal magnitude difference between the in-flowing blood and the stationary tissue at depth is possible only with the use of smaller RF flip angles.

Figure 17-28 demonstrates the depth effect associated with applying different RF flip angles in 3D TOF MRA. At a very low flip angle of 10° (Fig. 17-28A), very good depth penetration is observed in the sagittal MIP reconstructed image. Secondary and tertiary branches are visible, and slow flow vessels are depicted. However, poor overall contrast between all the vessels and the stationary tissue background is seen. Even at the immediate entry to the inferior side of the slab, where high contrast might be expected from in-flow enhancement, delineation of the internal cerebral artery is poor with the use of such a low flip angle. With 20° (Fig. 17-28B), substantial improvement in overall contrast is apparent. Depth penetration is still maintained, and smaller vessels can easily be seen. No preferential directionality to the vessels apparent in 2D TOF MRA applications occurs, since vessels that traverse laterally in the volume with a long path length still sustain good flow-related enhancement.

If the flip angle is further increased to 40° (Fig. 17-28C), in-flow enhancement begins to suffer deep in the imaging volume. Lateral structures that have long path

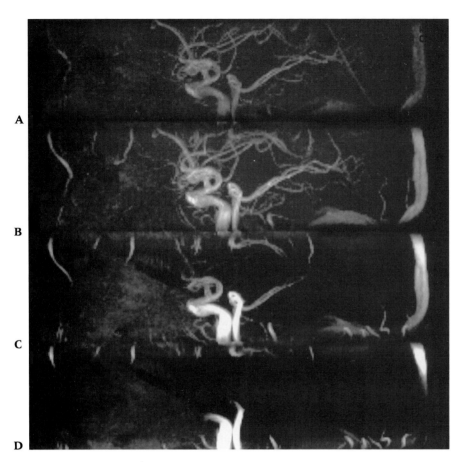

Fig. 17-28 RF flip angle dependence of 3D TOF MRA. A transverse 3D acquisition was obtained (TR/TE = 30/7, 256 × 256 matrix, 210-mm FOV, 52-mm slab thickness, 64 partitions, TA = 8:14 min). Sagittal MIP views are shown on data acquired with (*A*) 10°, (*B*) 20°, (*C*) 40°, and (*D*) 80° RF flip angles. Good depth penetration but low overall contrast are seen at the lowest flip angle. Poor depth penetration with high in-flow enhancement at the immediate entry to the slab is observed at the highest flip angle.

lengths from the entry to the slab are lost, and nearly all secondary vessels vanish. Only the primary large vessels with faster flow are visible. Directionality of the vessels also becomes apparent, similar to 2D TOF methods. Note that high-contrast arterial vessels are selectively seen at the inferior entry to the slab, whereas venous flow is observed entering the volume superiorly. Increased background signal from tissue also occurs at 40°, since this flip angle is close to the value that would generate maximum signal in the steady-state based on the T_1 of the tissues and the TR used. Finally, at an even larger flip angle of 80° (Fig. 17-28D), in-flow enhancement of vessels at the immediate entry to the slab is very high. However, only the vessels with the fastest flow penetrate the volume to any degree.

The very short path length of visible vessels with very high contrast at larger flip angles clearly suggests its potential utility in thin section 2D TOF MRA applications. However, in 3D techniques that employ thick slabs of excitation, RF flip angles should be kept small to attain sufficient depth penetration. Nevertheless, the

flip angle should not be so small as to lose overall contrast between vascular structures and the surrounding background tissue. In general, only a range between 15° and 25° is used, depending on the TR.

The need to use a low RF flip angle to achieve good flow-related enhancement at large depths in a 3D TOF MRA application results in less than optimal signal from in-flowing blood. Therefore, maintaining this signal in every way is crucial to the success of this technique. Short TE is a necessity. Lengthening the TE by even several milliseconds can severely compromise vessel contrast due to intravoxel phase dispersion in the blood signal, as discussed in the section "Spin Dispersion (Phase)." Figure 17-29 demonstrates the effect of TE and its importance in 3D TOF MRA. Coronal MIP images are shown from acquisitions using a TE ranging from 6 msec (Fig. 17-29A) to 24 msec (Fig. 17-29D). Clearly, at the largest echo times the voxel phase dispersion is extensive, resulting in significant vessel degradation and loss. Note, however, that even with a TE of 12 msec (Fig. 17-29B), a substantial reduction in the depiction of vascular structures is ob-

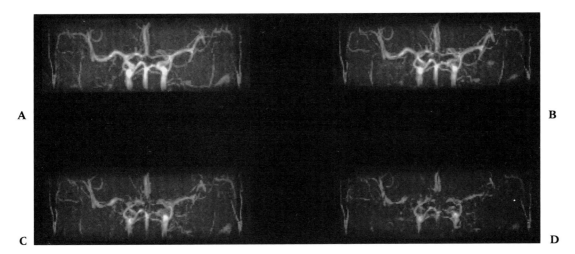

Fig. 17-29 TE dependence of 3D TOF MRA. A 3D scan was axially acquired (TR/FA = 38/20°, 256 × 256 matrix, 208 mm FOV, 51-mm slab thickness, 64 partitions, TA = 9:07 min). Coronal MIP images were processed from data acquired with a TE of (A) 6 msec, (B) 12 msec, (C) 18 msec, and (D) 24 msec. Poor contrast with substantial vessel loss is apparent at large TE values due to voxel phase dispersion and signal incoherence in the blood. Significant reduction in vascular contrast is even seen at a TE of 12 msec, even though most vessels are present.

served even though few vessels voids exist. Therefore, achieving a TE as short as possible is absolutely necessary for the success of 3D TOF MRA. The primary challenge lies in the ability to accomplish this while still incorporating gradient moment nulling to maximize the phase coherence of the moving spins in the blood.

A main advantage of 3D techniques is their ability to achieve high spatial resolution in all three physical directions. In conventional MRI, the signal/noise ratio will be linearly proportional to the voxel size. The temptation to obtain the highest spatial resolution possible is usually confounded by the associated reduction in signal/noise ratio, accompanied by significant loss in image quality. However, the inherent vessel contrast in a TOF MRA technique is based on in-flow effects, and good image quality of the vascular structures will not necessarily be related to the signal/noise ratio alone. Voxel phase dispersion, for example, can lead to subtle signal losses in the moving blood which would not otherwise be a consideration in conventional 3D MRI applications. In Fig. 17-30, the effect of voxel size and spatial resolution is demonstrated for 3D TOF MRA techniques. With a high isotropic spatial resolution of 0.8 mm (Fig. 17-30A), excellent overall depiction of the vasculature is observed, with good delineation of very small secondary and tertiary vessels. This level of resolution and voxel size would rarely be used in a conventional 3D MRI examination due to poor image quality

from the significant loss in signal/noise ratio. At 1 mm (Fig. 17-30B) and 1.2 mm (Fig. 17-30C) isotropic spatial resolution, overall vessel contrast is maintained but substantial loss in detail is seen. Note that subtle degradations also occur in smaller vessels.

Therefore, acquiring very high spatial resolution with 3D TOF MRA, particularly in the third dimension, is not only possible but desirable in visualizing smaller vascular structures. Compromises may be made, however, in terms of coverage and scan time. To ensure that a large slab of excitation becomes encoded with high resolution, many phase-encoded partitions in the third dimension are required. The number of 3D partitions is directly proportional to the imaging time, which may become prohibitively long. Conversely, to maintain a reasonable acquisition time, a compromise might be made in coverage if high spatial resolution in the third dimension is desired.

Although the large vascular contrast associated with 2D TOF MRA techniques cannot be achieved, 3D TOF MRA is usually the mode of choice, particularly for visualizing faster arterial flow, because of its superior spatial resolution in all three dimensions. Figure 17-31 shows a 3D TOF MRA acquisition depicting the circle of Willis obtained with 0.81 mm spatial resolution in all three directions in less than 8 min. High spatial resolution is attained in all MIP orientations. With the use of a low flip angle, short TE, small voxel size, and short

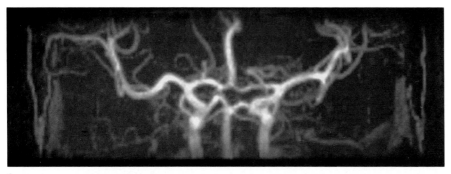

A

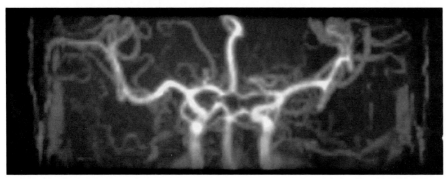

B

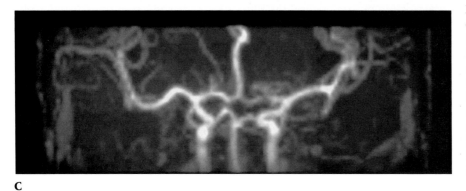

C

Fig. 17-30   Spatial resolution dependence of 3D TOF MRA. A transverse 3D acquisition was obtained (TR/TE/FA = 38/7/20°). Coronal MIP views are shown of data acquired with (*A*) 0.8 mm (*B*) 1.0 mm, and (*C*) 1.2 mm isotropic voxel dimensions. Superior spatial resolution and vessel depiction are observed at 0.8 mm. Progressive loss in vascular detail and subtle losses in small vessels are seen at lower spatial resolution.

TR, complete vascular structures of even small vessels can be visualized in any orientation, with examination times that usually do not exceed 10 min.

Advantages and Disadvantages
The inherently high spatial resolution in the third dimension that is possible with 3D TOF MRA techniques offers the advantage of depicting small structures in any orientation. Good depth penetration is achieved with the use of small flip angles, enabling large regions to be covered. However, due to the increased thickness of the excitation volume, it is usually more successful with imaging faster- rather than slower-flowing blood. Additionally, to maintain good in-flow enhancement

with a large slab, acquisitions tend to be restricted to the axial orientation. Although vessel contrast tends to be lower than with 2D TOF methods, high vascular conspicuity of even secondary and tertiary structures is attainable, provided that the TE is kept as short as possible without compromising gradient moment nulling.

3D Multislab TOF MRA[26,35–37]

Application
In 2D TOF MRA, where thin sections are acquired, the strategy is to use a large RF flip angle since depth penetration is not a major issue. Extremely high con-

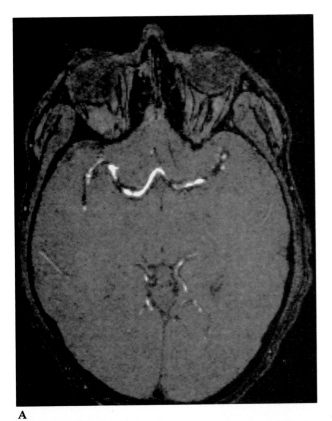

A

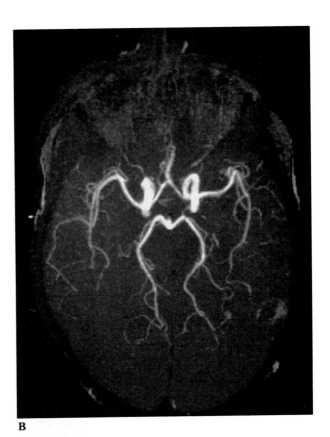

B

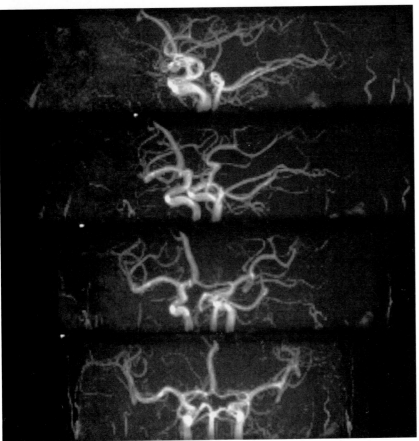

C

Fig. 17-31 High-resolution 3D TOF MRA of the circle of Willis. An axial scan was acquired (TR/TE/FA = 38/7/20°, 52-mm slab thickness, 64 partitions, 156 mm × 208 mm FOV, 192 × 256 matrix, TA = 7:49 min). Shown are (*A*) a representative transverse partition, (*B*) a transverse MIP, and MIP images incrementally rotated from sagittal to coronal orientation by (*C*) 0°, (*D*) 30°, (*E*) 60°, and (*F*) 90°. Superior spatial resolution and complete depiction of arterial structures can be seen at all orientations.

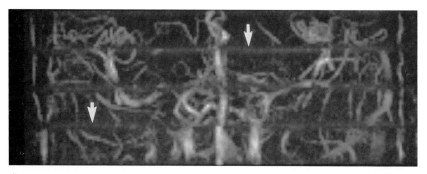

A

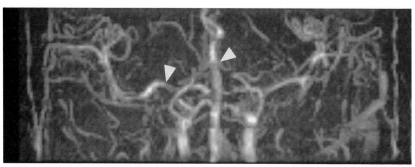

B

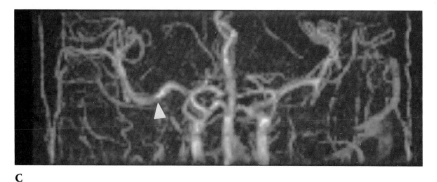

C

Fig. 17-32 Effect of slab overlap with 3D multislab TOF MRA at 25° RF excitation. Acquisitions were acquired axially (TR/TE/FA = 38/10/25°, 14-mm slab thickness, 16 partitions, 224-mm FOV, 256 × 256 matrix). Coronal MIP images are shown for (*A*) 0%, (*B*) 25%, and (*C*) 50% overlapping of the slabs. Striping in the background tissue (arrow) is observed in (*A*) due to imperfect slice excitation profiles. With overlapping this is circumvented, but vessel striping is also seen (arrowheads) based on differences in the in-flow enhancement at the entry to and exit from the slab volume. This is more prevalent at smaller degrees of overlap.

trast can be achieved but with poor spatial resolution in the third dimension. In 3D TOF MRA, thick slabs are used and the strategy is to acquire the data with a small RF flip angle for sufficient depth penetration. Comparably less vessel contrast is attained, but high spatial resolution is possible in the third dimension. The primary goal of 3D multislab TOF MRA is to take advantage of the high contrast in 2D applications and the good depth penetration and spatial resolution in 3D applications. To achieve this, *multiple thin-slab 3D acquisitions* are required. By keeping the slabs thinner than those normally used in 3D TOF MRA, a higher RF flip angle can be used without compromise in vessel loss at depth. This results in better overall vessel contrast. By acquiring it as 3D datasets, the spatial resolu-

tion of the third dimension can still be maintained. By acquiring multiple thin slabs that overlap to a certain degree, vessel continuity can be ensured while obtaining coverage of the vascular structures.

As with any TOF technique, choice of the RF flip angle is important. However, with 3D multislab methods, an additional factor must now be considered with respect to the percentage of overlap between the slabs to be employed. The optimum protocol must take into account how the flip angle varies with depth based on TR and vessel velocities, the slab thickness relative to this penetration depth, and the minimum slab overlap that can be used so that maximum coverage can be achieved with as few slabs as possible to minimize scan time.

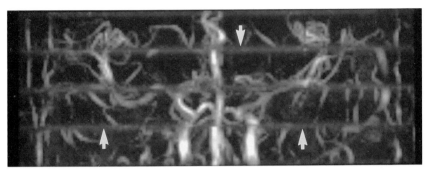

A

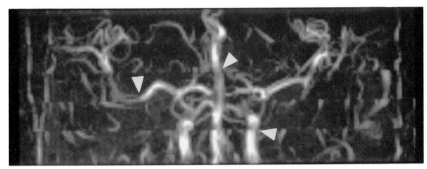

B

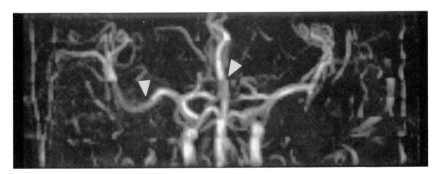

C

Fig. 17-33 Effect of slab overlap with 3D multislab TOF MRA at 50° RF excitation. Acquisitions were acquired axially (TR/TE/FA = 38/10/50°, 14-mm slab thickness, 16 partitions, 224-mm FOV, 256 × 256 matrix). Coronal MIP images are shown for (A) 0%, (B) 25%, and (C) 50% overlapping of the slabs. Striping in the background tissue (arrow) is observed in (A) due to imperfect slice excitation profiles to a larger degree than at 25° (Fig. 17-32A). With overlapping this is circumvented, but vessel striping is also seen (arrowheads) based on differences in the in-flow enhancement at the entry to and exit from the slab volume. This is more prevalent at smaller degrees of overlap but remains severe even at 50% overlap.

Figures 17-32 and 17-33 demonstrate the effect of overlapping the multiple slab regions with an RF flip angle of 25° and 50°, respectively. With a 0% overlap, complete coverage of the circle of Willis can be achieved with four 14 mm slabs. The same region requires five such slabs if overlapped by 25%. With a 50% overlap, seven slabs are necessary to attain the same coverage. Imaging time is increased by the number of slabs used in the total volume. Note the significant increase in overall visualization of vessel structures even with the use of a 25° flip angle compared to what can be obtained with a conventional single slab 3D TOF MRA application (Fig. 17-31F).

The primary concern with 3D multislab TOF MRA is a *striping phenomenon*. This manifests itself in several

ways. First, when a 0% overlap is used, the imperfect slab RF profile of excitation will be observed primarily in stationary background tissue (Figs. 17-32A and 17-33A). Due to finite RF pulse durations in any MRI technique, the RF flip angle through a slice is not a perfectly square profile. In other words, it would not excite a constant flip angle everywhere within the slab, with virtually no excitation outside of the slab. More typically, the excitation rolls out beyond the slab boundary that defines the thickness. As a result, when the multiple slabs are combined to generate a MIP, the edges from two adjacent sections will be added together, producing a visible stripe of background tissue across the image.

This problem can be solved by *overlapping* the multiple slabs to some degree so that the outermost partitions of each slab are not used in the MIP process. However, a second type of striping anomaly will still occur. Within each slab that is acquired, the use of a larger RF flip angle will cause a subtle difference in vessel contrast from the in-flow enhancement at the entry to the slab versus that at the exit. In a multislab situation, the entry to one slab will be the exit from another. The result is an inevitable striping phenomenon seen in the vessel structures as they pass through the slabs (Figs. 17-32B and 17-33B). This becomes less prevalent with a larger degree of overlap (Figs. 17-32C and 17-33C). However, with the use of a larger RF flip angle that possesses a greater change in vessel contrast with depth than does smaller flip angles, even with 50% overlap vessel striping can still be clearly seen (Fig. 17-33C).

Figure 17-34 shows a comparison between using 25° and 50° RF flip angles with a 50% overlap of the slabs in the axial and sagittal MIP images. Since the axial MIP is in the direction of the acquisition, no striping anomaly is observed in either case. Vessel contrast is higher at 50°, as expected (Fig. 17-34C), but a significant loss in secondary vessels is seen, indicating that 50° yields poor depth penetration and is too large an angle for the thickness of the slabs used. Contrast is lower at 25° (Fig. 17-34A), but numerous secondary and tertiary vessels are depicted. Comparing this to Fig. 17-31B, multislab techniques with slightly higher flip angles than those used with single-slab techniques might be more advantageous for visualizing secondary structures. In the sagittal MIP images, no striping of the vessels is observed at 25°, but it is seen at 50°.

Advantages and Disadvantages
By taking advantage of the high vessel contrast associated with 2D TOF MRA and the good depth penetration and 3D spatial resolution with 3D TOF MRA, multiple thin-slab 3D methods can yield improved vessel contrast while maintaining high spatial resolution. Smaller vessels can be visualized, and slower flow may be better depicted than with a single thick-slab technique. However, because the slab thicknesses are still relatively large, this application is mainly restricted to axial slab excitations. The primary drawback to this method is the striping phenomenon in the vessel structures even with overlapping of the slabs during the acquisition. This can be minimized with sufficient slab overlap in combination with an RF flip angle that is not too large, which may result in large depth changes of vessel signal and contrast. Increased overlap may also require a greater number of slabs to obtain proper

coverage and may increase the total scan time over that of a single-slab method. Since this is a multislab technique, it is also acquired in the same time sequential manner as 2D TOF MRA. Therefore, it may be prone to some of the same problems with vessel displacement due to patient motion during the examination.

Spatially Selective Flow Saturation[22,38–43]

Theory
Rapid RF pulsing, particularly with flip angles of 90° or more, is an effective way of suppressing transverse magnetization and signal. If the pulsing is sufficiently fast, little time is allowed for longitudinal or T_1 recovery of the magnetization, thereby providing little available magnetization to produce signal upon subsequent RF pulsing. Under normal imaging situations, this is not an optimal approach since it leads to overall poor image quality due to low signal/noise ratios. However, if the desire is to purposely suppress signal from certain tissues, such a strategy is quite effective and is routinely employed to spatially saturate body regions in many MRI protocols.[38,39]

Spatially selective saturation (SAT) pulsing can be incorporated in any MR imaging technique by simply preceding it with SAT pulsing.[41] Typically, there is very little technical difference between the standard RF pulsing used for imaging and spatially selective SAT pulsing. In effect, using the SAT pulsing is like acquiring another slice region, except that it is accomplished in such a way as to minimize rather than maximize the signal from that region. If the time between SAT pulsing and the imaging RF pulsing is nearly zero, so that no T_1 recovery of magnetization is allowed to occur, then the optimum flip angle for the SAT pulse is nearly 90°. However, if time is allowed between the pulsings, the flip angle that is necessary for maximum signal suppression in the region of SAT pulsing is increased above 90° to account for a certain degree of T_1 recovery during this time period. Although there are no special requirements for SAT pulses, their incorporation in an imaging technique adds time to the pulse sequence and may compromise rapid scan techniques that require very short TR values. The additional pulsing will also increase the RF absorption to the patient.

In general, SAT pulsing is used in two ways: *in-plane* (perpendicular to the imaging plane), and *out-of-plane* (parallel to the imaging plane). In-plane spatial saturation that is applied perpendicular to an imaging slice is used frequently to suppress in-plane signals from tissue regions in the image that typically move and generate

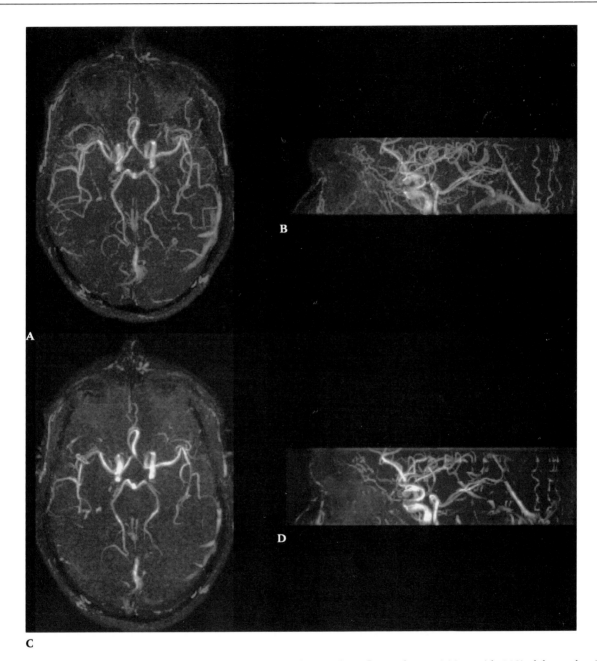

Fig. 17-34   3D multislab TOF MRA. MIP images are shown for a 25° RF flip angle acquisition with 50% slab overlap in the (*A*) axial and (*B*) sagittal planes, and for 50° RF flip angle in the (*C*) axial and (*D*) sagittal planes with a 50% overlap. All other imaging parameters are described in Figs. 17-32 and 17-33. Note the numerous secondary vessels associated with a 25° flip angle that are lost using a 50° flip angle, even though the large vessel contrast is higher. Vessel striping is not visible at 25° but is seen at 50°. Compared to a single-slab 3D TOF MRA technique (Fig. 17-31), multiple thin slabs may be superior for smaller vessel visualization.

ghosting artifacts that obscure areas of interest.[39] It might be employed, for example, to suppress signal from the beating heart, which may be in the plane of imaging but is not the area of interest, or to suppress the signal from abdominal fat in the imaging plane that is moving due to breathing.

A second use of SAT pulsing is out-of-plane spatial saturation that is applied parallel to the imaging slice. This is commonly used to suppress signal in the image coming from vessel blood that can typically generate pulsation artifacts in conventional MRI.[38,40] If a region of spatial saturation is applied above or below an imaging slice, magnetization from the blood coming from this region will be presaturated when it enters the imaging volume. Vessel lumens will be dark in the image due to minimal blood signal and therefore will create little or no ghosting artifact due to blood pulsation.

Application
Spatially selective SAT pulsing can also be used in certain TOF MRA applications.[22,42,43] In a very general way, blood that travels through vessels away from the direction of the heart can be considered arterial to a large degree, whereas vessels with blood flowing toward the heart are primarily venous. Specifically in the brain, although vessels are tortuous, blood flowing superiorly can be considered generally arterial, beginning at the middle cerebral and basilar arteries, and blood flowing inferiorly can be considered venous, draining through the sagittal sinus. In principle, if out-of-plane SAT pulsing parallel to the imaging volume is introduced in an MRA technique, it is possible to selectively saturate blood that is generally either arterial or venous, depending on whether the SAT pulsing is applied superiorly or inferiorly. Such techniques of SAT pulsing in MRA have been successfully employed to generate MR *venograms* as well as MR *arteriograms.*

Figure 17-35 shows sagittal MIP images that demonstrate both venous and arterial spatial saturation with a 3D TOF MRA application. With no SAT pulsing, all vascular structures are visible (Fig. 17-35A). When a SAT pulse is positioned superiorly at the top of the head so that venous drainage is saturated, no flowing blood generates signal. The arterial blood flow that enters the volume of excitation inferiorly remains intact (Fig. 17-35B). Note the total absence of the sagittal sinus. If, however, a SAT pulse is applied at the base of the volume, then in principle, venous structures entering from the top should become apparent. Other than the sagittal sinus, few vessels are seen (Fig. 17-35C). This can be attributed primarily to the fact that most venous blood flow is relatively slow, which is

difficult to accommodate using a 3D technique even with a small flip angle. As shown, 3D TOF MRA is mostly useful to effectively isolate arterial vessels with faster flow.

In order to achieve an MRA venogram, 2D TOF MRA can be used because of its ability to achieve good vessel contrast with slow flow.[43] Figure 17-36 shows a sagittal 2D TOF MRA acquisition without saturation (Figs. 17-36A,B) and with arterial saturation at the base of the brain (Figs. 17-36C,D). Better visualization of venous structures can be seen compared to a 3D technique. However, because the slices were acquired sagittally, much of the sagittal sinus, for example, traverses within one or two slices. In-flow enhancement relies on vessels that run through a region of excitation. Therefore, some vessel structures can be lost in a sagittal acquisition. If a 2D TOF MRA acquisition was obtained coronally or axially, then these vessels would traverse more orthogonally to the slices and become more easily visualized. Figure 17-37 shows sagittal MIP reversed displays of a 2D TOF MRA venogram acquired coronally (Fig. 17-37A) and axially (Fig. 17-37B), with SAT pulsing on both placed inferiorly at the base of the brain to selectively saturate arterial flow. Many more venous structures are visualized compared to a sagittal acquisition (Fig. 17-36), but due to the relatively thick slices used to ensure complete coverage of the brain, spatial resolution is reduced and preferential flow depiction along the respective directions of slice excitation is observed.

Advantages and Disadvantages
The advantage of applying spatially selective SAT pulses is the ability to isolate and visualize specific vessel structures. This can be implemented to observe flow in specific hemispheres, or it can be applied more globally to selectively visualize arterial or venous structures. With the need to incorporate an additional RF pulse into the technique, the minimum possible TR must be lengthened. Furthermore, the RF specific absorption rate (SAR) to the patient will be increased. The effectiveness of more global saturation will also rely on an unambiguous direction of in-flowing blood, which may be compromised in regions with tortuous vessels that traverse in all directions.

Magnetization Transfer[44-50]

Theory
In most tissues, water can be found in two distinct local molecular environments.[44] Water molecules can be freely mobile and unattached to other molecules, or

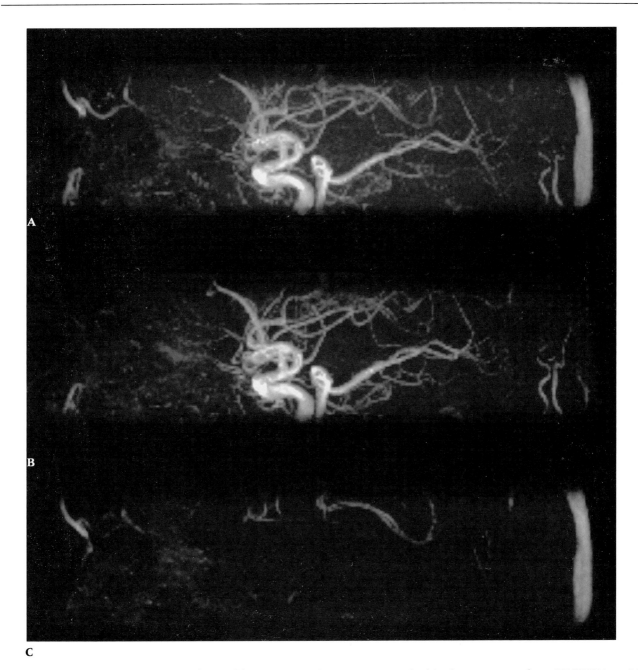

C

Fig. 17-35 Spatially selective SAT pulsing with 3D TOF MRA. Data were acquired in the transverse plane (TR/TE/FA = 36/7/20°, 52-mm slab thickness, 64 partitions, 210-mm FOV, 256 × 256 matrix). Sagittal MIP images demonstrate (*A*) no SAT pulsing, (*B*) venous SAT pulsing (superior), and(*C*) arterial SAT pulsing (inferior). All vessels are visualized as expected when no SAT pulsing is used. Only arterial structures are effectively observed when a SAT pulse is place superiorly to the volume of excitation. With arterial SAT, however, few venous structures are visible other than the sagittal sinus due to slow flow.

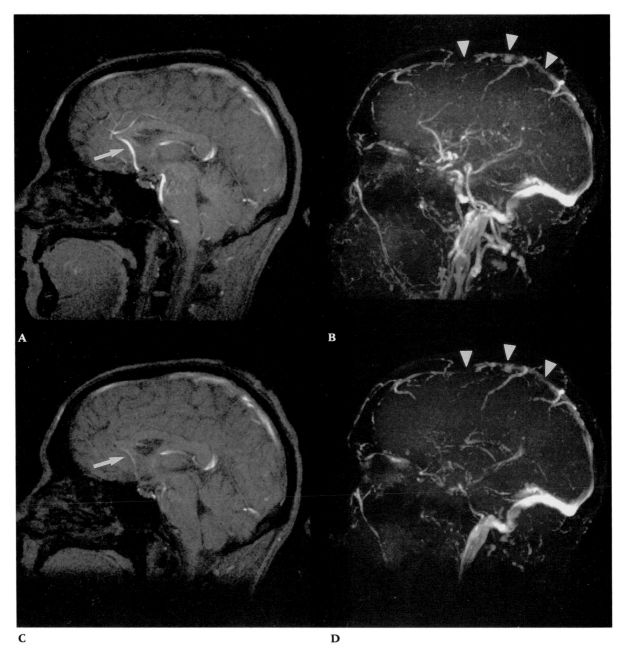

Fig. 17-36 Venography with 2D TOF MRA. Data were acquired in the sagittal plane (*A,B*) without arterior saturation and (*C,D*) with arterial saturation (TR/TE/FA = 39/10/30°, 5-mm thickness, 30% overlap, 230-mm FOV, 256 × 256 matrix). Individual slices (*A,C*) clearly exhibit the effect of flow saturation in arterial vessels (arrows). Corresponding sagittal MIP views (*B,D*) show the ability of 2D TOF MRA to depict the slower flow of venous structures. Note, however, the loss in vessel contrast from vessels that primarily traverse in plane with the sagittal orientation of the slices (arrowheads).

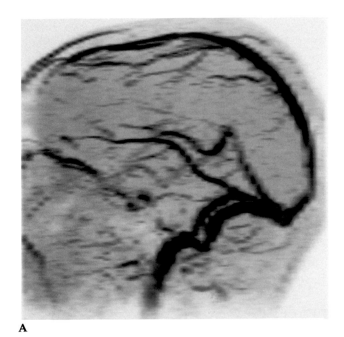

A

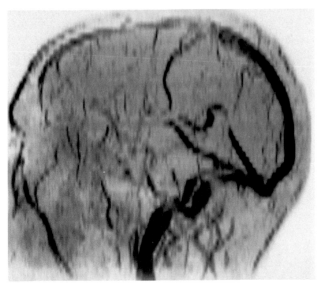

B

Fig. 17-37 Venography with 2D TOF MRA. Data were acquired in the (A) coronal and (B) axial planes (TR/TE/FA = 39/10/30°, 5-mm thickness, 30% overlap, 230-mm FOV, 256 × 256 matrix). Venous structures are visualized by spatially selective SAT pulsing of arterial flow placed inferiorly at the base of the brain. Sagittal MIP images are displayed in reverse gray scale. Note the loss of spatial resolution and directionality of vessel structures associated with the acquisition slice orientation that are characteristic of 2D methods. Nevertheless, slow flow of the venous structures is well depicted.

they can be highly restricted by being loosely or tightly bound to them. The NMR relaxation characteristics of the two distinct pools of free and bound water can be quite different. In particular, the T_2 of the bound or *restricted hydrogen pool* (H_r) is much shorter than that of the *free hydrogen pool* (H_f). This can be primarily attributed to the limited molecular motion of the H_r pool that gives rise to larger local magnetic field inhomogeneities, more rapid spin dephasing, and a resulting shorter T_2 relaxation time. Conversely, the freely moving H_f pool will experience fewer spin-spin interactions while, on the average, encountering a more homogeneous local magnetic field. This will result in a slower rate of spin dephasing and a longer T_2 relaxation time. The T_2 of the H_r pool may be on the order of microseconds, whereas that of the H_f pool can range from milliseconds to seconds for pure water.

Since the H_r pool possesses extremely short T_2 times, these hydrogen nuclei in the tissues are never observed in MRI because their transverse magnetization decays away before they can be detected. Even though pure, freely diffusible water is not necessarily found in all tissues, the signals obtained in all MRI techniques and displayed in the images come from the H_f pool, where the T_2 times are long enough to allow spatial encoding of the transverse magnetization before the signal is collected.

If RF can be applied in such a way as to affect only the magnetization of the H_r pool, it can be exchanged with the unaffected H_f pool through a *magnetization transfer (MT) process*. This, in turn, can alter the magnetization of the H_f pool. It has been found that the primary MT effect on the H_f pool is shortening of its T_1 relaxation time and reduction of its total available magnetization. MT has been used recently to indirectly study tissue distributions of the H_r pool by observing the degree of changes made in the H_f pool by the MT process. Clearly, if there is no bound water in the tissue, no H_r magnetization will become saturated, no transfer will occur, and the H_f magnetization will not be altered. On the other hand, if a large H_r pool exists in the tissue, large changes in H_f magnetization will be seen based on the MT effect.

In a basic MT experiment, the pulse sequence technique used normally to observe the H_f pool signal is immediately preceded by RF pulsing that is applied to specifically saturate the H_r pool.[45] Two basic approaches are used to ensure effective saturation of H_r while leaving H_f unaffected. The more common strategy is to apply an MT saturation pulse whose transmission frequency is several kilohertz off-resonance from the Larmor frequency of the H_f pool.[48] In this manner, since the RF field frequency does not match the Larmor frequency, the magnetization from the free water is unaffected. However, with such a short T_2 relaxation time, the bound water possesses a very wide frequency distribution that extends the spread of its Larmor frequencies to several kilohertz. Therefore, an off-resonance RF pulse will still saturate some of the H_r magnetization.

A limitation of *off-resonance MT pulsing* is that it is relatively inefficient and requires very long duration pulses of large RF amplitudes to achieve good saturation of the H_r pool.[48] This can severely restrict the use of rapid scanning techniques that employ very short TR values. In addition, the RF absorption to the patient from such pulsing can be quite large.

An alternative approach is to exploit the characteristically very short T_2 of the bound water pool.[46,47] Very rapid transmission of a series of on-resonance RF pulses can be applied that collectively result in a 0° RF flip angle. These "transparent," composite pulses will result in no effect on the H_f pool, provided that the RF pulse durations and times between the pulses are much shorter than T_1 and T_2 to minimize any relaxation during the transmission. A 90°–180°–90° combination, for example, adds up to an effective 360° or 0° flip angle, or a transparent pulse. However, if the T_2 of the H_r pool is short enough so that these same RF pulses can no longer be considered instantaneous, the net effect of the composite pulse will no longer be 0°, resulting in saturation of the magnetization. The inherently wide frequency bandwidth and short duration of the RF pulsing can ensure efficient H_r pool saturation for the MT process, with little compromise in TR for rapid scanning.

A main drawback of this *on-resonance MT pulsing* technique is that there may be partial saturation of the free water hydrogen, since it is transmitted on-resonance at the Larmor frequency, and it is not truly instantaneous, so that some relaxation will occur during pulsing. This method may also result in high RF absorption to the patient.

Application
The concept of using magnetization transfer in TOF MRA is relatively straightforward and has recently been introduced.[49,50] In TOF MRA, a major goal is to suppress the signal from stationary tissue as much as possible, and MT has been used to effectively reduce it by as much as 40%. If it can be assumed that the MT pulsing affects only the stationary tissue while minimally influencing the blood flowing into the imaging volume, then the MT process will shorten the T_1 and

reduce the available magnetization of the H_f pool from the stationary tissue. This latter effect can substantially reduce the background tissue signal and improve overall visualization of blood vessels. Both on-resonance and off-resonance MT pulsing have been successfully employed. Conventional TOF technique can be used, executing an MT pulsing scheme immediately in front of it.

Figure 17-38 shows a comparison between a 3D TOF MRA technique without (Figs. 17-38A,C) and with (Figs. 17-38B,D) MT pulsing. In this case, off-resonance pulsing was used. Overall signal suppression from background tissues is clearly visible, using MT pulsing without compromising in-flow enhancement from the blood (Fig. 17-38B,D). This results in better contrast and vessel conspicuity, particularly in smaller vessels. Note, however, that fat remains unaffected by the MT pulsing due to the lack of a restricted hydrogen pool.

Advantages and Disadvantages
MT is an effective way to further reduce background signal from stationary tissue without affecting the in-flow enhancement from blood. As a result, better visualization of the overall vasculature is possible, particularly in the smaller secondary and tertiary vessels. Similar to introducing SAT pulses, MT pulsing requires additional time and lengthens the minimum TR. It also increases, possibly in a substantial way, the RF SAR to the patient. Although in principle the blood should not be affected by an MT pulse, some saturation may occur, possibly with a slight reduction in the magnitude of the signal from flow. Fat may appear to increase. However, it remains unaffected by the MT pulse and retains its signal magnitude, thereby looking bright relative to the surrounding tissues. By presenting a nonuniform background, it may cause difficulty in interpretation of MIP images that incorporate the fat in its processing. With proper MIP targeting methods, however, this becomes a minor issue.

Spatially Varied Excitation[51–54]

Theory
In the theory of TOF MRA, the intrinsic contrast between moving blood and stationary tissues is primarily governed by the difference between the signal intensity of the moving blood and the steady-state signal intensity of the surrounding tissue. To maximize this difference, strategies are used to increase the intensity of the blood and/or reduce the steady-state signal of the stationary tissue.

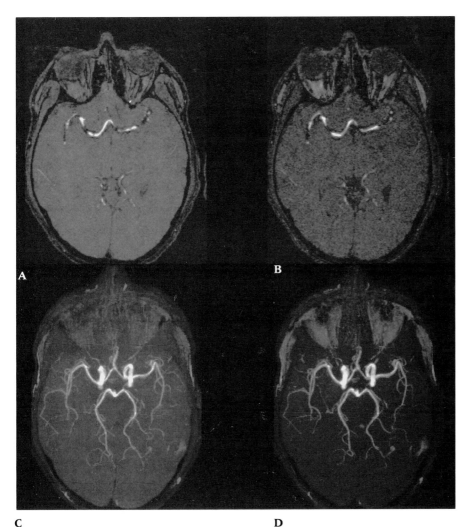

Fig. 17-38 Magnetization transfer in 3D TOF MRA. Data were acquired (*A*) without and (*B*) with off-resonance MT pulsing in the axial orientation (TR/TE/FA = 38/7/20°, 52-mm slab thickness, 64 partitions, 208-mm FOV, 256 × 256 matrix). Axial MIP images are also shown (*C*) without MT and (*D*) with MT. Substantial reduction in background stationary tissue is observed with the use of MT pulsing. No compromise, however, is seen from in-flowing blood. Better contrast and vessel delineation are demonstrated. Note that the fat remains unaffected by the MT pulsing.

Based on the Bloch solutions for the gradient echo techniques used for TOF MRA, a steady-state signal reaches a maximum when $\cos(\theta_{rf}) = \exp(-TR/T_1)$. This is the well-known Ernst angle relationship. For a typical TR of 40 msec used in a 3D TOF technique, and T_1 values ranging from 400 to 800 msec for tissue in the brain, the RF flip angle, θ_{rf}, that is expected to yield the greatest steady-state signal is anywhere from 20° to 25°. Therefore, to reduce the steady-state signal from stationary tissue in order to improve vessel visualization, this would require choosing a flip angle much less than 20° or much greater than 25°.

At very small flip angles, the steady-state signal is low. However, the total available magnetization that can yield a signal is proportional to $\sin(\theta_{rf})$, which means that even fresh blood entering the imaging volume that has never experienced a single RF excitation would also have very low signal. Although the inher-

ent depth penetration of blood is good at small flip angles, the blood signal is so small that the overall contrast is still compromised.

At very large flip angles, the steady-state signal is also very low. However, in this case, the total available magnetization for fresh blood entering the imaging volume is extremely large. Thus, the entry signal in vessels is very high, resulting in good vessel–stationary tissue contrast. Nevertheless, at very large flip angles, the depth penetration of the blood is poor and its signal quickly approaches the low steady-state value after experiencing only a few repeated RF excitations as it flows through the imaging volume.

In summary, small flip angles compromise overall signal and large flip angles compromise depth penetration. This is a primary dilemma in 3D TOF MRA, where relatively large imaging volumes are required that are excited by a uniform RF flip angle across the entire slab

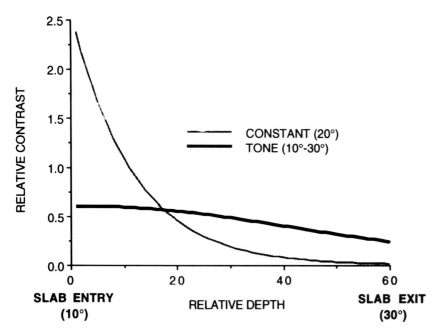

Fig. 17-39 Spatially varying RF excitation vs. constant RF excitation. Simulation of the depth penetration differences between a constant RF excitation of 20° and a spatially varying RF excitation (TONE) that varies from 10° at the entry to the slab to 30° at the exit of the slab. Better overall uniformity of TOF magnetization is seen with TONE pulsing.

thickness. If, however, small flip angles are used at the entry and larger flip angles are used deeper in the imaging volume, better depth penetration without too much of a compromise at the entry might be possible. This is the primary idea behind a *spatially varied excitation*, or *Tilted Optimized Nonsaturating Excitation* (TONE). Shown in Fig. 17-39 is a computer simulation of what would be expected of the vessel contrast from a spatially uniform 20° RF flip angle and TONE pulsing, with 10° at the entry and increasing linearly to 30° at the exit from the slab.

At the point at which blood first enters the imaging volume, it has experienced either no RF excitation or only a few repetitions of excitation. Therefore, the signal will be inherently large and far greater than the steady-state intensity. A small flip angle can be used without too much compromise in contrast with stationary tissue even though the overall signal may be low. A small flip angle at the entry into the imaging volume is important to ensure good depth penetration. As the blood continues into the volume of excitation and is hit with more successive RF pulsing, its magnetization begins to be saturated. However, unlike a uniform excitation situation, with TONE it will experience larger and larger flip angles of excitation as the blood penetrates deeper into the volume. This, in turn, leads to higher signal at the expense of less depth penetration. However, if this occurs at positions already deep within the imaging volume, depth penetration afforded by lower flip angles is no longer an important issue.

The end result of applying TONE is a more uniform depiction of vessels throughout the imaging volume, with improvement in vessel contrast at depth.

Application

In nearly all MRI techniques, whether 2D or 3D, the slice or slab thickness is excited with as uniform an RF flip angle distribution as possible. This is primarily because tissue contrast is directly related to the flip angle, regardless of the technique used, and a nonuniform excitation through the slice could lead to peculiar or unpredictable contrast. In TOF MRA, however, contrast among stationary tissues is not important, and uniformity and depth penetration of the blood improve with a spatially varied RF flip angle distribution through the slab. TONE can be incorporated into an MRA technique by simply replacing the RF pulsing by the specialized RF waveforms of the TONE pulsing.[51,54] Little or no compromise in TR is made, and little difference in RF absorption to the patient occurs.

Successful implementation of TONE consists largely of determining the slope, magnitude, and direction of the tilted RF excitation through the imaging volume.[52,53] In a 3D TOF MRA application where visualization of arterial structures is primary, applying a TONE pulsing that spatially increases from inferior to superior in the general direction of arterial in-flow is appropriate. If the RF flip angle is too small at the entry, in-flow enhancement at the base of the brain will be poor. As well, if the flip angle is too large within the

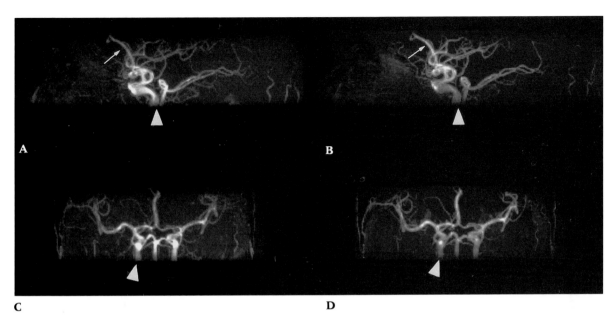

Fig. 17-40 Spatially varying excitation in 3D TOF MRA. MIP images are shown from data that were acquired (*A,C*) without and (*B,D*) with TONE pulsing in the axial orientation (TR/TE/FA = 38/7/20° and 10°–30° with TONE, 52-mm slab thickness, 64 partitions, 208-mm FOV, 256 × 256 matrix). Sagittal and coronal MIP comparisons demonstrate the reduction of in-flow enhancement at the immediate entry to the slab of excitation in the TONE images (arrowheads), with increased enhancement of deeply seated vessels (arrows).

volume of excitation, penetration will be reduced. It has been generally found that spatially varying the RF flip angle from 10° at the entry to 30° in the most superior boundary of an axial excitation affords the best uniformity of vessel contrast and the deepest penetration, as shown in simulations (Fig. 17-39).

Shown in Fig. 17-40 is a comparison between a standard 3D TOF MRA acquisition with a 20° uniform RF flip angle (Figs. 17-40A,C) and one that utilizes TONE with a spatially varying RF flip angle from 10° inferiorly to 30° superiorly (Figs. 17-40B,D). Although the conventional MRA technique depicts good contrast and vessel delineation, the TONE application shows subtle improvements. A slightly increased suppression of stationary tissue is observed with the use of TONE. This can be attributed to the fact that some of the tissues experience a lower flip angle than in the standard technique. Most notable is the increased depth penetration seen in the most deeply seated vessels with TONE. Other small vessels lying deep within the excitation volume can also be better visualized.

Advantages and Disadvantages
Spatially varying RF excitation, or TONE, can easily be implemented with any TOF technique, but it is most useful in single-slab 3D excitations where the slab

thickness is large and depth penetration becomes difficult to maintain. TONE affords better overall vessel uniformity and improved visualization of vessels at depth. Compromise with in-flow enhancement may occur at the immediate entry to the imaging volume on the side of the TONE excitation with the lowest flip angle. This, however, may also lead to a further slight reduction in the background tissue. One potential drawback to TONE is that the spatial variation is unidirectional, capable of varying the flip angle in only one physical direction. Therefore, vessel uniformity and better depth penetration will occur only with vessels that traverse in the direction of increasing flip angle.

PHASE CONTRAST MRA

Theory

Aside from TOF techniques, *phase contrast (PC) MRA* is the other major method used to visualize vascular structures. In TOF applications, the origin of vessel contrast is based on signal magnitude differences between stationary tissue and flowing blood. With PC MRA, the primary source of vessel contrast lies in the differences between their *signal phase*. Unlike TOF, where numerous strategies and techniques exist to suppress background signal and to improve in-flow enhancement and depth penetration, there exists very little in the conceptual approach to achieving vessel contrast with PC applications.

Most of the developments in PC MRA have focused primarily on ways to minimize the total scan time required to collect the data. Whereas a 3D TOF technique may take approximately 10 min, a 3D PC technique may take as long as 30 min. Different data acquisition strategies have reduced this time by as much as a factor of 2, but based on the type and wealth of information acquired, it will inevitably take more time to collect. Nevertheless, PC techniques offer the unique and clinically relevant ability to obtain quantitative and directional information of the flow they detect, something that TOF techniques cannot accomplish to the same degree. The fundamental principles of how signal phase is generally affected in flowing blood were presented in the section "Theoretical Concepts in Flow Imaging" and will not be discussed here. Rather, based on this knowledge, the practical concepts of how PC MRA is implemented will be described.

Transverse magnetization that is perpendicular to the direction of the main magnetic field will precess about this direction at the Larmor frequency. According to the Larmor equation (eq. 17-8), this precessional frequency is directly proportional to the strength of the magnetic field experienced in the region of transverse magnetization. If the field changes, the frequency will change accordingly. If two regions of transverse magnetization sense two different magnetic field strengths, then the magnetization will precess at different frequencies. Over time, the phases of the two regions of magnetization will diverge relative to each other.

In general, the main external magnetic field is purposely made to be as homogeneous as possible. In other words, it will possess little spatial variation in its strength. Magnetic field gradients, however, are pulsed to alter this field so that a linearly varying magnetic field is generated in space. The primary purpose of these gradients is to spatially encode the transverse magnetization so that an image can be produced from the MRI signal that is detected. Moving tissue, such as blood, will experience a total effective magnetic field that is fundamentally different from that of stationary tissue when gradients are applied. This is because it will sense a continually changing field strength as it moves along the direction of the spatially varying gradient. As a result, the net phase of the transverse magnetization from blood will be different from that of stationary tissue. This phase behavior was shown in Fig.

17-15 and described in detail in the section "Spin Dispersion (Phase)."

The application of a single gradient pulse will cause a net phase dispersion of all transverse magnetization and result in a complete loss of signal, regardless of whether it comes from moving blood or stationary tissue. This is because the transverse magnetization is a bulk macroscopic phenomenon based on the collective effect of the many hydrogen nuclei magnetic dipole moments that make up the tissue, each experiencing its own external magnetic field. In the presence of a gradient field that is spatially varied in a continuous manner, no two nuclei sense the same field. Therefore, they will all precess at different frequencies. The effect is a collective phase dispersion, with a corresponding decrease in the net transverse magnetization and signal.

If, however, two gradient pulses of equal duration and strength but opposite polarity are pulsed as a *bipolar pair*, the net phase effect on the transverse magnetization from stationary tissues will be zero. On the other hand, the transverse magnetization from blood that is flowing through vessels in the direction of the gradient pulses will possess a nonzero net phase at the end of

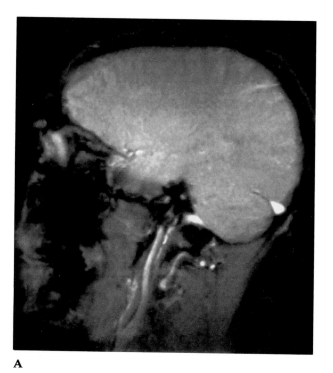

A

Fig. 17-41 The basic phase contrast MRA experiment. A 2D acquisition was obtained, retaining images of (*A*) signal magnitude and signal phase.

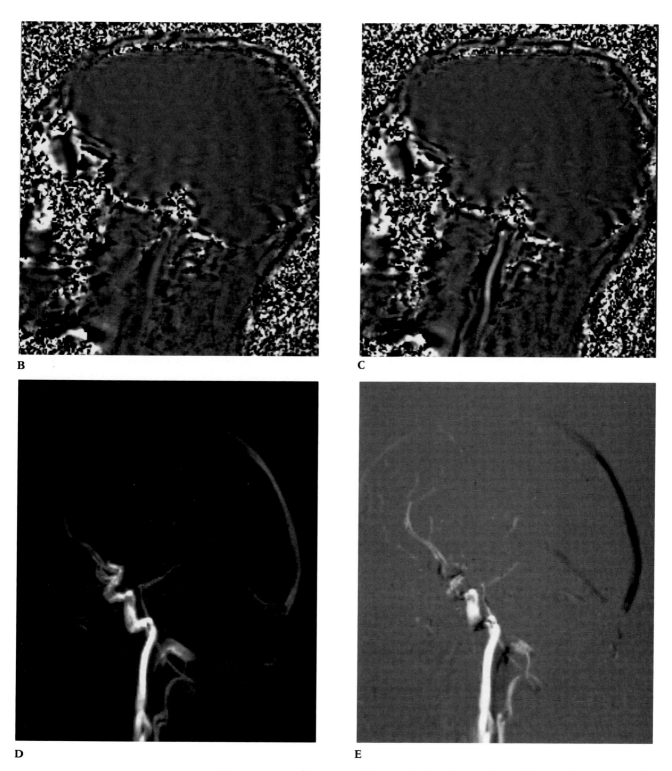

B

C

D

E

Fig. 17-41 (*B*) A second 2D dataset of the same type was acquired, but with a bipolar gradient pulse pair that sensitizes the signal to flowing blood. Only the phase image is shown (*C*). By subtracting the two phase images (*B*) and (*C*), a phase difference mapping can be processed that reveals only phase shifts that are due to blood. The results from a stack of slices can further be processed as a MIP that displays the magnitude of the phase differences (*D*). Directional MIP images that retain the sign of the phase difference can also be processed (*E*) that now reflect flow direction. White pixels are inferior-to-superior flow, and black pixels are superior-to-inferior flow.

the pulsing. It can also be shown that this phase, whose value is dictated by the specific characteristics of the bipolar gradient pulsing, will be directly proportional to the velocity of the blood. The essence of PC MRA lies in its ability to detect the phase difference between the signal from the blood and the surrounding stationary tissue. This phase contrast phenomenon was shown in Fig. 17-17 and discussed in detail in the section "Spin Dispersion (Phase)."

Equation 17-17 describes the quantitative relationship between signal phase and blood flow velocity based on pulsing of a *gradient bipolar pair*. First, it is a linear relationship, which means that the phase associated with the flowing blood will be directly proportional to the velocity. Faster flow will produce a greater phase shift relative to stationary tissue. Second, there exists an inherent directionality in that the phase of blood which flows in the opposite direction will possess a negative sign. Therefore, blood that moves in a given direction may generate a positive phase shift, whereas blood moving in the opposite direction will have a negative phase shift. Their amplitudes will be equal if their velocity amplitudes are equal.

Figure 17-41 demonstrates the kind of information that can be obtained in a typical PC imaging experiment. Every signal detected in an image is directly related to the transverse magnetization. Since the magnetization possesses both a magnitude and a phase, the signal also has a characteristic magnitude and phase. In nearly all conventional MRI techniques, only the magnitude is displayed in the image, as shown in Fig. 17-41A. In PC MRA, the important information lies in the *phase image,* as shown in Fig. 17-41B. The pixel intensity displayed in a phase image is related to the actual phase angle of the signal associated with that pixel position. The unique range of values that this angle can have is between $-180°$ and $+180°$. Therefore, the brightest pixels correspond to a phase angle of $+180°$, and the darkest pixels correspond to $-180°$. A phase angle of $0°$ lies in between at a gray level. Note that nearly all of the signal phases coming from the tissues are gray, indicating that they are all near zero. Since no signal from air exists, the phase is random and resembles "salt and pepper" in the phase image.

If a bipolar gradient pulse is applied as part of the data acquisition to induce a phase shift in any moving tissue, the corresponding phase image should reflect the nonzero phase. In Fig. 17-41C, a conspicuous phase shift can be seen in the carotid artery that is directly related to the movement of the blood in this vessel. Comparing this to Fig. 17-41B, which is not velocity encoded with a bipolar gradient pulse, other regions of more subtle phase change are also apparent. However, on careful inspection, it is apparent that the vast majority of the tissue phase has not changed. This is expected, since most of the tissue is not moving and the net effect of the bipolar gradient pair on the transverse magnetization of stationary tissue is zero.

This information can be further processed to isolate the structures that produce a *net phase difference* between images that were acquired with bipolar gradient encoding and those that were not. By subtracting the phase images, all stationary tissues should cancel out and only the vessels with flowing blood should remain. (In actuality, the phase difference is weighted by the signal magnitude unless quantitative information is desired. There are also different methods of subtraction. This is discussed in more detail in the section "Processing and Display.") Any pixel with a nonzero phase difference can then be mapped as a pixel intensity whose brightness is directly proportional to the phase difference. This can then be further processed into a MIP (see the section "Processing and Display" for further discussion) if a series of slices were acquired. An example of this is shown in Fig. 17-41D. Clearly, the fastest flow can be expected from the carotid artery. Its associated phase shift should be the largest and therefore should possess the brightest pixel intensity on the MIP image of the phase difference.

One major point that should be noted is that by obtaining vessel contrast from the signal phase difference, stationary tissue will, by definition, be canceled out since its phase difference will be at or close to zero. This is clearly observed in Fig. 17-41D, where no information is apparent other than the vessel structures. This is quite different from TOF MRA, where much effort is made to suppress stationary tissue signal. Unless a subtraction method is used, there will always be at least some background from stationary tissue in TOF techniques. In PC MRA, background is only a minor issue that may possibly be associated with systematic phase errors.

Mapping the magnitude of the phase difference, either in an individual slice or in a MIP of a stack of slices, discards an important piece of information that is also computed on subtraction: the mathematical sign of the phase difference. Blood that flows in one direction will have an opposite sign in the phase difference from blood that flows in the opposite direction. As shown in Fig. 17-41E, a *directional MIP* can also be displayed that retains the sign of the phase difference. In this case, bright pixels indicate inferior-to-superior flow, such as in the carotid, and dark pixels indicate superior-to-inferior flow, such as in the sagittal sinus.

Velocity Encoding in PC MRA

As shown in eq. 17-17, *flow velocity* is proportional to net phase after the application of a bipolar gradient pulse pair. With precise knowledge of the pulse timing and the gradient amplitudes that are used, flow can be quantified. The actual pixel intensities shown in Figs. 17-41E and 17-41F are digital representations of the actual phase difference angles between stationary and moving tissue. Since the amplitude of the angle of stationary tissue is in principle zero, pixel intensity should reflect the velocity of blood flow in the vessels. If the exact characteristics of the bipolar pair are known, then they can be directly converted into a velocity, according to eq. 17-17, and are the basis for *flow quantification* with phase contrast imaging.

Since vascular structures possess a wide range of flow velocities, the pixel intensities in a phase difference map will also cover a large range. This range can easily be manipulated by changing either the bipolar pulse timing or, more simply, the gradient amplitude. Equation 17-17 states that the phase shift is also directly proportional to the gradient amplitude. Therefore, velocity encoding to different phase shifts for a given velocity can be accomplished by changing the gradient amplitude of the bipolar pulsing in data acquisition.

One of the most important decisions in a PC MRA application is to determine what *degree of velocity encoding* is desired. By convention, a "velocity encoding of 50 cm/sec", for example, represents the fact that velocities of ±50 cm/sec will generate a phase difference equal to ±180°, respectively. The consequences of using different degrees of encoding are demonstrated. Sagittal MIP images of the phase difference magnitude are displayed in Fig. 17-42, with a velocity encoding ranging from 15 to 100 cm/sec. With 100 cm/sec encoding (Fig. 17-42A), the vessel contrast is relatively poor, with mainly primary vessels of faster flow being visualized. This is because blood flow with velocities at or near 100 cm/sec will have 180° phase shifts and be bright, but slower blood flow will possess small phase shifts and be close to the background pixel intensity. As velocity encoding is decreased, the slower flow becomes encoded with a larger phase shift and begins to generate contrast. At 15 cm/sec encoding, significant phase shifts are produced even in secondary and tertiary vessels (Fig. 17-42D) and good overall vascular contrast occurs. Therefore, the best vessel delineation is seen at the smallest velocity encoding attainable.

However, if flow directionality is retained in processing, as depicted in the sagittal MIP images shown

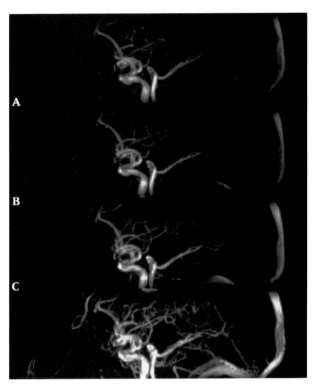

D

Fig. 17-42 Velocity encoding in PC MRA (magnitude display). Sagittal MIP images of the magnitude of the phase difference are shown for PC MRA acquisitions with (*A*) 100 cm/sec, (*B*) 50 cm/sec, (*C*) 30 cm/sec, and (*D*) 15 cm/sec velocity encoding. At large encoding (*A*), contrast is poor and smaller vessels with slower flow are not seen. At small encoding (*D*), contrast is superior even in vessels with slow flow, with numerous secondary and tertiary vessels visualized.

in Fig. 17-43, a significant artifact is observed that was not readily apparent in Fig. 17-42 with magnitude display. As velocity encoding is decreased, the vessels with faster flow will produce larger and larger phase shifts. Eventually, a situation will be reached where the phase differences in these vessels exceed the limit of 180° (Figs. 17-43C,D). This results in a phenomenon commonly seen in PC MRA when directional information is retained known as *phase aliasing*. It gives a "salt and pepper" appearance to the vessels, and leads to erroneous velocity amplitudes and direction if flow quantification is desired as part of the examination. This artifact is discussed in more detail in the section "MRA Artifacts."

It is therefore apparent that if PC MRA is used simply to visualize the vascular structures, a small encoding velocity may be helpful so that smaller vessels or slower

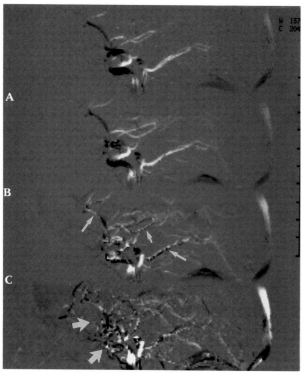

Fig. 17-43 Velocity encoding in PC MRA (directional display). Sagittal MIP images of the signed phase difference are shown for PC MRA acquisitions with (*A*) 100 cm/sec, (*B*) 50 cm/sec, (*C*) 30 cm/sec, and (*D*) 15 cm/sec velocity encoding. With smaller encoding (*C,D*), phase aliasing of faster flowing blood occurs (arrows).

flow can be better seen. On the other hand, if directional or quantitative information is required, then a larger velocity encoding must be used. The dilemma lies in the fact that if this unique aspect of PC MRA applications is exploited, it cannot be done simultaneously on both fast flow and slow flow. Fast flow in a technique with a small velocity encoding that is required to visualize slow flow will suffer from phase aliasing. Conversely, if aliasing is avoided in fast flow by using a large velocity encoding, slow flow will not be seen.

Data Acquisition in PC MRA

As previously mentioned, one of the main focuses of continued development in PC MRA is reduction of the scan time. A PC examination may take three to four times as long as its TOF counterpart. The primary rea-

son is that the phase shift flow information is based solely on the direction in which the bipolar gradient pulse velocity encoding is applied. Therefore, to encode the flow in all three directions, at least three separate datasets of directional velocity encoding must be acquired. In actuality, at least a fourth dataset must be obtained as a reference map of the phase so that phase difference computations can be performed. In TOF applications, only one dataset is collected that contains the vessel contrast from the magnitude of the flow signal in all three directions. Only in some 2D TOF MRA applications will a directional dependence with flow occur, as shown in Figs. 17-24 to 17-26.

Phase shifts due to blood flow will exist only when flow travels in the direction in which the magnetic field changes. Pulsed gradient fields can be generated in any of the three physical directions. Therefore, when a bipolar gradient pulse pair is applied to encode a phase shift in the signal from blood, only the flow moving in the direction of the bipolar pulsing will be sensitized. In Fig. 17-41, only the *z*-direction (anatomically, superior to inferior) was sensitized to flow. Comparing Figs. 17-41B and 17-41C, the carotid artery that runs along the *z*-direction clearly shows a phase difference due to the bipolar flow encoding in that direction. However, in the specific anatomical slice that is shown, the transverse sinus shows no phase shift because its direction of flow is through the slice and is perpendicular to the velocity encoding gradient direction. In the MIP images that show a more complete picture of the vascular structures (Figs. 17-41D,E), only the vessels that run superior to inferior are depicted since flow encoding was only in the *z*-direction.

A pair of independent data acquisitions that are used to compute a phase difference mapping of flow in one direction is sometimes referred to as a *two-point PC acquisition.*[55] The simplest way to acquire 3D flow information is to extend this to a *six-point acquisition,* or two acquisition pairs for each of the three directions of flow encoding. However, the scan time will increase proportionally, being six times that of a single acquisition. For a 2D application that obtains slices in a time sequential way, this may be marginally acceptable if the number of slices is kept to a minimum. However, it is apparent that if a 3D scan is performed to cover a large region of the brain that would normally take 10 min, a full six-point PC dataset to encode the flow in all three directions would take upward of 1 hr. This would clearly be prohibitive in a routine MRI examination.

It should be plausible that if three datasets are necessary to encode three separate directions of flow, then it should take only a fourth reference dataset, used repeatedly, to perform the necessary operations for a phase difference mapping in all directions. This is the basic concept behind the currently used *four-point PC acquisition* scheme. Several different four-point strategies have been studied and are beyond the scope of this discussion.[56-58] However, it is sufficient to say that to encode flow information in all directions in a PC technique, using either a 2D or 3D approach, at least four separate data acquisitions are required.

Still, a PC application will take four times as long as a TOF application if the TR is the same. In TOF MRA, the TR and the RF flip angle can profoundly affect the vessel contrast due to their integral role in generating the signal magnitude differences between in-flowing blood and stationary tissue. However, since the signal magnitude is not the source of vessel contrast in PC MRA, the TR is not crucial to its success. As long as some signal magnitude exists from the flowing blood, the signal phase will be measurable. Therefore, to further reduce the scan time in PC MRA methods, the TR can be chosen to be as short as that attainable by the MRI scanner while still maintaining the desired velocity encoding. In practice, the TR can be as short as half of the TR used in a TOF MRA technique. A PC MRA technique that covers the comparable region of interest thus may take only two to three times as long as its TOF MRA counterpart.

2D PC MRA[55,59-62]

Application
Strategies used to implement 2D and 3D TOF MRA exist. To attain optimal contrast from in-flow enhancement, significantly different methods of acquisition are used. However, this is not the case with PC MRA. Velocity encoding will be the same whether a thin 2D slice or a thicker 3D slice is acquired. Yet, there is a fundamental difference between the time sequential collection of a series of 2D-slice datasets that are separated in time versus a single time-averaged 3D dataset, regardless of the technique.

In a 2D application of PC MRA, one can acquire either one slice or many slices. If a small region of interest is desired, then only a few slices will be needed. Because scan time in 2D is directly proportional to the number of slices, the necessary flow information from the region can be acquired in only a few minutes. In addition, 2D PC MRA can provide accurate *quantitative analysis* of both flow velocity and flow direction. In a given slice, the primary image information will be collected in a few tens of milliseconds. Most of the remaining acquisition time is used to gather spatial in-

formation that adds resolution and edge definition to small structures. Therefore, snapshots in time of vessel flow information can be obtained. If multiple slices are acquired in the same anatomical position in a time sequential manner, one can depict the time dependence of blood flow at a given physical location. Synchronizing data acquisition with the cardiac cycle may allow detailed analyses of the flow in any vessel in relation to physiological or hemodynamic disorders.

The degree of velocity encoding for quantitative or even relative flow studies must be carefully chosen to avoid phase aliasing in the vessels. To yield sufficient phase differences in smaller vessels or slower flow, low-velocity encoding (<20 cm/sec) must be used. However, faster flow phase differences will become aliased and difficult to interpret. Keeping the velocity encoding high enough so that no phase aliasing occurs in the vessels with the fastest flow (>50 cm/sec) will inevitably cause smaller vessels and slower flow to disappear due to insufficient signal phase shifts. If directional and velocity information about the vascular flow is desired, then the choice of velocity encoding is crucial and depends on the vessels to be studied.

With the use of 2D TOF MRA, the choice of the RF flip angle and the slice thickness may be crucial. Time-of-flight effects in flow-related enhancement of the signal magnitudes are directly influenced by both factors, and an improper selection may lead to loss of both vessel contrast and delineation. In 2D PC MRA, the amount of signal phase shift from blood in a vessel that leads to the vascular contrast is based entirely on the interaction of flow magnetization with the gradient magnetic fields from a velocity encoding bipolar pulsing. The RF flip angle that is used will significantly alter the signal magnitude but will have no effect on the signal phase shift seen in moving blood. Therefore, it has little or no influence on vessel contrast with a 2D PC MRA acquisition, provided that a flip angle is used that will generate sufficient signal to measure the phase shift.

The thickness of the slice is also a relatively minor issue in 2D PC MRA, although it can be a factor. Whether a thin or thick section is excited, all blood flow in the vessels will generate the same phase shift that leads to contrast if their velocities and trajectories are identical. In this respect, slice thickness is not important. However, partial voluming with thick slice excitations may lead to a reduction in vessel contrast. A pixel in a slice represents the average signal magnitude and phase through the entire thickness. Therefore, if a vessel that traverses the slice at an angle is substantially smaller than the thickness, the majority of the signal

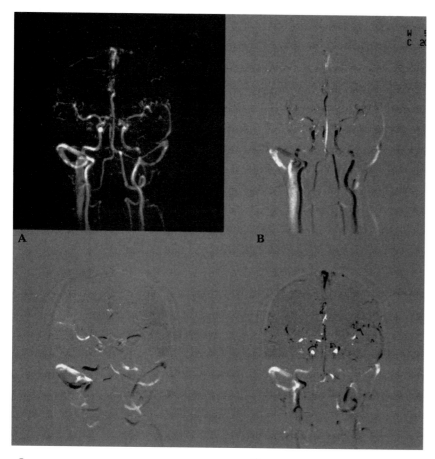

Fig. 17-44 A 2D phase contrast MRA (coronal acquisition). A four-point acquisition was obtained with velocity encoding of 50 cm/sec in all three directions (TR/TE/FA = 30/12/20°, 230-mm FOV, 256 × 256 matrix, 6-mm thickness, 33% overlap). A coronal magnitude MIP of complete flow is shown in (A), and directional MIP images are shown for the individual components of (B) inferior–superior, (C) left–right lateral, and (D) anterior–posterior flow. White pixels represent flow traveling inferiorly in (B), right laterally in (C), and anteriorly in (D).

phase in the pixel may be associated with stationary tissue, which in principle will have a phase shift of zero during velocity encoding. Even though the blood flow itself may possess a large phase shift, the resulting pixel of the signal phase will be more indicative of the stationary tissue. This could possibly lead to degradation in the depiction of smaller vessels. It may also depend on the type of data subtraction processing that is used to achieve the contrast.

If the thickness is larger still, so that multiple vessels overlap within the slice such that the pixel becomes a representation of their collective phases, it is conceivable that destructive phase interference or even complete phase cancellation can occur, so that the net phase shift in the pixel is at or near zero. Therefore, even though the choice of thickness may not alter the effects of velocity encoding of the vessels, it may influence the total phase that ends up representing a pixel. In turn, when the phase difference to achieve the phase contrast is computed, thick slices may lead to regional vessel voids, contrast reduction, and loss of entire structures of smaller vessels. If the thickness of the section is kept sufficiently thin so that the majority of the vessel dimensions are comparable in size, then these issues become far less important.

Figures 17-44 and 17-45 demonstrate some of the unique capabilities of 2D PC MRA. Velocity encoding was 50 cm/sec in both cases, and a four-point acquisition was used. The images in Fig. 17-44 were obtained from slices acquired in the coronal plane, whereas those in Fig. 17-45 were collected in the sagittal plane. Visualization of complete vascular structures with 2D TOF MRA techniques which rely on fresh, unsaturated magnetization from in-flowing blood into the slice volume can be severely compromised by the orientation of the slices, as seen in Figs. 17-24 to 17-26. However, provided that the 2D PC MRA acquisition is velocity encoded in the three directions, the slice orientation is irrelevant other than for the purpose of covering the region of interest.

Figs. 17-44 and 17-45 also show the different types of information that can be gleaned from 2D PC MRA. The series of slices that were obtained can be processed and displayed as a magnitude MIP of all of the phase

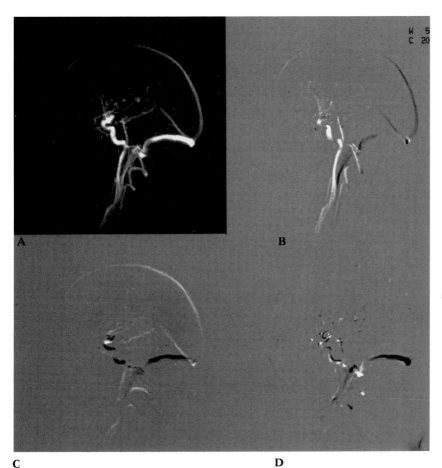

A

B

C

D

Fig. 17-45 A 2D phase contrast MRA (sagittal acquisition). A four-point acquisition was obtained with velocity encoding of 50 cm/sec in all three directions (TR/TE/FA = 30/12/20°, 230-mm FOV, 256 × 256 matrix, 6-mm thickness, 33% overlap). A sagittal magnitude MIP of complete flow is shown in (*A*), and directional MIP images are shown for the individual components of (*B*) inferior–superior, (*C*) anterior–posterior, and (*D*) left–right lateral flow. White pixels represent flow traveling superiorly (*B*), posteriorly (*C*), and left laterally (*D*).

differences that become generated from the flow in the different directions so that a complete picture of the vasculature can be interpreted (Figs. 17-44A and 17-45A). In addition, flow information can be separated into MIP displays of their individual directional components. In Figs. 17-44B and 17-45B, superior-to-inferior flow is shown. Carotid arteries in Fig. 17-44B are shown as black pixels indicating an upward flow, whereas in Fig. 17-45B they are shown as white pixels indicating the same direction of flow.

This shows that *negative* or *positive phase differences* from flow do not necessarily indicate an absolute physical direction, but only a relative direction with respect to other vessels. First, the mathematical sign of the phase shift will depend on the flow direction as it becomes influenced by the bipolar gradient pulsing. The sign of the phase shift of blood flow from a (+ −) pulsing will be the opposite of the sign of the phase shift from a (− +) pair. Second, the sign of the phase difference that results from subtraction depends on which dataset is subtracted from the other. Finally, the

way in which the phase shift is displayed in the image may depend entirely on the user. The important information that is retained is that the phase difference from flow in one direction will have the opposite sign of the phase difference from flow in the opposite direction. The relative directionality of the flow with respect to other vessels is preserved.

Since only the inferior-to-superior flow in Fig. 17-44B is depicted, information from the middle cerebral arteries that flow in the perpendicular direction are not observed. However, if these data are displayed as in Fig. 17-44C, these vessels are now seen and the carotid arteries are not. Here, white pixels indicate flow to the left and black pixels indicate flow to the right. The same directional flow information is shown in Fig. 17-45D, but it is acquired and displayed in the sagittal orientation. Figures 17-44D and 17-45C both demonstrate anterior-to-posterior flow.

In principle, the PC MRA technique has the advantage of superb background suppression from stationary tissues. Since stationary tissues have no velocity component, their signal phase shift from a velocity encoding bipolar pulsing should effectively be zero, which should lead to a zero phase difference after processing. Bulk patient motion that can produce a wholesale phase shift from signal in the entire head is one possible source of error that could lead to a nonzero tissue background. This problem can be easily avoided by properly securing the head. However, systematic errors such as eddy current fields can also generate signal phase errors, as observed in Fig. 17-44. They are particularly noticeable in the directional MIP images as a faint outline of the head. Eddy current fields are extraneous magnetic fields induced in surrounding conductive materials in the magnet upon gradient pulsing. These eddy current fields, in turn, may perturb the actual gradient pulsing so that a perfect velocity encoding bipolar pulsing will not occur. Any imperfection in this pulse pair will result in a finite phase shift from stationary tissue and yield a nonzero background. Compensating for eddy current fields or even preventing them from distorting the gradient pulsing with shielded gradients is therefore advantageous to ensure optimal background suppression in PC MRA.

Advantages and Disadvantages
One of the main issues with PC MRA is scan time. Since 2D PC MRA obtains images in a time sequential fashion, it allows the scan time to be reduced significantly by acquiring only the number of slices that are necessary for sufficient coverage of the region of interest. In contrast to 2D TOF MRA techniques, which rely heavily on TR, RF flip angle, and thickness for in-flow enhancement, these acquisition parameters are less crucial in 2D PC MRA. Thicker sections can be used without severe compromise in vessel contrast, particularly with larger vessels. Therefore, complete coverage is possible with fewer slices than with TOF methods. In addition, 2D PC MRA can be performed in any acquisition plane, with no reduction in vessel conspicuity, unlike its TOF counterpart. Scan time can be further reduced by keeping the TR as short as possible. If only one direction of flow is of interest, two-point acquisitions can be performed in only a few minutes.

PC MRA in general offers the unique capability of visualizing velocity and direction. In addition, 2D PC MRA allows absolute quantitation of these flow characteristics. In a single-slice experiment that is repeated in time at the same anatomical position, evolving flow can be studied in individual vessels. This can also be synchronized with the cardiac cycle for more accurate physiological evaluation. One of the primary advantages and uses of 2D PC MRA is for the study of blood flow characteristics.

Since 2D PC MRA is a slice technique, it possesses many of the disadvantages of any 2D application. First, if the slice thickness is much larger than the dimensions of the vessels, partial voluming effects may occur that will degrade the vascular contrast due to averaging with surrounding tissues. Phase cancellation from multiple overlapping small vessels can also result in regional vessel voids. In general, secondary and tertiary vasculature will be more difficult to visualize with 2D PC MRA. Second, the third dimension of slice excitation will typically have significantly lower spatial resolution than in-plane dimensions, as determined by the slice thickness. Therefore, any display, such as a MIP that is processed perpendicular to the plane of acquisition, will demonstrate poor spatial resolution. Finally, because 2D MC MRA is acquired sequentially in time, vessel displacement can occur due to bulk patient motion.

3D PC MRA[63-66]

Application
Basically, 3D PC MRA possesses the same type of information as a 2D application, provided that the velocity encoding is performed to the same degree and in the same directions. However, several major differences exist. In a 3D acquisition, the spatial resolution in the third dimension will be improved because of the additional spatial encoding in this direction. Thickness of the slab becomes an issue only with coverage and spatial resolution of the voxel. No partial voluming or effects of vessel overlap will occur, as in 2D PC MRA, provided that the spatial encoding in the third dimension is sufficient. Therefore, 3D PC MRA lends itself well to the visualization of smaller vessels.

Spatial information in a 3D acquisition is encoded in all three directions. The overall signal phase difference information in the vasculature will be representative of the flow taken over a period of time that may be as long as 20–30 sec. Therefore, absolute velocity and directional information in the processed PC images will be an average over this time interval. Synchronizing it with the cardiac cycle is not feasible in the 3D mode due to scan time. Thus, unlike its 2D counterpart, 3D PC MRA can only obtain gross average information about the blood flow in vessels and is not quantitative. Therefore, 3D PC MRA applications are primarily useful in visualizing complete vascular structures at high resolution in all three directions. If directional and velocity information is not of interest where the danger of phase aliasing exists in faster flow, the smallest velocity encoding (<20 cm/sec) is desirable, so that the smallest vessels and the slowest flow will be encoded with a

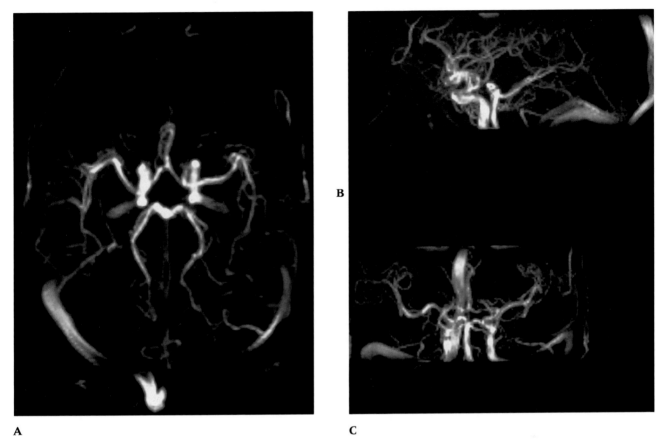

A   **C**

Fig. 17-46 High-resolution 3D PC MRA of the circle of Willis. An axial four-point acquisition was obtained with a velocity encoding of 15 cm/sec in all three directions (TR/TE/FA = 20/12/20°, 64-mm slab thickness, 64 partitions, 256-mm FOV, 256 × 256 matrix, TA = 21:50 min). Shown are magnitude MIP images in the (A) transverse (B) sagittal, and (C) coronal orientations. High spatial resolution can be seen at all orientations. Small vessels and slow flow are well visualized, with superb background suppression.

sufficient phase difference that enables them to be observed.

A four-point 3D PC MRA technique will inevitably require a long examination for complete coverage. Two of the three directions of spatial encoding contribute to the overall imaging time (phase encoding in one of the in-plane directions and in the third dimension). Therefore, spatial resolution may become limited from a scanning point of view. Since TR is not a primary factor in PC MRA, the shortest TR allowed by the scanner should be used in most cases. A TR greater than 25 msec will result in a scan time longer than 20 min for high-resolution studies with a four-point acquisition.

A high-resolution 3D PC MRA scan in the region of the circle of Willis is shown in Fig. 17-46. The velocity encoding was 15 cm/sec, and a four-point acquisition was used to encode flow in all three directions. Magni-

tude MIP images were processed. In comparison to a high-resolution 3D TOF MRA in the same region (Fig. 17-31), higher contrast from slow flow deep within the imaging volume and from more secondary and tertiary vessels is observed. Background from stationary tissue is also significantly reduced relative to the TOF technique, providing better contrast. However, several drawbacks exist. The isotropic spatial resolution in Fig. 17-31 for the TOF technique was 0.81 mm and the total imaging time was 7:49 min. To achieve a 1.0-mm isotropic resolution in Fig. 17-46 with 3D PC MRA, a scan time of 21:50 min was required.

Although flow directionality may be *time-averaged* and unquantifiable, the information still exists and can be processed so that the velocity components in all three directions can be displayed. This is demonstrated in Fig. 17-47. Here 3D PC MRA data were acquired directly in both the sagittal orientation (Figs. 17-

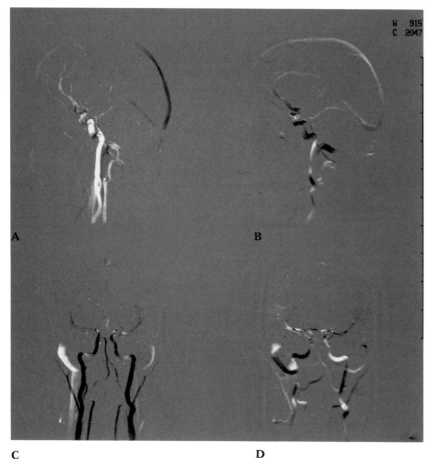

Fig. 17-47 Directional 3D PC MRA. Four-point (A,B) sagittal and (C,D) coronal acquisitions were obtained with a velocity encoding of 50 cm/sec in all three directions (TR/TE/FA = 20/12/20°, 64-mm slab thickness, 64 partitions, 256-mm FOV, 256 × 256 matrix). Sagittal directional MIP images are shown for the individual velocity components of (A) inferior–superior and (B) anterior–posterior flow. Coronal directional MIP images are shown for(C) inferior–superior and (D) left–right lateral flow. Note the reversed pixel intensity of the inferior–superior flow of the two acquisitions (A,C). This indicates display ambiguity, not the accuracy of the flow information, and is described in the section "2D PC MRA." Comparisons with 2D PC MRA (Figs. 17-44 and 17-45) of the same anatomical regions indicate consistent directional flow information with superior small vessel visualization.

47A,B) and the coronal orientation (Figs. 17-47C,D), with a velocity encoding of 50 cm/sec in all three directions. Different directions of acquisition are easily possible with PC MRA since they do not rely on time-of-flight in-flow enhancement for vessel contrast. Comparisons with 2D PC MRA in the same regions of coverage (Figs. 17-44 and 17-45) demonstrate that similar directional information can be obtained with 3D techniques. Furthermore, on closer scrutiny, better overall contrast and smaller vessels can be seen with 3D PC MRA because of the higher spatial resolution in the third dimension.

Advantages and Disadvantages

The primary advantage of any 3D technique is its higher resolution in the third dimension of spatial encoding. This enables better visualization of smaller vessels with 3D PC MRA even when the velocity encoding is the same as in 2D PC MRA. Phase differences in flowing blood do not rely on in-flow enhancement. Therefore, 3D PC MRA can be directly acquired in any

orientation, unlike 3D TOF MRA. However, selective localized flow suppression to study isolated arterial or venous structures, which is possible in TOF applications with the use of saturation pulses, is not an alternative unless complete suppression of the flow is achieved so that its signal magnitude is near zero.

Since the majority of the phase contrast information is acquired over much longer periods of time than with a 2D application, it represents time-averaged flow characteristics. Directional information is therefore not quantifiable, as it is in 2D MRA, yet it may still be useful to study average flow directionality. In this mode, however, velocity encoding levels must be kept large enough so that phase aliasing does not occur, thereby decreasing the chances of observing smaller vessels and slower flow. On the other hand, if 3D PC MRA is used to visualize complete vascular structures, the lowest levels of velocity encoding will allow high-resolution depiction of small vessels and slower flow not easily attainable with TOF applications. Coupled with good background tissue suppression, 3D PC MRA offers superior contrast of secondary and tertiary vasculature.

The 3D PC MRA examination is longer than the 3D TOF MRA. Although shorter TR can be used to reduce the scan time, the procedure may still be as much as three times longer. This can indirectly limit the attainable spatial resolution. Whereas a 512 matrix acquisition is possible with 3D TOF MRA in approximately 10 min, the imaging time with this large a matrix in 3D PC MRA would be prohibitive.

PROCESSING AND DISPLAY

Maximum Intensity Projection[27,67–70]

In both TOF and PC MRA, data are acquired either as phase-encoded partitions in a 3D application or as a series of slices in a 2D application. Individual images depict flow information, but vessel structures are difficult to visualize from image to image. A postprocessing aid to allow the display of the complete vasculature in one image is known as *maximum intensity projection (MIP)*. Alternative methods have been and continue to be studied along with variants of MIP processing. All of these attempt to better display vessels that might otherwise be difficult to process due to fundamental shortcomings of the acquisition method. Still other methods have been developed to display vessels from information different from that acquired with TOF and PC techniques. Their descriptions are beyond the scope of this chapter. The most widely used and accepted form of processing to facilitate interpretation of the vasculature obtained from MRA applications is the MIP.

The information obtained with TOF MRA consists of contrast between signal magnitudes from moving blood in the vessels and surrounding stationary tissue. This is achieved by exploiting the time-of-flight phenomenon of in-flow enhancement. The result is high signal from the blood against low signal from static tissue. In PC MRA, the contrast is based on the signal phase difference between moving blood and surrounding tissue. Large phase shifts are observed with flow, and stationary tissues exhibit near-zero phase shifts. In either MRA application, the flow information coming from the vessels is a large-valued quantity. Therefore, pixels associated with the vasculature in the acquired images will have bright intensity upon display.

The primary concept of MIP processing is to project onto a plane only those pixels that contain the highest intensities. This can be accomplished in a systematic way by employing *ray tracing* methods. A stack of 2D slices or 3D partitions make up a volumetric cube of data. The digital representation of its smallest dimensional piece of information is a voxel, the 3D equivalent of an image pixel. The third dimension of a voxel from a single 2D slice is simply its thickness. In a ray tracing procedure, if this volume of data can be envisioned as a cube in space, a ray or line can be passed through it that ends up at a defined pixel location in the projected MIP plane on the other side of the volume. This is analogous to an x-ray beam passing through a 3D object and impinging on a photographic plate. Once this ray through the volume has been defined, the intensity of each voxel that it passes through is examined. The intensity that is eventually assigned to the projected MIP plane is the maximum one along the ray. This procedure is then carried out repeatedly until each pixel in the MIP has been assigned a maximum intensity that came from the volume. In principle, if the largest intensity values came only from the vessels, then the MIP will be a projection of only the vascular structure.

Figure 17-48 shows a typical MIP result from a 3D TOF MRA acquisition. In this axial projection, note the complete depiction of the vasculature from the circle of Willis. Although it may be desirable to achieve a MIP image with only the vessel structures, in TOF applications suppression of stationary tissue is rarely complete and MIP processing will retain some of this information. Therefore, background can still be seen. Most notable is the fat in the region of the eyes. Since all of the data are digital, it is sometimes advantageous to negate the display so that vessels appear dark against a bright background (Fig. 17-48B). This should not be misinterpreted as a minimum-intensity projection, a similar ray tracing procedure that looks for minimum voxel intensities along the ray instead of maximums. The data in Fig. 17-48B are still based on maximum intensities. The MIP display is simply inverted.

A MIP image does not have to be projected only in the plane in which the data were acquired. Since this is a digital image processing procedure, MIPs can be computed along any angle of orientation. In the computation, the ray tracing is rotated to the desired angle, so that it now passes obliquely through the volume of the acquisition data. The process of attaining the projection of the maximum intensities from the volume is the same. Figure 17-49 demonstrates MIP views at different angles through the same original data, rotating from an axial projection to a coronal projection. Note that the background in the coronal view is slightly higher than in the other views. This is because the slightly brighter regions from fat are now in the same line as the vessels.

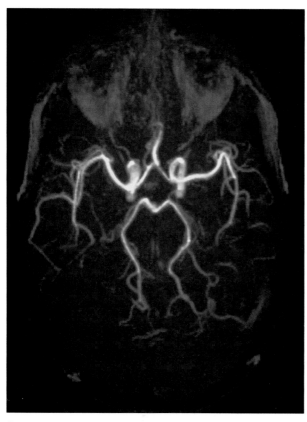

A

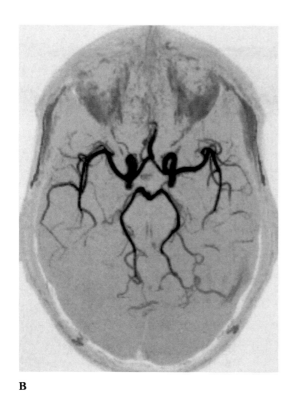

B

Targeting (Masking)

One potential drawback of a projection display is that everything from a volumetric dataset is essentially collapsed into the projection. Therefore, in an MRA application, if many vessels are highlighted in the acquisition, the MIP will project them all into one plane. Overlapping of the vessels may then occur, making it difficult to interpret important structures or areas of interest. Additionally, if regions of stationary tissues are bright in the acquired data due to shortcomings of the technique and its inability to suppress them, then these regions will also be incorporated in the MIP image possibly obscuring the vasculature. In these situations, *targeting (or masking)* only part of the volume of data to isolate the structures of interest for subsequent MIP processing can prove advantageous.

Shown in Fig. 17-50 is a sagittal MIP with various targeted regions of interest for further processing. Corresponding coronal MIP displays are also shown that demonstrate the effectiveness of this postprocessing tool. In Fig. 17-50A, a coronal MIP was processed from the full dataset. Note the high degree of vessel overlap, particularly from the sagittal sinus. By targeting only the arterial vasculature, the sagittal sinus is masked from the MIP processing, resulting in a coronal targeted MIP with less ambiguity (Fig. 17-50B). More localized targeting can be done to further isolate specific vascular structures, such as the internal, middle, and anterior cerebral arteries (Fig. 17-50C) and the basilar and posterior cerebral arteries (Fig. 17-50D). Targeting can also prove effective in masking regions of stationary tissue such as fat to improve vessel contrast and delineation in the MIP.

Directional MIP

PC MRA has the unique ability to measure both the velocity and direction of blood flow. Although individual images can be studied, the ability to display this information in terms of complete vascular structures can greatly enhance interpretation. After phase difference mapping is performed on each PC image in a data-

Fig. 17-48 MIP. A 3D MRA dataset was obtained in the region of the circle of Willis. In the acquired data, vessels have large signal intensities. Using ray tracing algorithms, the complete vascular structure can be visualized by selecting only the largest signal intensities and projecting them onto a plane. (*A*) Positive and (*B*) negative display of the axially projected MIP is shown.

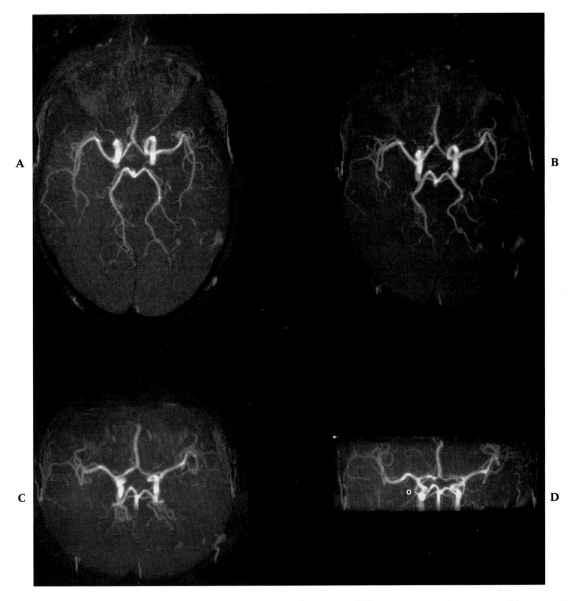

Fig. 17-49 Rotational MIP views. Due to the digital nature of the acquired data, a MIP can be processed in any orientation. Views are shown rotat-ing from an axial to a coronal orientation at (*A*) 0°,(*B*) 30°, (*C*) 60°, and (*D*) 90° angles. Background in the coronal view (*D*) is associated with the slightly brighter fat.

set, the magnitude or intensity of the phase difference can be processed as a MIP by conventional maximum intensity ray tracing, as shown in Fig. 17-51A.

However, if the mathematical sign of the phase difference is retained in MIP processing, then flow directionality will be preserved. Here, two maximum intensities values, the most positive and most negative, are effectively searched for in the ray tracing procedure. The end result will be a MIP with the direction of flow retained. *Directional MIP views*, however, must be processed on the PC dataset only after it has been separated into three more datasets that represent the three orthogonal directions of flow. Processing the information simultaneously would lead to a confusing MIP with ambiguity as to which of the three directions the flow is traversing. Therefore, one PC MRA dataset can yield a magnitude MIP and three directional MIPs, each displaying the vessel structures that possess flow only

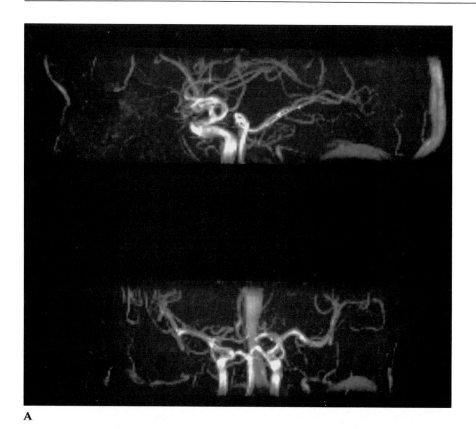

A

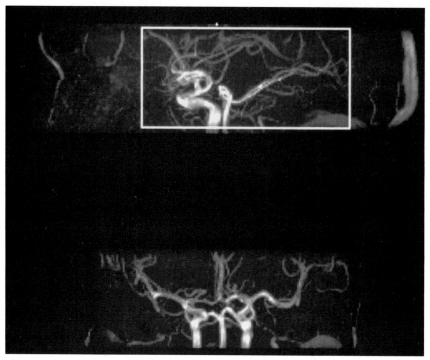

B

Fig. 17-50 MIP targeting (masking). Sagittal MIP views of various targeted regions are shown with corresponding coronal MIP views of (*A*) complete vasculature, (*B*) arterial vessels without the sagittal sinus.

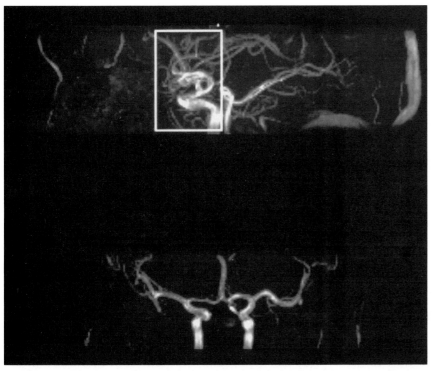

C

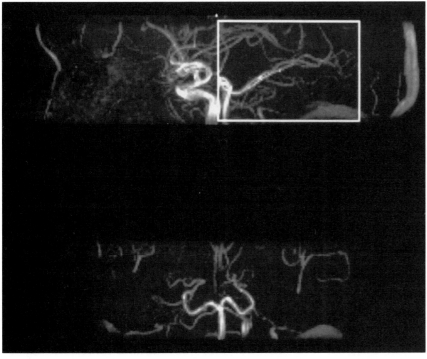

D

Fig. 17-50 (*C*) internal, middle, and anterior cerebral arteries, and (*D*) basilar and posterior cerebral arteries.

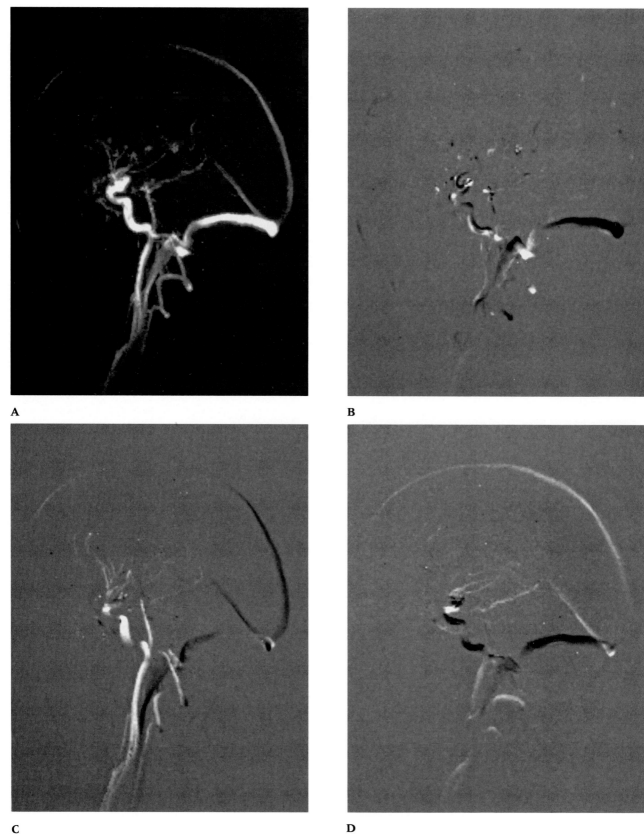

A

B

C

D

in that respective direction. An additional three MIP images can be generated that display the magnitude of the flow associated with each of the three directions, but this serves little purpose if the corresponding directional MIP images are computed.

Figures 17-51B through 17-51D are directional MIP images in the three physical directions of the same data that are displayed as a magnitude of all three directions of blood flow combined in Fig. 17-51A. Left-right lateral (Fig. 17-51B), inferior-superior (Fig. 17-51C), and anterior-posterior (Fig. 17-51D) flows are demonstrated. Black pixels represent a negative phase difference and white pixels represent a positive difference. The actual direction of flow that these differences are associated with will depend on the way the velocity was encoded in the originally acquired data, as discussed in the section "2D PC MRA." Air and background that possess approximately zero phase difference will be seen as a gray level, exactly halfway between a zero pixel value that becomes windowed in the display as black and the most positive pixel value that is capable of being displayed by the viewing hardware.

PC Processing[57,71,72]

In TOF MRA, once the data are acquired, little is done to the dataset to process the information further before a MIP is performed to view the vascular structures. However, it is worthwhile to discuss briefly the computation of phase differences in PC MRA processing that are necessary to achieve final vessel contrast before any MIP processing. Two-point data acquisition methods that velocity encode one direction and six-point methods that encode all three directions can be directly processed by the simplest algebraic manipulations. However, several different four-point acquisition methods have been studied, some of which simultaneously encode two different velocity directions. These require

Fig. 17-51 Directional MIP views. Specifically associated with PC MRA, information about the flow direction is acquired. Blood flow traversing in one direction will have a phase difference that is the negative of flow moving in the opposite direction. If the mathematical sign of the phase difference is retained, directional MIP views are possible. Shown are (*A*) a magnitude MIP of flow in all three directions, and directional MIPs of (*B*) left–right lateral flow, (*C*) inferior–superior flow, and (*D*) anterior–posterior flow. White pixels denote one direction and black pixels represent the opposite direction. The actual direction will depend on the acquisition and velocity encoding.

more complex computations to isolate the flow information from a given direction. Nevertheless, there are primarily three different ways to compute the phase difference information in PC MRA data.

The first and most straightforward method is to simply take two phase image datasets, such as those described in Fig. 17-41, and subtract one from the other. The resulting *phase difference mapping* will then be a direct reflection of the velocity of blood flow. This computation can only be performed on a two-point, four-point, or six-point method that encodes the different directions of velocity independently. Other four-point methods that combine directions of flow encoding cannot use this simple procedure. Such a method, however, is necessary for direct flow quantification where absolute velocities are desired. One drawback to this direct phase subtraction is that background from air will retain its random phase characteristics seen in Figs. 17-41B and 17-41C. Two datasets with random pixel values that are subtracted from each other will result in simply another arrangement of random pixel values. The end result is a PC image that has a "salt and pepper" background. Aside from being distracting to the eye, it makes it virtually impossible to process a MIP, since large random phase differences in the air will eventually make their way into the MIP image.

The second and third ways to obtain phase difference information are the only ways that will yield computed PC data that can be further processed to generate a MIP. Recall that the signal has both a magnitude and a phase associated with it. The directly computed phase difference mapping described above can then be weighted by the magnitude of the signal by multiplying the phase difference in each pixel by the average signal magnitude from the two datasets. Since air, by definition, has a zero signal magnitude, its weighted phase difference will be zero even if it has a large actual phase difference. This *magnitude-weighted phase subtraction* method can then be used to do MIP processing.

The third and final way to compute the phase contrast data is to do what is known as a *complex phase subtraction*. Signal can either be represented as a magnitude and phase, or it can be split into a real and an imaginary signal that possess both a magnitude and a phase contribution. Complex subtraction is performed by subtracting the two real signals from each other, then subtracting the two imaginary signals from each other, and finally combining the two results. The end result is slightly different from that achieved with the second method (in actuality, the complex difference is proportional to the trigonometric sine of the phase difference), but it is nevertheless weighted by the effec-

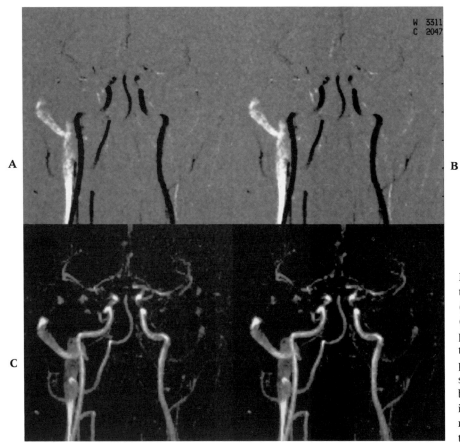

Fig. 17-52 Methods of PC computation. Coronal directional MIP images (A,B) and magnitude MIP images (C,D) are shown for PC MRA data processed by (A,C) complex subtraction and (B,D) magnitude-weighted phase subtraction. Little difference is seen in the directional MIP display, but a subtle reduction in background is observed in the magnitude MIP with magnitude-weighted phase subtraction (D).

tive signal magnitude of both datasets. Therefore, it can also be used to do MIP processing.

The differences between magnitude-weighted phase subtraction and complex subtraction are subtle and are beyond the scope of this discussion. However, it is worthwhile to demonstrate the comparative outcome of both. Figure 17-52 shows coronal directional MIP and magnitude MIP images from a PC acquisition where the phase difference information was computed by both methods. In the directional MIP comparison (Figs. 17-52A,B), little or no difference between the two processing methods is seen. However, in the magnitude MIP comparison (Figs. 17-52C,D), a subtle but noticeable reduction in the background is observed with magnitude-weighted phase subtraction (Fig. 17-52D). For PC applications with low vessel contrast, such as in small vessels or very slow flow, it may be more advantageous to use this subtraction method over the other.

MRA ARTIFACTS

In TOF and PC MRA, several different anomalies arise for a variety of reasons. Most types of artifacts can be categorized as being a result of the directly acquired data and of the shortcomings of the technique used, or due to certain aspects of the postprocessing used to visualize the complete vascular structure.

The importance of careful protocol selection for data acquisition cannot be overemphasized with MRA techniques. The optimal method used to image slow-flowing blood is quite different from that used to visualize fast-flowing blood and tortuous vessels. An incorrect decision may lead to major artifacts that can either compromise the study or lead to erroneous conclusions. One primary concern is vessel dropout and questionable vessel depiction. Clearly, a complete void in a region of vasculature that mimics an occlusion presents a serious danger of misdiagnosis. Although much improvement of the acquisition methodology has led to more robust techniques and increased reader confidence, care must still be taken not to rule out the possibility of an artifact. This becomes a far more important issue, for example, in grading the degree of stenoses or partial occlusions.

Although not necessarily intuitively obvious, artifacts may also occur due to the postprocessing technique used to assist in visualizing vessels. Based on the ability to project or reconstruct a plane of digital data in virtually any direction or at any angle, artifacts not related to the data acquisition can appear in postprocessing. In such cases, it is usually recommended that vascular regions that depict abnormalities in a processed image be cross-correlated with the actual acquired images to avoid the possibility of misinterpretation.

In this section, some of the more common artifacts associated with TOF and PC MRA are presented. Note, however, that most of these are either avoidable or easily identified. This is primarily because they were obtained on a normal, healthy volunteer. The examples shown here were chosen to accentuate such artifacts for the purposes of demonstration, and in some cases they are far more severe than the artifacts that would be experienced with state-of-the-art techniques. Other, far more subtle errors of similar origins, however, may occur in patients with vascular abnormalities.

Vessel Void: Pulsatility

Regional signal losses and vessel voids are one of the most common problems encountered with MRA techniques where magnitude of the blood signal is the primary origin of vessel contrast. One source of signal loss can be attributed to *blood flow pulsatility* and is shown in Fig. 17-53. In certain regions of the vasculature, pulsatility is more prevalent than in other areas and can result in localized vessel voids. Under most circumstances in TOF MRA, gradient moment nulling is sufficient to minimize pulsation artifacts. However, in some situations, this higher-order motion associated with acceleration is severe enough for these artifacts to occur. Some MRA techniques are also more prone to

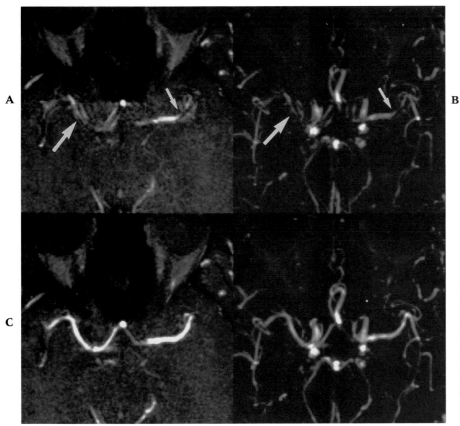

Fig. 17-53 A 2D TOF MRA depicting vessel voids due to pulsatility artifacts. The preprocessed acquisition image (*A*) shows ghosting in regions with high pulsatility resulting in vessel voids (arrows) in the corresponding MIP image (*B*) due to insufficient gradient moment nulling. Without pulsation, preprocessed (*C*) and MIP (*D*) images show good delineation of the vessels.

pulsatility than others. For example, one technique may use only first-order moment nulling (velocity correction), whereas another may incorporate second-order moment nulling as well (acceleration correction). In general, higher-order moment nulling requires more time to perform and typically lengthens the minimum possible TE. Using a longer TE may accentuate this error. Higher-order moment nulling is therefore a trade-off with TE and at some point reaches a point of diminishing returns. If TE is kept as short as possible, typically less than 7 or 8 msec, then first-order moment nulling is most likely sufficient to prevent this artifact. Note that in PC MRA, where velocity motion is necessarily encoded rather than nulled to obtain vessel contrast, pulsatility artifacts may sometimes be more severe.

With standard MRI techniques, pulsatility can be avoided by the use of electrocardiographic triggering and synchronizing of the data acquisition with the cycle of the pulsation of the blood. However, this is not a feasible alternative with MRA since the scan time would be prohibitively long. This artifact can also usually be easily identified as a ghosting artifact in a conventional scan and is shown in the preprocessed MRA data in Fig. 17-53A. However, on MIP processing, the artifact can become less apparent (Fig. 17-53B). Such an example supports the recommendation that a MIP should not necessarily be evaluated by itself. Images without pulsation artifacts under otherwise identical conditions are shown for comparison (Figs. 17-53C,D).

Vessel Void: Phase Dispersion

Another source of regional vessel voids in MRA is *phase dispersion*. In a TOF application, signal from moving blood is maximized by using gradient moment nulling to induce maximum spin phase coherence over and above time-of-flight in-flow effects. However, if the moment nulling is not sufficient, phase incoherence of the transverse magnetization within a voxel of spatial encoding leads to a reduction in the magnitude of the signal in that voxel. Although the endpoint of vessel loss is the same, the primary difference between this artifact and losses due to pulsatility is that the signal losses from phase dispersion are within the boundaries of a given voxel. Pulsatility usually induces signal losses in the vessel by displacing the blood signal outside of the voxel of origin to a different region through visible ghosting in the acquired image. With phase dispersion, ghosting is not prevalent and only regional signal loss in the vessel is observed. This artifact occurs primarily in areas of fast flow where moment nulling cannot

completely accommodate the large phase changes that result from the moving spins.

Figure 17-54 demonstrates voxel phase dispersion and subsequent regional vessel voids. In the preprocessed acquired image (Fig. 17-54A), losses are seen mainly in the middle cerebral artery. However, no visible ghosting associated with pulsatility is seen. Slower-flowing vessels are clearly observed. In the corresponding sagittal MIP (Fig. 17-54B), these regional phase dispersions are also demonstrated. Under otherwise identical acquisition conditions, images with no signal losses due to phase dispersion are shown for comparison (Figs. 17-54C,D).

The occurrence of such an artifact can be minimized in several ways. The signal magnitude or intensity that represents a voxel is the average of the transverse magnetization within the physical dimensions of the voxel. Therefore, if the voxel is large, there is a greater chance that the spins of the moving blood within the voxel will become dispersed in their phases even if moment nulling is employed. Keeping the voxel size sufficiently small will minimize this artifact. Spatial resolution will be maintained; however, the signal/noise ratio as well as the imaging time may be compromised. Another factor that may lead to this artifact is the echo time, TE. From the time the RF is applied and the transverse magnetization is created, the phase of the moving spins of the blood begins to evolve. If the TE is too long, voxel phase dispersion will be more prevalent even with moment nulling. Using as short a TE as possible will reduce the occurrence of this artifact, provided that moment nulling can still be applied.

Vessel voids due to voxel phase dispersion are primarily associated with TOF MRA techniques. In PC MRA, where the main source of vessel contrast is not related to the magnitude of the blood signal but is based on the phase difference, this artifact will be less important.

Vessel Stepping

An advantage of 2D TOF MRA is its ability to image slower flow compared to 3D techniques. The advantage of 2D PC MRA is that the acquisition can substantially reduce the scan time over a 3D application by acquiring slices only in the region of interest. However, the slice thickness of a 2D technique may typically be large; this is one of the drawbacks over a 3D method. If the thickness is large enough, a processed MIP of the slices in an orthogonal plane to the acquired data can demonstrate a *vessel stepping* artifact, as shown in Fig. 17-55. In this example, 5-mm 2D sections from a TOF

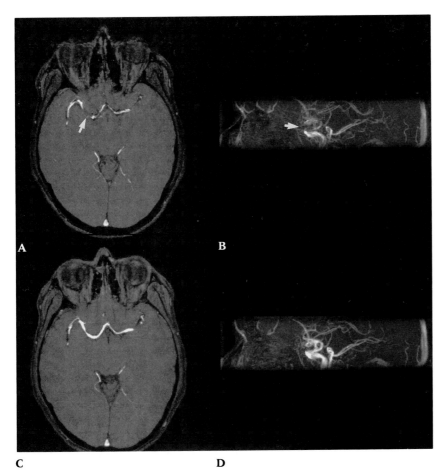

Fig. 17-54 A 3D time-of-flight MRA depicting vessel voids due to phase dispersion artifacts. Signal loss is seen on the preprocessed acquired image (*A*) in the region of the middle cerebral artery (arrows) and in the corresponding sagittal MIP image (*B*). These vessel voids are not seen on similar acquired (*C*) and MIP (*D*) images, where voxel phase dispersion was minimized by reducing the echo time.

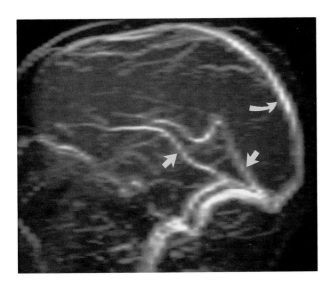

Fig. 17-55 Vessel stepping artifact associated with a 2D MRA technique. In this TOF venogram, 5-mm slices were acquired with a 33% overlap in the coronal plane and postprocessed as a MIP in the sagittal orientation. Stepping is most obvious in vessels that traverse from superior to inferior (arrows). Such an artifact will occur with 2D PC methods as well. If thick sections are necessary for regional coverage, processing the MIP with additional interpolation that more smoothly connects vessels from slice to slice will minimize this artifact.

venogram were obtained in the coronal plane and pro-cessed to produce a MIP image in the sagittal orienta-tion. Even with 33% overlapping of the slices, vessel stepping is observed, which is most prevalent in vessels that traverse from superior to inferior. Regardless of the type of information acquired, a 2D MRA application that uses thick slices is prone to this type of artifact. Therefore, this artifact can occur on a 2D PC acquisition as well.

Vessel stepping can be avoided by acquiring the data with thinner sections. Spatial resolution in the third dimension will also be improved. However, thick slices in a 2D acquisition may be required to obtain sufficient coverage of the region of interest. As well, since slices are acquired sequentially in time, a larger number of thin slices would be necessary to cover the same area, thereby increasing the scan time proportionally, and may not be desired. Increasing the degree of overlap between slices may also reduce the stepping, but it is still necessary to increase the number of slices for more coverage. In such cases, specific MIP postprocessing techniques can help minimize this artifact. Stepping in the MIP is a demonstration of the discreteness of a 2D acquisition of stacked slices even when overlapping of the slices appears to be sufficient. Simple MIP pro-cessing in an orientation that is orthogonal to the plane of acquisition will show this stacking. By applying in-terpolation algorithms in processing the data, smooth-ing of the discrete boundaries of the slices can be at-tained to connect the vessels more continuously from slice to slice.

Vessel Displacement

Another potential artifact that exists with a 2D MRA technique is a *wholesale vessel displacement* that can be observed in the processed MIP image. During data acquisition, slices are acquired in a time sequential manner. Since the total exam may take several min-utes, it is possible that the patient will move from slice to slice, causing a complete shift or rotation in the ana-tomical position. If this movement occurs only briefly, then no motion artifacts within a slice acquisition will be observed. However, physical shifts in the positions of the vessels associated with the slice or slices will be generated. This artifact is difficult to visualize in the individually acquired images of the sections. However, it is clearly demonstrated when a MIP of entire vascular structures is processed, as shown in Fig. 17-56.

If the physical movement did not occur in the projec-tion plane of the MIP, then such an artifact may be difficult to detect. This is seen in the sagittal MIP (Fig. 17-56A), where only one obvious region shows vessel displacement, particularly in the sagittal sinus. How-ever, coronal MIP images (Figs. 17-56C,D) demon-strate numerous large displacement artifacts that indi-cate that the patient's movement was anatomically from left to right, which is not observable in a sagittal MIP. With targeting of the MIP processing, the arterial structures of the circle of Willis (Fig. 17-56C) and of the venous structures associated with the sagittal sinus (Fig. 17-56D) can be isolated to further demonstrate the possible severity of vessel displacement artifacts.

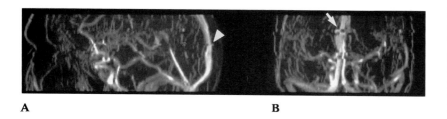

A   B

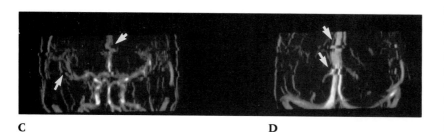

C   D

Fig. 17-56 Vessel displacement artifact associated with a 2D MRA technique. Wholesale shifts in vessel structures occur due to brief patient movements between the acquisitions of slices taken in a time sequential manner. The images shown here were obtained with a TOF technique. However, this artifact will also occur with 2D PC MRA. No motion-related artifacts will be observed, and the artifact is difficult to detect on the directly acquired images. With postprocessing, vessel displacement is clearly seen in a sagittal MIP (*A*), full coro-nal MIP (*B*), and targeted coronal MIP im-ages of the arterial structures in the circle of Willis (*C*) and venous structures in the sagittal sinus (*D*). The artifacts are most prevalent when the movement occurred in the projection plane of the MIP.

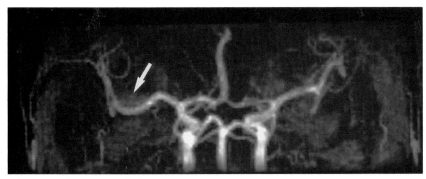

A

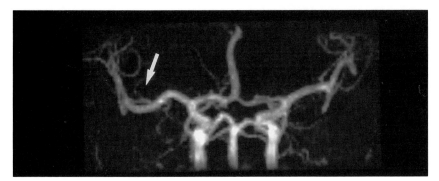

B

Fig. 17-57 Tissue obstruction artifact in processed MIP images. Since MIP images are projections onto a plane of the maximum signal through a set of acquired images, a MIP through the full dataset (*A*) may project stationary tissues with sufficient signal such as fat. This may obscure or lower the contrast of the vessels (arrow). Targeting of the MIP to a selected subvolume in the dataset can either minimize or eliminate this artifact (*B*). Shown are coronal MIP images obtained from a 3D TOF MRA acquisition employing magnetization transfer that suppresses most stationary tissues except fat. This artifact is not seen in PC techniques.

Since this anomaly is a result of patient movement, the entire slice or slices of acquisition will shift and will not be selective of particular vasculature. In Fig. 17-56D two large regions of discrete vessel displacement are observed. Yet, in Fig. 17-56C, these areas are not as obvious even though they exist.

In any 2D MRA application that acquires the slice data sequentially, whether TOF or PC, it is possible that vessel displacement artifacts will arise. This can be avoided by properly securing the patient's head so that lateral movements are minimized.

Tissue Obstruction

MIPs facilitate visualization of complete vascular structures. Postprocessing of the MIP entails ray tracing algorithms that assigns a given signal intensity to a pixel in the projection plane based on the maximum intensity along the ray that traces through the 3D data, whether a 2D stack of slices or a direct 3D acquisition. In TOF MRA, the strategy is to maximize the signal intensity from vessels while minimizing it from stationary tissues. In this manner, the MIP should project only the vessels. However, in some situations, surrounding

tissues have enough signal magnitude to become incorporated into the processed MIP, thereby obscuring vessels. Artifacts from *tissue obstruction* are primarily associated with TOF techniques, since stationary tissue signal can never be completely eliminated. By contrast, PC methods use signal phase differences to achieve vessel contrast rather than signal magnitude. As long as there is a sufficiently different degree of motion between moving blood and background tissue, the phase contrast of the vessels will be enough to delineate vascular structures in a MIP.

Figure 17-57 demonstrates tissue obstruction in a coronal MIP from a 3D TOF MRA acquisition using magnetization transfer to suppress stationary tissue. In Fig. 17-57A, a MIP is processed with the full 3D dataset. Heterogeneous areas throughout the projection are associated with relatively high signal of surrounding fat from subcutaneous regions and around the optic nerve. Signal from fat is not reduced with the use of magnetization transfer and can commonly obscure or reduce the contrast of vascular structures in a MIP image. Depending on the protocol of acquisition, other tissues may also contribute to this artifact. With appropriate targeting of the MIP, however, tissue obstruction can

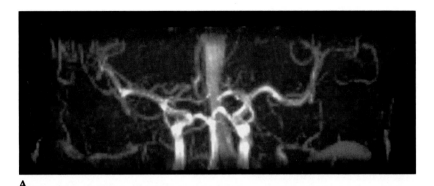

A

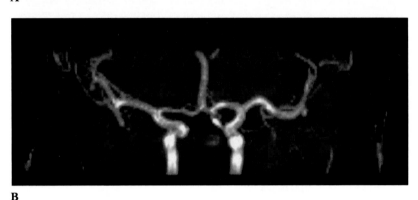

B

Fig. 17-58 Vessel overlap in processed MIP images. Vessel information that occupies the same region in the plane of projection in a MIP image generates overlapped regions of redundancy, even though it may occur at different depths in the data. This will occur with both TOF and PC MRA techniques. Shown are full (*A*) and targeted (*B*) coronal MIP images acquired with 3D TOF MRA. By selectively processing the MIP without the sagittal sinus, the circle of Willis is better differentiated and more easily interpreted.

usually be significantly reduced or even eliminated, as shown in Fig. 17-57B. Investigations of more sophisticated postprocessing methods, such as vessel connectivity algorithms that attempt to process only the signal associated with vessels, are also underway. With these methods, targeting would not be necessary to minimize this artifact.

Vessel Overlap

Another consequence of displaying MIP images is vessel overlap. If two or more vessels cross common paths in the plane of projection, even though they traverse at different levels in the acquired image dataset, they will occupy the same position in the MIP. This redundancy in processing may cause obscuring or loss of vessel contrast in the resulting MIP display. Since the MRA information (signal magnitude or signal phase difference) is overlapped, this will occur with both TOF and PC techniques in MIP postprocessing. A common source of *vessel overlap* occurs when coronal MIP images are displayed with inclusion of the large sagittal sinus, as shown in Fig. 17-58A from a 3D TOF MRA.

One method of eliminating signal from at least the sagittal sinus and other venous structures is to employ selective saturation techniques in TOF applications. In this manner, no signal will be generated from venous flow due to saturation and will not contribute to vessel overlap. Such strategies are not usually possible with PC since the phase difference from venous flow will still be present to produce vessel contrast. If, however, the signal magnitude can be completely eliminated, it may prove effective even in PC applications. A simpler and more general method that can be used with both TOF and PC is targeted MIP processing. Focusing only on the vascular region of interest, such as the circle of Willis, a targeted coronal MIP that does not include the sagittal sinus from the posterior portion of the dataset can yield well-delineated vessels, with little or no overlap, as demonstrated in Fig. 17-58B.

Finally, more complex postprocessing and display techniques are currently being studied. These introduce either depth information or vessel boundary delineation in the projected vessel data so that overlapped regions can be more easily identified and correctly interpreted.

Oblique Projections

Postprocessing such as MIP provides the ability to view vascular structures in any orientation and at any angle. This is particularly useful with 3D applications that employ isotropic spatial encoding where the voxel dimensions in all three physical directions are the same. However, several consequences arise when *projecting obliquely* through the 3D dataset. First, since an encoded voxel is a cube, cutting through it at an angle with ray tracing that is used in MIP processing will project the vessel information with larger pixel dimensions in the MIP image. The worst case is at an angle of 45°, where the pixel size is increased by 1/sin45°, or a factor of 1.41, above the dimension originally encoded in the data acquisition. As a result, the oblique MIP image will have reduced spatial resolution and will look blurred compared to an orthogonal MIP image of the same data.

A second, more subtle consequence of oblique processing may be an artifact that produces a splotchy or jagged appearance of the vessels, as shown in Fig. 17-59. In this example, MIP images were obtained at 45° from the orientation of acquisition in an isotropic 3D TOF technique. With simple, *nearest-integer postprocessing* the vessels in the image appear jagged (Fig. 17-59A). By using *interpolative procedures* that more smoothly connect neighboring voxels, this phenomenon disappears, without significant loss of spatial resolution (Fig. 17-59B).

Since these anomalies are consequences only of digital postprocessing of oblique projections, they will occur with both TOF and PC applications. Aside from using alternative approaches to the postprocessing procedure, little can be done to minimize these problems through data acquisition.

Phase Aliasing[73-75]

In PC MRA, vessel contrast is generated by phase shifts in the signal associated with the flowing blood. These phase shifts will occur only if the blood moves through different magnetic fields. By using linear magnetic field gradients, the blood can be encoded with phase shifts that are directly proportional to the gradient strength

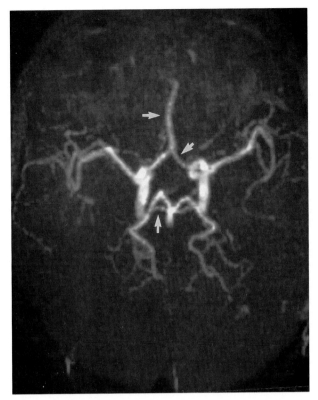

A

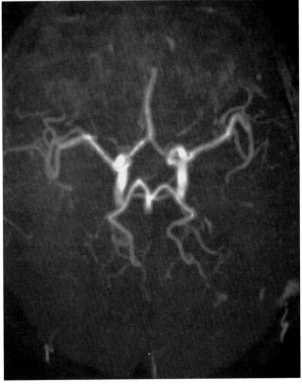

B

Fig. 17-59 MIP anomalies associated with oblique projections. Digitally processing MIP images at oblique angles to the orientation of data acquisition can yield a loss of spatial resolution up to a factor of 1.41 and blurring. In addition, nearest-integer processing (*A*) can give a splotchy, jagged appearance (arrows). With more appropriate interpolation routines (*B*), this can be minimized without significant additional blurring. MIP images are at 45° angles to the data acquired isotropically with 3D TOF MRA. This will also occur in PC methods since it is purely a postprocessing phenomenon.

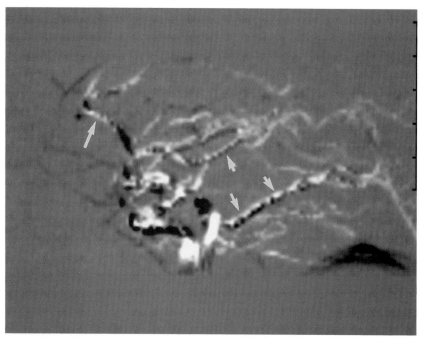

A

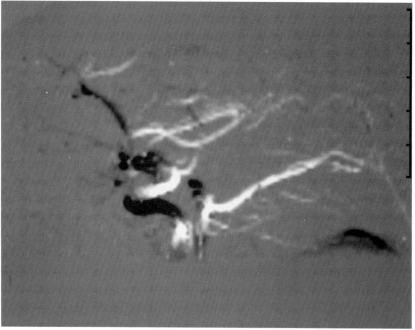

B

Fig. 17-60 Phase aliasing artifact in PC MRA. Sagittal MIP images with directional display were acquired with 3D PC MRA at encoding velocities of (*A*) ±30 cm/sec and (*B*) ±50 cm/sec. Velocity encoding was from anterior to posterior. Phase aliasing of faster flow in major arterial vessels is seen in (*A*), where phase shifts exceed the range of ±180° (arrows). One consequence of aliasing is a change in the sign of the phase shift angle so that flow appears to move in the opposite direction. Minimal aliasing is seen in (*B*), where white vessels indicate flow from anterior to posterior and black vessels indicate flow in the reverse direction. Note the loss of tertiary vessels due to reduced velocity encoding in order to eliminate aliasing.

and the velocity of flow. If, however, the velocity is too fast or the applied velocity encoding gradients are too large, the phase shift associated with the blood will exceed the maximum limit, and a *phase aliasing* artifact will occur in the PC processed images.

Any phase is a cyclic phenomenon that repeats every 360°. A phase of 0° is the same as a phase of 360° and −360°; a phase of 180° is the same as a phase of −180°. Therefore, it can be seen that if a phase is to be displayed as a pixel intensity, the unique range lies between −180° and 180°. In PC MRA, the pixel intensity is directly proportional to the phase shift associated with the moving blood. If this phase exceeds the range in which it can be uniquely identified, then an aliasing of its value will occur. For example, based on a given gradient strength of velocity encoding and a given blood flow velocity, the actual phase shift might possibly be 200°. However, this is mathematically the same as −160°. Since 200° lies outside of the unique range that can be displayed, it will be assigned and portrayed with a value of −160°, which lies within this range.

Furthermore, PC processing has the unique ability to show flow direction based on whether the phase shift is positive or negative. A 0° phase shift is associated with stationary tissue. A negative phase shift will indicate flow in one direction, and a positive phase phase shift will indicate flow in the opposite direction. The magnitude of the phase value will, of course, be related to the actual velocity. Reassigning a phase shift of 200° to a value of −160° due to aliasing will change not only the amplitude of the phase but also the sign of the angle, resulting in an erroneous display of flow going in the opposite direction.

Figure 17-60 demonstrates PC aliasing artifact in a sagittal MIP with directional display of a 3D PC MRA dataset. Velocity encoding is anterior to posterior. In Fig. 17-60A, the velocity encoding was set so that velocities of ±30 cm/sec would be encoded with phase shifts of ±180°, respectively. As a consequence, any velocities exceeding 30 cm/sec would generate an aliasing artifact. Although magnitude MIP images that do not retain the direction of flow appear quite normal (not shown), the directional MIP image in Fig. 17-60A shows numerous regions of phase aliasing where the sign of the phase shift angle becomes reversed. Note that slower flows in tertiary arterial vessels and the sigmoid sinus have velocities that do not exceed the phase limits. In Fig. 17-60B, the velocity encoding was ±50 cm/sec. In nearly all areas, phase aliasing does not occur since a much greater range of velocities are encoded within ±180°. The compromise that is made is that slower flow is proportionally associated with less of a phase shift and tertiary vessels are lost. Note the intensity reduction seen in the sigmoid sinus.

Since this is purely a phase-related phenomenon, it occurs only with PC MRA techniques, not with TOF MRA. However, the directional flow information associated with PC is also not available with TOF. Phase aliasing is an inevitable consequence of this ability. To avoid phase aliasing, knowledge of the ranges of flow velocities in the regions of interest can greatly assist in determining the appropriate degree of velocity encoding to be used in the acquisition. The trade-off is that to visualize slower flow, the probability of phase

aliasing with faster flow will increase. Conversely, eliminating phase aliasing of the major vessels that exhibit fast flow may possibly result in a loss of vessels with slower flow.

REFERENCES

1. Hahn EL. Spin echoes. *Phys Rev* 1950;80:580–594.
2. Carr HY, Purcell EM. Effects of diffusion on free precession in nuclear magnetic resonance experiments. *Phys Rev* 1954;94:630–638.
3. Singer JR. Blood flow rates by nuclear magnetic resonance measurements. *Science* 1959;130:1652–1653.
4. Stejskal EO. Use of spin echoes in a pulsed magnetic-field gradient to study anisotropic, restricted diffusion and flow. *J Chem Physical Phys* 1965;43:3597–3603.
5. Grover T, Singer JR. NMR spin-echo flow measurements. *J Appl Phys* 1971;42:938–940.
6. Shultz CL, Alfidi RJ, Nelson AD, et al. The effect of motion on two dimensional Fourier transform magnetic resonance images. *Radiology* 1984;152:117–121.
7. Bradley WG, Waluch V. Blood flow: Magnetic resonance imaging. *Radiology* 1985;154:443–450.
8. Ehman RL, McNamara MT, Brasch RC, et al. Influence of physiologic motion on the appearance of tissue in MR images. *Radiology* 1986;159:777–782.
9. Bryant DJ, Payne JA, Firmin DN, et al. Measurement of flow with NMR imaging using a gradient pulse and phase difference technique. *J Comput Assist Tomogr* 1984;8:588–593.
10. Constantinesco A, Mallet JJ, Bonmartin A, et al. Spatial or flow velocity phase encoding gradients in NMR imaging. *Magn Reson Imaging* 1984;2:235–240.
11. Von Schulthess GK, Higgins CB. Blood flow imaging with MR: Spin-phase phenomena. *Radiology* 1985;157:687–695.
12. Haacke EM, Tkach JA. Fast MR imaging: Techniques and clinical applications. *Am J Roentgenol* 1990;155:951–964.
13. Singer JR. NMR diffusion and flow measurements and an introduction to spin phase graphing. *J Phys E* 1978;11:281–291.
14. Haacke EM, Lenz GW. Improving MR image quality in the presence of motion by using rephasing gradients. *Am J Roentgenol* 1987;148:1251–1258.
15. Pattany PM, Phillips JJ, Chiu LC, et al. Motion artifact suppression technique (MAST) for MR imaging. *J Comput Assist Tomogr* 1987;11:369–377.
16. Elster AD. Motion artifact suppression technique (MAST) for cranial MR imaging. *Am J Neuroradiol* 1988;9:671–674.
17. Quencer RM, Hinks RS, Pattany PH, et al. Improved MR

imaging of the brain by using compensating gradients to suppress motion-induced artifacts. *Am J Neuroradiol* 1988;9:431−438.

18. Szeverenyi NM, Kieffer SA, Cacayorin ED. Correction of CSF motion artifact on MR images of the brain and spine by pulse sequence modification: Clinical evaluation. *Am J Neuroradiol* 1988;9:1069−1074.

19. Colletti PM, Raval JK, Benson RC, et al. The motion artifact suppression technique (MAST) in magnetic resonance imaging: Clinical results. *Magn Reson Imaging* 1988;6:293−299.

20. Gullberg GT, Wehrli FW, Shimakawa et al. MR vascular imaging with a fast gradient refocusing pulse sequence and reformatted images from transaxial sections. *Radiology* 1987;165:241−246.

21. Keller PJ, Drayer BP, Fram EK, et al. MR angiography with two-dimensional acquisition and three-dimensional display. *Radiology* 1989;173:527−532.

22. Edelman RR, Wentz KU, Mattle HP, et al. Intracerebral arteriovenous malformations: Evaluation with selective MR angiography and venography. *Radiology* 1989;173:831−837.

23. Litt AW, Eidelman EM, Pinto RS, et al. Diagnosis of carotid artery stenosis: Comparison of 2DFT time-of-flight MR angiography with contrast angiography in 50 patients. *Am J Neuroradiol* 1991;12:149−154.

24. Heiserman JE, Drayer BP, Fram EK, et al. Carotid artery stenosis: Clinical efficacy of two-dimensional time-of-flight MR angiography. *Radiology* 1992;182:761−768.

25. Finn JP, Goldmann A, Edelman RR. Magnetic resonance angiography in the body. *Magn Reson Q* 1992;8:1−22.

26. Lewin JS, Laub G. Intracranial MR angiography: A direct comparison of three time-of-flight techniques. *Am J Neuroradiol* 1992;12:1133−1139.

27. Laub GW, Kaiser WA. MR angiography with gradient motion refocusing. *J Comput Assist Tomogr* 1988;12:377−382.

28. Haacke EM, Masaryk TJ, Wielopolski PA, et al. Optimizing blood vessel contrast in fast three-dimensional MRI. *Magn Reson Med* 1990;14:202−221.

29. Ruggieri PM, Laub GA, Masaryk TJ, et al. Intracranial circulation: pulse-sequence considerations in three-dimensional (volume) MR angiography. *Radiology* 1989;171:785−791.

30. Masaryk TJ, Modic MT, Ross JS, et al. Intracranial circulation: Preliminary clinical results with three-dimensional (volume) MR angiography. *Radiology* 1989;171:793−799.

31. Marchal G, Bosmans H, Van fraeyenhoven L, et al. Intracranial vascular lesions: Optimization and clinical evaluation of three-dimensional time-of-flight MR angiography. *Radiology* 1990;175:443−448.

32. Masaryk TJ, Modic MT, Ruggieri PM, et al. Three-dimensional (volume) gradient-echo imaging of the ca-

rotid bifurcation: Preliminary clinical experience. *Radiology* 1989;171:801−806.

33. Ross JS, Masaryk TJ, Modic MT, et al. Intracranial aneurysms: Evaluation by MR angiography. *Am J Neuroradiol* 1990;11:449−456.

34. Masaryk AM, Ross JS, DiCello MC. 3DFT MR angiography of the carotid bifurcation: Potential and limitations as a screening examination. *Radiology* 1991;179:797−804.

35. Parker DL, Yuan C, Blatter DD. MR angiography by multiple thin slab 3D acquisition. *Magn Reson Med* 1991;17:434−451.

36. Blatter DD, Parker DL, Robinson R. MR angiography with multiple overlapping thin slab acquisition. *Radiology* 1991;179:805−811.

37. Davis WL, Warnock SH, Ric Harnsberger H, et al. Intracranial MRA: Single volume vs. multiple thin slab 3D time-of-flight acquisition. *J Comput Assist Tomogr* 1993;17:15−21.

38. Felmlee JP, Ehman RL. Spatial presaturation: A method for suppressing flow artifacts and improving depiction of vascular anatomy in MR imaging. *Radiology* 1987;164:559−564.

39. Edelman RR, Atkinson DJ, Silver MS, et al. FRODO pulse sequences: A new means of eliminating motion, flow, and wraparound artifacts. *Radiology* 1988;166:231−236.

40. Ehman RL, Felmlee JP. Flow artifact reduction in MRI: A review of the roles of gradient moment nulling and spatial presaturation. *Magn Reson Med* 1990;14:293−307.

41. Mugler JP, Brookeman JR. The design of pulse sequences employing spatial presaturation for the suppression of flow artifacts. *Magn Reson Med* 1992;23:201−214.

42. Edelman RR, Mattle HP, O'Reilly GV, et al. Magnetic resonance imaging of flow dynamics in the circle of Willis. *Stroke* 1990;21:56−65.

43. Mattle HP, Wentz KU, Edelman RR, et al. Cerebral venography with MR. *Radiology* 1991;178:453−458.

44. Wolff SD, Balaban RS. Magnetization transfer contrast (MTC) and tissue water proton relaxation in vivo. *Magn Reson Med* 1989;10:135−144.

45. Balaban RS, Ceckler TL. Magnetization transfer contrast in magnetic resonance imaging. *Magn Reson Q* 1992;8:116−137.

46. Yeung HN, Aisen AM. Magnetization transfer contrast with periodic pulsed saturation. *Radiology* 1992;183:209−214.

47. Hu BS, Conolly SM, Wright GA, et al. Pulsed saturation transfer contrast. *Magn Reson Med* 1992;26:231−240.

48. Hajnal JV, Baudouin CJ, Oatridge A, et al. Design and implementation of magnetization transfer pulse sequences for clinical use. *J Comput Assist Tomogr* 1992;16:7−18.

49. Pike GB, Hu BS, Glover GH, et al. Magnetization transfer time-of-flight magnetic resonance angiography. *Magn Reson Med* 1992;25:372–379.

50. Edelman RR, Ahn SS, Chien D, et al. Improved time-of-flight MR angiography of the brain with magnetization transfer contrast. *Radiology* 1992;184:395–399.

51. Purdy D, Cadena G, Laub G. The design of variable tip angle slab selection (TONE) pulses for improved 3-D MR angiography. *Proc 11th Ann Mtg SMRM* 1992;1:882.

52. Hardy P, Zelch M, Lammert G, et al. Improved uniformity of vessel contrast in 3D (volume) MRA. *Proc 11th Ann Mtg SMRM* 1992;2:3110.

53. Tkach JA, Masaryk TJ, Ruggieri PM, et al. Use of tilted optimized nonsaturating excitation (TONE) RF pulses and MTC to improve the quality of MR angiograms of the carotid bifurcation. *Proc 11th Ann Mtg, SMRM* 1992; 2:3905.

54. Matsuda T, Morii I, Kohno F, et al. An asymmetric slice profile: Spatial alteration of flow signal response in 3D time-of-flight NMR angiography. *Magn Reson Med* 1993; 29:783–789.

55. Dumoulin CL, Hart HR. Magnetic resonance angiography. *Radiology* 1986;161:717–720.

56. Dumoulin CL, Souza SP, Darrow RD, et al. Simultaneous acquisition of phase-contrast angiograms and stationary-tissue images with Hadamard encoding of flow-induced phase shifts. *J Magn Reson Imaging* 1991;1:399–404.

57. Pelc NJ, Bernstein MA, Shimakawa A, et al. Encoding strategies for three-direction phase-contrast MR imaging of flow. *J Magn Reson Imaging* 1991;1:405–413.

58. Hausmann R, Lewin JS, Laub G. Phase-contrast MR angiography with reduced acquisition time: New concepts in sequence design. *J Magn Reson Imaging* 1991;1: 415–422.

59. Huston J, Rufenacht DA, Ehman RL, et al. Intracranial aneurysms and vascular malformations: Comparison of time-of-flight and phase-contrast MR angiography. *Radiology* 1991;181:721–730.

60. Tsuruda JS, Shimakawa A, Pelc NJ, et al. Dural sinus occlusion: Evaluation with phase-sensitive gradient-echo MR imaging. *Am J Neuroradiol* 1991;12:481–488.

61. Pelc NJ, Herfkens RJ, Shimakawa A, et al. Phase contrast cine magnetic resonance imaging. *Magn Reson Q* 1991;7: 229–254.

62. Marks MP, Pelc NJ, Ross MR, et al. Determination of cerebral blood flow with a phase-contrast cine MR imaging technique: Evaluation of normal subjects and patients with arteriovenous malformations. *Radiology* 1992; 182:467–476.

63. Dumoulin CL, Souza SP, Walker MF, et al. Three-dimensional phase contrast angiography. *Magn Reson Med* 1989;9:139–149.

64. Wagle WA, Dumoulin CL, Souza SP, et al. 3DFT magnetic resonance angiography of carotid artery and basilar artery disease. *Am J Neuroradiol* 1989;10:911–919.

65. Napel S, Lee DH, Frayne R, et al. Visualizing three-dimensional flow with simulated streamlines and three-dimensional phase-contrast MR imaging. *J Magn Reson Imaging* 1992;2:143–153.

66. Pernicone JR, Siebert JE, Potchen EJ, et al. Three-dimensional phase-contrast MR angiography in the head and neck: Preliminary report. *Am J Neuroradiol* 1990;11: 457–466.

67. Laub G. Displays for MR angiography. *Magn Reson Med* 1990;14:222–229.

68. Brown DG, Riederer SJ. Contrast-to-noise ratios in maximum intensity projection images. *Magn Reson Med* 1992; 23:130–137.

69. Anderson CM, Saloner D, Tsuruda JS, et al. Artifacts in maximum-intensity-projection display of MR angiograms. *Am J Roentgenol* 1990;154:623–629.

70. Lin W, Haacke EM, Masaryk TJ, et al. Automated local maximum-intensity projection with three-dimensional vessel tracking. *J Magn Reson Imaging* 1992;2:519–526.

71. Bernstein MA, Ikezaki Y. Comparison of phase-difference and complex-difference processing in phase-contrast MR angiography. *J Magn Reson Imaging* 1991;1: 725–729.

72. Conturo TE, Robinson BH. Analysis of encoding efficiency in MR imaging of velocity magnitude and direction. *Magn Reson Med* 1992;25:233–247.

73. Pettigrew RI, Dannels W, Galloway JR, et al. Quantitative phase-flow MR imaging in dogs by using standard sequences: comparison with in vivo flow-meter measurements. *Am J Roentgenol* 1987;148:411–414.

74. Duerk JL, Pattany PM. In-plane flow velocity quantification along the phase encoding axis in MRI. *Magn Reson Imaging* 1988;6:321–333.

75. Axel L, Morton D. Correction of phase wrapping in magnetic resonance imaging. *Med Phys* 1989;16:284–287.

18

Magnetic Resonance Angiography: Intracranial Clinical Applications

Amir A. Zamani, M.D.

Magnetic resonance angiography (MRA) has undergone significant improvement in recent years. Although the technique still lags behind conventional angiography in spatial resolution, MRA is now capable of producing clinically adequate vascular images in a large percentage of patients. The advantages are many: MRA is noninvasive, does not usually need contrast injection, and allows simultaneous delineation of cervical and intracranial vessels. The accompanying MRI demonstrates the effect of vascular disease on the brain itself.

Ultrasonography, widely employed in evaluation of cervical vessels, is also noninvasive, but it does not yet provide adequate information regarding intracranial vessels. Transcranial Doppler is not universally available and does not provide simultaneous images of the brain.

Angiography is highly diagnostic in the majority of cases, but it is invasive, involves injection of contrast material, and carries specific risks of morbidity and mortality.[1,2]

Spiral computed tomography (CT) of intracranial vessels is in its infancy. Experience with this technique is limited, and its help in evaluating intracranial vascular pathology cannot be assessed until large-scale studies become available.[3]

TECHNICAL CONSIDERATIONS

In the forseeable future, a single MRA technique is unlikely to become the ideal method for assessment of the wide variety of intracranial vascular pathology. For the time being, judicial use of the available techniques in combination is necessary.

Three-dimensional time-of-flight (3D TOF) MRA is perhaps the most commonly used technique. Although data acquisition takes more time compared to two-dimensional (2D) TOF, spatial resolution is much better. In addition, the 3D data base can be manipulated into images in multiple planes for surgical planning. Its major drawback is its relative insensitivity to slow flow due to saturation of slowly moving spins while they traverse the imaging volume. Strategies to overcome this problem (e.g., to demonstrate the slow-flow component of an arteriovenous malformation) include intravenous injection of contrast and multiple overlapping thin slabs.[4,5]

Magnetization transfer contrast (MTC), described by Edelman and others,[6,7] improves delineation of small vessels on maximum-intensity projection (MIP) images. The 2D and 3D phase contrast (PC) techniques are widely used to subtract stationary tissues from the images, leaving vessels as the only structures shown.

These techniques are more sensitive to slow flow than is the 3D TOF technique. In addition, assessment of the direction of flow and flow rate, now becoming commercially available, is possible only with PC techniques. One major disadvantage is that PC techniques are time-consuming. The increased length of the study leads to image degradation due to patient movement.

Postprocessing techniques and MIP combined allow depiction of vessels in such a way that they resemble the scans of conventional angiography. In addition, one can view a vessel without significant overlap by other vessels. A price must be paid by employing these strategies, however, and the prudent radiologist should review the source images in any difficult case, lest important infomation be lost. Such a review provides better appreciation of the relationship of an aneurysm to the parent vessel and adjacent brain. Such relationships may not be as clearly depicted on MIP angiograms.

CLINICAL APPLICATION OF INTRACRANIAL MRA

Demonstration of Normal Anatomy

MRA can demonstrate major intracranial vessels with a high degree of accuracy. The volume studied by 3D imaging (either the TOF or PC) technique can be chosen to include the carotid siphons, A_1 and M_1 segments of the anterior and middle cerebral arteries, and proximal portions of the A_2 and M_2 segments. This same volume demonstrates the distal basilar artery and its branches. By shifting the volume inferiorly and obtaining 1-mm thick slices, one can include the vertebrobasilar system from the junction of the two vertebral arteries to the bifurcation of the basilar artery.

Within these boundaries, the major intracranial vessels are demonstrated fairly well with 3D TOF technique. If contrast injection is employed, the smaller vessels become visible, but enhancement of the stationary tissues may decrease the signal/noise ratio. Blatter et al. report that with multiple overlapping thin slab acquisition (MOTSA), arteries as small as 0.9 mm in diameter can be demonstrated.[5] Perforating arteries are not usually visible.

In 3D PC imaging, one can select the vessels to be demonstrated by choosing different velocity encoding (VENC) gradients. For example, a VENC of 100 cm/sec will provide optimal delineation of major intracranial arteries. A VENC of 20 cm/sec will provide better depiction of veins and venous sinuses. Different VENC val-

ues will illustrate different components of a vascular malformation.

Vascular Displacement

Intracranial vessels can be displaced by mass lesions such as tumors, as well as by edema associated with infarcts, hematoma, and abscesses. These displacements, as well as their causative lesions, can be demonstrated well with MRA and accompanying magnetic resonance imaging (MRI) (Fig. 18-1).

Infarction

Thromboembolic disease is present in the great majority of these patients. At least 20% of infarctions result from emboli of cardiac origin. Another 20% are lacunar infarcts seen in the basal ganglia and basis pontis, especially in patients with hypertension.

Evaluation of young patients with embolic disease and a probable cardiac source is rarely necessary. Here the patient's history and presumed lack of inherent atherosclerotic disease make emboli the most likely cause of the infarction. In older patients, particularly those with hypertension and diabetes, atherosclerotic disease of intracranial and extracranial vessels probably exists. Here differentiation of vessel occlusion as a result of thrombosis superimposed on an area of atherosclerotic narrowing from vessel occlusion caused by an embolic process may be more difficult.

Regardless of whether such differentiation is clinically relevant, a radiologist is often asked to help resolve this diagnostic dilemma. Most emboli eventually find their way to branches of the middle and posterior cerebral arteries. Later, they lodge in the distal small vessels. These occluded small vessels are usually hard to identify with current MRA techniques. Occasionally an embolic occlusion of a large proximal vessel is diagnosed on MRA by a sudden change in the vessel caliber and an abrupt decrease in the intensity of the vessel distal to this point of change (Fig. 18-2). One may also observe a decreased number of branches arising from the occluded parent vessel. To determine whether the embolic material arose from the heart or the carotid artery bifurcation, MRA of extracranial vessels is most helpful.

In addition to embolic disease, narrowing or occlusion of intracranial vessels may result from atherosclerotic changes. Stenosis and occlusion of these vessels also occur in a variety of other conditions, including moyamoya disease,[8] in response to radiation, phakomatosis, sickle cell disease, antiphospholipid antibody

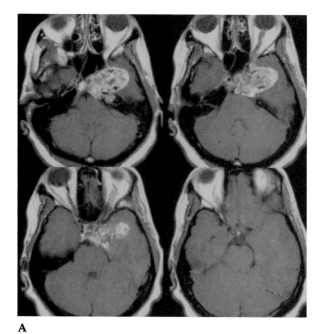

A

B

Fig. 18-1 Vascular displacement. (*A*) A homogeneous mass (chordoma) is seen in the left parasellar region. It involves the left cavernous sinus and left petrous apex. (*B*) MRA (3D TOF) demonstrates displacement of the petrous and cavernous portions of the left internal carotid artery. The artery is probably encased by the tumor.

syndrome, fibromuscular dysplasia, dissection,[9] arteritis,[10] spasm secondary to subarachnoid hemorrhage (SAH) or trauma, and brain tumors. Atherosclerotic disease is the dominant etiology however.

Narrowing of the intracranial vessels secondary to artherosclerosis may be seen in the carotid siphon, in the horizontal portion of the middle cerebral artery, in the middle or distal portion of the basilar artery, and in distal vertebral arteries just before the two arteries join.

Evaluation of siphon disease by MRA is difficult because the complex S-shaped anatomy and fast, turbulent flow cause signal loss even when no real narrowing is present. With experience, the radiologist generally becomes accustomed to the usual patterns of flow signal seen in the region with the technique being used. Reviewing source images in any difficult or confusing case is also helpful. The significance of siphon disease may be controversial, but there is little doubt that a diseased siphon may give rise to embolic material that will lodge distally.

Narrowing of the middle cerebral arteries and basilar arteries[11] pose less of a diagnostic problem. Here 3DF TOF imaging usually demonstrates the narrowing and its extent, although this technique may overestimate the degree of stenosis (Fig. 18-3). The precavernous and supraclinoid portions of the internal carotid arteries were the sites of frequent over- and underestimation of stenosis in the Heiserman et al. series.[12] Decreasing the voxel size and echo time (TE) can reduce the error. Theoretically, slower flow in a posterior circulation affected by atherosclerosis may also pose problems for 3D TOF imaging because of the relative insensitivity of this technique to slower flow,[13] necessitating the use of 2D TOF or phase contrast techniques. In our experience, this has not been a problem.

MRA is very helpful in evaluation of intracranial vascular occlusions seen in patients with sickle cell disease and moyamoya disease.[8] The progressive nature of the disease makes repeated contrast angiography burdensome. MRI and MRA demonstrate not only the vascular occlusions but also the resulting intracranial abnormalities (e.g., infarcts, hemorrhage). In these diseases, MRA will identify the resulting collateral pathways. PC techniques can provide information regarding the direction of flow in communicating arteries. Delineation of pial and dural collateral vessels may be more difficult.

Current MRA techniques poorly delineate small perforating vessels. Occlusion of these vessels leads to lacunar infarctions. MRA can help evaluate these patients. For example, in a patient with a pontine lacunar

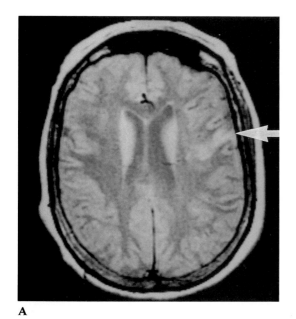

A

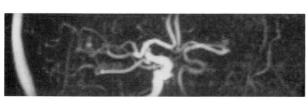

B

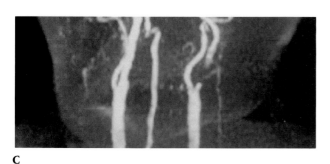

C

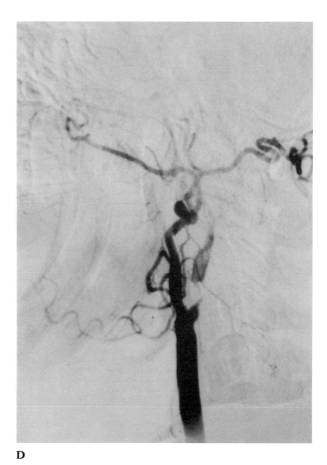

D

Fig. 18-2 Embolic occlusion. (*A*) An area of increased intensity is seen on this intermediate spin-echo image in the left midconvexity frontal region. (*B*) MRA (3D PC) demonstrates the sudden cutoff of the left middle cerebral artery. (*C,D*) MRA (2D TOF) and a conventional angiogram demonstrate significant stenosis of the proximal left internal carotid artery.

infarct, MRA may show significant disease of the basilar artery, presumably causing the infarct either by occlusion of the perforators at their origins or by embolic occlusion of these vessels.

Intracranial Aneurysms

The majority of aneurysms are berry aneurysms arising predominantly about the arterial circle. Of these, aneurysms arising at the origin of the posterior communicating artery, anterior communicating artery, and bifurcation of the middle cerebral artery are most common. About 15–20% of aneurysms are multiple, and 10% are related to the vertebrobasilar system.

In a patient with suspected SAH, imaging studies usually include a CT scan to document the presence and extent of hemorrhage and to document the possible site of aneurysm. Patients then usually undergo conventional angiography to demonstrate the lesion. In these acute circumstances, MRA is rarely used. The patient may be too unstable to be put in the magnetic environment. MRA techniques also suffer from a variety of shortcomings in this evaluation. The most important ones are: poor visibility of the neck and difficulty in assessing the exact size of an aneurysm due to thrombosis or flow in larger aneurysms. An aneurysm causing SAH may not be visible by MRA (e.g., due to its small size, adjacent SAH causing spurious blood

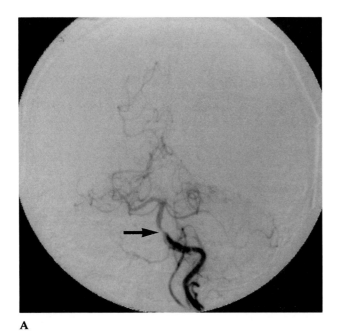

A

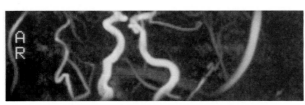

B

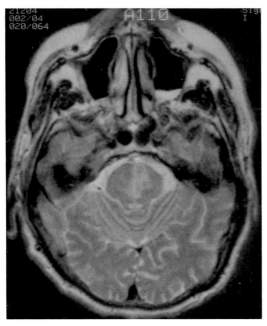

C

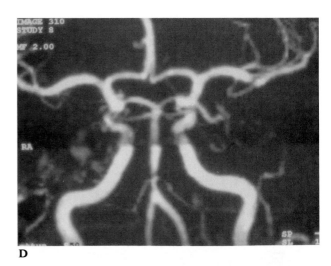

D

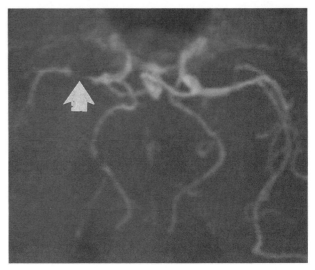

E

Fig. 18-3 Arterial narrowing. (*A*) Conventional angiography in this patient showed significant narrowing of the mid-basilar artery. (*B,C*) MRA (3D PC) and MRI images of the same patient a few months later. The patient had been lost to follow-up in the interval. The basilar artery was not visualized on MRA and was presumed to be occluded. An extensive brain stem infarction had resulted. (*D,E*) Different patients demonstrate proximal basilar and proximal right middle cerebral artery stenoses.

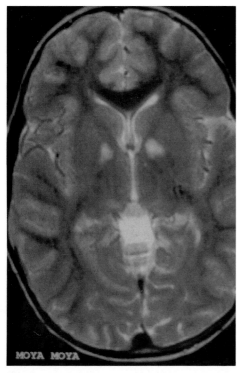

F

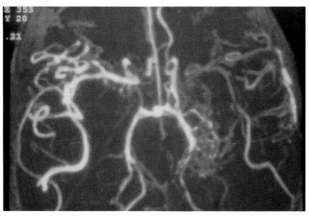

G

Fig. 18-3 (*F, G*)   Bilateral basal ganglionic infarcts in a child with moyamoya disease (*F*). MRA shows absent internal carotid arteries, a prominent left posterior communicating artery, and a middle meningeal–middle cerebral artery anastomosis. Prominent left medial temporal collaterals are also seen (*G*).

signals, spasm, and peripheral location outside of the imaging volume).

Most of these limitations can be overcome by studying both the MRI and MRA images; by screening the source images to appreciate the location of the neck; and by decreasing the voxel size and TE, which will decrease signal loss due to phase dispersion. Adding phase contrast images, which do not have some of these limitations, will also help but will add considerably to the length of the study. With all of these limitations, MRA plays a secondary role in patients with SAH. The contributions of MRA, however, may be important in a different way. For example, catheterization of vertebral arteries to rule out any vertebrobasilar aneurysm may prove very difficult or impossible. If a good-quality MRA scan does not show any abnormality in this system, the need for such a risky catheterization may be less acute.

MRA has proven to be quite sensitive in the detection of aneurysms. Using overlapping thin-section acquisitions, Blatter et al. detected 18 out of 19 aneurysms. The anatomy of the neck and the size of the aneurysm were correctly shown in 17 of the 19 patients.[5] In a study of 14 aneurysms in 12 patients utilizing both 3D TOF and 3D PC techniques, Huston et al. reported that MRA showed all 14 aneurysms.[14] According to these authors, aneurysms between 3 and 15 mm were shown equally well with both techniques. Aneurysms larger than 15 mm were better shown with the 3D PC technique. The overall impression is that aneurysms larger than 3–4 mm will be reliably demonstrated (Fig. 18-4).

Perhaps a solid indication for MRA is detection of aneurysms in patients at risk for harboring them who have not had SAH. Such patients include those with a familial history of aneurysms, polycystic kidney disease, or coarctation of the aorta. In these patients, as well as those with Ehlers-Danlos syndrome, for whom angiography could be dangerous, screening MRA may be indicated.

Special consideration should be given to patients with giant intracranial aneurysms. These lesions, with their complex luminal flow, mural thrombi, and peripheral hemosiderin, pose special problems for MRA. A single imaging technique is unlikely to provide all of the necessary information for optimal evaluation and surgical planning. Review of static MR images and a combination of 3D PC and 3D TOF are necessary.

A word of caution is in order regarding the imaging of patients who have undergone clipping of intracranial aneurysms. Although the newer clips are made of nonferromagnetic material, a reported death in a patient

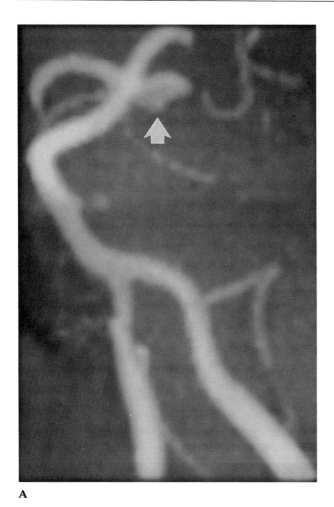

A

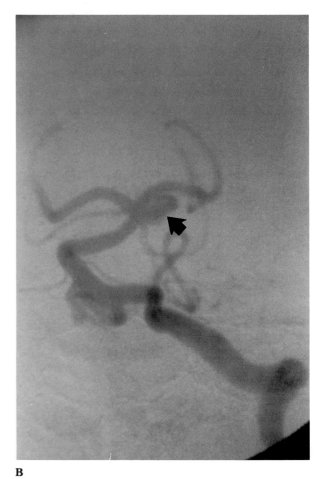

B

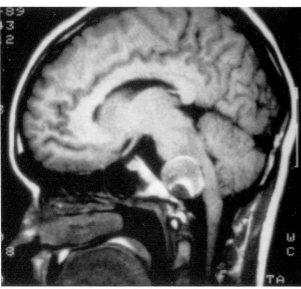

C

Fig. 18-4   Aneurysm. (*A,B*) A basilar artery–superior cerebellar artery aneurysm is demonstrated by MRA and conventional angiography. (*C*) MRI of a giant basilar artery aneurysm. The eccentric, inferiorly located flow void represents the patent lumen. Incomplete rings of different thickness and intensity surround it.

with a supposedly safe clip who underwent an MRA study is a potent reminder that such a study may not be as safe as was once believed. FDA has recently issued a warning regarding MR examination in these patients.[15]

Vascular Malformations

McCormick classified vascular malformations into five categories:

1. Arteriovenous malformations or fistulas
2. Venous angiomas
3. Cavernous angiomas
4. Capillary telangiectasias
5. Varices

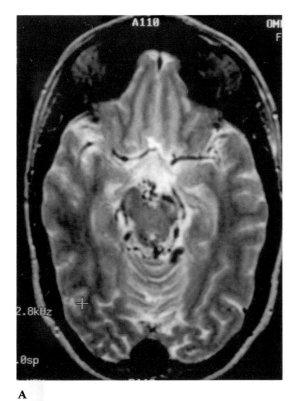

A

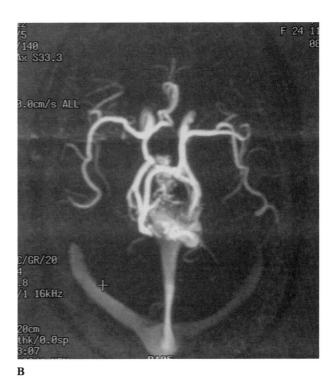

B

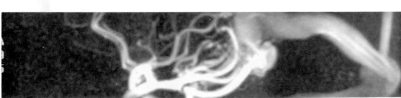

C

Fig. 18-5 AVM. (*A*) A perimesencephalic AVM is demonstrated by MRI. (*B*) MRA (3D PC) demonstrates a tuft of small vessels in the interpeduncular cistern. A second collection of vessels is noted behind the midbrain. (*C*) A distended vein of Galen and straight sinus drain this complex AVM.

Of these, only the first two have characteristic MRA findings.[1] The roles of imaging in a study of vascular malformations, whether by conventional angiography or MRA, are to demonstrate (1) the nidus, (2) the feeding arteries and draining veins, (3) the effects of the malformation on the adjacent brain, and (4) its relation to the brain parenchyma. An MRI–MRA study is a very strong tool in such an endeavor.

The technique of 3D TOF angiography is capable of demonstrating the nidus and the arterial feeders (Fig. 18-5). Occasionally a multicentric or multicompetent nidus is noted. To demonstrate the component with slow flow, contrast enhancement may be helpful. High-flow aneurysms on the feeding arteries or within the nidus are found in 10% of these patients. Intranidal aneurysms are associated with an increased risk of hemorrhage.[16] Other MRA features related to an increased risk of hemorrhage are a central location and central venous drainage.

Feeding arteries may be studied by 3D TOF MRA. The volume is selected based on the location of the nidus, as seen on MRI. This focus is put in the center or near the inferior edge of the imaging volume. Occasionally two different volumes have to be studied separately to delineate both the nidus and the vessels.

Identification of draining veins and slow components of the nidus may be difficult with the 3D TOF technique. A 2D TOF technique, which is more sensitive to slow flow, may be necessary. Alternatively, one may choose a 3D PC technique with flow sensitization chosen so that venous channels with slower flow are accentuated (e.g., with a VENC of 20 cm/sec). Marchal et al. suggest obtaining adjacent and slightly over-lapping 30-mm-thick slabs and gadolinium enhancement to overcome these problems.[17]

Different components of an arteriovenous malformation (AVM) may be fed from different sources. Careful placement of saturation bands can sequentially delin-

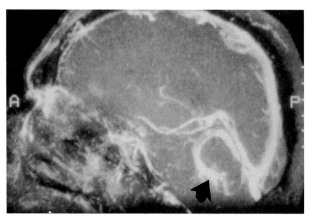

A

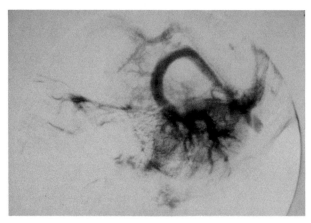

B

Fig. 18-6 Venous angioma. Typical appearance of a cerebellar venous angioma is demonstrated by 2D TOF MRA (*A*) and conventional angiography (*B*).

eate the different components. In a sense, this process is similar to identifying different components of an AVM by sequentially catheterizing the various arteries that feed it.

Obtaining directional flow information and measuring the flow rates are possible only with the 3D PC technique. Adequate delineation of a complex AVM thus may need a detailed study with both TOF and PC components.

Venous angiomas are perhaps the most common intracranial vascular malformations. The current understanding is that these anomalous venous channels rarely cause hemorrhage and that they have the normal function of draining brain tissues. The simultaneous occurrence of cavernous and venous angiomas has been recently described by Rigamonti et al.[18] Radiographically, these malformations are usually in the

periventricular white matter, where multiple small medullary veins come together. From here a venous channel begins and extends to the surface. The caliber of the vessel may diminish as it extends out (Fig. 18-6).

The imaging volume should be carefully selected after reviewing the MRI images. According to Marchal et al.,[17] the accuracy of MRA in detecting and demonstrating these lesions increases by utilizing multiple, slightly overlapping thick (30-mm) slabs and gadolinium enhancement.

REFERENCES

1. Caplan LR. Stroke neuroimaging. *Neuroimaging* 1993;3: 48–54.
2. Edelman RR, Mattle HP, Atkinson DJ, et al. MR angiography. *AJR* 1990;154:937–946.
3. Schwartz R, Tice HM, Hooton S, et al. Evaluation of cerebral aneurysms with helical CT: correlation with conventional angiography and magnetic resonance angiography. *Radiology* 1994;192:711–722.
4. Blatter DD, Parker DL, Robinson RO. Cerebral MR angiography with multiple overlapping thin slab acquisition Part I. Quantitative analysis of vessel visibility. *Radiology* 1991;179:805–811.
5. Blatter DD, Parker DL, Ahn SS, et al. Cerebral MR angiography with multiple overlapping thin-slab acquisition. Part II. Early clinical experience. *Radiology* 1992;183: 379–389.
6. Edelman RR, Ahn SS, Chien D, et al. Improved time-of-flight angiography of the brain with magnetization transfer contrast. *Radiology* 1992;184:395–399.
7. Lin W, Tkach JA, Haacke EM, et al. Intracranial MR angiography: Application of magnetization transfer contrast and fat saturation to short gradient-echo, velocity-compensated sequences. *Radiology* 1993;186:753–761.
8. Yamada I, Matsushima Y, Suzuki S. Moyamoya disease: Diagnosis with three dimensional time-of-flight MR angiography. *Radiology* 1992;184:773–778.
9. Levy C, Laissy JP, Raveau V, et al. Carotid and vetebral artery dissections. Three dimensional time-of-flight MR angiography and MR imaging versus conventional angiography. *Radiology* 1994;190:97–103.
10. Greenan TJ, Grossman RI, Goldberg HI. Cerebral vasculitis: MR imaging and angiographic correlation. *Radiology* 1992;182:65–72.
11. Wentz KU, Rather J, Schwartz A, et al. Intracranial vertebrobasilar system: MR angiography. *Radiology* 1994;190: 105–110.
12. Heiserman JE, Drayer BP, Keller PJ, et al. Intracranial vascular stenosis and occlusion: Evaluation with three-dimensional time-of-flight MR angiography. *Radiology* 1992;185:667–673.

13. Keller PJ, Dreyer BP, Fram EK, et al. MR angiography with two-dimensional acquisition and three-dimensional display. *Radiology* 1989;173:527–532.

14. Huston J III, Rufenacht DA, Ehman R, et al. Intracranial aneurysms and vascular malformations: Comparison of time-of-flight and phase-contrast MR angiography. *Radiology* 1991;181:721–730.

15. Klucznik RP, Carrier DA, Pyka R, et al. Placement of a ferromagnetic intracerebral aneurysm clip in a magnetic field with a fatal outcome. *Radiology* 1993;187:855–856.

16. Marks MP, Lane B, Steinberg GK, et al. Hemorrhage in intracerebral arteriovenous malformations: Angiographic determinants. *Radiology* 1990;176:807–813.

17. Marchal G, Bosmans H, Fraeyenhoven LV, et al. Intracranial vascular lesions: Optimization and clinical evaluation of three-dimensional time of flight MR angiography. *Radiology* 1990;175:443–448.

18. Rigamonti D, Spetzler RF. The association of venous and cavernous malformations: Report of four cases and discussion of the pathophysiological, diagnostic and therapeutic implications. *Acta Neurochir* 1988;92:100–105.

19

Intracranial Venous Magnetic Resonance Angiography

Ay-Ming Wang, M.D.

INTRODUCTION

The clinical utility of intracranial venous magnetic resonance angiography (MRA)[1–7] depends on its excellent visualization of the dural venous sinuses noninvasively and on its multiplanar display capability. In addition to visualization of the major dural sinuses, the present techniques of intracranial venous MRA allow visualization of many large deep and superficial cerebral veins. Familiarization with the normal intracranial venous anatomy and its normal variants, as well as pitfalls and artifacts, is crucial to correct interpretation of intracranial venous MRA.

TECHNIQUES, NORMAL ANATOMY, PITFALLS, AND ARTIFACTS

Techniques

Intracranial venous MRA is usually performed using two-dimensional sequential time-of-flight (TOF) technique, with application of arterial flow saturation band, and reconstructed with a maximal-intensity projection algorithm in multiple planes (Table 19-1).[1–2,4] Three (coronal, oblique sagittal, and axial) planes of acquisitions can be obtained, depending upon the area of interest; the most commonly used acquisition plane is the coronal plane. To obtain maximal signal intensity

of venous flow in the brain, the MRA acquisition plane should be perpendicular to the blood flow. Gadolinium-DTPA can be administered intravenously for evaluation of tumor. Phase contrast MRA[2,3] can be used when there is increased signal intensity on T_1-weighted images due to the presence of methemoglobin in the occluded dural sinuses.

Normal Anatomy and Normal Variants of Major Dural Venous Sinuses and Cerebral Venous Systems

Dural venous sinuses are an endothelium-lined separation between the two layers (inner and outer dural lamina) of cranial dural matter. They are located primarily in the junction and free edges of the major dural folds (e.g., the falx cerebri and the tentorium cerebelli). They surround the brain, receiving numerous contributions from the superficial and deep venous systems. The major dural venous sinuses, including the superior sagittal sinus (SSS), transverse sinus (TS), sigmoid sinus (Sig S), and straight sinus (SS), are routinely visualized on intracranial venous MRA (Fig. 19-1A).[5] Smaller dural sinuses such as the sphenoparietal sinus (SP S), inferior sagittal sinus (ISS), superior petrosal sinus (SPS), inferior petrosal sinus (IPS), and cavernous sinus (CS) are sometimes apparent on intracranial venous MRA (Fig. 19-1B).

The SSS typically begins rostrally at the foramen ce-

TABLE 19-1 Two-Dimensional Sequential TOF
Technique (Siemens 1.5 T Magnetom SP)

Acquisition plane	Oblique sagittal/coronal/axial, depending on the area of interest
Slice thickness	1.5 to 3 mm
Slice interval	1.5 mm or 33% overlap between slices
Number of slices	60–110 (cover the area of interest)
Field of view	20 cm
Repetition time (TR)	32 msec
Echo time (TE)	10 msec
Flip angle	40°
Flow compensation	First order
Saturation band	Inferior
Matrix	256 × 256
Number of excitations	One
Time	6–11 min

cum of the frontal bone, from which it may receive a cerebral emissary vein. It then travels in the midline of the dorsal fold of the falx cerebri; follows the concave surface of the skull, to which it is attached; and proceeds in a caudal direction toward the internal occipital protuberance. The SSS is triangular in shape, and its base is attached to the inner table of the cranial vault. At the internal occipital protuberance, the SSS usually turns more or less directly to terminate in the right transverse sinus. Its anterior portion may normally be atretic to the level of the coronal suture. From its origin to its termination, the SSS grows larger, receiving venous outflow from the lateral lacunal (lateral lakes) and the superior cerebral veins. The posterior one-third of the SSS may be duplicated (Fig. 19-1C).

The ISS courses above the corpus callosum in the free edge of the falx cerebri. It receives numerous veins that drain the roof of the corpus callosum, the cingulate gyrus, and the adjacent medical hemisphere. It joins the great cerebral vein of Galen (GVG). It is usually small and not well visualized on intracranial venous MRA.

The SS originates behind the splenium of the corpus callosum. It is formed chiefly by the union of the ISS and the GVG. The superior cerebellar vein and the basal veins also contribute to the formation of the SS. It may communicate with the SSS and, together with the two TSs, forms a large tocular Herophili (TH) or confluence of sinuses. It may be occasionally dupli-

cated (Fig. 19-1D). The SS usually terminates in the left TS (Fig. 19-1E).

The TS is usually a communication between the SSS, SS, and occipital sinus (OS) (Fig. 19-1F) near the internal occipital protuberance. The association between these sinuses is the TH. There are four major configurations of the sinuses forming the TH: the common pool (9%), the plexiform (56%), the ipsilateral (31%), and the unilateral (4%). From their origin, the TSs pass laterally and anteriorly to the base of the petrous portion of the temporal bone. Each TS courses along the attached margin of the tentorium cerebelli and along the groove of the squamous portion of the temporal bone. In addition to carrying venous blood from both the deep and superficial cerebral venous systems, the TSs drain surrounding structures throughout their course. A large portion of the cerebellum is drained by the TS. Near the petrous temporal bone, the TS receives blood from the SPS, thus establishing a communication with the cavernous sinus.

The Sig S is continuous with the TS. It originates at the posterior portion of the petrous temporal bone. It traverses the jugular foramen, where it becomes continuous with the internal jugular vein (IJV). The SPS commonly drains into the proximal portion of the Sig S. Throughout its course the Sig S receives inconstant veins from the cerebellum, the lateral pons, and the medulla. The IPS may enter the most distal segment of the Sig S, although it usually drains directly into the IGV. The presence of a well-formed Sig S draining the SPS or IPS, in the absence of a TS, is a development anomaly.

Deep and Superficial Cerebral Venous Systems
The following deep cerebral veins can be visualized on intracranial venous MRA. Running posteriorly from the foramen of Monro, the paired internal cerebral veins (ICVs) lie on either side of the midline within the velum interpositum and above the third ventricle. A number of subependymal veins join to form the ICV. The thalamostriate vein (TSV) is the largest of the lateral group of subependymal veins formed by the anterior caudate vein that drains the head of the caudate nucleus and the terminal vein that runs between the thalamus and the body of the caudate nucleus. The septal vein (SV) is the largest of the medial group of the subependymal vein; it runs in a paramedian location along the septum pellucidum. The SV and TSV join together to form the ICV at the foramen of Monro. The basal vein of Rosenthal (BVR) is formed in the sylvian fissure from the anterior and deep middle cerebral veins. It drains portions of the temporal lobe, the

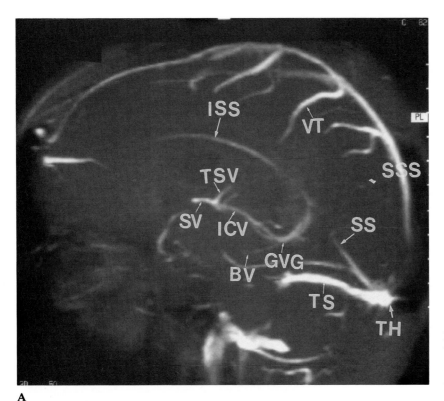

A

Fig. 19-1 (*A*) Normal sagittal view of two-dimensional (2D) TOF venous MRA. (*B*) Normal axial view of 2D TOF venous MRA.

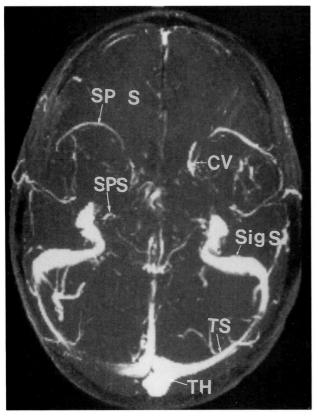

B

insula, the inferior basal gaglia, and the cerebral peduncles. It joins the contralateral BV and ICVs to form the great cerebral GVG with the ISS to drain to the SS.

The superficial cerebral veins are the most variable of the cerebral venous structures. The three largest, which are variably present, are the vein of Labbe (VL), the vein of Trolard (VT), and the superficial middle cerebral vein (SMCV) or sylvian vein. These veins drain the cortex and a portion of the underlying white matter. Numerous small, superficial cortical veins drain over the superior convexities into the SSS.

Deep and superficial veins in the posterior fossa are not commonly visualized on MRA. The OS is occasionally visualized on MRA; it is a posterior structure that runs in the midline at the attachment of the falx cerebelli. It drains superiorly, extending from the foramen magnum to the TH. As a variant of normal anatomy, the OS may represent a major path of drainage from the TH to the internal jugular veins.

Pitfalls and Artifacts

Pitfalls (Fig. 19-2) and artifacts (Fig. 19-3) in intracranial venous MRA and their solutions are listed in Tables 19-2 and 19-3.

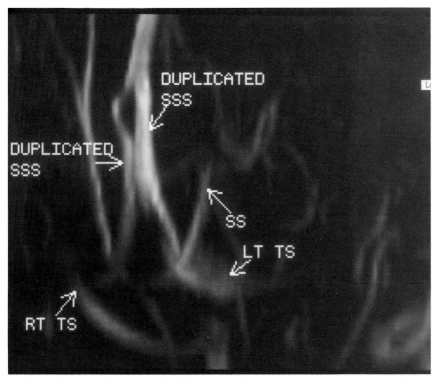

C

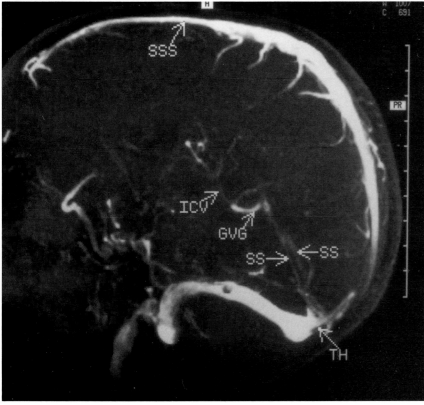

D

Fig. 19-1 (*C*) Oblique coronal view of 2D TOF venous MRA shows a duplicated SSS. (*D*) Sagittal view of 2D TOF venous MRA shows a duplicated SS.

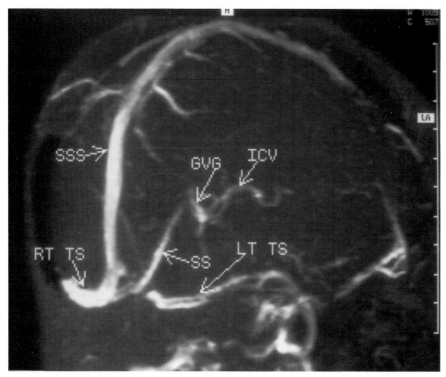

E

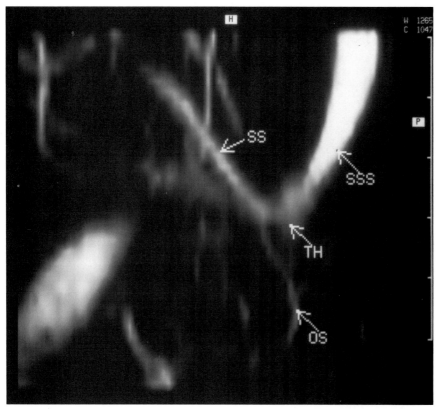

F

Fig. 19-1 (*E*) Oblique coronal view of 2D TOF venous MRA shows an SSS terminated in the right TS and an SS terminated in the left TS. (*F*) Sagittal view of 2D TOF venous MRA shows the OS connected to the TH.

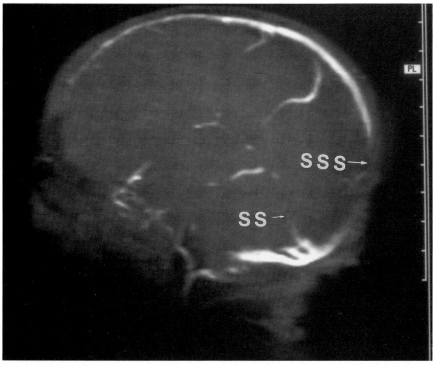

A

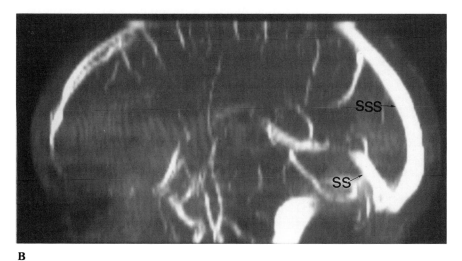

B

Fig. 19-2 Pitfalls of 2D TOF venous MRA. (*A*) Sagittal view of a 2D venous MRA scan obtained in the oblique sagittal plane. The posterior inferior SSS and SS are partially visualized, mimicking occlusion. (*B*) Sagittal view of 2D venous MRA scan obtained in the axial plane in the same patient shows intensive flow through the posterior inferior SSS and SS.

CLINICAL APPLICATIONS

Cerebral Venous and Dural Sinus Thrombosis

MRA is a noninvasive MR study for evaluation of the blood flow of the cerebral venous system and dural sinuses in multiple planes. It is particularly useful in pediatric and high-risk patients. It provides reliable in-

formation[1–4,6] for identification of the dural sinuses and thrombosis of the major cerebral venous systems. It also delineates the venous drainage patterns and dural sinus occlusion by the tumor before surgery (Fig. 19-4). It provides excellent information[4] for planning and follow-up of endovascular thrombolytic treatment for cerebral venous and dural sinus thrombosis (Fig. 19-5).

Numerous conditions can cause or predispose to ce-

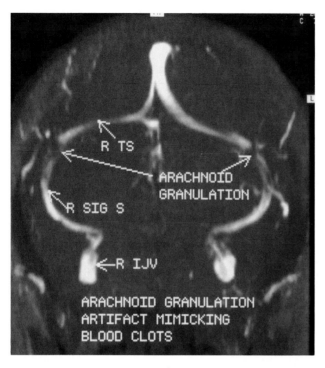

Fig. 19-3 Coronal view of a 2D TOF venous MRA scan shows arachnoid granulation mimicking blood clots.

TABLE 19-2 Pitfalls in Intracranial Venous MRA

Pitfall	Reason	Solution
Partial visualization of posterior SSS and SS	Signal loss due to in-plane flow saturation	Axial or coronal acquisition
Partial visualization of TS	Signal loss due to in-plane flow saturation	Oblique sagittal or coronal acquisition

TABLE 19-3 Artifacts in Intracranial Venous MRA

Artifact	Reason	Solution
Abnormal hyper-intensity	Fat or hemorrhage (spoiled gradient used for TOF MRA providing T_1 weighting; Fat or extracellular methemoglobin producing T_1 shortening)	Phase contrast MRA Review individual slice and/or Spin echo imaging
Defect mimicking blood clot	Arachnoid granulation	Become familiar with normal anatomy

rebral venous and dural sinus thrombosis (Table 19-4).[6] Infective and noninfective causes are the two most common ones; however, the incidence of cases of unknown etiology remains between 20% and 35%.

Although the incidence of septic cerebral venous and dural sinus thrombosis has greatly diminished recently, cavernous sinus thrombosis is still the most common form of septic thrombosis. In young women, cerebral venous and dural sinus thrombosis occur more frequently during the puerperium than pregnancy and remain very common in developing countries. In neonates and children, the incidence of cerebral venous and dural sinus thrombosis is higher than we predicted, and the etiology is characterized by frequent region infections (otitis, mastoiditis), neonatal asphyxia, severe dehydration (Fig. 19-6), and congenital heart disease.

Venous Angioma

Venous angioma of the brain consists of multiple, radially oriented, dilated medullary veins with the appearance of caput medusae that drain into a transparenchymal venous stem. It is probably the most common anomaly of the intracranial vasculature and is usually an incidental finding on neuroimaging studies. It has many appearances, ranging from a small, single draining vein, involving at most one small portion of the brain, to a large hemispheric venous anomaly draining an entire hemisphere. It can occur almost anywhere; favored sites include the frontal lobes (Fig. 19-7A) and the posterior fossa (Fig. 19-7B). Intracranial venous MRA[1,7] reliably identifies this venous anomaly and its drainage noninvasively. In complicated cases of venous angioma associated with hemorrhage, three-dimensional TOF MRA is needed to exclude an arterial component of vascular malformation in addition to a venous angioma.

SUMMARY

Intracranial venous MRA is an easily performed, noninvasive, reliable MRI technique utilized to evaluate intracranial large venous systems and dural sinuses. It is particularly useful in demonstrating the location of intracranial venous and dural sinus thrombosis and their relationship to the patent venous system on a multiplanar display. This facilitates successful endovascular thrombolytic treatment and provides precise information regarding the success of the treatment. It also demonstrates the relationship of a brain tumor to the surrounding dural venous compartment. Finally, it

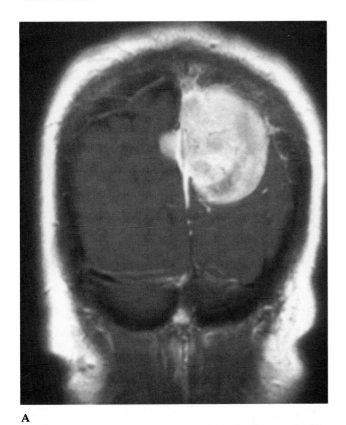

A

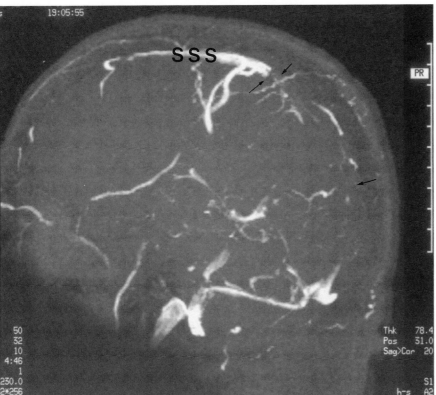

B

Fig. 19-4 A large parietal parasagittal meningioma causing complete occlusion of the posterior SSS. (*A*) T$_1$-weighted contrast coronal image shows a large left parietal parasagittal meningioma extending to the right. (*B*) Sagittal view of 2D TOF venous MRA scan shows occlusion of the posterior SSS (arrows).

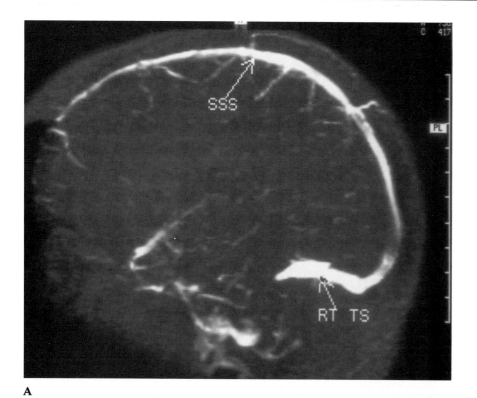

A

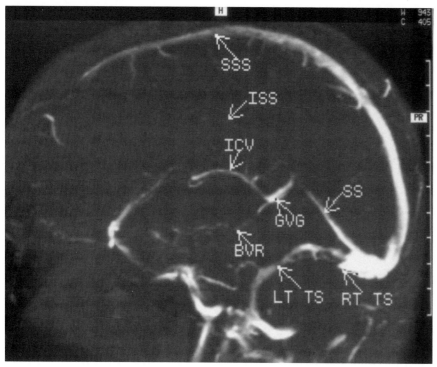

B

Fig. 19-5 A 22-year-old female developed severe headache and lethargy 2 months postpartum. (*A*) Sagittal view of a 2D TOF venous MRA scan shows occlusion of the deep cerebral venous system, SS, and left TS. (*B*) After endovascular thrombolytic treatment with urokinase, the patient completely recovered. This follow-up sagittal view of a 2D TOF venous MRA scan shows recanalization of the occluded deep cerebral venous system, SS, and left TS.

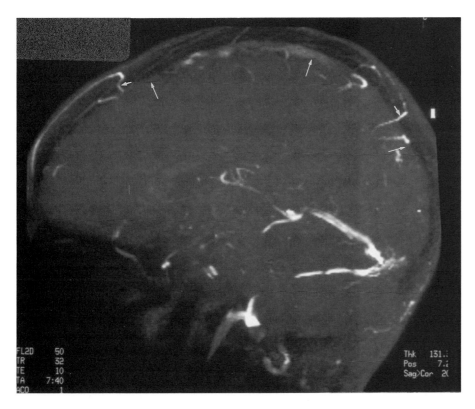

Fig. 19-6 A 13-year-old boy developed headache and seizures after dehydration from diarrhea. This sagittal view of a 2D TOF venous MRA scan shows occlusion of the SSS (white arrows) with development of collateral emissary venous drainage (small white arrows).

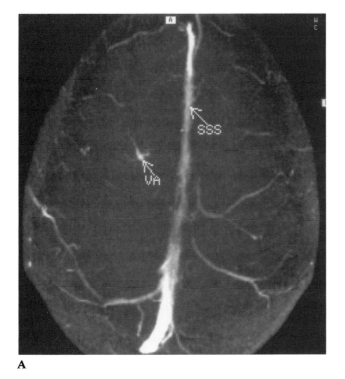

A

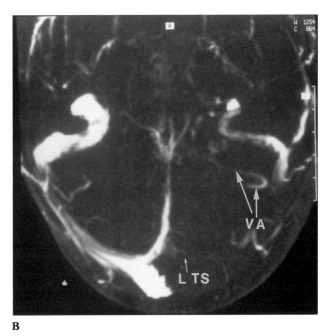

B

Fig. 19-7 Venous angioma. (*A*) Axial view of a 2D TOF venous MRA scan shows a venous angioma (VA) at the right frontal lobe, with hypoplasia of the right frontal cortical veins. (*B*) Axial view of a 2D TOF venous MRA scan shows a VA in the left cerebellum (arrows), with hypoplasia of the left TS.

TABLE 19-4 Causes of Factors Predisposing to Cerebral Venous and Dural Sinus Thrombosis

Infectious causes
    Local causes
        Direct septic trauma
        Intracranial infection
        Regional infection
    General causes
        Bacterial, viral, parasitic, and fungal infections
Noninfectious causes
    Local causes
        Head injury, neurosurgical procedure, brain infarctions and hemorrhages, brain tumors or masses, catheterizations and infusions into the internal jugular vein
    General causes
        Operation; pregnancy and puerperium; medical causes including cardiac disorders, malignancies, red blood cell disorders, coagulation disorders, severe dehydration, connective tissue disorders
Idiopathic causes

demonstrates the venous angioma and its drainage. Familiarity with the wide variation in the venous anatomy, as well as the pitfalls and artifacts of intracranial venous MRA, is necessary to interpret the scan correctly.

REFERENCES

1. Mattle PM, Wentz KU, Edelman RR, et al. Cerebral venography with MR. *Radiology* 1991;178:453–458.
2. Johnson BA, Fram EK. Cerebral venous occlusive disease: Pathophysiology, clinical manifestations, and imaging. *Neuroimag Clin North Am* 1992;2(4):769–783.
3. Rippe DJ, Boyko OB, Spritzer CE, et al. Demonstration of dural sinus occlusion by the use of MR angiography. *AJNR* 1990;11:199–201.
4. Yuh WTC, Simonson TM, Wang AM, et al. Venous sinus occlusive disease: MR findings. *AJNR* 1994;15:309–316.
5. Lindan CE, Wallace RC. Cerebrovascular anatomy on magnetic resonance angiography. *Neuroimag Clin North Am* 1992;2(4):743–752.
6. Ameri A, Bousser MG. Cerebral venous thrombosis. *Neurol Clin* 1992;10(1):87–111.
7. Truwit CL. Venous angioma of the brain: History, significance, and imaging findings. *AJR* 1992;159:1299–1307.

20

Magnetic Resonance Angiography: Extracranial Clinical Applications

Amir A. Zamani, M.D.

In the evaluation of extracranial vessels, like that of intracranial vessels, different imaging modalities are employed. Here Doppler ultrasound is a strong diagnostic tool. Ultrasound is noninvasive, inexpensive, easy to obtain, and fairly accurate. Its major shortcomings are (1) its inability to study the origin of the carotid arteries, and (2) its inability to study the intracranial vasculature, and (3) its operator dependency. Transcranial Doppler is not yet a very dependable means of evaluating the intracranial vessels. Despite these drawbacks, and in view of the fact that narrowing of the carotid arteries affects predominantly the carotid bifurcation, ultrasound in experienced hands remains the first imaging modality employed. Ultrasound can measure wall thickness and demonstrate with 90% accuracy those lesions that are more than 50% stenotic.[1]

High-resolution, contrast-enhanced spiral computed tomography (CT) of the carotid bifurcations is improving rapidly. Its ability to demonstrate calcification and large ulcers, and to demonstrate the bifurcations at different angles of rotation about the vertical axis, are its major advantages.[2] The necessity for contrast injection is a problem, and postprocessing of the data is time-consuming. The field of imaging, by necessity, is small, is confined to the carotid bifurcations and their vicinity. Viewing another site (e.g., the siphon) necessitates another study and another contrast injection. In a recent study, Dillon et al. found that in 50 bifurcations, CT angiography and conventional angiography agreed in estimating stenosis in 82% of studies.[3]

Conventional angiography is considered the gold standard in the evaluation of carotid artery disease. The method is accurate in estimating bifurcation narrowing and successful in demonstrating tandem lesions (such as carotid siphon disease and occasional middle cerebral artery narrowing). A small but definite risk of neurological complications and a reaction to the contrast are the two most important deterrents of its routine use. In addition, the patient requires a period of hospital observation after the procedure.

Magnetic resonance angiography (MRA) has improved significantly in recent years. Today the procedure (1) is fairly accurate, (2) can detect tandem lesions, (3) does not need contrast injection, and (4) is almost risk free. In addition, the accompanying magnetic resonance imaging (MRI) allows visualization of the resultant brain lesions. The problem of accuracy is most important. Even an MRA study of optimal quality leaves doubts as to whether the degree of stenosis has been correctly estimated.

We explore the merits and disadvantages of these tests in the following pages, but this discussion focuses primarily on MRA of extracranial vessels.

MRA TECHNIQUE

Two-dimensional time-of-flight (2D TOF) and 3D TOF are the most commonly used techniques. The differences between them have been discussed in chapter 18. Essentially, the 3D technique offers better spatial resolution, but it is more prone to degradation by patient movement and cannot differentiate very slow flow from occlusion. The 2D TOF technique is more sensitive to slow flow and can differentiate subocclusive narrowing from total occlusion. It is easier to obtain than the 3D TOF scan.

Occasionally 2D phase contrast slabs are used as scout views to localize the bifurcation. Most centers now use a combination of 2D and 3D TOF sequences.

Delineation of Normal Anatomy

Usually MRA offers excellent demonstration of the two common carotid arteries, the internal and external carotid arteries, and the two vertebral arteries (Fig. 20-1). To differentiate the internal from the external carotid artery, the images must include the skull base. Hypoplasia of the vertebral artery is rare. Sometimes one of the two vertebral arteries is quite small. Here differentiation from pathological proximal narrowing may be difficult and can be important if the patient is suffering from a vertebrobasilar insufficiency syndrome (e.g., Wallenberg's lateral medullary infarction). A vertebral artery of small caliber can be a normal variant or can be due to a constricting lesion at the origin of the vertebral artery. Differentiation of the two possibilities requires observation of the junction of the two vertebral arteries and the initial course of the basilar artery. Usually the junction is on the side of the congenitally smaller artery, and the basilar artery begins its ascent from there.

Vascular Displacement

A large unilateral mass can displace the ipsilateral carotid artery. The displacement is easy to detect if one uses the collapsed view or a perfect lateral view in which the two carotid arteries normally overlap.

Splaying of the internal and external carotid arteries develops in patients with carotid body tumors (Fig. 20-2). If it is sizable enough, this splaying will be demonstrated by MRA.

Carotid Stenosis

Atherosclerosis is the most common cause of carotid artery stenosis. In the carotid arteries, atherosclerosis affects the region of bifurcation more than any other site. Narrowing at the origin of the brachiocephalic vessels is said to be rare. According to one study, arch disease is found in only 1.8% of patients with significant bifurcation disease.[4] The same study estimates the inicidence of tandem siphon disease at 6%. With relatively low frequency of atherosclerosis at other sites, it is no surprise that evaluation of bifurcation disease is

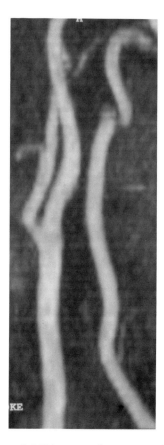

Fig. 20-1 Normal MRA scan of extracranial vessels using the 2D TOF technique: excellent visualization of the common, external, internal carotid, and vertebral arteries. Normal bifurcation.

paramount in the workup of patients with cerebrovascular disease.

An immense literature has accumulated on this subject. The role of imaging has received increasing attention with the publication of results from the North American Symptomatic Carotid Endarterectomy Trial in 1991.[5] This study reported that patients with more than a 70% diameter stenosis at the bifurcation and without tandem lesions benefited from endarterectomy. Also, the more severe the narrowing, the greater the benefit. In this study, conventional angiography and digital subtraction arterial angiography were utilized, and narrowing of the artery was measured by comparing the diameter of the artery at the point of maximal stenosis with the diameter of the internal carotid artery well beyond the bifurcation.[6] The study also reported a perioperative rate of major stroke and mortality of 2.1% (including 0.6% mortality). A problem with this study is that it did not consider the risks of angiography. Because the benefits of endarterectomy

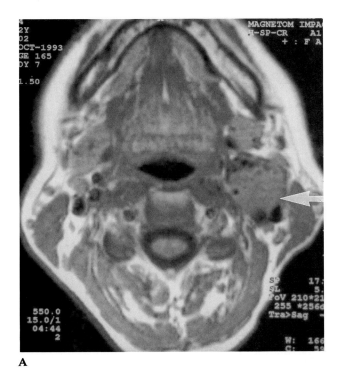

A

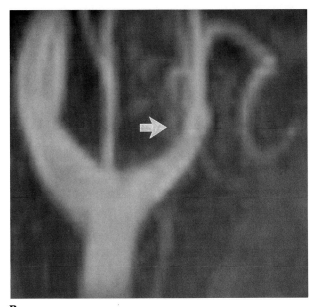

B

Fig. 20-2 Vascular displacement. (*A*) A carotid body tumor is demonstrated (arrow). Note the separation of the external and internal carotid arteries by this mass. (*B*) There is splaying of the external and internal carotid arteries. A few of the larger feeders are demonstrated (arrows).

in patients with stenosis of less than 70% are not clear, the authors suggest utilizing ultrasonography as a screening method to separate these patients and spare them the risks of catheter angiography.

An important outcome to this study is that there is now a clear definition of significant narrowing: 70%. In the future, when different imaging modalities are compared, the comparison will be based on how accurately they can measure stenosis above 70% and how accurately they can separate insignificant stenoses from significant ones. Although the significance of a tandem lesion is hotly debated,[7] the ability to demonstrate co-existing siphon disease simultaneously with bifurcation disease will be an important consideration for the foreseeable future.

Numerous studies have compared MRA, Doppler ultrasound, and conventional angiography in subocclusive disease at the bifurcation. Heiserman et al. reported in 1992 that MRA (2D TOF) reliably separated mild narrowing from severe narrowing and discriminated between severe narrowing and occlusion.[8] They also reported that 2D TOF MRA of moderately stenotic vessels (50–75%) frequently overestimated and rarely underestimated the degree of stenosis. Huston et al. reported similar results in 1993.[9] These authors compared color duplex flow ultrasound and 2D TOF MRA with conventional angiography in 50 patients with symptomatic hemispheric ischemia. In their study, a signal void on the maximum intensity projection (MIP) images corresponded to 70% or more stenosis in 17 of 20 arteries (Fig. 20-3). They concluded that the accuracy of MRA at this stage equals that of ultrasound, but they believed MRA was a poor replacement for conventional angiography.

Polak et al. in 1992 compared color Doppler sonography and 2D TOF MRA, using conventional angiography as the standard in 23 patients. They concluded that a combination of these two tests was useful in detecting and grading the stenosis.[10] Finally, in 1993, Polak et al. reported that in up to 79% of cases, the combined use of Doppler sonography and MRA can replace angiography in preoperative assessment of patients likely to undergo carotid endarterectomy.[11] This approach was criticized by Masaryk et al., who found scant data to show that combined use of color Doppler and MRA is a sufficient replacement for catheter angiography in these patients.[12,13]

Complete Occlusions of Carotid Arteries

Differentiation of a complete occlusion from a subocclusive severe stenosis has always been difficult with

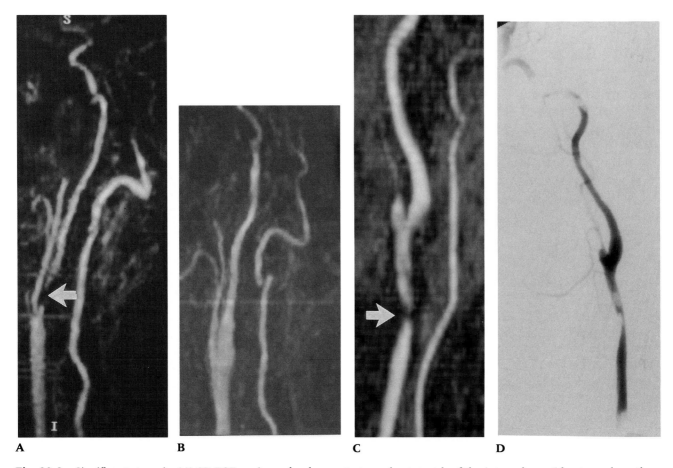

A   B   C   D

Fig. 20-3 Significant stenosis. (*A*) 2D TOF angiography demonstrates a short stretch of the internal carotid artery where there is no signal. Although this usually correlates with significant stenosis, at times moderate stenosis is associated with this phenomenon. (*B*) MRA: postendarterectomy appearance. (*C,D*) MR angiogram and conventional angiogram of a postradiation stenosis of the common carotid artery.

ultrasonography. Although large-scale studies are not yet available, evidence so far points to the accuracy of 2D TOF MRA in diagnosing complete occlusion. Anderson et al., in a study of 50 bifurcations with MRA (2D and 3D), color flow Doppler ultrasound, and angiography, found no instances in which MRA misidentified slow flow and occlusion.[14] Heiserman et al.[8] reported similar results with 2D TOF studies (Fig. 20-4).

Arterial Dissection

Arterial dissection usually involves the carotid artery in its midcervical portion. The lesion can extend superiorly to involve the petrous carotid artery, can cause luminal narrowing, and can lead to thrombosis. Embolic materials arising from dissected arteries can travel distally to cause branch occlusion.

Dissection can begin in the proximal, middle, or distal vertebral artery. Trauma is the usual cause; it may at times be very mild and unnoticeable (such as sneezing and coughing). MR images obtained with the spin echo technique can demonstrate blood in the wall of the artery. MRA may demonstrate luminal narrowing, which may be smooth and concentric or irregular and eccentric; complete occlusion may occur. In a recent study, Levy et al. compared 3D TOF MRA of cervical vessels to MR imaging and conventional angiography in 18 patients (19 extracranial internal carotid arteries and 5 vertebral arteries). They concluded that MRA had 95% sensitivity and 99% specificity for carotid dissections. MRA was therefore reliable in the diagnosis of internal carotid artery dissection. For vertebral artery dissection, conventional angiography was more helpful.[15]

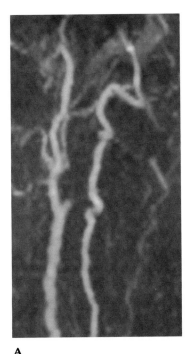

A

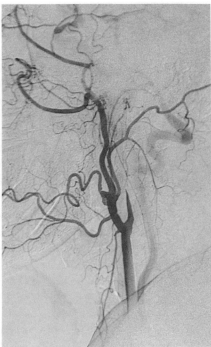

B

Fig. 20-4 Complete occlusion of the internal carotid artery. 2D TOF MR angiography demonstrates complete occlusion (*A*), which was confirmed by conventional angiography (*B*).

MRA of Arterial Narrowing as a Result of Arteritis

MRA is capable of demonstrating the vascular anatomy in this condition. Large-scale studies are not yet available, and the sensitivity of this technique has not been evaluated. Vascular occlusion in a patient with Takayasu arteritis was successfully demonstrated in a recent report[16] (Fig. 20-5).

Alterations of Flow in Vertebral Arteries Induced by Head Rotation

Reduction of flow, and even occlusion, in the upper cervical vertebral artery with head rotation (and hyperextension) is a common observation made by any angiographer. That these temporary alterations can, if continued, result in posterior circulation ischemia and stroke in the elderly has recently been reported. Dynamic MRA in these cases demonstrated the vascular changes with head rotation and hyperextension.[17]

SUMMARY

With renewed interest in carotid endarterectomy, the need for an effective, accurate, low-risk evaluation of the carotid arteries has become evident. As Masaryk points out, such a study must meet four essential criteria: (1) it must be accurate; (2) it must be able to differentiate between complete occlusion and subocclusive narrowing; (3) it must be able to demonstrate tandem lesions; and (4) it must be able to accomplish the above with low risk to the patient. Clearly, none of the imaging modalities available today meet all of these criteria.

Angiography, although fairly accurate, is invasive and is subject to significant interobserver and intraobserver variation. CT angiography suffers from the inability to demonstrate tandem lesions. Its value in differentiating complete occlusion from significant narrowing has not been tested in a large-scale study. Sonography suffers from some of the same shortcomings.

MRA has improved significantly during the past few years. Although it is safe and can demonstrate tandem lesions, it both overestimates and underestimates carotid stenosis. Although this may not matter if one considers a 90% stenosis demonstrated by MRA, it is important when moderate narrowing (less than 70%) is overestimated, putting the lesion in a more severe category.

It is clear that a large-scale prospective study com-

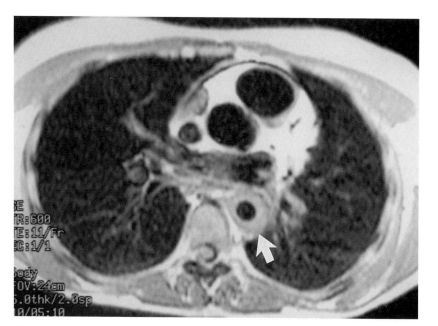

A

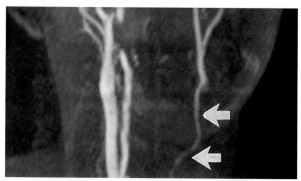

C

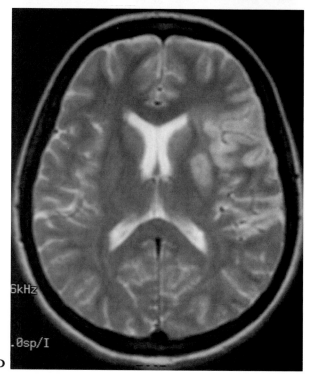

B

D

Fig. 20-5 Takayasu's arteritis. (*A*) Thickening of the wall of the aorta. (*B*) Occlusion of the left common carotid and vertebral arteries demonstrated by arch aortography. (*C*) MRA demonstrates occlusion of the left common carotid artery. A collateral channel crosses the anterior neck from right to left and superiorly, reconstituting the bifurcation. Because of a superior saturation band, the left vertebral artery (filling in a retrograde fashion on a conventional angiogram) is not seen. (*D*) MR scan demonstrates infarction in the left basal ganglia and the midfrontal region.

paring all imaging modalities is necessary. In the present era of cost containment, however, this may be too difficult to achieve or even justify. It is likely that in each institution, based on the available local expertise and the level of tolerable uncertainty, the radiologist, with his or her clinical colleagues, will devise imaging protocols acceptable to that particular institution. This process has already begun in many hospitals across the nation. Adopting an imaging package which utilizes Doppler sonography with MRA, and which uses angiography when results from these two studies are discordant, is one strategy. In the future, we will observe more of these combined protocols.

REFERENCES

1. Polak JF, O'Leary DH, Kronmal RA. Sonographic evaluation of carotid artery atherosclerosis in the elderly: Relationship of disease severity to stroke and transient ischemic attack. *Radiology* 1993;188:363–370.

2. Schwartz RB, Jones KM, Chernoff DM, et al. Common carotid artery bifurcation: Evaluation with spiral CT (work in progress). *Radiology* 1992;185:513–519.

3. Dillon EH, Van Leeuven MS, Fernandez MA, et al. CT angiography: Application to the evaluation of carotid artery stenosis. *Radiology* 1993;189:211–219.

4. Akers DL, Markowitz IA, Kerstein MD. The evaluation of the aortic arch in the evaluation of cerebrovascular insufficiency. *Am J Surg* 1987;154:230–232.

5. NASCET Collaborations. Beneficial effect of carotid endarterectomy in symptomatic patients with high-grade carotid stenosis. *N Engl J Med* 1991;325:445–453.

6. Fox AJ. How to measure carotid stenosis. *Radiology* 1993; 186:316–318.

7. Moore W. Does tandem lesion mean tandem risk in patients with carotid artery disease? *J Vasc Surg* 1988;7: 454–455.

8. Heiserman JE, Drayer BP, Fram EK. Carotid artery stenosis: Clinical efficacy of two-dimensional time-of-flight MR angiography. *Radiology* 1992;182:761–768.

9. Huston J, Lewis BD, Weibers DO, et al. Carotid artery: Prospective blinded comparison of two-dimensional time-of-flight MR angiography with conventional angiography and Doppler ultrasound. *Radiology* 1993;186: 339–344.

10. Polak JF, Bajakian RL, O'Leary DH, et al. Detection of internal carotid stenosis: Comparison of MR angiography, color Doppler sonography and arteriography. *Radiology* 1992;182:35–40.

11. Polak JF, Kalina P, Donaldson MC, et al. Carotid endarterectomy: Preoperative evaluation of candidates with combined Doppler sonography and MR angiography. (work in progress). *Radiology* 1993;186:333–338.

12. Masaryk TJ, Obuchowski NA. Noninvasive carotid imaging: Caveat emptor. *Radiology* 1993;186:325–329.

13. Polak JF. Noninvasive carotid evaluation: Carpe diem. *Radiology* 1993;186:329–331.

14. Anderson C, Saloner D, Lee R, et al. Assessment of carotid artery stenosis by MR angiography: Comparison with x-ray angiography and color-coded Doppler ultrasound. *AJNR* 1992;13:989–1003.

15. Levy C, Laissy JP, Raveau V, et al. Carotid and vertebral artery dissection: Three dimensional time-of-flight MR angiography and MR imaging versus conventional angiography. *Radiology* 1994;190:97–103.

16. Oneson SR, Lewis JS, Smith AS. Case report. MR angiography of Takayasu arteritis. *J Comput Assist Tomogr* 1992; 16(3):478–480.

17. Weintraub MI. Beauty parlor stroke syndrome. Report of five cases. *JAMA* 1993;269(16):2085–2086.

21

Magnetic Resonance Imaging Assessment of Diffusion and Perfusion

Charles R.G. Guttmann, M.D., Ferenc A. Jolesz, M.D.

INTRODUCTION

Magnetic resonance imaging (MRI) contrast can easily be manipulated to reflect a variety of physico-chemical and physiological properties of the tissues and organs studied. The purpose of this chapter is to introduce the reader to the clinical applications of diffusion- and perfusion-weighted MRI. These methods assess physiological or pathophysiological parameters in superposition to highly resolved anatomical information. Both diffusion and perfusion MRI depict the motion of water molecules.

Water *self-diffusion* in tissues refers to molecular-scale diffusive movements of interstitial as well as intracellular water, which may be influenced by the presence, permeability characteristics, and spatial distribution of structures such as membranes and other cellular components.

Perfusion is a combination of different phenomena, which include capillary flow and transcapillary exchange of water and solutes (oxygen and nutrients) between the parenchyma and intravascular spaces. The water molecules within and around the capillaries are subject to coherent (flow) as well as incoherent (diffu-

sive) motion. It is useful to distinguish these two components because two conceptually different MRI approaches to measure perfusion have been proposed.[1,2]

DIFFUSION IMAGING

In diffusion-weighted MRI, contrast is provided by local differences in the self-diffusion (Brownian motion) of water molecules. In self-diffusion the mean displacement of the water molecules is null and the motion is called *incoherent*. This is in contrast to *coherent motion*, with a net velocity, that is, flow phenomena.

Magnetic field gradients can be added to a variety of pulse sequences in such a way as to cause net dephasing of incoherently moving but not stationary or flowing spins. This causes signal attenuation when incoherently moving spins are present in a measured voxel.[3]

Since the measurement of diffusion involves water mobility, motion-related artifacts are a major limitation of diffusion-weighted imaging.[4] Ultrafast echo-planar imaging (EPI) with diffusion-sensitive gradients has been proposed to overcome this problem.[5]

Four main applications of diffusion-weighted imaging in the brain are currently under investigation.

1. The assessment of cerebral ischemia and the differentiation among various stages in the course of an insult (acute, subacute, or chronic).

Extensive efforts have been made to characterize experimental ischemic insults in animal brains.[6-8] It has been suggested that diffusion weighting can detect early ischemic changes in brain tissue with higher sensitivity than T_2-weighted imaging.[6,8] Results in humans confirmed these animal results by demonstrating lower diffusion (relative to control regions) in areas with a normal appearance on T_2-weighted images in the early hours after the onset of ischemic symptoms[9,10] (Fig. 21-1). Multiple pathogenetic factors, including reduced brain pulsation, localized hypothermia, and cytotoxic (intracellular) edema, have been suggested to participate in the slowing of diffusive water motion in acutely ischemic tissue, but no conclusive demonstration of their relative contributions has been presented.[11] These results indicate that diffusion-weighted imaging may play a major role in the early management and therapeutic evaluation of ischemic insults of the brain.

2. The differentiation among different components of a tumor (neoplastic cells, edema, necrosis, vascularity).

It would be useful to be able to distinguish the various features of a tumor, thus enabling the monitoring of drug effects on distinct features (e.g., edema, necrosis, neoplastic elements). The limitations and possibilities of this approach for gliomas have been discussed extensively.[12] Using diffusion-weighted imaging, Tsuruda et al. have evaluated its use in the characterization of extra-axial tumors.[13,14] They have pointed to a potential benefit in the noninvasive differential diagnosis among various pathologies, such as arachnoid cysts and epidermoid tumors. Steen has proposed the use of diffusion weighting to evaluate regional differences in tumor-associated edema for the purpose of indirectly estimating tumor perfusion.[15] Characterization of primary neoplasms of the human central nervous system (CNS) with diffusion-weighted imaging has been attempted but is in the preliminary stages[16-18] (Fig. 21-2).

3. The determination of the spatial orientation of white matter (WM) tracts in the brain (assessment of WM anisotropy).

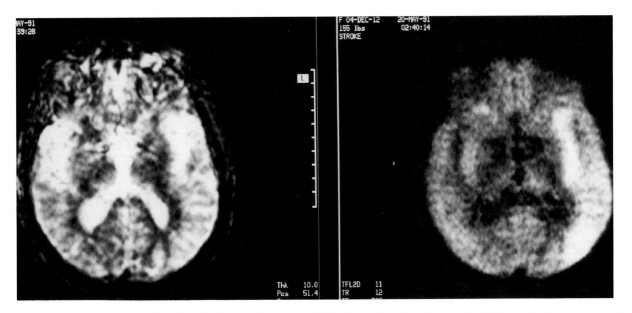

Fig. 21-1   Diffusion imaging of stroke. The images show an axial brain section 6 hr after a left middle cerebral artery occlusion, as seen with diffusion imaging on conventional MRI hardware (Siemens Magnetom, 1.5 Tesla). Left: turbo STEAM sequence with no additional diffusion gradients. Right: same pulse sequence with the addition of diffusion gradients (9 mT/m, $b = 372$ s/mm^2) in x, y and z directions. A hyperintense area indicative of lower diffusion is present in the left temporoparietal region. (Courtesy of Dr. Steven Warach, Beth Israel Hospital, Boston)

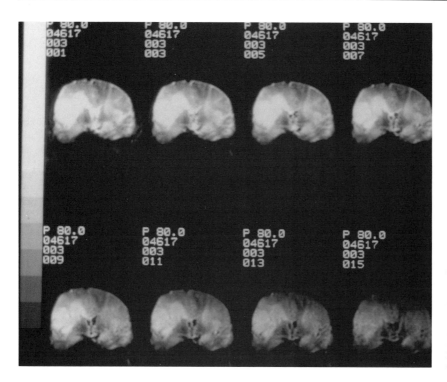

Fig. 21-2 Diffusion EPI of tumors. A coronal slice at the level of a tumor in a human brain was repeatedly assessed with varying diffusion-sensitizing gradient strengths (the lowest to highest gradient strength is from top left to bottom right). The effect of the gradient strength on image contrast can be appreciated. A pixel-by-pixel map of diffusion coefficients can be computed (see an example of a calculated diffusion image from a different subject in Fig. 21-3). (Courtesy of Dr. Denis Le Bihan, NIH, Bethesda, MD)

In the WM, it can be expected that water diffusion will be constrained by the directionality of the myelinated nerve fibers. The degree of signal attenuation (darkening in the image) will then depend on the relationship (angle) between the orientation of the fibers and that of the magnetic field gradient (Fig. 21-3). Several groups have shown the feasibility of this approach and are currently developing tridimensional anisotropy maps of the brain.[19,20] In terms of clinical application, this approach has already been used to assess varying degrees of myelination in CNS development,[21] as well as WM disorders such as leukomalacia, multiple sclerosis, and leukodystrophy associated with muscular distrophy.[22,23] These efforts may lead to a better understanding of the course and effects of myelination in humans. They may also prove useful for diagnosis and characterization, as well as for treatment evaluation of these or other myelin-related pathologies, including Wallerian degeneration and dysmyelinations. Because expansive and invasive processes in infection or neoplasia can disrupt the directionality of water diffusion in WM fiber tracts, images mapping anisotropy could prove useful in the assessment of such processes.[24,25]

4. Temperature monitoring.

The use of MRI to monitor thermal as well as structural changes during minimally invasive interventional

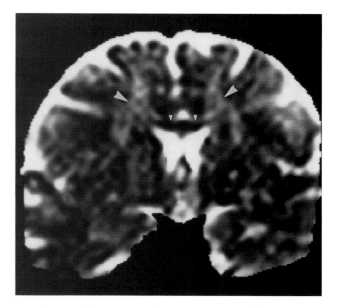

Fig. 21-3 Diffusion EPI of white matter anisotropy. Calculated diffusion image of a coronal brain slice. The diffusion-sensitizing gradient was applied in the z direction. Higher diffusion in the z direction is seen in white matter tracts that are parallel to the z-axis (large arrowheads), while in the corpus callosum (small arrowheads), where fibers are perpendicular to the z-axis, diffusion in the z direction is low. (Courtesy of Dr. Denis Le Bihan, NIH, Bethesda, MD)

procedures in the brain, using hyperthermia, laser-thermia, cryosurgery, and focused ultrasound heating, is currently being evaluated.[26–28] T_1- as well as diffusion-weighted imaging has been used. The feasibility of monitoring and controlling the deposition of disruptive energy and its effects on target tissues and their surroundings, using high-resolution images, has been demonstrated.[29–31] Interventions currently considered too hazardous may become applicable with MRI guidance.

IMAGING OF PERFUSION

Tracer Methods

Several authors have suggested a number of MRI tracer methods analogous to non-MRI tracer methods for perfusion measurement. Deuterated and ^{17}O water have been used to assess tissue washout.[32,33] Fluorine uptake experiments have been performed.[34] Inflow has been estimated by using gadolinium- or dysprosium-based contrast agents as tracers and echoplanar MRI for detection.[35,36] Finally, radiofrequency labeling of spins has been proposed.[37]

Currently, the most readily available MRI method uses a bolus of a contrast agent, which affects magnetic susceptibility (by causing local magnetic field gradients between intra- and extravascular spaces due to its intravascular compartmentalization), thus affecting T_2^*-weighted images and/or longitudinal (T_1) relaxation times.[36,38] The dynamics of contrast enhancement in the brain are monitored with fast imaging techniques such as EPI[36,38,39] (Fig. 21-4).

Blood volume maps can be obtained by surface integration of the curves representing signal intensity versus time in each pixel of an image. This measurement does not reflect transcapillary diffusion (the tracers used remain in the intravascular compartment under physiological conditions) and is therefore not really a measurement of perfusion. The mean transit time of these intravascular tracers can be accurately calculated only when the arterial input function (time course of the arterial concentration of the tracer) is known.[36]

Tumor Vascularization
Dynamic MRI tracer measurements in tumors may simultaneously provide an index of tumor vascularity and blood–brain barrier permeability.[16,36,40]

The differentiation of three phases in the uptake of a contrast agent by a brain tumor has been proposed using dynamic T_1-weighted EPI:[38]

1. The vascular phase (indicative of tumor vascularity).
2. The diffusive phase (indicative of vascular permeability, i.e., the degree of blood–brain barrier impairment).
3. The washout phase (indicative of vascular permeability).

In a study using susceptibility-sensitive, contrast-enhanced, dynamic MRI, a trend to higher blood volume values has been reported for high-grade primary brain tumors compared to low-grade ones.[41] This study also highlighted the presence of marked heterogeneity in the blood volume maps of the tumors, particularly those of high-grade lesions.

MRI-based estimates of tumor vascularity may reflect histological findings. This method has the potential to differentiate necrotic areas from more viable neoplastic components of a heterogeneous mass and may also provide information about potential drug delivery to areas of neoplasia.[40]

Cerebral Ischemia and Infarction
Contrast-enhanced, susceptibility-sensitive, dynamic MRI has proven useful in detecting early alterations of the brain in the course of an ischemic insult in animals and humans.[41–44] It also holds promise in the detection and delineation of reversible cerebral ischemia (ischemic penumbra) accompanying a large number of diseases, as well as in the evaluation of therapeutic approaches to stroke-like pathologies.[41]

Functional Imaging
Blood volume maps show changes due to functional cortical activation.[45] However, most recently, the feasibility of studies of cortical activation has also been demonstrated with nonenhanced, native susceptibility-sensitive MRI methods.[46,47] The latter appear to be more practical for most potential applications, although the limitations as well as the potential uses of both techniques need to be determined more extensively.

Pseudodiffusion Measurements

Le Bihan et al., using the assumption that the measured voxels contain capillary segments with random orientation and therefore random flow direction, proposed using diffusion-weighted MRI techniques to assess the water motion aspects of capillary perfusion.[48] This measurement has also been referred to as *slow flow* or *pseudodiffusion measurement*.

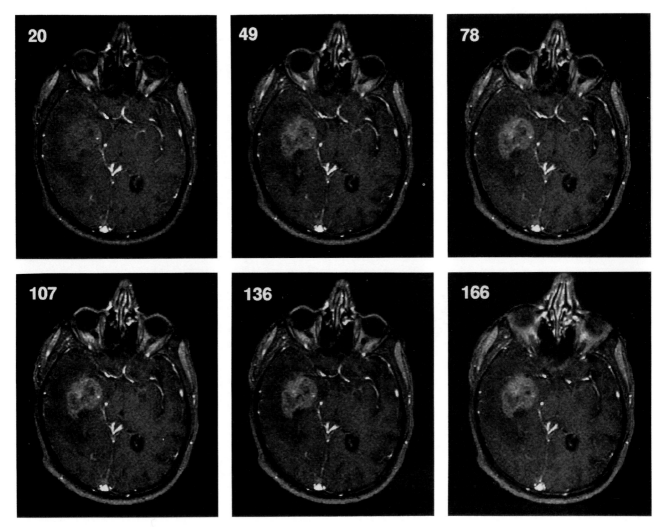

Fig. 21-4 Dynamic contrast-enhanced imaging of tumors. Repeated T_1 measurements with a gradient-echo technique were performed on an axial slice through a right hemispheric tumor after an IV bolus injection of 10 ml 0.1 mM gadolinium-DTPA (Magnevist, Berlex). The slice is shown at six time points (the number of seconds after the injection of the contrast agent is noted for each image). Contrast accumulation is seen, and a pixel-by-pixel computation of contrast accumulation can be performed. (Courtesy of Dr. Richard B. Schwartz, Brigham and Women's Hospital, Boston)

Depending on the strength and duration of the gradients applied, different motion amplitude ranges can be targeted. When the measured voxel is large enough compared to the capillary size, capillary flow may be viewed as incoherent motion. In addition, the discrimination of signal loss due to self-diffusion of water in tissue, as opposed to that caused by slow capillary flow, may be feasible. The relative fractions of these two components are calculated assuming that the function relating signal intensity to the so-called gradient b-factor (which reflects gradient strength and duration) will contain two distinguishable exponential components.[48,49] The images can reflect these two parameters qualitatively and perhaps quantitatively,[48] although serious criticism to the latter has been voiced.[50]

SUMMARY

MRI can provide significant information about the mobility of water molecules in the brain, with no or minimal invasivity. A variety of potential applications of these measurements of water diffusion and brain "perfusion" has been described. Although some of them hold significant promise for the diagnosis, characterization, and management of cerebral disease, further evaluation is needed to establish their clinical value.

REFERENCES

1. Le Bihan D. Magnetic resonance imaging of perfusion. *Magn Reson Med* 1990;14:283–292.

2. Henkelman MR. Does IVIM measure classical perfusion? *Magn Reson Med* 1990;16:470–475.

3. Le Bihan D, Turner R, Douek P, et al. Diffusion MR imaging: Clinical applications. *AJR* 1992;159:591–599.

4. Chenevert TL, Pipe JG. Effect of bulk tissue motion on quantitative perfusion and diffusion magnetic resonance imaging. *Magn Reson Med* 1991;19:261–265.

5. Turner R, Le Bihan D, Chesnick AS. Echo-planar imaging of diffusion and perfusion. *Magn Reson Med* 1991;19:247–253.

6. Moseley ME, Cohen Y, Mintorovitch J, et al. Early detection of regional cerebral ischemia in cats: Comparison of diffusion- and T_2-weighted MRI and spectroscopy. *Magn Reson Med* 1990;14:330–346.

7. Kucharczyk J, Mintorovitch J, Asgari HS, et al. Diffusion/perfusion MR imaging of acute cerebral ischemia. *Magn Reson Med* 1991;19:311–315.

8. Berry I, Gigaud M, Manelfe C. Experimental focal cerebral ischaemia assessed with IVIM*-MRI in the acute phase at 0.5 tesla. *Neuroradiology* 1992;34:135–140.

9. Chien D, Kwong KK, Gress DR, et al. MR diffusion imaging of cerebral infarction in humans. *AJNR* 1992;13:1097–1102.

10. Warach S, Chien D, Li W, et al. Fast magnetic resonance diffusion-weighted imaging of acute human stroke. *Neurology* 1992;42:1717–1723 (see also erratum in *Neurology* 1992;42:2192).

11. Sevick RJ, Kanda F, Mintorovitch J, et al. Cytotoxic brain edema: Assessment with diffusion-weighted MR imaging. *Radiology* 1992;185:687–690.

12. Jolesz FA, Schwartz RB, Guttmann CRG. Diagnostic imaging of intracranial gliomas, in Black PMcL, Lampson LA (eds): *Astrocytomas: Diagnosis, Treatment, and Biology.* Cambridge: Blackwell Scientific, 1993, pp 37–49.

13. Tsuruda JS, Chew WM, Moseley ME, et al. Diffusion-weighted MR imaging of the brain: Value of differentiating between extraaxial cysts and epidermoid tumors. *AJNR* 1990;11:925–931.

14. Tsuruda JS, Chew WM, Moseley ME, et al. Diffusion-weighted MR imaging of extraaxial tumors. *Magn Reson Med* 1991;19:316–320.

15. Steen RG. Edema and tumor perfusion: Characterization by quantitative ^{1}H MR imaging. *AJR* 1992;158:259–264.

16. Le Bihan D, Douek P, Argyropoulou M, et al. Diffusion and perfusion magnetic resonance imaging in brain tumors. *Top Magn Reson Imaging* 19;5:25–31.

17. Gazit IE, Aronen HJ, Davis TJ, et al. Diffusion, rCBV and T2 correlation in primary human CNS malignancies. *Proc SMRM 1993* 1993;1:487.

18. Hooper J, Rajan S, Rosa L, et al. Application of diffusion imaging to monitor tumor growth and response to chemotherapy. *Book of Abstracts SMRM 1990* 1990;1:371.

19. Davis TL, Wedeen VJ, Weisskoff RM, et al. White matter tract visualization by echo-planar MRI. *Proc. SMRM 1993* 1993;1:289.

20. Basser PJ, Mattiello J, Le Bihan D. MR imaging of fiber-tract direction and diffusion in anisotropic tissues. *Proc SMRM 1993* 1993;1:288.

21. Sakuma H, Nomura Y, Takeda K, et al. Adult and neonatal human brain: Diffusional anisotropy and myelination wih diffusion-weighted MR imaging. *Radiology* 1991;180:229–233.

22. Rutherford MA, Cowan FM, Manzur AY, et al. MR imaging of anisotropically restricted diffusion in the brain of neonates and infants. *JCAT* 1991;15:188–198.

23. Larsson HBW, Thomsen C, Fredericksen J, et al. In vivo magnetic resonance diffusion measurement in the brain of patients with multiple sclerosis. *Magn Reson Imag* 1992;10:7–12.

24. Doran M, Hajnal JV, Van Bruggen N, et al. Normal and abnormal white matter tracts shown by MR imaging using directional diffusion weighted sequences. *JCAT* 1990;14:865–873.

25. Hajnal JV, Doran M, Hall AS, et al. MR imaging of anisotropically restricted diffusion of water in the nervous system: Technical, anatomic, and pathologic considerations. *JCAT* 1991;15:1–18.

26. Bleier AR, Jolesz FA, Cohen MS, et al. Real-time magnetic resonance imaging of laser heat deposition in tissue. *Magn Reson Med* 1991;21:132–137.

27. Delannoy J, Chen C-N, Turner R, et al. Noninvasive temperature imaging using diffusion MRI. *Magn Reson Med* 1991;19:333–339.

28. Cline HE, Schenck JF, Hynynen K, et al. MR-guided focused ultrasound surgery. *JCAT* 1992;16:956–965.

29. Higuchi N, Bleier AR, Jolesz FA, et al. Magnetic resonance imaging of the acute effects of interstitial neodymium: YAG laser irradiation on tissues. *Invest Radiol* 1992;27:814–821.

30. El-Ouahabi A, Guttmann CRG, Hushek SG, et al. MRI guided interstitial laser therapy in a rat malignant glioma model. *Las Surg Med* 1993;13:503–510.

31. Matsumoto R, Selig AM, Colucci VM, et al. MR monitoring during cryotherapy in the liver: Predictability of histologic outcome. *JMRI* 1993;3:770–776.

32. Ackerman JJH, Ewy CS, Becker NN, et al. Deuterium nuclear magnetic resonance measurements of blood flow

and tissue perfusion employing ^2H_2O as a freely diffusible tracer. *Proc Natl Acad Sci. USA* 1987;84:4099–4102.

33. Kwong KK, Hopkins AL, Belliveau JW, et al. Proton NMR imaging of cerebral blood flow using $H_2{}^{17}O$. *Magn Reson Med* 1991;22:154–158.

34. Ewing JR, Branch CA, Helpern JA, et al. Cerebral blood flow measured by NMR indicator dilution in cats. *Stroke* 1989;20:259–267.

35. Kucharczyk J, Roberts T, Moseley ME, et al. Contrast-enhanced perfusion-sensitive MR imaging in the diagnosis of cerebrovascular disorders. *JMRI* 1993;3:241–245.

36. Rosen BR, Belliveau JW, Vevea JM, et al. Perfusion imaging with NMR contrast agents. *Magn Reson Med* 1990;14:249–265.

37. Zhang W, Williams DS, Koretsky AP. Measurement of rat brain perfusion by NMR using spin labeling of arterial water: In vivo determination of the degree of spin labeling. *Magn Reson Med* 1993;29:416–421.

38. Gowland P, Mansfield P, Bullock P, et al. Dynamic studies of gadolinium uptake in brain tumors using inversion-recovery echo-planar imaging. *Magn Reson Med* 1992;26:241–258.

39. Moseley ME, Sevick R, Wendland MF, et al. Ultrafast magnetic resonance imaging: Diffusion and perfusion. *Can Assoc Radiol J* 1991;42:31–38.

40. Aronen HJ, Cohen MS, Belliveau JW, et al. Ultrafast imaging of brain tumors. *Top Magn Reson Imaging* 1993;5:14–24.

41. Rosen BR, Belliveau JW, Aronen HJ, et al. Susceptibility contrast imaging of cerebral blood volume: Human experience. *Magn Reson Med* 1991;22:293–299.

42. Kucharczyk J, Roberts T, Moseley ME, et al. Contrast-enhanced perfusion-sensitive MR imaging in the diagnosis of cerebrovascular disorders. *JMRI* 1993;3:241–245.

43. Kucharczyk J, Mintorovitch J, Asgari HS, et al. Diffusion/perfusion MR imaging of acute cerebral ischemia. *Magn Reson Med* 1991;19:311–315.

44. Warach S, Wei L, Ronthal M, et al. Acute cerebral ischemia: Evaluation with dynamic contrast-enhanced MR imaging and MR angiography. *Radiology* 1992;182:41–47.

45. Belliveau JW, Kennedy DN, McKinstry RC, et al. Functional mapping of the human visual cortex by magnetic resonance imaging. *Science* 1991;254:716–719.

46. Ogawa S, Lee T-M, Nayak AS, et al. Oxygenation-sensitive contrast in magnetic resonance image of rodent brain at high magnetic fields. *Magn Reson Med* 1990;14:68–78.

47. Kwong KK, Belliveau JW, Chesler DA, et al. Dynamic magnetic resonance imaging of human brain activity during primary sensory stimulation. *Proc Natl Acad Sci USA* 1992;89:5675–5679.

48. Le Bihan D, Breton E, Lallemand D, et al. Separation of diffusion and perfusion in intravoxel incoherent motion MR imaging. *Radiology* 1988;168:497–505.

49. Turner R, Le Bihan D, Maier J, et al. Echo-planar imaging of intravoxel incoherent motion. *Radiology* 1990;177:407–414.

50. King MD, van Bruggen N, Busza AL, et al. Perfusion and diffusion MR imaging. *Magn Reson Med* 1992;24:288–301.

22

Proton Magnetic Resonance Spectroscopy of the Human Brain

R. Gilberto González, M.D.

INTRODUCTION

The routine clinical application of proton nuclear magnetic resonance spectroscopy (^{1}H MRS) for the study of the brain is imminent. I believe that clinical MRS will follow a course similar to that of MR angiography, that is, it will be applied as an add-on sequence to routine MRI examinations. For practical reasons, the proton will be the nucleus studied in the first widespread applications of MRS. Most important, no new MR hardware is needed. Also, the proton is the most sensitive MR nucleus that allows an adequate signal/noise ratio of a small volume.

Any new diagnostic tool must meet two basic requirements. First, it must provide clinically important information that will significantly aid the diagnosis, prognosis, and/or therapy; this information must be unattainable by other means, or competing methods must be less safe or more costly. Second, the new method must be practical in the clinical setting. In the case of proton MRS, simple methods for water suppression, shimming, and automated analysis of the MR spectrum are needed. Recent advances have fulfilled all of these requirements.

THE PROTON MR SPECTRUM

The proton MR spectrum provides qualitative and quantitative chemical information. The underlying physics of the method is identical to that of MRI. Figure 22-1 shows an axial T_2-weighted image of the brain. If we choose to collect the MR signal (from the voxel designated in the figure) in basically the same manner that we collect the MRI data, but with the exception that we turn off the gradients after the voxel is excited by radiofrequency (RF) pulses, we will get the spectrum shown in Fig. 22-1. This is a simple spectrum consisting of a single resonance; it is the spectrum of water. The position of the resonance along the horizontal axis allows us to make this chemical identification. Molecules other than water would have resonances that occur in different positions along the horizontal axis. The area under the peak is directly proportional to the water concentration. Thus, qualitative and quantitative information is provided. This example reminds us that MR images are spatially encoded MR spectra of water.

The water spectrum is not very informative. Can we obtain any more information about brain chemistry? Yes, but we need to suppress the water resonance to see these other chemicals. This suppression is required because other MR-observable brain molecules have concentrations that are 1/1,000th to 1/10,000th the concentration of water. If we selectively suppress water, we will obtain the spectrum shown in Fig. 22-2. As is readily apparent, with water suppression we obtain a complex spectrum teeming with brain chemistry. I would like to emphasize that this spectrum was acquired on a commercial magnetic resonance imaging

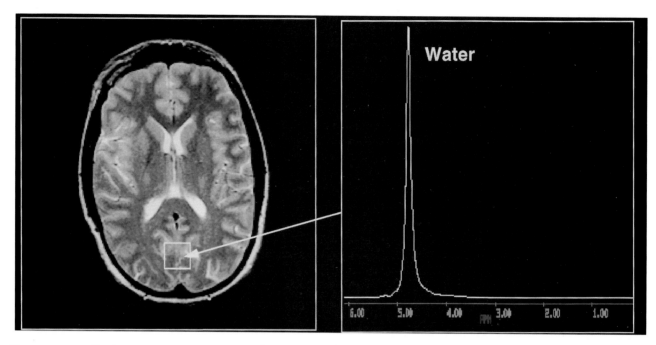

Fig. 22-1 Localized proton MR spectroscopy. The image on the left is a single slice from an axial T2 weighted image set acquired from a normal volunteer. The proton MR spectrum shown on the right was acquired from a single voxel in the location specified by the box in the image on the left.

(MRI) scanner in less than 5 min. Note the largest resonance, labeled "NAA," which stands for *n*- acetylaspartic acid. NAA is a very interesting molecule because it occurs in high concentrations and it is localized exclusively in neurons. Thus it may be an excellent marker of neuronal death or dysfunction.

AN EXAMPLE FROM ANIMAL EXPERIMENTS

I will illustrate the potential benefits of MRS by describing experimental work performed on rats in our laboratory by Alex Guimaraes.[1] In these experiments we introduced a small amount of excitotoxin into the rat striatum on one side. After 2 or 3 weeks, we performed MRI and proton MRS on these animals. The spectroscopy was in the form of spectroscopic images (also known as *chemical shift images* and *metabolite maps*). That is, we suppressed the water and then spatially encoded the remaining resonances. In this fashion, we can make images of different molecules—an image of NAA, for example.

Figure 22-3 shows the brain T_2-weighted water MRI image and the NAA spectroscopic image of a rat that was lesioned in the right striatum with an excitotoxin.

Great damage was induced, as is evident on the MRI scan. The spectroscopic image shows asymmetry at the level of NAA. This shows that there is neuronal loss and/or dysfunction in the right hemisphere of the rat. A more illuminating example is shown in Fig. 22-4. Once again, we lesioned the right striatum, but with a very low dose of excitotoxin. The MRI image reveals no abnormality; the NAA spectroscopic image clearly shows a loss of NAA on the right side. This animal was sacrificed, and biochemical measurements were made which showed that there was indeed neuronal loss in the right hemisphere. This example shows how MRS can provide information not available by MRI.

TECHNICAL ADVANCES

The routine application of MRS requires rapid, automated shimming (which makes the magnetic field as homogeneous as possible), water suppression, and spectral processing. Important advances have been made in these areas. Before describing these advances, I will discuss the issues of field strength and spatial localization. Most of the MRS work on humans has been performed at 1.5 Tesla. There are two advantages of higher field strength: there is an improved signal/

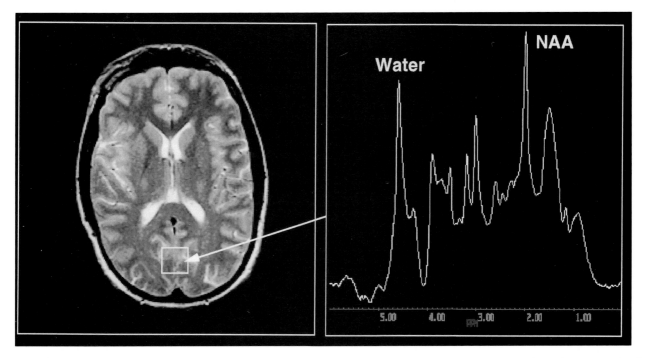

Fig. 22-2 Water suppressed localized MR spectroscopy. The spectrum shown on the right was obtained from the same individual as in Fig. 22-1 and from the same location. The difference between this spectrum and that of Fig. 22-1 is that the water resonance has been suppressed using frequency selective RF pulses followed by gradient crushers.

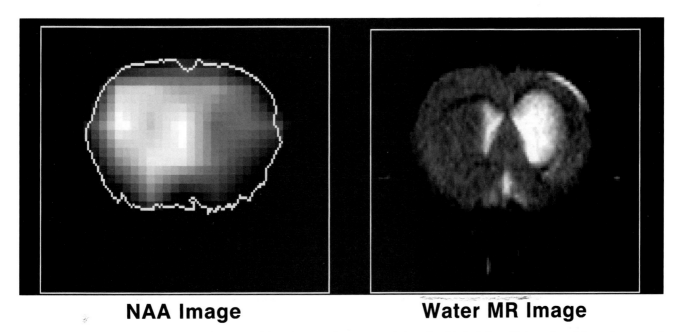

Fig. 22-3 Chemical shift imaging of neuronal loss in rat. The rat was injected with kainic acid into the right striatum and imaged several weeks later. The image on the right is a T2 weighted transaxial cut through the level of the injured corpus striatum. On the left is a chemical shift image of the neuron specific molecule, NAA. The relative depletion of NAA is demonstrated by decreased signal intensity in the right hemisphere.

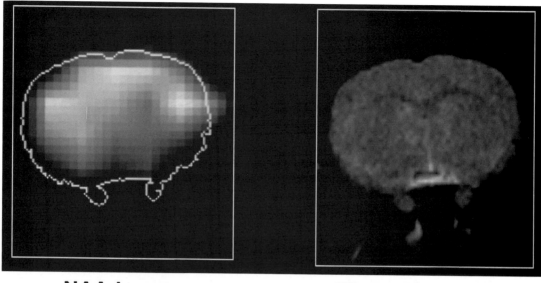

NAA Image   **Water MR Image**

Fig. 22-4 Chemical shift imaging of neuronal loss in a rat treated with NMDA. The animal was injected with n-methyl-d-aspartic acid (NMDA), a milder excitotoxin than kainic acid, into the right striatum. The T2 weighted image on the right does not reveal a significant lesion. The chemical shift image on the left demonstrates loss of NAA.

noise ratio, and there is greater spectral dispersion at higher fields which better separates different resonances. Thus, it is very likely that clinical MRS will be confined to systems of at least 1.5 Tesla.

Spatial localization with proton MRS is achieved by single-voxel selection or spectroscopic imaging. Single-voxel localization is simple and may be easily appended to a routine MRI study. However, only one location can be sampled at a time. In spectroscopic imaging, a relatively large area is selected and phase encoding with magnetic field gradients is used to spatially encode the spectra in one or two dimensions. The resulting data may then be reconstructed into separate images for each region of the spectrum. The disadvantage of this approach is that it is substantially more time-consuming than the single-voxel methods. For this reason, it is unlikely that proton CSI will become incorporated as an add-on sequence. However, the situation may change rapidly if a clear diagnostic role for spectroscopic imaging is demonstrated.

Proton MRS is far more demanding than standard MRI in its requirement for high magnetic field homogeneity and water suppression. Shimming to achieve high field homogeneity and water suppression can be performed manually, but this can be very time-consuming and, thus, impractical. However, recently, Webb, Hurd, and colleagues, under the direction of Wedmid in the MRS group at General Electric, have developed auto-

mated shimming and water suppression algorithms that are very robust.[2] Importantly, they have bundled their shimming and water suppression algorithms together. Thus, a single command results in the automated shimming and water of a voxel chosen from a scout MR image. The method takes less than 5 min to perform, so it is competitive timewise for the most experienced operators. We routinely use this method at the MGH Imaging Center for acquiring MR spectra during routine brain MRI examinations. The spectrum shown in Fig. 22-2 was acquired in this fashion.

The automation of spectral processing will have a role in the rapid dissemination of clinical MRS. Currently, the processing of MRS spectra acquired during a busy schedule is performed off-line on a separate workstation or during off hours. The task requires experience and judgment by the operator. However, the processing can also be automated, as demonstrated by Ross.[3] A commercial version of this process will soon be available. Thus, the major technical obstacles to the routine acquisition of proton MRS spectra in a clinical setting have been overcome.

CLINICAL APPLICATIONS

As I stressed in the Introduction, clinical proton MRS must provide information that is diagnostically or ther-

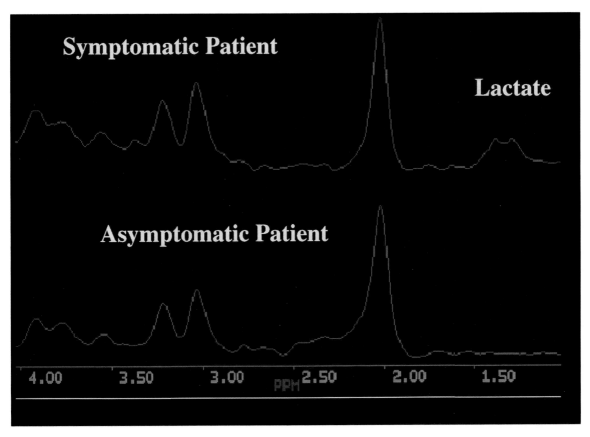

Fig. 22-5 Single voxel, water suppressed proton MR spectra from patients with Huntington's disease. The spectra were acquired from occipital cortex of a symptomatic patient (top) and an asymptomatic patient (bottom). Note the presence of lactate visible only in the symptomatic patient spectrum. (Spectra courtesy of Dr. Bruce Jenkins).

apeutically valuable and must be more cost effective than other methods. Potential clinical areas which have been investigated can be grouped into neurodegenerative, ischemic/hypoxic, neoplastic, and metabolic diseases. I will briefly cover a portion of these topics.

To date, many proton MRS studies have been conducted on adult neurodegenerative disorders including Alzheimer's disease, the AIDS dementia complex, and multiple sclerosis.[4-7] In the majority of cases, neuronal loss and/or dysfunction, as measured by a decline in the level of NAA relative to other compounds, have been amply demonstrated. In multiple sclerosis, Arnold has shown that areas of plaque have decreased NAA. In Alzheimer's disease and the AIDS dementia complex, a generalized decrease in NAA has been shown. In these latter two dementias, it has also been observed that there is an elevation in the concentration of myo-inositol in the brain which occurs late in the dementing process. The role of myo-inositol in the brain is unknown; the reason it is abnormally elevated is similarly unclear.

The group of ischemic/hypoxic disorders, stroke, near-drowning, and similar insults may be studied with proton MRS. Ross and his colleagues have demonstrated that in near-drowning events, the MR spectrum can provide important prognostic information. If the spectrum is normal, full recovery is expected; if, on the other hand, there is a substantial decrease in NAA, there will be significant neurological deficits if the victim survives. The study of stroke and head trauma by MRS has also been shown to be of value.

There are many other examples of the clinical utility of MRS wich I cannot discuss in this short review. I would like to conclude with an example of a neurodengenerative disorder, Huntington's disease, which is also a metabolic disorder. Figure 22-5 shows two spectra obtained by Dr. Bruce Jenkins at the Massachusetts General Hospital's NMR Center.[8] Both spectra were acquired from the occipital lobes. The top spectrum is from a symptomatic patient, and the lower one is from an asymptomatic individual. The symptomatic spectrum has a detectable resonance from lactic acid which is not normally observed. This indicates an abnormality in brain oxidative metabolism in this patient. Based on this and other data, patients are now being treated with agents that improve mitochondrial function, and the therapy is being monitored with MRS.

We have entered a new era in neuroradiology. Through the application of proton MRS, we are now able to provide previously unattainable chemical information about the human brain which can be beneficial to patients. This has been made possible by recent technical advances which allow high-quality MR spectra to be acquired during a routine brain MRS examination. The ultimate utility of this method in clinical practice remains to be defined. It is my hope that readers of this chapter have gained sufficient understanding of the method to be able to follow the development of MRS intelligently.

REFERENCES

1. Guimaraes AR, Carr CA, Schwartz P, et al. Quantitative in vivo 1H MRS of excitotoxicity in rats. *Proc Soc Mag Res* 1994;1413.

2. Webb P, Sailasuta N, Kohler S, et al. Automated single-voxel proton MRS: Technical development and multisite verification. *Magn Reson Med* 1994;31:365–373.

3. Kreis R, Ross BD, Farrow NA, et al. Metabolic disorders of the brain in chronic hepatic encephalopathy detected with H-1 MR spectroscopy. *Radiology* 1992;182:19–27.

4. Miller BL, Moats RA, Shonk T, et al. Alzheimer disease: Depiction of increased cerebral myo-inositol with proton MR spectroscopy. *Radiology* 1993;187:433–437.

5. Meyerhoff DJ, MacKay S, Bachman L, et al. Reduced brain N-acetylaspartate suggests neuronal loss in cognitively impaired human immunodeficiency virus-seropositive individuals. *Neurology* 1993;43:509–515.

6. Jarvik JG, Lenkinski RE, Grossman RI, et al. Proton MR spectroscopy of HIV-infected patients: Characterization of abnormalities with imaging and clinical correlation. *Radiology* 1993;186:739–744.

7. Arnold DL, Matthews PM, Francis G, et al. Proton magnetic resonance spectroscopy of human brain *in vivo* in the evaluation of multiple sclerosis: Assessment of the load of disease. *Magn Res Med* 1990;14:154–159.

8. Jenkins BG, Koroshetz WJ, Beal MF, et al. Evidence for impairment of energy metabolism in vivo in Huntington's disease using localized 1H NMR spectroscopy. *Neurology* 1993;43:2689–2695.

23

Nuclear Medicine: Single Photon Emission Computed Tomography

Wei-Jen Shih, M.D., Hans J. Biersack, M.D., Benjamin M.W. Tsui, Ph.D.

INTRODUCTION

Conventional brain imaging relies on the breakdown of the blood–brain barrier (BBB), allowing nondiffusible tracers to cross the BBB, localizing in the lesion(s) in the brain. The BBB is a unique arrangement of capillary endothelial cells having a large surface area of lipid bilayer which serves to isolate and protect the brain from extraneous chemical or bacterial influences.

Changes in the BBB occur in brain lesions, permitting nondiffusible radiopharmaceuticals to cross. In addition to breakdown the BBB, localization of radiopharmaceuticals in the brain tumor include abnormal permeability, increased vascularity, pinocytosis, cerebral edema, increased size of the extracellular space, and/or direct intracellular uptake. Nondiffusible radiotracers include Tc-99m diethylene triamine pentaacetic acid (DTPA) and Tc-99m glucohepatonate. A conventional brain study should include a radionuclide angiogram, immediate blood pool images, and delayed (1- to 3-hr) images. A cerebral flow study is an integral part of conventional brain imaging.

A radionuclide cerebral angiogram can detect the absence/decrease in flow in the carotid arteries and/or cerebral arteries that are not demonstrable with a static brain image or with computed tomography (CT) or magnetic resonance imaging (MRI). Compared with static brain images, a cerebral angiogram can easily show arteriovenous malformations, infarcts, subdural and epidural hematomas, and cerebral brain death. A flow study can be completed within 1 min.

Cerebral death in a flow study is marked by absence of internal carotid arterial and/or cerebral flow; subdural or epidural hematomas cause displacement of the middle cerebral artery medially. Cerebral infarction may demonstrate diminished middle or anterior cerebral artery flow in the arterial phase. Static brain images may not become positive for 7–14 days following the onset of symptoms.

As a result of the widespread availability of CT and MRI, the utilization of conventional brain imaging has been reduced. Conventional brain imaging is used most often in a complementary role when a CT or MRI scan is negative, equivocal, or contraindicated. However, certain intracranial disease processes, including infectious processes such as herpes encephalitis, can be detected in the first few days after onset of the illness, and conventional brain imaging may be more sensitive than CT.[1] Some tumors (isodensity lesions) may be detected by conventional brain imaging, which is especially helpful when intravenous contrast use is contraindicated.[2] Motion degradation of the images, an artifact due to the presence of high-density material (e.g., metal clips), may give false-negative or otherwise unsatisfactory results by CT.

Current diagnostic brain imaging may be divided into morphological/structural imaging and functional imaging. While CT and MRI provide information on anatomical/structural changes due to disease processes in the brain, single-photon emission computed tomography (SPECT) and/or positron emission tomography (PET) enables assessment of the functional/physiological processes in the brain.[3] Functional abnormalities can usually be detected prior to anatomical changes. The usage of brain SPECT in evaluation of cerebrovascular disease, dementia, and psychiatric disorders has relied on recent advances in two areas: radiopharmaceuticals and instrumentation.

For example, lipophilic radiopharmaceuticals such as I-123 iodoamphetamine (IMP) and Tc-99m hexamethyl-propylene-amine oxime, (HMPAO) cross the intact BBB, localizing in the normal neurons. The regional cerebral distribution of Tc-99m HMPAO and the earlier phase of I-123 IMP compare quite well with that of the labeled microsphere. The information on regional blood flow provided by these agents is concordant with metabolic data reported with the PET technique; the regional blood flow detected by these agents is an indirect measurement of cerebral metabolism. Thus, evaluation of cerebrovascular disease, dementia, epilepsy trauma, or psychiatric disorders can be performed by brain SPECT, demonstrating the functional status of a disease process.[4]

Recent advances in instrumentation have also played an important role in the development of brain SPECT imaging. Multidetector and ring SPECT systems have gained widespread acceptance in nuclear medicine clinics. These systems provide a significant improvement in terms of detection efficiency and/or spatial resolution compared with conventional single-detector SPECT systems. New collimator designs such as fan-beam, cone-beam, and astigmatic collimators provide a better trade-off between spatial resolution and detection efficiency compared with the conventional parallel-hole collimator design. In addition, continued improvements in scintillation cameras have resulted in better uniformity, linearity, stability, intrinsic and energy resolution. These advances in instrumentation, combined with those in radiopharmaceuticals and in image reconstruction methods, have contributed to the improved quality and quantitative accuracy of brain SPECT images.

RADIOPHARMACEUTICALS

Cerebral blood flow varies to meet the metabolic requirements of the brain, regional cerebral blood flow of gray matter being four to five times higher than that of white matter.[5] Normal cerebral blood flow has been found to be about 20 ml/100 g/min for white matter and 80 ml/100 g/min for gray matter. The transport of substances across the BBB occurs by either passive diffusion or active transport. Criteria for a brain flow imaging agent are (1) the ability to cross the intact BBB, (2) high first-pass extraction, (3) prolonged retention in the brain, (4) activity representing regional flow, and (5) little or no metabolism.[5] The agents, such as Tc-99m HMPAO, Tc-99m ethyl cysteinate dimer (ECD), or I-123 IMP, have for the most part, fulfilled these requirements. Lipid-soluble tracer such as HMPAO or IMP molecules can cross the BBB by passive diffusion. To be passive diffusible, the molecular size should be less than 600 daltons; the HMPAO molecule is less than 500 daltons and well fits the criterion.[5] Cerebral blood flow agents such as Tc-99m HMPAO or I-123 IMP localize in the brain proportionally to the blood flow. The distribution of radioactivity in brain parenchyma is therefore the estimation of rCBF, resumable a radiolabeled microspheres model,[6] O-15-labeled CO_2 for PET, or F-18-labeled fluoromethane PET.[7–10]

Tc-99m HMPAO

Tc-99m HMPAO, a lipophilic agent and the only Food and Drug Administration (FDA)-approved Tc-99m-labeled compound for brain flow imaging, crosses the intact BBB and remains in neurons of the brain in proportion to tissue perfusion[11,12]; approximately 3.5–7% of the injected dose is localized in the brain, and the radiotracer is retained in brain parenchyma following conversion of lipophilic Tc-99m HMPAO to a poorly diffusible, hydrophilic compound form. A postulated mechanism of Tc-HMPAO retention in the neurons without redistribution is that Tc-HMPAO interacts with glutathione.[13] Those crossing BBB property and non-redistributionable retained in the neurons, Tc-99m HMPAO behaves like a "chemical microsphere." The mechanism appears not to be affected by metabolic disturbances such as those caused by uremia, hepatic encephalopathy, anoxia, severe sepsis, high-dose diazepam, or barbiturates, and hypothermia.[14]

Because it is fixed in the neurons, the radiopharmaceutical can be injected during seizure attacks, for example, permitting freezing of the seizure status then

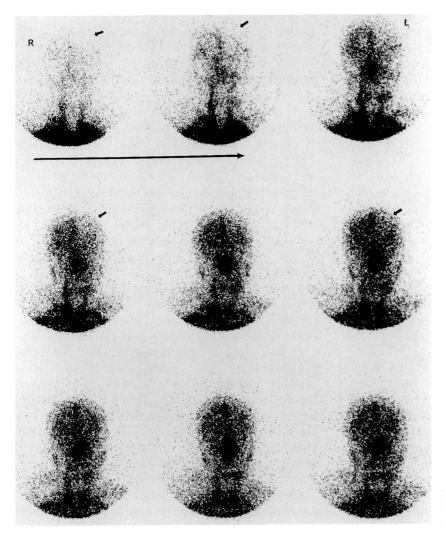

Fig. 23-1 First-pass cerebral flow study with 2 sec per image shows decreased flow in the left cerebral hemisphere (arrow).

the patient may send to the nuclear medicine service for imaging later. The pattern of brain SPECT revealed represents the rCBF at the time of tracer injection.[15] Because HMPAO is labeled by Tc-99m 10–30 mCi of the radiopharmaceutical can be used for cerebral dynamic study, monitoring the passage of carotid and cerebral arterial flow (Fig. 23-1) to delineate asymmetrical cerebral flow, for example, in a stroke patient or total absence of cerebral flow in a brain death patient. The disadvantage of Tc-99m HMPAO is that it possesses limited in vitro chemical stability, and it must be used within 30 min following reconstitution of the kit.[11] The instability of the reconstituted kit is characterized by the tendency of the lipophilic complex content to diminish with time, producing a less lipophilic complex and free pertechnetate. A method of stabilizing the kit of HMPAO by the addition of 200 μg cobalt chloride hexahydrate in 2 ml of water has been described.[16] The

addition of this solution can extend the shelf life of the reconstituted kit to at least 5 hr postreconstitution. The presence of cobalt chloride greatly extends (up to 4 hr) the period over which Tc HMPAO can be used after reconstitution to generate images of CBF distribution in normal and ischemic tissue.[17] Once the method of in vitro stability is approved by the FDA, its clinical usage will be more convenient.

I-123 IMP

Although I-123 IMP was the first radiopharmaceutical approved by the FDA (in 1988), after approval of HMPAO by the FDA, its clinical usage became less popular. After IV administration of I-123 IMP, 6–7% of the injected dose remains in the brain for 20 min. The I-123 IMP is taken up by the brain by simple diffusion. Following initial uptake, the amines are retained in the brain, possibly by the following mechanisms or sites: amine metabolism, nonspecific sites, pH shift, and/or specific binding sites of the brain. The retention mechanism in the disease state may also be changing, and the pattern of distribution may also be changed due to the differences in the retention mechanism.[5] Brain SPECT should be performed immediately after I-123 IMP administration.

In addition to brain uptake, there is significant uptake in the lungs and liver and rapid excretion by the urine. Brain SPECT should be performed immediately after administration. Due to a high level of activity in the lungs, there is a significant amount of residual activity in the blood circulation later. This residual blood level may contribute to what is termed redistribution of initial hypoperfusion area(s).[5] Brain distribution of IMP changes over time and redistribution changes significantly by 3–4 hr,[18] so brain distribution no longer represents perfusion at the time of injection.[18] I-123 IMP may be contaminated with higher energy and a longer half-life, resulting in a high radiation dose. I-123 IMP back diffusion or redistribution has been considered a disadvantage of this imaging agent. However, the redistribution phenomenon has been used as a prognostic predictor of cerebrovascular disease.[19,20] In a comparative study, brain SPECT with I-123 IMP showed higher lesion contrast than Tc-99m HMPAO.[21]

Tc-99m ECD

ECD is a neutral lipophilic complex that crosses the BBB and is trapped in the brain by conversion to polar acid products through a specific enzymatic pathway.[22]

ECD is radiochemically pure and stable[23] for an extended period. Background radioactivity from facial structures, blood, and lungs clears rapidly, leading to improved image quality compared to Tc-99m HMPAO.[24,25] Uptake in the brain is 6.5 ± 1.9% within 5 min of the IV injection.[24,26] Optimal imaging time is 1 hr or more after injection.[6,15] Lung uptake and retention of the ECD is negligible because it is excreted rapidly by the kidneys.[23] Tc-99m ECD brain SPECT produces a high-quality image, resulting from the optimal physical characteristics of Tc-99m and favorable biodistribution. ECD is a promising tracer for evaluation of rCBF.[22–25,27] In a comparative study of stroke, in the cerebral cortex, cerebellum, and white matter, I-123 IMP showed higher lesion uptake than TC-99m ECD and Tc-99m HMPAO. In the striatum and thalamus, Tc-99m ECD and I-123 IMP showed higher lesion sensitivity than Tc-99m HMPAO. I-123 IMP showed highest lesion contrast in the cerebral cortex and cerebellum. Tc-99m ECD showed the highest contrast in

the thalamus and striatum. In all regions, Tc-99m ECD showed higher lesion contrast than Tc-99m HMPAO.[27]

INSTRUMENTATION

Single-photon emission computed tomography (SPECT) is designed to take advantage of the principles of computed tomography to produce three-dimensional images of the distribution of radiopharmaceuticals. The first SPECT system was the MARK IV system developed by Kuhl and Edwards[28–30] over two decades ago. Since then, a number of SPECT system designs have been developed. In particular, clinical SPECT instrumentation has evolved from those based on a single rotating camera,[31,32] dual cameras,[33] and triple cameras[34,35] to ring detector[36] designs. The development of new SPECT systems is guided by the demands for reduced acquisition time, improved image quality in terms of spatial resolution and detection efficiency, and higher quantitative accuracy. Multiple cameras or ring detector–based SPECT systems offer distinct advantages over single-camera systems, including reduction of acquisition time, which is important in imaging uncooperative or clinically unstable patients. Increased detection efficiency can also be traded off for improved spatial resolution. When combined with advances in image reconstruction methods, substantial improvement in both the quality and quantitative accuracy of SPECT images are realized.

Camera-based SPECT systems allow acquisition of two-dimensional (2D) projection data which can be reconstructed to give multiple transaxial image slices or three-dimensional (3D) image data. Since they can be used in both planar and SPECT studies, they have become the most popular design for commercial SPECT systems. A limitation of camera-based SPECT systems is the dead time loss at high counting rates. Also, for systems based on a single rotating camera, single-slice sensitivity is low. However, the latter limitation is reduced with new SPECT systems which are based on multiple cameras.

Triple-camera SPECT systems have gained acceptance as all-purpose nuclear medicine imaging device for brain, cardiac, and whole body SPECT studies (Fig. 23-2A–C). These systems provide full 360° data acquisition with 120° rotation, thus reducing the acquisition time by a factor of 3 compared with single-camera SPECT systems. Using the capability of rapidly reversing the direction of rotation, the entire data acquisition of the triple-camera system can be divided into several subsegments (e.g., eight segments in the Picker Prism SPECT system). Each subsegment consists of

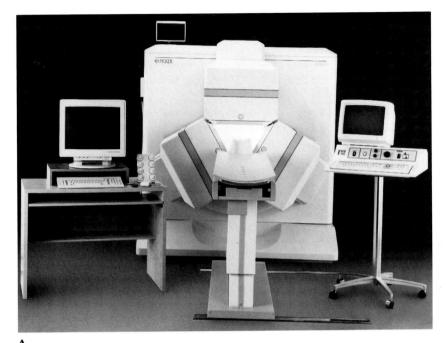

Fig. 23-2 (*A*) Three-head camera system of the Prism Picker. (Courtesy of Picker International, Nuclear Medicine Division, Bedford Heights, OH) (*B*) Three-head camera system of the Triad SPECT. (Courtesy of Trionix Research Laboratory, Inc., Twinsburg, OH) (*C*) Three-head system of Siemens. (Courtesy of Siemens Medical Systems, Inc., Hoffman Estates, IL)

A

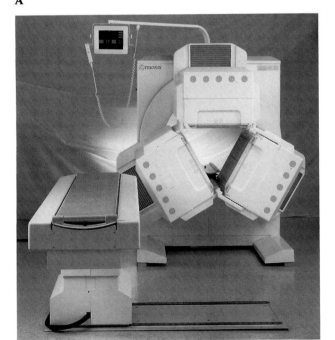

B

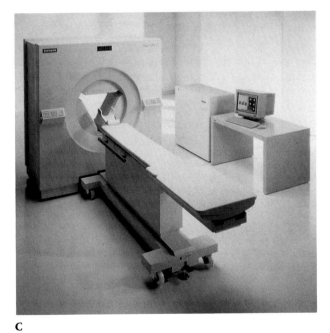

C

120° clockwise and counterclockwise rotations. The capability allows discarding of specific segments of the data acquisition due to patient motion for improved reconstructed image quality.

Large-field-of-view dual-camera SPECT systems have also gained popularity for use in both whole body scanning and SPECT studies. Currently, most commercial nuclear medicine system manufacturers are producing dual-camera SPECT systems. Dual cameras arranged at a 90° angle have also been developed by commercial manufacturers (GE, Sohpa, and ADAC Laboratory). These systems are particularly well suited for cardiac SPECT studies where 180° projection data can be acquired with 90° detector rotation, thus reducing the normal acquisition time by a factor of 2. A dedicated brain SPECT system is available which is based on a unique stationary ring detector geometry design.[36,37] The system consists of a cylindrical scintillator. Projection data from different views are acquired by rotating a ring collimator which is fitted inside the detector ring, thus eliminating the need to rotate the bulky detector assembly.

Special collimator designs have also been developed for use in camera-based SPECT to improve the trade-off between detection efficiency and spatial resolution compared to the conventional parallel-hole design. Fan-beam collimators[38,39] have been proposed for brain SPECT studies. The holes of a fan-beam collimator are focused to a point in a transverse image plane and are parallel across the image slices. Depending on the particular design parameters, fan-beam collimators provide approximately a 50% increase in detection efficiency compared with parallel-hole collimators with the same spatial resolution. The trade-off is a limited field of view. The limitation restricts the application of fan-beam collimators to brain studies[38,39] and, more recently, cardiac studies.[40]

Other collimator designs for SPECT include cone-beam[41,42] and astigmatic[43] collimators. The collimator holes of a cone-beam collimator are focused to a point. They provided approximately a 2-fold increase in detector efficiency compared with parallel-hole collimators with the same spatial resolution. As with the fan-beam collimator design, the trade-off is a limited field of view. Cone-beam collimators have also been applied to brain studies[40,41] and cardiac[44] studies. The astigmatic collimator consists of collimator holes which are focused to two separate points. The resulting field of view is designed to match the shape of the head. In addition, a collimator design with increased detection efficiency toward the central part of the source distribution has been proposed.[36,45] The design provides an improved signal/noise ratio toward the center of the reconstructed image, where the counting statistics are lower.

SPECT systems based on multiple detector arrays have also been developed and commercialized. The earlier system designs allow acquisition from a single image slice.[46] A single-slice dedicated brain system based on 12 large single detectors, each fitted with a highly focused collimator, has been developed.[47,48] Each of the 12 detectors moves tangentially and radially such that the focal points scan over the image space. Though the system provides good spatial resolution within the transaxial image slices, it has poor axial resolution, which affects its overall image quality. More

recently, multiple-slice systems have become available from Medimatic. These systems consist of one-dimensional (1D) bar scintillation cameras[49,50] and have much higher count rate detection capability than camera-based systems. They are designed with high detection efficiency and corresponding poor spatial resolution for dynamic brain perfusion studies using Xe-133.

Novel SPECT system designs have also been developed in various research laboratories. One design is based on a stationary array of detectors arranged in a ring. Projection data are acquired using a rotating slit[51] or focused collimators.[52,53] A stationary hemispherical SPECT imager is also being developed.[54] The system consists of a number of small modular cameras arranged in a hemispherical fashion around the patient's head.[55] Projection data are acquired from a set of stationary pinhole collimators fitted inside the detector array. Three-dimensional images can be reconstructed from the projection data, and high detection efficiency can be achieved by this system.

More recently, several SPECT instrumentation developments have been spurred by specific clinical needs. For example, a scintillation camera can be designed to detect the 511-kEv photons emitted by positron-emitting radiopharmaceuticals. This can be achieved by increasing the crystal thickness and designing high-energy collimators for the 511-kev photons. A triple-head camera system has been developed for imaging with positron-emitting F-18 fluoro-2-deoxyglucose (FDG).[56] The system provides a cost-effective alternative positron emission tomography (PET) in imaging positron-emitting radiopharmaceuticals. There is also increased interest in imaging two radiotracers, such as Tc-99m and I-123, with different photon emissions simultaneously. This requires SPECT systems equipped with simultaneous data acquisition from multiple energy windows and methods to eliminate cross-contamination between photons from different radionuclides into various energy windows.

Methods for coregistering and fusing images from different imaging modalities have been under active investigation.[57] They can be achieved by using fiducial markers placed on the surface of the patient or anatomical markers identifiable in the images themselves. When the functional SPECT images are combined with anatomical images from computed tomography (CT) and magnetic resonance imaging (MRI), increased information can be obtained which allow physicians to make more accurate clinical diagnoses.

In summary, substantial advances have been made in SPECT instrumentation in the last several years.

They have resulted from the increased recognition of SPECT as an important diagnostic tool and from the demand for improvement in both the quality and quantitative accuracy of clinical SPECT images. Combined with advances in new radiopharmaceuticals, image reconstruction methods, and clinical applications, SPECT imaging will continue to play an important role in diagnostic imaging for improved patient care.

IMAGING TECHNIQUES AND IMAGE INTERPRETATION

Most nuclear medicine services have three-head cameras and/or single-head cameras with SPECT capabilities. If a gamma camera does not have the ability to perform brain SPECT scanning, planar images can still detect abnormalities of cerebral[58–61] cerebellar[58] hemispheres, especially if the lesion is large.[60]

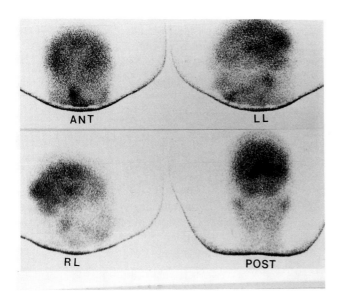

Fig. 23-3 Four views of planar images in a patient with Pick's disease showing diffuse hypoperfusion in the frontal lobes.

The following is an example for a nuclear medicine service having a three-head camera and using Tc-99m HMPAO as the radiopharmaceutical.

A rapid sequential cerebral flow study every 2 sec can be performed in either the sitting or supine position, with an IV injection of up to 30 mCi of Tc-99m HMPAO. One hour later, SPECT imaging is performed with either a triple-head or a single-head camera. The delayed hour allows clearance from the blood pool component to improve image contrast.

Patient motion will degrade SPECT imaging quality; therefore, avoidance of motion during acquisition is essential. It may be necessary to sedate uncooperative patients at the time of the actual imaging. Since sedation may decrease cerebral blood flow, it should be avoided before Tc-99m HMPAO administration.

Alternatively, planar brain imaging techniques can be applied. Using a large field-of-view (Siemens) gamma camera fitted with a low-energy collimator, four planar brain images (anterior, posterior, right lateral, and left lateral views) are obtained (Figs. 23-3, 23-4). In addition, planar brain imaging may apply in certain situations that preclude the use of SPECT: a psychological condition such as phobia to a gantry, patient weight of more than 250 lb, or the inability to lie down.[58] SPECT imaging is performed next, using the three-head gamma camera fitted with an ultra-high-resolution parallel (preferably fan-beam) collimator and interfaced with a 64-bit supercomputer. Imaging procedures are as follows: The patient is placed in the triple-head camera, with acquisition of SPECT data from 120 projections over 360°, with 30 sec per projection. Acquisition time for each brain SPECT is usually 22 min. The SPECT images, including transaxial, coronal, and sagittal sections, are reconstructed using a Butterworth filter (order of 4, cutoff 0.3), back-projection, and attenuation correction.[61]

Surface and volume three-dimensional images are reconstructed from transaxial SPECT data; processing time is 5 to 10 min. The surface three-dimensional threshold value is set at 50%; the volume 3D weighing factor is set at 0.1.[61]

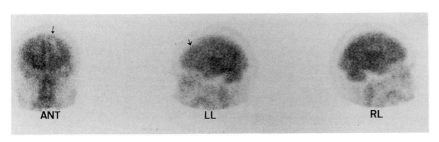

Fig. 23-4 Planar images show an area of slightly decreased activity in the left frontal lobe (arrow) in a stroke patient.

Since, as previously mentioned, patient motion will degrade SPECT imaging quality, avoidance of motion artifacts is essential. With an agitated patient, speed technique can be used—either a shortened or sequential, rapid acquisition sequence imaging procedure.

In the interpretation of the brain SPECT scan, one should assess the status of focal as well as global perfusion in the transaxial, coronal, and sagittal plane images. For transaxial and coronal sections, cerebral and cerebellar hemispheres and midline structures of the basal ganglia and thalami should have symmetrical uptake. The sagittal sections begin in the lateral aspect of the right temporal lobe and section continuously to the contralateral (left) temporal lobe. These sections provide excellent delineation of the anterior-to-posterior uptake gradient. Concurrent CT or MRI should be available for correlation.

Neurological development and maturational changes in the human brain continue beyond birth; until the end of the second month, there is marked predominant perfusion in the basal ganglion, thalamus, cerebral sensorimotor cortex, and cerebellum (Fig. 23-5), with very little in the remainder of the cerebral cortex.[62,63] At the beginning of the second year, adult-like pattern of frontal activity evolve. The rCBF changes correspond to behavioral evolution in infancy.[62]

One should be aware of these maturational change of the brain when interpreting brain SPECT scans of newborn babies.

VOLUME AND SURFACE 3D DISPLAYS

The brain is a nonhomogeneous organ with a complex structure including cortical gray and white matter, basal ganglia, and ventricles. Regional cerebral blood flow of gray matter is four to five times higher than that of white matter of the brain.[64] Evaluation with SPECT imaging improves image contrast by separating the overlapping structures.[65–68] When evaluating a lesion or lesions in SPECT images, the interpreter has to bring all slices of the transaxial, coronal, and sagittal sections together to make a whole for accurate localization of the lesion(s). Volume (Fig. 23-6) and surface (Fig. 23-7) 3D displays provide tomographic information: (1) 3D perception by motion appears to be an inherent characteristic of human visual perception, enhancing continuity of structures and understanding of spatial relationships; (2) a 3D display exactly localizes the lesion in relation to normal structures; and (3) volume and surface 3D displays view the brain from all angles.[65–67] As shown in Fig. 23-8, the location and extension of lesion(s) in the brain were easier to appreciate and to interpret.

These displays have been routinely applied to stroke patients. It has been concluded that surface and volume 3D displays equally enhance and simplify SPECT interpretation.[67–69] The volume 3D display does demonstrate crossed cerebellar diaschisis (CCD).[68] One limitation is that basal ganglia abnormalities cannot be delineated by surface or volume 3D displays. This is because the basal ganglia are deep-seated in the brain, and interpretation of abnormalities is hampered by the normal perfusion activity of the cerebral cortex.[68] Surface 3D display technique has been also used in patients with stroke,[68] slowly progressive apraxia to detect cortical lesions,[69] and chronic hypnosedative use,[70] as well as in a Diamox-augmented cerebral perfusion study.[71] Dementia patients can certainly be examined with this technique.

CEREBROVASCULAR DISEASE

Acute Ischemia

Tc-99m HMPAO brain SPECT is able to detect acute cerebral infarcts before radiographic CT.[72] Brain SPECT imaging is more sensitive than CT; brain SPECT detection rates are 88–95%,[72–74] while CT detection rates are only 20–63%.[75,76] The defects seen on SPECT (by I-123 IMP) are also larger than those seen on early CT. In one study, 47% of the patients with positive CT scans had larger defects on SPECT.[77] The discrepancy in defect size may result from neuronal dysfunction of the peripheral zone of infarction, from edema, from diaschisis, or from a lag time between functional and structural changes.[78–80] Absent perfusion or hypoperfusion of the cerebral cortex (Fig. 23-8A–D) and putamen (Fig. 23-8E) are readily demonstrated by Tc-99m HMPAO brain SPECT images.

Hemorrhagic Stroke

Hemorrhagic strokes are generally divided into three groups: subarachnoid hemorrhage (SAH), intracerebral hemorrhage (ICH), and arteriovenous malformation. Though CT and MRI are well established as basic diagnostic tools for the evaluation of ICH, very little data have been reported regarding brain SPECT in the assessment of ICH.[79]

The most common cause of SAH (accounting for approximately one-half of all hemorrhagic strokes) is the rupture of a congenital aneurysm (berry aneurysm). Posthemorrhage neurological deficits that appear within 2 weeks are the most common consequences of vasospasm.[81] The resulting delayed cerebral ischemia/infarction makes vasospasm an equally important fac-

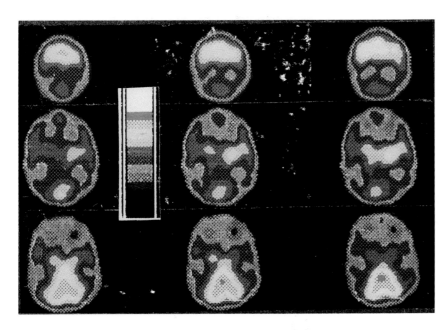

Fig. 23-5 Brain SPECT scan of a newborn (4 days old) shows normal prominent perfusion in the thalamus, basal ganglion, cerebral sensomotor cortex, and cerebellum.

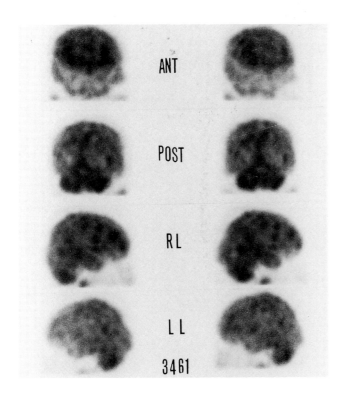

Fig. 23-6 A normal-volume three-dimensional display showing homogeneous perfusion in the cerebral and cerebellar hemispheres.

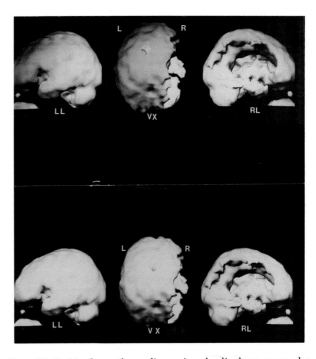

Fig. 23-7 Surface three-dimensional displays may be viewed at different projections and angles: a large perfusion defect in the right hemisphere extending from the frontal, parietal, and temporal lobes to the occipital lobes is easily delineated. RL = right lateral; LL = left lateral; VX = vertex.

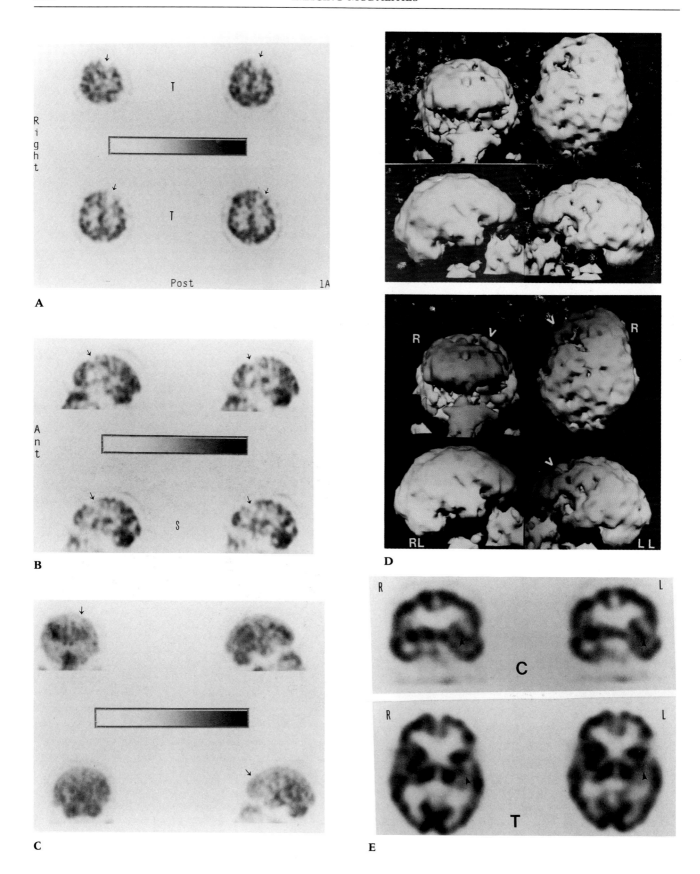

tor in recurrent hemorrhage causing the morbidity and mortality of SAH.[82,83] Compared with angiography and transcranial Doppler,[84] brain SPECT provides a more direct measure of hemodynamic significance in observed vasospasm, and it may help to differentiate vasospasm from other causes of neurological deterioration following SAH.[82]

Arteriovenous Malformation

Brain SPECT with HMPAO or IMP demonstrates reduced tracer uptake, while SPECT with Xe-133 gave a high flow.[82] Xe-133 SPECT dynamic studies have shown a high incidence of steel (region of hypoperfusion).[85,86] Recently, acetazolamide (ACZ)-enhanced rCBF SPECT to predict the risk to patients with arteriovenous malformation (AVM) has been evaluated.[87,88] Abnormally enhanced vasodilatation from ACZ stimulation was noted in these threatened territories in AVM, resulting in a poor outcome.[87]

Transient Ischemia Attacks

Most transient ischemia attack patients (82%) have normal CT scans, and 12% of patients with abnormal CT scans show only the nonspecific finding of atrophy.[89] Brain SPECT may identify patients at highest risk for subsequent infarction. Persistent focal hypoperfusion at or beyond 24 hr is significant in patients with a recent transient ischemic attack. In patients with a normal SPECT scan in one study, none progressed to infarction in the following weeks.[90] Thus brain SPECT may distinguish patients at higher risk for the development of progressive disease.

Transient global amnesia is considered to be transient ischemia in the medial temporal lobe or thalamus, as supported by the neuropsychological dysfunction[91–93] and evident by brain SPECT.[94–97] Brain SPECTs demonstrates bitemporal hypoperfusion at 7 hr after the ictus,[93] hypoperfusion in the territory of the posterior cerebral artery,[95] and perfusion defects in both thalami.[96] While brain CT, EEG, and duplex carotid artery scans were normal,[97] sequential Tc-99m HMPAO brain SPECT scans performed at 6 hr, 3 days, and 28 days after the onset of transient global amnesia demonstrated partial resolution of hypoperfusion involving the occipital lobes, left medial temporal lobe, and left thalamus on the third day and complete resolution by 28 days. These SPECT findings are concordant with the neuropsychological assessment.[97]

Prognostic Prediction by Brain SPECT in Ischemia

Prognostic and/or predictive values in acute ischemic stroke have been evaluated by brain SPECT.[98–100] The study of Hanson et al.[101] showed a strong association between the severity of an ischemic insult, as demonstrated by SPECT performed within 6 hr of symptom onset, and clinical presentation, long-term outcome, and the complications of cerebral edema and hemorrhagic conversion of ischemic stroke. Redistribution is one of the phenomena that is judged by comparing an early and a delayed SPECT imaging using I-123 IMP. Hypoperfusion area(s) of brain SPECT studies performed at 15 min were compared with those on brain SPECT studies 3–5 hr after injection of I-123 IMP. Redistribution (filling in) of the area of hypoperfusion is assumed to reflect metabolic activity in viable cerebral tissue, indicating a favorable clinical outcome in patients with cerebrovascular diseases. Evaluation is done visually[102] and quantitatively.[103] Redistribution on delayed SPECT is based on the low blood flow of a reversible ischemic lesion (peri-infarct area).

In the Odano et al.[103] study, supratentorial cerebral blood flow and the ratio of gray matter to white matter in normal subjects were 52.7 ± 5.0 ml/100 g/min and 2.34, respectively. The cerebral flow of the infarct and peri-infarct areas was 9–20 and 22–41 ml/100 g/min, respectively. After bypass of blood flow, the Odano et al. study[103] indicated that the redistribution phenomenon depends on the maintenance of minimal blood flow to sustain cellular function. The peri-infarct area, extended around the infarct zone, would show normal density on CT[104] but redistribution on delayed SPECT.[103] These findings were explained by functional inactivation of the peri-infarct area[104,105] and/or neuronal disconnection.[106]

Fig. 23-8 (*A,B*) A 66-year-old man had a history of several acute episodes of right arm and right leg numbness. A first-pass cerebral flow study, as in Fig. 23-1, shows decreased flow in the left cerebral hemisphere (arrow). Tc-99m HMPAO brain SPECT scans show decreased perfusion in the left hemisphere (T = transaxial; S = sagittal). (*C*) Volume three-dimensional displays show relative hypoperfusion in the left frontal lobe (arrow). (*D*) Surface three-dimensional displays show multiple perfusion defects in the left frontoparietal region. A concurrent carotid duplex study and a contrast angiogram show complete occlusion of the left internal carotid artery. (*E*) Hypoperfusion in the left putamen (arrowheads) is demonstrated by Tc-99m HMPAO brain SPECT images (C = coronal section; T = transaxial section; R = right; L = left).

Diaschisis

When localized injury to the brain occurs, depression of function results not only in the primarily affected site of damage, but also in remote areas that appear structurally intact. These remote injuries of neuronal function are termed *diashisis*.[107] Two common types of diaschisis resulting from cerebrovascular disease are crossed cerebellar diasachisis[108–113] and intrahemispheric thalamic diaschisis.[114,115] Hypoperfusion of the cerebellar hemisphere contralateral to the lesion of the cerebrum is called *crossed cerebellar diaschisis* (CCD). Intrahemispheric thalamic diaschisis consists of metabolic/perfusion depression in the thalamus ipsilateral to unilateral infarction in the territory of the middle cerebral arteries. These two types of diaschisis may be observed simultaneously in a stroke patient[115] (Fig. 23-9). In comparison with Tc-99m HMPAO and I-123 IMP, Tc-99m ECD brain SPECT showed an apparent decrease in activity in the thalamus, providing the highest lesion contrast.[116]

Crossed Cerebellar Diaschisis
Crossed cerebellar diaschisis (CCD), which is documented by positron emission tomography (PET), was initially defined as decreased blood flow resulting from contralateral cerebral damage[108,109] in the otherwise normal cerebellar hemisphere. Subsequently, CCD was demonstrated by brain SPECT,[110,111] and about 50–60% of patients with cerebral infarct were found to be positive for this phenomenon.[112,113] CCD occurs preferentially with large infarcts involving the internal capsule/basal ganglia or the frontoparietal lobes.[113,117]

Cerebrocerebellar disconnection is responsible for this CCD[112,113] when the cerebrum has been damaged by an infarct, for example, resulting in interruption of the cerebro-ponto-cerebellar pathways. The interruption deactivates cerebellar hemispheric metabolism. Decreased activity of the cerebellar hemisphere contralateral to the infarcted cerebrum is reflected by decreased I-123 HIPDM or Tc-99m HMPAO activity (Fig. 23-9). An alternative explanation of CCD is as follows: When infarction of a cerebral hemisphere occurs, the impulses of the pyramidal tracts to the contralateral spinal cord are absent. Consequently, the signal originating from the spinal cord through the spinocerebellar tract to the cerebellum (contralateral to the cerebral infarct) is eliminated.[113] It is assumed that the requirement of metabolism/blood flow in the cerebellum contralateral to the cerebral infarct is decreased, even though the structure appears intact, as seen on the CT scan. The diminished signal to stimulate the contralateral cerebellum results in low consumption of oxygen

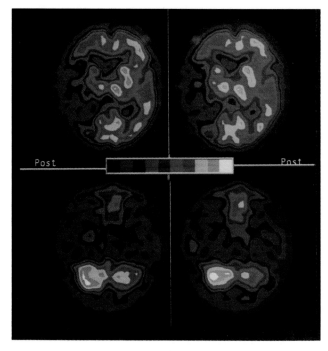

Fig. 23-9 Tc-99m HMPAO brain SPECT images show a stroke patient with a large perfusion defect in the right cerebral hemisphere, hypoperfusion in the right (ipsilateral) thalamus and basal ganglia, and marked hypoperfusion in the left (contralateral) cerebellum: crossed cerebellar diaschisis and intrahemispheric thalamic diaschisis.

and glucose, leading to a reduction of CO_2 production in the area of diaschisis. Due to the shortage of CO_2, the arterioles in the area of diaschisis are relatively constricted, resulting in decreased uptake on brain SPECT.[115]

Recently, in addition to hypoperfusion of the contralateral cerebellum, decreased ipsilateral pontine function has been documented.[117] Thus, CCD may indicate disruption of the cerebrocerebellar interconnections.[109,118,119] Despite decreased blood flow, the area of diaschisis preserves the regional vascular reserve (vasoreactivity). This has been demonstrated by AZT Tc-99m HMPAO brain SPECT imaging,[115] in which all six patients with intrahemispheric thalamic diaschisis, and five of eight patients with CCD, had significantly augmented perfusion after ACZ administration.[115] The degree of response to ACZ demonstrates that the vasodilatory reserve capacity of the cerebellar diaschisis area is more than that of the thalamic diaschisis area.[115] The supratentorial lesion resulting in CCD is located in the motor cortex, basal ganglia, and/or internal capsule relating to the territory of the middle cerebral artery.[113] A large cerebral lesion located in the posterior parietal region was not demonstrable by CCD.[121] CCD may appear within 1 day and may persist as long as there is structural damage of the descending cortico-ponto-cerebellar pathway.[113]

In the Wada test (intracrotid injection of amobarbital to examine the laterality of speach, injection on the dominant side abolishes the power of speech temporarily) test, CCD occurred immediately and disappeared when the primary insult resolved.[119]

When CCD was considered as a physiological phenomenon, cerebellar atrophy was observed in 8 of 26 patients with CCD shown on MRI. Those patients were generally younger than those with or without atrophy and had significant contralateral supratentorial hemispheric atrophy.[122]

In addition to cerebral strokes and the WADA test, other conditions that induce CCD include spinocerebellar degeneration,[123] Alzheimer's disease,[124] progressive supranuclear palsy,[125] brain tumor,[126–129] tuberous sclerosis,[130] Sturge-Weber syndrome,[131] hydrocephalus,[132] and brain stem lesions.[133]

Recently, Frazekas et al.[134] reported that a brain stem infarct caused hypoperfusion both infratentorially (CCD) and supratentorially (ipsilateral to the area of cerebral hemispheric diaschisis). Damage to the corticopontocerebellar pathways is responsible for CCD.[135] Cerebellocerebral disruption may explain ipsilateral cerebral hemispheric diaschisis.[134]

Crossed Cerebello-Cerebral Diaschisis (CCeCD)
CCD can be observed in opposite direction; for example, hypoperfusion of the contralateral cerebral hemisphere may be seen in patients with unilateral cerebellar lesion.[135–139] This phenomenon is called *crossed cerebello-cerebral diaschisis:* functional alterations of the cerebral cortex induced by a cerebellar lesion. Supratentorial hypoperfusion contralateral to the cerebellar lesion has been demonstrated by Tc-99m HMPAO SPECT imaging.[135–141] The absence of a cerebral cortical lesion and the presence of a cerebellar insult have been documented by CT and/or MRI. Damage to the fiber tracts of the cerebrocerebellar loop is the most likely explanation of the diaschisis.[131]

The locations of supratentorial hypoperfusion include the motor cortex;[141] the premotor-temporal,[137] fronto-parieto-temporal,[139] and prefrontal areas;[140] and the lateral basal ganglia.[138]

The cerebellar lesions include cerebellar softening,[136] ischemia,[137–138] hematoma,[137] and primary neoplasm.[140]

As in CCD, areas of supratentorial hypoperfusion in CCeCD result from transneuronal metabolic depression through nervous tracts of anatomical connections. The cerebellum has two levels of organization. The lower

level sends signals to the motor area for manipulating muscles; the higher level contributes to mental and language skills by applying signals to the prefrontal areas.[138–142] The close anatomical and physiological relationship between the cerebellar hemisphere and the frontal and prefrontal areas results in transneuronal metabolic depression. The dentate nucleus of the cerebellar hemisphere projects to the motor area (area 4) and the premotor area (area 6) through the dento-thalamo-cortex pathway. The ventroanterior and ventrolateral nuclei constitute thalamic relays for the nerve fibers directed to areas 6 and 4, respectively. For prefrontal abnormalities, dentate nucleus projections, and thalamic relay to the associated prefrontal cortex,[110] this hypothesis is supported by (1) neuropsychological reports suggesting a possible role of the cerebellum in frontal cognitive processes[142,143] and (2) the fact that a cerebellar lesion can cause subtle cognitive defects.[138–143]

Tc-99M HMPAO BRAIN SPECT AND INTERVENTIONAL STUDIES

Intervention studies with Tc-99m HMPAO brain SPECT can be induced by chemical (pharmacological), physiological, and mechanical methods.[144] As mentioned in the "Radiopharmaceuticals" section, Tc-99m HMPAO has excellent retention in brain tissue within a few minutes after IV injection, with minimal redistribution for a long period of time. This property allows evaluation of cerebral blood flow changes during short intervention periods. The usefulness of HMPAO brain SPECT for the detection of brain perfusion changes is well documented.[144] The established intervention tests include acetazolamide (Diamox)[145] for assessment of vascular reserve, the Wada test for epilepsy (unilateral intracarotid arterial injection of sodium amytal),[146] the Matas test (compression of the common carotid artery on the affected side),[147] yohimbine (for panic disorder),[148] L-acetyl-carptine,[149] physiostigmine for Alzheimer's disease,[150] the balloon occlusion test,[151] and the hyperventilation test.[152] Acetazolamide intervention for cerebrovascular reserve, the balloon occlusion test, and the hyperventilation test will be detailed in the following subsections.

Tc-99m HMPAO SPECT Brain Imaging Using Acetazolamide (Diamox)

Acetazolamide (ACZ) (Diamox) with Tc-99m HMPAO SPECT imaging allows detection of diminished cerebral perfusion reserve; this cannot be done without ACZ.[144,145] ACZ inhibits carbonic anhydrase of erythrocytes and other tissue and is a potent vasodilator of the cerebral vessels, and increases rCBF. Possible mechanisms include inhibition of carbonic anhydrase in the brain parenchyma and/or cerebral vessels, as well as in the smooth muscle of the cerebral vasculature.

Cerebral autoregulation compensates for decreased cerebral perfusion pressure by vasodilatation until further response is impossible. Patients with cerebral or carotid artery disease may show a blunted or absent response to ACZ. The autoregulation capacity may be exhausted by reduction of perfusion pressure distal to the stenosis of the carotid or cerebral artery and poor collateral circulation. Patients with cerebral or carotid artery stenosis may show a decreased perfusion in the cerebral hemisphere distributed by stenotic carotid or cerebral artery due to an absent or decreased response to ACZ.[144,145,153-161] This procedure provides an objective evaluation of the hemodynamic effects of the carotid stenosis.[153,159]

The procedure is as follows: Twenty-five minutes after an injection of 1 g ACZ, 20–30 mCi Tc-99m HMPAO is injected IV. Then the standard SPECT imaging procedure is performed. IV of ACZ should be done slowly over 1–2 min; the side effects include numbness around the mouth or fingers, lightheadedness or blurred vision, and flushing of the face and neck.

Except for patients with an allergy to sulfa drugs or with active (transient) attacks, the clinical indications are as follows:

1. Pre- and postcarotid endarterectomy for patients with transient ischemic attacks, recent stroke (within 6–8 weeks) and amaurosis fugax.[145]

2. Evaluation of cerebral flow reserve in the patient with significant cerebrovascular occlusive disease.[145,159-161]

3. Objective evaluation of normalcy of restored flow after carotid reconstruction.[154]

4. Evaluation of vasoreactivity in areas with intrahemispheric thalamic diaschisis and cross-cerebellar diaschisis.[155]

5. Evaluation of vasoreactivity in SAH: deterioration of vasoreactivity by vasospasm due to angiography, intracerebral hematoma, surgical intervention, or severe intracranial pressure.[156]

6. Prognosis for postoperative outcomes of AVM.[157] Visual interpretation includes hemispheric uptake

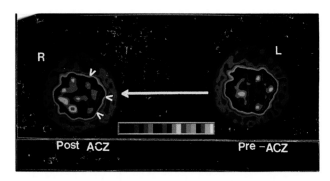

Fig. 23-10 Diamox Tc-99m HMPAO brain SPECT scan shows compromised perfusion reserve in a 61-year-old man with left internal carotid artery occlusion and 80% left vertebral artery stenosis (open arrowheads) in post-ACZ image compared with pre-ACZ images.

symmetry, focal area of absent or decreased uptake, and the response to ACZ.

7. Monitoring of cerebral vasospasm after aneurysmal SAH. Serial brain SPECT scans with ACZ are useful for monitoring the development of cerebral vasospasm to determine the most appropriate time for aneurysm surgery.[158]

The results of the assessment can be classified as follows:[145,153]

1. Normal: symmetrical uptake and no change in the distribution between the baseline and ACZ SPECT scans.

2. Compromised perfusion reverse: normal baseline study and focal or hemispheric asymmetry on ACZ SPECT (Fig. 23-10). These patients are most likely to benefit from medical or surgical efforts to augment blood flow delivery.[145]

3. Chronic ischemia with compromised perfusion reverse: focal or hemispheric asymmetry at the baseline is increased further on ACZ SPECT.

4. Decreased baseline with augmentation of the post-ACZ injection. The findings may be explained either by adequate collateral circulation or by an intact vasodilatory reserve.[145] These patients are probably not good candidates for vascular reconstructive surgery.

Tc-99m HMPAO Brain SPECT with the Balloon Occlusion Test

Permanent occlusion of the internal carotid artery may be required for en bloc resection of a neoplastic lesions in the neck or skull base or to treat certain intracerebral aneurysms (cavernous aneurysm).[162] The risk of ischemic infarct is usually assessed with carotid balloon test occlusion.[151,163–170] Up to 20% of patients have delayed neurological sequelae after permanent occlusion despite tolerance of a 15- to 30-min test occlusion without symptoms.[151,162]

In a typical procedure, the balloon is kept inflated for 15–45 min; then HMPAO is injected.[163,168] SPECT images are performed 1–6 hr later. Tc-99m HMPAO SPECT in conjunction with the balloon test can show clinically silent areas of decreased perfusion. Such patients are at increased risk of permanent sequelae after permanent carotid occlusion.[165] It is essential to assess collateral cerebral perfusion prior to performing external carotid/internal artery bypass so that the complications of stroke can be reduced.[165] Timing of HMPAO injection at the duration of the inflated balloon is the key to an abnormal perfusion finding in asymptomatic patients. The delayed injection of Tc-99m HMPAO may demonstrate collateral flow more clearly because it may take time for collateral perfusion to develop.[163] The duration of balloon inflation should be further evaluated. Nevertheless, Tc-99m HMPAO brain SPECT should be an integral part of the balloon occlusion examination.

Hyperventilation Test

The cerebrovascular response to the reduction of carbon dioxide is well known. Cerebral blood flow during voluntary hyperventilation in man is known to decrease by 30–40%.[171–173] Decreased cerebral blood flow is primarily due to cerebral vasoconstriction caused by hypocapnia, with little influence by any accompanying change in blood pressure.[174] Terada et al.[152] reported a patient with repeated attacks of transient left hemaparesis who underwent a hyperventilation test resulting in vasospasm of the right anterior cerebral artery. The reduction of cerebral flow by 67–78% was demonstrated by brain SPECT. The concurrent angiogram confirmed this finding.[152] The most important information regarding flow alteration obtained from the hyperventilation test is the capillary level. This information is easily provided by brain SPECT scans showing perfusion defects. The hyperventilation test appears to be useful for detecting alterations in regional brain perfusion due to vasospasm during a brief intervention period.

Upright Stress Test

Postural cerebral hypotension can lead to transient neurological deficits during postural change.[174] Patients with cerebrovascular disease have been studied by comparing brain SPECT scans after upright and supine injection of Tc-99m HMPAO. The hypoperfusion visualized on the upright scans may relate to silent cerebral ischemia.[176]

HEAD TRAUMA

Certain imaging techniques are useful in the diagnostic evaluation of closed intracranial injury. MRI is more useful than CT in the evaluation of small lesions, chronic lesions, and isointense subdural hematomas.[177] In mild head trauma, CT and MRI may not be helpful in demonstrating structural changes. Functional brain SPECT imaging has been used in head traumas and appears to be very promising.[178]

Tc-99m HM-PAO SPECT shows functional abnormalities triggered by head trauma, even when the CT or MRI images are normal. In 14 patients with normal CT or MRI scans all brain SPECT scans showed abnormal cerebral perfusion, which correlated with clinically detected abnormalities.[178] These abnormalities may have resulted from altered regional cerebral flow regulation, either as a direct consequence of head trauma or as a secondary result of metabolic abnormalities.[179,180] In one study, intracerebral hematomas (>1.5 cm) were always surrounded by a zone of ischemic tissue, as shown by severe reduction of perfusion on SPECT scans, and by pyknotic dead neurons; vasospasm was not shown in the periphery of these lesions. Focal hyperemia was seen in the normal tissue (as judged by CT and/or MRI) adjacent to or contralateral to the focal lesion; it lasted for up to 2 weeks after injury.[181]

SPECT abnormalities are larger than those noted on CT,[180,182,183] with decreased tracer retention in the ipsilateral hemispheres.[182] Brain SPECT is significantly more sensitive than CT in the detection of both minor and major head injuries.[184] Defects on SPECT scans have been correlated with focal neurological deficits[185] that were not explained by CT or MRI. SPECT may complement the clinical evaluation in assessment of the outcome after head injury, executive function, and memory disturbance.[185] In addition, posttraumatic behavioral and affective disorders, as well as the locations of decreased perfusion in Tc-99m HMPAO brain SPECT scans, have been assessed.[186,187]

BRAIN DEATH

The definition of brain death is total and irreversible cessation of brain function. Clinical diagnosis of brain death is based on the presence of deep coma, absence of spontaneous respiration, and absence of brain stem reflexes.[188] Available diagnostic methods for brain death include contrast cerebral angiography, EEG, Doppler sonography, and scintigraphy. Two kinds of radionuclide scintigraphy are available for brain death. One is conventional brain imaging using Tc-99m DTPA or Tc-99m glucohepatonate; the other is a cerebral flow study using Tc-99m HMPAO or I-123 IMP. Brain death is rapidly followed by cerebral edema and increased intracranial pressure. The intracranial pressure eventually exceeds the cerebral arterial pressure and cerebral perfusion ceases, resulting in absence of cerebral flow by contrast or radionuclide cerebral angiography. Using a cerebral perfusion agent such as Tc-99m HMPAO, absent uptake reflects nonviability of parenchyma of the brain. Presence of uptake in the brain reflects viability of brain tissue.

Diagnosis of Brain Death Using Conventional Brain Scintigraphy

Brain scintigraphy using a Tc-99m DTPA or Tc-99m glucohepatonate cerebral angiogram and static brain imaging aids in the diagnosis of brain death.[189-192] The scintigraphy technique is as follows: (1) the images are obtained with either a stationary or a portable gamma camera; (2) 20–30 mCi of Tc-99m DTPA or Tc-99m glucohepatonate is IV injected; (3) a cerebral angiogram is recorded at a rate of 2 sec/frame; (4) the static blood pool obtained immediately after flow is studied. The scintigraphic criteria of brain death are the absence of cerebral artery flow on the cerebral angiogram, absence of a sagittal venous sinus on the cerebral angiogram, and static brain images.[191] A ''hot'' nose may also be visualized in brain death patients.[191] In conventional radionuclide brain imaging, this is due to an increase in collateral blood flow from the external carotid artery through the facial and ophthalmic arteries. The presence of hot nose has been reported in 73% of brain death cases.[191] It is considered a secondary, nonspecific scintigraphic sign used only to support a diagnosis of brain death.[191]

Absence of superior sagittal sinus (SSS) activity is not diagnostically definitive of brain death. Frequently scintigraphic patterns show no cerebral arterial flow with SSS visualization. The following are explanations of SSS activity despite absence of cerebral flow:

1. Filling of venous sinuses through emissary veins via the external carotid artery.
2. Supply through a collateral vein.

3. Supply by the external carotid artery system through rich flax and tentorium vascular structures.
4. Existing perforated communication between the internal and external carotid circulations.

Lee et al.[192] report that the mere presence of SSS in the absence of cerebral artery flow is not clinically significant and does not contradict the diagnosis of brain death. There has been no report of patient survival in the absence of detectable intracranial blood flow with the presence of SSS activity.[191]

Absence of cerebral arterial flow is the most reliable criterion used to confirm brain death. Absent cerebral flow is explained as increased intracranial pressure exceeding systolic blood pressure. Cessation of internal carotid artery flow at the siphon is due to the increase in intracranial pressure, not to intraluminal obstruction; however, hemodynamic effects are similar in patients with true intraluminal obstruction of the internal carotid artery(ies).

False-negative reports of brain death can result from cerebral radionuclide flow studies. Visible normal intracerebral blood flow in the presence of clinical brain death has been observed in patients with a ventricular drain[193] or open skull fracture.[194]

Diagnosis of brain death depends on arrest of the carotid circulation at the base of the skull, as well as absence of cerebral perfusion due to the edema and consequent increase in intracranial pressure exceeding the level of systolic arterial pressure. Adjustment in the arterial blood pressure and in the intracranial pressure gradient, either by an increase in arterial blood pressure or a decrease in intracranial pressure, permits cerebral blood flow. A skull defect or an intraventricular drain producing decompression allows cerebral blood flow even neuronal death of the brain. After severe ischemia, reperfusion at the microvascular level does not occur. In this event, planar imaging using Tc-99m is better than a TC-99m DTPA or Tc-99m glucohepatonate cerebral flow study. Normal Tc-99m HMPAO brain imaging depends not only on regional cerebral blood flow but also on the normal neuronal capacity to localize Tc-99m HMPAO.

Diagnosis of Brain Death Using a Cerebral Perfusion Agent

Tc-99m HMPAO or I-123 IMP, a lipophilic perfusion agent, crosses the intact blood–brain barrier and accumulates in the neurons of the brain parenchyma and glial cells. The uptake and retention in the neurons are equal to cellular viability. Because of its properties, the tracer is particularly well suited to examination of brain death. Tc-99m HMPAO allows the use of 10–30 mCi to perform a cerebral first-pass study to examine the carotids and middle cerebral arteries similar to performing conventional brain scintigraphy. Planar/SPECT images, as well as a cerebral flow study, can be completed within 15–20 min. The criteria for brain death using Tc-99m HMPAO are straightforward: (1) absent flow through the internal carotid, middle cerebral, and anterior cerebral arteries and (2) absence of uptake in the cerebrum and cerebellum. Hot nose may also be seen (Fig. 23-11). Usually cerebral uptake disappears before cerebellar uptake[195–198] unless massive cerebellar bleeding occurred.[199] Patients with suprainfratentorial blood flow dissociation, lack of supratentorial perfusion, and preservation of infratentorial perfusion cannot be considered dead, although the prognosis is poor and death may occur within a short time.[198] Tc-99mm HMPAO imaging is as simple and convenient as conventional radionuclide angiography but provides more certain evidence for a diagnosis of brain death.

Advantages and Disadvantages of Tc-99m HMPAO

The advantages of the Tc-99m HMPAO cerebral flow study for brain death are as follows: (1) a dynamic first-pass study can be done; (2) it allows visualization of the posterior fossa (cerebellum), as well as the cerebral hemispheres; (3) it does not depend on an adequate bolus injection to determine brain death; and (4) it does not require consideration of dural venous sinus activity.

The disadvantages are as follows: (1) Tc-99m HMPAO is more expensive than Tc-99m DTPA or Tc-99m glucohepatonate and (2) there is chemical instability after reconstruction.

Epilepsy

The electroencephalogram (EEG) is the gold standard for evaluation of epilepsy. Adjunctive tests include MRI and CT (structural evaluation) and SPECT and PET (functioning imaging). The changes in cerebral perfusion are not always accompanied by structural changes detectable by CT or MRI imaging. EEG can determine the patient's functional status during an attack, but it has significant limitations in lateralizing or localizing

the origin of the seizure or determining the severity and extent of the underlying cerebral involvement.

Effective surgical treatment of patients with epileptic seizures depends on accurate preoperative seizure focus localization. In addition to precise focus localization, estimation of the postoperative outcome in regard to seizure frequency and memory function is the goal of presurgical studies.[200] Noninvasive assessment of brain function is becoming increasingly important when evaluating epileptic patients for surgical treatment. Brain SPECT using Tc-99m HMPAO or I-123 HIPDM has become a valuable diagnostic procedure for the lateralization and localization of epileptic foci,[201–204] especially in patients without morphological lesions by CT or MRI.[205] Rowe et al. concluded that Tc-HMPAO brain SPECT is a useful noninvasive technique for independent confirmation of EEG seizure localization.[203]

Seizures with pronounced changes in regional cerebral flow (rCBF) and metabolic (glucose) shown by PET,[206] rCBF and metabolism are associated. Since Tc-99m HMPAO localizes in brain parenchymal cells, with virtually no washout, the pattern of brain SPECT reveals the rCBF at the time of tracer injection.[15] Blood flow revealed by SPECT reflects the ictal or postictal status of brain metabolism. Hyperperfusion or increased tracer uptake within the epileptic focus in the temporal or extratemporal areas occurs during seizure attack. In the interictal period between seizure attacks, the focus of increased uptake in ictal phase becomes decreased uptake or cold area.[207] Interictal images are usually obtained following the ictal study, with a minimum period of 24 hr after the last seizure.[206]

Tc-99m HMPAO brain SPECT is more suitable for use in epileptic seizure patients than PET since the greater complexity of PET imaging and the ultra-short half-life of the isotopes used make such ictal studies more difficult to obtain.[206] Injection of Tc-99m HMPAO during seizures provides the findings of dramatic perfusion changes than that of studies injection by interictal and postictal.[208] For ictal SPECT, the radiopharmaceutical should be injected as soon as possible after seizure onset. If IV injection of the tracer is done within 15 min[202] or 30 min[203] of seizure onset (optimal time of injection is less than 1 min), either ictal or postictal brain SPECT images will be obtained. The SPECT images can be obtained 1–2 hr after cessation of the seizure, revealing the rCBF at the time of tracer (HMPAO) injection (Fig. 23-12). Ictal or postictal Tc-99m HMPAO brain SPECT is more valuable than interictal images, having 73% for ictal vs. 43% interictal[202] respectively. Simultaneous interpretation of ictal (or postictal) and interictal brain SPECT images im-

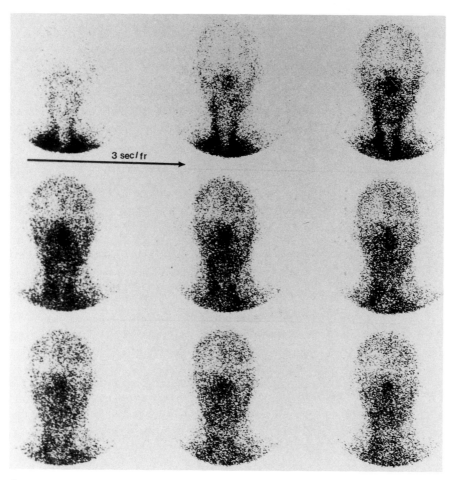

A

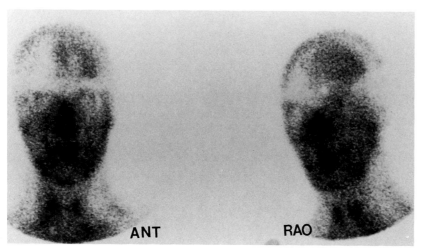

B

Fig. 23-11 (*A*) Thirty-six hours after a motor vehicle accident, a 19-year-old man was referred for evaluation of brain death. He had left skull fracture and laceration of the scalp with sutures. A first-pass cerebral flow study shows absence of middle and anterior cerebral flow bilaterally. There is gradual buildup of activity in the scalp/skull, with increased activity on the left side of the head due to the left scalp laceration and skull fracture. (*B*) Immediately anterior planar brain scan image shows absent perfusion in the cerebral and cerebellar hemispheres. The activity on the left side of the head is due to scalp and skull lesions and should not be mistaken for cerebral uptake.

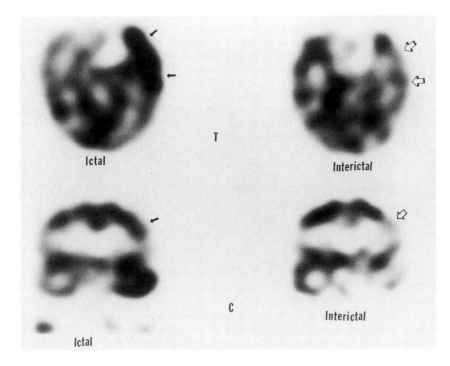

Fig. 23-12 Tc-99m HMPAO brain SPECT scans in an epilepsy patient show hyperperfusion (solid arrow) in the ictal images and hypoperfusion in the interictal images (open arrows). T = transaxial section; C = coronal section.

proves localization of the epileptogenic area,[202–204] and ictal/postictal brain SPECT is reliable for presurgical localization of a complex partial seizure.[209] Postictally, a typical pattern consists of temporolateral hypoperfusion and temporomesial hyperperfusion in temporal lobe epilepsy.

A method for rapid preparation (reconstitution) of Tc-99m HMPAO and optimal deployment of the radiopharmaceutical during seizures in the video-EEG monitoring suite has been reported.[210] The clinical results in patients with temporal lobe epilepsy show that ictal studies (97% correct lateralization of focus, 0% incorrect) are more sensitive and accurate than interictal ones (48% correct, 10% incorrect.)[210]

To improve the diagnostic accuracy of brain SPECT in epilepsy, interventional techniques may be used to detect ictal hyperfusion. HMPAO can be injected during EEG monitoring and videotaping; then the patient can be transported to the nuclear medicine service for study. Interventional methods include (1) asking questions to stimulate the seizure in patients with epileptic/psychogenic seizures, (2) hyperventilation tests, and (3) reduction of medication. Interventional brain SPECT allows normally perfused or hypoperfused areas interictally to become hyperperfused. Brain SPECT can be used in the evaluation of posttemporal lobectomy to confirm the lesion.[15] The Wada test (unilateral hemispheric anesthesia) is also used in patients with temporal lobe epilepsy to determine the vulnerability of speech centers.[211] Recently, the imaging of benzodi-

azepine receptors by ^{123}I-iomazenil has been used to localize the focus in temporal lobe epilepsy. In some cases, it has been more sensitive than blood flow imaging.[212]

DEMENTIA

Alzheimer's Disease

Diagnosis of probable Alzheimer's disease is made by a combination of characteristic clinical findings when normal laboratory studies reveal no structural or metabolic cause of the dementia. A definitive diagnosis, however, can only be made with brain tissue examination. PET scanning reveals parietotemporal decreases in cerebral blood flow and glucose metabolism that differentiate Alzheimer's disease from normal aging and from multi-infarct dementia.[213–215]

As with PET, the appearance of Alzheimer's disease on brain SPECT consists of bilateral posterior temporal and/or parietal perfusion defects. The degree of abnormality on SPECT scans correlates with the severity of dementia.[216] Alzheimer's disease produces regional perfusion and metabolic abnormalities without corresponding abnormalities on CT or MRI images.[217,218] In addition to Alzheimer's disease, the scintigraphic defects in the parietal and temporal regions (Fig. 23-13B) include decreased cortical thickness in the temporoparietal cortex[219] and a reduction in neuron number.[220]

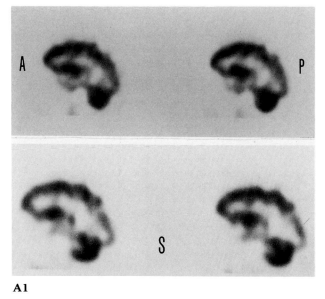

A1

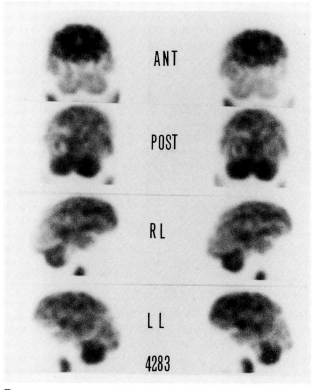

B

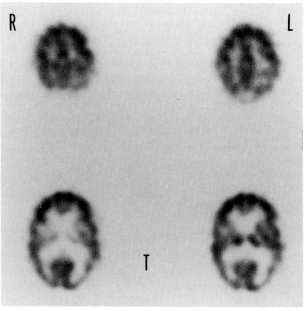

A2

Fig. 23-13 (*A*) Alzheimer's disease with posterior cortical hypoperfusion bilaterally in a 69-year-old man (PI 4283) with increased difficulty with short-term memory. T = transaxial; S = sagittal. (*B*) Volume three-dimensional displays show diffuse hypoperfusion in the posterior cerebral cortices.

The scintigraphic appearance of Alzheimer's disease has been divided into six patterns.[217] The predictive value of these patterns is as follows: The probability of Alzheimer's disease is 82% with bilateral temporal and/or parietal defects, 77% with bilateral temporal and/or parietal cortex defects together with additional defects, 57% with unilateral temporoparietal defects, 43% with frontal defects only, 18% with other large (>1 cm) defects, and 0% with multiple small (≤1 cm) cortical defects.[217,218] Thus, the predominant finding of bilateral posterior temporal/parietal defects in these patients is highly predictive Alzheimer's disease.[217,218] A method

of quantitative brain SPECT analysis in comparison with the pattern of normal aging has been developed. This method has proved accurate in distinguishing Alzheimer's disease patients from elderly controls.[221]

Bilateral posterior cortical defects may not be a specific pattern of Alzheimer's disease. Cortical defects may also appear in Parkinson's disease,[222,223] hypoglycemia,[224] carbon monoxide poisoning,[223] vascular dementia,[225] mitochondrial encephalopathy,[226] and obstructive hydrocephalus.[227]

In general, different types of degenerative dementia exhibit distinct patterns of Tc-99m HMPAO localization;[228] however, in Alzheimer's disease, decreased uptake is prominent in the parietal and temporal lobes. Hypoperfusion is significant only in the superior and inferior parts of the frontal lobes, most likely due to Pick's disease (Fig. 23-14). Patients with progressive supranuclear palsy exhibit a slight but significant re-

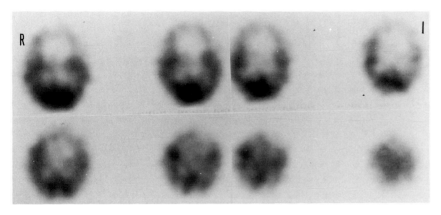

Fig. 23-14 Transaxial brain SPECT scans in Pick's disease: diffuse hypoperfusion involving both frontal lobes and hypoperfusion extending to the left temporal lobe.

duction in perfusion in the superofrontal cortex (Fig. 23-15). In patients with Parkinson's disease, significant decreases in uptake in the parietal, temporal, and occipital cortices occur.[228]

Dementia of Parkinson's Disease

Dementia in Parkinson's disease is thought to be attributable not only to subcortical lesions but also to cortical alterations. Dementia occurs in 10–40% of patients with Parkinson's disease.[229] Cortical perfusion defects[230–232] and basal ganglia perfusion abnormalities[216]

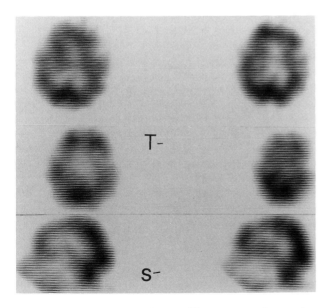

Fig. 23-15 Transaxial and sagittal brain SPECT images in a patient with progressive supranuclear palsy: hypoperfusion in the suprafrontal cortices.

demonstrated by brain SPECT have been reported. As in Alzheimer's disease, demented patients with Parkinson's disease had significant reduction in the parietal, temporal,[231,233] and occipital cortices.[231] Three patterns of cortical involvement have been described: (1) hypoperfusion of the frontal lobe in 3 of 4 patients, (2) hypoperfusion of the frontal and parietal lobes in 8 of 13 patients, and (3) hypoperfusion of the parietal lobe in 1 of 13 patients;[223] Frontal hypoperfusion was present in 12 of the 13 dementia patients.[228] These abnormalities have been successfully detected by Tc-99m HMPAO brain spect (Fig. 23-16).

Schizophrenia

Gross brain structure in patients with psychiatric disorders is preserved on structural images. Functional imaging shows abnormal brain function related to disturbance in perfusion or metabolism. In brain SPECT imaging of schizophrenia, there are three groups of findings: (1) frontal lobe hypoperfusion, (2) altered basal ganglia perfusion, and (3) altered temporal lobe perfusion.[234]

Hypoperfusion in the frontal lobe has been shown in a female schizophrenic patient and in schizoaffectives[235] with some evidence of greater impairment in the left frontal lobe compared to the right.[236] Schizophrenic patients with auditory hallucinations have been found to have increased uptake in the left superior temporal lobe of the primary and secondary auditory centers on brain SPECT.[237–240] Patients with acute paranoid schizophrenia with paranoid delusions, auditory hallucinations, and/or destructive behavior may show increased uptake in the caudate nuclei and right superior temporal region, possibly associated with decreased uptake in the frontal lobes.[237,240]

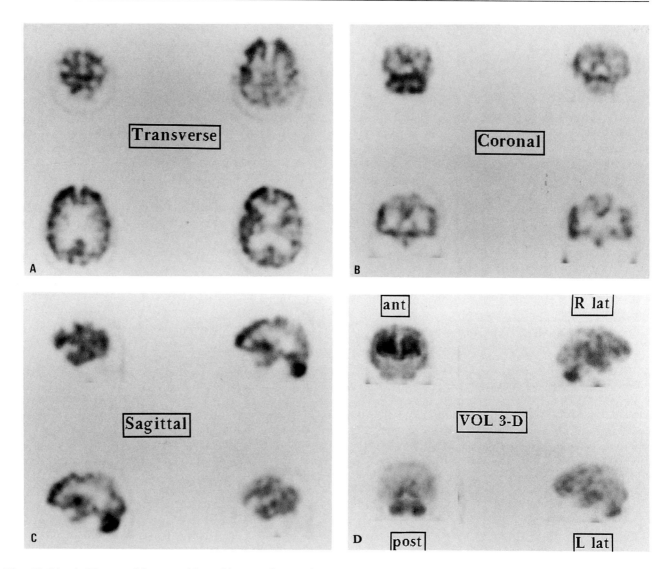

Fig. 23-16   A 78-year-old man with Parkinson's disease for 10 years developed confusion and dementia. Transaxial (*A*), coronal (*B*), and sagittal (*C*) sections show hypoperfusion in the bitemporal-parietal region (worse on the left side) and asymmetrical uptake (decreased on the left side). Volume three-dimensional displays (*D*) show decreased uptake in the posterior cortices. Surface three-dimensional displays

Affective Disorders

The unipolar depressed patient typically shows generalized decreased cortical tracer uptake, especially in the frontal lobes.[241] Cerebral perfusion in 115 patients with mood and behavior disorders has been studied by Tc-99m HMPAO brain SPECT; 40 of 52 patients with abnormal brain SPECT scans had temporal hypoperfusion (27 on the right, 22 on the left, 2 on both); 11 patients had hypoperfusion in the basal ganglia; in the frontal, parietal, or occipital lobes; or in the thalamus.[242]

Obsessive-Compulsive Disorder

Obsessive-compulsive disorder apparently occurs more frequently than schizophrenic disorders, mania, and panic disorders.[240] The proposed dysfunctional areas in the disorder include the frontal lobes and basal ganglia.[243,244] In brain SPECT studies,[245–247] there was significantly increased Tc-99m HMPAO uptake in the left posterofrontal cortex, in the orbital frontal cortex (medial frontal),[242] and in the high dorsal parietal cortex bilaterally.[247] There was also significantly decreased

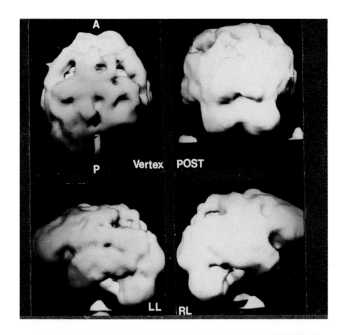

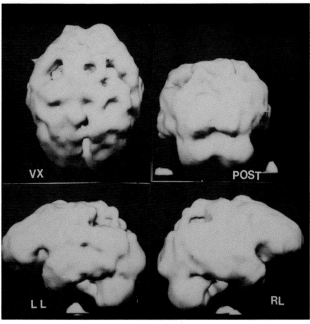

E

Fig. 23-16 (*E*) show multiple perfusion defects in the parietal-temporal region bilaterally.

uptake in the head of the caudate nucleus bilaterally. These results provide additional support for the involvement of specific cortical areas and caudate nucleus and help to clarify the pathophysiology of this illness.[247]

Chronic Fatigue Syndrome

Chronic fatigue syndrome is a disabling illness with both somatic and neuropsychological symptoms of uncertain etiology. Physical and laboratory findings are usually unremarkable. The rCBF of the cortical/cerebellar ratio has been studied in chronic fatigue syndrome. Compared with normal subjects, chronic fatigue syndrome patients showed significantly lower cerebral perfusion ratios in the frontal (63% of cases), parietal (53%), temporal (35%), and occipital (38%) regions. Brain SPECT provides objective evidence for functional impairment of the brain and may play an important role in clarifying the pathophysiology of the disease.[247]

HIV Infection

Tc-99m HMDP brain SPECT of HIV-infected patients showed focal defects in 6 of 30 and diffuse perfusion defects in 9 of 30.[248] There was a significant correlation between perfusion defects and the presence of anticardiolipin antibodies.[249]

BRAIN SPECT IN SUBSTANCE ABUSE

Various effects on the central nervous system due to chronic ethanol intake have been demonstrated, including reduction of cerebral gray matter observed by MRI.[250] Hypometabolism in the medial frontal region of the cerebral cortex has been detected by PET using F-18-2-fluoro-2 deoxy-*d*-glucose in alcoholic patients.[251] Impairment of rCBF has also been observed.[252,253] An alcohol- and diazepam-abusing patient had a fronto-temporo-parietal defect on the left side on a brain SPECT scan, which was also demonstrated by three-dimensional displays.[254] A long history of alcoholism results in hypoperfusion in both hemispheres, especially involving the left fronto-temporo-parietal region (Fig. 23-17A,B).

In a study of asymptomatic patients with chronic alcoholism, 65% showed significant hypoperfusion mainly in the frontal and temporal lobes, with only 25% exhibiting morphometric evidence of frontal lobe atrophy on CT.[255] A group of 10 alcoholics underwent another SPECT scan after 2 months of alcohol abstinence; the rCBF ratio of the frontal lobes normalized in 8 of them. It has been concluded that asymptomatic chronic alcoholics frequently showed reversible frontal lobe hypoperfusion related to recent ethanol intake.[255]

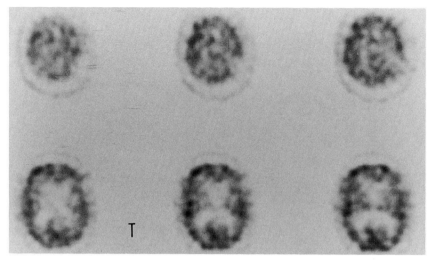

A

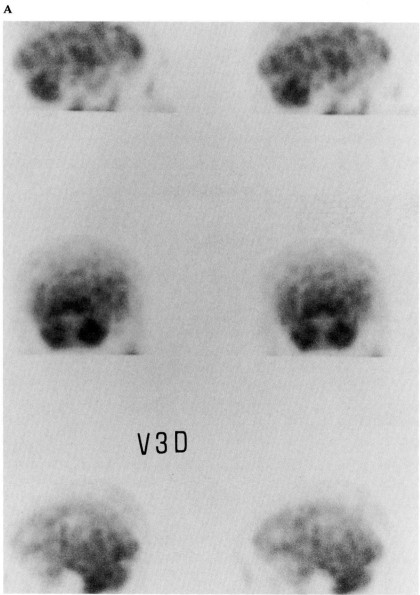

B

Fig. 23-17 A 58-year-old man (SR 3288) with chronic alcoholism complicated by Korsakoff's psychosis (gross defect of memory for recent events associated with disorientation). Brain SPECT scans show global hypoperfusion with prominent hypoperfusion on the left. (*B*) Three-dimensional volume displays demonstrate hypoperfusion involving especially the left fronto-temporo-parietal region.

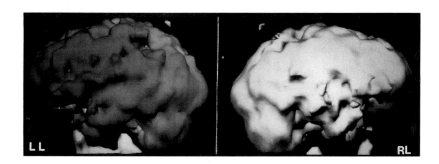

Fig. 23-17 (*C*) Three-dimensional surface displays demonstrate a perfusion defect in the left hemisphere involving the fronto-temporo-parietal region.

C

Two possible forms of brain damage are exhibited by chronic alcoholics: (1) a subacute effect on the cerebral microcirculation and (2) a more chronic effect on the cortical or subcortical structures. The subacute effect on the microcirculation of the brain may be explained by the hypoperfusion of the frontal lobes resulting from recent ethanol intake. The chronic effect on cortical or subcortical structures may play a part in the origin of the cerebral atrophy which correlates with the total lifetime consumption of ethanol.[255] It is also suggested that chronic hypnosedative abuse may lead to local neuronal alteration that attenuates the neuronal capacity to localize Tc-99m HMPAO, resulting in the cerebral defects.[254] This is similar to the condition of patients with Creutzfeldt-Jakob disease or Alzheimer's disease who had no observable changes in brain tissue density, as shown by CT or MRI, but who demonstrated cerebral perfusion defects on brain SPECT.[256–259]

Cocaine causes many serious medical problems affecting metabolism and function in the brain, heart, lung, and other tissues.[260–263] The neurovascular complications lead to cerebral infarct, subdural and intracerebral hemorrhage, cerebral ischemia, vascular spasm, and cerebral vasculitis.[261,262,264,265] Brain SPECT scans of cocaine users showed perfusion defects,[264–267] though these patterns are often indistinguishable from those in early AIDS dementia complex.[255] The perfusion defects in Tc-99m HMPAO brain SPECT observed in chronic cocaine polydrug users improved with short-term treatment.[267]

An I-123 IMP brain SPECT study of crack users showed that the rate of cerebral uptake averaged 23% less than that of a control group over the first 25 min after tracer injection; the foci of abnormally reduced uptake were found mainly in the frontal and parieto-occipital cortices. Focal defects observed 6/21 in crack users with filled-in on 4-hr images in four of six patients.[268] Neurovascular complications and/or neuronal changes associated with cocaine use are responsible for the SPECT findings.

Neuropsychogenic complications have been associated with amphetamine abuse. Amphetamine-related necrotizing angiitis, vasculitis, and hemorrhage has been described.[269,270] The Tc-99m HMPAO brain SPECT study in amphetamine abusers has been evaluated;[271] the results demonstrated that 20/21 (95%) patients had small defects and 15/21 (71%) patients had multiple defects in the cerebral hemispheres.

Tc-99m HMPAO brain SPECT scans in heroin abusers have been studied.[272] Like PET studies, Tc-99m HMPAO brain SPECT scans showed decreased perfusion in the right temporal lobe and gyrus post centralis of heroin abusers.[272] The density of opiate receptors was high in the right temporal lobe.[272]

REFERENCES

1. Go RT, Aba Yousef MM, Jacoby CG. The role of radionuclide brain imaging and computerized tomography in the early diagnosis of herpes simplex encephalitis. *CT* 1979;3:286–296.

2. Shih WJ, DeLand FH. Equivocal findings on cranial CT but apparent lesion(s) on conventional radionuclide imaging. *Clin Nucl Med* 1987;12:219–222.

3. Van-Heertum RL, O'Connell RA. Functional brain imaging in evaluation of psychiatric illness. *Semin Nucl Med* 1991;21:24–39.

4. Lim CB, Walker R, Pinkstaff C, et al. Triangular SPECT system for 3-D organ volume imaging: Clinical prototype and dynamic potential. *J Nucl Med* 1985;26(5):P11.

5. Kung HF, Ohmomo Y, Kung MP. Current and future radiopharmaceutical for brain imaging with SPECT. *Semin Nucl Med* 1990;20:290–302.

6. Pupi A, Bisi G, Sciagra R, et al. The comparison of brain distribution of HMPAO and microspheres in humans. *J Cereb Blood Flow Metab* 1989;9:S411.

7. Yonekura Y, Nishizawa S, Mukai T, et al. SPECT with Tc-HMPAO compared with regional cerebral blood

flow measured by PET: Effects of linearisation. *J Cereb Blood Flow Metab* 1988;8:S82–S89.

8. Inugami A, Kanno I, Uemura K, et al. Linearisation correction of Tc-labelled HMPAO image in terms of regional CBF distribution: Comparison to C-15-O₂ inhalation steady-state method measured by positron emission tomography. *J Cereb Blood Flow Metab* 1988; 8:S52–S60.

9. Gemmell HG, Evans NTS, Besson JAO, et al. Regional CBF imaging: A quantitative comparison of 99mTc-HMPAO SPECT with C-15-O₂ PET. *J Nucl Med* 1990;31: 1595–1600.

10. Heiss W-D, Herholz K, Podreka I, et al. Comparison of 99mTc HMPAO SPECT with [18F]fluoromethane PET in cerebrovascular disease. *J Cereb Blood Flow Metab* 1990;10:687–697.

11. Neirinckx RD, Canning LR, Piper IM, et al. Technetium-99m d, 1-HM-PAO: A new radiopharmaceutical for SPECT imaging of regional cerebral blood perfusion. *J Nucl Med* 1987;28:191–202.

12. Sharp PF, Smith FW, Gemmell HG, et al. Technetium-99m HMPAO stereoisomers as potential agents for imaging regional cerebral blood flow: Human volunteer studies. *J Nucl Med* 1986;27:171–177.

13. Neirinckx RD, Burke JF, Harrison RC, et al. The retention mechanism of Tc-99m HMPAO: Intracellular reaction with glutathione. *J Cereb Blood Flow Metab* 1988;8: S4–S12.

14. Laurin NR, Driedgar AA, Hurwitz GA, et al. Cerebral perfusion imaging with Tc-99m HMPAO in brain death and severe central nervous system injury. *J Nucl Med* 1989;30:1627–1635.

15. Biersack JH, Brunwald F, Reichmann K, et al. Functional brain SPECT imaging with Tc-99m HMPAO. *Nucl Med Ann* 1990 (Ed. Freeman LM);59–93. Raven Press, NY

16. Weisner PS, Bower GR, Dollimore LA, et al. A method for stabilizing Tc-99m exametazime prepared from a commercial kit. *Eur J Nucl Med* 1993;20:661–666.

17. Gartshore G, Bannan P, Patterson J, et al: Evaluation of Tc-99m exametazine stabilized with cobalt chloride as a blood flow tracer in focal cerebral ischemia. *Eur J Nucl 1944,* 21:913–923.

18. Holman BL, Lee RGL, Hill TC, et al. A comparison of two cerebral blood flow tracers in I-123 IMB and I-123 HIPDM in humans. *J Nucl Med* 1984;25:25–30.

19. Moretti JL, Cinotti L, Cesaro P, et al. Amines for brain tomoscintigraphy. *Nucl Med Commun* 1987;8:581–595.

20. Odano I, Tsuchiya T, Nishihara M. Regional cerebral blood flow measured with I-123 IMP and its redistribution in ischemic cerebrovascular disease. *Stroke* 1993; 24:1167–1172.

21. Matsuda H, Li YM, Higashi S, et al. Comparative SPECT

study of stroke using Tc-99m ECD, I-123 IMP, and Tc-99m HMPAO. *Clin Nucl Med* 1993;18:754–758.

22. Walovitch RC, Franceschi M, Picard M, et al. Metabolism of Tc-99m L,L-ethyl cysteinate dimer in healthy volunteers. *Neuropharmacology* 1991;30:283–292.

23. Leveille J, Demonceau G, De Roo M, et al. Characterization of technetium-99m-L,L-ECD for brain perfusion imaging: Part 2. Biodistribution and brain imaging in humans. *J Nucl Med* 1989;30:1902–1911.

24. Holman BL, Hellman RS, Goldsmith SJ, et al. Biodistribution, dosimetry, and clinical evaluation of technetium-99m ethyl cysteinate dimer in normal subjects and in patients with chronic cerebral infarction. *J Nucl Med* 1989;30:1018–1024.

25. Leveille J, Demonceau G, Walovitch RC: intrasubject comparison between technetium-99m-ECD and technetium-99m-HMPAO in healthy human subjects. *J Nucl Med* 1992;33:480–484.

26. Vallabhajosula S, Zimmerman RE, Picard M, et al. Technetium-99m ECD: A new brain imaging agent: In vivo kinetics and biodistribution studies in normal human subjects. *J Nucl Med* 1989;30:599.

27. Matsuda H, Li YM, Higashi S, et al. Comparative SPECT study of stroke using Tc-99m ECD, I-123 IMP, and Tc-99m HMPAO. *Clin Nucl Med* 1993;18:754–758.

28. Kuhl DE, Edwards RQ. Image separation radioisotope scanning. *Radiology* 1963;80:653–662.

29. Kuhl DE, Edwards RQ. Cylindrical and section radioisotope scanning of the liver and brain. *Radiology* 1964; 83:926–935.

30. Kuhl DE, Edwards RQ. Reorganizing data from transverse section scans of the brain using digital processing. *Radiology* 1968;91:975–983.

31. Jaszczak RJ, Murphy PH, Huard D, et al. Radionuclide emission computed tomography of the head with ⁹⁹ᵐTc and a scintillation camera. *J Nucl Med* 1977;18: 373–380.

32. Keyes JW Jr, Orlandea N, Heetderks WJ, et al. The Humogotron—A scintillation-camera transaxial tomography. *J Nucl Med* 1977;18:381–387.

33. Jaszczak RJ, Chang LT, Stein NA, et al. Whole-body single-photon emission computed tomography using dual, large-field-of-view scintillation cameras. *Phys Med Biol* 1979;24:1123–1143.

34. Lim CB, Chang LT, Jaszczak RJ. Performance analysis of three camera configurations for single photon emission computed tomography. *IEEE Trans Nucl Sci* 1980; NS-27:559–568.

35. Lim CB, Gottschalk S, Walker R, et al. Triangular SPECT system for 3-D total organ volume imaging: Design concept and preliminary imaging results. *IEEE Trans Nucl Sci* 1985;NS-32:741–747.

36. Genna S, Smith A. The development of ASPECT, an

annular single crystal brain camera for high efficiency SPECT. *IEEE Trans Nucl Sci* 1988;NS-35:654–658.

37. Smith AP, Genna S. Imaging characteristics of ASPECT, a single-crystal ring camera for dedicated brain SPECT. *J Nucl Med* 1988;30:796–802.

38. Jaszczak RJ, Chang LT, Murphy PH. Single photon emission computed tomography using multi-slice fan beam collimators. *IEEE Trans Nucl Sci* 1979;NS-26:610–619.

39. Tsui BMW, Gullberg GT, Edgerton ER, et al. Design and clinical utility of a fan beam collimator for SPECT imaging of the head. *J Nucl Med* 1986;27:810–819.

40. Gullbert GT, Christian PE, Datz FL, et al. Cardiac SPECT imaging with fan beam collimators. *J Nucl Med* 1990;31:1590. Abstract

41. Jaszczak RJ, Floyd CE, Manglos SM, et al. Cone beam collimation for single photon emission computed tomography: Analysis, simulation, and image reconstruction using filtered backprojection. *Med Phys* 1987;13:484–489.

42. Jaszczak RJ, Greer KL, Coleman RE. SPECT using a specially designed cone beam collimator. *J Nucl Med* 1988;29:1398–1405.

43. Hawman EG, Hsieh J. An astigmatic collimator for high sensitivity SPECT of the brain. *J Nucl Med* 1986;27:930. Abstract

44. Gullberg GT, Zeng GL, Christian PE, et al. Single photon emission computed tomography of the heart using cone beam geometry and noncircular detector rotation, in Ortendahl DA, Llacer J (eds): *Information Processing in Medical Imaging*. XIth IPMI International Conference, Berkeley, California, June 19–23. New York, Wiley-Liss, 1989, pp 123–138.

45. Nohara N, Murayama H, Tanaka E. Single photon emission tomography with increased sampling density at central region of field-of-view. *IEEE Trans Nucl Sci* 1987;NS-34:359–363.

46. Hirose Y, Ikeda Y, Higashi Y, et al. A hybrid emission CT Headtome II. *IEEE Trans Nucl Sci* 1982;NS-29:520–523.

47. Stoddart HF, Stoddart HA. A new development in single gamma transaxial tomography Union Carbide focused collimator scanner. *IEEE Trans Nucl Sci* 1979;NS-26:2710–2712.

48. Moore SC, Doherty MD, Zimmerman RE, et al. Improved performance from modifications to the multidetector SPECT brain scanner. *J Nucl Med* 1984;25:688–691.

49. Stokely EM, Sveinsdottir E, Lassen NA, et al. A single photon dynamic computer assisted tomography (DCAT) for imaging brain function in multiple cross-sections. *J Comput Assist Tomogr* 1980;4:230–240.

50. Lassen NA, Sveinsdottir E, Kanno I, et al. A fast moving single photon emission tomograph for regional cerebral blood flow studies in man. *J Comput Assist Tomogr* 1978;2:661–662.

51. Rogers WL, Clinthorne NH, Shao L, et al. SPRINT II: A second generation single photon ring tomograph. *IEEE Trans Med Imag* 1988;7:291–297.

52. Chang W, Li S, Williams JJ, et al. A position sensitive bar detector for multi-slice brain SPECT (abstract). *J Nucl Med* 1988;29:760.

53. Chang W, Huang G, Wang L. A multi-detector cylindrical SPECT system for phantom imaging, in *Conference Record of the 1990 Nuclear Science Symposium*, Vol 2, IEEE. Piscataway, NJ, 1990, pp 1208–1211.

54. Rowe RK, Barrett HH, Chen J, et al. A stationary, hemispherical SPECT imager for 3D brain imaging. *J Nucl Med* 1993;34:474–480.

55. Milster TD, Aarsvold JN, Barrett HH, et al. A full-field modular gamma camera. *J Nucl Med* 1990;31:632–639.

56. Drane WE, Nicole M, Mastin ST, et al. FDG SPECT: Cost-effective alternative to PET (abstract). *Radiology* 1993;189:303–304.

57. Pelizzari CA, Chen GTV, Spelbring DR, et al. Accurate 3-dimensional registration of CT, PET and/or MR images of the brain. *J Comput Assist Tomogr* 1989;13:20–26.

58. Shih WJ, Coupal JJ, Magoun S, et al. I-123 HIPDM planar brain images demonstrating crossed cerebellar diaschisis. *Clin Nucl Med* 1990;15:34–37.

59. Lee RGL, Hill TC, Holman BL, et al. Comparison of N-isopropyl-^{123}I-p-iodamphetamine brain scans using Anger camera scintigraphy and single-photon emission tomography. *Radiology* 1982;145:789–793.

60. Shih WJ, Hartman RS, McQuade BH, et al. A cystic lesion in the left posterior parietal region demonstrated by Tc-99m HMPAO brain SPECT imaging. *Clin Nucl Med* 1992;17:54–55.

61. Shih WJ, Schleenbaker R, Stipp V, et al. Surface and volume three-dimensional displays of Tc-99m HMPAO brain spect images in stroke patients by three-headed gamma camera. *Clin Nucl Med* 1993;18:945–949.

62. Rubinstein M, Denay R, Ham HR, et al. Functional imaging of brain maturation using I-123 iodoamphetamine and SPECT. *J Nucl Med* 1989;30:1982–1985.

63. Fockele DS, Baumann RJ, Shih WJ, et al. Tc-99m HMPAO SPECT of the brain in the neonate. *Clin Nucl Med* 1990;15:175–177.

64. Park CH, Madsen MT, McLellan T, et al. Iofetamine Hcl I-123 brain scanning in stroke: A comparison with transmission CT. *Radiographics* 1988;8:305–326.

65. Wallis JW, Miller TR. Volume rendering in three-dimensional display of SPECT images. *J Nucl Med* 1990;31:1421–1428.

66. Wallis JW, Miller TR. Three-dimensional display in nu-

clear medicine and radiology. *J Nucl Med* 1991;33: 534–546.

67. Ishimura J, Fukuchi M. Clinical application of three-dimensional surface of display in brain imaging with Tc-99m HMPAO. *Clin Nucl Med* 1991;16:343–351.

68. Shih WJ, Schleenbaker RE, Stipp V, et al. Surface and volume three-dimensional displays of Tc-99m HMPAO SPECT images in stroke patients by three-head gamma camera. *Clin Nucl Med* 1993;18:945–949.

69. Okuda B, Tachibana H, Kawabata K, et al. Three-dimensional surface display with I-123 IMP of slowly progressive apraxia. *Clin Nucl Med* 1993;18:85–87.

70. Shih WJ, Hyatt M. Volume and surface three-dimensional displays of Tc-99m HMPAO brain SPECT imaging in a chronic hypnosedative abuser. *Clin Nucl Med* 1993;18:506–509.

71. Holman BL, Devous MD. Functional brain SPECT: The emergence of a powerful clinical method. *J Nucl Med* 1993;33:1888–1904.

72. Van Heertum RL, Pile-Spellman J, Miller SH, et al. The current role of cerebral SPECT imaging. *Appl Radiol* 1993;(June):22:35–44.

73. Podreka I, Suess E, Goldenberg G, et al. Initial experience with technetium-99m HMPAO brain SPECT. *J Nucl Med* 1987;28:1657–1666.

74. DeRoo M, Morteimans L, Devos P, et al. Clinical experience with Tc-99m HMPAO high-resolution SPECT of the brain in patients with cerebrovascular accidents. *Eur J Nucl Med* 1989;15:9–15.

75. Fieschi G, Argentino C, Lenzi GL, et al. Clinical and instrumental evaluation of patients with ischemic stroke within the first six hours. *J Neuro Sci* 1989;91: 311–322.

76. Rango M, Candelise L, Perani D, et al. Cortical pathophysiology and clinical neurological abnormalities in acute cerebral ischemia. *Arch Neurol* 1989;46: 1318–1322.

77. Hill TC, Magistretti PL, Holman BL, et al. Assessment of regional cerebral blood flow (rCBF) in stroke using SPECT and *N*-isopropyl-(I-123)-*p*-iodoamphetamine (IMP). *Stroke* 1984;15:40–45.

78. Yeh SH, Liu RS, Hu HH, et al. Brain SPECT imaging with Tc-99m HMPAO in the early detection of cerebral infarction: Comparison with transmission computed tomography. *Nucl Med Comm* 1986;7:873–878.

79. Brott TC, Gelfand MJ, Williams CG, et al. Frequency and patterns of abnormality detected by iodine-123 amine emission CT after cerebral infarction. *Radiology* 1986;158:729–734.

80. Fight PQ, Brass LM. Single photon emission computed tomography in cerebrovascular disease. *Curr Conc Cerebrovasc Dis Stroke* 1991;26:7–12.

81. Voldby B. Alterations in vasomotor reactivity in suba-rachnoid hemorrhage, In Wood JH (ed): *Cerebral Blood Flow*. New York, McGraw-Hill, 1987, pp 402–412.

82. Holman BL, Devous MD. Functional brain SPECT: The emergence of a powerful clinical method. *J Nucl Med* 1992;33:1888–1904.

83. Davis S, Andrews J, Lichtenstein M, et al. A single-photon emission computed tomography study of hypoperfusion after subarachnoid hemorrhage. *Stroke* 1990; 21:252–259.

84. Caplan LR, Brass LM, DeWitt LD, et al. Transcranial Doppler ultrasound. Present status. *Neurology* 1990;40: 696–700.

85. Batjer HH, Devous MD Sr, Meyer YJ, et al. Cerebrovascular hemodynamics in arteriovenous malformation complicated by normal perfusion pressure breakthrough. *Neurosurgery* 1988;22:503–509.

86. Batjer HH, Devous MD Sr, Seibert GB, et al. Intracranial arteriovenous malformation. Relationship between clinical factors and surgical complications. *Neurosurgery* 1989;24:74–79.

87. Batjer HH, Devous MD Sr. The use of acetazolamide-enhanced rCBF measurement to predict risk to AVM patients. *Neurosurgery* 1992;31:213–218.

88. Davis S, Andrews J, Lichtenstein M, et al. A single photon emission computed tomography study of hypoperfusion after subarachnoid hemorrhage. *Stroke* 1990;21: 252–259.

89. Crow W, Guinto FC Jr. Limitations of CT in the evaluation of transient ischemic attacks. *Tex Med J* 1982;78: 65–71.

90. Bogousslavski J, Delaloye-Bischof A, Regli F, et al. Prolonged hypoperfusion and early stroke after transient ischemic attack. *Stroke* 1990;21:40–46.

91. Regard M, Landis T. Transient global amnesia: Neuropsychological dysfunction during attack and recovery of two "pure" cases. *J Neurol Neurosurg Psychiatry* 1984; 47:668–672.

92. Wilson RS, Koller W, Kelly MP. The amnesia of transient global amnesia. *J Clin Neuropsychol* 1980;2: 259–266.

93. Hodges JR, Ward CD. Observations during transient global amnesia: A behavioral and neuropsychological study of five cases. *Brain* 1989;112:595–620.

94. Stillhard G, Landis T, Schiess R, et al. Bitemporal hypoperfusion in transient global amnesia: 99m-Tc-HMPAO SPECT and neuropsychological findings during and after an attack. *J Neurol Neurosurg Psychiatry* 1990; 53:339–342.

95. Tanabe H, Hashikawa K, Nakagawa Y, et al. Memory loss due to transient hypoperfusion in the medial temporal lobes including hippocampus. *Acta Neurol Scand* 1991;84:22–27.

96. Goldenberg G, Podreka I, Pfaffelmeyer N, et al. Tha-

lamic ischemia in transient global amnesia: A SPECT study. *Neurology* 1991;41:1748–1752.

97. Lin KN, Liu RS, Yeh TP, et al. Posterior ischemia during an attack of transient global amnesia. *Stroke* 1993;24: 1093–1095.

98. Limburg M, van Royen EA, Hijdra A, et al. rCBF-SPECT in brain infarction: When does it predict outcome? *J Nucl Med* 1991;32:382–387.

99. Giubilei F, Lenzi GL, DiPiero V, et al. Predictive value of brain perfusion single-photon emission computed tomography in acute stroke. *Stroke* 1990;21:895–900.

100. Limburg M, van Royen EA, Hijdra A, et al. Single-photon emission computed tomography and early death in acute ischemic stroke. *Stroke* 1990;21: 1150–1155.

101. Hanson SK, Grotta JC, Rhoades H, et al. Value of single photon emission-computed tomography in acute stroke therapeutic trials. *Stroke* 1993;24:1322–1329.

102. Moretti JL, Cinotti L, Cesaro P, et al. Amines for brain tomoscintigraphy. *Nucl Med Commun* 1987;8:581–595.

103. Odano I, Tsuchiya T, Nishihara M, et al. Regional cerebral blood flow measured with I-123 IMP and its redistribution in ischemic cerebrovascular disease. *Stroke* 1993;24:1167–1172.

104. Lassen NA, Olsen TS, Hojgaad K, et al. Incomplete infarction: A CT-negative irreversible ischemic brain lesion. *J Cereb Blood Flow Metab* 1983;3(Suppl 1): S602–S603.

105. Mies G, Auer LM, Ebhardt G, et al. Flow and neuronal density in tissue surrounding chronic infarction. *Stroke* 1983;14:22–27.

106. Nedergaard M, Astrup J, Klinken L. Cell density and cortex thickness in the border zone surrounding old infarcts in the human brain. *Stroke* 1984;15:1033–1039.

107. Meyer JS, Hata T, Imai A. Clinical and experimental studies of diaschisis, in Wood JH (ed): *Cerebral Blood Flow.* New York, McGraw-Hill, 1987, pp 481–501.

108. Baron JC, Bousser MG, Comar D, et al. Crossed cerebellar diaschisis in human supratentorial brain infarction. *Ann Neurology* 1980;105:459–8:p128 (Abstract).

109. Patano P, Baron JC, Samson J, et al. Crossed cerebellar diaschisis: Further studies. *Brain* 1986;109:677–694.

110. Meneghetti S, Vorstrup B, Mickey B, et al. Crossed cerebellar diaschisis in ischemic stroke: A study of regional cerebral blood flow by Xe-133 inhalation and single photon emission computerized tomography. *J Cereb Blood Flow Metab* 1984;4:235–240.

111. Fazio F, Gerundini P, Lenzi G, et al. Evaluation of cerebrovascular disorders using the brain imaging agent (I-123) HIPDM and SPECT. *J Nucl Med* 1983;24:P5 (Abstract).

112. Brott TG, Gelfand MJ, Williams CC, et al. Frequency and patterns of abnormality detected by I-123 amine emission CT after cerebral infarct. *Radiology* 1986;158: 729–734.

113. Shih WJ, DeKosky ST, Coupal JJ, et al. I-123 HIPDM cerebral blood flow imaging demonstrating transtentorial diaschisis. *Clin Nucl Med* 1990;15:623–629.

114. Kuhl DE, Phelps ME, Kowell AP, et al. Effects of stroke on local cerebral metabolism and perfusion: Mapping by emission computed tomography of F-18 DG and N-13 H3. *Ann Neurol* 1980;8:47–60.

115. Matsuda H, Tsuji S, Sumiya H, et al. Acetazolamide effect on vascular response in areas with diaschisis as measured by Tc-99m HMAO brain SPECT. *Clin Nucl Med* 1992;17:581–586.

116. Matsuda H, Li MY, Higashi S, et al. Comparative SPECT study of stroke using Tc-99m ECD, I-123 IMP and Tc-99m HMPAO. *Clin Nucl Med* 1993;18:754–758.

117. Fulham M, Brooks RA, Hallett M, et al. Cerebellar diaschisis revisited: Pontine hypometabolism and dentate sparing. *Neurology* 1992;42:2267–2273.

118. Allen GI, Tsukahara N. Cerebrocerebellar communication system. *Physiol Rev* 1974;54:957–1006.

119. Brodal A. Cerebrocerebellar pathways: Anatomical data and some functional implications. *Acta Neurol Scand* 1972;51(Suppl):153–195.

120. Biersak HJ, Stefan H, Reichmann K, et al. HM-PAO brain SPECT and epilepsy. *Nucl Med Commun* 1987;8: 513–518.

121. Shih WJ, Hartman RS, McQuaide BH, et al. A large cystic lesion in the left posterior parietal region demonstrated by Tc-99m HMPAO brain SPECT imaging. *Clin Nucl Med* 1992;17:54–55.

122. Tien RD, Ashdown BC. Crossed cerebellar diaschisis and crossed cerebellar atrophy: Correlation of MR findings, clinical symptoms, and supratentorial diseases in 26 patients. *AJR* 1992;158:1155–1159.

123. Mori Y, Abe T, Goto H, et al. Evaluation of spinocerebellar degeneration by SPECT using I-123 IMP. 5th Congress World Federation of Nuclear Medicine 809. *Eur J Nucl Med* 1990;16:5(Abstract) 187.

124. Akiyama H, Harrop R, McGeer PL, et al. Crossed cerebellar and uncrossed basal ganglia and thalamic diaschisis in Alzheimer's disease. *Neurology* 1989;39: 54–548.

125. D'Antona R, Baron JC, Samson Y, et al. Subcortical dementia, frontal cortex hypometabolism detected by PET in patients with progressive supranuclear palsy. *Brain* 1985;108:787–799.

126. Patronas NJ, Dichiro G, Smith BH, et al. Depressed cerebellar glucose metabolism in supratentorial tumors. *Brain Res* 1984;291:93–101.

127. Rozenthal JM, Levine RL, Nickle RJ, et al. Cerebral diaschisis in patients with malignant glioma. *J Neurooncol* 1990;8:153–161.

128. Fukuyama H, Kameyama M, Harada K, et al. Thalamic tumors invading the brain stem produce crossed cerebellar diaschisis demonstrated by PET. *J Neurol Neurosurg Psychiatry* 1986;49:524–528.

129. Lindegaard MW, Skretting A, Hager B, et al. Cerebral and cerebellar uptake of 99mTc-(*d,l*)-hexamethylpropyleneamine oxime (HM-PAO) in patients with brain tumor studied by single photon emission computerized tomography. *Eur J Nucl Med* 1986;12:417–420.

130. Sieg KG, Harty JR, Simmons M, et al. Tc-99m HMPAO SPECT imaging of the central nervous system in the tuberous sclerosis. *Clin Nucl Med* 1991;16:665–667.

131. Yoshikawa H, Fueki N, Sakuragawa N, et al. Crossed cerebellar diaschisis in the Sturge-Weber syndrome. *Brain Dev* 1990;12:535–537.

132. Abe M, Kanaoka N, Nonomura K, et al. Crossed cerebellar diaschisis in hydrocephalus. A case report. *No To Shinkei* 1989;41:1085–1090.

133. Michikawa M, Takahashi M, Kishida S, et al. Crossed cerebellar diaschisis and crossed cerebellar diaschisis and crossed cerebellar atrophy in a patient with a lesion in brainstem. *Rinsho Shinkeigakuk* 1991;32:44–48.

134. Fazekas F, Payer F, Valetitsch ?, et al. Brain stem infarction and diaschisis. A SPECT cerebral perfusion study. *Stroke* 1993;24:1162–1166.

135. Botez MI, Leveille J, Lambert R, et al. Single photon emission computed tomography (SPECT) in cerebellar disease: Cerebellocerebral diaschisis. *Eur Neurol* 1991;31:405–412.

136. Rousseaux M, Steinling M. Crossed hemispheric diaschisis in unilateral cerebellar lesions. *Stroke* 1992;23:511–514.

137. Baron JC, Bousser MG, Comar D, et al. Crossed cerebellar diaschisis in human supratentorial brain infarction. *Trans Am Neurol Assoc* 1980;8:120–135.

138. Leveille J, Botez MI, Botez T, et al. Tc-99m HMPAO SPECT imaging: Comparison with neuropsychological findings in patients with cerebellar damage, in Schmidt HAE, Chambron J (eds): *Nuclear Medicine.* Proceedings of the Congress of the European Association of Nuclear Medicine, Strasbourg, 1989. Stuttgart: Schattauer, 1990, pp 355–357.

139. Attig E, Botez MI, Hublet C, et al. Cerebral crossed diaschisis caused by cerebellar lesion: Role of the cerebellum in mental functions. Rev Neurol 1991;147:200–207.

140. Perrone E, Tofani A, Maini CL. Crossed cerebellocerebral diaschises: A SPECT study. *Nucl Med Commun* 1992;13:824–831.

141. Dierckz R, Fidlers L, Dobbeleir A, et al. High spatial resolution Tc-99m HMPAO brain SPECT in cerebellar embolic infarction. *Clin Nucl Med* 1993;1991;8:83–84.

142. Decety J, Sjoholm H, Ryding E, et al. The cerebellum participates in mental activity: Tomographic measurements of regional cerebral blood flow. *Brain Res* 1990;535:313–317.

143. Leiner HC, Leiner AL, Dow RS. Cerebro-cerebellar learning loops in apes and humans. *Ital J Neurol Sci* 1987;8:425–436.

144. Tikofsky RB, Hellman RS. Brain SPECT: New activation and intervention studies. *Semin Nucl Med* XXI 1991;21:40–57.

145. Matsuda H, Higashi S, Kinuya K, et al. SPECT evaluation of brain perfusion reserve by the acetazolamide test using Tc-99m HMPAO. *Clin Nucl Med* 1991;16:572.

146. Biersack HJ, Linke D, Brassel F, et al. Technetium-99m HM-PAO brain SPECT in epileptic patients before and during unilateral hemispheric anesthesia (Wada test): Report of three cases. *J Nucl Med* 1987;28:1763–1767.

147. Matsuda H, Higashi S, Neshandar I, et al. Evaluation of cerebral collateral circulation by Tc-99m HMPAO brain SPECT during Matas test: Report of three cases. *J Nucl Med* 1988;29:1724–1729.

148. Woods SW, Koster K, Krystal JK, et al. Yohimbine alters regional cerebral blood flow in panic disorder. *Lancet* 1988;2:678.

149. Battistin L, Pizzolato G, Dam M, et al. Single photon emission computed tomography studies with ⁹⁹ᵐTC-hexamethylpropyleneamine oxime in dementia: Effects of acute administration of L-acetylcarnitine. *Eur Neurol* 1989;29:261–265.

150. Geaney DP, Soper N, Shepstone BJ, el al. Effect of central cholinergic stimulation on regional cerebral blood flow in Alzheimer disease. *Lancet* 1990;335:1484–1487.

151. Gonzalez CF, Moret J. Balloon occlusion of the carotid artery prior to surgery for neck tumors. *AJNR* 1990;11:649–652.

152. Terada H, Kuwajima A, Hiramatsu Y, et al. Demonstration of focal brain ischemia induced by hyperventilation using Tc-99m HMPAO SPECT. *Clin Nucl Med* 1993;18:405–408.

153. Cikric D, Burt RM, Dalsing MC, et al. Acetazolamide enhanced single photon emission computed tomography (SPECT) evaluation of cerebral perfusion before and after carotid endarterectomy. *J Vasc Surg* 1992;15:747–753.

154. Lord RSA, Yeates M, Fernandes V, et al. Cerebral perfusion defects, dysautoregulation, and carotid stenosis. *J Cardiovasc Surg* 1988;29:670–675.

155. Matsuda H, Tsuji S, Sumiya H, et al. Acetazolamide effect on vascular response in areas with diaschisis as measured by Tc-99m HMPAO brain SPECT. *Clin Nucl Med* 1992;17:581–586.

156. Shinoda J, Kimura T, Funakoshi T, et al. Acetazolamide reactivity on cerebral blood flow in patients with subarachnoid hemorrhage. *Acta Neurchiv* 1991;109:102–108.

157. Batjer HH, Devous MD Sr, Seibert GB, et al. Intracranial

arteriovenous malformation. Relationships between clinical and radiographic factors and ipsilateral steal severity. *Neurosurgery* 1988;23:322–328.

158. Dinh YRT, Lot G, Benrabath R, et al. Abnormal cerebral vasodilatation in aneurysmal subarachnoid hemorrhage; use of serial Xe-133 cerebral blood flow measurement plus acetazolamide to assess cerebral vasospasm. *J Neurosurg* 1993;79:490–493.

159. Burt RW, Witt, RM, Cikrit D, et al. Increased brain retention of Tc-99m HMPAO following acetazolamide administration. *Clin Nucl Med* 1991;16:568–571.

160. Burt RW, Witt RM, Cikrit DF, et al. Carotid artery disease: Evaluation with acetazolamide-enhanced Tc-99m HMPAO SPECT. *Radiology* 1992;182:461–466.

161. Yudd AP, Van Heertum RL, Masdeu JC. Interventions and functional brain imaging. *Semin Nucl Med* 1991;21:153–158.

162. De Vries EJ, Sekhar LN, Horton JA, et al. A new method to predict safe resection of the internal carotid artery. *Laryngoscope* 1990;100:85–88.

163. Mathews D, Walker BS, Purdy PD, et al. Brain blood flow SPECT in temporary balloon occlusion of carotid and intracerebral arteries. *J Nucl Med* 1993;34:1239–1243.

164. Monsein LH, Jeffery PJ, van Heerden BB, et al. Assessing adequacy of collateral circulation during balloon test occlusion of the internal carotid artery with ^{99m}Tc-HMPAO SPECT, *AJNR* 1991;12:1045–1051.

165. Simonson TM, Ryals TJ, Yuh WTC, et al. MR imaging and HMPAO scintigraphy in conjunction with balloon test occlusion: Value in predicting sequelae after permanent carotid occlusion. *AJR* 1992;159:1063–1068.

166. Eckard DA, Purdy PD, Bonte FJ. Temporary balloon occlusion of the carotid artery combined with brain blood flow imaging as a test to predict tolerance prior to permanent carotid sacrifice. *AJNR* 1992;12:1565–1569.

167. Peterman SB, Taylor A, Hoffman JC. Improved detection of cerebral hypoperfusion with internal carotid balloon test occlusion and ^{99m}-Tc-HMPAO cerebral perfusion SPECT imaging. *AJNR* 1991;12:1035–1041.

168. Askienazy S, Lebtahi R, Meder JF. SPECT HMPAO and balloon test occlusion: Interest in predicting tolerance prior to permanent cerebral artery occlusion. *J Nucl Med* 1993;34:1243–1245.

169. Palestro CJ, Sen C, Muzinic M, et al. Assessing collateral cerebral perfusion with Tc-99m-HMPAO SPECT during temporary internal carotid artery occlusion. *J Nucl Med* 1993;34:1235–1238.

170. Moody EB, Dawson RC III, Sandler MP. ^{99m}Tc-HMPAO SPECT imaging in interventional neuroradiology: Validation of balloon test occlusion. AJNR 1991;12:1043–1044.

171. Fazekas JF, Bessman AN, Cotsonas NJ, et al. Cerebral

hemodynamics in cerebral arteriosclerosis. *J Geront* 1953;8:137–145.

172. Wasserman AJ, Patterson JL. The cerebral vascular response to reduction in arterial carbon dioxide tension. *J Clin Invest* 1961;40:1297–303.

173. Sokoloff L. The action of drugs on the cerebral circulation. *Pharmacol Rev* 1959;11:1–85.

174. Gotoh F, Meyer JS, Takagi Y. Cerebral effects of hyperventilation. *Arch Neurol* 1965;12:410–423.

175. Ziegler MG. Postural hypotension. *Ann Rev Med* 1980;31:239–245.

176. Hayashida K, Hirose Y, Kaminage T, et al. Detection of postural cerebral hypoperfusion with Tc-99m HMPAO brain SPECT in patients with cerebrovascular disease. *J Nucl Med* 1993;34:1931–1935.

177. Isaka Y, Imaizumi M, Itoi Y, et al. Cerebral blood flow imaging with technetium-99m-HMPAO SPECT in a patient with chronic subdural hematoma: Relationship with neuropsychological test. *J Nucl Med* 1992;33:246–250.

178. VanHeertum RL, Miller SH, Mosesson RE. SPECT brain imaging in neurologic disease. *Radiol Clin North Am* 1993;31:881–907.

179. Goncalves JM, Vaz R, Cerejo A, et al. HMPAO SPECT in head trauma. *Acta Neurochir* 1992(Suppl):55:11–73.

180. Yamakami I, Yamaura A, Isobe K. Types of traumatic brain injury and regional cerebral blood flow assessment by 99mTc-HMPAO SPECT. *Neurol Med Chir* 1993;33(1):7–12.

181. Bullock R, Sakas D, Patterson J, et al. Early posttraumatic cerebral blood flow mapping: Correlation with structural damage after focal injury. *Acta Neurochir* 1992(Suppl);55:14–17.

182. Abdel-Dayem HM, Sadek SA, Kouris K, et al. Changes in cerebral perfusion after acute head injury: Comparison of CT with Tc-99m HMPAO SPECT. *Radiology* 1987;165(1):221–226.

183. Choksey MS, Costa DC, Iannotti F, et al. 99m Tc-HMPAO SPECT studies in traumatic intracerebral hematoma. *J Neurol Neurosurg Psychiatry* 1991;54:6–11.

184. Gray BG, Ichise M, Chung DG, et al. Technetium-99m-HMPAO SPECT in the evaluation of patients with a remote history of traumatic brain injury: A comparison with x-ray computed tomography. *J Nucl Med* 1992;33:52–58.

185. Newton MR, Greenwood RJ, Britton KE, et al. A study comparing SPECT with CT and MRI after closed head injury. *J Neurol, Neurosurg Psychiatry* 1992;55(2):92–94.

186. Oder W, Goldenberg G, Spatt J, et al: Behavioural and psychosocial sequelae of severe closed head injury and regional cerebral blood flow: A SPECT study. *J Neurol, Neurosurg Psychiatry* 1992;55:475–480.

187. Goldenberg G, Oder W, Spatt J, et al. Cerebral corre-

lates of disturbed executive function and memory in survivors of severe closed head injury: A SPECT study. *J Neurol, Neurosurg Psychiatry* 1992;55:362–368.

188. Report of the Harvard Medical School. A definition of irreversible coma: Report of the ad hoc committee of the Harvard Medical School to examine the definition of brain death. *JAMA* 1986;205:337–340.

189. Roine RO, Launes J, Lindroth L, et al. ^{99m}Tc-hexamethylpropyleneamine oxime scans to confirm brain death. *Lancet* 1986;2:1223–1224.

190. Schoober O, Galaske R, Heyer R. Determination of brain death with ^{123}I-IMP and ^{99m}Tc-HM-PAO. *Neurosurg Rev* 1987;10:19–22.

191. Galaske RG, Schober O, Heyer R. ^{99m}Tc-HM-PAO and ^{123}I-iodoamphetamine cerebral scintigraphy: A new, noninvasive method in determination of brain death in children. *Eur J Nucl Med* 1988;14:446–452.

192. Lee VW, Hauck RM, Morrison MC, et al. Scintigraphic evaluation of brain death: Significance of sagittal sinus visualization. *J Nucl Med* 1987;28:1279–1283.

193. Hansen AVE, Lavin PJM, Moody EB, et al. False-negative cerebral radionuclide flow study, in brain death, caused by a ventricular drain. *Clin Nucl Med* 1993;18:502–505.

194. Alvarez LA, Lipton RB, et al. Brain death determination by angiography in setting of a skull defect. *Arch Neurology* 1988;45:225–227.

195. Weiteo H, Marohl K, Kaiser KP, et al. Tc-HMPAO cerebral scintigraphy a reliable non-invasive method for determination of brain death. *Clin Nucl Med* 1993;18:104–109.

196. Laurin NR, Driedger AA, Hurwitz GA, et al. Cerebral perfusion imaging with technetium-99m HM-PAO in brain death and severe central nervous system injury. *J Nucl Med* 1989;30:1627–1635.

197. Reid RH, Gulenchyn KY, Ballinger JR. Clinical use of technetium-99m HMPAO for determination of brain death. *J Nucl Med* 1989;30:1621–1626.

198. Valle G, Citrella P, Bonetti MG, et al. Considerations of brain death on a SPECT cerebral perfusion study. *Clin Nucl Med* 1993;18:953–954.

199. Schauwecker DS. Tc-99m HMPAO brain survival study reveals flow to the cerebrum but none to the cerebellum. *Clin Nucl Med* 1993;18:984–985.

200. Grunwald F, Durwen HF, Bockisch A, et al. Technetium-99m-HMPAO brain SPECT in medically intractable temporal lobe epilepsy: A postoperative evaluation. *J Nucl Med* 1991;32:388–394.

201. Rowe CC, Berkovic SF, Austin MC, et al. Patterns of postictal cerebral blood flow in temporal lobe epilepsy: Qualitative and quantitative analysis. *Neurology* 1991;41:1096–1103.

202. Adams C, Hwang PA, Gilday DL, et al. Comparison of SPECT, EEG, CT, MRI, and pathology in partial epilepsy. *Pediatr Neurol* 1992;8:97–103.

203. Rowe CC, Berkovic SF, Benjamin ST, et al. Localization of epileptic foci with postictal single photon emission computed tomography. *Ann Neurol* 1989;26:660–668.

204. Lee BI, Markland ON, Wellman HN, et al. HIPDM-SPECT in patients with medically intractable complex seizures. Ictal study. *Arch Neurol* 1988;45:397–402.

205. Stefan H, Bauer J, Feistel H, et al. Regional cerebral blood flow during focal seizures of treating focal seizures of temporal and frontocentral onset. *Ann Neurol* 1992;27:162–166.

206. Editorial. SPECT and PET in epilepsy. *Lancet* 1989;19; 1:135.

207. Marks DA, Katz A, Hoffer P, et al. Localization of extratemporal epileptic foci during ictal single photon emission computed tomography. *Ann Neurol* 1992;3:250–255.

208. Newton MR, Berkovic SF, Austin MC, et al. Ictal, postictal and interictal SPECT in laterization of temporal lobe epilepsy. *Eur J Nucl Med* 1994;21:1067–1071.

209. Duncan R, Patterson J, Roberts R, et al. Ictal/postictal SPECT in the presurgical localization of complex partial seizure. *J Neurol Neurosurg Psychiatry* 1993;56:141–148.

210. Newton MR, Austin MC, McKay J, et al. Ictal SPECT using Tc-99m HMPAO: Methods for rapid preparation and optimal deployment of tracer during spontaneous seizures. *J Nucl Med* 1993;34:666–670.

211. Biersack HJ, Linke D, Brassel F, et al. Technetium-99m HMPAO brain SPECT in epileptic patients before and during unilateral hemispheric anesthesia (Wada test): Report of 3 cases. *J Nucl Med* 1987;28:1763–1767.

212. Bartenstein P, Ludolph A, Schober O, et al. Benzodiazephine receptors and cerebral blood flow in partial epilepsy. *Eur J Nucl Med* 1991;18:111–118.

213. Haxby JV, Duara R, Grady CL, et al. Relations between neuropsychological and cerebral metabolic asymmetries in early Alzheimer's disease. *J Cereb Blood Flow Metab* 1985;5:93–200.

214. Duara R, Grady C, Haxby J, et al. Positron emission tomography in Alzheimer's disease. *Neurology* 1986;37:879–887.

215. Foster NL, Chase TN, Mansi L, et al. Cortical abnormalities in Alzheimer's disease. *Ann Neurol* 1984;16:649–654.

216. DeKosky ST, Shih WJ, Schmitt FA, et al. Assessing utility of SPECT in Alzheimer disease: correlation with cognitive severity. *Alzheimer's Dis Associated Disorders* 1990;4:14–23.

217. Holman BL, Johnson KA, Garada B, et al. The scintigraphic appearance of Alzheimer's disease: A prospective study using technetium-99m HMPAO SPECT. *J Nucl Med* 1992;33:181–185.

218. Holman BL, Devous MD. Functional Barin SPECT: The emergence of a powerful clinical method. *J Nucl Med* 1992;33:1888–1904.

219. Herscovitch P, Auchus AP, Gado M, et al. Correction of positron emission tomography data for cerebral atrophy. *J Cereb Blood Flow Metab* 1986;6:120–124.

220. Brun A, Englund E. Regional pattern of degeneration in Alzheimer's disease: Neuronal loss and histopathological grading. *Histopathology* 1981;5:549–564.

221. Johnson KA, Kijewski MF, Becker JA, et al. Qualitative brain SPECT in Alzheimer's disease and normal aging. *J Nucl Med* 1993;34:2044–2048.

222. Sawada H, Udaka F, Kameyama M, et al. SPECT findings in Parkinson's disease associated with dementia. *J Neurol Neurosurg Psychiatry* 1992;55:960–963.

223. Spampinato U, Habert MO, Mas JL, et al. (99mTc)-HMPAO SPECT and cognitive impairment in Parkinson's disease: A comparison with dementia of the Alzheimer type. *J Neurol Neurosurg Psychiatry* 1991;54:787–792.

224. Kuwabara Y, Ichiya Y, Otsuka M, et al. Differential diagnosis of bilateral parietal abnormalities in I-123 IMP SPECT imaging. *Clin Nucl Med* 1990;15:893–899.

225. Launes J, Sulkava R, Erkinjuntti T, et al. Tc-99m HMPAO SPECT in suspected dementia. *Nucl Med Commun* 1991;12:757–765.

226. Grunwald F, Zierz S, Broich K, et al. HMPAO-SPECT imaging resembling Alzheimer-type dementia in mitochondrial encephalomyopathy with lactic acidosis and stroke-like episodes (MELAS). *J Nucl Med* 1990;31:1740–1742.

227. Dierckx RA, Appel B, Saerens J, et al. Tc-99m HMPAO brain SPECT in dementia due to transitory obstructive hydrocephalus. *Clin Nucl Med* 1993;18:245–246.

228. Habert MO, Spampinato U, Mas JL, et al. A comparative Tc-99m HMPAO SPECT study in different types of dementia. *Eur J Nucl Med* 1991;18:3–11.

229. Mayeux R, Stern Y, Rosenstein R, et al. An estimate of the prevalence of dementia in idiopathic Parkinson's disease. *Arch Neurol* 1988;45:260–262.

230. Sawada H, Udaka F, Kameyama M, et al. SPECT findings in Parkinson's disease associated with dementia. *J Neurol Neurosurg Psychiatry* 1992;55:960–963.

231. Spampinato U, Habert MO, Mas JL, et al. (99mTc)-HMPAO SPECT and cognitive impairment in Parkinson's disease: A comparison with dementia of the Alzheimer type. *J Neurol Neurosurg Psychiatry* 1991;54:787–789.

232. Liu RS, Lin KN, Wang SJ, et al. Cognition and 99Tcm-HMPAO SPECT in Parkinson's disease. *Nucl Med Commun* 1992;13:744–748.

233. Sawada H, Udaka F, Kameyama M, et al. SPECT findings in Parkinson's disease associated with dementia. *J Neurol Neurosurg Psychiatry* 1992;55:960–963.

234. Woods SW. Regional cerebral blood flow imaging with SPECT in psychiatric disease: Focus on schizophrenia, anxiety disorders, and substance abuse. *J Clin Psychiatry* 1992;53(11 Suppl):20–25.

235. Hawton K, Shepstone B, Soper N, et al. Single-photon emission computerized tomography (SPECT) in schizophrenia. *Br J Psychiatry* 1990;156:425–427.

236. Schuckit MA. Introduction and overview to clinical applications of neuro SPECT in psychiatry. *J Clin Psychiatry* 1992;53(11 Suppl):3–6.

237. O'Connell RA, Van Heertum RL, Billick SB, et al. Single photon emission computed tomography (SPECT) with [^{123}I]IMP in the differential diagnosis of psychiatric disorders. *J Neuropsychiatry* 1989;1:145–153.

238. Matsuda H, Gyobu T, Ti M, et al. Iodine-123 iodoamphetamine brain scan in a patient with auditory hallucination. *J Nucl Med* 1988;29:558–560.

239. Matsuda H, Gyobu T, Ii M, et al. Increased accumulation of *N*-isopropyl-(I-123)*p*-iodamphetamine in the left auditory area in schizophrenic patient with auditory hallucinations. *Clin Nucl Med* 1988;13:53–55.

240. Van-Heertum RL, O'Connell RA. Functional brain imaging in evaluation of psychiatric illness. *Semin Nucl Med* 1991;21:24–34.

241. Robins LM, Helzer JE, Weissman MM, et al. Lifetime prevalence of specific psychiatric disorders in three sites. *Arch Gen Psychiatry* 1984;41:949–958.

242. Akin EA, Stein MH, Atkins FB, et al. Cerebral perfusion in psychiatric outpatients with paroxysmal mood and behavior disorders. *Radiology* 1993;189(P):115.

243. Khanna S. Obsessive-compulsive disorder: Is there a frontal lobe dysfunction? *Biol Psychiatry* 1988;24:602–613.

244. Wise SP, Rapoport JL. Obsessive-compulsive disorder: Is it basal ganglia dysfunction, in Rapoport JL (ed): *Obsessive-Compulsive Disorder in Children and Adolescents.* Washington, DC, American Psychiatric Press, 1989, pp 327–344.

245. Rubin RT, Villaneuva-Meyer J, Ananth J, et al. Regional xenon 133 cerebral blood flow and cerebral technetium 99m HMPAO uptake in unmedicated patients with obsessive-compulsive disorder and matched normal control subjects: Determination by high-resolution single-photon emission computed tomography. *Arch Gen Psychiatry* 1992;49:695–702.

246. Machlin SR, Harris GJ, Pearlson GD, et al. Elevated medial-frontal cerebral blood flow in obsessive-compulsive patients: A SPECT study. *Am J Psychiatry* 1991;148:1240–1242.

247. Harris GJ, Pealson GD, Hoehn-Saric R. Single photon emission computed tomography in obsessive-compulsive disorders. *Arch Gen Psychiatry* 1993;50:498–501.

248. Ichise M, Salite IE, Abbey SE, et al. Assessment of re-

gional cerebral perfusion by Tc-99m HMPAO SPECT in chronic fatigue syndrome. *Nucl Med Commun* 1993;13: 767–772.

249. Bock E, Rubbert A, Feistel H, et al. HMPAO-SPECT in HIV infected patients: Correlation between cerebral perfusion defects and the presence of anticardiolipin antibodies. *Eur J Nucl Med* 1993;20:848.

250. Jernigan TL, Butters N, DiTraglia G, et al. Reduced cerebral grey matter observed in alcoholics using magnetic resonance imaging. *Alcohol Clin Exp Res* 1991;15: 418–427.

251. Gilman S, Adams K, Koeppe RA, et al. Cerebellar and frontal hypometabolism in alcoholic cerebellar degeneration studied with positron emission tomography. *Ann Neurol* 1990;28:775.

252. Matew RJ, Wilson WH. Substance abuse and cerebral blood flow. *Am J Psychiatry* 1991;148:292–305.

253. Melgaard B, Henriksen L, Danielsen UT, et al. Regional cerebral blood flow in chronic alcoholics measured by single photon emission computerized tomography. *Acta Neurol Scand* 1990;82:87–93.

254. Shih WJ, Hyatt M. Volume and surface three-dimensional displays of Tc-99m HMPAO brain SPECT imaging in a chronic hypnosedative abuser. *Clin Nucl Med* 1993;18:506–509.

255. Nicolas JM, Catafau AM, Estrach R, et al. Regional cerebral blood flow—SPECT in chronic alcoholism: Relation to neuropsychological testing. *J Nucl Med* 1993;34: 1452–1459.

256. Shih WJ, Markesberry WR, Clark DB, et al. I-123 HIPDM brain imaging findings in subacute spongiform encephalopathy (CJD). *J Nucl Med* 1987;28:1484–1487.

257. Gennell HG, Sharp PF, Evans NTS, et al. Simple photon emission tomography with I-123 isopropylamphetamine in Alzheimer's disease and multi-infarct dementia. *Lancet* 1984;2:1348.

258. Biersack HJ, Reichmann X, Winkler C, et al. Tc-99m labeled hexamethylpropyleneamine oxime photon emission scans in epilepsy. *Lancet* 1985;2:1436–1437.

259. Ell PJ, Jarritt PH, Cullum I, et al. Regular cerebral blood flow mapping with Tc-99m labelled compound. *Lancet* 1985;2:50–51.

260. Gregler LL, Mark H. Medical complications of cocaine abuse. Special report. *N Engl J Med* 1986;315:1495–1500.

261. Jacobs IG, Rosler MH, Kelly JK, et al. Cocaine abuse: Neurovascular complications. *Radiology* 1989;170:223–227.

262. Brown E, Prager J, Lee H-Y, et al. CNS complications of cocaine abuse; prevalence, pathophysiology, and neuroradiology. *Am J Roentgenol* 1992;159:137–147.

263. Levine SR, Brust JCM, Futrell N, et al. Cerebrovascular complications of the use of "crack" form of alkaloidal cocaine. *N Engl J Med* 1990;323:699–704.

264. Holman BL, Carvalho PA, Mendelson JH, et al. Brain perfusion is abnormal in cocaine dependent polydrug users; a study using ^{99m}Tc-HM-PAO and ASPECT. *J Nucl Med* 1991;32:1206–1210.

265. Holman BL, Garada B, Johnson KA, et al. A comparison of brain perfusion SPECT in cocaine abuse and AIDS dementia complex. *J Nucl Med* 1992;33:1312–1315.

266. Tumeh SS, Nagel JS, English RJ, et al. Cerebral abnormalities in cocaine abusers: Demonstration by SPECT perfusion brain scintigraphy. *Radiology* 1990;176:821–824.

267. Holman BL, Mendelson J, Garada B, et al. Regional cerebral blood flow improves with treatment in chronic cocaine polydrug users. *J Nucl Med* 1993;34:723–727.

268. Weber DA, Franceschi D, Ivanovic M, et al. SPECT and planar brain imagings in crack abuse: I-123 IMP uptake and localization. *J Nucl Med* 1993;34:899–907.

269. Citron BP, Halpern M, McCarron M, et al. Necrotizing angiitis associated with drug abuse. *N Engl J Med* 1970; 283:1003–1011.

270. Salanova V. Taubner R. Intracerebral hemorrhage and vasculitis secondary to amphetamine use. *Postgrad Med J* 1984;60:429–430.

271. Kao CH, Wang SJ, Yeh SH. Presentation of regional cerebral blood flow in amphetamine abusers by Tc-99m HMPAO brain SPECT. *Nucl Med Commun* 1994;15: 94–98.

272. Klemm E, Grunwald F, Danus P, et al. Tc-99m HMPAO analysis of rCBF changes in heroin abuse: involvement of the temporal lobe. *Eur J Nucl Med* 1993;20:848.

24

Brain Positron Emission Tomography

Wei-Jen Shih, M.D., Abass Alavi, M.D.

Positron emission tomography (PET) is a technique that utilizes positron-emitting radiopharmaceuticals to reveal the regional physiology, biochemistry, hemodynamics, and pharmacology of the living human body.[1-3] Three types of PET studies involve (1) regional blood flow; (2) substrate metabolism; and (3) chemical recognition sites, receptors, and enzymes. PET provides function or biochemical data or images of disease in the brain and other organs.[3-5]

POSITION-EMITTING ISOTOPES

Unlike gamma-emitting radionuclides, whose decay results directly in emission of gamma photons, decay of positron-emitting isotopes results in emission of a positron. A positron, an energetic, positively changed particle with the same mass as an electron, travels in tissue until it meets an electron. Positron–electron collision is called an *annihilation event;* during the event, the mass and energy of the positron and electron combine to form two 511-keV photons 180° opposite to each other.[6]

This distinguishing characteristic of positrons is integral to the design of PET imaging devices. The detection of an annihilation pair of photons by opposing detectors forms the basis for a PET scanner's coincidence concept. A PET scanner's coincidence concept is defined as two high-energy photons resulting from a positron emission. Annihilation is detected by two radiation detectors that are connected by an electronic coincidence circuit. A decay event is recorded as a coincidence line between the detectors, only when both photons are detected almost simultaneously. The coincidence concept is unique to PET scanning and is fundamental to the modality's ability to achieve a high spatial resolution and quantitative measurements.[6]

POSITRON-EMITTING RADIOPHARMACEUTICALS

PET imaging utilizes radionuclides of basic elements of the organic compounds carbon (C-11), oxygen (0-15), nitrogen (N-13), and fluorine (F-18) (substituting hydrogen, H). Synthesizing physiologically relevant compounds labeled with positron-emitting radionuclides is therefore easier. Because the half-lives of positron-emitting radionuclides are ultrashort, ranging from a few seconds to 110 min, operation of the PET system requires a cyclotron as a stand-by in the hospital, with the exception of F-18.[3-5] However, the PET examina-

TABLE 24-1   Characteristics of Positron-Emitting Radionuclides Used in Brain Imaging

Radionuclide	Source	Half-Life	Examples of Compounds
Carbon-11	Cyclotron	20.3 min	C-11 carfentanil, C-11 diprenophine, C-11 glucose, C-11 methionine, C-11 aminoisobutyric acid, C-11-pyruvate, C-11 putrescine
Nitrogen-13	Cyclotron	9.97 min	N-13H, N-13 cisplatin
Oxygen-15	Cyclotron	2.03 min	$C-15O_2$, $^{15}O_2$, $C^{15}O$, ^{15}O-butanol
Fluorine-18	Cyclotron	1.83 hr	F-18 L-dopa, F-18 DG, F-18 spiperone, F-18 GBR
Gallium-68	Generator	1.13 hr	Ga-68 EDTA, ionic species
Rubidium-82	Generator	1.258 min	Rb-82 chloride, ionic species

tion can be performed without installing a cyclotron in a hospital, using (1) F-18 2-fluorodeglucose (FDG) provided by the local institute's cyclotron or a regional radiopharmacy system and/or (2) utilizing radionuclide from a system's generator-produced positron emitter; such a generator can be used for 4–6 months.

Table 24-1 summarizes the positron-emitting radionuclides and presents examples of compounds (radiopharmaceuticals) used in brain single-photon emission computed tomography (PET).[1–4,7–19] For decades, O-15-labeled water, carbon dioxide, carbon monoxide, and oxygen gas have been used in conjunction with PET to measure cerebral flow, blood volume, and oxygen utilization. Positron-emitting, radioisotope-labeled substrates, substrate analogs, drugs, ligands, and other biochemical active compounds have been developed and are in the process of clinical evaluation. F-18-L-dopa has been used to evaluate presynaptic dopamine terminally, and C-11- and F-18-labeled analogs of spiperone and raclopride have been used to study postsynaptic dopamine receptors.[9] These compounds potentially have important clinical applications in neurology.

Clinical Indications for PET

Researchers in a small number of academic medical centers have used PET for many years; now PET is emerging in clinical applications. Clinical indications for PET include three areas: cardiological, oncological, and neurological.[10] In neurological applications of cerebrovascular disease, PET has been studied in the physiology of cerebral infarct, cerebral blood flow, the regional metabolic rate for oxygen, and regional cerebral volume; however, PET has not been used to gather data for the clinical management of patients with cerebrovascular disease. Clinical neurological indications for PET will now be discussed.

Localization of Seizure Foci in Patients with Refractory Seizure Disorders

During the interictal period, the seizure focus is usually characterized by hypometabolism. By contrast, during a seizure, there is increased glucose metabolism at the site of origin, which propagates throughout the brain.[20–22]

Patients with uncontrolled seizures of presumed focal origin who are candidates for epilepsy surgery may benefit from FDG-PET imaging. The detection of unilateral temporal hypometabolism ipsilateral to the EEG, focus found 60–80% of patients with complex partial seizures. Localization of the seizure focus is valuable for epilepsy surgery.[21–24] For localization of the focus, PET is more sensitive than magnetic resonance imaging (MRI) or computed tomography (CT).[25–27] PET findings will help the clinician plan and reduce the scope of invasive electrode evaluation.

To detect the ictal phase of the seizure attack, Tc-99m hexamethyl-propylene-amin oxime (HMPAO) brain SPECT is more practical and convenient than PET. Tc-99m HMPAO is retained in neurons of the brain that will be "frozen" in the brain tissue. Although Tc-99m HMPAO brain SPECT offers only regional, not metabolic, cerebral blood flow, localization of the seizure focus on ictal or postictal SPECT studies has increased to about 90%.[28,29]

Dementia

Dementia is a term denoting cognitive and behavioral impairment secondary to dysfunction of the brain. MRI or CT provides structural information, which show normal structures in the early stage of dementia and nonspecific changes in later stages of the disease. However, PET using FDG or O-15 labeled compounds demonstrates functional changes which allow the early differential diagnosis of dementia.[30–33] These dementias include Alzheimer's disease, Parkinson's disease, Huntington's disease, progressive supranuclear palsy, and multi-infarct dementia.[31] Patients with Alzheimer's disease exhibit decreased glucose, reduction of cerebral blood flow, and reduction of oxygen utilization typically involving the bilateral superior parietal lobes and extending to the inferior parietal and temporal lobes.

Reduction of cerebral flow or hypometabolism in patients with multi-infarct (vascular) dementia produces focal defects that are often wedge-shaped, relating to arterial territories. Based on their PET patterns, Alzheimer's disease and vascular dementia can be differentiated.

FDG-PET has been utilized to evaluate absolute whole brain metabolism. The absolute amount of glucose metabolism of the whole brain was found to be significantly different ($p < 0.001$) in Alzheimer's disease patients (29.96 $\pm$ 7.90 mg of glucose per 100 cc brain tissue per min) and control groups (30.1 $\pm$ 7.0) on examination. It has been concluded that decreased absolute whole brain metabolism provides a sensitive correlation for cognitive dysfunction in Alzheimer's disease.[34]

In Parkinson's disease, FDG uptake is normal in the basal ganglia, but there is a marked reduction of F-18 fluoro dopa, which is consistent with the marked loss of putamen dopaminergic terminals in this disease. Parkinson's disease causes bilateral temporoparietal hypometabolism.[35,36]

Huntington's disease is a hereditary disease with a developing subcortical dementia, as well as involuntary movements and psychiatric disturbances. FDG-PET shows metabolic changes in the caudate nuclei before the onset of structural changes in symptomatic patients. Hypometabolism in the caudate and putamen has been shown to correlate with the degree of locomotor disability.[37–41] Progressive supranuclear palsy (PSP) is due to neurodegenerative changes in the specification throughout the neuraxis, especially in the globus pallidus, substantia nigra, Meynert's nucleus, and the subthalamic nucleus. FDG-PET shows marked frontal hypometabolism.[42,43] The frontal hypometabolism in PSP is thought to be due to loss of afferent input to the frontal cortex from subcortical changes.[43]

Brain Tumors
The most commonly used positron-emitting radiopharmaceutical for cancer patients is FDG, which accumulates avidly in most cancers, including tumors of the central nervous system.[1,10,12,44–50] FDG enters (cancer) cells and is phosphorylated by hexokinase to form 2DG-6-phosphate. FDG is trapped inside the cells since it lacks the 2-hydroxyl group and cannot be further

metabolized via the glycolytic pathway. FDG-PET offers a unique in vivo study of local glucose utilization in tumor tissue. Three areas of PET study for brain tumors are (1) detection of the degree of malignancy, (2) determination of recurrent tumor from necrosis after therapy, and (3) prognostic usefulness.[3,10,44,45,47–49]

1. *Detection of the degree of malignancy:* Measurement of the rate of F-18-FDG uptake is helpful for histological grading of brain tumor malignancy.[10,46,48] Local cerebral metabolic rates for glucose correlate with the degree of malignancy in gliomas, differentiating low-grade from high-grade disease. Patients with hypermetabolic tumors have a median survival of 7 months, whereas those with normal-accumulation lesions have a median survival of 33 months. Patients with meningiomas have been evaluated with FDG-PET to determine the aggressiveness of the tumors and to predict postsurgical recurrence. There is a significant correlation between the rate of growth of meningiomas and their glucose metabolic rate.[48,49]

2. *Differentiation of recurrent tumor from necrosis after irradiation- and/or chemotherapy-induced necrosis:* Recurrent tumor and necrosis have similar appearances and are essentially indistinguishable on CRT or MRI images. Radiation necrosis is measured as an area of hypometabolism, and recurrent hypermetabolism is measured on the FDG-PET study.[10,50] Patients with necrosis secondary to intra-arterial chemotherapy also demonstrate hypometabolism.

3. *Prognostic usefulness:* FDG-PET provides important prognostic information on all types of primary brain tumors; high FDG uptake indicates a poor prognosis regardless of the histological diagnosis or previous therapy.[1,10,44]

F-18 FDG-PET is now the most commonly used clinical method for studying patients with brain tumors. However, increased uptake of FDG has also been demonstrated in inflammatory diseases, brain hematoma, and/or cerebral fungal infection.[51,52] This suggests that FDG-PET of the brain may produce false-positive results.

PET using C-11 methionine has also been used for brain tumors.[13–18,53–56] C-11 methionine uptake increases in brain tumors, including gliomas and one case of gliomatosis cerebri.[14,16] Tumor accumulation was 1.2–3.5 times greater than normal brain accumulation. Uptake in high-grade tumors tended to be greater than in low-grade tumors. PET C-11 methionine demonstrates increased uptake of the tracer in 80–90% of malignant brain tumors and has been successfully applied to grading and delineation of gliomas.[15] Similar to FDG, however, C-11 methionine has occasionally been seen in necrotic areas secondary to radiation therapy of brain tumors, brain abscesses, and areas surrounding cerebral hematomas.[57,58] We should be aware of these potential false-positive results and realize that C-11 methionine or FDG-PET does not always differentiate between neoplastic and nonneoplastic causes.

Other potential positron emission radiopharmaceuticals for brain PET include O-15 water, O-15 oxygen, O-15 carbon monoxide, C-11 aminoisobutyric acid, C-11 pyruvate, C-11 putrescine, C-11 tyrosine, N-13 cisplatin, and analogs of chemotherapeutic agents such as F-18 fluorouracil and fluorestradiol, Rb-82 chloride, and gallium-68 EDTA.[13,55]

PET, once used only to map regional brain metabolism and blood flow, is now being used to measure neurotransmitters, transmitter uptake sites, neurotransmitter receptors, and enzymes that metabolize neurotransmitters. For example, presynaptic L-dopa and postsynaptic analogs of spiperone and reclopride positron emission pharmaceuticals have been used to study movement disorders and to evaluate psychiatric disorders.[9] Seizure patients had been studied by mu and non-mu opiate receptors and by benzodiazepine receptors.[8]

The advantages of PET over SPECT include greater sensitivity (10 times that of SPECT), resolution (spatial resolution less than 5 mm, to resolve one-half the size of SPECT), attention correction, and demonstration of biological subtracts. Clinical utility of PET, however, is limited by its limited availability and high cost. Recently, a triple-head or dual gamma camera dedicated to the use of the positron-emitting radiopharmaceutical F-18 FDG has been developed. To handle the 511-keV positron emission from F-18 FDG, the gamma camera may be upgraded by using a thicker crystal in the detectors or by using specially designed high-energy collimators. Currently, the special high-energy collimator appears to be more popular. Using F-18 FDG, SPECT studies can be performed in cardiology, neurology, and oncology patients to obtain glucose metabolic information, but the usefulness and quality of SPECT study never equal those of the PET study.[59] Using positron-emitting pharmaceuticals, radiochemists learn how to improve and develop gamma-emitting pharmaceuticals. SPECT will follow in the footsteps of PET and will be used to carry out certain functional imaging studies.[60]

REFERENCES

1. Wagner HN Jr, Conti PS. Advances in medical imaging for cancer diagnosis and treatment. *Cancer* 1991;67: 1121–1128.
2. Strauss LG, Conti PS. The application of PET in clinical oncology. *J Nucl Med* 1991;21:623–648.
3. Wagner HN. Clinical PET: Its time has come. *J Nucl Med* 1991;32:561–564.
4. Therapeutics and Technology Assessment Subcommittee of the American Academy of Neurology. Assessment: Positron emission tomography. *Neurology* 1991;41: 163–167.
5. Conti PS, Keppler JS, Halls JM. Positron emission tomography: A financial and operational analysis. *AJR* 1994;162:1279–1286.
6. Reba RC. PET and SPECT opportunities and challenges for psychiatry. *J Clin Psychiatry* 1993;54:26–32.
7. Alavi A, Ferris S, Wolf A, et al. Determination of cerebral metabolism in senile dementia using F-18 FDG and positron emission tomography. *J Nucl Med* 1980;21:21–25.
8. Frost JJ, Mayberg HS, Fisher RS, et al. Quantification of mu and non-mu opiate receptors in temporal lobe epilepsy using positron emission tomography. *Ann Neurol* 1991;30:3–11.
9. Savic I, Persson A, Roland P, et al. In vivo demonstration of reduced benzodiazepine receptor binding in human epileptic foci. *Lancet* 1988;2:863–866.
10. Coleman RE. Clinical PET: A technology on the brink. *J Nucl Med* 1993;34:2269–2271.
11. Frost JJ. Receptor imaging by positron emission tomography and single-photon emission computed tomography. *Invest Radiol* 1992;27:554–558.
12. Pruim J, Willemsen ATM, Van Waarde A, et al. Visualization of brain tumors and quantitation of the protein synthesis rate with C-11-tyrosine. *J Nucl Med* 1994; 35:p28.
13. Ericson K, Lija A, Bergstrom M, et al. Positron emission tomography with ([^{11}C]methyl)-L-methionine, [^{11}C]D-glucose, and [^{68}Ga]EDTA in supratentorial tumors. *J Comput Assist Tomogr* 1985;8:683–689.
14. Mineura K, Sasajima T, Suda Y, et al. Early and accurate detection of primary cerebral gliomas with interfibrillary growth using ^{11}C-L-methionine positron emission tomography. *J Med Imaging* 1989;3:192–196.
15. Wong FCL, Kim EE, Korkmaz M, et al. Semiquantitative using C-11 methionine and F-18 FDG. *J Nucl Med* 1993; 34:206p.
16. Mineara K, Sasakima T, Kowada M, et al. Innovative approach in the diagnosis of gliomatosis cerebri using C-11-L-methionine PET. *J Nucl Med* 1991;323:726–728.
17. Coleman RE, Hoffman JM, Hanson MW, et al. Clinical

application of PET for evaluation of brain tumors. *J Nucl Med* 1991;32:616–622.

18. Derlon JM, Bourdet C, Bustany P, et al. [^{11}C]L-methionine uptake in gliomas. *Neurosurgery* 1989;25:720–728.

19. Engel J Jr, Rausch R, Lieb JP, et al. Correlation of criteria used for localizing epileptic foci in patients considered for surgical therapy of epilepsy. *Ann Neurol* 1981;9:215–224.

20. Engel J Jr, Brown WJ, Kuhl DE, et al. Pathological findings underlying focal temporal lobe hypometabolism in partial epilepsy. *Ann Neurol* 1982;12:518–528.

21. Engel J Jr. The use of PET in epilepsy. *Ann Neurol* 1984;15(Suppl):S180–S191.

22. Engel J Jr, Kuhl DE, Phelps ME, et al. Comparative localization of epileptic foci in partial epilepsy by PET and EEG. *Ann Neurol* 1982;12:529–537.

23. Abo-Khalil BW, Siegel GJ, Sackellares JC, et al. Positron emission tomography studies of cerebral glucose metabolism in chronic partial epilepsy. *Ann Neurol* 1987;22:480–486.

24. Henry TR, Mazziotta JC, Engel J, et al. Quantifying interictal metabolic activity in human temporal lobe epilepsy. *J Cereb Blood Flow Metab* 1990;11:748–757.

25. Theodore WH, Dorwart R, Holmes M, et al. Neuroimaging in refractory partial seizures. Comparison of PET, CT and MRI. *Neurology* 1986;36:750–759.

26. Theodore WH, Katz D, Kufta C, et al. Pathology of temporal lobe foci; correlations with CT, MRI, and PET. *Neurology* 1990;40:799–803.

27. Engel J Jr, Henry TR, Risinger MW, et al. Pre-surgical evaluation for partial epilepsy: Relative contributions of chronic depth electrode recordings versus FDG-PET and scalp sphenoidal ictal. EEG. *Neurology* 1990;40:1670–1677.

28. Shen W, Lee BI, Park HM, et al. HIPDM-SPECT brain imaging in the presurgical evaluation of patients with intractable seizures. *J Nucl Med* 1990;31:1280–1284.

29. Rowe CC, Berkovic SF, Sia STB, et al. Localization of epileptic foci with postictal single photon emission computed tomography. *Ann Neurol* 1989;26:660–668.

30. Duara R, Grady C, Haxby J, et al. Positron emission tomography in Alzheimer's disease. *Neurology* 1986;36:879–887.

31. Chase TN, Burrows GH, Mohr E. Cortical glucose utilization patterns in primary degenerative dementias of the anterior and posterior type. *Arch Gerontol Geriatr* 1987;6:289–297.

32. Grady CL, Haxby JV, Schlageter NL, et al. Stability of metabolic and neuropsychological asymmetries in dementia of the Alzheimer type. *Neurology* 1986;36:1390–1392.

33. Mueller-Gaertner HW, Mayberg HS, Ravert HT, et al.

Mu opiate receptor binding in amygdala in Alzheimer's disease: In vivo quantification by IC carfentanil and PET. *J Cereb Blood Flow Metab* 1991;11(Suppl):S20.

34. Alavi A, Newberg AB, Souder E, et al. Quantitative analysis of PET and MRI data in normal aging and Alzheimer's disease: Atrophy weighted total brain metabolism and absolute whole brain metabolism as reliable discriminators. *J Nucl Med* 1993;34:1681–1687.

35. Garnet ED, Nahmias C, Firnua G. Central dopaminergic pathways in hemiparkinsonism examined by PET. *Can J Neurol Sci* 1984;11:174–179.

36. Brooks DJ, Salmon EP, Mathias CJ, et al. The relationship between locomotor disability, autonomic dysfunction and integrity of the striatal dopaminergic system in patient with multiple system atrophy, pure autonomic failure, and Parkinson's disease studied with PET. *Brain* 1990;113:1539–1552.

37. Kuhl DR, Phelps ME, Markham CH, et al. Cerebral metabolism and atrophy in Huntington's disease determined by 18-FDG and computed tomographic scan. *Ann Neurol* 1982;12:425–434.

38. Hayden MR, Martin WRW, Stoessl AJ, et al. Positron emission tomography in the early diagnosis of Huntington's disease. *Neurology* 1986;36:888–894.

39. Mazziotta JC. Huntington's disease: Studies with structural imaging techniques and positron emission tomography. *Semin Neurol* 1989;9:360–369.

40. Young AB, Penny JB, Starosta-Rubenstein S, et al. PET scan investigations of Huntington's disease: Cerebral metabolic correlates of neurologic features and functional decline. *Ann Neurol* 1986;20:296–303.

41. Foster NL, Gilman S, Berent S, et al. Cerebral hypometabolism in progressive supranuclear palsy studies with positron emission tomography. *Ann Neurol* 1988;24:399–406.

42. Goffinet AM, DeVolder AG, Gidlain C, et al. PET demonstrates frontal lobe hypometabolism in progressive supranuclear palsy. *Ann Neurol* 1989;25:131–139.

43. Blin J, Baron JC, Dubois B, et al. PET study in progressive supranuclear palsy: Brain hypometabolism pattern and clinicometabolic correlations. *Arch Neurol* 1990;47:747–752.

44. Alavi JA, Alavi A, Chawluk J, et al. Positron emission tomography in patients with glioma: A predictor of prognosis. *Cancer* 1988;62:1074–1078.

45. Di Chiro G. Positron emission tomography using F-18 fluorodeoxyglucose in brain tumors: A powerful diagnostic tool. *Invest Radiol* 1987;22:360–371.

46. Di Chiro G, DeLaPaz RL, Brooks RA, et al. Glucose utilization of cerebral gliomas measured by [^{18}F]fluorodeoxyglucose and positron emission tomography. *Neurology* 1982;32:1323–1329.

47. Francavilla TL, Miletich RS, De Chiro G, et al. Positron

emission tomography in the detection of malignant degeneration of low grade gliomas. *Neurosurgery* 1989; 24:1–5.

48. Di Chiro G, Hatazawa J, Katz DA, et al. Glucose utilization by intracranial meningiomas as an index of tumor aggressitivity and probability of recurrence: A PET study. *Radiology* 1987;154:521–526.

49. Hoffman JM, Lowe VJ, Brown M, et al. The prognostic and diagnostic usefulness of FDG-PET in primary brain tumor management. *J Nucl Med* 1993;34:37p.

50. Goldberg IE, Pardo FS, Kennedy DN, et al. Multislice MRI CVD mapping of brain tumors: A comparison with PET studies using FDG and CO. *J Nucl Med* 1993;34: 208p–209p.

51. Lawerence S, Kessler RM. Hypermetabolic cerebral fungus infection with PET FDG studies. *J Nucl Med* 1993; 34:38p.

52. Reske SN, Fleischmann W, Brecht-Kraub BD, et al. Increased focal FDG uptake is a sensitive indicator of musculoskeletal inflammation. *J Nucl Med* 1994;35:113p.

53. O'Tuama LA, La France ND, Dannals RF, et al. Quantitative imaging of neutral amino acid transport by human brain tumors (abstract). *J Cereb Blood Flow Metab* 1987; 7(Suppl):5517.

54. Mineura K, Yasuda T, Kowada M, et al. Positron emission tomographic evaluation of histological malignancy in gliomas using oxygen-15 and fluorine-18-fluorodeoxyglucose. *Neurol Res* 1986;8:164–169.

55. Ericson K. PET studies of amino acid metabolism: Integration in clinical routine and current research on intracranial tumours, in Mazoyer BM, Heiss WD, Comar D (eds): *PET Studies on Amino Acid Metabolism and Protein Synthesis.* Dordrecht, the Netherlands, Kluwer, 1993, pp 215–221.

56. Mosskin M, VonHolst H, Bergstrom M, et al. Positron emission tomography of intracranial tumours compared with histopathologic examination of multiple biopsies. *Acta Radiol* 1987;28:673–681.

57. Ishii K, Ogawa T, Hatazawa J, et al. High L-methyl-[^{11}C]methionine uptake in brain abscess: A PET study. *J Comput Assist Tomogr* 1993;17:660–661.

58. Dethy S, Goldman S, Blecic S, et al. Carbon-11 methionine and fluorine-18 FDG PET study in brain hematoma. *J Nucl Med* 1994;35:1161–1166.

59. Drane WE, Abbott FD, Nicole MW, et al. Technology for FDG SPECT with a relatively inexpensive gamma camera. *Radiology* 1994;191:461–465.

60. Schober O. Nuclear medicine 2000. *Eur J Nucl Med* 1992; 19:1–5.

25

Appropriate Diagnostic Modalities and their Sequence for Evaluation of Cerebrovascular Disease

Calvin Rumbaugh, M.D., Ay-Ming Wang, M.D., Fong Y. Tsai, M.D.

FACTORS IN CHOOSING THE DIAGNOSTIC PROCEDURE

Almost any pathologic process involving the brain sometimes presents clinically with symptoms of stroke (sudden loss of a neurologic function). In addition to primary hemorrhage or infarction, stroke-like symptoms can result from tumor, infection, trauma and many other less common entities.

In evaluating the stroke patient, the detailed sequence of diagnostic studies will vary with the diagnostic facility and within each facility from time to time, depending upon the diagnostic equipment available, technologists available, skills of key personnel, patient load factors and scheduling options. (Immediate access to diagnostic facilities on an emergency basis 24 hr/day is essential for optimal care.)

Ideally, the procedures should be safe, with no risk of patient injury or death as a complication of the procedure. The risk of death or serious injury in angiography is probably less than 1% (0.1%, according to Mani et al.,[1] and 0.33%, according to Earnest et al.[2]). Computed tomography (CT), magnetic resonance imaging (MRI) and ultrasound are risk-free unless a contrast agent is administered in conjunction with the study. Even then, the risk is quite small, probably comparable to the risk from receiving a penicillin injection.

The procedures should also cause as little pain, discomfort and anxiety as possible. MRI produces severe claustrophobia in some patients; sedation may be required. Angiographic procedures also may require sedation to ease patient anxiety.

One of the most important considerations is the amount of useful, relevant diagnostic information provided. This is a significant factor when considering the monetary cost of the procedures. The cost effectiveness of a less expensive procedure which provides minimal relevant diagnostic information is low, particularly if one considers the time wasted and the resulting delay in establishing the diagnosis. Conversely, a relatively expensive diagnostic procedure such as MRI and magnetic resonance angiography (MRA) combined may be very cost-effective if it provides significant diagnostic information, enabling the physician to initiate a treatment program immediately.

Finally, since many stroke patients are confused and uncooperative during diagnostic studies, and, in particular, continue to move during the study, the study must be as brief as possible. Many of the new CT units have very short acquisition times for imaging data, which minimizes the problem of patient movement. Substantial progress is also being made in reducing data acquisition times for various MRI sequences.

Good medical practice and the patient's best interest require immediate efforts by the managing physician to determine the specific cause of a stroke, followed by appropriate treatment. Time is critical if the patient is to receive meaningful help. Stroke is a medical emergency, and most authorities in the field believe that treatment should be initiated within the first 6 hr or less following onset, when possible. "Brain attack" (stroke) should be addressed with the same urgency as heart attack.

In most imaging departments, CT should be the initial diagnostic procedure for the majority of stroke patients and should be done as soon as possible. CT will usually place the patient in one of three categories: hemorrhagic stroke, ischemic stroke or other (tumor, infection, posttrauma, etc.). Also, most of the time, CT permits identification of ischemic stroke patients with significant hemorrhagic infarction in the acute phase. However, the initial CT study in the ischemic stroke patient may be negative in the first 6 hr (and even in the first 24 hr or more). In these patients, MRI of the brain and MRA of the neck and circle of Willis branches, along with diffusion MRI to confirm the diagnosis of ischemic stroke, are probably the next diagnostic options. Spiral CT and/or ultrasound studies of the neck and circle of Willis branches are other important options at this stage. Echocardiography may be considered to rule out a cardiac source of emboli to the brain.

Some diagnostic departments which have state-of-the-art MRI equipment readily available and experienced neuroradiologists to evaluate hemorrhagic components in the stroke patient, whatever the age, could start immediately with MRI and MRA and omit the initial screening CT study.

Readers may find Figure 25-1 useful.

COMMENTS

Computed Tomography

Advantages
- In the acute and subacute stroke patient, usually good for discriminating between ischemic and hemorrhagic stroke.
- Good for differentiating between acute intracerebral hematoma and infarction.
- Good for demonstrating acute subarachnoid hemorrhage (SAH).
- Good for identifying the acute hemorrhagic infarct.
- Usually can exclude tumor, brain abscess, and subdural and/or epidural hematoma (all may present initially as a nonspecific stroke).
- Good for evaluation of bony changes.
- Good for identification of calcifications.

Disadvantages
- Often not good for posterior fossa disease due to bone artifact.
- In the subacute and chronic stages of hematoma formation, CT is less specific than in the acute stage.

Magnetic Resonance Imaging

Advantages
- Very sensitive in detecting the disease process but not very specific, although more specific than CT.
- Good for the early diagnosis of infarcts (between 30 min and 4 hr in experimental animals) (diffusion MRI in particular).
- Infarcts enhance in 3–7 days (after breakdown of the blood–brain barrier).
- Specific for cryptic vascular malformations.
- Especially good for posterior fossa disease (bone gives no signal), in contrast to CT.
- Good for SAH (subacute) after 1 week—bright on T_1 images (debatable).
- In patients with multiple aneurysms, a small hematoma often identifies the bleeding site.

Disadvantages
- Acute intracerebral hematoma is difficult to diagnose.
- Acute SAH is often not seen.

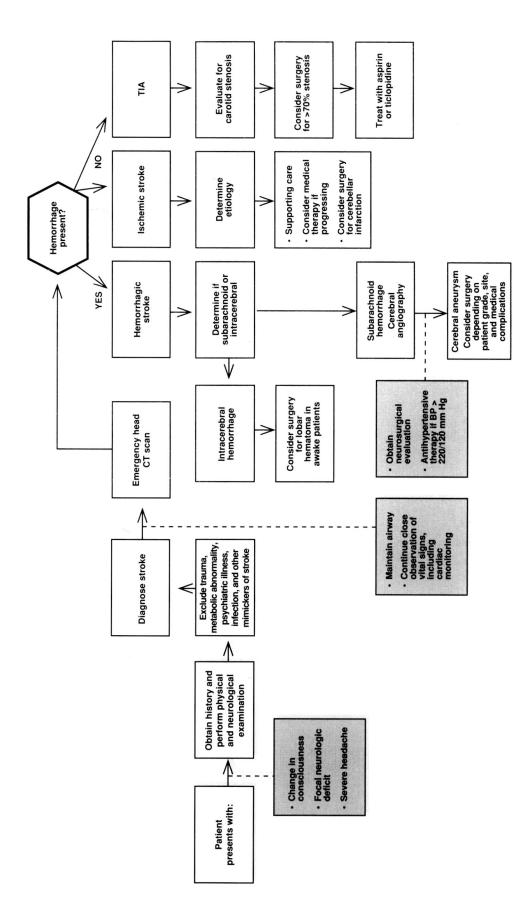

Fig. 25-1 Stroke: the first 6 hr: National Stroke Association consensus recommendations. (From ref. 3)

- If an acute infarct is hemorrhagic, this component often is not recognized.
- Calcium is not well demonstrated.
- Bony structures are not well defined.

Magnetic Resonance Angiography

Advantages
- Good for evaluation of major vessels in the neck and head.
- Good screening method for aneurysms.
- Good for treatment planning for arteriovenous malformations (AVMs).
- Non technologist dependent.
- MRI and MRA can often be combined at little additional cost. Although this is more expensive than CT and takes longer for most examinations, it usually provides more relevant information regarding the patient's diagnosis and/or treatment options.

Disadvantages
- Resolution poor at times, usually due to patient motion.

Doppler-Carotid Studies (Color)

Advantages
- Relatively inexpensive.
- Usually readily available on an emergency basis.
- Fast.

Disadvantages
- Technologist dependent.
- Requires special equipment and transducers (need color).

PREVENTION

The most effective treatment of stroke is prevention. This involves good general preventive medicine and is discussed in Chapter 1. There the following are emphasized:

1. Prevention and/or treatment of high blood pressure.

2. Prevention and/or treatment of heart disease.
3. Prevention and/or treatment of diabetes.
4. Prevention and/or treatment of hyperlipidemia.
5. Prevention and/or treatment of uricemia.
6. Prevention and/or treatment of hypothyroidism.
7. Prevention and/or treatment of obesity.
8. Stopping smoking.
9. Moderate alcohol intake.
10. Prevention and/or treatment of the hypercoagulable state.

This treatment requires the responsible individual to consult a physican on a regular basis and to follow his advice. The most important steps can only be taken by the patient. This decision cannot be made by the doctor, by government, or by parents or friends. Only the individual can make the decision to adopt and remain committed to healthy lifestyle choices. These choices include not smoking, avoiding alcohol and drug abuse, controlling fat intake, getting adequate exercise and operating motor vehicles in a sensible manner.

Finally, screening methods are being developed for use in the patient who is in the high-risk category for stroke. These methods include ultrasound (single photon emission computed tomography) (SPECT), positron emission tomography, MR diffusion and perfusion studies, proton MR spectroscopy, CT, MRI, MRA, and ocular imaging.

Not only are these modalities being used for screening, but ultimately they should have significant value in monitoring responses to therapy, particularly with some of the new drug treatments, with thrombolysis, growth factor, and so on.

REFERENCES

1. Mani RL, Eisenbery RL, McDonald EJ, et al. Complications of cerebral angiography: Analysis of 5000 procedures: I Criteria and incidence. *AJR* 1978;131:861.
2. Earnest F, Forbes G, Sandok BA, et al. Complications of cerebral angiography: Prospective assessment of risk. *AJNR* 1983;4:1191.
3. Grotta JC (ed). Stroke. *Clinical Updates* Special Edition, Vol IV, Issue 1, May 1993, p. 9.

Section 3

Endovascular Treatment of
Cerebrovascular Diseases

26

Introduction to Neurointerventional Treatment for Cerebrovascular Diseases

Fong Y. Tsai, M.D.

Neurointerventional procedures began to evolve slowly three decades ago. The most significant part of this evolution has occurred in the past 15 years and has achieved rapid acceptance. The development of angiographic equipment, catheters, embolic agents, and contrast material has advanced the study of neurovascular anatomy and physiology.[1-8] Neurointerventional procedures began with embolization, first extracranial, then intracranial. Following embolization, techniques expanded to include thrombolysis and angioplasty. Over the past two decades, a whole spectrum of neurointerventional procedures has been developed in the treatment of cerebrovascular disorders. I was fortunate to have been in the mainstream during a period of many exciting developments.

The basic requirements for neurointerventional endovascular procedures are optimal skills, a commitment to patient care, and a dedicated, interrelated multidisciplinary team. A specific goal and a comprehensive treatment plan should be thoroughly discussed and established with the primary team prior to the procedure.[9-11] The patient and family should be fully informed about the nature of the disease and the details of the procedure, including the risks, benefits, and al-ternatives. Institutional approval through an investigative committee may be necessary to accredit your skills. At the institution, approval must be granted by a review board for major endovascular and neurointerventional procedures, such as balloon embolization, balloon angioplasty, and direct thrombolytic treatment.

ANGIOGRAPHIC ROOM

The modern neuroangiographic room should be equipped with state-of-the-art digital equipment with high-resolution capabilities, road mapping, live digital subtraction, fluoroscopy, and fast imaging rates; biplane or C-arm apparatus allow for rapid and flexible positioning in multiple planes.[12,13] Patient-monitoring equipment should have automatic, continuous monitoring for blood pressure, cardiac, and pulmonary functions. Transducers should be available for endovascular pressure measurements during embolization, angioplasty, and thrombolysis.[14] The neuroangiographic suite should be spacious enough to accommodate extra equipment for EEG or anesthesiology.[15-18]

PREPROCEDURE PATIENT MANAGEMENT[19-23]

Patient control and cooperation are very important for the success of the procedure. A detailed explanation of the procedure and its risks is necessary for informed consent. Sufficient time should be allowed for the patient to ask questions and make the decision to proceed. Pain management with moderate amounts of local and intravenous neuroleptic medication calms the patient and limits unwanted motion. We routinely use a short-half-life agent such as fentanyl (Sublimaze) or midazolam (Versed). Narcan (Naloxone) should be available to reverse the effects of fentanyl if necessary. It is important to routinely reexamine the patient after IV sedation for potential adverse effects. Most procedures are performed with the patient awake; however, general anesthesia may be used to ensure patient control and adequate oxygenation.

ANGIOGRAPHIC CATHETERS

Femoral Introducer Sheath

We prefer to place a femoral introducer sheath to reduce unnecessary trauma to the femoral artery at the puncture site. It will deter the reflux of blood and facilitate catheter exchanges. The introducer sheath should be connected with a continuous infusion of heparinized saline (5,000 units in 1,000 cc) to prevent clot formation during the procedure.

Diagnostic Catheters

The 5F double-curved catheter is used routinely for all cerebral diagnostic angiography. A long, soft-tip guidewire is used as a standard in diagnostic angiography. However, the Glidewire (Terumo) may be used for a tortuous artery.

Guiding Catheters

Guiding catheters are thin-walled and nontapered, ranging from 5F to 10F. They should be used in conjunction with an introducer sheath and may be advanced coaxially to the desired location with smaller angiographic catheters or independently. These guiding catheters are well suited for the introduction of microcatheters for embolization, thrombolysis, or angioplasty. They are available from several manufacturers, such as Cook (Bloomington, IN), Interventional Therapeutic Corporation (ITC) (San Francisco, CA), and MediTech (Watertown, MA).

SPECIAL CATHETERS FOR SPECIAL NEEDS

Embolization Catheters

Large Interventional Catheters

Tracker 38 This can be used as a guiding catheter for a small microcatheter in a very tortuous neck vessel. It has two different sizes. The Tracker 38 NL is a 4F catheter that takes a 0.022-in. guidewire. The regular Tracker 38 has a 5.3F shaft tapering to 4.7F distally and takes a regular 0.038-in. guidewire.

Tracker 25 This has a proximal 4F shaft tapering to 3.6F distally and takes a 0.025-in. guidewire.

Both catheters can be used for large particulate agents and large microcoils.

Microcatheters

Flow-Directed Microcatheters[24-28] These are progressive in suppleness, with a proximal stiff shaft of 3.2F, tapering to a very soft, floppy distal (1.5 to 2.5 cm) end with silastic material. These catheters are carried by blood flow to the target site once the catheter is introduced into the vessel. They are used to deliver liquid embolic agents such as NBCA but are not used for particulate agents. These catheters are available as the Magic (Balt, Montmorency, France), Mini-Torquer (Ingenor, Paris, France) and Zephyr (Target Therapeutics, Fremont, CA). Although these flow-directed microcatheters are not intended for a guidewire, they may be used with caution with guidewire (0.01–0.014 in.) to improve pulsability.

Non-Flow-Directed/Guidewire-Directed Microcatheters[29-32] The most popular type of catheter in this group is the Tracker catheter (Target Therapeutics, Fremont, CA). It has a 3F shaft tapering to a 2.2F tip distally; it requires a guidewire for advancement. Various types of microcatheters are also available through Cordis (Miami, FL) and Microvena (Vandnais Heights, MN). Microvena produces the Microferret, a stiffer microcatheter made for use in extracranial vessels. A large variety of microguidewires ranging from 0.014 to 0.0018 in. in diameter with varying degrees of stiffness are available from manufacturers such as Target Therapeutics (Fremont,

CA), Advanced Cardiovascular (Temecula, CA), Cordis (Miami, FL), and Microvena (Vandnais Heights, MN) for use with these microcatheters. These catheters are used for liquid, particulate, and microcoil embolization. The Tracker 10, with a 2.6F shaft tapering to 2F distally and a 0.010-in.-diameter wire, is a miniature of the original Tracker 18. It is used to deliver liquid embolic agents, smaller particulates up to 250 mm, and specially designed platinum microcoils.

Open-Ended Guidewire[33,34] The open-ended guidewire was formerly used for small particulate embolization and thrombolytic infusion. It has been replaced by the Tracker catheter.

Catheters for Thrombolysis[35–38]

In the extracranial vessels, a regular angiographic catheter may be used for thrombolysis. However, the intracranial vessels require a microcatheter for thrombolytic infusion. Thrombolytic agents may be delivered with a regular Tracker 18 or with a multiple side-hole infusion catheter. For superselective catheterization of the ophthalmic artery, we prefer to use either a Tracker 18 with an extended 2.2F tip or a Tracker 10.[38] Side-hole infusion catheters are preferred for thrombolytic treatment of superior sagittal sinus thrombosis or basilar artery occlusion. Target Therapeutics, Cordis, and Cook have developed side-hole and end-hole catheters for intracranial thrombolysis. There are two types of side-hole infusion catheters from Tracker.

Microsoft Stream Infusion Catheter
This catheter has a 3F shaft tapering to 2.5F distally, which can go through a regular 5F thin-walled angiographic catheter for intracranial infusion. This catheter takes a 0.014-in. to ~0.016-in. guidewire.

Regular Soft Stream Infusion Catheter
This catheter has a larger 3.5F shaft tapering to a 3F distal tip. It may need a 6F thin-walled catheter for coaxial delivery. This catheter can take a 0.014-in. to ~0.016-in. guidewire.

Catheters for Angioplasty

Extracranial Portion[39–45]
Many angioplasty balloon catheters are available. To avoid distal embolization complications, different types of balloons are designed to fit supra-aortic arteries during angioplasty. The balloon has been modified with a short side-hole tip catheter, and the balloon is folded

to provide a very low profile (Fig. 26-1). The material is softer than normal, which allows stenosis dilation with slow inflation and rapid deflation. This modified balloon catheter is available from MediTech and Cordis. A single large 9F guiding catheter taking both the angioplastic catheter and the distal protection catheter was described by Theron et al.[44] During balloon inflation, transient ischemia frequently occurs due to the interruption of cerebral blood flow caused by the balloon dilitation rather than emboli.[45]

Intracranial Portions[36,43,46–51]
Although there are many small balloon catheters designed for extracranial angioplasty, a tortuous, stenotic artery may prevent the use and advancement of the ordinary small, stiff-tipped balloon. Nondetachable silicone micro-balloons (ITC) or nondetachable latex micro-balloons (Ingenor, Balt) mounted on a variety of 2F microcatheters are available for intracranial angioplasty. They are designed for spasmatic arterial angioplasty. The pressures generated by silicone and latex balloons are different; less than 1 atm is generated with the silicone balloon, but two to three times more pressure is generated with latex. However, balloon diameter cannot be controlled during inflation. This disadvantage does not exist with the Stealth (Target) balloon catheter, on which the inflated balloon will conform to the curve of the artery rather than straighten it. We prefer to use the Stealth catheter (Fig. 26-2) for distal carotid and vertebral arteries as well as intracranial arteries.[36,46] The Stealth catheter is navigated with a steerable microcatheter guidewire. Once the balloon is in position, this guidewire is exchanged for a special dilatation guidewire (with a ball at its extremity). The ball of the dilatation guidewire blocks the distal outlet of the balloon to allow inflation. Target Therapeutics recommends that pressure not exceed 5.4 atm. We prefer to inflate the balloon slowly. This balloon catheter may be used to treat not only spastic artery but also atherosclerotic stenosis.

Detachable Balloon Catheters[51–68]

The detachable balloon technique was initially developed in Russia by Serbinenko, Romadanov, and Scheglov. This technique was further refined by Debrum et al. and Hieshima et al. The Hieshima silicone balloon is available from ITC (Fremont, CA), and the latex balloon is available from Ingenor and Balt. Both types of balloons have self-sealing valves to prevent premature deflation after detachment from the microcatheter. Silicone balloons are softer and have larger expansion

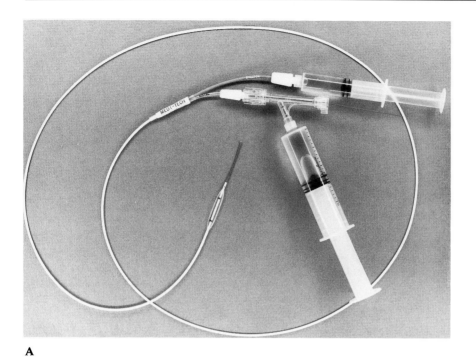

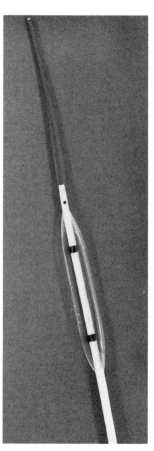

A

Fig. 26-1 Extracranial angioplasty catheters. (*A*) A set of angioplastic catheters assembled with two syringes. The small one is for balloon inflation. The large one is for injection of heparinized arterial blood. (*B*) Magnified view of a balloon and tip with side holes. The side holes enhance the injection rate of heparinized arterial blood and suction during deflation of the balloon.

B

capabilities than latex balloons. The silicone membrane is semipermeable and is inflated with iso-osmolar solution or HEMA (2 hydroxyethyl methacrylate) to avoid premature deflation.[62,63,66–68] However, HEMA is no longer available.

The detachable balloon is delivered coaxially on a 2F Tracker catheter through a thin-walled, nontapering

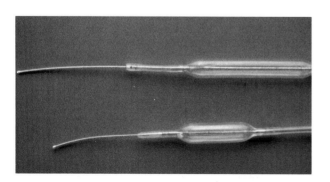

Fig. 26-2 Intracranial angioplastic catheter. Magnified view of the Stealth catheter tip with an inflated balloon.

guiding catheter at least 7F in size. A micro-guidewire is then placed inside the microcatheter to add torque and help achieve balloon placement at the target site without the need for blood flow or inflation. The detachable balloon can also be advanced through a 4F catheter before introduction through the 7F thin guiding catheter.

EMBOLIC MATERIALS

A wide variety of embolic materials have been used. However, no single embolic agent can be utilized in all circumstances. The choice of embolic material must be based on the desired result, the vascular anatomy, and the delivery system. The risk of the procedure must be considered one of the most important factors. Despite the advances in interventional techniques and materials, the ideal embolic material is yet to be discovered. Each center should have its own embolic materials, which can be mastered in any situation to achieve the best result. In general, the more efficient the devascularization of the microvascular beds and plexiform niduses, the better the embolization results. Embolic materials may be categorized into several different types.

Particulates

Silastic beads were used for embolization in the early years, but they were relegated to history after the development of microcatheters.

Polyvinyl Alcohol (PVA or Ivalon) Sponge or Powdered PVA

This is the most commonly used particulate embolic material in the United States.[69-84] Although PVA particulates are permanent embolic material, recanalization may occur after embolization. Small pieces of sponge measure 1 × 1.5 mm or 1 × 2 mm, and powder ranges from 200-mm to 1,000-mm particles. These are available from ITC (Fremont, CA), Biodyne (El Cajon, CA), Balt (Paris, France), Ingenor (Montmorency, France), and Ivalon (San Diego, CA).

Gelfoam Sponge and Powder[85-87]

Gelfoam is an excellent temporary embolic material, either alone or mixed with PVA powder. It is available from Upjohn (Kalamazoo, MI).

Microfibrillar Collagen (Avitene)[88-93]

This is a hemostatic material which is utilized topically to stop local bleeding. It is a microcrystalline polymer product prepared from purified bovine collagen. It is available from Medchem Products (Woburn, MA). Avitene is considered a temporary embolic material with medium duration, much longer than that of Gelfoam. It can be suspended and administered in contrast material. Another form of microfibrillar collagen is Angiostat (glutaraldehyde cross-limbed microfibrillar collagen), which is available from Collagen Corporation (Los Angeles, CA). Angiostat is different in that it produces mechanical arterial occlusion without any coagulation or thrombus formation. Avitene produces platelet agglutination to promote hemostatic occlusion from early granulomatous arteritis.

Surgical Sutures (Silk or Polytene)[94,95]

Surgical sutures can be cut to different lengths, 3 to 10 mm or longer. They are then injected through a Tracker catheter as particulate embolic material.

Embolic Cocktails[96,97]

A combination of PVA, Avitene, silk sutures, and ethanol has been used as an embolic cocktail. It has the combined advantages of each of its components.

Liquid Embolic Materials

Cyanoacrylates[98-108]

NBCA (N-butyl-2-cyanoacrylate) has replaced the old IBCA (isobutyl-2-cyanoacrylate) in the past 5 years. NBCA is a vinyl monomer of the alky-2-cyanoacrylate and functions as a tissue adhesive. It is available from Tri-point Medical (Raleigh, NC) as Avacryl and from B Braun (Melsungen, Germany) as Histoacryl.

Extensive training is required before using this liquid embolic material because of its potential risks. The catheter must be thoroughly flushed with 5% dextrose solution before injection of NBCA mixture to avoid polymerization in the catheter. The mixture of NBCA with Pantopaque may delay the polymerization from 0.2 to 5 sec.

Ethanol[109-114]

Dehydrated 96% ethanol is available from Abbott Laboratories (North Chicago, IL) as a strong sclerosing and thrombogenic agent in a vessel. Great care must be taken to avoid injecting it into a normal vessel. Ethanol can be used as part of a particulate embolic cocktail or alone with nonionic contrast materials.

Other Materials

There are many liquid embolic materials but they are rarely used.

1. Sotradecol[115] (sodium tetradecyl sulfate) (Elkins, Sinn, Cherry Hill, NJ).
2. Ethabloc[116-118] (Ethicon, Hamburg, Germany).
3. Eval, a mixture of ethylene vinyl alcohol copolymer and metrizamide powder dissolved in DMSO (dimethyl sulfoxide[119]), which must be delivered through a metallic hub because DMSO causes plastic to deteriorate.

Discrete Materials

Stainless Steel Coils[120-126]

Dacron fibers attached to stainless steel coils (Fig. 26-3) are responsible for thrombogenic development. These coils need to be delivered through a regular angiographic 5F or larger interventional embolization catheter with ID 0.035 in. to ~0.038 in.

Microcoils[127-131]

Microcoils of many types and shapes were designed to aid endovascular embolization for an AVM, fistula, or aneurysm.

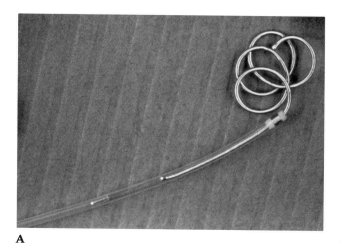

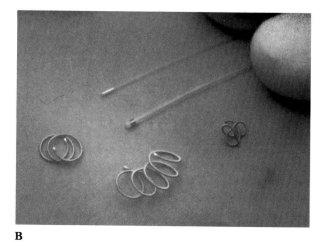

A   B

Fig. 26-3   Stainless steel coil pushed out of the delivery catheter. (*A*) Larger coil. (*B*) Smaller coils.

1. Platinum microcoils (Figs. 26-4 and 26-5) are available from Target Therapeutics and Cook. Two kinds of occlusion coil are available from Target Therapeutics: a braided occlusive device and fibered platinum coils. A coil pusher is required to deliver these microcoils but, using caution, they may also be detached with saline injection.

2. Detachable platinum coils[130,131] (Fig. 26-6) were developed by Guglielmi et al. for the treatment of aneurysms. They may be used to treat arteriovenous fistula or arteriovenous malformation. They are now available from Target Therapeutics. This soft microcoil is soldered at the end of an insulated stainless steel micro-guidewire and is detached by direct current in an electrolytic process. Detachable platinum coils can achieve better packing in the aneurysm than the regular platinum micro-coils.

FUTURE DEVELOPMENT

Despite the numerous variety of embolic agents and catheters available for neurointerventional procedures, none are ideal in all conditions and situations. Further development and new ideas will continue, although the current regulatory situation in the United States makes it difficult to develop and distribute embolic materials and create new methodology.

Stents[132,133]

Although stents (Fig. 26-7) have been widely used in the field of peripheral vascular intervention, they have

been used in the cerebrovascular system only on rare occasions. Stents have been used in the treatment of vascular stenosis or dissection independently or as adjuncts to PTA, as well as for the treatment of aneurysms, specifically giant traumatic aneurysm with a wide-based neck. Available are the Wallstent (Schneider, MN) and Palmaz stents (Johnson & Johnson, New Brunswick, NJ). The limitation for intracranial use in currently available stents is due to their inadequate flexibility for passing through the tortuous segment of the distal cervical or intracranial vessels.

Atherectomy

Though many types of atherectomy devices have been used in the treatment of peripheral vascular stenosis, only one was developed for carotid artery stenosis; previously, it was used only experimentally in animals.[134] A heavily calcified plaque is not suitable for PTA but is ideal for atherectomy. The use of atherectomy to treat cerebrovascular stenosis definitely requires further study in order to know the feasibility and to lower the expense.

Snares[135]

Complications may result when dislodging embolic material or a microcoil or when a catheter becomes fragmented. It may be retrieved by a newly available Microsnare from Target (Fremont, CA) and Microvena (Vandnais Heights, MN) which comes with microcatheters and micro-guidewire snares.

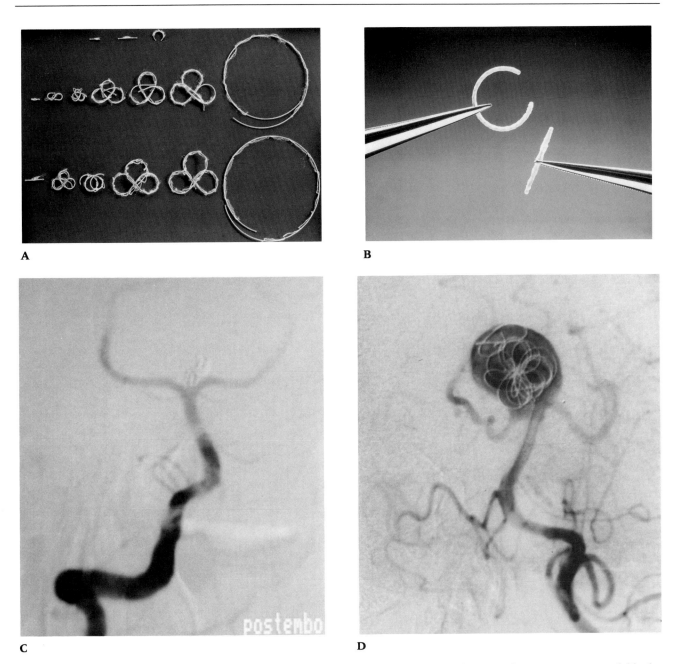

Fig. 26-4 Platinum microcoils. (*A*) Fibered platinum microcoils of many different shapes and sizes are now available for different embolization purposes. (*B*) Braided occlusive microcoils. (*C*) Platinum microcoils were placed into a small basilar arterial tip aneurysm with complete obliteration. (*D*) Multiple platinum microcoils were placed into a giant aneurysm of the basilar artery tip. Complete packing cannot be achieved as easily with platinum coils as with GDC coils.

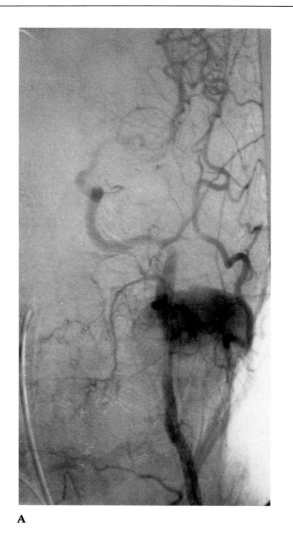

A

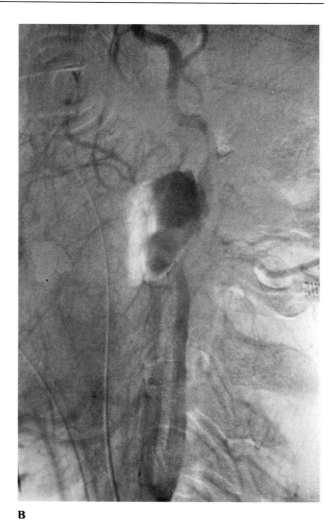

B

C

Fig. 26-5 Giant traumatic aneurysm. A 16-year-old male presented with active bleeding from the mouth 3 months after a gunshot injury. (*A,B*) Frontal and lateral views of the left common carotid artery angiogram showed a giant traumatic aneurysm from a high cervical internal carotid artery. (*C*) Simultaneous placement of a detachable balloon and a Tracker catheter in the side of the aneurysm. The balloon served as an anchor to block the wide-based neck of the pseudoaneurysm in order to prevent migration of coils and to stop blood flow to the aneurysm, which has a leak, inducing active bleeding from the mouth.

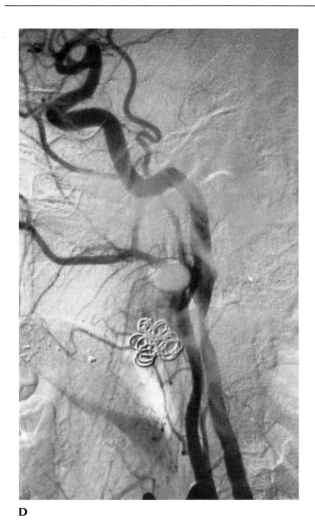

D

Fig. 26-5 (*D*) Postembolization angiography showed that the coils stayed at the deep end of the aneurysm and that the balloon detached at the base of the aneurysm. There was a thrombus formation between the coils and the balloon.

Treatment for Arterial Spasm from SAH[136–138]

The etiology of and treatment for spastic intracranial artery had been uncertain until recently. Transluminal angioplasty has now shown some promising results. The potential arterial injury from transluminal angioplasty has led neurointerventionalists to use papaverine for intra-arterial infusion. Recent reports have suggested more superselective injections into individual arteries to gain better results. A pulsed-dye laser angioplasty technique was reported recently, which creates cavitation within the catheter and emits a high pressure fluid wave to dilate the spastic artery.

Microcoils[139–141]

Collagen-coated microcoils and polyurethane-coated GDC coils have been recently reported to increase thrombogenicity. Metallic fragments from electrolytic detachable coils (Gugliemi-GDC) during electrolysis may induce infarcts. The relationship between stroke and the metallic fragments remains unknown. It may warrant further study.

CONCLUSION

The current widespread acceptance of neurointerventions is the result of the tireless effort of the pioneers in this field. Their work is not yet finished, however. Continuous research and further development are needed to offer the safest interventional treatment to our patients.

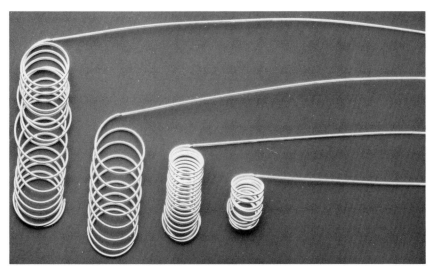

Fig. 26-6 Detachable platinum GDC coils. Different lengths of GDC coils are available for different aneurysm sizes or vascular malformations.

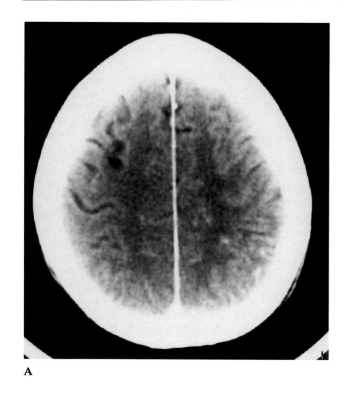

A

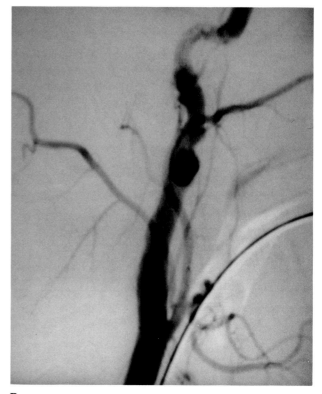

B

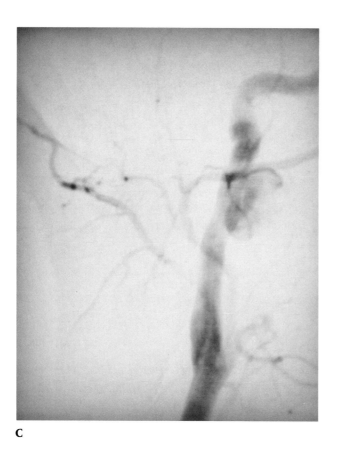

C

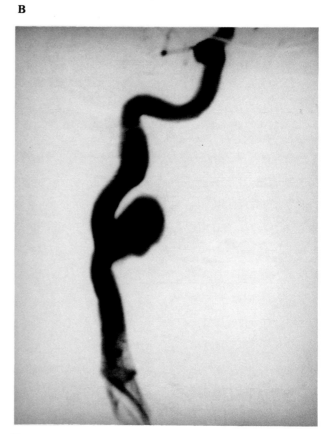

D

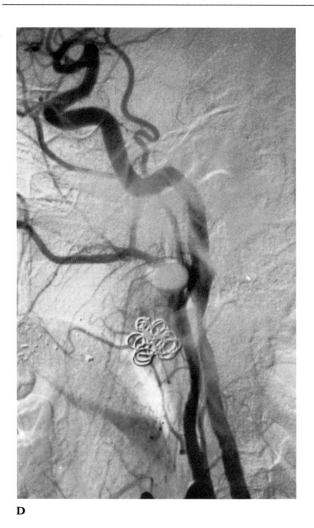

D

Fig. 26-5 (*D*) Postembolization angiography showed that the coils stayed at the deep end of the aneurysm and that the balloon detached at the base of the aneurysm. There was a thrombus formation between the coils and the balloon.

Treatment for Arterial Spasm from SAH[136–138]

The etiology of and treatment for spastic intracranial artery had been uncertain until recently. Transluminal angioplasty has now shown some promising results. The potential arterial injury from transluminal angioplasty has led neurointerventionalists to use papaverine for intra-arterial infusion. Recent reports have suggested more superselective injections into individual arteries to gain better results. A pulsed-dye laser angioplasty technique was reported recently, which creates cavitation within the catheter and emits a high pressure fluid wave to dilate the spastic artery.

Microcoils[139–141]

Collagen-coated microcoils and polyurethane-coated GDC coils have been recently reported to increase thrombogenicity. Metallic fragments from electrolytic detachable coils (Gugliemi-GDC) during electrolysis may induce infarcts. The relationship between stroke and the metallic fragments remains unknown. It may warrant further study.

CONCLUSION

The current widespread acceptance of neurointerventions is the result of the tireless effort of the pioneers in this field. Their work is not yet finished, however. Continuous research and further development are needed to offer the safest interventional treatment to our patients.

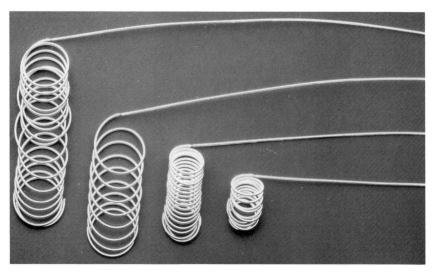

Fig. 26-6 Detachable platinum GDC coils. Different lengths of GDC coils are available for different aneurysm sizes or vascular malformations.

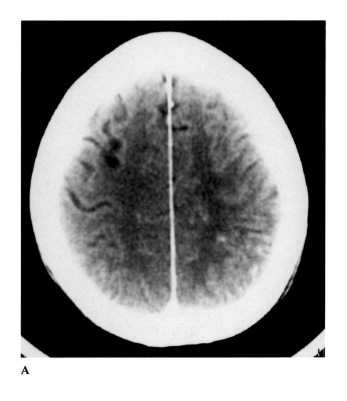

A

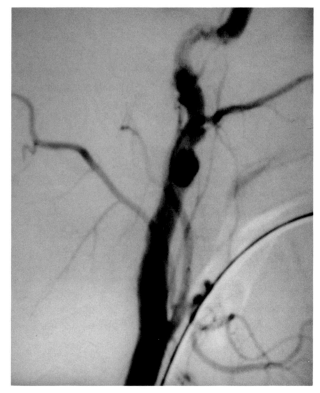

B

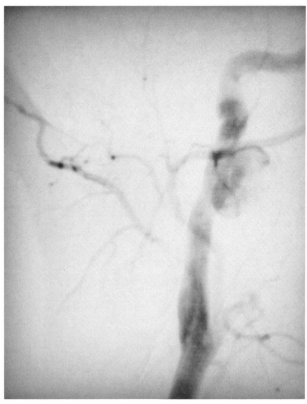

C

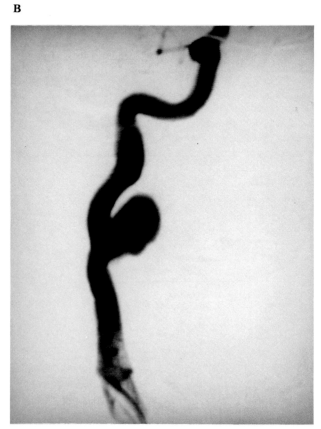

D

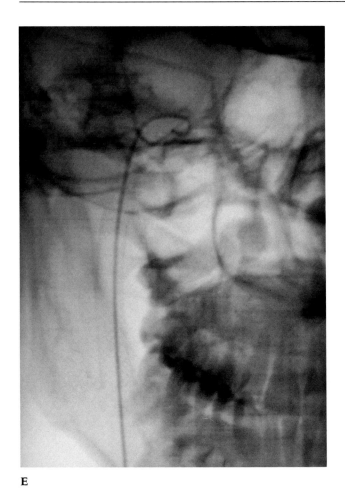

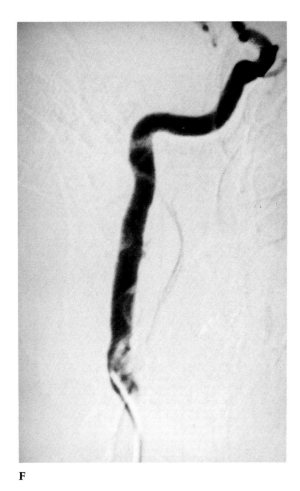

E

F

Fig. 26-7 A 30-year-old female presented with left-sided weakness following a motor vehicle accident. The weakness eventually resolved, but further workup revealed bilateral carotid artery dissections. There was healing of the left-sided dissection but enlargement of a pseudoaneurysm from the right internal carotid artery dissection. Because surgical treatment of a high cervical internal carotid artery aneurysm was felt to be difficult, the physician decided to treat it with a stent. (*A*) Enhanced heat CT scan 1 month following the trauma shows low density in the right frontoparietal region consistent with a small infarct. (*B*) Right common carotid arteriogram shows irregularity of the upper cervical internal carotid artery, with a pseudoaneurysm seen en face. (*C*) Three-month follow-up right common carotid arteriogram shows enlargement of the pseudoaneurysm. (*D*) Right internal carotid arteriogram immediately prior to stent placement better defines the broad neck of the pseudoaneurysm. (*E*) A stent was successfully placed across the pseudoaneurysm. (*F*) Right internal carotid arteriogram 3 months following stent placement shows that the pseudoaneurysm is almost completely gone. The patient did well following stent placement.

In a recent survey, neuroradiology procedures were rated the second highest focus of malpractice litigation.[142] Only angiographic procedures were litigated more often. In neuroradiology cases, complaints arose mainly from intervention following stroke and its complications. Thus, careful planning for patient management is essential to minimize the frequency of these disputes and achieve the best results for our patients.

Please refer to the individual chapters for detailed discussions of techniques and statistical information regarding interventional procedures for cerebrovascular diseases.

REFERENCES

1. Vinuela F, Dion J, Lylyk P, et al. Update on interventional neuroradiology. *AJR* 1989;153:23–33.
2. Vinuela F, Fox AJ. Interventional neuroradiology and

the management of arteriovenous malformations and fistulas. *Neurol Clin* 1983;1:131–154.

3. Eskridge JM. Interventional neuroradiology. *Radiology* 1989;172:992–1006.

4. Halbach VV, Higashida RT, Hieshima GB. Interventional neuroradiology. *AJR* 1989;153:467–476.

5. Gerlock AJ, Mirfakhraee M. Embolization procedure in neuroradiology, in *Essentials of Diagnostic and Interventional Angiographic Techniques*. Philadelphia, WB Saunders, 1985, pp 131–173.

6. Gerlock AJ, Mirfakhraee M. Materials and techniques for peripheral visceral embolization, in *Essentials of Diagnostic and Interventional Angiographic Techniques*. Philadelphia, WB Saunders, 1985, pp 209–236.

7. Luessenhop AJ. Interventional neuroradiology: A neurosurgeon's perspective. *AJNR* 1990;11:625–629.

8. Luessenhop AJ, Spence WT. Artificial embolization of cerebral arteries. Report of use in a case of arteriovenous malformation. *JAMA* 1960;172:1153–1155.

9. Rigamonti D, Spetzler RF, Johnson PC, et al. Cerebral vascular malformations. *BNI Q* 1987;3:18–28.

10. McCormick WS. Pathology of vascular "arteriovenous" malformations. *BNI Q* 1987;3:18–28.

11. McCormick WS. Pathology of vascular malformations of the brain, in Wilson CB, Stein BM (eds): *Intracranial Arteriovenous Malformations*. Baltimore, Williams & Wilkins, 1984, pp 44–63.

12. Martin NA, Bentson J, Vinuela F, et al. Intraoperative digital subtraction angiography and the surgical treatment of intracranial aneurysms and vascular malformations. *J Neurosurg* 1990;73:526–533.

13. Hieshima GB, Reicher MA, Higashida RT, et al. Intra-operative digital subtraction neuroangiography: Diagnostic and therapeutic tool. *AJNR* 1987;8:759–768.

14. Duckwiler G, Dion J, Vinuela F, et al. Intravascular microcatheter pressure monitoring, experimental results and early clinical evaluation. *AJNR* 1990;11:169–175.

15. Nuwer MR, Jordan SE, Ahn SS. Evaluation of stroke using EEG frequency analysis and topographic mapping. *Neurology* 1987;37:1153–1159.

16. John ER, Chabot RJ, Prichep LS, et al. Real time intraoperative monitoring during neurosurgical and neuroradiological procedures. *J Clin Neurophysiol* 1989;6:125–158.

17. Hacke W, Zuemer H, Berg-Danner E. Monitoring of hemispheric or brain stem functions with neurophysiologic method during interventional neuroradiology. *AJNR* 1983;4:382–384.

18. Bernstein A, Young W, Ransohoff J, et al. Somatosensory evoked potentials during spinal angiography and therapeutic transvascular embolization. *J Neurosurg* 1984;60:777–785.

19. Diament MG, Stanley P. The use of midazolam for sedation of infants and children. *AJR* 1988;150:377–378.

20. Miller DL, Wall RT. Fentanyl and diazepam for analgesia and sedation during radiologic special procedures. *Radiology* 1987;162:195–198.

21. Cragg AH, Smith TP, Berbaum KS, et al. Randomized double-blind trial of midazolam/placebo and midazolam/fentanyl for sedation and analgesia in lower extremity angiography. *AJR* 1991;157:173–176.

22. Stevenson GW, Pathria MN, Lamping DL, et al. Driving ability after intravenous fentanyl or diazepam. A controlled double-blind study. *Invest Radiol* 1986;21:717–719.

23. Erba M, Jungreis CA, Horton JA. Nitorpaste for prevention and relief of vascular spasm. *AJNR* 1989;10:155–156.

24. Dion JE, Duckwiler GR, Lylyk P, et al. Progressive suppleness pursil catheter: A new tool for superselective angiography and embolization. *AJNR* 1989;10:1068–1070.

25. Kerber CW. Balloon catheter with calibrated leak. *Radiology* 1976;120:574–577.

26. Bank WO, Trainer FG, Edwards MS, et al. Arterial injury during intracerebral manipulation of intracerebral microcatheters. *Neuroradiology* 1982;22:274.

27. Debrun GM, Vinuela FV, Fox AJ, et al. Two different calibrated-leak balloons: Experimental work and application in humans. *AJNR* 1982;3:407–414.

28. O'Reilly GV, Kleefield J, Forrest MD, et al. Calibrated leak balloon: Accurate placement of leak. *AJNR* 1985;6:90–91.

29. Russell EJ, Levy JM. Direct catheter redirection of a symptomatic intracranial silastic sphere embolus. *Radiology* 1987;165:631–633.

30. Kikuchi Y, Strother CM, Boyer M. New catheter for endovascular interventional procedures. *Radiology* 1987;165:870–871.

31. Tsai FY, Higashida RT, Matovich VB, et al. Acute thrombosis of the intracranial dural sinus—direct thrombolytic treatment. *AJNR* 1992;13:1137–1141.

32. Nelson N. A versatile, steerable, flow-guided catheter for delivery of detachable balloons. *AJNR* 1989;10:155–156.

33. Encarnacion CE, Kadir S, Malone RD Jr. Subselective embolization with gelatin sponge through an open-ended guidewire. *Radiology* 1990;174:265–267.

34. Jungreis CA, Berenstein A, Choi IS. Use of open-ended guidewire: Steerable microguidewire assembly system in surgical neuroangiographic procedures. *AJNR* 1987;8:237–242.

35. Wolpert SM, Kwan ESK, Heros D, et al. Selective delivery of chemotherapeutic agents with a new catheter system. *Radiology* 1988;166:547–549.

36. Tsai FY, Matovich VB, Berberian B, et al. PTA adjunct to thrombolysis for acute MCA rethrombosis. *AJNR* 1994;15:1823–1829.

37. Tsai FY, Berberian B, Lavin M, et al. Thrombolytic treatment of acute middle cerebral arterial occlusion. ASNR annual meeting Nashville, TN. May 1–7, 1994.

38. Tsai FY, Wadley D, Angle JF, et al. The implication of superselective ophthalmic angiography. *AJNR* 1990;11:1203–1204.

39. Tsai FY, Matovich VB, Hieshima GB, et al. Percutaneous transluminal angioplasty of carotid artery. *AJNR* 1986;7:349–358.

40. Tsai FY, Matovich VB, Hieshima GB, et al. The practical aspects of percutaneous transluminal angioplasty for the treatment of carotid artery stenosis. *Acta Radiol* 1986;369(Suppl):127–130.

41. Higashida RT, Hieshima GB, Tsai FY, et al. Transluminal angioplasty of the subclavian and vertebral arteries for vertebrobasilar insufficiency. *Acta Radiol* 1986;(Suppl)369:124–126.

42. Higashida RT, Hieshima GB, Tsai FY, et al. Transluminal angioplasty of the vertebral and basilar artery. *AJNR* 1987;8:745–749.

43. Higashida RT, Tsai FY, Halbach, VV et al. Transluminal angioplasty for atherosclerotic disease of the vertebral and basilar arteries. *J Neurosurg* 1983;78:192–198.

44. Theron J, Courtheoux P, Alachkar S, et al. New triple coaxial catheter system for carotid angioplasty with cerebral protection. *AJNR* 1990;11:869–874.

45. DeMonte F, Peerless S, Rankin RN. Carotid transluminal angioplasty with evidence of distal embolization. Case report. *J Neurosurg* 1989;70:138–141.

46. Higashida RT, Halbach VV, Tsai FY, et al. Intravascular balloon dilatation for intracranial arterial spasm: Patient selection, technique and clinical results. *Neurosurg Rev* 1992;15:89–95.

47. Zubkov YN, Nikiforov BM, Shustin VA. Balloon catheter technique for dilatation of constricted cerebral arteries after aneurysmal SAH. *Acta Neurochir (Wein)* 1984;70:65–79.

48. Newell DW, Eskridge JM, Mayberg MR, et al. Angioplasty for the treatment of symptomatic vasospasm following subarachnoid hemorrhage. *J Neurosurg* 1989;71:654–660.

49. Higashida RT, Halbach VV, Dormandy B, et al. New microballoon device for transluminal angioplasty of intracranial arterial vasospasm. *AJNR* 1990;11:233–238.

50. Higashida RT, Halbach VV, Cahan LO, et al. Transluminal angioplasty of intracranial vessels for treatment of intracranial arterial vasospasm. *J Neurosurg* 1989;71:648–653.

51. Serbinenko SA. Balloon catheterization and occlusion of major cerebral vessels. *J Neurosurg* 1974;41:125–128.

52. Brothers MF, Holgate RC. Intracranial angioplasty for treatment of vasospasm after subarachnoid hemorrhage: Technique and modifications to improve branch access. *AJNR* 1990;11:239–248.

53. Zubkov YN, Nikiforov BM, Shustin VA. Balloon catheter technique for dilatation of constricted cerebral arteries after aneurysmal SAH. *Acta Neurochir (Wein)* 1984;70:65–79.

54. Romodanov AP, Scheglov VI. Intravascular occlusion of saccular aneurysms of the cerebral arteries by means of a detachable balloon, in Krayenbuhl H (ed): *Advances and Technical Standards in Neurosurgery.* Vienna, Springer-Verlag, 1982, pp 25–49.

55. Debrun G, Lacour P, Caron J. Detachable balloon and calibrated-leak balloon techniques in the treatment of cerebral vascular lesions. *J Neurosurg* 1978;49:635–639.

56. Tsai FY, Hieshima GB, Mehringer CM, et al. Delayed effects in the treatment of carotid cavernous fistulas. *AJNR* 1983;4:357–361.

57. Hieshima GB, Higashida RT, Wapenski J, et al. Balloon embolization of a large distal basilar artery aneurysm. *J Neurosurg* 1986;65:413–416.

58. Kaufman SL, Strandberg JD, Barth KH, et al. Therapeutic embolization with detachable silicone balloons, long term effects in swine. *Invest Radiol* 1979;14:156–161.

59. White RI, Kaufman SL, Barth KH, et al. Therapeutic embolization with detachable silicone balloons. Early clinical experience. *JAMA* 1979;241:1257–1260.

60. O'Reilly GV, Kleefield J, Forrest MD, et al. Fabrication of microballoons for interventional neuroradiology: Preliminary report. *AJNR* 1984;5:625–628.

61. Hawkins TD, Szaz KF, The permeability of detachable latex rubber balloons. An in-vitro study. *Invest Radiol* 1987;22:969–972.

62. Higashida RT, Halbach VV, Dowd CD, et al. Intracranial aneurysms: Interventional neurovascular treatment with detachable balloons: Results in 215 cases. *Radiology* 1991;178:663–670.

63. Higashida RT, Halbach VV, Dormandy B, et al. Endovascular treatment of intracranial aneurysms with a new silicone microballoon device: Technical considerations and indications for therapy. *Radiology* 1990;174:687–691.

64. Burrows P, Lasjaunias P, Terbrugge KG. 4-F Coaxial catheter system for pediatric vascular occlusion with detachable balloons. *Radiology* 1989;170:1091–1094.

65. Taki W, Handa H, Niyake H, et al. New detachable balloon technique for traumatic carotid-cavernous fistulae. *AJNR* 1985;6:961–964.

66. Goto K, Halbach VV, Hardin CW, et al. Permanent inflation of detachable balloons with a low viscosity, hydrophilic polymerizing system. *Radiology* 1988;169:787–790.

67. Taki W, Handa H, Yamagata S, et al. Radiopaque solidifying liquids releasable balloon technique: A technical note. *Surg Neurol* 1980;13:140–142.

68. Monsein LH, Debrun GM, Chazaly JR. Hydroxyethyl methylacrylate and latex balloons. *AJNR* 1990;11: 663–664.

69. Berenstein A, Kricheff II. Catheter and material selection for transarterial embolization: Technical considerations. II. Materials. *Radiology* 1979;132:631–639.

70. Kunstlinger F, Brunelle F, Chaumont P, et al. Vascular occlusive agents. *AJR* 1981;136:151–156.

71. Berenstein A, Kricheff II. Microembolization techniques of vascular occlusion: Radiologic, pathologic and clinical correlation. *AJNR* 1981;2:261–268.

72. Wright K, Anderson JH, Gianturco C, et al. Partial splenic embolization using polyvinyl alcohol foam, dextran, polystyrene, or silicone. An experimental study in dogs. *Radiology* 1982;142:351–354.

73. Chuang VP, Tsai CC, Soo CS, et al. Experimental canine hepatic artery embolization with polyvinyl alcohol foam particles. *Radiology* 1982;45:21–25.

74. Tsai FY, Hieshima GB, Mehringer CM, et al. Arterial digital subtraction angiography with particulate intravascular embolization and angioplasty. *Surg Neurol* 1984;11:104–212.

75. Scialfa G, Scotti G. Superselective injection of polyvinyl alcohol microemboli for the treatment of cerebral arteriovenous malformations. *AJNR* 1985;6:957–960.

76. Purdy PD, Samson D, Batjer HH, et al. Preoperative embolization of cerebral arteriovenous malformations with polyvinyl alcohol particles: Experience in 51 adults. *AJNR* 1990;11:501–510.

77. Jack CR Jr, Forbes G, Dewanjee MK, et al. Polyvinyl alcohol sponge for embolotherapy: Particle size and morphology. *AJNR* 1985;6:595–597.

78. Berenstein A, Graeb DA. Convenient preparation of ready-to-use articles in polyvinyl alcohol foam suspension for embolization. *Radiology* 1982;145:846.

79. Herrera M, Rysavy J, Kotula S, et al. Ivalon shavings: Technical considerations of a new embolic agents. *Radiology* 1982;144:638–640.

80. Szwarc IA, Carrasco CH, Wallace S, et al. Radiopaque suspension of polyvinyl alcohol foam for embolization. *AJR* 1986;146:591–592.

81. Kerber CW, Bank WP, Horton JA. Polyvinyl alcohol foam: Prepacking emboli for therapeutic embolization. *Radiology* 1988;130:1193–1194.

82. Horton JA, Marano GD, Kerber CW, et al. Polyvinyl alcohol foam/Gelfoam for therapeutic embolization: A synergistic mixture. *AJNR* 1983;4:143–148.

83. Repa I, Moradian GT, Dehner LP, et al. Mortalities associated with use of a commercial suspension of polyvinyl alcohol. *Radiology* 1989;170:395–399.

84. White RI, Strandberg JD, Gross JS, et al. Therapeutic embolization with long-term occluding agents and their effects on embolized tissues. *Radiology* 1977;125: 677–687.

85. Matsumoto AH, Suhocki PV, Barth KH. Technical note: Superselective Gelfoam embolotherapy using a highly visible caliber catheter. *Cardiovasc Intervent Radiol* 1988; 11:303–304.

86. Berenstein A, Russell E. Gelatin sponge in therapeutic neuroradiology: A subject review. *Radiology* 1981;141: 105–112.

87. Barth KH, Strandberg JD, White RI. Long-term follow-up of transcatheter embolization with autologous clot, Oxycel and Gelfoam in domestic swine. *Invest Radiol* 1977;12:273–280.

88. Kumar A, Kaufman SI, Patt J, et al. Preoperative embolization of hypervascular head and neck neoplasms using microfibrillar collagen. *AJNR* 1982;3:163–168.

89. Kaufman SL, Strandberg JD, Barth KH, et al. Transcatheter embolization with microfibrillar collagen in the swine. *Invest Radiol* 1978;13:200–204.

90. Daniels JR, Kerland RK, Dodds L, et al. Peripheral hepatic arterial embolization with cross-linked collagen fibers. *Invest Radiol* 1987;22:126–131.

91. Strother CM, Laravuso R, Rappe A, et al. Glutaraldehyde cross-linked collagen (GAX): New material for therapeutic embolization. *AJNR* 1987;8:509–516.

92. Lee DH, Wriedt CH, Kaufmann JCE, et al. Evaluation of three embolic agents in pig rete. *AJNR* 1989;10: 773–776.

93. Lylyk P, Vinuela F, Vinters H, et al. Use of a new mixture for embolization of intracranial vascular malformations: Preliminary experimental experience. *Neuroradiology* 1990;32:304–310.

94. Benati A, Beltramello A, Colombari R, et al. Preoperative embolization of arteriovenous malformations with polylene threads: Techniques with wing microcatheter and pathologic results. *AJNR* 1989;10:579–586.

95. Eskridge JM, Hartling RP. Preoperative embolization of brain AVMs using surgical silk and polyvinyl alcohol (abstract). *AJNR* 1989;10:882.

96. Mehta BA, Sanders WP, Malik G, et al. Detroit cocktail: New embolic agent for embolization of cerebral AVMs (abstract). *AJNR* 1989;10:902.

97. Hilal SK, Michelsen JW. Therapeutic percutaneous embolization for extra-axial vascular lesions of the head, neck and spine. *J Neurosurg* 1975;43:275–287.

98. Cromwell LD, Freeny PC, Kerber CW, et al. Histologic analysis of tissue response to bucrylate-pantopaque mixture. *AJR* 1986;147:627–631.

99. Berenstein A, Hieshima GB. Clinical versus experimental use of isobutyl-2-cyanoacrylate (letter to the editor). *J Neurosurg* 1987;67:318–319.

100. Goldman ML, Philip PK, Sarrafizadeh MS, et al. Transcatheter embolization with bucrylate (in 100 patients). *Radiographics* 1982;2:340–375.

101. Vinuela F, Fox AJ, Debrun G, et al. Pre-embolization superselective angiography: Role in the treatment of brain arteriovenous malformations with isobutyl-2-cyanoacrylate. *AJNR* 1984;5:765–769.

102. Klara PM, George ED, McDonnell D, et al. Morphological studies of human arteriovenous malformation. Effects of isobutyl-2-cyanoacrylate embolization. *J Neurosurg* 1985;63:421–425.

103. Kish KK, Rapp SN, Wilner HI, et al. Histopathologic effects of transarterial bucrylate occlusion of intracerebral arteries in mongrel dogs. *AJNR* 1983;4:385–387.

104. Marck PA, Cummins JE, Galil K, et al. Weak mutagenicity of isobutyl-2-cyanoacrylate tissue adhesive. *J Dent Res* 1982;61:288–292.

105. Brothers MF, Kaufmann JCE, Fox AJ, et al. N-Butyl-2-cranoacrylate: Substitute for IBCA in interventional neuroradiology—histopathologic and polymerization time studies. *AJNR* 1989;10:777–786.

106. Cromwell LD, Kerber CW. Modification of cyanoacrylate for therapeutic embolization: Preliminary experience. *AJR* 1979;132:799–801.

107. Spiegel SM, Vinuela F, Goldwasser MJ, et al. Adjusting polymerization time of isobutyl-2-cyanoacrylate. *AJNR* 1986;7:109–112.

108. Rao VRK, Mandalam KR, Gupta AKM, et al. Dissolution of isobutyl-2-cyanoacrylate on long term follow-up. *AJNR* 1989;10:135–142.

109. Yakes WF, Leulthke JM, Parker SH, et al. Ethanol embolization of vascular malformations. *Radiographics* 1990;10:787–796.

110. Yakes WF, Haas DK, Parker SH, et al. Symptomatic vascular malformations: Ethanol embolotherapy. *Radiology* 1989;170:1059–1066.

111. Ellman BA, Parkhall BJ, Markus PB. Renal ablation with absolute ethanol: Mechanism of action. *Invest Radiol* 1984;19:416–422.

112. Pevsner PH, Klara P, Doppman J, et al. Ethyl alcohol: Experimental agent for interventional therapy of neurovascular lesions. *AJNR* 1983;4:388–390.

113. Choi IS, Berenstein A, Scott J. Use of ethyl alcohol in the treatment of malignant tumors. *AJNR* 1985;6:462.

114. Berenstein A, Choi IS. Treatment of venous angiomas by direct alcohol injection (abstract). *AJNR* 1983; 4:1144.

115. Chow KJ, Williams DM, Brady TM, et al. Transcatheter embolization with sodium tetradecyl sulfate. Experimental and clinical results. *Radiology* 1984;153:95–99.

116. Wright KC, Bowers T, Chuang VP, et al. Experimental evaluation of Ethibloc for non-surgical nephrectomy. *Radiology* 1982;145:339–342.

117. Rohrbach R, Friedburg H. Capillary embolization with Ethibloc: New embolization concept tested in dog kidneys. *AJR* 1981;137:1163–1168.

118. Dubois JM, Sebag GH, De Prost Y, et al. Soft tissue venous malformations in children: Percutaneous sclerotherapy with Ethibloc. *Radiology* 1991;180:195–198.

119. Taki W, Yonekawa Y, Iwata H, et al. A new liquid material for embolization of arteriovenous malformations. *AJNR* 1990;11:163–168.

120. Rao BR, Mandalam RK, Joseph S, et al. Embolization of large saccular aneurysms with Gianturco coils. *Radiology* 1990;175:407–410.

121. Chuang VP, Wallace S, Gianturco C, et al. Complications of coil embolization: Prevention and management. *AJR* 1981;137:809–813.

122. Braun IS, Hoffman JC Jr, Casarella WJ, et al. Use of coils for transcatheter carotid occlusion. *AJNR* 1985;6: 953–956.

123. McLean GK, Stein EJ, Burke DR, et al. Steel occlusion coils: Pretreatment with thrombin. *Radiology* 1986;158: 549–550.

124. Hanner JS, Quisling RG. Transtorcular embolization of vein of Galen aneurysm: Technical aspects. *Radiographics* 1988;8:935–946.

125. Spickler E, Dion JE, Lufkin R, et al. The MR appearance of endovascular embolic agents in vitro with clinical correlation. Computerized medical imaging and graphics. *Comput Med Imag Graph* 1990;14:415–423.

126. Morse SS, Clark RA, Puffenbarger A. Platinum microcoils for therapeutic embolization: Non-neuroradiologic applications. *AJR* 1990;155:401–403.

127. Graves VB, Partington CR, Rufenacht DA, et al. Treatment of carotid artery aneurysms with platinum coils: An experimental study in dogs. *AJNR* 1990;11:249–252.

128. Yang PJ, Halbach VV, Higashida RT, et al. Platinum wire: A new transvascular embolic agent. *AJNR* 1988; 9:547–550.

129. Hilal SK, Khandji AG, Chi TL, et al. Synthetic fiber-coated platinum coils successfully used for endovascular treatment of arteriovenous malformations, aneurysm and direct arteriovenous fistulas of CNS (abstract). *AJNR* 1988;9:1030.

130. Guglielmi G, Vinuela F, Sepetka I, et al. Electrothrombosis of saccular aneurysms via endovascular approach. Part 1: Electrochemical basis technique and experimental results. *J Neurosurg* 1991;75:1–7.

131. Gugliemi G, Vinuela F, Dion JE, et al. Electrothrombosis of saccular aneurysms via endovascular approach. Part 2: Preliminary clinical experience. *J Neurosurg* 1991;75:8–14.

132. Theron J. Angioplasty of brachiocephalic vessels, in Vinuela F, Halbach VV, Dion JE (eds): *Interventional Neuroradiology*. New York, Raven Press, 1992, pp 167–180.

133. Mark MP, Dabe MD, Love B, et al. Stent placement for arterial and venous cerebral disease: Preliminary clinical experience. Presented at the Western Neuroradiology Society annual meeting, 1993, Pasadena, CA.

134. Tsai FY, Nakashima H, Wadley D, et al. IVT atherectomy with suction for treatment of carotid stenosis: Experimental study. *Neuroradiology* 1991;33(Suppl): 63–65.

135. Smith T, Graves VB, Halbach VV et al. Microcatheter retrieval device for intravascular foreign body removal. *AJNR* 1993;14:809–811.

136. Eskridge JM, Newell DW, Pendleton GA. Transluminal angioplasty for treatment of vasospasm. *Neurosurg Clin North Am* 1990;1:2:387–399.

137. Numaguchi Y, Clouston J, Zoarski G, et al. Intraarterial infusion for cerebral vasospasm. Presented at the annual meeting of ASNR, May 1994, Nashville, TN.

138. Choi IS, McAulliffe DJ, de la Torre R, et al. Angioplasty of SAH-induced vasospasm with pulsed dye laser. Presented at the annual meeting of ASNR, May 1994, Nashville, TN.

139. Halbach VV, Dowd CF, Higashida RT, et al. Metallic fragment emboli resulting from treatment with electrolytically detachable coils (GDC). Presented at the annual meeting of ASNR, May 1994, Nashville, TN.

140. Halbach VV, Higashida RT, Dowd CF, et al. Factors that influence the production of metallic fragments during electrolysis of electrolytically detachable coils. Presented at the annual meeting of ASNR, May 1994, Nashville, TN.

141. Gribenko V, Perl J II, Rappe AA, et al. The effect of polyurethane coating on thrombogenicity of the GDC coil: An experimental study in canines. Presented at the annual meeting of ASNR, May 1994, Nashville, TN.

142. Editorial. Angiography: Frequent source of malpractice cases, survey reports. *Radiology Today* 1994;11:5–17.

27

Interventional Therapy for Intracranial Arteriovenous Malformations

Kenneth Fraser, M.D., Randall T. Higashida, M.D., Van V. Halbach, M.D.,
Christopher F. Dowd, M.D., Grant B. Hieshima, M.D.

INTRODUCTION

Interventional treatment of cerebral arteriovenous malformations (AVMs) was introduced by Luessenhop and Spence in 1960.[1] Methyl methacrylate spherical emboli were directly injected into the surgically exposed cervical internal carotid artery. These emboli were carried by flow to the AVM and occluded the feeding arterial pedicles.[2,3] Newton and Adams in 1968 and Doppman in 1971 described transfemoral embolization of spinal cord vascular malformations.[4,5] Hilal et al. in 1970 described embolization of an external carotid artery AVM by a transfemoral approach.[6] In 1972, Kricheff et al. introduced transfemoral catheterization for embolization of intracerebral AVMs.[7] These techniques pioneered the field of interventional therapy of both intracranial and extracranial vascular malformations.

CLASSIFICATION

Vascular malformations have been classified in order to understand their behavior and their propensity to produce neurologic symptoms, as well as to define those patients best suited for treatment.[8–12] The simplest classification is based on the arterial supply to an AVM and is divided into pial, dural, and mixed pial-dural.[13] Other classification systems are based on histological and angiographic characteristics and include arterial, arteriovenous, venous, capillary, and cavernous (cryptic) malformations, capillary telangiectasia, and varix.[10]

An understanding of the hemodynamics, angioarchitecture, and different compartments of an AVM is important for treatment planning. The three components of an AVM are the feeding arteries, the nidus, and the draining veins. The AVM nidus consists of 50- to 2,000-μm-diameter vessels with rudimentary communication of low resistance and high-flow shunting vessels.[4] The arteries directly supplying the AVM are characterized by low intrinsic pressure secondary to the low resistance of the nidus. These arteries lack autoregulation and have inherently poor reactivity to normal vasoactive stimuli.[14–16]

The arteries may have terminal vessels directly connecting with the AVM nidus or may have "en passage" arteries. En passage arteries possess low intravascular pressures, supply the AVM nidus, and nourish normal adjacent brain parenchyma. The intravascular pressure of the en passage vessels progressively decreases with downstream arborization.[17]

Abrupt occlusion of the afferent AVM arteries, by either endovascular or microsurgical methods, may acutely redistribute previously shunted blood to hypoperfused regions supplied by either en passage or adjacent vessels.[18] This abrupt increased pressure may subject previous areas of hypoperfusion to normal perfusion pressure. This may lead to brain edema or hemorrhage due to the inability of these vessels to readapt to the physiological changes. This occurrence has been termed *normal perfusion pressure breakthrough*.[15,19–25]

NATURAL HISTORY

The natural history of cerebral AVMs has been well documented in a number of reports.[26–37] The incidence of a spontaneous intracranial hemorrhage is 2–4% per year.[31,35] Following a hemorrhage, the risk of rehemorrhage in the first year is 6%. A 10–15% mortality is associated with each hemorrhage.[37] Death related to hemorrhage occurs in 29% of patients with cerebral AVMs. Permanent neurological injury ranges between 10% and 15% per episode of hemorrhage.[28]

In terms of location, cerebral AVMs are supratentorial in 90% and infratentorial in 10% of cases. AVMs involving the ependymal and intraventricular regions account for 4–13% of cases.[38–41] In regard to AVM hemodynamics, there are rare case reports of spontaneous thrombosis or regression of AVMs, as well as AVM enlargement.[29,34,42–45]

CLINICAL PRESENTATION

The clinical presentation of AVM patients includes headaches, seizures, vascular steal, and hemorrhage. Headaches may be the only presenting symptom in 16% of patients with an AVM and may be a concomitant complaint with other symptoms in 57%.[46] Headaches related to an AVM often improve and rarely worsen following embolization. A change in the hemodynamics secondary to venous outflow restriction, hemorrhage, thrombosis of cortical veins, and recruitment of the dural arterial supply may alter the symptoms of headache.[3,47–49]

Seizures are the second most common presentation of patients with cerebral AVMs. Seizures related to AVMs are more common in the frontal, temporal, and Rolandic regions. Seizures are usually due to gliosis of the adjacent margins surrounding the AVM, but venous hypertension and arterial steal may also contribute to the underlying pathophysiology.[50] Seizures may be the only manifestation of small peri-AVM hemorrhages.[51] The surgical literature reports a decrease in seizures after resection of AVMs.[52] Berenstein et al. reported his series correlating seizure activity in 257 patients who underwent embolization of their cerebral AVMs.[47] Of these patients, 137 (52%) had documented seizure activity prior to embolization. Ninety-one of these patients (68%) were seizure-free after embolization. The development of new-onset seizures occurred in only 8 of 123 patients (6%).

Symptoms of progressive neurological deficit are usually referable to cerebral vascular steal.[14,19,53–56] The underlying pathophysiology of steal is the existence of high-flow arteriovenous shunts within the AVM which siphon blood from adjacent vascular territories with normal neuronal function. Constantino and Vinters performed an autopsy on a patient after surgical resection of an occipital AVM.[57] They identified diffuse, marked neuronal loss and gliosis in all cell layers in the hippocampus, presumably from vascular steal, which was distant from an occipital AVM but shared the same vascular supply. Other causes of progressive neurological deficit may be venous hypertension from elevated pressures causing edema and mass effect secondary to the enlarged veins on adjacent brain tissue.[58]

Cerebral hemorrhage is the most devastating presentation of patients with a cerebral AVM. Factors that have been identified as increasing the risk of hemorrhage include venous outflow restriction and associated arterial aneurysms. Venous outflow restriction secondary to draining vein stenosis may increase the risk of hemorrhage[59–61] (Fig. 27-1A,B). Viñuela studied 50 patients with deep cerebral AVMs.[58] Seventy-seven percent of these patients presented with an intracranial hemorrhage. The basal vein of Rosenthal provided the dominant venous drainage pattern in all patients with either occlusion or outflow restriction at the level of

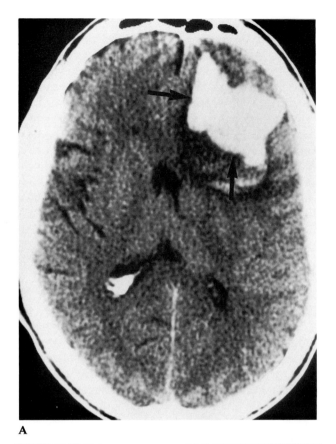

A

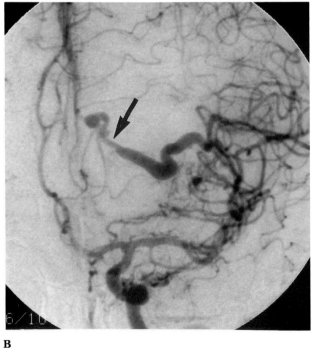

B

Fig. 27-1 (*A*) Large intracerebral hemorrhage (arrows) from a frontal lobe AVM. (*B*) Note the severe cortical venous restriction (arrow) from the vein draining the AVM.

the vein of Galen or straight sinus. Miyasaka et al. also studied the risk of hemorrhage in cerebral AVMs by analyzing venous drainage patterns.[62] In 18 patients with venous outflow restriction, a hemorrhagic rate of 94% was identified. Additional risk factors for hemorrhage were a cerebral AVM that possessed only deep venous drainage or the existence of only a single draining vein.

The association of aneurysms with AVMs has also been extensively studied. An aneurysm can be flow related and can develop on the arterial pedicle supplying the AVM.[47] (Fig. 27-2). Flow-related aneurysms can be subdivided into proximal and distal. Proximal arterial aneurysms are located near the base of the brain in the second-order vessels. Hayashi et al. noted that 77% of aneurysms in patients with AVMs were located with a hemodynamically related feeding artery.[63] In one case, a patient had three aneurysms arising from the anterior cerebral artery supplying a left frontal AMV. Two of these aneurysms were not treated prior to excision of the AVM. This patient was followed with serial angiography in the postoperative period and had documented regression of the two aneurysms over a 6-month period. Lasjaunias et al. reported on the evaluation of 101 patients with cerebral AVMs, of whom 23 had 37 associated arterial aneurysms.[64] Of the 23 patients with associated aneurysms, endovascu-

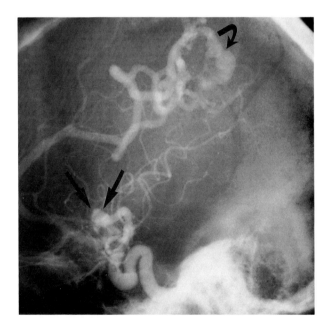

Fig. 27-2 Large flow-related aneurysm (straight arrow) arising from the proximal anterior cerebral artery. The distal anterior cerebral artery supplies a high-flow AVM (curved arrow) in the posterior frontal lobe region.

lar treatment of the cerebral AVM was performed in 16. There were no permanent complications, and treatment of the cerebral AVM resulted in diminution or secondary disappearance of the associated aneurysms.

Distal aneurysms are described as being close to or within the AVM nidus and are usually classified as dysplastic. Intranidus aneurysms or pseudoaneurysms can be identified in 6–23% of AVMs[65] (Fig. 27-3). Pseudoaneurysms were identifed within ruptured AVMs in 8% of 189 patients studied retrospectively by Garcia-Monaco et al.[66] Nine of the pseudoaneurysms were arterial and six were venous. A female predominance (5 : 1) has been noted with remote or dysplastic aneurysms.

There is an increased incidence of associated aneurysms with AVMs in relation to age. In patients less than 25 years of age there is an 8% incidence; between 25 and 50 years there is a 24% incidence; and over 50 years there is a 37% incidence. The neurosurgical literature has cited different approaches for treating patients with cerebral AVMs associated with arterial aneurysms.[63,64,67–72] Yasargil suggests simultaneous treatment of the aneurysm and the AVM.[41] Miyasaka et al. recommend treatment of the aneurysm prior to resection of the AVM.[65] Some reports have documented regression or disappearance of flow-related aneurysms after surgical resection of the AVM.[64] Therefore, a consensus does not exist, and follow-up angiography is necessary to document the course of any associated aneurysm with an AVM following treatment.

INDICATIONS FOR TREATMENT

The selection of patients for treatment depends on a number of factors, including the initial presentation; current neurological status; age of the patient; size, site, and angioarchitecture of the AVM with its associated risk factors; and the desires of the patient and family. The major current indications for endovascular treatment include preoperative embolization prior to definitive surgical resection or radiosurgery, and palliation of progressive neurological symptoms and/or refractory seizures, severe headaches, and hemorrhage.[27,47,52,54,73–84]

In planning for preoperative interventional therapy, deep or surgically difficult arterial pedicles to an AVM are usually treated first. Superficial branches and those easily accessible by surgery may not require preoperative occlusion. However, if the draining veins of the AVM overlie the surgical access to the nidus, embolization may be warranted. If the AVM is large, staged embolization in several sessions is indicated to decrease the risk of intraoperative or periembolization hyperemic complications.[79,80,83,85,86] Staged embolization to gradually redistribute previously shunted blood to the normal adjacent brain is safer in these cases. If there is a single draining vein, staged embolization may be necessary to avoid sudden stasis of flow within the vein, which may lead to thrombosis, resulting in hemorrhage.

A cerebral AVM in an eloquent location, or one which is considered too large for surgical resection, may also be treated by embolization. Reduction of the size of the nidus can change the surgical classification and allow reevaluation for subsequent surgery or radiosurgery.

The treatment of cerebral AVMs during pregnancy has been controversial.[87–91] Debate exists as to whether pregnant patients are at increased risk for hemorrhage

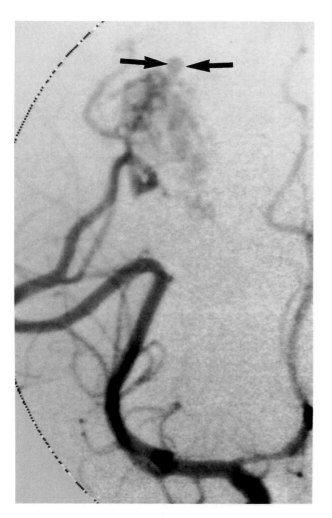

Fig. 27-3 Large intranidus aneurysm within an AVM (arrows). These aneurysms are frequently associated with the site of hemorrhage.

during pregnancy and delivery. Yasargil and Berenstein have not found an increase of hemorrhage in pregnant patients with AVMs.[41,47]

EMBOLIZATION MATERIALS

The ideal embolic agent should be easily controlled during injection, safe to adjacent tissues, radiopaque, permanent, nonbiodegradable, and easily manipulated during operative excision.[92] Multiple agents have been utilized, including liquid adhesives (isobutyl cyanoacrylate [IBCA]; normobutyl cyanoacrylate [NBCA]), silk suture, polyvinyl alcohol foam particles (PVA or Ivalon), microfibrillar collagen (Avitene), platinum coils, detachable latex and silicone balloons, and alcohol.

Particulate agents, such as PVA, are available in a variety of sizes ranging from 100 to 1000 μm and can be individually cut into small pledgets from an Ivalon block to be delivered through a microcatheter[47,93–98] (Fig. 27-4A,B). Selection of particle size is based on the size of the shunts within the AVM. Optimally, the embolic material should penetrate the nidus without passing through the AVM and going into the venous circulation. PVA provides occlusion of the arterial pedicle by adhesion to the wall of the vessel, with subsequent angionecrosis.[93,99] The disadvantage of using PVA is the lack of passage of some of the particles into the AVM nidus. In addition, PVA is not radiopaque, and it recanalizes over several days to weeks. Therefore, PVA is usually utilized for embolization prior to definitive surgical resection. Following embolization, surgery should be performed within 2 to 3 weeks to avoid recanalization or recruitment of collateral vessels, which can make the surgery more difficult. Viñuela et al. have reported on the rapid recruitment of transdural, leptomeningeal, and transmedullary collateral arteries by an AVM if timely surgery is not performed following embolization therapy.[100]

Silk suture for intravascular embolization is also being used as an embolic material.[101] Surgical silk (4-0 to 6-0) of various lengths can be injected through the microcatheter. Silk is highly thrombogenic and induces an intense foreign body reaction in the feeding pedicle, which may produce a postprocedural fever with leukocytosis. Silk suture can be used alone or in combination with other embolic agents. It is often used to close large fistulas associated with cerebral AVMs in combination with other agents, such as platinum microcoils and PVA. A major disadvantage of this material is that it is nonradiopaque.[102]

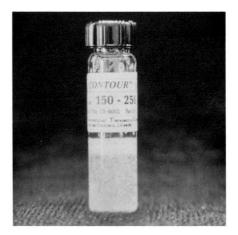

A

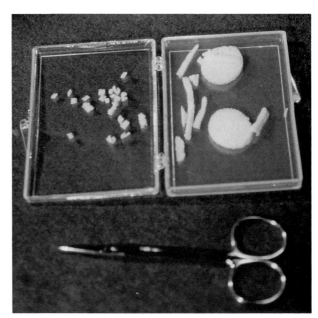

B

Fig. 27-4 (*A*) Polyvinyl alcohol foam particles, which are available in specific sizes ranging from 100 to 1,000 μm. (*B*) Larger sheets of polyvinyl alcohol foam sponges are available and can be cut into larger-diameter pieces to occlude larger shunt lesions.

Liquid adhesive agents utilized in embolization of cerebral AVMs include isobutyl 2-cyanoacrylate (IBCA) and normobutyl-cyanoacrylate (NBCA)[103–108] (Fig. 27-5). Berenstein and Lasjaunias have advocated the use of liquid tissue adhesives, with the goal of permanent cure without operative resection for certain AVMs. The safe use of NBCA requires extensive experience and training due to the rapid polymerization time, which can result in significant morbidity if improperly

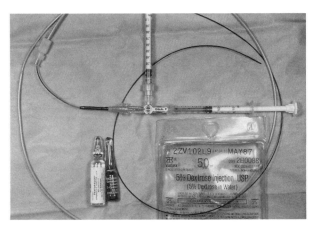

Fig. 27-5 Liquid tissue adhesive cyanoacrylates are available as liquid embolization agents. The cyanoacrylates need to be used in conjunction with a material to allow opacity and flushed with a nonionic material such as D5W prior to injection.

injected. NBCA polymerizes on contact with an ionic solution. Polymerization time of the adhesive is adjusted by the ratio of NBCA to pantopaque (Ethiodol) or glacial acetic acid[109] (Fig. 27-6A–C). Ethiodol provides radiopacity for visualization during injection and decreases the polymerization time. Tantalum powder may also be added to the mixture to improve radiopacity. The major risks of liquid adhesive agents are premature polymerization of the glue, causing adhesion of the delivery catheter; reflux of glue into normal proximal arteries; delayed polymerization with passage of the glue through the nidus, with subsequent occlusion of the venous drainage; and nontargeted embolization of small normal vessels below the visual resolution of fluoroscopy. The liquid tissue adhesives, although longer-lasting than polyvinyl alcohol particles, may also recanalize. Rao et al. reported on 8 patients with large intracerebral AVMs incompletely embolized with IBCA in 17 patients.[110] Follow-up plain film and angiographic studies identified resorption of the glue cast and reconstitution of the AVM 6–20 months postembolization. Other reports have also demonstrated recanalization of IBCA in intracerebral AVMs.[100,111]

Platinum microcoils can be delivered through microcatheters; may be thrombogenic, depending on their coating; are magnetic resonance imaging (MRI) compatible; and are available in a variety of shapes, lengths, and sizes[96,112] (Fig. 27-7). These coils can be placed by controlled delivery or may be injected. Inadvertently placed coils may be retrieved with the newer microsnare devices in the larger proximal arteries.[113,114] In

some cases, occlusion of proximal flow-related aneurysms can be accomplished with electrolytic platinum coils prior to embolization of an AVM.[115,116]

The liquid, nonadhesive embolic agent ethylene vinyl alcohol copolymer (EVAL) can be injected through microcatheters; it forms an elastic cast within the nidus and feeding arterial pedicle. It polymerizes on contact with blood. The advantages are its nonadhesive properties and its lack of an inflammatory reaction within the vessel. This method is being used in Japan but is not currently approved in the United States.[117]

Ethyl alcohol is also being investigated for embolization of cerebral AVMs. Pevsner et al. used absolute alcohol to experimentally occlude cerebral arteries in six rhesus monkeys.[118] They demonstrated thrombosis of the middle cerebral artery, which was injected with 0.2 ml of absolute ethyl alcohol within 2 cm of the catheter tip. Until further investigation is performed with this agent, it is not recommended for use in the intracranial vasculature.

RADIOLOGICAL IMAGING

Computed tomography (CT) and magnetic resonance imaging (MRI) can provide information regarding location, size, shape, mass effect, associated edema, and identification of prior hemorrhage of an AVM (Fig. 27-8A–C). Kumar et al. studied 60 patients with unruptured cerebral AVMs with high-resolution CT scans. Thirty-three patients demonstrated edema with mass effect and compression, displacement, and distortion of adjacent anatomical structures.[119] CT is optimal in patients suspected of having acute hemorrhage, intubated patients, and patients who are claustrophobic. However, Batjer et al. reported only 8 of 23 patients (35%) with posterior fossa AVMs and clinical symptoms of hemorrhage who had blood identified by CT.[120] Thus, with a high clinical suspicion of a bleed, lumbar puncture should be performed for examination of the cerebrospinal fluid if the CT scan is negative.

MRI is useful for identifying the three-dimensional anatomical relationships for optimal surgical therapy and for identifying prior hemorrhage.[121–123] Yousem et al. studied 29 patients with cerebral AVMs by MRI.[124] Twenty patients (69%) demonstrated MRI evidence of acute hemorrhage; 4 (14%) demonstrated evidence of remote hemorrhage but raised no clinical suspicion of a prior intracranial bleed; and 6 (21%) had a clinical history consistent with previous hemorrhage, without MRI findings correlating with a bleed.

Cerebral angiography is required for pretreatment

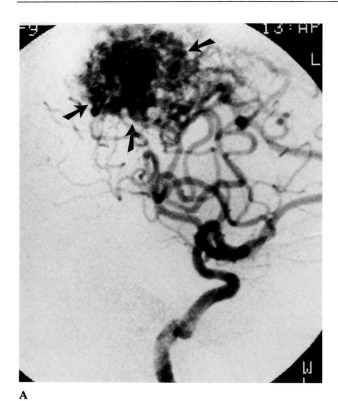

A

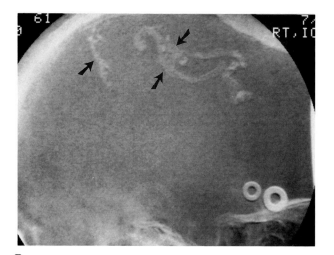

B

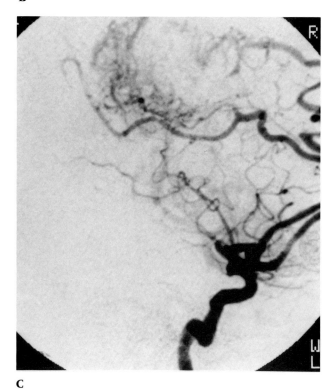

C

Fig. 27-6 (*A*) Large frontal AVM in a patient presenting with vascular steal symptoms, intractable seizures, and progressive hemiparesis. (*B*) Following selective catheterization of the anterior cerebral artery feeders and embolization with cyanoacrylate, a cast of the AVM nidus could be visualized. (*C*) Postembolization arteriogram demonstrating a marked decrease in flow to the AVM.

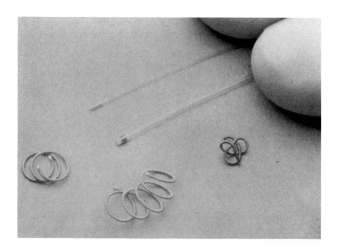

Fig. 27-7 Platinum microcoils with diameters of 0.015 and 0.010 in. are available in a wide variety of shapes and sizes for neurovascular embolization.

evaluation (Fig. 27-9). High-speed film acquisition during the arterial phase, and an extended period of filming to assess deep and superficial cortical drainage patterns, should be utilized. Rapid filming is recommended to identify associated arterial aneurysms, intranidus aneurysms, and arteriovenous shunts. Evaluation of the draining veins identifies risk factors for hemorrhage such as venous outflow restriction, venous aneurysms, venous drainage patterns, and the number and location of venous outflow pedicles in anatomical

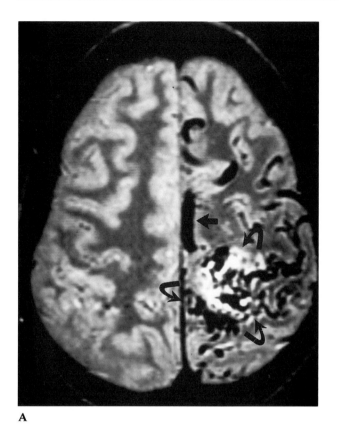

A

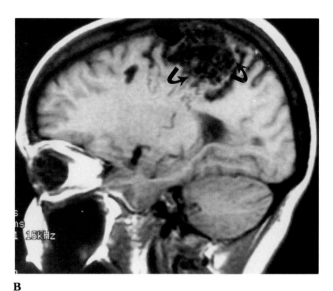

B

Fig. 27-8 MRI scans in the axial (*A*) and sagittal (*B*) planes are extremely useful to define the AVM nidus (curved arrows), draining veins (straight arrow), and relationship of the AVM to adjacent normal cortical structures.

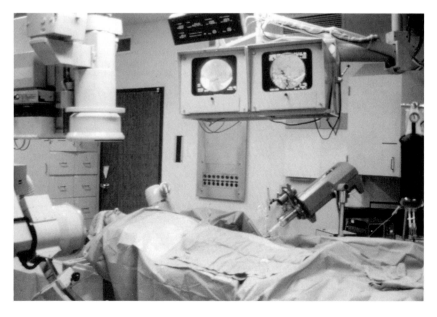

Fig. 27-9 Interventional neurovascular angiography suite where embolization procedures are performed. Ideally, a bi-plane room with high-resolution, rapid-filming, digital subtraction angiography capability should be available for these procedures.

relationship to arterial pedicles for determining the operative approach.[58,62,125]

FUNCTIONAL TESTING

Functional testing prior to embolization should be performed in the vessel to be treated.[126,127] The original test, described by Wada and Rassmussen in 1960, utilized sodium amytal injected into the internal carotid artery for evaluation of lateralization of speech prior to surgical procedures within the brain.[128] Rauch et al. in 1992 reported their experience with 109 superselective amytal tests performed in 33 patients undergoing preoperative staged embolization of AVMs prior to surgical removal.[129,130] The use of 30-mg injections of amytal was correlated with clinical and EEG monitoring (Fig. 27-10). Of the 23 positive amytal tests, only 12 (52%) demonstrated a positive clinical deficit; the remainder had abnormal EEG findings. Three of the positive amytal tests did not demonstrtate any changes with EEG monitoring. Rauch et al. also reported a 10% neurological complication rate in 147 embolizations in 30 patients despite amytal testing. They concluded that the repeated use of amytal testing with serial embolization could reduce unanticipated neurological deficits. When a high-flow arteriovenous shunt exists within the pedicle being treated, repeated amytal testing should be performed when there is visible slowing of the shunt angiographically. Newton and Cronquist reported on involvement of the dural arteries with intracranial AVMs.[13] If collateral or recruitment of the dural or leptomeningeal-pial arterial supply from external carotid branches is identified, amytal should be used to check neurological function prior to embolization therapy[131] (Fig. 27-11).

Recently, the use of a shorter-acting barbiturate, sodium methohexital (Brevital), has been described for intra-arterial testing. Peters et al. reported on 30 patients having 66 vascular pedicles with cerebral AVMs undergoing preoperative embolization.[132] When patients were injected with 1–6 mg of a 1% Brevital solution, altered neurological function identified functional territories of the vascular pedicle, with clearing of the transient deficit within 2 min in all patients. None of the patients experienced seizures or permanent deficits associated with the Brevital injection. Brevital must be used in a concentration of 1%, since higher concentrations may induce vasospasm, vascular necrosis, and possibly permanent deficits.

Other techniques involving functional evaluation include on-line or Fourier-transformed EEG analysis, somatosensory-evoked potentials, and brain stem acoustic-evoked potentials.[133] These additional monitoring techniques are especially useful in patients under general anesthesia.

The arterial pedicles which supply high-flow AVMs possess lower pressures, by 40–80 mm Hg, compared to systemic arterial pressures.[17] Measurement of intravascular pressures by microcatheters may provide clues to dynamic pressure changes occurring during the embolization procedure.[134] Duckwiler et al. demonstrated the feasibility of measuring the mean intravascular pressures with several microcatheters, compared to the larger guiding catheters, measured in experimental animals, as well as in two patients undergoing intracranial embolization.[135]

ANATOMICAL CONSIDERATIONS

Prior to performing embolization and occlusion of the arterial supply to an AVM, the anatomical and functional anatomy should be thoroughly understood. It is important to perform a complete baseline neurological

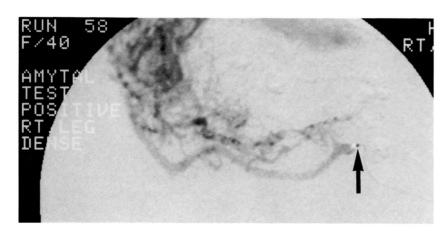

Fig. 27-10 Superselective amytal testing of the distal pericallosal artery. Note the tip of the microcatheter (arrow) in relation to the AVM. Injection of amytal from this position produced a dense paresis in the right leg. Therefore, this vessel cannot be safely embolized from this location.

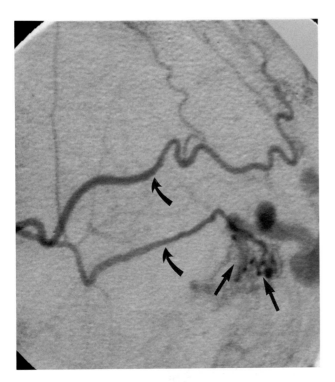

Fig. 27-11 Enlarged branches of the middle meningeal artery (curved arrows), arising from the external carotid artery, that supply a frontal lobe AVM (straight arrows).

examination. Following selective catheterization of the arterial vessels to be treated, functional testing with pharmacological agents should be performed, and a focused neurological examination of the area to be treated should be performed to detect gross and subtle deficits.

Occipital Lobe and Visual Pathway

Occipital lobe AVMs derive their arterial supply mainly from the posterior cerebral artery and occasionally may recruit transmastoid perforating branches of the occipital artery.[136,137] The posterior cerebral artery divides at the P3 segment into the parieto-occipital artery, the calcarine artery, and the posterior temporal artery, in a superior-to-inferior relationship in the lateral projection. The calcarine artery supplies the occipital pole visual cortex in a variety of anatomical combinations, and can divide into branches supplying the superior and/or inferior striate cortex. Occipital branches of the middle cerebral artery may also provide collateral leptomeningeal anastomoses with the occipital cortex.[46]

The terminal branches of the posterior cerebral artery supply the medial surface of the inferior temporal lobe, the occipital lobe visual cortex, and the splenium of the

corpus callosum (Fig. 27-12A–C). Therefore, patients with an occipital lobe AVM involving the posterior cerebral artery should be evaluated for contralateral homonymous hemianopsia prior to embolization. The arterial supply to the splenium should be tested for alexia, since occlusion can result in disruption of the connection between the primary visual cortex of the nondominant hemisphere and the language areas of the dominant hemisphere.[138]

Supratentorial AVMs within the temporal or parietal lobes can disrupt the optic radiation, resulting in a complete or partial incongruous homonymous defect. The middle cerebral artery supplies the deep white matter tracts of the temporal and parietal lobes. The posterior temporal artery supplies the visual radiation of the geniculocalcarine tracts. It is divided into an upper optic radiation in the parietal white matter and a lower optic radiation in the temporal white matter. The visual disturbance is worse in the upper quadratic field when Meyer's loop is affected in the temporal white matter. Visual disturbance is greater in the lower quadratic field with the involvement of the parietal white matter.

Other branches of the middle cerebral artery can affect visual pathways directly or indirectly. The posterior parietal artery and angular artery should be tested for contralateral hemianopsia, as well as for mild sensory deficits such as visual and verbal aphasia and agraphia in the dominant hemisphere. The anterior parietal artery should be tested for contralateral astereognosis.

Temporal Lobe

Temporal lobe AVMs are generally supplied by branches of the middle and posterior cerebral arteries. Mesial temporal AVMs may also derive their arterial supply from the anterior choroidal artery. Inferior and posterior temporal lobe AVMs may receive their supply from temporal branches of the posterior cerebral artery, as well as from the middle cerebral artery. The posterior temporal artery should be tested for hemianopsia, as well as auditory receptive aphasia (Wernicke's) in the dominant hemisphere if the superior temporal gyrus is involved.

Frontal Lobe

Frontal lobe AVMs can be divided into inferior, posterior, and lateral. Inferior frontal lobe AVMs often are supplied by the M1 and M2 branches of the middle cerebral artery and the A1 and A2 branches of the anterior cerebral artery. If the AVM is near the orbital region, ethmoidal and anterior falcine branches of the

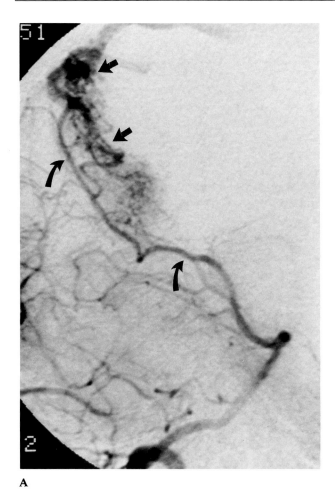

A

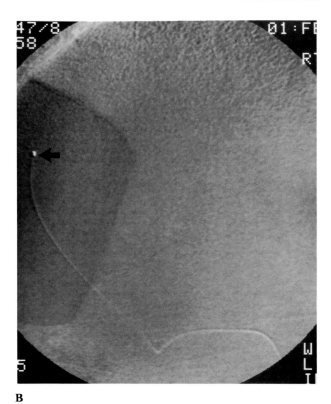

B

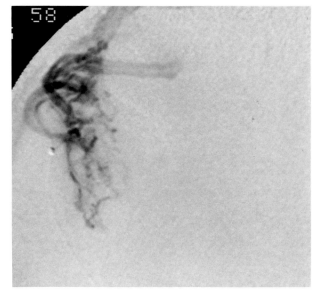

C

Fig. 27-12 (*A*) Posterior parietal-occipital AVM (straight arrows) supplied by the distal posterior cerebral artery (curved arrows). (*B*) Selective catheterization of the distal posterior cerebral artery with the microcatheter at the nidus (arrow). (*C*) Selective injection demonstrates only nidus filling, without normal branches. Embolization was performed preoperatively with polyvinyl alcohol particles.

ophthalmic artery can be recruited. Lateral frontal lobe AVMs are primarily supplied by cortical branches from the middle cerebral artery.[47]

The callosomarginal arterial branches supply the central Rolandic sulcus with branches to the precentral gyrus motor area. Posterior frontal AVMs are supplied by middle cerebral artery branches including the lenticulostriate arteries. The primary motor cortex of the posterior frontal lobe receives blood supply from branches of the middle and anterior cerebral arteries. The anterior cerebral artery branch to the central sulcus, the Rolandic artery, supplies the precentral, postcentral, and adjacent gyri. Over the convexity, the cen-

tral sulcus artery anastomoses with middle cerebral artery branches at the upper third of the convexity. These anterior cerebral artery branches to the superior margin of the convexity, including the superior frontal gyrus and parts of the pre- and postcentral gyri, provide vascular supply for primary motor and sensory areas of the contralateral leg. Fox et al. presented three patients undergoing embolization for large Rolandic AVMs.[139] All three patients had significant reversal of progressive neurological deficits with respect to limb function after embolization therapy. The improvement was attributed to the reduction of vascular steal from the precentral gyrus.

In 95% of right-handed and 70% of left-handed persons, the left cerebral hemisphere is the center of speech and language. Occlusion of the left main trunk or upper division of the middle cerebral artery results in global dysfunction of language, as well as other deficits.[104]

The right cerebral hemisphere is usually the non-dominant side supplied by the right middle cerebral artery. The right hemisphere is dominant for different aspects of attention such as directed, focused, and vigilant attention. Deficits secondary to right middle cerebral artery occlusion include inattention secondary to neglect, extinction, and impersistence (Fig. 27-13A–C).

Broca's Area

Broca's area resides within the dominant hemisphere operculum of the inferior frontal gyrus of the frontal lobe, anterior to the primary motor and premotor cortices. The primary arterial supply to this region is from the prefrontal arterial branches of the anterior or upper division of the middle cerebral artery. The operculofrontal branches supply the inferior and middle frontal gyri which represent Broca's and the premotor areas. Testing of the orbitofrontal and precentral arteries should evaluate the patient's ability for paresis of the contralateral face and tongue in the dominant hemisphere. Broca's (motor) aphasia is a consequence of occlusion of the main trunk or branches of the upper division[47,64] of the middle cerebral artery.

Wernicke's Area

Wernicke's area is related to the caudal portion of the superior temporal gyrus between the angular gyrus and the primary auditory cortex. This area is primarily in the vascular distribution of the posterior temporal artery, a branch of the middle cerebral artery. Wernicke's (sensory) aphasia may be a consequence of occlusion of the posterior temporal artery or lower division branches of the middle cerebral artery.

Anterior Choroidal Artery

AVMs with supply from the anterior choroidal artery require special consideration. Cerebral AVMs of the temporal and parietal lobes, basal ganglia, internal cap-

sule, and vessels closely associated with the lateral ventricle can recruit supply from the anterior choroidal artery. Surgical resection of AVMs with supply from the anterior choroidal artery are difficult to treat.[141]

The anterior choroidal artery usually arises from the posteromedial aspect of the internal carotid artery, distal to the posterior communicating artery. It can also arise directly from the posterior communicating artery, the middle cerebral artery, or the terminal internal carotid bifurcation.[142]

Functionally, the anterior choroidal artery supplies the optic tract, optic radiation, lateral geniculate body, part of the lateral thalamus, subthalamus, medial globus pallidus, tail of the caudate nucleus, middle third of the cerebral peduncles of the midbrain, substantia nigra, posterior limb of the internal capsule, portions of the medial temporal lobe including the amygdala, uncus and pyriform cortex, as well as the choroid plexus of the inferior aspect of the temporal horn and the atrium of the lateral ventricle. There may be collateral blood flow from the lateral posterior choroidal artery, posterior communicating artery, and posterior cerebral artery to this vascular distribution.

Functional testing should always be performed with close attention to contralateral motor strength, contralateral sensory acuity, visual fields, and memory. During embolization of the anterior choroidal artery, it is important to place the tip of the catheter beyond the plexal point. The plexal point is where the artery enters the choroidal fissure to supply the choroid plexus of the temporal horn. Proximal occlusion of the plexal point may result in the triad of hemiplegia, homonymous hemianopsia, and hemianesthesia.

Retrograde thrombosis of the anterior choroidal artery may also occur if the arterial flow is taken to complete stasis. Dowd et al. reported significant reduction of blood flow in 14 of 15 patients with cerebral AVMs supplied by the anterior choroidal artery using particulate embolization.[143] One permanent and three transient neurological deficits occurred in the 15 patients. Hodes et al. reported on six patients with temporal lobe AVMs who underwent selective embolization of the anterior choroidal artery.[144] One of these patients (16.7%) developed fixed neurological deficits during selective embolization of the anterior choroidal artery using liquid tissue adhesives.

INFRATENTORIAL AVMs

Infratentorial AVMs account for 10–25% of intracranial AVMs. Posterior fossa AVMs are predominantly located in the cerebellum (71–86%), cerebellum and

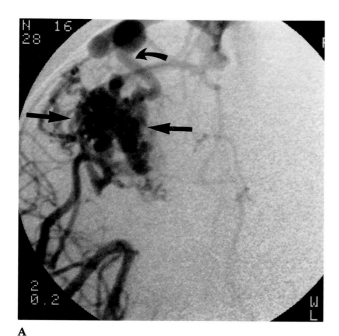

A

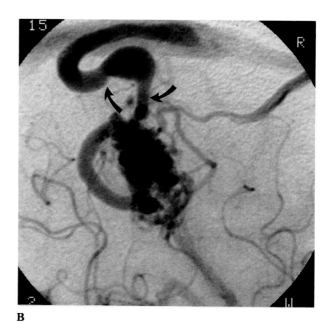

B

Fig. 27-13 (*A*) Large midfrontal AVM (straight arrows), frontal view, supplied by branches of both the anterior and middle cerebral arteries. There is evidence of venous restriction (curved arrow). (*B*) The lateral view clearly demonstrates evidence of venous outflow restriction (curved arrows). Notice the sudden change in caliber of the draining veins. (*C*) Following selective catheterization and embolization of both the anterior and middle cerebral artery branches to the AVM (arrows), there is more than a 90% reduction in filling.

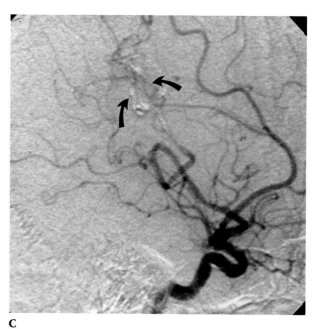

C

brain stem (< 30%), and brain stem alone (5–14%).[145] The clinical presentation is usually secondary to hemorrhage since seizures are rare in this location. Brain stem AVMs present more commonly with neurological symptoms because of their eloquent location. Hemorrhage is higher with infratentorial versus supratentorial AVMs, with an incidence of 72–92%. This may be due to the presentation rather than the true incidence, since infratentorial AVMs are less likely to present with other symptoms.[120,146,147]

Embolization of infratentorial versus supratentorial AVMs is technically more difficult. The effect of hemorrhage or acute thrombosis of draining veins in this area can compromise vital control centers of respiration, consciousness, limb function, and control of ocular movements. Occlusion and ischemia in the region of the pons, medulla, midbrain, cerebellum, and posterior cerebral artery which supplies the visual cortex is particularly hazardous. Neurological deficits which can occur with unilateral lesions in the cerebellar cortex in-

clude ipsilateral ataxia, atonia, and intention tremor. Ischemia involving the cerebellar peduncles can result in disabling ataxia and intention tremor. If the flocculonodular region is injured, disorders of equilibrium and nystagmus will occur.[120,147]

Arterial supply to infratentorial AVMs is via the posterior circulation, except in rare fetal persistence from the anterior circulation. AVMs around the tentorium are predominantly supplied by the superior cerebellar artery, with additional branches from the posterior choroidal arteries. Cerebellar AVMs are supplied by branches from the superior, anterior inferior, and/or posterior inferior cerebellar arteries.

The superior cerebellar artery (SCA) is the most common artery supplying cerebellar AVMs. The SCA supplies the superior aspect of the cerebellum, including the cerebellar nuclei, the superior and middle cerebellar peduncles, and the lateral tegmentum of the pons and midbrain. Occlusion or ischemia of this artery can result in ipsilateral cerebellar asynergy with hypotonus, involuntary choreiform or choreoathetoid movements, and ipsilateral Horner's syndrome. Contralateral loss of sensation of pain and temperature on the face and trunk, central facial palsy, and partial deafness can result from occlusion of the branches supplying the spinothalamic tract and the secondary ascending tract of the fifth cranial nerve, which is also supplied by the SCA.

The anterior inferior cerebellar artery (AICA) supplies parts of the cerebellum, the lower and middle cerebellar peduncles, the flocculus, and the inferior surface of the cerebellum. The lower pons and upper medullary lateral tegmentum are also supplied by branches of the AICA. In 85% of patients, the inner ear and acoustic nerve are supplied by a branch of the AICA, the artery to the internal auditory canal.[142] Occlusion of the AICA can result in ipsilateral cerebellar asynergy, loss of pain and temperature, diminished light touch of the face, and Horner's syndrome, with peripheral facial palsy and deafness. Incomplete contralateral limb and trunk loss of pain and temperature can also occur.

The posterior inferior cerebellar artery (PICA) supplies the inferior cerebellar peduncle, the inferior surface of the cerebellum, and the dorsolateral tegmentum of the medulla. Occlusion can result in injury to the nucleus ambiguus with emerging fibers to the ninth and tenth cranial nerves, descending tract and nucleus of the fifth nerve, descending sympathetic pathways, inferior cerebellar peduncle, afferent spinocerebellar tracts, and lateral spinothalamic tracts. Clinically, this results in a lateral medullary or Wallenberg's syndrome, with ipsilateral paralysis of the soft palate, pharynx, and larynx, resulting in dysphonia and dysphagia, ipsilateral anesthesia of pain and temperature on the face, depression of the corneal reflex, ipsilateral Horner's syndrome, cerebellar asynergy, and hypotonus ipsilateral to the lesion, with contralateral trunk and extremity loss of pain and temperature. Dysfunction of the sixth, seventh, and eighth cranial nerves may also occur.[147]

Fox et al. reported the results of endovascular treatment of 38 patients with intracranial AVMs.[139] Five of these patients had cerebellar AVMs and one had a midbrain AVM. All patients were embolized with IBCA, with moderate obliteration of the nidus. Two patients suffered complications. One patient with a vermian cerebellar AVM had worsening of her preoperative deficit. The other patient with a large vermian cerebellar AVM developed mild ataxia after treatment. Of the other four patients, only one underwent complete surgical resection. None of these patients developed postembolization neurological deficits.

INTRAOPERATIVE EMBOLIZATION AND ANGIOGRAPHY

Intraoperative embolization began before transfemoral techniques were well established. Intraoperative embolization was previously performed due to difficulty in catheterizing the supplying arterial pedicles from the transfemoral route. Current improvements in guiding and microcatheters, micro-guidewires, and embolization materials have largely eliminated the use of intraoperative embolization.

Intraoperative angiography, however, is being performed with increasing frequency following surgical resection of an AVM to ensure complete excision and to help localize the exact site of the nidus during the surgical exposure.[148,149] Prior to the craniotomy, a sheath is placed into the common femoral artery. The patient should be placed in a radiolucent head frame, and on a radiolucent operating room table, to allow adequate visualization of the area of interest. A portable fluoroscopic unit with rapid-sequence filming and digital subtraction angiography should be used.

EMBOLIZATION AND RADIATION THERAPY

The results of conventional radiation therapy of cerebral AVMs has been poor. Redekop et al. reported on a series of 15 patients with cerebral AVMs, measuring 1.5–6.5 cm, treated with 4,000–5,000 cGy delivered in 15–28 fractions, with conventional radiation therapy.[150] These patients were followed for a mean of 8.1 years (range, 1.5–21 years) and had a hemorrhage rate of 3.3% per year. The angiographic cure rate in this group was only 20%. Due to these poor results, other forms of radiosurgery were developed, focusing on the nidus and deemphasizing the nontargeted areas. These methods included a multisource cobalt-60 gamma unit, Bragg ionization peak proton beams, heavy-charged-particle Bragg peak radiation, and modified linear accelerator methods.[76,151–153]

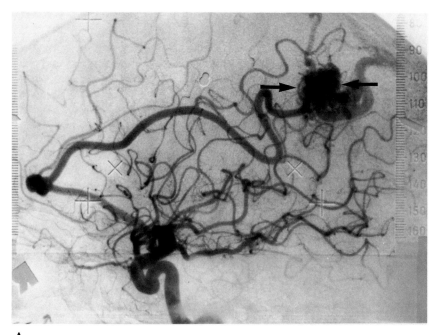

A

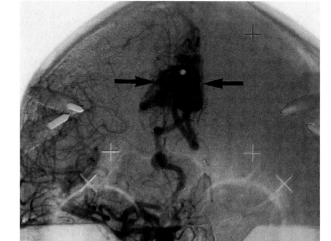

B

Fig. 27-14 (A) Focal, compact AVM (arrows); lateral view, located adjacent to the motor cortex. These lesions near eloquent territories can be effectively treated by stereotactic radiation therapy. (B) Frontal view of the AVM demonstrating supply predominantly by the pericallosal artery and its branches.

The factors used to evaluate patients for radiation therapy include the size, volume, and location of the AVM; previous hemorrhage; feeding arterial aneurysms; intranidus aneurysms; venous outflow restriction; and age of the patient. A period of 24–36 months is usually required to induce thrombosis and occlusion of an AVM using radiation therapy (Fig. 27-14A,B).

In patients with increased risk factors for bleeding, such as intranidus or feeding artery aneurysms, embolization to occlude these aneurysms may need to be performed prior to radiation treatment. The dural supply to an AVM should also be embolized, since recruitment by these vessels may occur after radiosurgery of the pial vascularity. For large AVMs, embolization using permanent embolic agents to decrease the size and volume may be performed to increase the effectiveness of radiation therapy. Resorbable embolic materials should not be used since recanalization or recruitment may occur, leading to recanalization of the AVM by areas outside of the targeted focus of radiation.[154,155]

Embolization may also be used in cases where radiation therapy has failed. Marks et al. reported on five of six patients who underwent radiation therapy, had residual AVM nidus, and then underwent embolization therapy. There was a mean decrease in AVM volume by 74% following embolization. Three of these patients subsequently underwent surgical cure, one was cured by embolization alone, and the other two underwent a second course of radiotherapy.[156]

POTENTIAL COMPLICATIONS

The risk of iatrogenic stroke or hemorrhage from embolization of cerebral AVMs is approximately 5%, with a permanent neurological deficit occurring in approximately 2% in one large reported series.[46] The recognition and immediate correction of complications can mean the difference between a mild versus a severe neurological deficit or death.[157]

Hemorrhage may occur during or after the procedure and can be due to perforation of a vascular pedicle during manipulation of the guidewire or microcatheter. It may also occur from changing hemodynamic flow patterns, normal perfusion pressure breakthrough, or occlusive hyperemia following embolization of an AVM. Postembolization occlusive hyperemia usually occurs in larger AVMs with high flow, due to thrombosis or a sudden increase in the pressure of the draining veins.[158]

Arterial injury, including perforation and vasospasm, may occur to vessels supplying the AVM due to the underlying high-flow arteriopathic changes already existing within the arterial wall.[17,159,160] Vascular perforations during the procedure require expedient treatment. Halbach et al. described 15 vascular perforations occurring during 1,200 endovascular procedures.[161] Treatment included immediate reversal of anticoagulation, placement of coils across the perforation site, temporary inflation of a balloon across the perforation, and immediate institution of medical therapy, including protamine sulfate to reverse the effects of heparin, anticonvulsants, and steroids if necessary.[162] Arterial vasospasm may occur during catheter manipulation if the embolization is performed relatively early after a hemorrhage. Thrombosis secondary to spasm, with proximal occlusion of normal vessels, can result in stroke. Prophylactic medications to decrease the incidence of spasm include nifedipine and nitropaste.[163-166]

CONCLUSION

Neurointerventional therapy for the treatment of cerebral AVMs requires extensive training and experience. A close working relationship with the neurosurgeon, radiation therapist, neurologist, and neurological intensive care unit is required. As advances are made in delivery systems, embolic materials, anatomical imaging, and functional testing, overall patient therapy and outcome will continue to improve.

REFERENCES

1. Luessenhop AJ, Spence WT. Artificial embolization of cerebral arteries. Report of use in a case of arteriovenous malformation. *JAMA* 1960;172:1153–1155.
2. Wolpert SM, Stein BM. Factors governing the course of emboli in the therapeutic embolization of cerebral arteriovenous malformations. *Radiology* 1979;131:125–131.
3. Wolpert SM, Barnett FJ, Prager RJ. Benefits of embolization without surgery for cerebral arteriovenous malformations. *AJNR* 1981;2:535–541.
4. Doppman J. The nidus concept of spinal cord arteriovenous malformations. A surgical recommendation based upon angiographic observations. *Br J Radiol* 1971;44:758–763.
5. Newton TH, Adams JE. Angiographic demonstration and nonsurgical embolization of spinal cord angiomas. *Radiology* 1968;91:873–876.
6. Hilal S, Mount L, Correll J, et al. Therapeutic embolization of vascular malformation of the external carotid circulation: Clinical and experimental results. IX Symposium Neuroradiologicum, Göteberg, Sweden, Aug 24–29, 1970.
7. Kricheff II, Madayag M, Braunstein P. Transfemoral catheter embolization of cerebral and posterior fossa arteriovenous malformations. *Radiology* 1972;103:107–111.
8. Luessenhop AJ. AVM grading in assessing surgical risk. *J Neurosurg* 1987;66:637–642.
9. Luessenhop AJ, Gennarelli TA. Anatomical grading of supratentorial arteriovenous malformations for determining operability. *Neurosurgery* 1977;1:30–35.
10. McCormick WF. The pathology of vascular (arteriovenous) malformations. *J Neurosurg* 1966;24:807–816.
11. Pasqualin A, Barone G, Cioffi F, et al. The relevance of anatomic and hemodynamic factors to a classification of cerebral arteriovenous malformations. *Neurosurgery* 1991;28:370–379.
12. Spetzler RF, Martin NA. A proposed grading system for arteriovenous malformations. *J Neurosurg* 1986;65:476–486.
13. Newton TH, Cronqvist S. Involvement of dural arteries in intracranial arteriovenous malformations. *Radiology* 1969;93:1071–1078.
14. Leblanc R, Little JR. Hemodynamics of arteriovenous malformations. *Clin Neurosurg* 1983;36:299–317.
15. Muraszko K, Wang HH, Pelton G, et al. A study of the reactivity of feeding vessels to arteriovenous malformations: Correlation with clinical outcome. *Neurosurgery* 1990;26:190–200.
16. Tarr RW, Johnson DW, Horton JA, et al. Impaired cerebral vasoactivity after embolization of arteriovenous malformations: Assessment with serial acetazolamide challenge xenon CT. *AJNR* 1991;12:417–423.
17. Nornes H, Grip A. Hemodynamic aspects of cerebral arteriovenous malformations. *J Neurosurg* 1980;53:456–464.
18. Stehbens WE. Blood vessel changes in chronic experimental arteriovenous fistula. *Surg Gynecol Obstet* 1968;127:327–331.

19. Batjer HH, Purdy PD, Giller CA, et al. Evidence of blood flow redistribution during treatment for intracranial arteriovenous malformation. *Neurosurgery* 1989;25: 599–605.

20. Hassler W, Steinmetz H. Cerebral hemodynamics in angioma patients: An intraoperative study. *J Neurosurg* 1987;67:822–831.

21. Lindegaard K, Grolimund P, Aaslid R, et al. Evaluation of cerebral AVMs using transcranial Doppler ultrasound. *J Neurosurg* 1986;65:335–344.

22. Rosenblum BR, Bonner RF, Oldfield EH. Intraoperative measurement of cortical blood flow adjacent to cerebral AVMs using laser Doppler velocimetry. *J Neurosurg* 1987;66:396–399.

23. Spetzler RF, Wilson CB, Weinstein P, et al. Normal perfusion pressure breakthrough theory. *Clin Neurosurg* 1978;25:651–672.

24. Spetzler RF, Hargraves RW, McCormic PW, et al. Relationship of perfusion pressure and size to risk of hemorrhage from arteriovenous malformations. *J Neurosurg* 1992;76:918–923.

25. Young WL, Prohovnik I, Ornstein E, et al. Monitoring of intraoperative cerebral hemodynamics before and after arteriovenous malformation resection. *Anesth Analog* 1988;67:1011–1014.

26. Abad JM, Alvarez F, Manrique M, et al. Cerebral arteriovenous malformations: Comparative results of surgical vs. conservative treatment in 112 cases. *J Neurosurg Sci* 1983;27:203–210.

27. Aminoff MJ. Management of unruptured cerebral arteriovenous malformations. *Clin Neurosurg* 1986;33: 177–185.

28. Brown RD, Wiebers DO, Forbes G, et al. The natural history of unruptured intracranial arteriovenous malformations. *JNS* 1988;68:352–357.

29. Crawford PM, West CR, Chadwick DW, et al. Arteriovenous malformations of the brain: Natural history in unoperated patients. *J Neurol Neurosurg Psychiatry* 1986; 49:1–10.

30. Forster DMC, Steiner L, Hakanson S. Arteriovenous malformations of the brain. A long term clinical study. *J Neurosurg* 1972;37:562–570.

31. Graf CJ, Perret GE, Torner JC. Bleeding from cerebral arteriovenous malformations as part of their natural history. *J Neurosurg* 1983;58:331–337.

32. Jane JA, Kassel NF, Torner JC, et al. The natural history of aneurysms and arteriovenous malformations. *J Neurosurg* 1985;62:321–323.

33. Michelsen WJ. Natural history and pathophysiology of arteriovenous malformations. *Clin Neurosurg* 1979;26: 307–313.

34. Minakawa T, Tanaka R, Koike T, et al. Angiographic follow-up study of cerebral arteriovenous malformations with reference to their enlargement and regression. *Neurosurgery* 1989;24:68–74.

35. Ondra SL, Troupp H, George ED, et al. The natural history of symptomatic arteriovenous malformations of the brain: A 24-year follow-up assessment. *J Neurosurg* 1990;73:387–391.

36. Steinmeier R, Schramm J, Müller HG, et al. Evaluation of prognostic factors in cerebral arteriovenous malformations. *Neurosurgery* 1989;24:193–200.

37. Wilkins RH. Natural history of intracranial vascular malformations. A review. *Neurosurgery* 1985;16:421–430.

38. Kaplan HA, Aronson SM, Browder EJ. Vascular malformations of the brain: An anatomical study. *J Neurosurg* 1961;18:630–635.

39. Samson DS, Batjer HH. Surface lesions: Lobar arteriovenous malformations, in Appuzo MLJ (ed): *Brain Surgery*. Churchill Livingstone, 1993, pp 1142–1175.

40. Uh S. Microsurgical excision of paraventricular arteriovenous malformations. *Neurosurgery* 1985;16:293–303.

41. Yasargil MG. Pathologic considerations, in Yasargil MG (ed): *Microneurosurgery, AVM of the Brain: History, Embryology, Pathologic Considerations, Hemodynamics, Diagnostic Studies, Microsurgical Anatomy*, Vol 3A. New York, Thieme, 1987, pp 49–211.

42. Conforti P. Spontaneous disappearance of cerebral arteriovenous angioma: Case report. *J Neurosurg* 1971;34: 432–434.

43. Eisenman JL, Alekoumbides A, Pribram H. Spontaneous thrombosis of vascular malformations of the brain. *Acta Radiol (Diagn) (Stockh)* 1972;13:77–85.

44. Marconi F, Parenti G, Puglioli M. Spontaneous regression of intracranial arteriovenous malformation. *Surg Neurol* 1993;39:385–391.

45. Wakabayashi SI, Ohno K, Shishido T, et al. Marked growth of a cerebral arteriovenous malformation: Case report and review of the literature. *Neurosurgery* 1991; 29:920–923.

46. Kupersmith MJ, Berenstein A. Vascular malformations of the brain, in Kupersmith MJ, Berenstein A (eds): *Neurovascular Neuro-ophthalmology*. New York, Springer-Verlag, 1993, pp 301–349.

47. Berenstein A, Lasjaunias P. Indications and objectives in the treatment of brain arteriovenous malformations, in *Surgical Neuroangiography* Vol. 4 P, Berlin, Springer-Verlag, 1992, pp 107–188.

48. Troost BT, Newton TH. Occipital lobe arteriovenous malformations. Clinical and radiographic features in 26 cases with comments on differentiation from migraine. *Arch Ophthalmol* 1975;93:250–256.

49. Troost BT, Mark LE, Maroon JC. Resolution of classic migraine after removal of an occipital lobe AVM. *Ann Neurol* 1979;5:199–201.

50. Crawford PM, West CR, Shaw MDM, et al. Cerebral arteriovenous malformations and epilepsy: Factors in the development of epilepsy. *Epilepsia* 1986;27:270–275.

51. Yeh HS, Kashiwagi S, Tew JM, et al. Surgical management of epilepsy associated with cerebral arteriovenous malformations. *J Neurosurg* 1990;72:216–223.

52. Yeh HS, Tew JM, Gartner M. Seizure control after surgery on cerebral arteriovenous malformations. *J Neurosurg* 1993;78:12–18.

53. Batjer HH, Devous MD Sr, Seibert GB, et al. Intracranial arteriovenous malformation: Relationship between clinical and radiographic factors and ipsilateral steal severity. *Neurosurgery* 1988;23:322–328.

54. Hachinski V, Norris JW, Cooper P, et al. Symptomatic intracranial steal. *Arch Neurol* 1977;34:149–153.

55. Marks MP, Lane B, Steinburg G, et al. Vascular characteristics of intracerebral arteriovenous malformations in patients with clinical steal. *AJNR* 1991;12:489–496.

56. Morgan MK, Johnson I, Besser M, et al. Cerebral arteriovenous malformations, steal and the hypertensive breakthrough threshold. *J Neurosurg* 1987;66:563–567.

57. Constantino A, Vinters HV. Pathologic correlate of the steal phenomenon in a patient with cerebral arteriovenous malformation. *Stroke* 1986;17:103–106.

58. Viñuela F, Nombela L, Roach MR, et al. Stenotic and occlusive disease of the venous drainage system of deep brain AVMs. *J Neurosurg* 1985;63:180–183.

59. Al-Rodhan NAF, Sundt TM Jr, Piepgras DG, et al. Occlusive hyperemia: A theory for the hemodynamic complications following resection of intracerebral arteriovenous malformations. *J Neurosurg* 1993;78:167–175.

60. Duckwiler GR, Dion JE, Viñuela F, et al. Delayed venous occlusion following embolotherapy of vascular malformations of the brain. *AJNR* 1992;13:1571–1579.

61. Willinsky R, Lasjaunias P, Terbrugge K, et al. Brain arteriovenous malformations: Analysis of the angioarchitecture in relationship to hemorrhage (based on 152 patients explored and/or treated at the hospital de Bicêtre between 1981 and 1986). *J Neuroradiol* 1988;15:225–237.

62. Miyasaka Y, Yada K, Ohwada T, et al. An analysis of the venous drainage system as a factor in hemorrhage from arteriovenous malformations. *J Neurosurg* 1992;76:239–243.

63. Hayashi S, Arimoto T, Itakura T, et al. The association of intracranial aneurysms and arteriovenous malformations of the brain. *J Neurosurg* 1981;55:971–975.

64. Lasjaunias P, Piske R, Terbrugge K, et al. Cerebral arteriovenous malformations and associated arterial aneurysms. *Acta Neurochir* 1988;91:29–36.

65. Miyasaka K, Wolpert SM, Prager RJ. The association of cerebral aneurysms, infundibulum and intracranial arteriovenous malformations. *Stroke* 1982;13:196–203.

66. Garcia-Monaco R, Rodesch G, Alverez H, et al. Pseudoaneurysms within ruptured intracranial arteriovenous malformations: Diagnosis and early endovascular management. *AJNR* 1993;14:315–321.

67. Batjer HH, Suss RA, Samson D. Intracranial arteriovenous malformations associated with aneurysms. *Neurosurgery* 1986;18:29–35.

68. Brown RD, Wiebers DO, Forbes G. Unruptured intracranial aneurysms and arteriovenous malformations: Frequency of intracranial hemorrhage and relationship of lesions. *J Neurosurg* 1990;73:859–863.

69. Cunha E SA MJ, Stein BM, Solomon RA, et al. The treatment of associated intracranial aneurysms and arteriovenous malformations. *J Neurosurg* 1992;77:853–859.

70. Hunt B, Suss RA, Samson D. Intracranial arteriovenous malformations associated with aneurysms. *Neurosurgery* 1986;18:29–35.

71. Okamoto S, Hand H, Hashimoto N. Location of intracranial aneurysms associated with cerebral arteriovenous malformations: Statistical analysis. *Surg Neurol* 1984;22:335–340.

72. Suzuki J, Onuma T. Intracranial aneurysms associated with arteriovenous malformations. *J Neurosurg* 1979;50:742–746.

73. Cromwell LD, Harris AB. Treatment of cerebral arteriovenous malformations: A combined neurosurgical and neuroradiological approach. *J Neurosurg* 1980;52:705–708.

74. Lasjaunias P, Manelfe C, Chiu M. Angiographic architecture of intracranial vascular malformations and fistulas—pretherapeutic aspects. *Neurosurg Rev* 1986;9:253–263.

75. Leblanc R, Feindel W, Ethier R. Epilepsy from cerebral arteriovenous malformations. *Can J Neurol Sci* 1983;10:91–95.

76. Lunsford LD, Kondziolka D, Flickinger JC, et al. Stereotactic radiosurgery for arteriovenous malformations of the brain. *J Neurosurg* 1991;75:512–524.

77. Luessenhop AJ, Rosa L. Cerebral arteriovenous malformations. Indications for and results of surgery, and the role of intravascular techniques. *J Neurosurg* 1984;60:14–22.

78. Murphy MJ. Long-term follow-up of seizures associated with cerebral arteriovenous malformations. *Arch Neurol* 1985;42:477–479.

79. Pasqualin A, Scienza R, Cioffi F, et al. Treatment of cerebral arteriovenous malformation with a combination of preoperative embolization and surgery. *Neurosurgery* 1991;29:358–368.

80. Spetzler RF, Martin NA, Carter LP, et al. Surgical management of large AVMs by staged embolization and operative excision. *J Neurosurg* 1987;67:17–28.

81. Stein BM, Wolpert SM. Arteriovenous malformations of the brain. I. Current concepts and treatment. *Arch Neurol* 1980;37:1–5.

82. Stein BM, Wolpert SM. Arteriovenous malformations of the brain. II. Current concepts and treatment. *Arch Neurol* 1980;37:69–75.

83. Viñuela F, Fox AJ, Peltz D, et al. Combined endovascular embolization and surgery in the management of cerebral arteriovenous malformations: Experience with 101 cases. *J Neurosurg* 1991;75:856–864.

84. Yamada S, Brauer FS, Knierim DS. Direct approach to arteriovenous malformations in functional areas of the cerebral hemispheres. *J Neurosurg* 1990;72:418–425.

85. Andrews BT, Wilson CB. Staged treatment of arteriovenous malformations of the brain. *Neurosurgery* 1987;21:314–323.

86. Lasjaunias P, Manelfe C, Terbrugge K, et al. Endovascular treatment of cerebral vascular malformations. *Neurosurg Rev* 1986;9:265–275.

87. Carmel PW, Swift DM. Spontaneous intracranial hemorrhage occurring during pregnancy, in Kauffman HH (ed): *Intracerebral Hematomas*. New York, Raven Press, 1992, pp 117–125.

88. Dias MS, Sekhar LN. Intracranial hemorrhage from aneurysms and arteriovenous malformations during pregnancy and puerperium. *Neurosurgery* 1990;27:855–866.

89. Horton JC, Chambers WA, Lyons SL, et al. Pregnancy and the risk of hemorrhage from cerebral arteriovenous malformations. *Neurosurgery* 1990;27:867–872.

90. Robinson JL, Hall CJ, Sedzimir CB. Arteriovenous malformations, aneurysms and pregnancy. *J Neurosurg* 1974;41:63–70.

91. Weir B. Management of intracranial aneurysms and arteriovenous malformations during pregnancy, in Wilkens RH, Rengechary SS (eds): *Neurosurgery Update, Vol II*. New York, McGraw-Hill, 1991, pp 119–125.

92. Kerber CW. Catheter therapy: Fluoroscopic monitoring of deliberate embolic occlusion. *Radiology* 1977;125:538–540.

93. Castaneda-Zuniga WR, Sanchez R, Amplatz K. Experimental observations on short and long term effects of arterial occlusion with Ivalon. *Radiology* 1978;126:783–785.

94. Horton JA, Marano GD, Kerber CW, et al. Polyvinyl alcohol foam-Gelfoam for therapeutic embolization: A synergistic mixture. *AJNR* 1983;4:143–149.

95. Jack CR, Forbes G, Dewanjee MK, et al. Polyvinyl alcohol sponge for embolotherapy: Particle size and morphology. *AJNR* 1985;6:595–600.

96. Nakstad PH, Bakke SJ, Hald JK. Embolization of intracranial arteriovenous malformations and fistulas with polyvinyl alcohol particles and platinum fibre coils. *Neuroradiology* 1991;33:101–105.

97. Schumacher M, Horton JA. Treatment of cerebral arteriovenous malformations with PVA. Results and analysis of complications. *Neuroradiology* 1991;33:101–105.

98. Tadavarthy SM, Moller HJ, Amplatz K. Polyvinyl alcohol foam (Ivalon): A new embolic material. *AJNR* 1975;125:609–616.

99. Herrera M, Rysavy J, Kotula F, et al. Polyvinyl shavings: Technical considerations of a new embolic agent. *Radiology* 1982;144:638–640.

100. Viñuela F, Fox AJ, Peltz D, et al. Angiographic follow-up of large cerebral AVMs, incompletely embolized with isobutyl-2-cyanoacrylate. *AJNR* 1986;7:919–925.

101. Benati A, Belltramello A, Maschio A, et al. Combined embolization of intracranial AVMs with multi-purpose mobile wing microcatheter system: Indications and results in 71 cases. *AJNR* 1987;8:938–945.

102. Halbach VV, Higashida RT, Hieshima GB, et al. Transarterial occlusion of solitary intracerebral arteriovenous fistulas. *AJNR* 1989;10:747–754.

103. Berenstein AB, Krall R, Choi IS. Embolization with *n*-butyl-cyanoacrylate in the management of CNS lesions (abstract). *AJNR* 1989;10:883.

104. Brothers MF, Kaufmann JCE, Fox AJ, et al. *N*-butyl 2-cyanoacrylate-substitute for IBCA in interventional neuroradiology: Histopathologic and polymerization time studies. *AJNR* 1989;10:777–786.

105. Debrun G, Viñuela F, Fox AJ, et al. Embolization of cerebral arteriovenous malformations with bucrylate: Experience in 46 cases. *J Neurosurg* 1982;56:615–627.

106. Pelz DM, Fox AJ, Viñuela F, et al. Preoperative embolization of brain AVMs with isobutyl-2-cyanoacrylate. *AJNR* 1988;9:757–765.

107. Vinters HV, Galil KA, Lundie MJ, et al. The histotoxicity of cyanoacrylates: A selective review. *Neuroradiology* 1985;27:279–291.

108. Viñuela F, Fox AJ, Debrun GM, et al. Preembolization superselective angiography: Role in the treatment of brain arteriovenous malformations with isobutyl-2-cyanoacrylate. *AJNR* 1984;5:765–769.

109. Cromwell LD, Kerber CW. Modification of cyanoacrylate for therapeutic embolization: Preliminary experience. *AJR* 1979;132:799–801.

110. Rao VRK, Mandalam KR, Gupta AK, et al. Dissolution of isobutyl 2-cyanoacrylate on long term follow-up. *AJNR* 1989;10:135–141.

111. Vinters HV, Lundie MJ, Kaufmann JCE. Long term pathological follow-up of cerebral arteriovenous malformations treated by embolization with bucrylate. *N Engl J Med* 1986;314:477–483.

112. Hilal SK, Khandji AG, Chi LT, et al. Synthetic fiber-coated platinum coils successfully used for the endovascular treatment of arteriovenous malformations, aneurysms, and direct arteriovenous fistulas of the CNS (abstract). *AJNR* 1988;9:1030.

113. Graves VB, Rappe AH, Smith TP, et al. An endovascular retrieving device for use in small vessels. *AJNR* 1993; 14:804–808.

114. Smith TP, Graves VB, Halbach VV, et al. Microretrieval device for intravascular foreign body removal. *AJNR* 1993;14:809–811.

115. Gugliemi G, Viñuela F, Sepetka I, et al. Electrothrombosis of saccular aneurysms via endovascular approach. Part 1: Electrochemical basis, technique, and experimental results. *J Neurosurg* 1991;75:1–7.

116. Gugliemi G, Viñuela F, Dion J, et al. Electrothrombosis of saccular aneurysms via endovascular approach. Part 2: Preliminary clinical experience. *J Neurosurg* 1991; 75:8–14.

117. Terada T, Nakamura Y, Nakai K, et al. Embolization of arteriovenous malformations with peripheral aneurysms using ethylene vinyl alcohol copolymer. Report of three cases. *J Neurosurg* 1991;75:655–660.

118. Pevsner PH, Klara P, Doppman J, et al. Ethyl alcohol: Experimental agent for interventional therapy of neurovascular lesions. *AJNR* 1983;4:388–390.

119. Kumar AJ, Viñuela F, Fox AJ, et al. Unruptured intracranial arteriovenous malformations do cause mass effect. *AJNR* 1985;6:29–32.

120. Batjer HH, Samson D. Arteriovenous malformations of the posterior fossa. Clinical presentation, diagnostic evaluation, and surgical treatment. *J Neurosurg* 1986; 64:849–856.

121. Kucharczyk W, Lemme-Pleghos L, Uske A, et al. Intracranial vascular malformations: MR and CT imaging. *Radiology* 1985;56:383–389.

122. Noorbehesht B, Fabrikant JI, Enzmann DR. Size determination of supratentorial arteriovenous malformations by MR, CT, and angiography. *Neuroradiology* 1987;29:512–518.

123. Smith HJ, Strother CM, Kikuchi Y, et al. MR imaging in the management of supratentorial intracranial AVMs. *AJR* 1988;150:1143–1153.

124. Yousem DM, Flamm ES, Grossman RI. Comparison of MR and clinical history in the identification of the incidence of hemorrhage in cerebral arteriovenous malformations. *Am J Neuroradiol* 1989;10:1151–1154.

125. Albert P, Salgado H, Polaina M, et al. A study of the venous drainage of 150 cerebral arteriovenous malformations as related to haemorrhagic risks and size of the lesion. *Acta Neurochir (Wein)* 1990;103:30–34.

126. Horton JA, Kerber CW. Lidocaine injection into external carotid branches: Provocative tests to preserve cranial nerve function in therapeutic embolization. *AJNR* 1986;1:105–108.

127. Viñuela F. Functional evaluation and embolization of intracranial arteriovenous malformations, in Viñuela F, Halbach VV, Dion JE (eds): *Interventional Neuroradiology: Endovascular Therapy of the Central Nervous System.* New York, Raven Press, 1992, pp 77–86.

128. Wada J, Rasmussen T. Intracarotid injection of sodium amytal for the lateralization of cerebral speech dominance. *J Neurosurg* 1960;17:266–282.

129. Rauch RA, Viñuela F, Dion J, et al. Preembolization functional evaluation in brain arteriovenous malformations: The superselective amytal test. *AJNR* 1992;13: 303–308.

130. Rauch RA, Viñuela F, Dion J, et al. Preembolization functional evaluation in brain arteriovenous malformations: The ability of superselective amytal test to predict neurologic dysfunction before embolization. *AJNR* 1992;13:309–314.

131. Ahn HS, Kerber CW, Deeb ZL. Extra- to intracranial anastomoses in therapeutic embolization: Recognition and role. *AJNR* 1980;1:71–75.

132. Peters KR, Quisling RG, Gilmore R, et al. Intraarterial use of sodium methohexital for provocative testing during brain embolotherapy. *AJNR* 1993;14:171–174.

133. Hacke W, Zeumer H, Berg-Dammer E. Monitoring of hemispheric or brainstem functions with neurophysiologic methods during interventional neuroradiology. *AJNR* 1983;4:382–384.

134. Jungreis CA, Horton JA, Hecht ST. Blood pressure changes in feeders to cerebral arteriovenous malformations during therapeutic embolization. *AJNR* 1989;10: 575–577.

135. Duckwiler GR, Dion JE, Viñuela F, et al. Intravascular microcatheter pressure monitoring: Experimental work and early clinical evaluation. *AJNR* 1990;11:169–175.

136. Kattah JC, Luessenhop AJ, Kolsky M, et al. Removal of occipital arteriovenous malformations with sparing of the visual fields. *Arch Neurol* 1981;38:307–309.

137. Martin NA, Wilson CB. Medial occipital arteriovenous malformations. Surgical treatment. *J Neurosurg* 1982; 56:798–802.

138. Jack CR Jr, Nichols DA, Sharbrough FW, et al. Selective posterior cerebral artery amytal test for evaluating memory function before surgery for temporal lobe seizure. *Radiology* 1988;168:787–793.

139. Fox AJ, Girvin JP, Viñuela F, et al. Rolandic arteriovenous malformations: Improvement in limb function by IBCA embolization. *AJNR* 1985;6:575–582.

140. Ojemann G, Ojemann J, Lettich E, et al. Cortical language localization in left, dominant hemisphere. An electrical stimulation mapping investigation in 117 patients. *J Neurosurg* 1989;71:316–326.

141. Rhoton AL Jr, Fujii K, Fradd B. Microsurgical anatomy of the anterior choroidal artery. *Surg Neurol* 1979;12: 171–187.

142. Osborn AG. The anterior choroidal artery, in *Introduction to Cerebral Angiography*. Philadelphia, Harper & Row, 1980, pp 167–184.

143. Dowd CF, Halbach VV, Barnwell SL, et al. Particulate embolization of the anterior choroidal artery in the treatment of cerebral arteriovenous malformations. *AJNR* 1991;12:1055–1061.

144. Hodes JE, Aymard A, Casasco A, et al. Embolization of arteriovenous malformations of the temporal lobe via the anterior choroidal artery. *AJNR* 1991;12:775–780.

145. Silber MH, Sandok BA, Earnest F. Vascular malformations of the posterior fossa. Clinical and radiologic features. *Arch Neurol* 1987;44:965–969.

146. Drake CG, Friedman AH, Peerless SJ. Posterior fossa arteriovenous malformations. *J Neurosurg* 1986;64:1–10.

147. Solomon RA, Stein BA. Management of deep supratentorial and brainstem arteriovenous malformations, in Barrow DL (ed): *Intracranial Vascular Malformations*. Park Ridge, IL, AANS, 1990, pp 125–140.

148. Bauer BL. Intraoperative angiography in cerebral aneurysm and AV malformation. *Neurosurg Rev* 1984;7: 209–217.

149. Foley KT, Cahan LD, Hieshima GB. Intraoperative angiography using a portable digital subtraction unit: Technical note. *J Neurosurg* 1986;64:816–818.

150. Redekop GJ, Elisevich KV, Gaspar LE, et al. Conventional radiation therapy of intracranial arteriovenous malformations: Long-term results. *J Neurosurg* 1993; 78:413–422.

151. Kjellberg RN, Davis KR, Lyons S, et al. Bragg peak proton beam therapy for arteriovenous malformations of the brain. *Clin Neurosurg* 1983;31:248–290.

152. Kjellberg RN, Hanamura T, Davis KR, et al. Bragg peak proton-beam therapy for arteriovenous malformations of the brain. *N Engl J Med* 1983;309:269–274.

153. Steinberg GK, Fabrikant JI, Marks MP, et al. Stereotactic heavy-charged particle Bragg-peak radiation for intracranial arteriovenous malformations. *N Engl J Med* 1990;323:96–101.

154. Dawson RC, Tarr RW, Hecht ST, et al. Treatment of arteriovenous malformations of the brain with combined embolization and stereotactic radiosurgery: Results after 1 and 2 years. *AJNR* 1990;11:864–877.

155. Steiner L. Radiosurgery in cerebral arteriovenous malformations, in Fein JM, Flamm ES (eds): *Cerebrovascular Surgery*, Vol IV. New York, Springer-Verlag, 1985, pp 1161–1215.

156. Marks MP, Lane B, Steinberg GK, et al. Endovascular treatment of cerebral arteriovenous malformations following radiosurgery. *AJNR* 1993;14:297–303.

157. Dion JE, Gates PC, Fox AJ, et al. Clinical events following neuroangiography: A prospective study. *Stroke* 1987;4:269–280.

158. Wilson CB, Hieshima GB. Occlusive hyperemia: A new way to think about an old problem. *J Neurosurg* 1993; 78:165–166.

159. Fry DL. Acute vascular endothelial changes associated with increased blood velocities gradients. *Circ Res* 1968; 22:165–197.

160. Pile-Spellman J, Baker KF, Liszczak TM, et al. Highflow angiopathy: Cerebral blood vessel changes in experimental chronic arteriovenous fistula. *AJNR* 1986;7: 811–815.

161. Halbach VV, Higashida RT, Dowd CF, et al. Management of vascular perforations that occur during neurointerventional procedures. *AJNR* 1991;12:319–327.

162. Purdy PD, Batjer HH, Samson DS. Management of hemorrhagic complications from preoperative embolization of arteriovenous malformations. *J Neurosurg* 1991;74:205–211.

163. Debrun GM, Viñuela FV, Fox AJ. Aspirin and systemic heparinization in diagnostic and interventional neuroradiology. *AJNR* 1982;3:337–340.

164. Kaku Y, Yonekawa Y, Tsukahara T, et al. Superselective intra-arterial infusion of papaverine for the treatment of cerebral vasospasm after subarachnoid hemorrhage. *J Neurosurg* 1992;77:842–847.

165. Kassell NF, Helm G, Simmons N, et al. Treatment of cerebral vasospasm with intra-arterial papaverine. *J Neurosurg* 1992;77:848–852.

166. Scott JA, Berenstein A, Blumenthal D. Use of the activated coagulation time as a measure of anticoagulation during interventional procedures. *Radiology* 1986;158: 849–850.

28

Interventional Treatment of Intracranial Aneurysms

Randall T. Higashida, M.D., Fong Y. Tsai, M.D., Van V. Halbach, M.D., Christopher F. Dowd, M.D., Grant B. Hieshima, M.D.

INTRODUCTION

Interventional neurovascular treatment of intracranial aneurysms was pioneered in the early 1970s by the Russian neurosurgeon Serbinenko.[1,2] He described the use of fixed and detachable latex balloons, which were used in the diagnosis and management of complex cerebral vascular disorders including arteriovenous malformations, carotid cavernous sinus fistulas, and intracranial aneurysms. Treatment was performed by proximal occlusion of the aneurysm and parent vessel via direct puncture of the cervical internal carotid artery.

Over the past decade, this field has rapidly expanded due to the development of high-resolution fluoroscopy, newer materials for aneurysm occlusion, and improved screening modalities for the diagnosis of cerebrovascular diseases.[3] These developments have made it feasible to place detachable balloons, coils, polymers, and other embolic materials directly into an aneurysm for obliteration, with preservation of the parent vessel.[4,5] Computed tomography (CT) and magnetic resonance imaging (MRI) have improved the diagnostic efficacy in screening patients with suspected vascular disorders.

This chapter discusses the various technical and therapeutic modalities currently utilized to treat patients with ruptured and unruptured intracranial aneurysms by endovascular techniques.

ANEURYSM INCIDENCE

Cerebrovascular disease is the third leading cause of death in North America. Various reports estimate that as many as 5 million individuals in North America have or will develop an intracranial aneurysm. Each year in the United States, 28,000 people present with an acute subarachnoid hemorrhage (SAH) from aneurysm rupture.[6,7]

The incidence of intracranial aneurysm in the general population is 1.5% to 8.0%. Seventy-seven percent of acute subarachnoid bleeding is due to aneurysm rupture. Aneurysm rupture usually occurs between the fifth and seventh decades of life. In terms of size, only 2% of aneurysms less than 5 mm in diameter tend to bleed, whereas more than 40% of aneurysms between 6 mm and 10 mm have already bled when they are discovered. Multiple aneurysms occur in approximately 20% of patients.[7,8]

In terms of the incidence of an aneurysm, females, at 56%, have a slightly higher preponderance than males, at 44%. The Cooperative Aneurysm Study in 1981 studied 249 patients admitted with an acute SAH due to aneurysm rupture.[9] Overall there was a 36.2% mortality rate and a 17.9% morbidity rate with serious neurological sequelae; only 46% of patients had a favorable outcome at 90 days. Intracranial aneurysms therefore remain a leading cause of significant morbidity and mortality among cerebrovascular disorders in the general population.[10,11]

EMBOLIZATION MATERIALS

Detachable Balloons

Currently, two types of balloons are utilized for treatment of intracranial aneurysms: silicone and latex. The ITC silicone detachable balloon, developed in the United States, was specifically designed for treatment of cerebrovascular disorders (Interventional Therapeutics Corporation [ITC], South San Francisco, California)[12] (Fig. 28-1). The ITC balloon is made from a blended, biocompatible, nonbiodegradable, silicone elastomer. This provides the balloon with enhanced elongation and expansion characteristics while maintaining a soft, low-tension shell. Blended silicone was chosen since it provides a high degree of conformational structure and allows the balloon to be placed in restrained areas, with minimal damage to the surrounding vessel wall or aneurysm. Its isotropic expansion capabilities allow the balloon shell to respond with gradual enlargement when inflated with fluid, in contrast to latex balloons, which retain a pressure buildup and then suddenly expand. Latex balloons will also degrade with time in the intravascular system, whereas silicone will not, unless placed under unusual stress.

The balloon is attached to a 2.0 French polyethylene catheter by sliding the catheter tip through the base of the valve. To aid in navigation, the distal catheter tip can be curved into a variety of shapes over steam. Ad-

ditionally, an 0.014- or 0.016-in. steerable guidewire may be used in conjunction with the catheter and placed proximal to the base of the balloon. The balloon and catheter are filled with an iso-osmotic contrast material such as metrizamide, at a concentration of 200 mg% iodine for opacification. The balloon is guided by flow into the distal intracranial circulation to the site of occlusion. It is then inflated to produce occlusion and detached by gentle traction on the catheter. The balloon has a self-sealing, internal miter valve to prevent deflation when detached.[13]

Latex balloons have also been used for aneurysm occlusion therapy (Ingenor Corp., Paris; Balt Inc., Montmorency, France).[14,15] Latex balloons have a higher expansion coefficient and therefore can be inflated to larger sizes. These balloons are also available with internal valves. However, since latex will degrade over time, a polymerization material such as hydroxyethyl methacrylate is needed to fill the balloon if permanent occlusion within an aneurysm is desired.[16,17]

Generally, balloons are used for parent vessel occlusion for ectatic, fusiform aneurysms without a well-defined neck.[18] Although balloons have been utilized for direct aneurysm occlusion, newer techniques and devices have supplanted balloons as the device of choice for intra-aneurysmal occlusion.

Thrombogenic Coils

Microcoils composed of platinum and tungsten, with and without Dacron fibers to increase thrombogenicity, have recently been investigated for use in aneurysms as an embolic material (Cook Inc, Bloomington, IN; Target Therapeutics Corp., Fremont, CA; Balt Corp., Montmorency, France)[19–22] (Fig. 28-2). These coils measure 0.010–0.016 in. in diameter, are placed through microcatheters, and are highly radiopaque. These microcoils have been demonstrated to be efficacious in promoting thrombosis and occlusion of small aneurysms (<15 mm) with narrow necks. The coils must be tightly packed within the aneurysm, since loose packing may cause shifting of the coils and recanalization may occur.

The disadvantages of this technique are that the coils are not useful for larger, broad-necked aneurysms. The coils are also not retrievable. Once the coil is deployed outside the catheter, if it shifts or migrates outside the aneurysm, a separate procedure to retrieve the coil from its undesired location is necessary. In addition, these coils are relatively stiff and noncompliant; therefore, during deployment, they may cause inadvertent vessel perforation or aneurysm rupture.

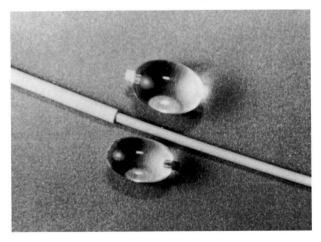

Fig. 28-1 The ITC silicone detachable balloon used for treatment of intracranial aneurysms. The balloon has an internal miter valve to prevent deflation when detached. It is placed on a 2.0 French guiding catheter.

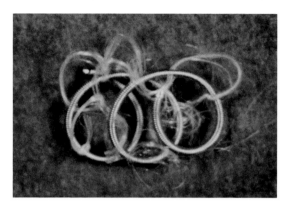

Fig. 28-2 Platinum microcoil with Dacron thrombogenic fibers used for aneurysm and vessel occlusion. These coils are available in various configurations, diameters, and lengths.

Electrolytic Detachable Coils

In 1991, the Guglielmi Detachable Coil (GDC) system was introduced.[23,24] This technique employs either 0.010- or 0.015-in.-diameter platinum coils, fixed to a stainless steel guidewire by a solder connection. The coil is introduced into the aneurysm and, when properly placed, an electrical current is applied to the proximal end of the guidewire, using a battery-operated generator. The positive charge of the platinum coil attracts the negatively charged white blood cells, red blood cells, platelets, and fibrinogen, inducing thrombus formation. At the same time, the current acts to electrolyze and dissolve the solder junction, resulting in detachment. The platinum coils are a packing material that holds the intra-aneurysmal thrombus, preventing its displacement and clot fragmentation. Multiple coils of various diameters and sizes can be introduced into an aneurysm until complete packing of the aneurysm is achieved.[25]

The two major advances this technique offers over other embolic materials are (1) the ability to place a coil into an aneurysm and withdraw it if the coil migrates into an undesired location and (2) the ability to promote thrombus within an aneurysm to produce a stable clot.

This technique is now being investigated at various institutions in North America, Europe, and Japan. Preliminary reports indicate that the GDC system is efficacious for small and large aneurysms (<15 mm) with narrow necks. Larger aneurysms (>15 mm) with wide necks (>6–10 mm) are harder to treat by this technique due to difficulty in producing a stable mesh across the neck which induces permanent clotting.

Since these coils are extremely soft and pliable, they tend to "compact" and reposition themselves within a large aneurysm. This results in subtotal occlusion and the possibility for recanalization of the aneurysm requiring retreatment. Therefore, long-term follow-up for all of these patients is mandatory to ensure complete, lasting obliteration of the aneurysm by this technique.

Liquid Embolic Materials

Rapidly polymerizing liquid embolic agents have been investigated for use in aneurysm treatment. This technique requires temporary occlusion across the neck of an aneurysm, with delivery of a rapidly polymerizing material into it for obliteration. Berenstein and Lasjaunias described the use of isobutyl cyanoacrylate directly injected into an aneurysm for occlusion.[14] However, due to the technical difficulties of ensuring complete flow arrest during delivery, the preliminary reports resulted in parent artery occlusion, and this technique was abandoned.

In 1992, a second type of liquid polymer, cellulose acetate polymer, was investigated for use. A mixture of cellulose acetate polymer and bismuth trioxide was dissolved in dimethyl sulfoxide. On contact with blood, the dimethyl sulfoxide diffused out, and the cellulose acetate polymer formed a rapidly hardened material which conformed to the shape of the aneurysm. In animal studies and in a small preliminary group of six patients, this technique was employed.[26,27] Although a novel application, further investigative studies will be needed to demonstrate the safety and efficacy of utilizing these materials for intracranial aneurysm therapy.

METHODS

All procedures are performed using a transfemoral arterial approach under light neuroleptic anesthesia. Patients are therefore awake for the entire procedure, so that continuous neurological monitoring can be done by the interventional neuroradiologist or neurosurgeon performing the procedure.

Initially, a complete four-vessel cerebral arteriogram should be performed to determine the location, size, shape, dimensions, and width of the aneurysm's body and neck. In addition, it is important to determine if intraluminal thrombus is present and if there is associated vasospasm. In 20% of cases, more than one aneurysm may be present.

For fusiform, wide-necked aneurysms, a test occlusion of the parent artery proximal to the aneurysm should be initially performed. The patient is systemically anticoagulated with 72 units/kg of heparin, and a fixed balloon catheter is guided into the proximal parent artery. The balloon is inflated until there is complete cessation of blood flow, and test occlusion for 30 min is performed to determine if the patient will tolerate vessel occlusion. Ancillary studies that may assist in determining tolerance to vessel occlusion include Xenon CT scanning with a Diamox challenge, nuclear medicine blood flow studies to assess cerebral revascularization, and positron emission tomography (PET) to determine physiological changes with test occlusion of a major vascular territory. If the patient tolerates the test occlusion, permanent occlusion using detachable balloons across the aneurysm neck or just proximal to the inflow of the aneurysm can be performed for permanent occlusion[13,15] (Figs. 28-3, 28-4A–D).

For aneurysms with a well-defined anatomical neck, a microcatheter is initially placed directly into the central lumen of the aneurysm. The dimensions of the aneurysm body and neck are then measured, and appropriate-sized balloons or coils are chosen for placement (Fig. 28-5A, B). If the coil diameter is too large, excessive pressure against the thin-walled aneurysm during

deployment could result in rupture. If the coil diameter is too small, it may not be situated properly after deployment; this could result in its migration into the parent artery. Therefore, it is imperative to choose the correct size, shape, and length of coil to be deposited. During coil deposition, it is important to pack all of the interstices, and to occlude the base and neck of the aneurysm as completely as possible. Loose packing or subtotal occlusion may cause the coils to shift, which can result in thromboemboli, coil reformation, and the possibility of recanalization, possibly leading to delayed rupture or continued expansion of the aneurysm (Fig. 28-6A–C).

Following the procedure, systemic anticoagulation is reversed by giving protamine sulfate; 10 mg reverses the action of 1,000 units of heparin. The patient is rechecked neurologically. Close observation of the patient for 24–72 hr in the neurosurgical intensive care unit is required, to ensure that there are no delayed neurological problems. Patients should be seen for follow-up at 1–3 months and at 6–12 months for clinical and radiological assessment to ensure that the aneurysm remains completely treated. For parent vessel occlusion, a noninvasive CT or MRI scan is adequate to document continued aneurysm thrombosis. For direct aneurysm occlusion using coils, follow-up cerebral angiography is necessary to ensure continued obliteration of the aneurysm.

RESULTS OF ANEURYSM OCCLUSION THERAPY

Romodanov and Shchegelov in 1982 reported on the treatment of 119 patients by detachable balloon occlusion techniques.[28] In 93 cases (78.2%), occlusion of the aneurysm with preservation of the parent artery was achieved. In 96.7%, good to excellent results were obtained with complete aneurysm obliteration. Only 15 patients (12.6%) required parent artery occlusion. In 11 cases (9.2%), there was failure to occlude the aneurysm successfully by endovascular techniques.

In 1989, Shchegelov updated his series and reported on 617 patients treated by balloon occlusion therapy.[29] In his current series, 561 patients (91%) were reported as successfully treated in terms of primary occlusion of the aneurysm, with preservation of the parent artery. In 54 patients (9%), occlusion of the parent vessel was performed. The reported mortality rate was 1.7% of 338 patients treated in "fair" condition. The mortality rate was 22% for 71 patients in "poor" condition at the time of the procedure.

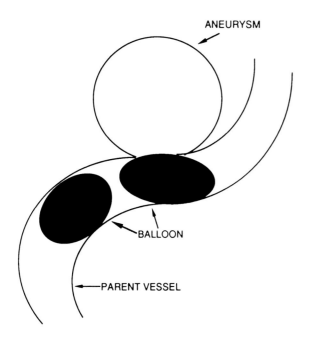

PROXIMAL BALLOON OCCLUSION

Fig. 28-3 Technique used for parent artery vessel occlusion of wide-necked aneurysms. The balloon is placed across or just proximal to the aneurysm neck for occlusion.

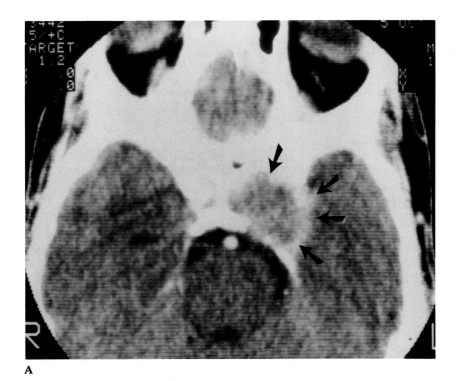

A

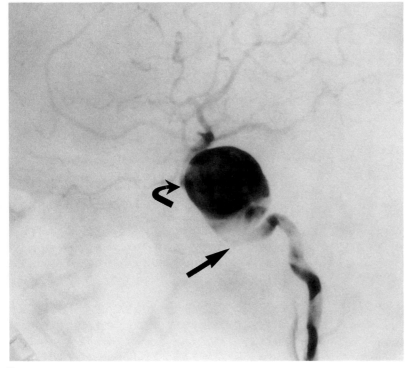

B

Fig. 28-4 (*A*) CT scan demonstrating a giant fusiform aneurysm of the left cavernous internal carotid artery (arrows). This patient presented with ophthalmoplegia and severe retro-orbital pain. (*B*) Cerebral angiogram demonstrates a giant ectatic aneurysm with separate inflow (straight arrow) and outflow (curved arrow) within the cavernous sinus. These aneurysms are best treated by occlusion of the parent vessel.

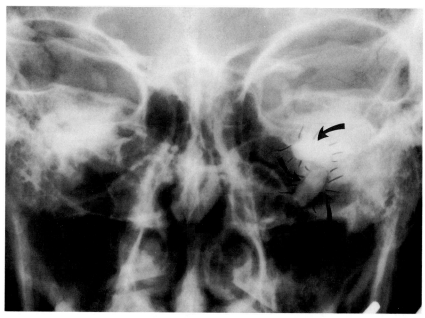

C

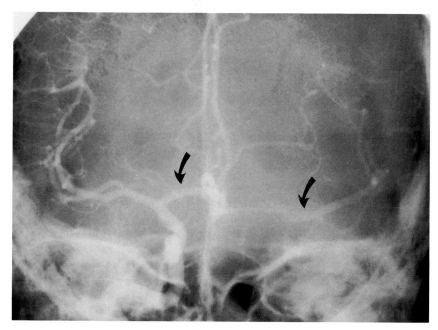

D

Fig. 28-4 (C) Following test occlusion, two detachable balloons are placed in the precavernous segment of the internal carotid artery for occlusion (arrows). (D) Angiogram of the contralateral carotid artery demonstrates excellent cross-filling from the right to left hemisphere (arrows).

In 1990, Moret reported on a series of 60 patients treated with saccular aneurysms by balloon occlusion therapy.[30] He reported a 10% rate of failure to treat the aneurysm via an endovascular approach, a 10% neurological complication rate, an 8% partial recanalization rate requiring retreatment, and a 4% mortality rate.

Higashida in 1991 reported on 215 patients treated by balloon occlusion techniques.[31] In 84 patients (39%) there was successful treatment by primary occlusion of the aneurysm, with preservation of the parent artery.[32] The distribution of the 84 aneurysms included 59 cases in the anterior circulation and 25 cases in the posterior circulation. The presenting symptom was mass effect in 45 cases (53.6%), SAH in 31 cases (36.9%), rupture of an intracavernous aneurysm resulting in a carotid

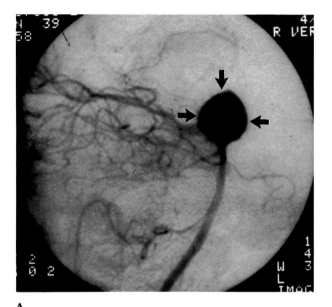

A

B

Fig. 28-5 (*A*) Large distal basilar artery aneurysm which recently ruptured, producing an SAH (arrows). (*B*) Following endovascular placement of detachable balloons within the aneurysm (arrows), there is total obliteration, with preservation of the distal posterior circulation vessels.

cavernous sinus fistula in 6 cases (7.1%), 1 case of traumatic pseudoaneurysm, and 1 patient presenting with symptoms of thromboemboli. Permanent complications from endovascular therapy included 15 deaths (17.9%) and 9 patients with a stroke (10.7%). Follow-up studies demonstrated that in 65 cases (77.4%)

there was complete aneurysmal obliteration, and in 19 cases (22.6%) there was subtotal occlusion of more than 85%.

Guglielmi in 1992 reported on the use of electrolytic detachable coils for direct aneurysm obliteration, with preservation of the parent artery.[23] He described a series of 46 patients ranging in age from 21 to 73 years. Twenty-four patients presented with SAH, and 14 with mass effect; 6 patients were asymptomatic, and 2 had other symptoms. In 45 cases (97.8%), Guglielmi reported 70–100% occlusion. There were three permanent and three transient complications (13.3%), with two reported mortalities due to acute and delayed aneurysm rupture.

DISCUSSION

Interventional neurovascular techniques for the treatment of intracranial aneurysms, is now being utilized in selected cases. At several centers, this has become the primary treatment of choice over conventional surgical clipping.[29,30] The advantage of this technique is that it can be performed under local anesthesia in an awake patient, allowing continuous neurological monitoring. This is extremely important for patients who present with fusiform, ectatic aneurysms without a

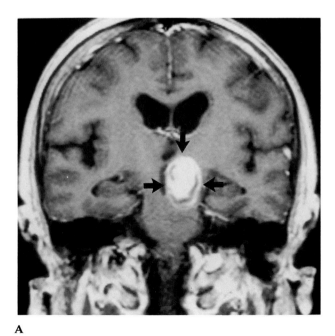

A

Fig. 28-6 (*A*) MRI scan demonstrates a large aneurysm arising from the distal basilar-proximal posterior cerebral artery junction (arrows).

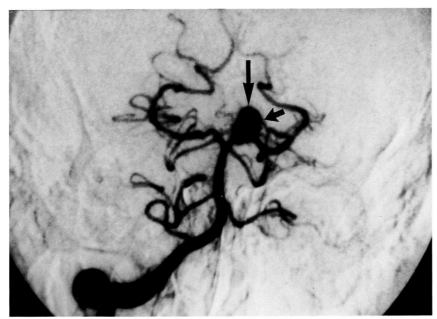

B

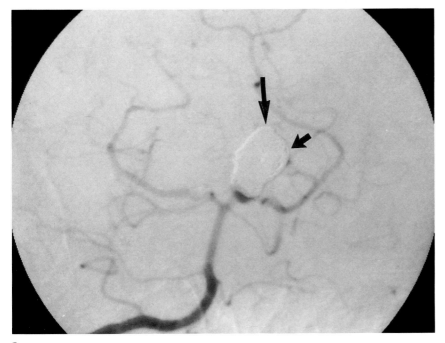

C

Fig. 28-6 (*B*) Cerebral angiogram confirms the irregularly shaped aneurysm (arrows). (*C*) Following treatment with electrolytic detachable coils placed directly into the aneurysm, there is obliteration of the aneurysm (arrows), with normal filling of the distal posterior cerebral artery.

well-defined neck in which parent vessel occlusion is to be performed. By testing patients using temporary balloon occlusion, one can assess collateral blood flow to the blocked vascular territory prior to permanent occlusion. If the patient fails the test occlusion, an extracranial-to-intracranial bypass graft can first be per-

formed to increase blood flow to the affected vascular territory.[18,33]

Direct occlusion of aneurysms is now being performed with detachable balloons, coils, and electrolytic detachable coils in controlled clinical trials. The preliminary results are encouraging for small aneurysms (<15 mm in diameter) with small (<5 mm) necks. By tightly packing off the aneurysm, thrombosis without recanalization, appears feasible. However, for larger aneurysms with wide necks, interventional treatment to completely thrombose the aneurysm is more difficult.

Another limitation of endovascular embolization therapy is that these procedures are performed with anticoagulation to avoid thrombus formation on the catheters and embolic materials. In the patient with an acutely ruptured aneurysm, anticoagulation may precipitate further bleeding. There is also the possibility of dislodging thrombus, which may already be present within an aneurysm, during placement of the occlusion device. Subtotal occlusion of an aneurysm may result in delayed hemorrhage or continued aneurysm growth.[34,35] The balloons or coils may shift or "compact" after placement, resulting in subtotal occlusion, parent vessel occlusion, or delayed embolic occlusion of normal vessels. Finally, long-term follow-up is required for patients treated by these interventional techniques.

CONCLUSION

Continued advances in the field of interventional neurovascular radiology have improved the safety, efficacy, and morbidity of patients with ruptured and unruptured intracerebral aneurysms. Newer devices and techniques are currently being investigated for treatment of aneurysms, including intravascular stents and lasers.[36-38] Improvements in microcatheters, high-resolution fluoroscopic imaging, improved radiographic screening modalities such as ultrafast CT and magnetic resonance angiography (MRA), and advances in intravascular occlusive devices will continue to broaden the indications for treatment of patients with complex cerebrovascular disorders.

REFERENCES

1. Serbinenko FA. Catheterization and occlusion of major cerebral vessels and prospects for the development of vascular neurosurgery. *Vopr Neirokhir* 1971;35:17–27.

2. Serbinenko FA. Balloon catheterization and occlusion of major cerebral vessels. *J Neurosurg* 1974;41:125–145.

3. Hieshima GB, Reicher MA, Higashida RT, et al. Intraoperative digital subtraction neuroangiography: A diagnostic and therapeutic tool. *Am J Neuroradiol* 1987;8(5):759–768.

4. Higashida RT, Halbach VV, Hieshima GB. Endovascular therapy of intracranial aneurysms, in *Interventional Neuroradiology: Endovascular Therapy of the Central Nervous System*. New York, Raven Press, 1992, pp 51–62.

5. Higashida RT, Halbach VV, Hieshima GB. Treatment of complex intracranial aneurysms by interventional techniques, in Margulis AR, Gooding CA, (eds): *Diagnostic Radiology 1989*. University of California Printing Services, San Francisco, 1989, pp 357–360.

6. Camarata PJ, Latchaw RE, Rufenacht DA, et al. Intracranial aneurysms. *Invest Radiol*, 1993;28(4):373–382.

7. Kassell NF, Torner JC. Epidemiology of intracranial aneurysms. *Int Anesthesiol Clin* 1982;20:13–17.

8. Weir B. Epidemiology, in Weir B (ed): *Aneurysms Affecting the Nervous System*. Baltimore, Williams & Wilkins, 1987, pp 1–53.

9. Adams HP Jr, Kassell NF, Torner JC, et al. Early management of aneurysmal subarachnoid hemorrhage: A report of the cooperative aneurysm study: *J Neurosurg* 1981;54:141–145.

10. Graf CJ. Prognosis for patients with nonsurgically-treated aneurysms. Analysis of the cooperative study of intracranial aneurysms and subarachnoid hemorrhage. *J Neurosurg* 1971;35:438–443.

11. Sundt TM. History of the recognition and management of intracranial aneurysms, in *Surgical Techniques for Saccular and Giant Intracranial Aneurysms*. Baltimore, Williams & Wilkins, 1990, pp xv–xxiii.

12. Higashida RT, Halbach VV, Dormandy B, et al. Endovascular treatment of intracranial aneurysms with a new silicone microballoon device: Technical considerations and indications for therapy. *Radiology* 1990;174:687–691.

13. Higashida RT, Hieshima GB, Halbach VV, et al. Intravascular detachable balloon embolization of intracranial aneurysms: Indications and techniques. *Acta Radiol* 1986;369:594–596.

14. Berenstein A, Lasjaunias P. Indications and results of endovascular treatment of aneurysms, in Berenstein A, Lasjaunias P (eds): *Surgical Neuroangiography*, Vol 5. New York, Springer-Verlag, 1992, 149–184.

15. Debrun G, Fox A, Drake C, et al. Giant unclippable aneurysms: Treatment with detachable balloons. *Am J Neuroradiol*, 1981;2:167–173.

16. Goto K, Halbach VV, Hardin CW, et al. Permanent inflation of detachable balloons with a low-viscosity, hydrophilic polymerizing system. *Radiology* 1988;169:787–790.

17. Taki W, Handa H, Yamagata S, et al. Radio-opaque solidifying liquids for releasable balloon technique: A technical note. *Surg Neurol* 1980;13:140–142.

18. Fox AJ, Vinuela F, Pelz DM, et al. Use of detachable balloons for proximal artery occlusion in the treatment

of unclippable cerebral aneurysms. *J Neurosurg* 1987;66: 40–46.

19. Higashida RT, Halbach VV, Dowd CF, et al. Interventional neurovascular treatment of a giant intracranial aneurysm using platinum micro coils. *Surg Neurol* 1991; 35(1):64–68.

20. Hilal S. Synthetic fiber coated platinum coils successfully used for the endovascular treatment of arteriovenous malformations, aneurysms, and direct arteriovenous fistulae of the central nervous system. Presented to the American Society of Neuroradiology. Chicago, May 15–20, 1988.

21. Moret JG, Boulin A, Mawad ME, et al. Adjustable and detachable tungsten spirales (MDS system) for treatment of intracranial aneurysms: Characteristics of the device, comparison with existing detachable coils, analysis of results (abstract). Presented to the 31st Annual Meeting of the American Society of Neuroradiology, Vancouver, May 16–20, 1993.

22. Yang PJ, Halbach VV, Higashida RT, et al. Platinum wire: A new transvascular embolic agent. *AJNR* 1983;9: 547–550.

23. Guglielmi G. Endovascular treatment of intracranial aneurysms, in Vinuela F, Dion J, Duckwiler G (eds): *Neuroimaging Clinics of North America: Interventional Neuroradiology*, Vol 2, No 2. Philadelphia, WB Saunders, 1992, 269–278.

24. Guglielmi G, Vinuela F, Duckwiler G, et al. Endovascular treatment of posterior circulation aneurysms by electrothrombosis using electrically detachable coils. *J Neurosurg* 1992;77:515–524.

25. Guglielmi G, Vinuela F, Sepetka I, et al. Electrothrombosis of saccular aneurysms via endovascular approach. Part I: Electrochemical basis, technique, and experimental results. *J Neurosurg* 1991;75:1–7.

26. Kinugasa K, Mandai S, Terai Y, et al. Direct thrombosis of aneurysms with cellulose acetate polymer. Part II: Preliminary clinical experience. *J Neurosurg* 1992;77: 501–507.

27. Mandai S, Kinugasa K, Ohmoto T. Direct thrombosis of aneurysms with cellulose acetate polymer. Part I: Results of thrombosis in experimental aneurysms. *J Neurosurg* 1992;77:497–500.

28. Romodanov AP, Shchegelov VI. Intravascular occlusion of saccular aneurysms of the cerebral arteries by means of a detachable balloon catheter, in Krayenbuhl H (ed):

Advances and Technical Standards in Neurosurgery, Vol 9. New York, Springer-Verlag, 1982, pp 25–49.

29. Shchegelov VI. Endovascular occlusion of saccular intracranial aneurysms: Results in 617 patients. Proceedings of the 27th Annual Meeting of the American Society of Neuroradiology, Orlando, FL, March 1989.

30. Moret J, Picard L, Mawad M, et al. A critical study on endosaccular treatment of berry aneurysm based on 60 cases. Proceeding of the 28th Annual Meeting of the American Society of Neuroradiology, Los Angeles, March 1990.

31. Higashida RT, Halbach VV, Dowd CF, et al. Intracranial aneurysms: Interventional neurovascular treatment with detachable balloons—results in 215 cases. *Radiology* 1991;178:663–670.

32. Higashida RT, Halbach VV, Barnwell SL, et al. Treatment of intracranial aneurysms with preservation of the parent vessel: Results of percutaneous balloon embolization in 84 patients. *AJNR* 1990;11:633–640.

33. Gelber BR, Sundt TM Jr: Treatment of intracavernous and giant carotid aneurysms by combined internal carotid ligation and extra- to intracranial bypass. *J Neurosurg* 1965;23:572–577.

34. Drake CG, Vanderlinden RG. The late consequences of incomplete surgical treatment of cerebral aneurysms. *J Neurosurg* 1967;27:226–238.

35. Ebina K, Suzuki M, Andoh A, et al. Recurrence of cerebral aneurysm after initial neck clipping. *Neurosurgery.* 1982;11:764–768.

36. Geremia G, Haklin M, Charletta D, et al. Embolization of experimentally created aneurysms with intravascular stent devices (abstract). 60th Annual Meeting of the American Association of Neurological Surgeons, San Francisco, April 11–16, 1992.

37. Marks MP, Dake M, Lane B, et al. Stent placement for arterial and venous cerebral vascular disease: Preliminary clinical experience (abstract). Presented at the 31st Annual Meeting of the American Society of Neuroradiology, Vancouver, May 16–20, 1993.

38. Szikora I, Guterman LR, Wells K, et al. Combined use of tantalum stents and electrically detachable coils in the endovascular treatment of giant wide necked aneurysms (abstract). Presented at the 31st Annual Meeting of the American Society of Neuroradiology, Vancouver, May 16–20, 1993.

29

Thrombolytic Treatment in the Setting of an Acute Stroke

Kenneth Alfieri, M.D., Fong Y. Tsai, M.D.

INTRODUCTION

In the setting of a progressive stroke, the goal of therapy is to minimize the volume of infarcted tissue and preserve as much of the ischemic neural tissue (the ischemic penumbra) as possible. This can be achieved with infusion of thrombolytic agents into the involved vessel. If this is accomplished in the appropriate time frame, neurologic deficits can be reversed. Systemic anticoagulation with heparin has been unsatisfactory in the setting of a stroke in progress.[1-3] The thrombolytic agents streptokinase, urokinase and tissue plasminogen activator have been applied with great success in the therapy of peripheral vascular thrombosis.[4-20] With the advent of microcatheter delivery systems, these agents can now be administered directly to arterial and venous thrombi within the central nervous system. The thrombolytic agents have a short intravascular half-life, induce rapid clot dissolution, and have acceptably low systemic hemorrhagic complication rates.

Ischemic Stroke

Thromboembolic insults to the arterial supply of the brain are the most common cause of ischemic strokes. These thromboemboli arise from the cardiac chambers (during an arrhythmia) or from atherosclerotic plaques in the carotid bifurcation or vertebral arteries. A stroke may also arise from an occlusion of a venous structure such as one of the dural sinuses. Complete anoxia will result in an infarct within a few minutes. An acute decrease in flow to 25% of normal perfusion can initiate an ischemic event.[21] The clinical course of an ischemic stroke is frequently progressive. This provides a window of opportunity for thrombolytic intervention which can halt the progression and prevent irreversible neuronal damage.

Spontaneous fibrinolysis can occur but may not do so early enough to avoid a permanent deficit. Angiography is not frequently performed earlier than 12 to 24 hr after an acute thromboembolic event, and the intrinsic fibrinolytic system may lyse the clot during this interval. This probably explains why cerebrovascular emboli are detected less than 50% of the time during angiography. However, if arteriography is performed earlier than 12 hr after the onset of an acute stroke, the causative occlusion can be identified in as many as 90% of cases.[22,23]

In addition to arterial ischemia, a stroke may result from a venous occlusion. Venous stroke, which has not received its share of medical attention until recently, is primarily the result of venous congestion rather than arterial ischemia. Dural sinus thrombosis is probably underrecognized clinically and may be associated with a variety of conditions, including dehydration, hyper-coagulable states, infections of the mastoids, disseminated intravascular coagulation (DIC), sickle cell disease, trauma, pregnancy, and neoplasms.[24]

The following is an overview of the approach to the patient with an acute arterial or venous thrombosis of the central nervous system and a description of patient selection, preparation, and postthrombolytic care. Also discussed is the optimal timing of thrombolysis and the complication rates associated with this intervention.

PRELIMINARY PATIENT EVALUATION

Before initiating thrombolytic treatment, the patient must be evaluated for risk factors for hemorrhagic complications. Baseline laboratory values and a coagulation profile must be obtained, including hemoglobin, hematocrit, platelet count, fibrinogen level, prothrombin time, and activated partial thromboplastin time.

Magnetic resonance imaging (MRI) and/or computed tomography (CT) are the modalities that are almost invariably utilized in patient evaluation before angiography is performed. A CT scan should be done immediately after complete physical and neurologic examinations. After the CT scan, the patient is transferred directly to a neuroangiographic room for cerebral angiography. The cerebral examination must include arch aortography, as well as extra- and intracranial carotid and vertebral angiography.

MRI is more sensitive than CT in the evaluation of a suspected cerebrovascular occlusion; however, MRI may not always be practical in the superacute stage of a stroke because the patient may be clinically unstable. Utilizing standard spin-echo techniques, MRI can demonstrate compromised arterial flow as an intraluminal signal within vessels that should normally show a signal void. This is particularly true in the internal carotid arteries and the Sylvian portions of the middle cerebral arteries as they are imaged in the transaxial plane. Unfortunately, this is a nonspecific finding, and spin-echo imaging cannot differentiate reliably between a stenosis and a complete occlusion. However, two-dimensional and three-dimensional time-of-flight MR angiography (MRA) can make this differentiation reliably. With MRA, a discontinuity in the vessel signal is a sign of decreased vessel caliber, whereas an occlusion is demonstrated as nonvisualization of distal vessel branches.[25] MRA is limited in that it cannot provide adequate information about small peripheral vessels. Small vessel visualization can be improved by adminis-

tration of the carbonic anhydrase inhibitor acetazolamide 20 min before the MRA.[26]

Contraindications to thrombolytic treatment include active hemorrhaging, recent cerebrovascular hemorrhage, and intracerebral tumor or vascular malformation. Relative contraindications are recent major surgery (less than 10 days ago), recent serious trauma, internal hemorrhage and severe uncontrolled hypertension.[27]

In an early pilot study utilizing systemic (rather than intra-arterial) urokinase in patients with completed strokes, a 25% intracerebral hemorrhage rate was observed, with no demonstrable therapeutic benefit.[28,29] Recent studies using microcatheter techniques and local infusions directly into the thrombus or between the thrombus and the wall of the vessel have demonstrated generally lower hemorrhagic complication rates (approximately 13%). The observed risk factors for intracerebral hemorrhagic complications were brain stem infarction, occlusion of lenticulostriate arteries, and late (beyond 6 hr) initiation of thrombolytic therapy.[30-34]

TECHNIQUES OF THROMBOLYSIS

With recent advances in catheter techniques, superselective local application of thrombolytic agents to the thromboembolus has become practical for extra- and intracranial vessels.

The procedure begins with a routine angiographic examination, usually by way of a transfemoral approach with a 5F catheter to delineate the location of the thrombus. By using a coaxial technique, a 2F or 3F Tracker catheter (Target Therapeutics—San Jose, CA) can be advanced into intracranial branches of the carotid or vertebrobasilar artery. The catheters utilized generally have multiple side holes, which enhance the thrombolytic effect.

If a cerebrovenous occlusion is suspected, a 5F catheter is advanced to the jugular bulb using the transfemoral vein approach. A Tracker catheter is introduced coaxially through the 5F catheter. The catheter is then navigated to the occluded dural sinus for direct dural sinus venography and thrombolysis.[35,36]

Once the occlusion or thrombus is identified, 5000 units of intravenous heparin is given; if necessary, an additional 1,000 units of heparin is given every hour. The infusion catheter is slowly advanced to the thrombosed area with a soft-tipped guidewire positioned just beyond the end of the catheter. The catheter and guidewire are then gently pushed into the thrombus. A thrombolytic agent is administered with intermittent injections rather than via a continuous infusion. We prefer to inject 250,000 IU immediately and then 80,000 IU every 15 min, in a concentration of about 8,000 IU/ml, until thrombolysis is completed.

THROMBOLYSIS AT SPECIFIC SITES

Extracranial Carotid Artery

Acute occlusion of the internal carotid artery usually is associated with a proximal stenosis which results in progressive propagation of clot and partial or complete occlusion. An occluded internal carotid artery may contain both fresh and aged thrombus. Segments of those clots may dislodge and occlude distal intracranial branches after the major thrombus is broken up. Routine intracranial angiography is needed to search for these distal occlusions. Thrombolysis is done after superselective catheterization of the involved intracranial vessels according to the technique described above (Fig. 29-1).

Middle Cerebral Artery (MCA)

The clinical symptoms of MCA occlusion may be somewhat different, depending upon the site of the occlusion and possible existence of collaterals. Dense hemiplegia usually results from the occlusion of lenticulostriate branches. The lenticulostriate territory has no collateral vasculature; therefore, the timing of thrombolysis is more urgent when these vessels are involved than with a distal MCA occlusion. Hemorrhage more commonly occurs when there has been a delay between the onset of stroke and the institution of thrombolytic treatment.[37,38]

As a general rule, satisfactory dissolution of a thrombus cannot be achieved if the tip of the catheter is not directly in the clot or between the clot and the vessel wall. If the catheter cannot be advanced into the clot for technical reasons, there is a real danger that the thrombolytic agent will not reach the clot and may instead perfuse proximal arterial branches that do not contain clot; hemorrhagic complications may then result (Figs. 29-2, 29-3).

The intermittent infusion technique allows incremental advancement of the catheter (if this is technically possible) as the clot dissolves. Frequent digital subtraction angiography (DSA) imaging can be used to monitor this process. We believe that this method minimizes both the infusion of uninvolved vessels and

the risk of hemorrhage. The risk of hemorrhage can be significant when treating thromboses of the lenticulostriate and thalamoperforator arteries. Since we have adopted the intermittent infusion technique, we have not experienced hemorrhagic complications in these territories.

Thrombosis of the MCA is frequently associated with an underlying stenosis (Fig. 29-4). Occasionally, angioplasty of the stenosis is required to prevent rethrombosis after thrombolysis is completed.[39]

Ophthalmic and Central Retinal Arteries

The occlusion of branches of the ophthalmic artery or the central retinal artery often leads to blindness if immediate treatment is not instituted. After our initial report of superselective ophthalmic angiography,[40] we applied thrombolytic techniques to those patients with acute visual loss due to occlusion of the central retinal artery. A 2F microcatheter is generally used in this setting (Fig. 29-5).

Vertebrobasilar Artery

Vertebrobasilar artery occlusion may be due to a dislodged embolus from the heart or a proximal vertebral artery stenosis with distal proliferation of the thrombus. Distal vertebral artery stenosis can lead to propagation of the thrombus, resulting in occlusion of the posterior inferior cerebellar artery (PICA). The coma center is supplied by thalamoperforators which are branches of the posterior cerebral artery. The comatose patient with a basilar artery occlusion may not regain consciousness if the occlusion of the thalamoperforators is not reopened (Fig. 29-6).

Dural Sinus Occlusion

Clinical and radiographic findings may be very nonspecific in the setting of an acute dural sinus thrombosis. This condition causes extensive morbidity and mortality by creating severe venous congestion, which can lead to a massive venous infarction.

Less is known about the natural history of occlusive disease involving the intracranial dural sinuses and veins than about arterial thrombosis. There is a wide variety of septic and aseptic etiologies for this condition, including tumors (meningiomas, meningeal metastasis, leukemia), trauma (subdural or epidural hematoma), infection (mastoiditis, subdural or epidural empyema, meningitis, encephalitis, brain abscess, sinusitis, DIC), low flow states and coagulopathies, as

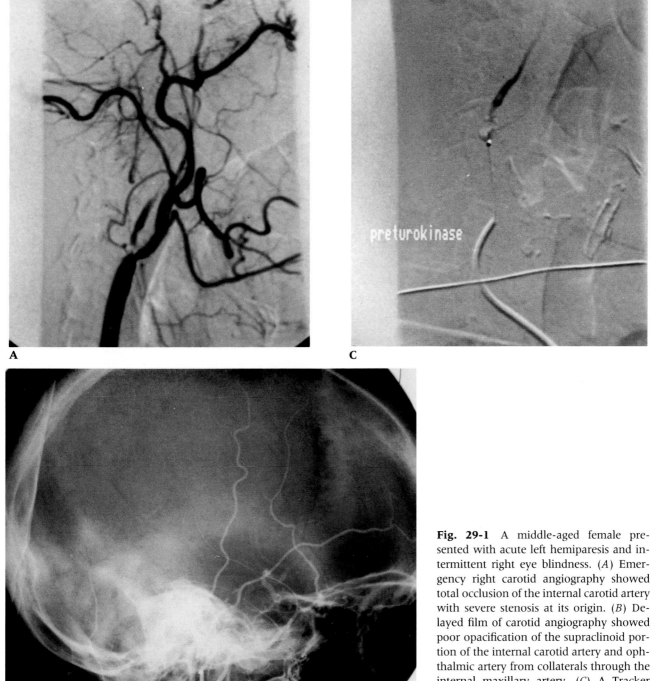

Fig. 29-1 A middle-aged female presented with acute left hemiparesis and intermittent right eye blindness. (*A*) Emergency right carotid angiography showed total occlusion of the internal carotid artery with severe stenosis at its origin. (*B*) Delayed film of carotid angiography showed poor opacification of the supraclinoid portion of the internal carotid artery and ophthalmic artery from collaterals through the internal maxillary artery. (*C*) A Tracker catheter was placed into the proximal internal carotid artery coaxially through a 5F angiographic catheter at the common carotid artery.

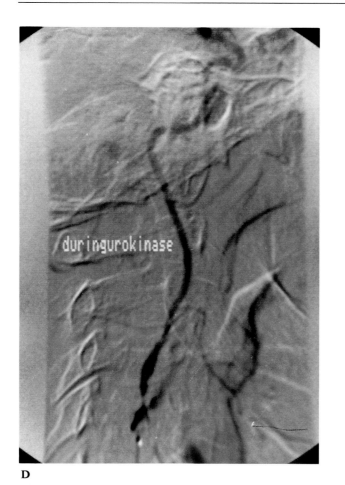

D

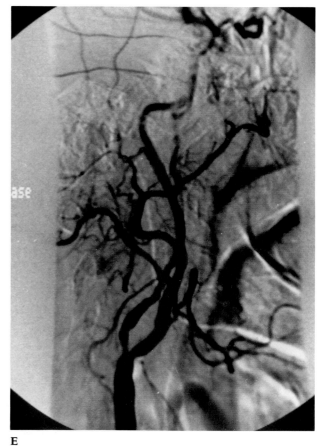

E

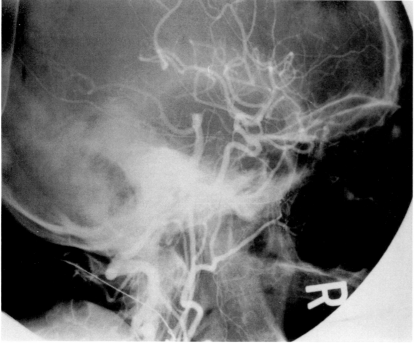

F

Fig. 29-1 (*D*) DSA of the right carotid artery. Injection during thrombolysis showed recanalization of the occluded internal carotid artery. (*E,F*) Right common carotid angiography showed recanalization of the extracranial and intracranial portions of the right internal carotid artery. The patient recovered without deficit and had an endarterectomy for carotid stenosis 3 months later.

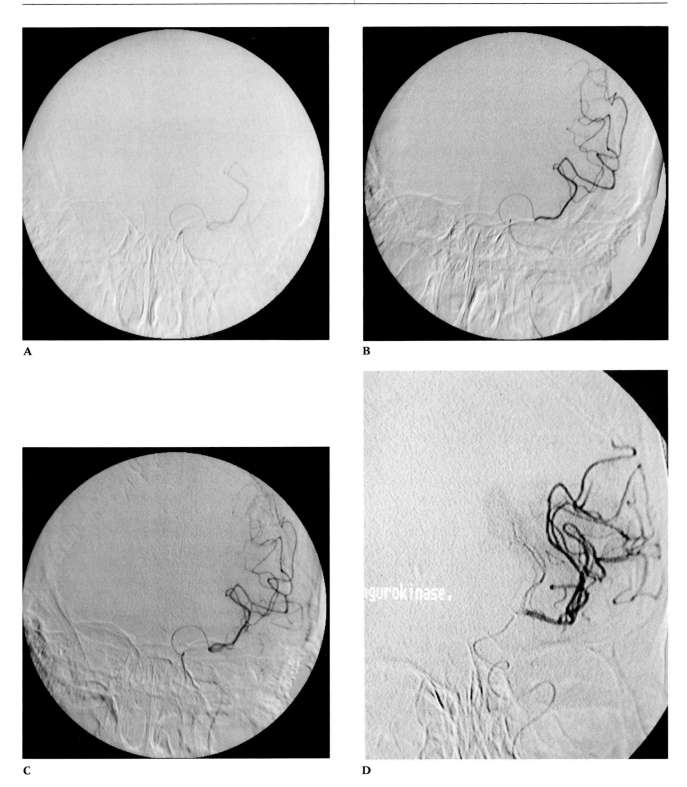

Fig. 29-2 (*A*) DSA of the left MCA showed the tip of the Tracker catheter at the M$_2$ segment with a distal occlusion. (*B,C*) Postthrombolytic DSA showed recanalization of the left MCA. (*D*) The tip of the Tracker catheter frequently stayed at the origin of the lenticulostriate artery. It is preferable to advance the tip of the catheter beyond the origin after good visualization of those arteries.

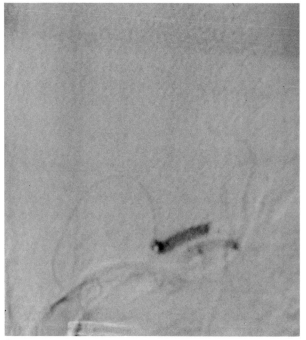

A

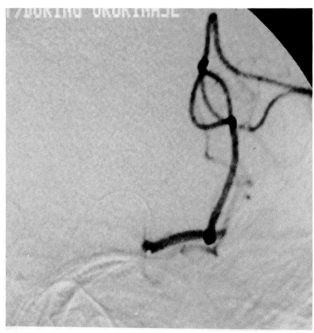

B

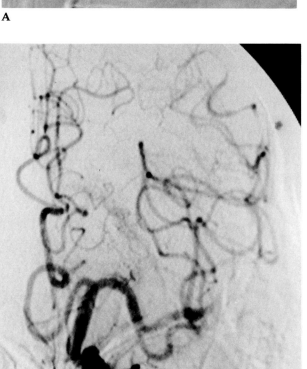

C

Fig. 29-3 (*A*) DSA of the left MCA showed complete occlusion of the posterior parietal artery. (*B*) DSA of the left MCA during thrombolysis showed recanalization of the left posterior parietal artery. (*C*) Left carotid angiography showed normal anterior and MCA arteries.

well as numerous miscellaneous conditions (diabetes, postoperative state, oral contraceptive use, pregnancy and the postpartum state, etc.). Venous sinus thrombosis can be diagnosed noninvasively with contrast-enhanced CT (by the "empty delta" sign, a triangular filling defect at the posterior confluence of the dural sinuses) and by a persistent loss of normal signal void in the involved dural sinus on MRI (an increased signal in the sinus lumen suggests the presence of slow, turbulent flow or thrombus in the vessel). It is estimated that parenchymal hemorrhages accompany approximately 20% of dural sinus thromboses.[41]

An acutely thrombosed dural sinus may have an isointense appearance on spin-echo MRI sequences. Therefore routine MRI might miss the finding of an intracranial acute dural sinus thrombosis. Thrombus in the superior sagittal sinus can be identified more easily than transverse sinus, sigmoid sinus or vein of Galen thromboses. The most common MRI finding in the setting of an acute dural sinus thrombosis is simply a mass effect, and frequently the mass effect is not associated with abnormal signal on T_2-weighted images. When abnormal signal is present on T_2-weighted images, it is less extensive than the mass effect. This signal may be reversible and is not necessarily a sign of an infarction; it probably represents interstitial edema. Abnormal parenchymal enhancement does not occur, and breakdown of the blood–brain barrier apparently does not

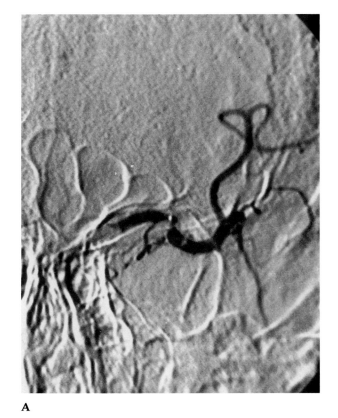

A

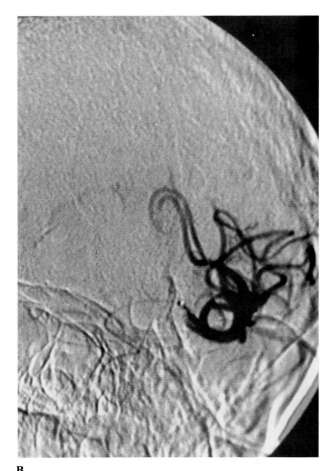

B

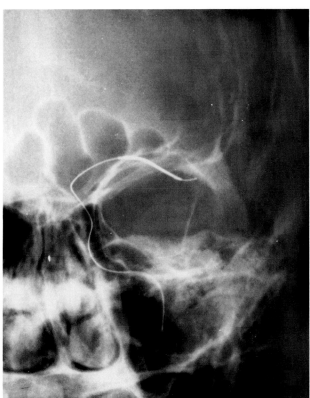

C

Fig. 29-4 *(A,B)* DSA showed stenosis of the MCA with re-thrombosis. *(C)* A Stealth catheter was placed at the MCA for angioplasty to prevent further rethromboses.

result from the venous occlusion.[42] Some investigators feel that time-of-flight venous MRA is the preferred method of evaluating patients suspected of having an acute venous occlusion. With this technique, flowing blood is conspicuous as high signal that stands out against a dark background. A fresh thrombus will manifest itself as a region of signal void.[43]

There are several reports of successful treatment of acute dural sinus thrombosis in adults and infants with urokinase. By using an approach through the femoral vein, a coaxial catheter system identical to the one used for arterial procedures can be employed to bring the tip of the microcatheter into the involved dural sinus. A typical dose of urokinase in this setting is 4,000 IU/hr until the clot is dissolved, which may take several hours. An intermittent injection technique of urokinase may be used as well. The microcatheter is repeatedly advanced into the remaining clot as lysis proceeds. Sys-

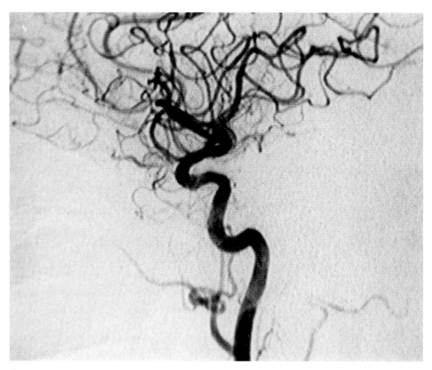

A

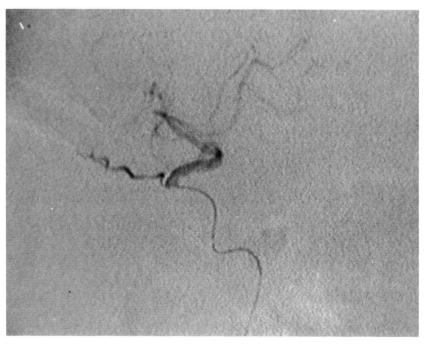

B

Fig. 29-5 Ophthalmic artery occlusion. (*A*) Carotid artery angiography showed acute occlusion of the distal two-thirds of the ophthalmic artery at the crossing point of the optic nerve (arrow). (*B*) DSA showed the tip of the Tracker catheter at the origin of the ophthalmic artery. Contrast refluxed into the internal carotid artery.

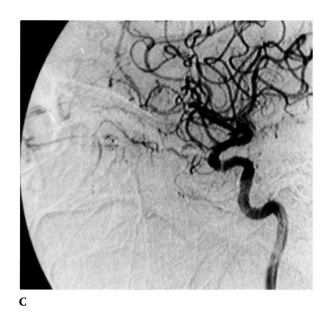

C

Fig. 29-5 (*C*) Postthrombolytic angiography showed recanalization of the whole ophthalmic artery with a choroidal blush.

temic anticoagulation with heparin is administered with the urokinase. At the conclusion of clot lysis, the catheter system may be removed from the venous access site, with little risk of local bleeding complications.[35,36,44-48] In the setting of dural venous thrombosis, the timing of thrombolytic therapy is very important. The optimal time of thrombolysis for an acute dural sinus thrombosis is at the first sign of clinical deterioration. If the patient's clinical condition deteriorates, thrombolysis must be initiated as soon as possible because the patient may suddenly lapse into a coma.[35] The dose of the thrombolytic agent for dural sinus thrombosis may be the same as that used for arterial thromboses. Systemic anticoagulation with heparin is given along with the thrombolytic treatment (Figs. 29-7, 29-8).

Correlation can be made between clinical symptoms, dural venous sinus pressure and CT/MRI findings. Five stages of dural venous thrombosis can be based on these parameters, and the prognosis becomes poorer with increasing stage.[49,50] Stage I patients have dural sinus pressures less than 20 mm Hg and no parenchymal changes on CT and/or MRI. Symptoms are headache, decreased mental status, drowsiness and papilledema. In stage II, dural sinus pressures are higher (20–25 mm Hg) and parenchymal changes are present: these are brain swelling, sulcal effacement, and a mass effect but no increased signal on MRI. Symptoms in-

clude double vision, seizures, and focal weakness, in addition to the stage I symptoms.

In stage III, patients are obtunded and unarousable and have moderate edema with areas of increased signal on MRI. These patients have dural sinus pressures of 32 to 38 mm Hg. Those with pressures of 42 to 51 mm Hg are comatose, and have dense hemiparesis with more severe brain swelling and small parenchymal hemorrhages (stage IV). Stage V patients are in a deep coma, with massive edema and hemorrhage; pressures in excess of 50 mm Hg are postulated to occur.

Up to stage III, the parenchymal changes can be reversible if thrombolytic therapy is instituted appropriately. Some stage IV patients have residual neurologic deficits, and all stage V patients have fatal outcomes (Figs. 29-9, 29-10).

COMPLICATIONS AND RESULTS

Most patients who receive local thrombolytic treatment have moderate or severe deficits at the end of thrombolysis. However, it is common for these patients to improve progressively. Frequently patients recover completely within a few days. Those patients with an early recovery usually have a better prognosis. Even if patients do not have a complete recovery, the thrombolytic treatment can be beneficial by halting clinical deterioration. Patients with dural sinus thrombosis have a much better prognosis than those with an arterial stroke. Generally, the earlier thrombolysis begins, the better the result will be. Earlier treatment also results in fewer complications.[30,31,46-52]

The main complication of arterial thrombolytic treatment is hemorrhage. Three patients in our series had hemorrhage during thrombolysis using a continuous infusion. This represents about 4% of all patients who received thrombolysis. Forty-nine percent of patients had partial or complete recovery. Thirty-three percent had moderate deficits, and 14% had severe deficits. No hemorrhagic complication was noted in those patients with dural sinus thrombosis. All of our patients with dural sinus thrombosis recovered completely, with one exception; this patient had a moderate deficit from a large cerebellar infarct. In this individual there was a 4-day interval between clinical deterioration and the institution of thrombolytic therapy.[35,36]

CT examinations are frequently performed on patients shortly after thrombolysis. It is not uncommon for these studies to demonstrate high-attenuation brain parenchymal lesions that are suggestive of an acute hemorrhage. These lesions are often seen in the basal

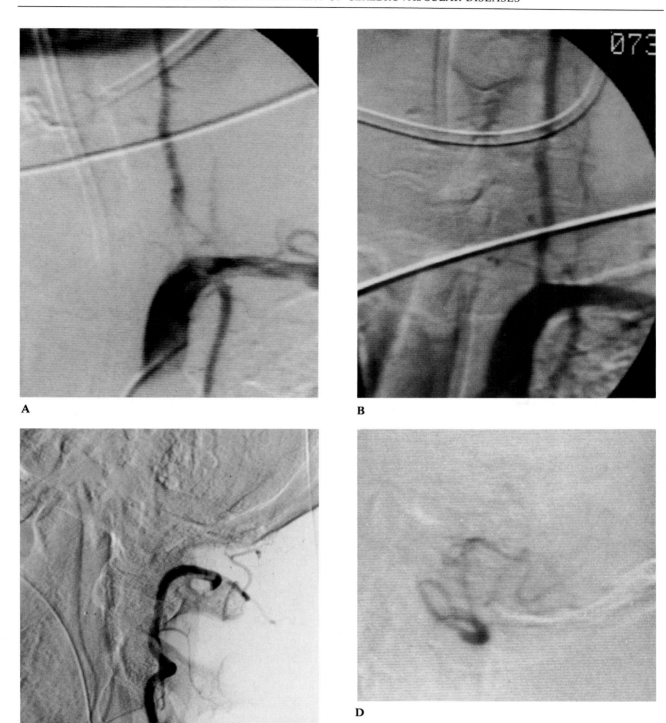

Fig. 29-6 Vertebral artery occlusion. (*A*) DSA of the left subclavian artery showing thrombosis of the proximal left vertebral artery. (*B*) Postthrombolytic angiography showed restoration of the left vertebral artery. (*C*) Left vertebral angiography showed occlusion of the distal vertebral artery at the C_1 level. (*D*) DSA during thrombolysis showed partial recanalization of the distal vertebral artery and left PICA.

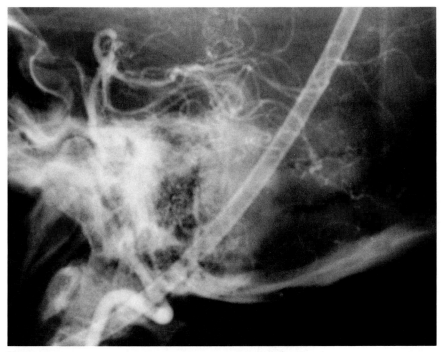

E

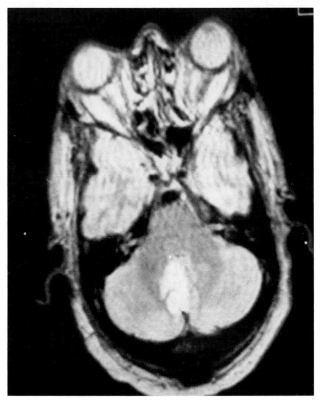

F

Fig. 29-6 (*E*) Postthrombolytic angiography showed complete restoration of posterior fossa circulation. (*F*) Follow-up MRI showed residual infarct at the inferior vermis.

ganglia that are ipsilateral to the vessel that received the urokinase infusion. The incidence of this finding varies widely; in one study involving a small number of patients, it was seen in 60% of the cases. Only 20% of the cases were associated with clinical deterioration. The remainder had clearing of the radiodense lesions within 24 hr, and these patients did not worsen clinically. These data suggest that CT evidence of an acute intraparenchymal hemorrhage soon after treatment is not necessarily a bad prognostic sign in all cases.[53]

DISCUSSION

The traditional treatment for acute cerebrovascular occlusion is anticoagulation. However, the results of anticoagulation have not been encouraging. Anticoagulation may enhance spontaneous lysis of a thrombus; however, the outcome is not predictably favorable.[1–3]

Ischemic stroke frequently results in catastrophic morbidity and is a leading cause of death in the United States. Effective early treatment of an acute stroke is essential to prevent devastating sequelae. This is especially important for patients whose stroke symptoms are progressive at the time of presentation. The use of heparin for the treatment of a progressive ischemic stroke has been widespread for the past 30 years. However, 25–36% of patients continue to deteriorate while receiving heparin treatment.[34]

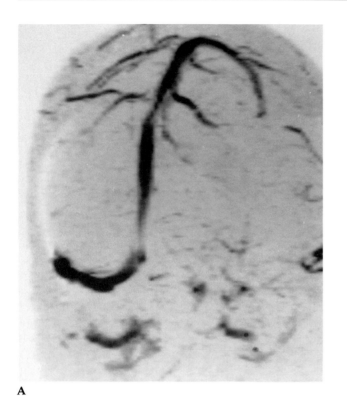

A

The demonstration of an acute thrombosis with angiography performed early in the process (within 12 hr) provides a theoretical basis for the use of thrombolytic agents in this setting. Thrombolytic agents increase perfusion to the infarct and adjacent cerebral tissue by dissolving the thrombus; they prevent thrombus propagation as well. Intravenous systemic thrombolytic therapy (as opposed to standard anticoagulation therapy) has been attempted to treat acute cerebrovascular thromboembolic disease for nearly 20 years; the results have not been satisfactory. High rates of morbidity and mortality are associated with intravenous therapy when high doses are used; when low doses are used, there is no apparent clinical benefit. As an example, a multicenter clinical study with intravenous recombinant tissue plasminogen activator (rt-PA) produced unsatisfactory clinical results and unacceptable hemorrhagic complication rates.[54] With recent improvements in catheter techniques, local intra-arterial or intradural sinus thrombolysis has become feasible. Urokinase is favored over streptokinase for local infusions because of its shorter half-life and fewer systemic effects. The timing of thrombolytic treatment of arterial occlusions is somewhat different from that of dural sinus throm-

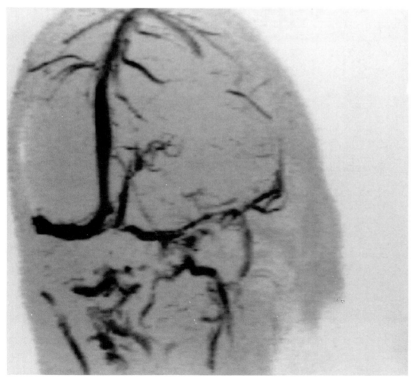

Fig. 29-7 Dural sinus thrombosis. (*A*) Two-dimensional time-of-flight MR venography showed occlusion of the straight sinus, torcular region, and Galenic venous system. (*B*) Postthrombolytic MR venography showed recanalization of the dural sinus and Galenic venous system.

B

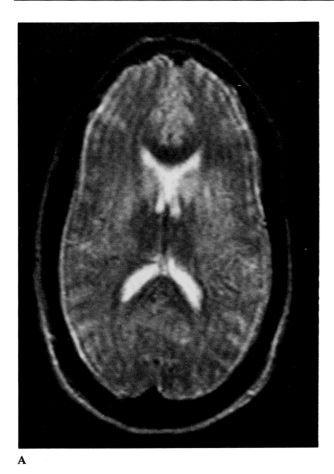

A

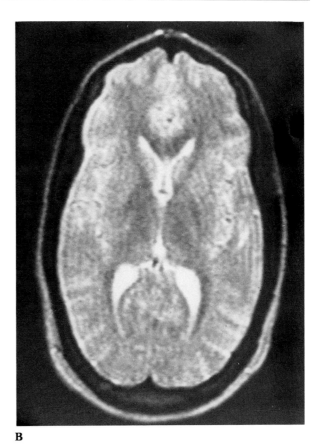

B

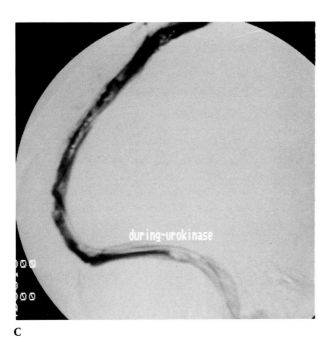

C

Fig. 29-8 Thrombolytic treatment of the superior sagittal sinus. (*A*) Lateral view of the skull showed a 4-cm-length multiple side hole Tracker catheter in the posterior half of the superior sagittal sinus. (Two arrows indicate the length with side holes.) (*B*) Dural sinus venography after administration of 6 million IU of urokinase showed some residual thrombosis in the superior sagittal sinus. (*C*) Dural sinus venography showed nearly complete dissolution of thrombosis after the administration of 1 million IU of urokinase.

bosis. The so-called "golden grace" period for an arterial stroke is a more critical factor than in venous occlusions.[30,31,35,36] In our experience, dural sinus thrombosis has a longer grace period before thrombolysis needs to be performed. The initial treatment for acute dural sinus thrombosis is anticoagulation, and thrombolysis is given only if clinical deterioration occurs. However, arterial ischemia requires immediate attention. Thrombolysis should be started within 6 hr in order to have an optimal effect.[28–34] Once there is obvious edema or hemorrhage, thrombolysis is contraindicated. This is not true with dural sinus thrombosis. Thrombolytic treatment in dural sinus thrombosis is not contraindicated if edema is seen on CT or MRI scans.

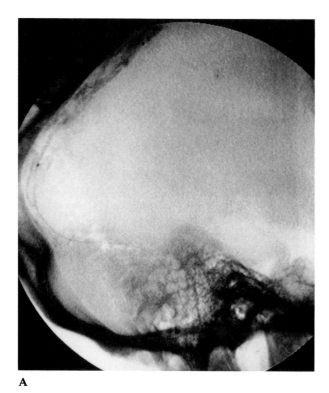

A

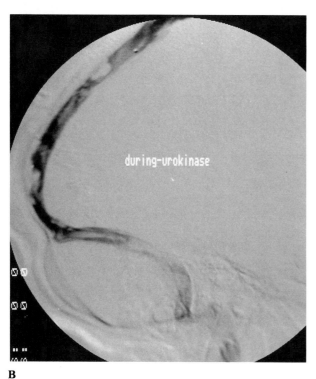

B

Fig. 29-9 (*A*) Spin-echo T$_2$-weighted MRI showed edema as high intensity at both basal ganglia from acute superior sagittal sinus thrombosis. (*B*) Postthrombolytic therapy MRI showed disappearance of edema.

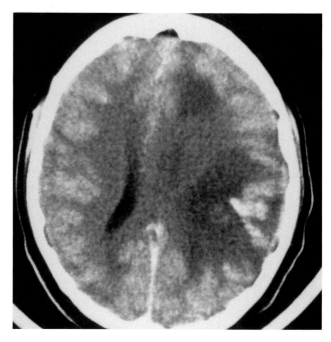

Fig. 29-10 Stage V of acute dural sinus thrombosis. Noncontrast CT scan showed hemorrhage and extensive edema of the left cerebral hemisphere from the straight and sagittal sinus thromboses. The dural sinus appeared as an area of high density on the noncontrast CT scan.

CONCLUSIONS

Until now, there has been little effective treatment for patients experiencing an acute ischemic stroke. Approximately 25% of patients with an acute stroke treated with heparin demonstrate progressive symptoms during therapy. With the advent of effective fibrinolytic agents and the development of suitable microcatheters, there now appears to be a beneficial treatment strategy available for ischemic stroke patients. It has been shown that in the setting of an evolving acute stroke, rapid intervention with local infusion of these agents can rescue neurons in the ischemic penumbra, reverse or halt the progression of clinical neurologic deficits, and do so with acceptable local and systemic complication rates. Thrombolytic therapy is clearly a major improvement over traditional anticoagulation with heparin.

REFERENCES

1. Duke RJ, Block RF, Turpie AG, et al. Intravenous heparin for the prevention of stroke progression in acute par-

tial stable stroke: A randomized controlled trial. *Ann Intern Med* 1986;105:825–828.

2. Haley EC, Kassell NF, Torner JC. Failure of heparin to prevent progression in progressing ischemic infarction. *Stroke* 1988;19:10–14.

3. Slivka A, Levy D. Natural history of progressive ischemic stroke in a population treated with heparin. *Stroke* 1990; 21:1657–1662.

4. Rentrop P, Blanke H, Karsch KR, et al. Selective intracoronary thrombolysis in acute myocardial infarction and unstable angina pectoris. *Circulation* 1981;63:307–317.

5. Ganz W, Buchbinder N, Marcus H, et al. Intracoronary thrombolysis in evolving myocardial infarction. *Am Heart J* 1981;101:4–13.

6. Timmis GC, Gangadharan V, Hauser AM, et al. Intracoronary streptokinase in clinical practice. *Am Heart J* 1982; 104:925–938.

7. Smalling RW, Fuentes F, Freund GC, et al. Beneficial effects of intracoronary thrombolysis up to eighteen hours after onset of pain in evolving myocardial infarction. *Am Heart J* 1982;104:912–920.

8. Kennedy JW, Ritchie JL, Davis KB, et al. Western Washington randomized trial of intracoronary streptokinase in acute myocardial infarction. *N Engl J Med* 1983;309: 1477–1482.

9. Leiboff RH, Katz RJ, Wasserman AG, et al. A randomized, angiographically controlled trial of intracoronary streptokinase in acute myocardial infarction. *Am J Cardiol* 1984;53:404–407.

10. TIMI Study Group. Special report: The thrombolysis in myocardial infarction (TIMI) trial. *N Engl J Med* 1985; 312:932–936.

11. Walsh P, Greenspan RH, Simon AL, et al. Urokinase-pulmonary embolism trial. *Circulation* 1978;67(Suppl II): 1–108.

12. Urokinase Pulmonary Embolism Trial Study Group. Urokinase-streptokinase embolism trial. *JAMA* 1974;229: 1606–1613.

13. Tibbutt DA, Javies JA, Anderson JA, et al. Comparison by controlled clinical trial of streptokinase and heparin in treatment of life-threatening pulmonary embolism. *Br Med J* 1974;1:343–347.

14. Mavor GE, Dhall DP. Streptokinase therapy in deep-vein thrombosis. *Br J Surg* 1973;60:468–474.

15. Kakkar VV, Lewis M, Sagar S. Treatment of deep-vein thrombosis with intermittent streptokinase and plasminogen infusion. *Lancet* 1975;1:674–676.

16. Seaman AJ, Common HH, Rosch J, et al. Deep vein thrombosis treated with streptokinase and heparin. A randomized study. *Angiology* 1976;27:549–556.

17. Serradimigni A, Bory M, Dijiane P, et al. Treatment of venous and pulmonary embolism by streptokinase. *Angiology* 1978:29:825–831.

18. D'Angelo A, Mannuci PM. Outcome of treatment of deep-vein thrombosis with urokinase: Relationship to dosage, duration of therapy, age of the thrombus and laboratory changes. *Thromb Haemostas* 1984;51: 236–239.

19. Agnelli G, Buchanan MR. A comparison of the thrombolytic and hemorrhagic effects of tissue-type plasminogen activator and streptokinase in rabbits. *Circulation* 1985; 72:178–182.

20. Risius B, Graor RA, Geisinger MA, et al. Recombinant human tissue-type plasminogen activator for thrombolysis in peripheral arteries and bypass grafts. *Radiology* 1986;160:183–188.

21. Larsen B, Lassen NA. Regulation of cerebral blood flow in health and disease. In Goldstein M, Bolis L, Fieschi C, et al (eds): *Advances in Neurology,* Vol 25. New York, Raven Press, 1979, pp 180–188.

22. Solis OJ, Roberson GR, Taveras JM, et al. Cerebral angiography in acute cerebral infarction. *Rev Interam Radiol* 1977;2:19–25.

23. Mohr JP, Caplan LR, Melski JW, et al. The Harvard Cooperative Stroke Registry. *Neurology* 1978;28:754–762.

24. Chuang S, Harwood-Nash D, Blaser S. Vascular occlusive disease: Veins and dural sinuses. In Taveras J, Ferrucci J (eds): *Radiology: Diagnosis, Imaging, Intervention.* Vol 2. Philadelphia, JB Lippincott Co, 1992, chap 49.

25. Fujita N, Hirabuki N, Fujii K, et al. MR imaging of middle cerebral artery stenosis and occlusion: Value of MR angiography. *AJNR* 1994;15:335–341.

26. Mandai K, Sueyoshi K, Fukunaga R, et al. Acetazolamide challenge for three-dimensional time-of-flight MR angiography of the brain. *AJNR* 1994;15:659–665.

27. Thrombolytic therapy in thrombosis. National Institutes of Health Consensus Development Conference, Vol 2, No. 1. *Stroke* 1981;12(1):17–21.

28. Fletcher AP, Alkjaersig N, Lewis M, et al. A pilot study of urokinase therapy in cerebral infarction. *Stroke* 1976; 7:135–142.

29. Hanaway J, Torak R, Fletcher A, et al. Intracranial bleeding associated with urokinase therapy for acute ischemic hemispheral stroke. *Stroke* 1976;7:143–146.

30. Siepmann G, Muller-Jensen M, Goossens H, et al. Local intraarterial fibrinolysis in acute middle cerebral artery occlusion. *Neuroradiology* 1991;33(Suppl):69–71.

31. Zeumer H, Freitag HJ, Knospe V. Intravascular thrombolysis in central nervous system cerebrovascular disease. *Neuroimaging Clin North Am* 1992;2:359–369.

32. Mori E, Tabuchi M, Yoshida T, et al. Intracarotid urokinase with thromboembolic occlusion of the middle cerebral artery. *Stroke* 1988;19:802–812.

33. Theron J, Courthroux P, Casasco A, et al. Local intra-arterial fibrinolysis in the carotid territory. *AJNR* 1989; 10:753–765.

34. Fieschi C, Argentino C, Lenzi GL, et al. Clinical and instrumental evaluation of patients with ischemic stroke within the first six hours. *J Neurol Sci* 1989;91:311–322.

35. Tsai FY, Higashida RT, Matovich V, et al. Acute thrombosis of the intracranial dural sinus: Direct thrombolytic treatment. *AJNR* 1992;13:1137–1141.

36. Tsai FY, Wang AM, Meoli C, et al. The optimal timing for thrombolytic treatment of acute cranial dural sinus thrombosis. Presented at the 30th annual meeting of the American Society of Neuroradiology, St Louis, MO, June 1–5, 1992.

37. Wolpert SM, Bruckmann H, Greenlee R, et al. Neuroradiologic evaluation of patients with acute stroke treated with recombinant tissue plasminogen activator. *AJNR* 1993;14:3–13.

38. Del Zoppo GJ, Poeck K, Pessin, MS, et al. Recombinant tissue plasminogen activator in acute thrombotic and embolic stroke. *Ann Neurol* 1992;32:78–86.

39. Tsai FY, Berberian B, Matovich V, et al. Percutaneous transluminal angioplasty adjunct to thrombolysis for acute MCA rethrombosis. *AJNR* 1994;15:1823–1829.

40. Tsai FY, Wadley D, Angle JF, et al. Superselective ophthalmic angiography for diagnostic and therapeutic use. *AJNR* 1990;11:1203–1204.

41. Rao CVK, Knipp HC, Wagner EJ. Computed tomographic findings in cerebral sinus and venous thrombosis. *Radiology* 1981;140:391–398.

42. Yuh WTC, Simonson TM, Wang AM, et al. Venous sinus occlusive disease: MR findings. *AJNR* 1994;15:309–316.

43. Vogl TJ, Bergman C, Villringer A, et al. Dural sinus thrombosis: Value of venous MR angiography for diagnosis and follow-up. *AJR* 1994;162:1191–1198.

44. Scott JA, Pascuzzi RM, Hall PV, et al. Treatment of dural sinus thrombosis with local urokinase infusion. *J Neurosurg* 1988;68:284–287.

45. Higashida RT, Helmer E, Halvach VV, et al. Direct thrombolytic therapy for superior sagittal sinus thrombosis. *AJNR* 1989;10:S4–S6.

46. Eskridge JM, Wessbecher FW. Thrombolysis for superior sagittal sinus thrombosis. *J Vasc Intervent Radiol* 1991;2:89–93.

47. Barnwell SL, Higashida R, Halbach VV, et al. Direct endovascular thrombolytic therapy for dural sinus thrombosis. *Neurosurgery* 1991;28:135–142.

48. Grotta JC. Current medical and surgical therapy for cerebrovascular disease. *N Engl J Med* 1987;317:1505–1516.

49. Tsai FY, Wang AM, Lavin M, et al. Correlation of venous pressure with MR brain parenchymal changes associated with acute dural sinus thrombosis. Accepted for publication by *AJNR*, 1994.

50. Tsai FY, Lavin M, Berberian B, et al. Brain parenchymal manifestations of acute cerebrovenous occlusion. Presented at the 32nd annual meeting of the American Society of Neuroradiology, Nashville, TN, May 3–7, 1994.

51. Del Zoppo GJ, Ferbert A, Otis S, et al. Local intra-arterial fibrinolytic therapy in acute carotid artery stroke. *Stroke* 1987;19:307–313.

52. Hacke W, Del Zoppo GJ, Harker LA. Thrombosis and cerebrovascular disease. In Poeck U, Ringelstein EB, Hacke W (eds): *New Trends in Diagnosis and Management of Stroke.* Berlin, Springer Verlag, 1987, pp 59–74.

53. Wildenhain S, Jungreis CA, Barr J, et al. CT after intracranial intraarterial thrombolysis for acute stroke. *AJNR* 1994;15:487–492.

54. The rt-PA Acute Stroke Study Group. An open safety/efficacy trial of rt-PA in acute thromboembolic stroke. Final report. *Stroke* 1991;22:153.

30

Angioplasty of the Supra-aortic Vessels

Donald A. Eckard, M.D., Edward L. Siegel, M.D., Solomon Batnitzky, M.D.

INTRODUCTION

Stroke is the third leading cause of death in the United States following ischemic heart disease and all forms of cancer.[1] The American Heart Association estimates that there are approximately 3 million survivors of stroke, most of whom are disabled. Prolonged nursing care is often required for those patients who survive the stroke. Therefore, it should come as no surprise that stroke is one of the most costly diseases in the United States. Approximately 15% of stroke survivors require institutional care, 30% are dependent in activities of daily living, and 60% have decreased socialization outside of the home.[2] The estimated cost of stroke-related care and lost productivity was $18 billion in 1993.[1] Stroke can occur as a result of either intracranial hemorrhage or tissue infarction. Eighty-five percent of all strokes are ischemic, mostly secondary to thromboembolic disease.[3,4] Of these, the majority are due to atherosclerotic narrowing of the supra-aortic blood vessels. While some strokes in these patients are due to reduced flow through the blood vessels, most are due either to emboli which form in areas of slow flow behind these stenotic lesions or to emboli which form

on the rough, denuded surface of the plaque. Recent studies have shown that in patients with greater than 70% stenosis (by diameter), endarterectomy dramatically reduces the incidence of stroke compared to management of these patients with medical therapy alone.[5,6] Although no studies have yet been done comparing angioplasty to endarterectomy, the studies which have been done regarding angioplasty are encouraging.[7-38]

Percutaneous transluminal angioplasty (PTA) using flexible dilators was first described by Dotter and Judkins in 1964 for the treatment of peripheral vascular disease.[39] Although the technique was successful, it was originally greeted with skepticism. Most vascular surgeons familiar with atherosclerotic disease considered it a dangerous technique. However, it was exported to Europe, where it was refined and widely utilized. After Grüntzig developed a soft, flexible, double-lumen balloon catheter, the procedure gained much more widespread acceptance.[40] Since then, it has become accepted as an effective method of treating arterial stenoses throughout most of the body.[41,42] Application to the supra-aortic vessels, though, has been slow and greeted with skepticism by most vascular surgeons due to fear of stroke from embolic discharge at the time of angioplasty. In 1968, Morris first reported dilatation of stenotic lesions in the head and neck region. He was able to use dilators at surgery to treat patients with fibromuscular dysplasia.[43] It was not until 1980 that the first reports of percutaneous carotid artery angioplasty were published by Mathias et al.[44] The number of cases of supra-aortic angioplasty performed is slowly increasing as the number of reports of its efficacy and relative safety grow. It is expected that the number of supra-aortic angioplasty procedures will continue to increase, spurred in part by the cost savings compared to surgical therapy. Improvements in the equipment used to perform the procedures (catheters, wires, stents, etc.) should continue, as well as improvements in the medical management of postangioplasty patients. These advances should make the procedure safer and more durable. The purpose of this chapter is to discuss the indications for supra-aortic angioplasty, the methods employed, and the results various operators have had using angioplasty. It is expected that even the excellent results reported to date will only get better in the future as improvements occur.

The mechanism of PTA involves stretching the arterial wall, with permanent widening of the arterial lumen.[45] Angioplasty has been described as a controlled injury to the arterial wall. Since atheromatous plaques are essentially noncompressible and nonelastic, this stretching is possible only after partial splitting and partial detachment of the plaque. This stretching also produces fissures in the intima, followed by distention and splitting of the media. When the media is freed from the restraints of the atherosclerotic intima, it expands and partially separates from the intima. The vessel remains stretched by the blood pressure and can even undergo further widening as the vessels adapt to the circulatory needs. The arterial wall then undergoes healing and remodeling, although the exact mechanism has not been clarified. The examinations of human arteries performed following PTA have revealed a neointima bridging the plaque ruptures and tears, similar to the healing process which takes place after surgical endarterectomy.[42]

INDICATIONS

Supra-aortic angioplasty should only be performed on symptomatic patients who have a severe stenotic lesion which corresponds to the symptomatology. Atherosclerotic lesions are the most common, but there are also reports in which patients with fibromuscular dysplasia/

hyperplasia, Takayasu's arteritis, and neointimal fibrosis from previous surgery or trauma have been successfully treated.[46] Symptoms may include transient ischemic attacks (TIAs), recurrent incomplete strokes or dizziness, and other ischemic signs secondary to subclavian steal. It is important that a good working relationship be established between the neurologists, neurosurgeons, vascular surgeons, and interventional neuroradiologists so that the best possible therapy can be given to each patient. Ideal patients for angioplasty are those who have failed attempted medical therapy; those who have underlying medical conditions precluding surgery; those with lesions that require difficult and risky surgical procedures; those with postoperative restenosis; and those with intracranial stenotic lesions not amenable to surgery.

Angioplasty should generally not be performed on patients with severely ulcerated plaques or on those with thrombus adherent to the plaque or in the artery distal to the plaque because of the risk of emboli. Future developments may someday make even these lesions safe to dilate. Heavily calcified plaques generally do not respond well to angioplasty.

PATIENT EVALUATION

The patient with atherosclerotic cerebrovascular disease needs a thorough evaluation. These patients often have other problems related to their atherosclerotic disease which may also need to be evaluated. A careful history should be performed, not only to evaluate the patient's cerebral problems but also to alert the operator to other health problems. A complete physical examination should also be performed on these patients, with attention to the neurological exam. The only blood work we routinely perform prior to angioplasty is a complete blood count, platelet determination, prothrombin time, partial thromoplastin time, blood urea nitrogen, creatinine, electrolyte evaluation, and serum glucose and cholesterol evaluations, unless other lab work is indicated after the patient's history and physical examination. An electrocardiogram is also recommended in these patients. We routinely perform magnetic resonance imaging (MRI) on all of our patients before angioplasty to evaluate for any sign of a recent infarct or hemorrhage, which may cause us to postpone the angioplasty procedure. Careful attention must also be paid to controllable risk factors such as hypertension, diabetes mellitus, hypercholesterolemia, a history of smoking, and diet. Attempts should be made to modify and improve on these risk factors as much as possible.

PATIENT PREPARATION

Angioplasty of the supra-aortic vessels is generally not performed in the same setting as the diagnostic arteriogram. This is mainly so that the patient can be properly prepared prior to the angioplasty procedure. Tsai et al. recommend oral or parenteral anticoagulation for 5 to 7 days before PTA to reduce the possibility of emboli at the time of angioplasty and dexamethasone (10 mg) given daily during the 48 hr prior to the procedure.[46] We do not use heparin prior to angioplasty unless the patient is experiencing multiple TIAs not controlled with aspirin. However, we do routinely start our patients on aspirin, and begin low molecular weight dextran, decadron, and nimodepine beginning 12 to 24 hr prior to the procedure. The low molecular weight dextran serves as a volume expander and makes the platelets less adhesive. Decadron and nimodepine are used because we believe that in the event of an embolus at the time of angioplasty, these drugs will exert a cerebral protective effect. As stated above, we also obtain an MRI scan with contrast prior to angioplasty to exclude a recent infarct or hemorrhage. If there is evidence of a recent large infarct or a hemorrhagic infarct, we may decide to postpone the procedure, depending on the individual patient's circumstances. For example, patients with impending stroke, such as those with crescendo TIAs in spite of full anticoagulation therapy, should be seriously considered for emergency angioplasty.

It is important to sit down with the patient and his or her family before the procedure to discuss the underlying problem, describe the procedure, discuss potential alternatives to angioplasty such as continued medical therapy or surgery, and consider possible risks.

EXTRACRANIAL CEREBRAL ARTERY ANGIOPLASTY

After the diagnostic tests and premedications discussed above have been given, the patient is brought to the angiographic suite. A sheath is generally placed into the femoral artery (or occasionally into the axillary artery for vertebral angioplasty), one of sufficient size to allow passage of the angioplasty catheter. The procedure is performed using local anesthesia with conscious sedation. An arteriogram of the artery of interest is then repeated and compared to the diagnostic study to exclude any changes in the appearance of the lesion that would suggest the presence of clot. Tsai now routinely infuses 250,000 units of urokinase into vessels that have irregular walls to lyse any potential clot prior to the angioplasty (Personal communication, Fong Tsai, M.D.). The procedure is then performed 30 min following the infusion. The lesion needs to be localized fluoroscopically and a bony landmark selected or a metal marker placed on the skin at the site of the stenosis. The artery to be dilated is then sized by measuring a normal segment of the artery near the region of the stenosis. Care must be taken not to mistake areas of poststenotic dilatation for the normal artery. The artery can be measured using either cut films with a radiopaque ruler, so that the artery can be accurately sized, or the digital algorithm included on some of the newer interventional systems, which relates the size of the artery to the size of the diagnostic catheter. An appropriate balloon catheter should then be selected. In general, we use a balloon sized to the inner diameter of the normal artery.

After performing the diagnostic portion of the angioplasty procedure, we administer heparin (5000 units IV) and give atropine (0.8 mg IV). A floppy guidewire or, in some cases, a hydrophilic guidewire is then gently passed across the lesion, followed by the diagnostic catheter. The wire is removed, and a small amount of contrast is injected to confirm the intraluminal position of the catheter. A rigid exchange guidewire is then passed through the catheter and the 5F catheter is withdrawn. An angioplasty balloon catheter of the appropriate diameter and length is passed over the wire and across the stenosis, with the center of the balloon positioned in the center of the stenosis. We do not purge the balloon of air prior to passing the angioplasty catheter beyond the stenosis because we have found that in most lesions which are very tight, this makes passage of the balloon much more difficult. For this reason, we are careful not to exceed the recommended inflation pressure of the balloon. The balloon is then gently inflated by hand with half-strength contrast until a waist is identified on the balloon which confirms the proper position. A balloon inflation device is then used to inflate the balloon. The balloon is inflated until the waist on the balloon disappears or until the maximum pressure of inflation is reached. The balloon is kept inflated for approximately 10 to 40 secs, depending on the response of the lesion and the patient, and then deflated. The balloon may be inflated one to three times, depending on the response of the lesion to angioplasty. The exchange wire is removed and replaced with an 0.018 inch diameter wire. The wire is passed into the artery distal to the stenosis, and the angioplasty catheter is pulled back proximal to the stenosis. Contrast is injected through the angioplasty catheter around the wire so that the angioplasty result can be evaluated. If the result appears adequate, the wire is removed and a final set of films is obtained. The heparin is not reversed with protamine following the procedure but is instead allowed to wear off over several hours. The sheath is then pulled from the femoral artery.

If the result is unsatisfactory, there are several options. The first option is to accept the unsatisfactory result. If the flow in the artery from an angioplasty-related dissection is slow, we recommend keeping the patient heparinized and giving coumadin for 3 months following the procedure. Angioplasty-related dissections generally heal, and although they may initially look distressing, the end result is often quite good.

The second option is to redilate the lesion or dilate it with a larger angioplasty balloon catheter. To redilate with a larger balloon catheter, the existing angioplasty balloon is first passed over the 0.018 wire across the stenosis. The 0.018 wire is then removed, and the rigid exchange wire is placed through the balloon catheter. The initial angioplasty catheter is then removed over the wire, and the larger balloon catheter is passed across the lesion. Angioplasty is then repeated using the technique described above.

The third option, which shows great promise, is to place an endovascular stent. To place the stent, the existing angioplasty balloon is passed over the 0.018 wire across the stenosis. The 0.018 wire is removed, and the rigid exchange wire is placed through the balloon catheter. The initial angioplasty catheter is then removed over the wire. At this point, it will probably be necessary to also remove the existing femoral artery sheath and place a sheath of sufficient size to accept the stent introducing catheter. The stent is then loaded onto an appropriate balloon, if necessary, or prepared in its introducer. The stent is loaded through an appropriate introducer catheter, and the entire assembly is passed over the wire and positioned across the lesion. The introducer sheath is pulled back, and the stent is deployed. The result is evaluated by injecting contrast through the introducer sheath. If a stent is placed, care must be taken not to cover normal branches, such as the vertebral artery, if placing a stent into the subclavian artery. Following stent placement, the patient should be restarted on heparin after removing the femoral sheath, and coumadin therapy should be initiated and continued for 3 months until the stent endothelializes.

We have described the method we use to perform angioplasty of the brachiocephalic and internal carotid arteries. We have not encountered any embolic or ischemic complications using this technique. However, some variations adapted by others are worth considering. Tsai et al. report a slightly different technique.[46] They remove the larger, more rigid exchange wire after passing the angioplasty balloon across the stenosis or, in some cases, replace it with a smaller diameter wire. Then approximately 40 ml of fresh arterial blood is withdrawn from the side port of the sheath into a heparinized syringe. This blood is then injected through the lumen of the balloon catheter while the balloon is slowly inflated with a 50% saline/contrast solution. The balloon remains inflated for a few seconds while the fresh blood is injected distally through the inner lumen of the balloon catheter. The balloon is then deflated while pulling back on the plunger of the syringe to possibly aspirate back plaque debris. Following this maneuver, the catheter is pulled back over a guidewire, and the result is evaluated as discussed previously.

Théron et al. have reported on a technique involving temporary occlusion of the internal carotid artery to prevent cerebral embolization during manipulation of ulcerated plaques.[47] Briefly, they position a guiding catheter in the artery just proximal to the stenosis. The angioplasty balloon is then passed up into the distal part of the sheath but not out of the sheath. A small, nondetachable latex balloon on a microcatheter is then passed through the angioplasty catheter and across the stenosis. The balloon is inflated, causing occlusion of the internal carotid artery distal to the stenosis. The angioplasty catheter is then passed across the stenotic lesion, and the angioplasty procedure is performed. After deflating the angioplasty balloon, the angioplasty catheter is withdrawn, leaving the small temporary occlusion balloon inflated. Potential atherosclerotic particles or clots that could have been dislodged during inflation of the angioplasty balloon are aspirated forcefully with a 20-ml syringe through the side arm of the guiding catheter. Saline is then forcefully injected after aspiration to push potential residual fragments toward the external carotid artery. The temporary occlusion balloon is then deflated, and an angiographic series is performed to evaluate the result of the angioplasty. Ferguson has described a similar technique using a large-lumen balloon occlusion catheter positioned proximal to the stenosis to occlude flow (personal communication, Robert D. G. Ferguson). The angioplasty balloon is then passed through the temporary balloon occlusion catheter and the procedure is performed, with aspiration of any potential emboli following the angioplasty.

RESULTS

Innominate Artery Stenosis

We believe that angioplasty is ideally suited for therapy of stenotic lesions in this artery (Fig. 30-1). Tsai et al. have performed innominate artery angioplasty in seven patients without complications, and others have also reported their results, which overall have been excellent.[15,46,48,49] Surgical intervention for innominate artery stenosis carries a high risk, with endarterectomy or transternal bypass procedures having a reported mortality rate as high as 6%.[24] The procedure was first reported in 1981 by Lowman et al., who performed intraoperative retrograde transluminal angioplasty through a right common carotid arteriotomy.[24] The first successful percutaneous transluminal angioplasty procedure was reported by Garrido and Garofola in 1983.[15]

Carotid Artery Stenosis (Extracranial)

Results of angioplasty in the extracranial internal carotid artery circulation are extremely encouraging (Fig. 30-2). Tsai et al. have reported performing extracranial internal carotid artery angioplasty on 111 patients, with a 98% rate of improvement and no permanent complications.[46] In a more detailed account in 1986, Tsai et al. reported on 27 of these patients with clinical follow-up ranging from 3 months to 4 years, without recurrent symptoms in any patients.[49] Théron et al. have reported on a total of 23 patients on whom they performed carotid artery angioplasty.[47,50] They reported significant angiographic improvement in 22 of these patients, with no complications. All patients were reported to be asymptomatic at follow-up, which ranged from 3 to 18 months in their series. However, 9 of the 23 patients were treated for severe but asymptomatic stenoses. Other authors have also reported excellent results with extracranial carotid artery angioplasty.[29,51–53]

Surgical endarterectomy is now the treatment of choice for patients with severe stenotic lesions located at the carotid bifurcation. This procedure is safe and effective. Various published reports show 0.8–19% morbidity and 1.9–19% mortality associated with carotid endarterectomy.[54–56] Differences in complication rates are due to a variety of factors, including the patient population treated, surgical technique, and lesion location. Patients with a poor preoperative medical status and those with lesions of the carotid artery proximal to the bifurcation should be candidates for PTA.

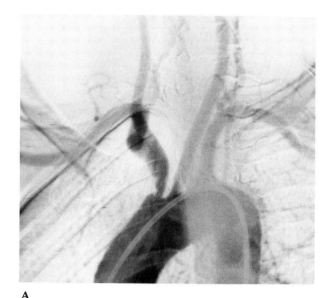

A

B

Fig. 30-1 A 50-year-old male who had right cerebral TIAs. (*A*) Arch angiography demonstrated severe stenosis at the origin of the innominate artery. (*B*) Following angiography, the stenosis was dilated to normal caliber.

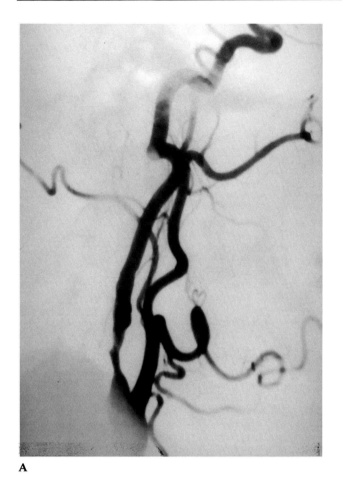

A

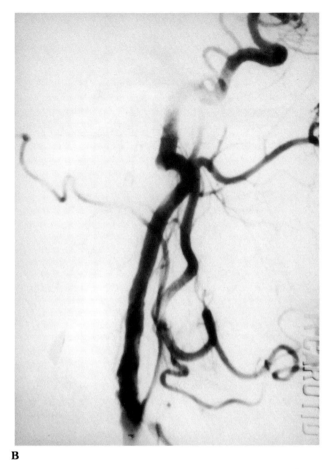

B

Fig. 30-2 A 60-year-old male who had a right carotid endarterectomy 6 years prior to presenting with left upper extremity TIAs. (*A*) There is a tight stenosis of the right internal carotid artery just above its origin. (*B*) Following angioplasty there is a marked improvement in the stenosis. The TIAs resolved following angioplasty.

Subclavian Artery Stenosis

Angioplasty for subclavian artery stenosis was first reported in 1977 by Zeitler and Holki with Backman and Kim and Mathias et al. the first to describe subclavian artery angioplasty in 1980 for subclavian steal.[7,57,58] Numerous reports in the literature now show that subclavian angioplasty has a low morbidity rate and a high technical success rate.[10,12,14,16,17,20,26–28,59–62] (Fig. 30-3). Nonsurgical treatment of subclavian stenotic disease is important because of the high risks associated with transthoracic vascular reconstruction and extrathoracic bypass. Various series have reported complication rates ranging from 4% to 23%.[63–66.]

Vertebral Artery Stenosis

Most stenotic lesions that involve the vertebral artery occur at the origin, but stenotic lesions can occur any-where along the course of the artery. Atherosclerotic disease of the vertebral artery carries a high risk of stroke. Recent data have shown that the incidence of stroke in patients with severe stenotic lesions of the vertebral artery is approximately 7% per year, with a cumulative risk ranging from 20% to 62% over 5 years.[11,67–69] In the past, intraoperative angioplasty or bypass of the origin of the vertebral artery has been the treatment of choice.[67–69] While up to 80% of patients show clinical improvement following surgery, about 10% show worsening of symptoms. The surgical bypass procedure itself is quite complex, with morbidity as high as 13% and mortality ranging from 1% to 3%.[67–69]

Several reports have now been published describing vertebral artery angioplasty with promising results. Mortarjeme et al. were the first to describe angioplasty of the origin of the vertebral artery.[70] In 1982 they reported on angioplasty of 13 vertebral arteries, with technical success in 11.[27] Two of the stenotic lesions

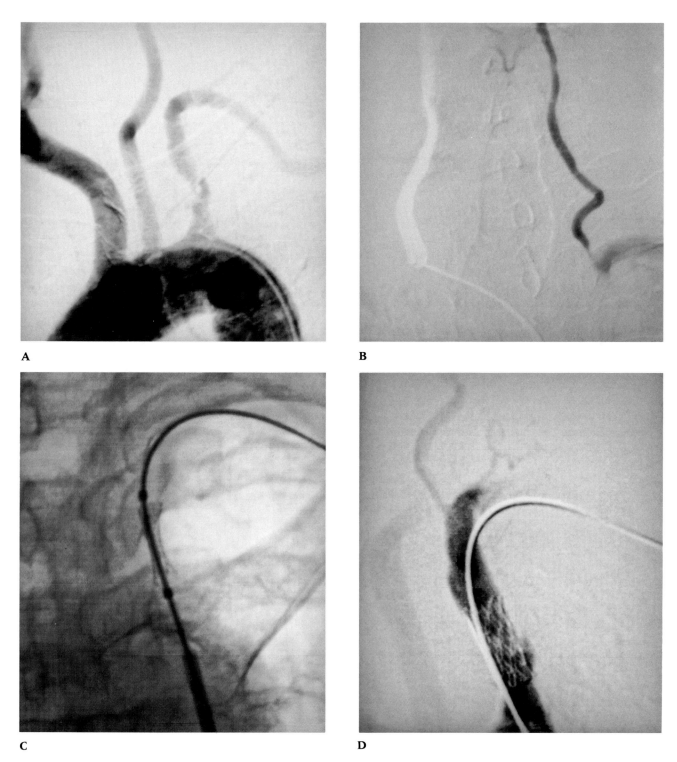

A

B

C

D

Fig. 30-3 An 80-year-old female with a 3-month history of increasing dizziness and falling to the left. (*A*) Aortic arch angiogram demonstrates a severe ulcerated stenosis of the proximal left subclavian artery. The left vertebral artery is not visualized. (*B*) Right vertebral arteriogram shows subclavian steal with retrograde flow down the left vertebral artery. (The subtracted image in this case was obtained by using a film with antegrade flow in the right vertebral artery as the mask. Thus, flow in the left vertebral artery shows up as white on this image). (*C*) Because of the ulceration, it was decided to place a stent to treat the stenosis. (*D*) Films following stent placement show marked improvement, with antegrade flow now seen in the left vertebral artery. Symptoms improved following angioplasty but did not completely resolve. Consideration is now being given to treating a severe stenosis of the distal left vertebral artery (not shown).

could not be reached secondary to vessel tortuosity. There were no complications from the procedure in their series. Higashida et al. have described angioplasty in the proximal and middle segments of the vertebral artery in 33 cases.[71] All patients showed angiographic improvement, and all but one had improvement in symptoms at follow-up, which ranged from 6 to 12 months. Further evaluation of the patient with continued symptoms suggested that the symptoms were secondary to cardiac disease. Although three patients experienced restenosis in less than 6 months, two of them were successfully redilated without problems and the third patient is being followed without recurrent symptoms. Other authors have reported similar encouraging results[46,72] (Fig. 30-4).

INTRACRANIAL ANGIOPLASTY

Percutaneous intracranial angioplasty is a new procedure made possible by the recent development of nondetachable microballoon catheters. Intracranial angioplasty was first described by Sundt et al. for angioplasty of the basilar artery via an operative approach.[30] The procedure was technically and clinically successful in two patients. The percutaneous approach to intracranial angioplasty was initially described for the treatment of vasospasm caused by aneurysmal subarachnoid hemorrhage by Zubkov et al. in 1984.[73] They reported on 105 dilatations in 33 patients with vasospasm from subarachnoid hemorrhage. They concluded that vasospasm could be effectively dilated, thereby improving cerebral perfusion. Higashida et al. have also reported a large number of intracranial dilatations primarily for vasospasm.[74] Intracranial angioplasty for vasospasm is indicated in selected patients with severe symptomatic vasospasm not responsive to the more traditional therapy of hypervolemia, hypertension, and hemodilution (Fig. 30-5). It is generally performed with the softer, nondetachable silicone microballoons.

Following reports of angioplasty for vasospasm and with the development of the Stealth catheter (Target Therapeutics, Fremont, CA), it is now possible to perform angioplasty of the distal vertebral and intracranial circulations for atherosclerotic disease. The Stealth catheter can also be used to perform angioplasty on the cervical portion of the internal carotid artery or vertebral artery in patients with tortuous vessels not amenable to therapy with the stiffer double-lumen angioplasty catheters. The Stealth catheter is a flexible, single-lumen catheter with the balloon incorporated into the distal portion. The balloon is inflated by first inserting a "valve" wire which has a bead near its distal tip. The bead occludes the distal tip of the catheter, causing the balloon to inflate when contrast is injected around the valve wire.

Patient preparation and diagnostic evaluation are similar to those of extracranial PTA. A 7F sheath is placed into the femoral artery. Heparin and atropine are given. The artery with the lesion is then selectively catheterized with a diagnostic catheter, and digital films are obtained. The diameter of the normal artery is then carefully measured and the stenotic lesion is carefully evaluated, as described in the previous section. We do not attempt to overdilate the intracranial vessels. If the stenosed segment is longer than 3 mm, irregular, or near a curve, we slightly underdilate the lesion. After assessing the lesion, the diagnostic catheter is exchanged over a stiff exchange wire for a 7F thin-walled, nontapered introducer catheter. After checking the position of the introducer catheter with a small amount of contrast, A Stealth catheter which has been preloaded with a 0.014 or 0.016 wire is passed in a coaxial fashion through the introducer catheter. We have found that the use of a hydrophilic coated wire facilitates the placement of the Stealth catheter. When the Stealth catheter is in position across the stenotic lesion, the guidewire is removed and exchanged for the tip-occluding valve wire, and the balloon is slowly inflated by injecting contrast around the valve wire. The operator must be very careful to ensure that no air bubbles are injected during inflation of the balloon, as these could enter the artery around the occluding bead during deflation of the balloon or in the event of balloon rupture. In order to avoid rupturing the balloon, we exert only gentle pressure on the inflating syringe. To better monitor inflation pressure, we usually use an inflation device with a pressure gauge. The balloon is

Fig. 30-4 A 70-year-old male with drop attacks (four-extremity weakness) and transient visual disturbances several times a day despite anticoagulant therapy. (A) Right subclavian arteriogram (through a right axillary approach) shows severe stenosis of the proximal right vertebral artery. The left vertebral artery was occluded. (B) Initial attempts to pass a double-lumen balloon angioplasty catheter were unsuccessful. Initial dilatation was performed with a Stealth catheter (2.5-mm-diameter balloon). (C) After preliminary dilatation with the Stealth catheter, a 4-mm-diameter × 4-cm-long double-lumen balloon catheter was passed across the stenosis and the lesion was dilated. (D) Postangioplasty arteriogram shows marked improvement, with much improved flow. The patient's neurological disturbances resolved, and he was discharged home on aspirin (325 mg every day).

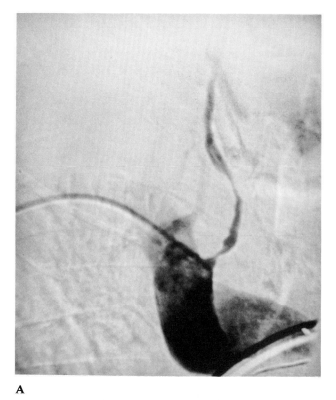

A

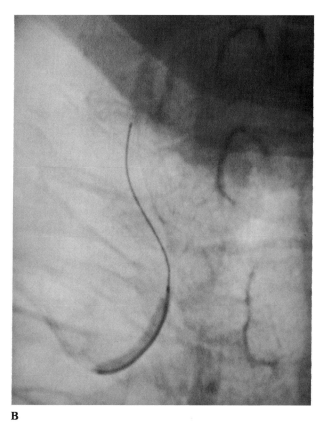

B

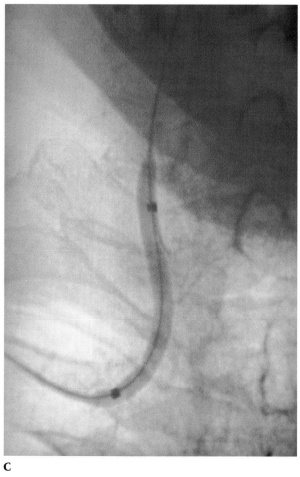

C

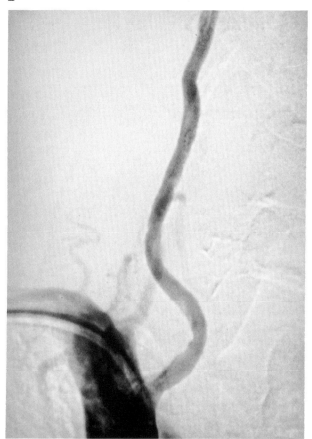

D

495

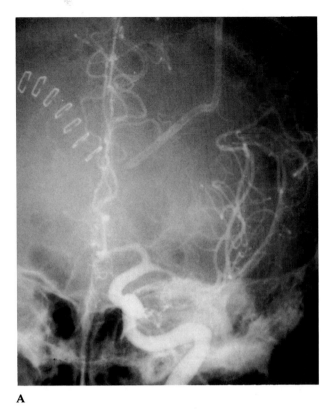

A

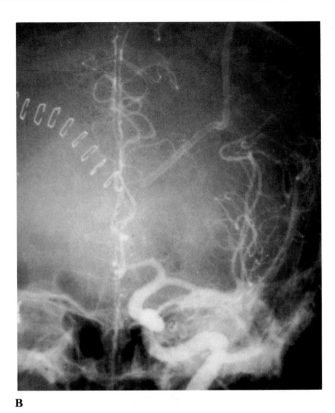

B

Fig. 30-5   A 66-year-old female with lethargy as well as expressive and receptive aphasia, following rupture and clipping of a right MCA aneurysm. (A) There is narrowing of the left M1 segment from vasospasm. (B) Following angioplasty of the left M1 segment, there was marked improvement in caliber and flow. The patient's symptoms improved following angioplasty.

generally inflated one to three times for 10 to 40 secs on each inflation, depending on the response of the patient and of the lesion. After the lesion appears to be adequately dilated, the balloon is deflated and contrast is injected around the Stealth catheter through the introducer catheter. The Stealth catheter is left in place across the lesion during this maneuver in order to avoid recrossing the lesion if further dilatation is necessary. If all looks well, the Stealth catheter is removed and contrast is injected through the introducer to evaluate the final result. The heparin is not reversed with protamine, but rather allowed to wear off over several hours before the sheath is removed.

At this time, there are very few reports of intracranial angioplasty for atherosclerotic disease. Purdy et al. reported dilatation of a middle cerebral artery, with improved blood flow on brain blood flow imaging following angioplasty.[75] Rostomily et al. reported on a patient with improvement in symptoms following angioplasty of the petrous portion of the internal carotid artery.[76] Follow-up of this patient at 24 months with an arteriogram showed an excellent result, with no evidence

of recurrent stenosis. The patient remained asymptomatic. We have performed intracranial internal carotid artery angioplasty on seven patients who presented with either TIA (five) or recurrent incomplete strokes (two) (Fig. 30-6). We have found no permanent neurological complications from these procedures. One patient had a very elastic lesion which could not be adequately dilated but his TIA's are much less frequent compared to before the angioplasty procedure. There have been no strokes, and none of the other six patients have had any TIAs since the procedure. Clinical follow-up in these patients now ranges from 1 to 24 months. Recent presentations by Hyogo et al., Barnwell et al., and McKenzie et al. also suggest that intracranial angioplasty is an effective therapy for TIAs and reducing stroke.[77–79]

POSTPROCEDURE CARE

Following angioplasty of the extracranial or intracranial cerebral circulation, the patient is monitored in the intensive care unit for 12 to 24 hr. The low molecular

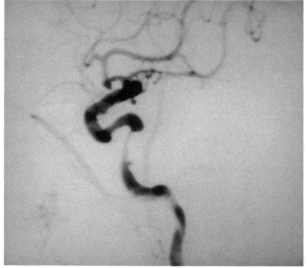

A

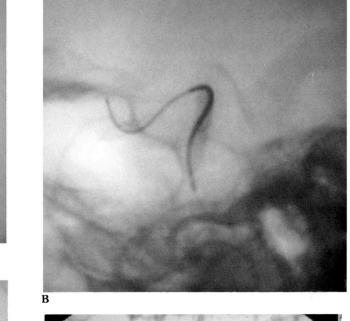

B

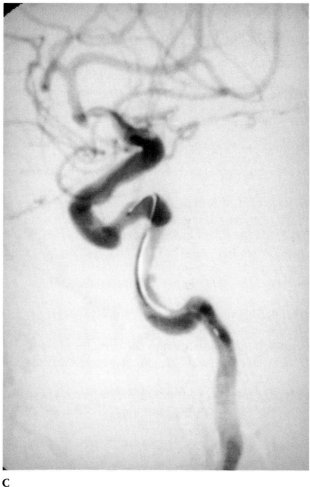

C

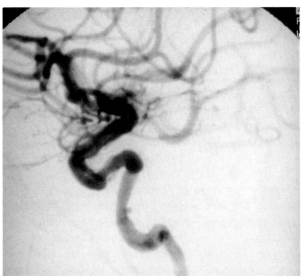

D

Fig. 30-6 A 79-year-old male with TIAs consisting of episodes of expressive aphasia and amorosws fugax. He also noted a decline in short-term memory over the last several months. MRI showed a small enhancing infarct in the left temporal lobe. (*A*) Left internal carotid arteriogram shows a severe stenosis of the distal petrous portion of the internal carotid artery. There is a small ulceration at the proximal end of the stenosis. (*B*) The Stealth catheter (3-mm-diameter balloon) is positioned across the stenosis, and the balloon is inflated. (*C*) Following dilatation, the result is evaluated by injecting contrast through the introducer catheter around the Stealth catheter. (*D*) Left internal carotid arteriogram performed following the angioplasty shows marked improvement, with much improved flow. The ulceration is not changed. The patient has had no further TIAs or strokes since the angioplasty procedure.

weight dextran, decadron, and nimodepine are continued for an additional 12 to 24 hr following the procedure. If no problems develop, the patient is transferred out of the intensive care unit the day following the procedure and monitored on the floor for an additional 24 to 48 hr. We discuss with the patient the importance of reducing any manageable risk factors for stroke, such as smoking, hypertension, diet, hypercholesterolemia, and diabetes control. We also have the patient take 325 mg aspirin every day following the procedure indefinitely. Tsai et al. also give methylprednisolone orally for 1 week following the procedure and believe it reduces the incidence of recurrent stenosis.[46] We generally see the patient back in our clinic at 2 weeks, 3 months, and 6 months. We maintain telephone contact with our patients thereafter at 3- to 6-month intervals. We also try to have the patient return for a follow-up noninvasive study (either ultrasound/Doppler or magnetic resonance angioplasty, depending on the location of the lesion) at approximately 6 months following the procedure.

COMPLICATIONS

Angioplasty has become an accepted and widely utilized procedure throughout the body except for the supra-aortic vessels. This is primarily related to the fear of stroke from the procedure. Experience to date suggests that this fear is exaggerated, since the incidence of stroke following angioplasty of the extracranial supra-aortic blood vessels ranges from zero to 4%.[46] However, only a small number of these procedures have been performed by a small number of individuals, and the true incidence of stroke is not yet known. Obviously, the procedure should be performed only by operators experienced with angioplasty and with a working knowledge of stroke. Future catheter developments and future developments in the field of cerebral protection should help to reduce the incidence of stroke.

Angioplasty is an invasive procedure; therefore, complications will occur. Many of these complications are minor and will resolve with conservative therapy. Other complications can be managed by the interventional radiologist, and a few may require surgical management. Complications related to angioplasty can occur at the puncture site or the angioplasty site or distal to the angioplasty site; alternatively, they may be systemic.

Puncture Site Complications

Complications related to the puncture site are the most frequent complications encountered when performing angioplasty.[42] Hematoma related to the puncture site is a frequent complication but is rarely of clinical significance. A large hematoma can result in a pseudoaneurysm. Femoral artery puncture should be performed below the level of the inguinal ligament, as a puncture above this level may not be adequately controlled with manual compression. Bleeding into the retroperitoneum, which may occur with puncture above the inguinal ligament, may not be suspected on physical examination. A high index of suspicion should be maintained in patients who develop unexplained tachycardia or hypotension following angioplasty. If the puncture is performed in the brachial artery, hematoma can compress the brachial plexus and cause damage to the nerve. Rarely, dissection and/or thrombosis of the artery can occur.

Angioplasty Site Complications

The most important complication occurring at the angioplasty site is acute occlusion of the vessel. Acute occlusion can be due to spasm, subintimal dilatation, intimal flaps, or thrombosis. If the patient is symptomatic, attempts should be made to reopen the artery. The supra-aortic arteries are prone to spasm, which, if severe, may result in occlusion. Since spasm will improve with vasodilators, we inject 100 μg or more of nitroglycerine into the artery, being careful to monitor the patient's blood pressure so that hypotension does not occur. If occlusion persists, the next maneuver is to try to redilate the lesion. We keep a wire across the lesion, as described earlier, in the event that this becomes necessary. Another option is to place an endovascular stent. Schwarten has successfully placed a stent for a patient with a traumatic dissection of the internal carotid artery, with resolution of symptoms (personal communication, Donald Schwarten, M.D.). Thrombosis of the vessel with acute occlusion is a potential complication. It may be possible to treat this complication successfully with intra-arterial thrombolytic agents.

Occlusion of branch vessels is a potential complication, especially when performing intracranial angioplasty. Occlusion of small brain stem perforators or lenticulostriate arteries may not be apparent at angiography. Careful neurological monitoring throughout the procedure is mandatory.

Rupture of the vessel is a very rare complication when performing angioplasty for atherosclerotic disease. If this complication occurs in the supra-aortic extracranial vessels, the bleeding can be controlled by reinflating the balloon, sealing the rupture site.[42] Depending on the location of the rupture site, the patient can then be taken to surgery. The vessel distal to the rupture can be partially perfused through the balloon catheter while it is inflated if the patient is symptomatic from ischemia.

While the result is not ideal, patients who develop acute occlusion or vessel rupture may also be treated with permanent balloon occlusion of the internal carotid artery or the vertebral artery. Of course, this assumes that the patient is asymptomatic from the acute occlusion. There are reports of internal carotid artery occlusion to arrest embolic discharge from stenotic lesions not amenable to surgery, with good results.[80]

Distal Complications

Distal embolization is potentially a very serious complication. As discussed earlier, some operators use cerebral protection devices to try to avoid it. Another way to reduce this complication in the future may be to use stents. We have found clinically significant embolization from angioplasty to be rare. When we select our patients, we are careful not to perform angioplasty in those with severely ulcerated lesions or in those with thrombus in the vessel. If this complication occurs, we attempt treatment with intra-arterial thrombolysis.

Intracranial hemorrhage is a potential complication, especially in patients with a recent infarct. We attempt to avoid this problem by evaluating patients with MRI prior to the procedure.

Other Complications

Systemic complications may occur or other problems may arise away from the angioplasty site. The operator should be prepared to deal with adverse reactions to contrast medium and/or other medications. Transient renal insufficiency can occur especially in patients with preexisting renal problems.

CONCLUSION

Extensive experience has conclusively demonstrated that angioplasty is an effective treatment for stenotic lesions below the neck. We believe that supra-aortic angioplasty is also an effective procedure to treat symptomatic, hemodynamically significant stenoses of the supra-aortic blood vessels. Appropriate patient selection is essential, as is a close working relationship with neurologists, neurosurgeons, and vascular surgeons. Although complications occur, they can be minimized with meticulous technique and often treated with good results. Advantages of PTA include the following: (1)

it is less costly than surgical alternatives; (2) the patient is awake during the procedure, which allows continuous neurological monitoring; (3) if a complication develops, it is immediately apparent and corrective measures can be taken; (4) it can be performed on patients who are not surgical candidates; and (5) intracranial stenotic lesions can be treated. The indications for PTA of the supra-aortic vessels are likely to become broader as more experience is gained in this field.

REFERENCES

1. American Heart Association. *1993 Stroke Facts.* Dallas, TX, American Heart Association, 1992.
2. Gresham GE, Phillips TF, Wolf PA, et al. Epidemiologic profile of long-term stroke disability: The Framingham Study. *Arch Phys Med Rehabil* 1979;60:487–491.
3. Cerebral Embolism Task Force. Cardiogenic brain embolism. *Arch Neurol* 1989;46:727–743.
4. Mohr JP, Caplan LR, Melski JW, et al. The Harvard Cooperative Stroke Registry: A prospective registry. *Neurology* 1978;28:754–762.
5. North American Symptomatic Carotid Endarterectomy Trial Collaborators. Beneficial effects of carotid endarterectomy in symptomatic patients with high-grade carotid stenosis. *N Engl J Med* 1991;325:445–453.
6. European Carotid Surgery Trialists' Collaborative Group. MRC European Carotid Surgery Trial: Interim results for symptomatic patients with severe (70–99%) or with mild (0–29%) carotid stenosis. *Lancet* 1991;337:1235–1243.
7. Backman DM, Kim RM. Transluminal dilatation for subclavian steal syndrome. *AJR* 1980;135:995–996.
8. Belan A, Vesela M, Vanek I, et al. Percutaneous transluminal angioplasty of fibromuscular dysplasia of the internal carotid artery. *Cardiovasc Intervent Radiol* 1982;5:79–81.
9. Bockenheimer SAM, Mathias K. Percutaneous transluminal angioplasty in arteriosclerotic internal carotid artery stenosis. *AJNR* 1983;4:791–792.
10. Courtheoux P, Théron J, Maiza D, et al. Endoluminal angioplasty for atheromatous stenosis of supra-aortic trunks. The brachiocephalic arterial trunk, subclavian arteries. *J Radiol* 1984;65(12):845–851.
11. Courtheoux P, Tournade A, Théron J, et al. Transcutaneous angioplasty of vertebral artery atheromatous ostial stricture. *Neuroradiology* 1985;27:259–264.
12. Damouth HD Jr, Diamond AB, Rapporport AS, et al. Angioplasty of subclavian artery stenosis proximal to the vertebral origin. *AJNR* 1983;4(6):1239–1242.
13. Freitag G, Freitag J, Koch RD, et al. Percutaneous angioplasty of carotid artery stenoses. *Neuroradiology* 1986;28:126–127.

14. Galich JP, Bajaj AK, Vine DL, et al. Subclavian artery stenosis treated by transluminal angioplasty: Six cases. *Cardiovasc Intervent Radiol* 1983;6(2):78–81.

15. Garrido E, Garofola J. Intraluminal dilatation of the innominate artery before extracranial-intracranial bypass. Case report. *Neurosurgery* 1983;12(5):581–583.

16. Gordon RL, Haskell L, Hirsch M, et al. Transluminal dilatation of the subclavian artery. *Cardiovasc Intervent Radiol* 1985;8(1):14–19.

17. Grote R, Greyschmidt J, Walterbusch G. Percutaneous transluminal angioplasty in proximal subclavian stenoses. *ROFO* 1983;138(6):660–664.

18. Hasso AN, Bird CR, Zinek DE, et al. Fibromuscular dysplasia of the internal carotid artery. Percutaneous transluminal angioplasty. *AJNR* 1981;2:175–180.

19. Higashida RT, Hieshima GB, Tsai FY, et al. Percutaneous transluminal angioplasty of the subclavian and vertebral arteries. *AJNR* 1986;369:124–126.

20. Hodgins GW, Dutton JW. Subclavian and carotid angioplasties for Takayasu's arteritis. *J Can Assoc Radiol* 1982;33(3):205–207.

21. Kerber CS, Cronwell LD, Lehden OL. Catheter dilatation of proximal carotid stenosis during distal bifurcation endarterectomy. *AJNR* 1980;1:348–349.

22. Kobinia G, Bergmann H Jr. Angioplasty in stenosis of the innominate artery. *Cardiovasc Intervent Radiol* 1983;6:82–85.

23. Levien LJ, Fritz VU. Intra-operative transluminal angioplasty in the management of symptomatic aortic arch vessel stenosis. *S Afr J Surg* 1985;23(2):49–52.

24. Lowman B, Queral L, Holbrook W, et al. The treatment of innominate artery stenosis by intraoperative transluminal angioplasty. *Surgery* 1981;5:565–568.

25. Lowman B, Queral L, Holbrook W, et al. The correction of cerebrovascular insufficiency by transluminal dilatation: A preliminary report. *Am Surg* 1983;49(11):621–624.

26. Moore TS, Russell WF, Parent AD, et al. Percutaneous transluminal angioplasty in subclavian steal syndrome: Recurrent stenosis and retreatment in two patients. *Neurosurgery* 1982;11(4):512–517.

27. Motarjeme A, Keifer JW, Zuska AJ. Percutaneous transluminal angioplasty of the brachiocephalic arteries. *AJR* 1982;138(3):457–462.

28. Motarjeme A, Keifer JW, Zuska AJ, et al. Percutaneous transluminal angioplasty for treatment of subclavian steal. *Radiology* 1985;155(3):611–613.

29. Namaguchi Y, Puyau FA, Provenza LJ, et al. Percutaneous transluminal angioplasty of the carotid artery. *Neuroradiology* 1984;26:527–530.

30. Sundt TM Jr, Smith HC, Campbell JK, et al. Transluminal angioplasty for basilar artery stenosis. *Mayo Clin Proc* 1980;55:673–680.

31. Théron J, Courtheoux P, Henriet JP, et al. Angioplasty of supra-aortic arteries. *J Neuroradiol* 1984;11(3):187–200.

32. Tievsky AL, Dray EM, Mardiat JG. Transluminal angioplasty in postsurgical stenosis of the extracranial carotid artery. *AJNR* 1980;1:348–349.

33. Tsai FY, Hieshima GB, Higashida RT. Percutaneous transluminal angioplasty for the treatment of stroke, in Fisher M (ed): *Medical Therapy of Acute Stroke*, New York, Marcel Dekker, 1989, pp 203–239.

34. Tsai FY, Higashida RT, Matovich V, et al. Seven years' experience with PTA of carotid artery. *Neuroradiology* 1991;33(Suppl):397–398.

35. Vitek JJ. Percutaneous transluminal angioplasty of the external carotid artery. *AJNR* 1983;4:796–799.

36. Vitek JJ. Subclavian artery angioplasty and the origin of the vertebral artery. *Radiology* 1989;170:407–409.

37. Wiggli U, Gratzl O. Transluminal angioplasty of stenotic carotid arteries: Case report and protocol. *AJNR* 1983;4:793–795.

38. Zeitler E, Berger G, Schemitt-Rutt R. Percutaneous transluminal angioplasty of the supra-aortic arteries, in Dotter CT, Gruntzig A, Schoop W, et al. (eds): Percutaneous Transluminal Angioplasty: Technique, Early and Late Results. Berlin, Springer-Verlag, 1983, pp 245–261.

39. Dotter CT, Judkins MP. Transluminal treatment of arteriosclerotic obstruction: Description of a new technique and preliminary report of its application. *Circulation* 1964;30:654–670.

40. Grüntzig A, Hopff H. Perkutane rekanalisation chronischer arterieller verschulusse mit einem neuren dilatationskatheter: Modifikation der Dotter-technik. *Dtsch Med Wochenschr* 1974;99:2502–2505.

41. Becker GJ, Katzen BT, Dake MD. Noncoronary angioplasty. *Radiology* 1989;170:921–940.

42. Tegtmeyer CJ. Percutaneous transluminal angioplasty, in Keats TE (ed): *Current Problems in Diagnostic Radiology,* Vol 16, part 2. Chicago, Year Book, 1987, pp 71–139.

43. Morris GC, Lechter A, DeBakey ME. Surgical treatment of fibromuscular disease of the carotid arteries. *Arch Surg* 1968;96:636–643.

44. Mathias K, Mitlermeyer C, Ensinger H, et al. Percutane katherdilatation von karotisstenosen. *Fortschr Roentgenstr* 1980;133:348–361.

45. Zollikofer CL, Cragg AH, Hunter DW, et al. Mechanism of transluminal angioplasty, in Castaneda-Zuniga WR, Tadararthy SM (eds): *Interventional Radiology.* Baltimore, Williams & Wilkins, 1992, pp 249–297.

46. Tsai FY, Higashida R, Meoli C. Percutaneous transluminal angioplasty of extracranial and intracranial arterial stenosis in the head and neck, in Vinuela F, Dion J, Duckwiler G (eds): *Neuroimag Clin North Am* 1992;2(2):371–384.

47. Théron J, Courtheoux P, Alachkar F, et al. New triple coaxial catheter system for carotid angioplasty with cerebral protection. *AJNR* 1990;11:869–874.

48. Kobinia G, Bergmann H Jr. Angioplasty in stenosis of the innominate artery. *Cardiovasc Intervent Radiol* 1983;6: 82–85.

49. Tsai FY, Matovich V, Hieshima G, et al. Percutaneous transluminal angioplasty of the carotid artery. *AJNR* 1986;7:349–358.

50. Théron J, Raymond J, Casasco A, et al. Percutaneous angioplasty of atherosclerotic and postsurgical stenosis of carotid arteries. *AJNR* 1987;8:495–500.

51. Belloni G, Bonaldi G, Moschini L, et al. Percutaneous angioplasty of atherosclerotic carotid arteries. *AJNR* 1989;10:898.

52. Smith CD, Smith LL, Hasso AN. Fibromuscular dysplasia of the internal carotid artery treated by operative transluminal balloon angioplasty. *Radiology* 1985;155:645–648.

53. Courtheoux P, Théron J, Tournade A, et al. Percutaneous endoluminal angioplasty of postendarterectomy carotid stenoses. *Neuroradiology* 1987;29:186–189.

54. West H, Burton R, Roon AJ, et al. Comparative risk of operation and expectant management for carotid artery disease. *Stroke* 1979;10:117–121.

55. Riles TS, Imparato AM, Mintzer R, et al. Comparison of results of bilateral and unilateral carotid endarterectomy five years after surgery. *Surgery* 1982;91:258–262.

56. Loftus CM, Quest DO. Current status of carotid endarterectomy for atheromatous disease. *Neurosurgery* 1983;12: 718–723.

57. Zeitler E, Holki B. Angiographische diagnostik, in Raithel D (ed): *Zerebrale insuffizienz durch extrakranielle gefabverschdusse.* Erlangen, Permid, 1977, pp 359–363.

58. Mathias K, Staiger J, Thron A, et al. Perkutane katheterangioplastik der arteria subclavia. *Dtsch Med Wochenschr* 1980;105:16–31.

59. Basche S, Ritter H, Gaerisch F, et al. Percutaneous transluminal angioplasty of the subclavian artery. *Zentralbl Chir* 1983;108(3):142–149.

60. Kichikawa K, Makagawa H, Yoshiya K, et al. Percutaneous transluminal angioplasty in a case of left subclavian and brachiocephalic artery stenosis due to aortitis syndrome. *Rinsho Hoshasen* 1985;30(1):121–124.

61. Pernes JM, Brenot P, Seuro M, et al. Percutaneous endoluminal angioplasty of the supra-aortic arterial trunks. Immediate and remote results. *Presse Med* 1984;12(17): 1075–1078.

62. Rabkin IKH, Matevosov AL, Shekhter IUI. X-ray endovascular dilatation of the subclavian artery. *Gruden Khir* 1984;2:76–78.

63. Dietrich EB, Garrett HB, Ameriso J, et al. Occlusive disease of the common carotid and subclavian arteries treated by carotid subclavian bypass. *Am J Surg* 1967; 114:800–808.

64. Crawford ES, DeBakey ME, Morris GC Jr, et al. Surgical treatment of occlusion of the innominate, common carotid and subclavian arteries. *Surgery* 1969;65:17–31.

65. Beebe HG, Start K, Johnson ML, et al. Choices of operation for subclavian-vertebral arterial disease. *Am J Surg* 1980;139:616–623.

66. Schlosser V. Subclavian steal syndrome: Correction by transthoracic or extra-anatomic repair. *Vasc Surg* 1984; 289–293.

67. Baker RN, Carroll-Ramseyer J, Schauartz WS. Prognosis in patients with transient ischemic attacks. *Neurology* 1968;18:1157–1165.

68. Cartlidge NEF, Whisnant JJP, Elveback LR. Carotid and vertebral basilar transient cerebral ischemic attacks. *Mayo Clin Proc* 1977;52:117–120.

69. Delos Reyes RA, Ausman JI, Diaz FG, et al. The surgical management of vertebrobasilar insufficiency. *Acta Neurochir* 1983;68:203–216.

70. Motarjeme A, Keifer JW, Zuska AJ. Percutaneous transluminal angioplasty of the vertebral arteries. *Radiology* 1981;139:715–717.

71. Higashida RT, Tsai FY, Halbach VV, et al. Transluminal angioplasty for atherosclerotic disease of the vertebral and basilar arteries. *J Neurosurg* 1993;78:192–198.

72. Schultz H, Yeung HP, Chin MC, et al. Dilatation of vertebral artery stenosis. *N Engl J Med* 1981;304:733.

73. Zubkov YN, Nikiforov BM, Shustin VA. Balloon catheter technique for dilatation of constricted cerebral arteries after aneurysmal SAH. *Acta Neurochir* 1984;70:665–679.

74. Higashida RT, Halbach VV, Cahan LD, et al. Transluminal angioplasty for treatment of intracranial arterial vasospasm. *J Neurosurg* 1989;71:648–653.

75. Purdy PD, Devous MD, Unwin DH, et al. Angioplasty of an atherosclerotic middle cerebral artery associated with improvement in regional cerebral blood flow. *AJNR* 1990;11:878–880.

76. Rostomily RC, Mayberg MR, Eskridge JM, et al. Resolution of petrous internal carotid artery stenosis after transluminal angioplasty. *J Neurosurg* 1992;76:520–523.

77. Hyogo T, Kataoka T, Nakamura J, et al. Balloon angioplasty for intracranial vertebral artery stenosis. Presented at the annual meeting of the ASNR, Vancouver, May 16–20, 1993.

78. Barnwell SL. Angioplasty of intracranial atheromatous lesions involving the vertebral, basilar, internal carotid, and middle cerebral arteries. Presented at the annual meeting of the ASNR, Vancouver, May 16–20, 1993.

79. McKenzie JD, Dean BL, Rand JC, et al. Intracranial angioplasty of vascular stenoses. Presented at the annual meeting of the ASNR, Vancouver, May 16–20, 1993.

80. Countee RW, Vijayanathan T, Hubschmann OR, et al. Carotid ligation for recurrent ischemia due to inaccessible carotid obstruction. *J Neurosurg* 1980;53:491–499.

31

Endovascular Treatment of Cerebral Dural Arteriovenous Fistulas

Graham K. Lee, M.D.

Cerebral dural arteriovenous fistulas (DAVFs) are abnormal arteriovenous shunts located within the dura overlying the brain. They occur predominantly near the major cerebral venous sinuses, with meningeal arteries shunting to dural sinuses, meningeal veins, or pial veins without an intervening nidus. The majority of cerebral DAVFs appear to be acquired, probably related to venous thrombosis or obstruction. Etiological factors predisposing to these conditions include cerebral trauma, craniotomy, meningiomas, infection, and the peripartum period.[1]

Some cerebral DAVFs are congenital, presenting in early childhood. An increased incidence of DAVFs in hereditary hemorrhagic telangiectasia (Osler-Weber-Rendu syndrome) is noted. (Fig. 31-1).

CLASSIFICATION OF CEREBRAL DAVFs

Cerebral DAVFs are classified either by their location, including the dural sinus with which they are associated, or by the venous drainage of the DAVF.[2] The various anatomical locations of the DAVF may result in different symptoms and clinical manifestations. To a large extent, this is related to the venous drainage patterns. Common locations for DAVFs include the ante-rior or posterior cavernous sinus, sigmoid and transverse sinuses, torcular and superior sagittal sinuses, basal or marginal tentorium, and anterior cranial fossa. The Djindjian classification of DAVFs by venous drainage (Table 31-1) is based on the finding that venous drainage to cerebral veins results in a high incidence of neurological complications.[3] Partial or complete occlusion of cerebral sinuses is frequently encountered in association with these lesions, which in some cases may be due to the primary initiating event (e.g., venous sinus thrombosis) or may occur secondary to the abnormally high flow through the sinus. The venous obstructions may result in venous hypertension or proximal venous dilatation, predisposing to hemorrhage or mass effect.

The natural history of cerebral DAVFs is not fully understood. Many of these lesions remain stable for years, with no change in appearance or occurrence of symptoms. Regression or disappearance of the DAVF has been documented in some instances, either spontaneously, following a hemorrhage or cerebral arteriography; compression therapy of the carotid arteries has been shown to produce occlusion in approximately one-third of patients. Many series have shown a high incidence of presentation with cerebral hemorrhage in DAVFs with cerebral venous drainage. Anatomical lo-

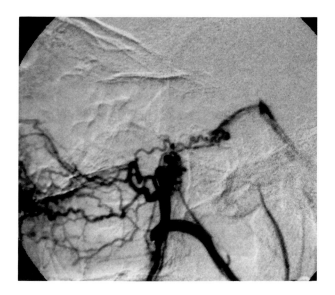

Fig. 31-1 Incidental middle cranial fossa cerebral DAVF in association with Osler-Weber-Rendu disease. A 63-year-old woman with profuse epistaxis was treated by embolization. Lateral view, internal maxillary arteriogram. Enlarged nasal branches of the sphenopalatine artery supplying nasal telangiectasis. Enlarged artery of the foramen rotundum with cerebral DAVF in the middle cranial fossa, with drainage to the inferior petrosal sinus.

cations related to a high incidence of hemorrhage include the anterior cranial fossa and marginal tentorial region, but this may be largely related to their cerebral venous drainage.

RADIOLOGICAL EVALUATION

Many cerebral DAVFs are diagnosed following complications, particularly cerebral hemorrhage (Fig. 31-2). Many others are detected due to specific neurological manifestations. Ophthalmic venous drainage, such as from cavernous DAVFs, generally presents with proptosis and chemosis with visual disturbance (Fig. 31-3). Some patients present with pulsatile tinnitus or headaches.

TABLE 31-1 Classification of Cerebral DAVFs

Type I	Drainage into a sinus (or meningeal vein)
Type II	Sinus drainage with reflux into cerebral veins
Type III	Drainage solely into cortical veins
Type IV	With a supra- or infratentorial venous lake

Source: Ref. 3.

Noncontrast computed tomography (CT) is relatively insensitive in detecting cerebral DAVFs, although it is extremely useful in the evaluation of cerebral hemorrhage. Contrast-enhanced CT may also detect distended pial veins and enlarged draining sinuses and venous pouches. Specific focal abnormalities such as venous infarcts can be detected.

Magnetic resonance imaging (MRI) and magnetic resonance angiography (MRA) may detect enlarged pial veins and show increased flow or obstruction of cerebral dural sinuses (Fig. 31-4). The resolution of MRA and MR venography is generally insufficient to allow precise determination of the fistula site, and arteriography is required for this purpose. MRA is usually negative in the absence of distended pial veins. MRI is useful in detecting complications such as venous infarct and cerebral hemorrhages.

Superselective arteriography is required for definitive diagnosis of most DAVFs, and is essential prior to surgery or endovascular therapy. This precisely localizes the site of the fistula, the arterial supply, and the venous drainage. Careful analysis of the angioarchitecture of the lesion is required prior to therapeutic consideration.

The angiographic protocol in evaluation of a cerebral DAVF is based on knowledge of the arterial supply of the dura. Bilateral internal carotid, vertebral, and multiple superselective external carotid artery injections may be required.

It is important to recognize that a normal MRI or CT scan does not exclude the presence of a DAVF. An awareness of the condition and high-quality arteriography are required to diagnose and fully evaluate these abnormalities.

CLINICAL MANIFESTATIONS

Cerebral DAVFs presenting in adult patients are generally slow flow. Their clinical presentation depends on their precise location and venous drainage. Cavernous sinus DAVFs present with ophthalmic venous hypertension, producing chemosis, proptosis, and increased intraocular pressure. This may result in papilledema, glaucoma, and retinal detachment. Involvement of oculomotor nerves results in diplopia, which may also be produced by the orbital venous engorgement.[4]

Pulsatile tinnitus is frequently noted and may be associated with an objective bruit on auscultation over the orbits or temporal bones. Venous hypertension related to the fistula may result in venous infarct or focal neurological signs (e.g., sensory or motor abnormality).

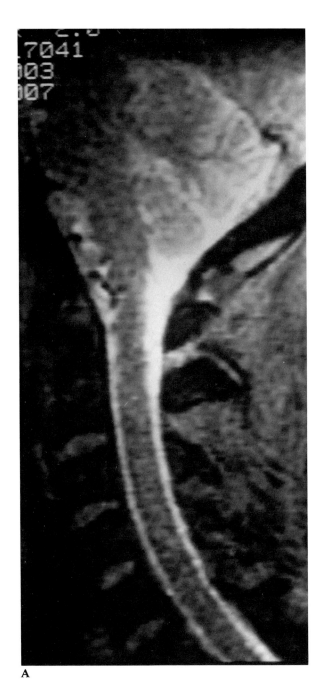

A

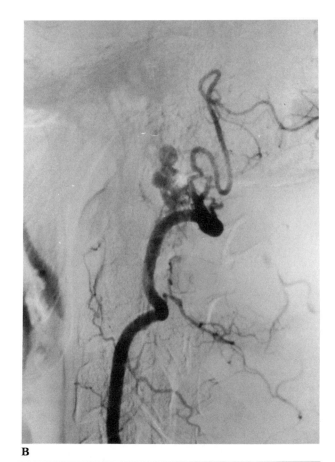

B

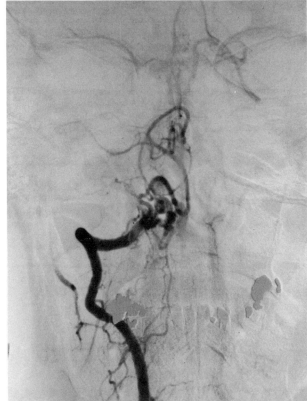

C

Fig. 31-2 A 42-year-old man with subarachnoid hemorrhage. Cerebral DAVF is seen at the margin of the foramen magnum. (*A*) Sagittal T_2-weighted MRI scan of the craniocervical junction shows signal void ventral to the medulla and signal abnormality along the clivus coresponding to subarachnoid hemorrhage. (*B*) Lateral view, right vertebral arteriogram. Cerebral DAVF at the margin of the foramen magnum with distended veins along the clivus. (*C*) AP view, right vertebral arteriogram. Vertebral artery primarily supplies no external carotid arterial supply to the fistula. Meningeal artery supply is too small to catheterize safely. The patient was treated surgically and cured.

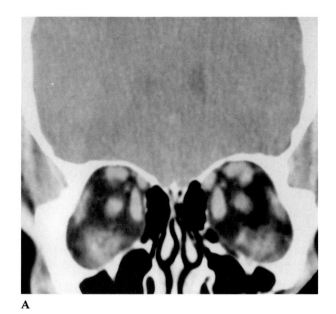

A

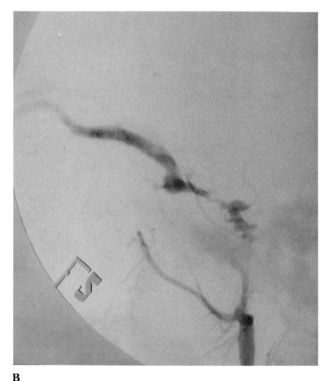

B

Fig. 31-3 A 36-year-old man with a 2-week history of left orbital chemosis and proptosis. Left middle meningeal artery to superior ophthalmic vein fistula. (*A*) Coronal CT scan demonstrates an enlarged left superior ophthalmic vein (arrow). (*B*) Left internal maxillary arteriogram, lateral view, shows an enlarged middle meningeal artery leading to a fistula draining to the superior ophthalmic vein. Cure was achieved with embolization utilizing NBCA.

Cranial nerve deficits may occur and may be due to relative ischemia, venous hypertension, or pressure effects. Cerebral pial venous drainage is generally present in patients with neurological deficits and in those presenting with hemorrhage. The hemorrhage may be subdural, subarachnoid, or intraparenchymal. This has been reported in 20 to 42% of patients in various series of patients with cerebral DAVFs.[2]

Venous thrombosis may alter the clinical picture. This may occasionally result in resolution of symptoms or even obliteration of the DAVF. Thrombosis may lead to rerouting of the venous drainage to pial venous structures, possibly resulting in focal neurological symptoms. Cerebro venous hypertension can result in deficits such as aphasia, weakness, sensory abnormalities, or seizures. Transient neurologic defects may occur due to fluctuation in pressure and possible venous thrombosis.

Venous hypertension due to extensive cerebral DAVFs may produce increased intracranial pressure with papilledema and visual disturbance (Fig. 31-5). Global cerebral changes, including dementia, may occur and can be reversed with therapy.

Special consideration must be given to cerebral DAVFs with venous drainage to the spinal cord, as the clinical manifestation of myelopathy may lead to the erroneous consideration of spinal cord abnormality (e.g., tumor, vascular malformation, or spinal DAVF).

Occasional instances of multiple cerebral DAVFs have been noted, particularly related to prior extensive dural venous thrombosis and in association with syndromes such as Osler-Weber-Rendu disease (hereditary hemorrhagic telangiectasia).

MANAGEMENT

The initial decision regarding management of cerebral DAVFs is whether or not treatment is indicated. DAVFs producing minimal symptoms and without cerebral pial or ophthalmic venous drainage have a low incidence of complications and may be followed clinically. Any change in the patient's condition could indicate thrombosis of the primary venous drainage and alternate pial venous drainage, which would require treatment. Focal neurological signs produced by a DAVF, such as paresis; sensory change, or changes due to the presence of a hemorrhage, are an indication for treatment. Pial venous drainage is an indication for treatment due to its high association with neurological complications.

Ophthalmic venous drainage, such as from a cavern-

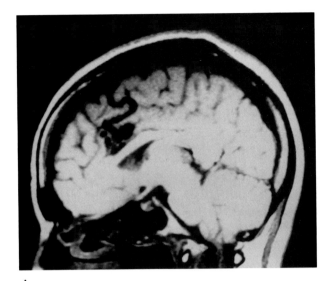

A

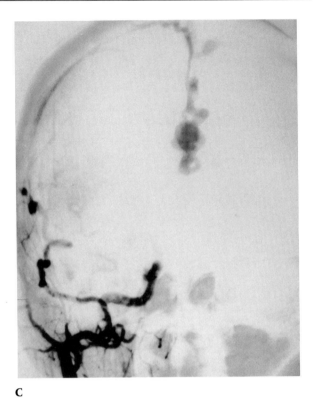

C

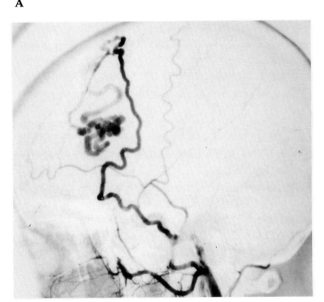

B

Fig. 31-4 Cerebral DAVF of the falx cerebri. (*A*) Sagittal T_1-weighted MRI scan shows dilated superficial veins in the frontal interhemispheric region draining to the superior sagittal sinus. (*B*) Lateral view, right external carotid arteriogram, demonstrates an enlarged middle meningeal artery supply to the falx DAVF and cerebral venous drainage. (*C*) AP view, right external carotid injection, shows an enlarged middle meningeal artery leading to the falx DAVF and the interhemispheric draining vein. Also present was a supply from the left middle meningeal artery (not shown). The patient was treated by NBCA embolization.

ous sinus DAVF, requires careful ophthalmological follow-up. The patient may tolerate the mild proptosis and conjunctival injection rather than accept the small risk of treatment. Visual deterioration or any increase in intraocular pressure unresponsive to medical therapy is an indication for treatment.

Cerebral DAVFs in certain anatomical locations generally require treatment, largely related to their strong association with pial venous drainage and hemorrhage. These include the anterior cranial fossa and marginal tentorial locations. Treatment options must be tailored to the specific type and location of the DAVF and include conservative clinical follow-up, compression therapy, or endovascular therapy.

Cavernous sinus DAVFs may undergo a trial of carotid-jugular compression therapy, which reduces arterial flow through the carotid artery and increases the venous pressure. The patient performs this procedure utilizing the contralateral hand, compressing the common carotid pulse for 10 sec at a time, four to six times an hour. The period of compression is gradually increased to 30 sec. This procedure is successful in approximately a third of patients with cavernous DAVF. In cases with a bilateral internal carotid artery supply to the cavernous DAVF, alternate compression of carotid arteries utilizing the contralateral hand at 5-min intervals between compressions is performed. Compression therapy is tried for 4 to 6 weeks. Carotid compression

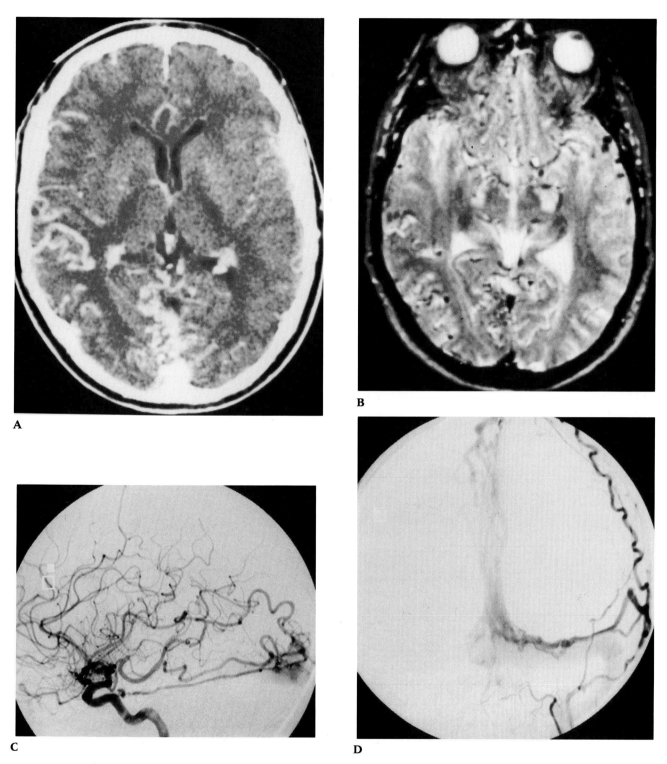

Fig. 31-5 A 65-year-old man with papilledema and dementia. There were multiple arteriovenous fistulas to the superior sagittal sinus, torcula, and transverse sinus. (*A*) Contrast-enhanced CT scan demonstrating multiple enlarged superficial cerebral veins and prominence of the torcula. (*B*) T² MRI scan shows flow void in dilated superficial cerebral veins over both hemispheres. (*C*) Lateral view of a right internal carotid artery injection shows an enlarged meningeohypophyseal artery dural supply to a torcula fistula, in addition to enlarged posterior cerebral artery branches leading to the fistula. (*D*) AP view of the left external carotid artery demonstrating enlarged middle meningeal artery feeders to the sagittal sinus and torcula fistulas.

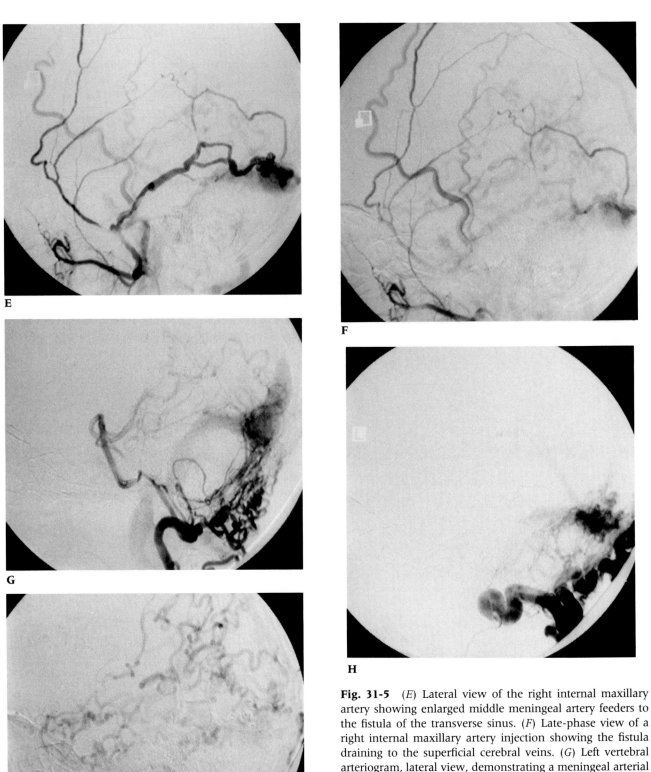

Fig. 31-5 (*E*) Lateral view of the right internal maxillary artery showing enlarged middle meningeal artery feeders to the fistula of the transverse sinus. (*F*) Late-phase view of a right internal maxillary artery injection showing the fistula draining to the superficial cerebral veins. (*G*) Left vertebral arteriogram, lateral view, demonstrating a meningeal arterial supply to the fistula at the torcula, in addition to the extracranial occipital artery supply. (*H*) Right occipital artery injection, lateral view, shows a markedly enlarged occipital artery and numerous transosseous branches supplying the fistula. (*I*) Late-phase right occipital artery injection demonstrating extensive superficial cerebral venous drainage from the fistula.

508

therapy is contraindicated in patients with severe carotid artery stenosis, as it may produce cerebral ischemia. This therapy is also contraindicated in patients with cerebral venous drainage, as compression of the jugular vein may elevate venous pressure and potentially predispose to cerebral hemorrhage.

Surgical management of cerebral DAVFs is undertaken in patients who are significantly symptomatic from the abnormality or who have undergone a complication from the DAVF. Surgery is indicated when treatment is required and endovascular therapy cannot be performed due to specific angioarchitectural features of the malformation which do not allow arterial or venous access to the lesion. Recurrent DAVF following incomplete embolization therapy may require surgery. The surgical procedure requires exposure of the fistula site, ligation of bridging veins leading from the fistula to the brain, and electrocoagulation or laser diathermy of the dura at the site of the malformation. Certain cases may warrant a combined open surgical procedure with cannulation of arterial feeders or draining veins and embolization therapy intraoperatively.

Radiosurgery may be performed in certain instances to obliterate the site of the DAVF. Potential complications related to nerve damage may limit the usefulness of this technique.

Endovascular therapy of cerebral DAVFs requires initial superselective arteriography to precisely define the feeding arteries, site of the fistula, and draining veins and dural sinuses. Certain arterial feeders, such as from the cavernous carotid artery, are often too small to catheterize or to achieve a stable position for embolization. Multiple distal small arterial feeders are frequently present and make embolization at the precise site of the fistula difficult in many cases. Occlusion of the precise fistula site with embolic material extending to the proximal venous drainage site is required to ensure permanent cure. Incomplete embolization is generally characterized by development of multiple small collateral arterial feeders and recurrence of symptoms. Arterial embolic agents include a variety of metallic coils, polyvinyl alcohol (PVA) particles, acrylic glues (N-butyl cyanoacrylate or isobutyl cyanoacrylate), and 95% ethanol. Coils are useful in large direct fistulas or to occlude the sinus; they should not be used to produce proximal arterial occlusion. While the small particles such as PVA 150–250 μm in diameter are generally safer than liquid embolic agents, their use is frequently complicated by proximal occlusion of arterial feeders, recurrence of the malformation, and potentially more difficult treatment of DAVF recurrence. Liquid embolic agents require specialized training and experience.

They also pose the risk of inadvertent damage to cranial nerves and inadvertent embolization on intracranial arteries via extra- to intracranial arterial anastomoses. Ethanol (95%) destroys the vascular endothelium and is effective in occluding multiple small dural arterial feeders. Its use produces significant pain, so good analgesia or anesthesia is necessary. Great care must be exercised in using it to avoid the cranial nerve's arterial supply, which may be damaged by unintended embolization.

Provocative testing with Lidocaine may be performed prior to arterial embolization.[5] This may result in a false-negative test result when Lidocaine flows through the fistula and does not penetrate the arterial supply to the cranial nerves. The flow situation may change during the embolization procedure, and unwanted passage of embolic material to cranial nerve arteries may result in a neurological deficit.

Transvenous embolization may be performed via the transfemoral approach or, in certain instances, by the direct approach (e.g., superior ophthalmic vein canalization via cutdown). Embolic agents utilized include fibered coils, silk thread, and occasionally detachable balloons. Transvenous catheterization and retrograde entry into the feeder may enable embolization of the feeders utilizing acrylic.

Platinum coils, detached either mechanically or by electronically, may be utilized in certain instances.[6] The initial strategy for embolization depends on the precise location and arterial supply of the DAVF. Certain cavernous sinus DAVFs may be treated by an initial transfemoral venous approach to the cavernous sinus via either the inferior petrosal sinus or the superior ophthalmic vein. Many cerebral DAVFs receive arterial supply from intracranial arteries (e.g., carotid or vertebral) in addition to the external carotid artery supply. In these patients, the external carotid artery feeders are generally approached first. If the site of the fistula can be reached through the external carotid artery feeders, the internal carotid artery feeders may regress. In some instances, this is not achieved and the fistula will continue with an internal carotid artery supply alone.

Recurrence of symptoms (e.g., vascular bruit or increased intraocular pressure) must be observed for, and several treatments may be required. Particular note must be made of the development of pial venous drainage following thrombosis of alternate venous drainage pathways.

Complications of endovascular treatment may be directly related to the embolization therapy or superselective catheterization or to indirect effects of the therapy. Direct complications include inadvertent embolization, particularly with liquid embolic agents, producing cranial nerve palsies. Inadvertent embolization of the central retinal artery via collaterals (e.g., middle meningeal artery or ethmoid artery branches) may produce blindness. Oculomotor palsies following embolization of the arterial supply to the third, fourth, and sixth cranial nerves tend to be less common with particle embolization and generally resolve. This complication is generally permanent with liquid embolic agents. Additional cranial nerve complications depend on the precise arteries embolized, such as seventh nerve palsy following embolization of the petrosal branch of the middle meningeal artery or the stylomastoid branch of the posterior auricular or occipital arteries. The ascending pharyngeal artery's neuromeningeal branch may produce abnormalities of the 9th, 10th, 11th, and 12th cranial nerves. Cerebral hemorrhage may occur following perforation of a venous sinus during catheterization, or as a consequence of venous thrombosis resulting in secondary hemorrhage. Thrombosis of draining veins and venous sinuses may occur following therapy. Superior ophthalmic vein thrombosis may result in transient worsening of proptosis, chemosis, and visual acuity, which generally resolve.

The risks of superselective angiography and subsequent endovascular treatment must be balanced against the risks to the patient of the untreated disease. A low-risk fistula without cerebral venous drainage, especially in an elderly patient, may indicate conservative follow-up rather than aggressive intervention.

DAVFs OF THE TRANSVERSE AND SIGMOID SINUSES

The transverse and sigmoid sinuses are the most common locations for cerebral DAVFs. The clinical manifestations depend on the location, quantity of arteriovenous shunting, and venous drainage. Pulsatile tinnitus is present in fistulas near the temporal bone. It is exacerbated by exercise, which increases arterial flow, and is reduced by jugular vein compression, which decreases flow through the fistula. Headaches may be the presenting symptom and may be exacerbated by exercise. Focal neurologic deficits are generally associated with cortical venous drainage and related venous hypertension, venous infarction, or hemorrhage. Occipital or cerebellar parenchymal hemorrhage, subarachnoid hemorrhage, or subdural hemorrhage may occur (Fig. 31-6). Additional focal signs include visual disturbances due to occipital cortical venous drainage or in-

creased intracranial pressure producing papilledema. Dementia and memory disturbance may occur.

The arterial supply to fistulas in this location is usually from occipital artery transosseous perforators, the posterior auricular artery, the middle meningeal artery, and the ascending pharyngeal artery (neuromeningeal division). There may be an internal carotid artery supply through the tentorial branches of the meningeohypophyseal trunk and a vertebral artery supply from posterior meningeal or falx cerebelli artery branches. Arterial supply from pial arteries may be present. Venous drainage may be through the ipsilateral sigmoid sinus to the internal jugular vein, to the contralateral transverse sinus, or to pial veins. Irregularity, stenosis, and occlusion of the sigmoid or transverse sinus may be present.

Management

Small fistulas of the transverse and sigmoid sinuses, without cortical venous drainage and minimal symptoms, may be followed clinically without therapy. Indications for therapy include neurological complications and pial venous drainage.

Compression therapy has been reported[6] to produce occlusion of the fistula in 27% of a small series of patients. Manual compression of the occipital artery for up to 30 min, repeated four to six times a day, was performed.

Transarterial embolization requires superselective catheterization of the feeding pedicles (Fig. 31-7). Microcatheters and use of road-mapping technique facilitate the procedure and enable detection of extra- to intracranial anastomosis during embolization. Embolization with PVA particles has a relatively low risk, but there is only a low incidence of permanent cure. Recur-

Fig. 31-6 A 47-year-old woman with acute right occipital cerebral hemorrhage. Right transverse sinus cerebral DAVF with drainage to the occipital lobe. (A) Noncontrast cranial CT scan demonstrates right occipital cerebral hemorrhage. (B) Contrast-enhanced cranial CT scan reveals abnormal vascular structures of the right occipital lobe in association with hemorrhage. (C) Right occipital artery injection, lateral view. Cerebral DAVF of the transverse sinus, with cerebral pial drainage to the occipital lobe and subsequently to the straight sinus. (D) Right occipital artery injection, AP view, shows a fistula and cerebral venous drainage. There is no arterial supply from the posterior cerebral artery. There is a minimal supply from the right middle meningeal artery (not shown). The patient was cured with embolization.

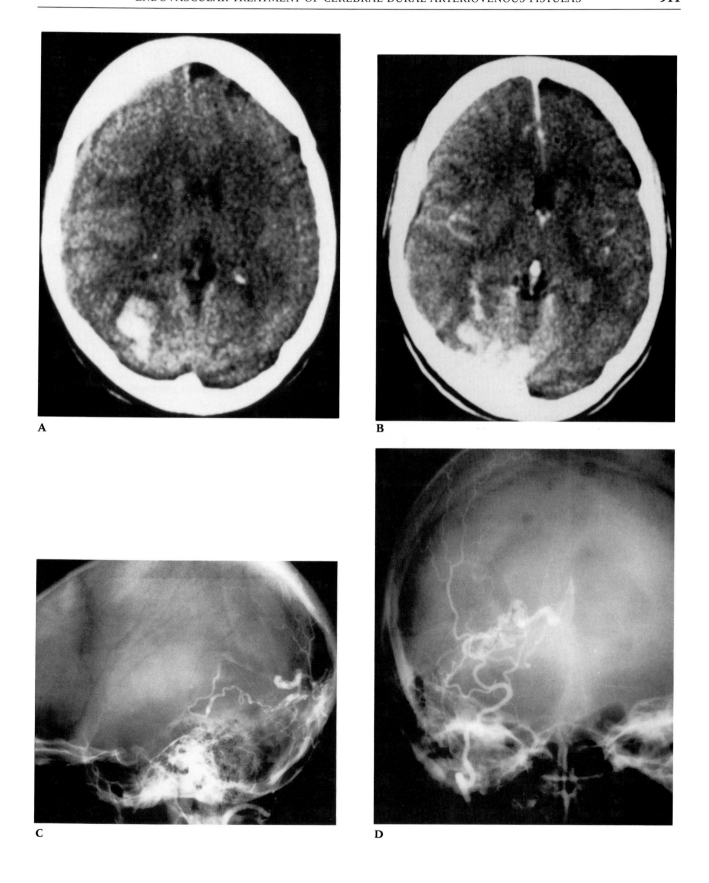

A

B

C

D

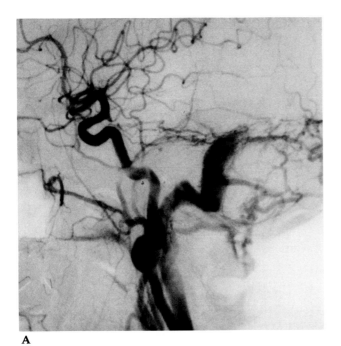

A

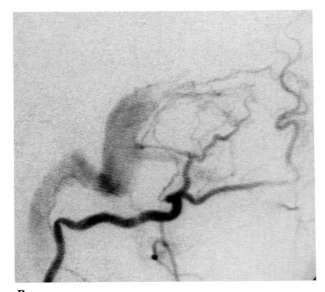

B

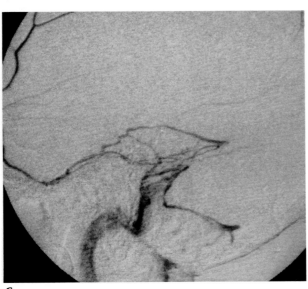

C

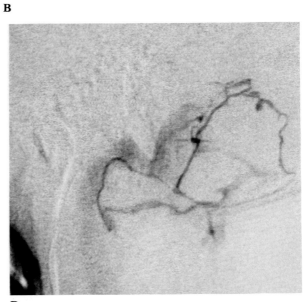

D

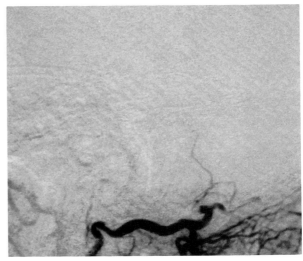

E

Fig. 31-7 A 55-year-old woman with pulsatile tinnitus and vertigo. Left transverse sinus cerebral DAVF. (*A*) Lateral view, left common carotid arteriogram, showing the supply to the transverse sinus DAVF from the meningeohypophyseal trunk of the internal carotid artery and occipital artery transmastoid feeders. (*B*) Left occipital arteriogram showing detail of the transmastoid artery supply to the transverse sinus fistula. (*C*) Left middle meningeal artery supply to the cerebral DAVF. (*D*) Injection of the neuromeningeal branch of the left ascending pharyngeal artery, lateral view. Posterior meningeal artery supply to the DAVF. (*E*) Left occipital arteriogram post-embolization of individual feeders with 95% ethanol. Occlusion of the fistula was confirmed. Follow-up arteriogram 6 months postprocedure showed no recurrence of the fistula.

rences with recanalization and development of collaterals are frequent. Liquid embolic agents, particularly acrylic glues and ethanol, have a higher success rate, with approximately 50% of patients cured, and a lower recurrence rate. Specific arterial territories, such as the neuromeningeal division of the ascending pharyngeal artery, may have a high risk of neurological complications. This division supplies the 9th, 10th, 11th, and 12th cranial nerves and has communications with the internal carotid and vertebral arteries. The occipital artery may supply the seventh cranial nerve via its stylomastoid branch and has anastomoses to the vertebral artery. The posterior auricular artery may supply the seventh nerve via its stylomastoid branch.

Prior to embolization therapy, provocative testing with Lidocaine may demonstrate an arterial supply to the cranial nerves and a potential risk of embolization with liquid embolic agents. The change that occurs in arterial circulation during embolization and the presence of the fistula diverting flow may result in false-negative provocative tests.

A transvenous approach to the fistula may be made via the transfemoral route,[7] with retrograde catheterization of the fistula and embolization using coils or acrylic, or with occlusion of the draining sinus using multiple coils or detachable balloons. This procedure is performed only after careful analysis of the venous drainage pathways, including that of normal brain. Reversal of venous flow in veins draining to the affected sinus may indicate that these veins can be occluded due to adequate collateral venous drainage in the involved brain. Veins with normal direction of flow to the sinus should not be occluded due to the risks of venous infarction and hemorrhage. Transvenous treatment is indicated in patients with cortical venous drainage from the segment of involved sinus and without normal cerebral venous drainage to the involved sinus.

Some situations require combined operative and endovascular treatment, with isolation of the involved sinus and direct puncture of the sinus. The fistula site should be occluded with acrylic or fibered coils. Silk thread may be utilized in addition. It is important not to leave segments of involved sinus patent, as continued drainage to the segment may result in cortical venous drainage and potential neurological deficit.

Combined arterial and transvenous embolization may be performed, either in the same procedure or in staged procedures. Transvenous embolization has been reported to result in 55% cure and 35% improvement in a fistula, with a 5% complication rate.[7] Unwanted occlusion of normal venous drainage pathways, including the sinus, may result in venous hypertension, including the sinus, may result in venous hypertension, in-

farction, or hemorrhage. Preoperative embolization may be performed in complex fistulas with multiple feeders. This reduces the number of arterial feeders, reducing intraoperative blood loss and enabling surgical stripping and ligation of multiple dural fistulas. Combined embolization and surgical excision has been reported to produce an 88% cure and a 12% improvement rate, with a 12% rate of complications.[8,9]

CAVERNOUS SINUS DAVFs

Cavernous sinus DAVFs generally present due to retrograde venous drainage through the ophthalmic veins, producing venous engorgement of the orbit and orbital veins. This results in proptosis, chemosis, and restriction of ocular motility. Increased intraocular pressure produces glaucoma and reduces visual acuity. Retinal detachment may occur. Involvement of the third, fourth, and sixth cranial nerves may produce diplopia.[4] Distention of the cavernous sinus may be present. Venous drainage via the coronary veins to the contralateral cavernous sinus may result in distention of the contralateral superior ophthalmic vein. This can produce bilateral orbital congestion. Thrombosis of the superior ophthalmic vein on the side of the fistula can result in venous congestion on the contralateral orbit, with an apparently normal eye on the side of the fistula.

The arterial supply to the fistula commonly arises from the internal carotid artery, primarily the inferolateral and meningeohypophyseal trunks. The external carotid arterial supply is generally from the distal internal maxillary artery (artery of the foramen rotundum), the middle meningeal and accessory meningeal arteries, and the ascending pharyngeal artery (clival branches of the neuromeningeal division). Venous drainage is via the superior and inferior ophthalmic veins, the emissary veins through the skull base to the pharyngeal veins, and posteriorly to the superior and inferior petrosal sinuses. Retrograde flow through the sphenoparietal sinus and cerebral cortical veins may be present, but if adequate additional venous drainage is present, this poses a relatively low risk of neurological dysfunction. Symptoms include headaches, hemorrhage, and focal neurological signs. Vascular tinnitus is related to drainage through the petrosal sinuses.

Cavernous sinus DAVFs must be differentiated from direct AV fistulas from the carotid artery, which are generally related to trauma or aneurysm rupture. Subtypes of cavernous sinus DAVFs are those with an arterial supply only from dural branches of the internal carotid artery, dural branches of the external carotid artery, and combined internal and external carotid artery supply. This is the most common group.

Management

Asymptomatic cavernous DAVFs may be followed clinically with careful ophthalmological supervision. Deteriorating vision, increased intraocular pressure unresponsive to medical management, or an unacceptable cosmetic appearance requires treatment of the DAVF.[10] Symptomatic cavernous DAVFs may be treated initially by carotid jugular compression. The patient compresses the common carotid artery with the contralateral arm for 10 sec per compression, four to six times an hour, increasing the compression duration to 30 sec. This is contraindicated in patients with severe carotid artery stenosis or cortical venous drainage due to the potential risk of elevating venous pressure and predisposing the patient to cerebral hemorrhage. Compression therapy has been reported to be successful only in up to 34% of patients.[8]

Endovascular occlusion of arterial feeders or transvenous embolization may be performed in symptomatic patients.

Transarterial embolization is performed initially to occlude external carotid artery feeders (Fig. 31-8). These include internal maxillary artery branches such as the artery of the foramen rotundum, accessory meningeal artery, and middle meningeal arteries. Internal carotid artery feeders, primarily involving the inferolateral trunk, are usually too small to catheterize. On occasion, these may be large enough to catheterize and safely embolize.[11] Embolization utilizing PVA particles is generally safer than with liquid embolic agents but has a higher rate of proximal occlusion and recurrence. Liquid embolic agents, primarily acrylic glues, result in higher cure and improvement rates, but are associated with an increased risk to cranial nerves and unintended

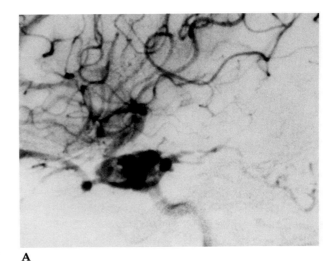

A

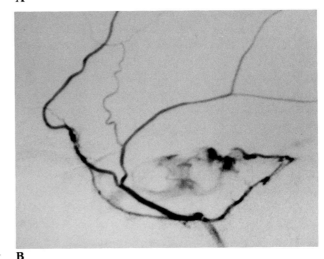

B

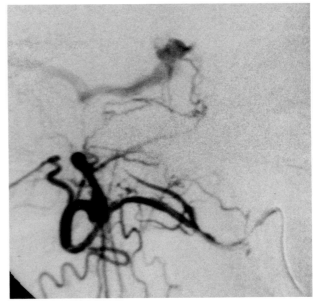

C

Fig. 31-8   A 68-year-old woman with proptosis and chemosis of the left orbit. Cerebral DAVF supplied by right and left internal carotid and left external carotid arteries. (*A*) Lateral view, left internal carotid arteriogram, shows an internal carotid fistula to the cavernous sinus and retrograde flow through the superior ophthalmic vein. (*B*) Left middle meningeal arteriogram with the fistula at the posterior aspect of the left cavernous sinus supplied by a marginal tentorial artery branch. (*C*) Left internal maxillary arteriogram shows supply to the cavernous DAVF via the artery of the foramen rotundum and the accessory meningeal artery. It was embolized with PVA particles.

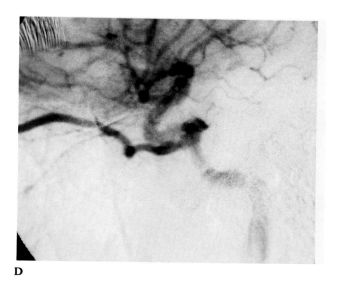

D

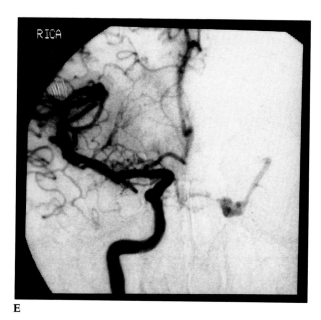

E

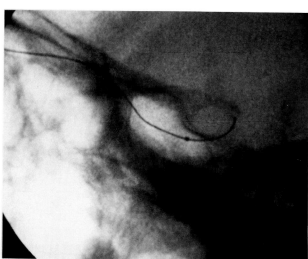

F

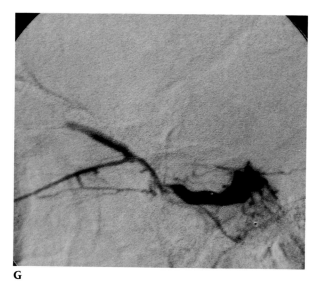

G

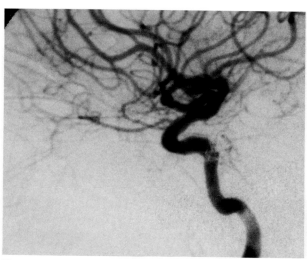

H

Fig. 31-8 (*D*) Recurrence of symptoms 2 months following treatment. Left internal carotid arteriogram shows dural branches supplying the fistula of the posterior cavernous sinus, with superior ophthalmic vein drainage. Partial thrombosis of the cavernous sinus has occurred. (*E*) Right internal carotid artery injection with filling of the left cavernous DAVF via right meningeohypophyseal artery branches. (*F*) Retrograde cannulation of the left superior ophthalmic vein following cutdown. (The inferior petrosal sinus was occluded.) A guidewire and microcatheter are in the cavernous sinus. (*G*) Cavernous sinus injection retrogradely fills the dural arterial feeders to the fistula. Embolization with microcoils was performed. (*H*) Left internal carotid arteriogram following embolization shows obliteration of the fistula.

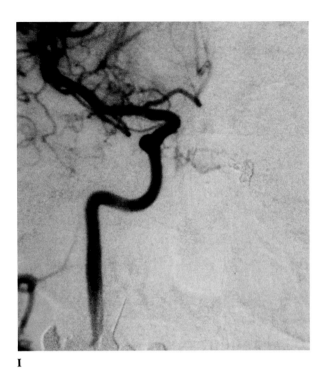

I

Fig. 31-8 (*I*) Right internal carotid arteriogram following embolization confirms the absence of the cavernous sinus fistula.

embolization of the internal carotid artery via unrecognized anastomoses. Liquid embolic agents can pass through minute arterial anastomoses. Complications include cranial nerve deficits of the third, fourth, fifth, sixth, and seventh cranial nerves. Unintended ophthalmic artery embolization can produce blindness. Transarterial embolization has been reported to produce a 78% cure rate and a 20% improvement rate in symptoms in the remaining patients.[8,12]

Transvenous embolization may be performed via transfemoral catheterization of the cavernous sinus through the inferior petrosal sinus or the facial vein to the superior ophthalmic vein (Figs. 31-9, 31-10).[13] Frequently, the inferior petrosal sinus appears occluded on arteriography, but it is possible to cannulate it. If the inferior petrosal sinus approach and transfemoral catheterization of the superior ophthalmic vein through the facial veins are unsuccessful, a cutdown on the superior ophthalmic vein may be performed to facilitate direct catheterization.[14] The cavernous sinus is packed with thrombogenic coils. Silk thread has also been utilized to produce sinus thrombosis.

Complications of the transvenous approach include perforation of the inferior petrosal sinus and thrombo-

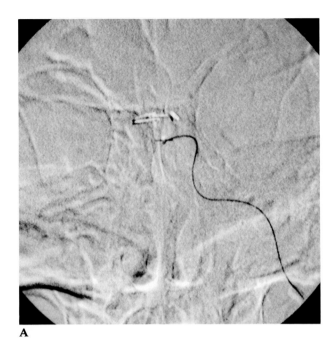

A

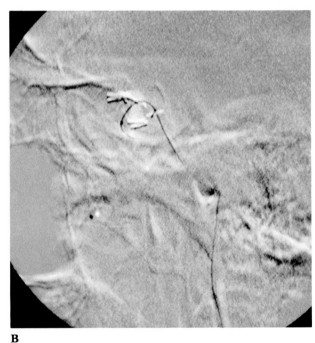

B

Fig. 31-9 (*A,B*) AP and lateral detail of transfemoral catheterization of the cavernous sinus via the inferior petrosal sinus and deposition of platinum coils.

sis of the superior ophthalmic vein. Occlusion of normal cerebral draining veins may occur, with resultant cerebral venous infarct or hemorrhage. Transvenous embolization of cavernous DAVFs has been reported to result in an 81% cure rate and a 19% improvement rate.[13]

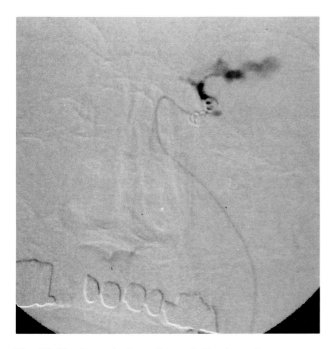

Fig. 31-10 Frontal view after embolization of a cavernous sinus dural malformation. The Tracker catheter was advanced from the internal jugular view to the facial vein (at the C_4 level), angular vein, and infraorbital vein to connect to the cavernous sinus.

Thrombosis of the cavernous sinus and superior ophthalmic vein may occur as a result of treatment, producing paradoxical worsening of symptoms. This generally resolves with conservative treatment.[15]

CEREBRAL DAVFs OF THE ANTERIOR CRANIAL FOSSA

These DAVFs are relatively rare, presenting in middle-aged to elderly patients, with a mean age of 55 years. The arterial supply is generally from ethmoid artery meningeal branches, with venous drainage to olfactory or inferior frontal cerebral veins. There is a high incidence of cerebral and subarachnoid hemorrhage.[16] Treatment of these fistulas is generally recommended due to the risks of neurological deficit. Most of these patients have undergone surgical resection and coagulation of a fistula site. Endovascular treatment is limited due to the potential risk of ophthalmic artery embolization, either by embolizing ethmoid artery branches or by direct catheterization of the ophthalmic artery. Ethmoid artery embolization through the internal maxillary arteries following surgical clipping of the ethmoid branches of the ophthalmic arteries has been reported.

CEREBRAL DAVFs AT OTHER SITES

Superior sagittal sinus DAVFs may be multiple and present with headaches, hemorrhage, dementia, papilledema, and nonfocal neurological changes. Multiple staged catheterization is frequently required.[17] Cerebral dural fistulas with spinal venous drainage may present with myelopathy. These may be confused clinically with spinal cord tumors or spinal DAVFs, but the distended spinal veins in the cervical region may be the clue to the diagnosis. Treatment is required and may consist of surgery or embolization therapy. This depends on the anatomical site of the fistula and the accessability of its arterial supply.

REFERENCES

1. Chaudhary M, Sachdev VP, Cho SH, et al. Dural arteriovenous malformation of the major venous sinuses: An acquired lesion. *AJNR* 1982;3:13–19.
2. Lasjaunias P, Berenstein A. *Surgical Neuroangiography. Functional Anatomy of Craniofacial Arteries.* Berlin, Springer-Verlag, 1987.
3. Djindjian R, Merland JJ. *Superselective Arteriography of the External Carotid Artery.* Berlin, Springer-Verlag, 1978.
4. Viñuela F, Fox AJ, Pelz DM, et al. Unusual clinical manifestations of dural arteriovenous malformation. *J Neurosurg* 1986;64:554–558.
5. Horton JA, Kerber CW. Lidocaine injection into the external carotid branches: Provocative test to preserve cranial nerve function in therapeutic embolization. *AJNR* 1986;7:105–108.
6. Sadato A, Taki W, Nishi S, et al. Treatment of a spontaneous carotid cavernous fistula using an electrodetachable microcoil. *AJNR* 1993;14:334–336.
7. Halbach VV, Higashida RT, Hieshima GB, et al. Transvenous embolization of dural fistulas involving the transverse and sigmoid sinuses. *AJNR* 1989;10:385–392.
8. Viñuela F, Halbach VV, Dion JE. *Interventional Neuroradiology: Endovascular Therapy of the Central Nervous System.* New York, Raven Press, 1992.
9. Halbach VV, Higashida RT, Hieshima GB, et al. Dural fistulas involving the transverse and sigmoid sinuses: Results of treatment in 28 patients. *Radiology* 1987;163:443–447.
10. Halbach VV, Hieshima GB, Higashida RT, et al. Carotid cavernous fistula: Indications for urgent therapy. *AJNR* 1987;8:627–633 and *AJR* 1987;149:587–593.
11. Halbach VV, Higashida RT, Hieshima GB, et al. Embolization of the dural branches arising from the cavernous internal carotid artery. *AJNR* 1989;10:143–150.

12. Halbach VV, Higashida RT, Hieshima GB, et al. Dural fistulas involving the cavernous sinus: Results of treatment in 30 patients. *Radiology* 1987;163:437–442.

13. Halbach VV, Higashida RT, Hieshima GB, et al. Transvenous embolization of dural fistulas involving the cavernous sinus. *AJNR* 1989;10:377–384.

14. Teng MM, Guo WY, Huang CI, et al. Occlusion of arteriovenous malformations of the cavernous sinus via the superior ophthalmic vein. *AJNR* 1988;9(3):539–545.

15. Sergott RC, Grossman RI, Savino PJ, et al. The syndrome of paradoxical worsening of dural cavernous sinus arteriovenous malformations. *Ophthalmology* 1987;94(3):205–212.

16. Kobayashi H, Hayashi M, Noguchi Y, et al. Dural arteriovenous malformations in the anterior cranial fossa. *Surg Neurol* 1988;30(5):396–401.

17. Halbach VV, Higashida RT, Hieshima GB, et al. Treatment of dural arterial venous malformations involving the superior sagittal sinus. *AJNR* 1988;9:337–343.

Index

Angle correction, Doppler sonography, 127
Arteriovenous fistula
  dural, 510–513
    anterior cranial fossa, 517
    cavernous sinus, 513–517
    classification of, 502–503
    clinical manifestations, 503–505
    management, 505–510
    radiological evaluation, 503
    of transverse/sigmoid sinuses, 510–513
  endovascular treatment, dural, 502–518
Arteriovenous malformation(s), 44–45, 242–244
  anatomical considerations, 447–450
  anterior choroidal artery, 450
  Broca's area, 450
  computed tomography, 173–178
  embolization materials, 443–444
  frontal lobe, 448–450
  functional testing, 447
  infratentorial, 450–452
  intra-arterial digital subtraction angiography, 114
  intracranial, interventional therapy for, 439–459
  intracranial hemorrhage, 242–244
  occipital lobe, 448
  radiological imaging, 444–447
  single photon emission computed tomography, 387
  temporal lobe, 448
  visual pathway, 448
  Wernicke's area, 450
Arteritis
  arterial narrowing, magnetic resonance angiography, extracra-
      nial, 361
  intra-arterial digital subtraction angiography, 104–105,
      109–111
Artery, *see also specific artery*
  circulation, retina, and fluorescein angiography, 63
  narrowing, arteritis, magnetic resonance angiography, extracra-
      nial, 361
  occlusion, 33–37
  spasm, neurointerventional treatment, 431
Artifacts, magnetic resonance angiography, 324–333
  intracranial, 346–350
Atherectomy, neurointerventional treatment, 428
Atherosclerosis
  disease, intra-arterial digital subtraction angiography, 101–
      103, 107–108
  lesions, ultrasound, 133–134
  plaque
    distribution, 133
    relationship to stroke, 133–134
Attenuation, ultrasound, 123
Autoregulation, failure of, 27

B
Bacterial aneurysm, 44
Balloon, detachable, aneurysm, 461
Balloon catheter, detachable, neurointerventional treatment,
    425–426
Balloon occlusion test, Tc-99m HMPAO brain single photon emis-
    sion computed tomography, 390–391
Bandwidth, ultrasound, 126
Basilar artery, anatomy, 17
Bloch equations, magnetic resonance imaging, 213–214
B-mode ultrasound, gray scale image, 121–123
Brain death
  cerebral perfusion agent, 392–393
  conventional brain scintigraphy, 392
  single photon emission computed tomography, 392–395

Brain positron emission tomography, 411–416
  brain tumors, 413–414
  dementia, 412–413
  localization of seizure foci, refractory seizure disorders, 412
  positron-emitting isotopes, 411
  radiopharmaceuticals, 411–414
  refractory seizure disorders, localization of seizure foci, 412
Brain tumors, positron emission tomography, 413–414
Broca's area, arteriovenous malformation, 450

C
Calcification, carotid arteries, extracranial, 136
Carotid artery
  cavernous fistula, 70
  color flow imaging, 121–147
  duplex imaging, 121–147
  endarterectomy, intraoperative sonography, 142
  extracranial
    aneurysm, 139
    atherosclerosis
      lesions, 133–134
      plaque
        distribution, 133
        relationship to stroke, 133–134
    calcification, 136
    clinical significance, threshold for, 136
    contralateral lesions, 139
    diagnostic criteria, 134–135
    dissection, 139
    imaging/waveform analysis, clinical applications, 133–139
    neoplasms, 139
    pathologies, 139
    plaque, sonographic classification of, 134
    pseudoaneurysm, 139
    radiation, 139
    stenoses, hemodynamically significant, 134–139
    stroke, acute, thrombolytic treatment, 472
    subtotal vs. total occlusion, 136–137
    tandem lesions, 137–139
    ultrasound, atherosclerotic lesions, 133–134
    vasculitis, 139
  internal
    anatomy of, 10–11
    cavernous segment of, aneurysm, intra-arterial digital sub-
        traction angiography, 106–107
    occlusion, magnetic resonance angiography, extracranial,
        359–360
    pathology, 33
    stenosis
      computed tomography, spiral, 189–194
      high-grade, altered flow with, 142
      magnetic resonance angiography, extracranial, 358–359
      supra-aortic vessel, angioplasty, 491
      ultrasound, 131
Carotid-vertebral disease, extracranial, intra-arterial digital subtrac-
    tion angiography,101–107
Catheter, *see also* Microcatheters
  angiographic, neurointerventional treatment, 424
  angioplasty, 425
  balloon, detachable, neurointerventional treatment, 425–426
  diagnostic, neurointerventional treatment, 424
  embolization, neurointerventional treatment, 424–425
  guiding, neurointerventional treatment, 424
  microsoft stream infusion, neurointerventional treatment, 425
  regular soft stream infusion, neurointerventional treatment,
      425
  for special needs, neurointerventional treatment, 424–426
  thrombolysis, neurointerventional treatment, 425

TOTAL WARMTH

The Complete Guide to Winter Well-Being

Total

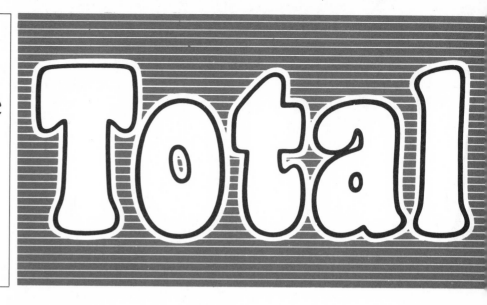

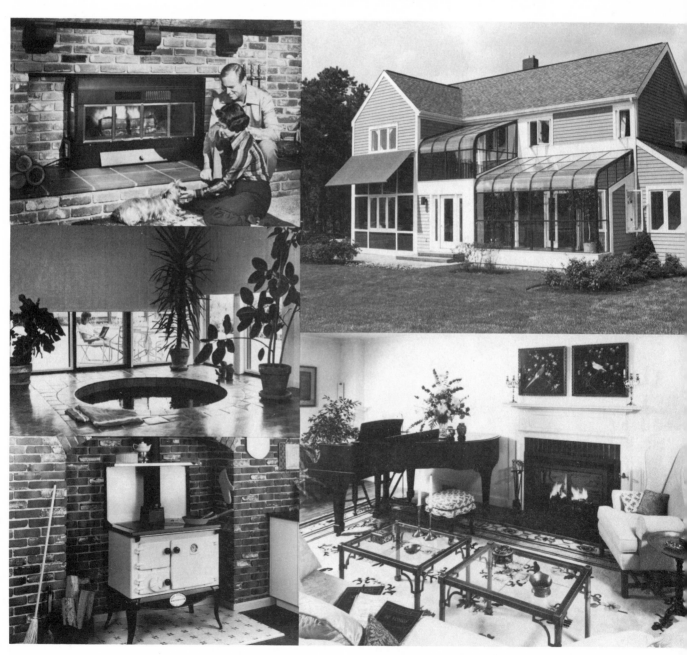

Warmth

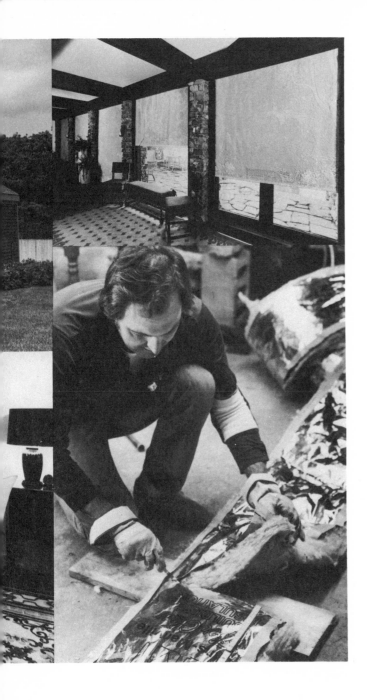

Geri Harrington

Barbara Shook Hazen

Michael deCourcy Hinds

Carolyn Jabs

Jonathan Leonard

L. Donald Meyers

Sandra Oddo

A. T. Perrin

Delores Wolfe

Macmillan Publishing Co., Inc.
New York

Collier Macmillan Publishers
London

Credits for Title Page Photos
Fireplace insert: The Free Heat Machine;
insulating curtain walls: Thermal Technology
Corporation; range: Waterford; solar greenhouse:
Brookhaven National Laboratory

Macmillan Publishing Co., Inc.
866 Third Avenue, New York, N.Y. 10022
Collier Macmillan Canada, Inc.

Library of Congress Catalog Card Number: 81-13722

ISBN 0-02-548460-5

10 9 8 7 6 5 4 3 2 1

The information given in this book is
intended solely as a guide of broad general
usefulness, and inclusion in this book does
not constitute a guarantee of a product or
its safety by the publisher.

Printed in the United States of America

Editor: Maron L. Waxman
Assistant: Jeffrey Neuman
Designer: Ron Farber

Contents

Contributors

An authority who frequently lectures on heating with wood and coal, Geri Harrington has written several books, including *The Wood-Burning Stove Book* and *Fireplaces, Stoves, Hearths, and Inserts.* Her most recent book is *Never Too Old: A Guide for the Over 50 Adult.*

Barbara Shook Hazen is the author of several books of household hints and many juvenile books, most recently *Tight Times.*

Michael deCourcy Hinds is the home energy reporter for the *New York Times.*

Carolyn Jabs is a frequent contributor to the *New York Times* and national magazines on home products. She is the author of the forthcoming book *HomEconomy: 2,133 Ways to Reuse and Recycle the Things You Usually Throw Away.*

Jonathan Leonard, a medical editor, writes for *Harvard* and scientific magazines.

The author of *Home Insulating, Home Wiring for Cowards,* and several other how-to books, L. Donald Meyers writes frequently for *Popular Science, Family Circle,* and *Popular Mechanics.*

Sandra Oddo, the coauthor with Peter Powell of *Solar for Existing Homes,* writes "Energy Answers" for *House & Garden* magazine, and was the founding editor of *Solar Age* magazine.

A. T. Perrin is the writer and compiler of *Explorers Ltd. Source Book.*

Delores Wolfe is the author of *Growing Food in Solar Greenhouses.*

Introduction: The Cold Facts

Barbara Hazen

The world is getting colder, and we may as well get used to it. We're running out of fossil fuels, especially oil, and many scientists predict that another Ice Age is on the way. For most of us—two-thirds of the world's population—coping with the cold is a major factor in our lives. In the face of these chilling facts, can we keep ourselves from going the way of the woolly mammoth?

Cold times are, of course, nothing new. The earth has been as warm as it is today for only about 10 percent of the past 100,000 years. Twenty thousand years ago, blizzards raged through most of the Northern Hemisphere. A huge ice sheet covered New York City, and arctic foxes and reindeer gamboled along the snow-banked shores of southern France.

In the past million years of world history, there have been eight major advances of ice sheets from the north, followed by eight warming trends. By the end of the fourth, 10,000 years ago, only one species of man was left on the earth—Homo sapiens. He overcame the limits of his fragile body by using his fertile mind. He built fires, made clothes from animal skins to compensate for his own inadequate fur, and, most importantly, became an efficient hunter by devising weapons and cooperating with his fellow man to hunt in groups.

THE WEATHER TODAY

During the 20th century, the global thermometer rose until 1950, when things started to get a little quirky. By the end of 1976, the United States National Academy of Science warned that a chilling change was in progress and that the cozy warmth of the first half of the century was "highly abnormal."

A year later, the secretary of agriculture ordered his department to stop assuming "normal" weather when making forecasts of agricultural production. That was the year it froze in Miami and snowed in Washington, while in Fairbanks, Alaska, a hockey game was canceled as a result of melting ice in 50° weather. Clearly, abnormal weather was fast becoming the norm.

SEVEN DANGER SIGNS OF THE COMING ICE AGE

1. Fog in California is increasing.
2. Freakish winter storms in the United States and Western Europe are on the rise.
3. Basically colder temperatures prevail, interspersed with occasional bouts of intense heat—these are the chill and fever symptoms of a planet catching cold.
4. The prevailing winds are changing.
5. Glaciers are advancing in Alaska, Canada, Iceland, and the Soviet Union.
6. Severe floods and drought in the United States indicate extreme weather to come.
7. Sea ice in the North Atlantic is increasing.

Scientists are studying these climate changes, using balloons, rockets, satellites, and all available expertise. They're learning about how to raise crops in the cold, conserve water, and hoard our remaining energy more carefully while seeking new sources. Homo sapiens is again trying to think his way through the coming cold.

STUDIES IN COLD

At two sites in New England, scientists are studying the dynamics of snow and ice. At the Army's Cold Regions Research and Engineering Laboratory (CRREL) in Hanover, New Hampshire, scientists brave indoor temperatures of 30° below zero in August to study winter problems, including how to handle snow loads, frost damage, and ice on airplane wings.

Atop Mount Washington, also in New Hampshire, meteorologists study what has been called the worst weather in the world. Wind gusts commonly hit 100 mph. When the thermometer's reading goes up, it's usually because the observatory's pet cat is snuggling up against it. The extreme conditions make it an ideal training ground for meteorologists. Remarked one staff weatherman, "I've seen more weather here in eighteen months than most meteorologists see in a lifetime."

COLD SPOTS

The coldest average yearly temperature in the United States: 9.6°F at Barrow, Alaska. (Summers average a swimless 37.7°.)

The coldest average yearly temperature in the continental United States: 27°F, atop Mount Washington in New Hampshire. (Summers are a balmy 47.2°)

The coldest temperature recorded in the United States: −79.8°F at Prospect Creek Camp, Alaska, on January 23, 1971.

The coldest temperature recorded in the continental United States: −70°F at Rogers Pass, Montana, on January 20, 1954.

The coldest temperature ever recorded in Hawaii: 14°F on January 2, 1961, at Huleakela Summit on Maui.

Fast falls: In Browning, Montana, in twenty-four hours on January 23–24, 1916, the temperature fell from 44°F to −56°F. In Rapid City, South Dakota, on January 12, 1911, the temperature fell from 49°F at 6 A.M. to −13°F at 8 A.M. In Spearfish, South Dakota, the temperature fell from 54°F to −4° in just twenty-seven minutes. Earlier in the day, the temperature had risen from −4° to 45° in just *two* minutes. (Imagine trying to dress for a day like that!)

The coldest inhabited place in the world: Polus Kholodo (Pole of Cold) in Soviet Siberia. Wolves roam the streets, tires rip open when they hit pot holes, and sheet metal snaps like a breadstick. But mayor Ivan Danielovich

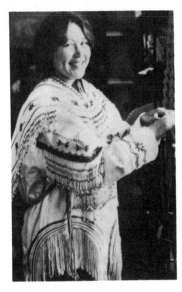

Eskimos have the ideal faces for cold weather, with short noses on flat faces. This keeps all the features in reach of the warming blood that flows to the brain and decreases the chance of frostbite. (TravelArctic)

Tcherov says, "Anyone can adapt to anything."

The coldest spot in the world: Vostok, also in Siberia, recorded a world record of −126.94°F on August 24, 1960.

SNOW NEWS IS GOOD NEWS

Even if you don't ski, can't stand the cold, and dislike the fluffy stuff, snow is essential to your life. Full reservoirs and a successful growing season depend on it. The more snow on the ground in winter, the more water in the ground that spring.

Snow is also an invaluable blanket for plants and burrowing animals. When it is 0°F on the snow's surface, it's as much as 20° warmer underneath.

Much snow lore is grounded in fact. While all snowflakes have six sides, it's true that no two are exactly alike. It's also true that if the first snowflakes are large, the snow will be a long one, since larger snowflakes are a result of very turbulent air blowing ice crystals against each other. Also, "if snow begins in the middle of the day, expect at least a foot to lay." Since midday air is warmer, it causes a lot of precipitation when it meets a cold front. Among the flakier winter notions are that if you melt snow on your stove, the number of rising bubbles will be the number of snows to come, or that the date of the first snowfall foretells the number of snow storms for the winter. These meth-

ods are notoriously unreliable, and you'll do better by leaving the forecasting to the groundhogs.

One thing you can't do is take snow lightly. A 10-inch snowfall over an acre weighs a total of 226,000 pounds. If your job is to remove 15 inches of snow from a 5 x 50-foot sidewalk, you'll have lifted a ton of snow by the time you finish—if you finish.

LUCKY STIFFS

Occasionally, the incredible happens—living people freeze and are revived.

In the 1950s, a hobo from Windsor Locks, Connecticut, named Crow Connors fell asleep during a severe snowstorm. When found, he was declared dead by the local doctor. He was taken to the nearest undertaker and stored in a wooden box, where he thawed. He awoke to find a man preparing a formaldehyde injection. "Howdy," was his greeting to the mortified undertaker.

In December 1980, a woman named Jean Hilliard was found outside the home of a friend following a night of −22° temperatures. Her car had stalled, and she was trying to get help when she collapsed. The friend, Wally Nelson, loaded her diagonally in the back of his car and took her to the hospital. Her temperature was too low to register on the thermometer, and her skin was too hard to pierce with a hypodermic needle. After slow and careful thawing,

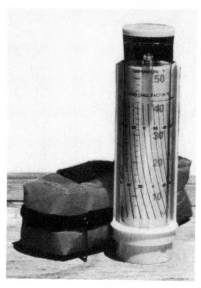

In winter, the wind has much more to do with how cold you feel than the temperature does. The wind chill factor, devised in the Antarctic in 1941 by Dr. Paul Siple, takes into account both temperature and wind velocity. This portable wind chill meter measures both to tell you at a glance how cold it really is. (The Nature Company)

she was successfully revived by doctors at the Fosston, Minnesota, hospital.

WHAT THE FORECAST MEANS: COLD WEATHER WORDS

Snow flurries: Intermittent snowfall for short periods of time. Not much accumulation, but visibility may be bad at times.

Drifting snow: Strong winds are likely to cause drifts, which are particularly hazardous to drivers.

Heavy snow: More than 4 inches are expected in 12 hours, or 6 inches in 24 hours.

Freezing rain: Ice on exposed surfaces, such as roads.

Heavy ice: The kind of ice that snaps power lines and bows branches. Give a quick look to your favorite tree.

Cold-wave warning: Expect a dramatic temperature fall within 24 hours. Be prepared: check the antifreeze in your car, wear a wooly cap, and take protective measures.

Livestock warning: Extreme cold, ice, and/or snow expected. Bring animals in out of the cold.

Traveler's warning: Blowing, falling, or drifting snow or freezing rain. Ice will make driving dangerous.

Winter storm watch: A storm has formed and is coming closer. Keep an ear to the radio and an eye on the television for further information.

Winter storm warning: A storm is imminent. Take the necessary steps to stay safe and snug and to protect property.

Blizzard warning: Expect low temperatures, strong winds, a lot of snow, and bad visibility.

Severe blizzard warning: Expect winds of 45 m.p.h. and a temperature of 10°F or lower.

THE COLD NATURALIST

For those who wish to pursue nature in the winter, there is a way. Here are a few good guides:

John R. Quinn, *The Winter Woods.* Greenwich, Connecticut: Chatham Press, 1976.
Donald W. Stokes, *A Guide to Nature in Winter: Northeast and North Central North America.* Boston: Little Brown, 1976.
Lauren Brown, *Weeds in Winter.* New York: Norton, 1976.
May Theilgaard Watts and Tom Watts, *Winter Tree Finder.* Berkeley, California: Nature Study Guild, 1970.

A BERG IN THE HAND . . .

Over two-thirds of the earth's fresh water is locked up in antarctic ice, in icebergs that pose a constant temptation to countries with chronic water shortages. One such country is Saudi Arabia, which has already spent close to

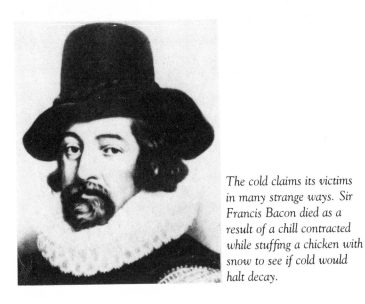

The cold claims its victims in many strange ways. Sir Francis Bacon died as a result of a chill contracted while stuffing a chicken with snow to see if cold would halt decay.

$2 million on research exploring the possibility of towing icebergs to its shores. The main problem is how to tow a berg to a southern port without its melting. Of course, that assumes it can be towed at all; even a powerful tug has less than 200 pounds of pull, and an individual iceberg has over 1,000 tons of resistance.

COLD HARD FACTS

A mere 5–7° drop in global temperatures will bring on another Ice Age.

Minus 40° is the one temperature that's exactly the same on both the centigrade and Fahrenheit scales.

If your house has a dozen double-hung windows and two doors with 1/16″ cracks, you are losing as much heat as if you had a foot-wide hole in your living-room walls.

The ideal situation for quick weight loss, according to Dr. Frank Katch, chairman of the Department of Exercise Science at the University of Massachusetts, is "a very overweight person wearing very little clothing in a very cold environment." Before you rush outside in your bikini undies, bear in mind that it's also an ideal situation for pneumonia.

The ideal temperature for health and mental alertness is 65 to 68° Fahrenheit. (A little lower if you exercise a great deal and eat a lot of protein.)

You're right if you've always thought that your feet were colder than the rest of you. The extremities get less body heat than the torso, and since warm air rises, the air at ground level is colder than the air you breathe. The difference may be as much as 20°, which is why feet are the body part most often frostbitten.

According to Planned Parenthood, the three months with the highest birth rates are August, September, and October. This means that many people still rely on the old-fashioned methods of generating heat in November, December, and January.

Birds migrate in the winter, or build up reserves of subcutaneous fat. Animals hibernate or grow thick fur coats. Fish seek warmer waters. Man is the only animal whose adaptations to cold weather are cultural rather than biological.

WHERE DO WE GO FROM HERE?

If meteorologists are right, it looks as if we will be facing the cold for a good long time; some say the next 4,000 years. This will, of course, sorely tax our ability to produce energy for heating. The gloomier estimates indicate that, at our present levels of consumption, we have only an eight-to-ten-year supply of oil. What can we do?

We can enhance oil discovery by developing new techniques to coax oil out of shale and bedrock.

We can search for oil in new places—under the Arctic icecap, perhaps.

We can turn to coal and natural gas, ignoring the fact that they, too, will someday run out.

We can make greater use of solar energy, which has only begun to realize its full potential.

One answer that few people like, but that many scientists see as the only long-range solution, is nuclear energy, which now provides 10 percent of the electricity for the United States. On one hand, it promises limitless energy; on the other hand, it offers the possibility of a global ecological disaster.

Then there are the solutions based on individual initiative, like wood stoves. They offer freedom from centralized energy sources but require a lot of work: chopping wood, hauling it, storing it, and so on.

The only answer is to recognize that there isn't any answer yet, but that we're looking in many promising directions. The best that we can do for now is to conserve the energy we've got and realize that there is no quick fix. Insulate, bundle up, stoke that stove, and get ready for the long, cold winter ahead.

TOTAL WARMTH

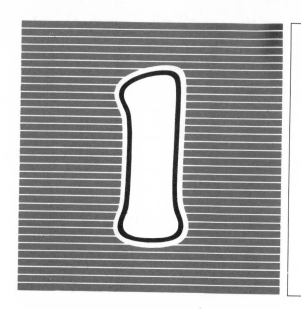

Back to Basics: Keeping Warm with Wood and Coal

Geri Harrington

HOW TO ENJOY CUTTING HOME HEATING COSTS

If your most recent home heating-oil or gas bill left you speechless, relieve your feelings with a couple of four-letter words—wood and coal. These old-fashioned fuels can not only cut those costs but also help you enjoy a warm, cozy home no matter how the winds blow or the temperature drops.

With wood and coal, you don't have to turn your thermostat down to the point of discomfort, and you don't have to feel guilty or go broke in order to have one of life's essentials —heat. And, best of all, it can really be fun to gain control of such an important part of your life. The satisfying sight of your wood or coal pile will generate a warm glow all by itself.

If you'd like to consider joining the millions of Americans who have already installed wood- or coal-burning stoves, read on and learn how easy it can be.

IS A WOOD OR COAL STOVE RIGHT FOR YOU?

Are you fed up with high home heating bills? Are you willing to try a better way of life? Are you open minded about new solutions to the energy problem? Are you looking for easy ways to exercise and to get in better physical shape? Are you tired of being cold and of risking hypothermia every time you sit down to read the paper or watch television? If the answer to these questions is "Yes!" what are you waiting for? A wood/coal stove is for you.

WHICH FUEL?

Wood or coal? Which is best? Each has its advantages and disadvantages.

AVAILABILITY

If you can't get it, you can't burn it, so your first job is to make sure the fuel of your choice is available in your area. Study the ads in your local paper and make a few phone calls. Talk to wood or coal stove owners. You won't go wrong with either fuel in terms of heat, but one might be much better than the other in terms of availability. It's hard to imagine, for instance, that a stove owner in Pennsylvania would not do better with coal than with wood —unless, of course, he owns his own woodlot. Of course, sometimes the rules may not hold. Maine, which is ninety percent forest and has a limitless supply of wood, has lately begun to burn a lot of coal.

> Coal is a portable climate.
> Ralph Waldo Emerson

COST

Both wood and coal will save you money over oil and electricity (and probably over gas), but wood is usually cheapest. Since many

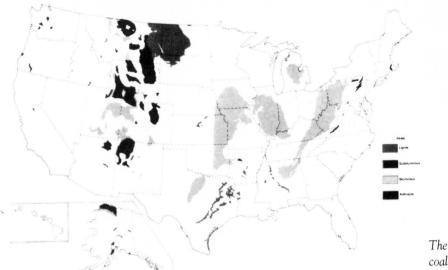

The location of America's coal resources.

of the coal mines are owned by oil companies, the price of coal may soon rise sharply as the demand for it increases. Further, coal dealers are just a step in the line of supply; they have to buy the product from the mines so, obviously, they have to add their markup to the original cost. Wood, on the other hand, is a cottage industry; wood dealers—mostly one- or two-man operations—usually own their own business and, frequently, cut their own wood to sell directly to the consumer.

Other cost factors are the production and distribution methods employed. Wood is easy to get at. About all anyone needs is a chain saw, some experience, and a lot of common sense. Wood tends to be used where it is most available; it could be distributed over long distances, but it isn't. So if there is wood in your area, you are the one who will benefit. Prices will vary from one wood seller to another and shopping around will get you the best price. Mining coal, on the other hand, requires expensive equipment, expensive labor, and an elaborate distribution network. Unfortunately, at the moment, such a network doesn't even exist, since the most efficient way to distribute coal is by rail, and the railways are no longer capable of delivering coal in any quanity—and won't be for many years. The fact is the United States coal industry has been kept alive through all these years of domestic oil and gas heating by the demand from foreign countries. Korea, France, and many other nations depend on American coal. The potential demand, as oil prices continue to rise, will, it is said, make the United States the "Saudi Arabia of coal." That's good for the economy but—here's the hitch—bad for the coal-stove owner, who will be taken care of only after foreign commitments have been met. The government may help change this situation. But, for the moment at least, domestic heating doesn't seem to be the government's first priority. After all, in spite of Washington's exhortations to the consumer to save oil, it still refuses to give a tax credit for a wood-burning stove—an obvious and efficient energy saver. This refusal to give a tax credit for what is surely no more of a frill than insulation, caulking, and storm windows—all of which do earn tax credits—is a real puzzle, and I wonder why consumers haven't spoken up and made more of a fuss about this injustice.

SUPPLY

Wood is a renewable resource, so we need never run out of it if we manage our forests and woodlots properly. Finland, a tiny country whose leading exports are wood and wood products, has proved this dramatically over the past hundred years. And now, in addition to its enormous exports of wood and its free domestic use of wood in construction, Finland is planning to make itself 40 percent self-sufficient in energy within the next ten years—50 percent in the long term—by using peat and wood. Its goal is to *halve* its dependence on Soviet oil.

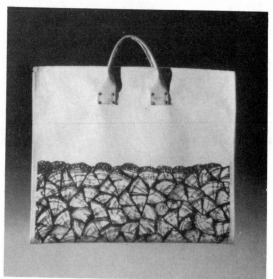

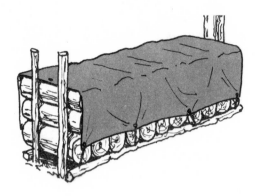

You can't chop wood with your bare hands, so why should you carry it in them? A canvas log carrier makes the long trek back from the woods much easier. (Hart Fireplace Furnishings) Once you've stacked your woodpile, you should cover it with a canvas top to help keep it dry. (Firl Industries, Inc.)

4

Coal is a fossil fuel and, while we have enough of it in the United States to last at least the next 200 years, we will eventually run out of it. It's not any more renewable than oil.

HOMEGROWN

Anyone with an acre of land can grow some wood of his own if he wants to. A properly managed one-acre woodlot will provide a cord of wood a year *forever*. Poplar is said to produce five cords of wood a year. And while I don't have any production figures for it, black locust, which grows as much as three feet in a single year, must also have a high rate of production. Both poplar and black locust are self-propagating. After the initial planting, you'll never have to plant another locust or poplar tree; in fact, you'll have trouble keeping them down. They send up shoots from their roots, often as much as 15 to 30 feet away from the parent tree. Every tree you cut down sends up shoots from the stump as well as increased shoots from the roots. Add to this the fact that black locust is one of the hardest domestic woods with one of the highest Btu-production rates, and you'll see a very encouraging woodlot picture.

No one can grow coal, any more than he can produce oil. The homeowner must depend on commercial sources for coal, as well as for most other fuels. Not everyone, however, is interested in growing his own wood, so this may not be a consideration.

HOW MUCH CHEAPER IS WOOD OR COAL?

You'll be amazed at how much you can save on your heating bills when you switch to wood and coal. They'll probably mean such a big saving that setting up for them will be worthwhile even if you use them only part of the time.

You'll see many different figures in books and articles claiming that oil and electric heat are really not comparatively expensive. If you examine those figures, you'll find they allow much less efficiency for wood and coal stoves than is generally the case and much higher efficiency for oil and electric heat than is realistic. They also throw in a lot of other "adjustments," and, invariably, wherever a range is given, use the most favorable figures for the fuel they are promoting and the least favorable for wood and coal.

Here are the facts for some common hardwoods, courtesy of the Cooperative Extension Services of the Northeast States, United States Department of Agriculture.

STORAGE

Both wood and coal take up a lot more room than a tank of oil, especially since, ideally, it's a good idea to lay in a year's supply at a time. This means several tons of coal or cords of wood to store, handy to the house and under cover. Of course, if you had to store a year's

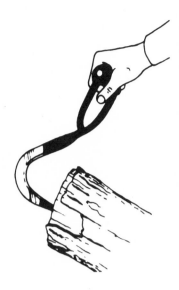

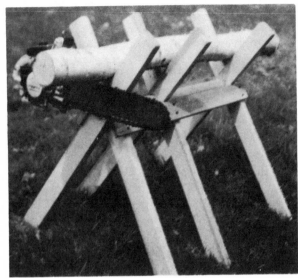

Any job is easier when you have the right tools. The pulp hook digs into the heart of the log, and the handle provides a firm grip and good leverage for maneuvering unwieldy logs. A saw buck will hold the logs while you cut them to a length suitable for your stove or fireplace. (L. L. Bean)

Wood (1 standard cord) [a]	Available heat of 1 cd. wood (Btus) [b]	Anthracite coal (tons) [c]	No. 2 fuel oil (gallons) [d]	Natural gas (100 cu. ft.) [e]
Apple	23,877,000	1.09	244	298
Ash, white	20,000,000	0.91	204	250
Beech, American	21,800,000	0.99	222	273
Birch, yellow	21,300,000	0.97	217	286
Elm, rock	23,488,000	1.07	240	294
Hickory, butternut	23,477,000	1.07	240	293
Hickory, shagbark	24,600,000	1.12	251	308
Ironwood (hardhack)	24,100,000	1.09	246	301
Locust, black	24,600,000	1.12	251	307
Maple, sugar	21,300,000	0.97	217	286
Oak, white	22,700,000	1.04	232	284

[a] One standard cord = 128 cubic feet wood and air; 80 cubic feet solid wood; 20% moisture content. One lb. of this wood contains 5780 Btus (British thermal units).

[b] It is assumed that available heat of wood is oven-dry, or calorific value, minus loss due to moisture, minus loss due to water vapor formed, minus loss due to heat carried away in dry chimney gas. Stack temperature 450° Fahrenheit. No excess air. Efficiency of burning unit—50 to 60%.

[c] Contains 28 million Btus per ton, but available heat is only 22 million Btus per ton. One lb. of coal contains 11,000 available Btus. Coal burned under similar conditions to wood.

[d] One gallon contains 140,000 Btus but is burned at 70% efficiency, providing 98,000 available Btus.

[e] One hundred cu. ft. = 1 therm = 100,000 Btus, but is burned at 80% efficiency, providing 80,000 available Btus.

supply of oil, that would take a lot of room, too. But you don't.

LABOR

Your labor, that is. Nothing beats the ease of turning up or down an oil-burner thermostat. Both wood and coal mean a certain amount of physical work.

The amount of labor involved in a wood stove depends in part on your inclinations. If you want to do it all yourself—cutting down, gathering, log splitting and so on—you're talking about a lot of work. Even if you aren't quite that ambitious, you'll still have to lug the wood indoors, feed the fire, and remove and dispose of the ashes. The more work you do, the better you'll probably feel physically. Working with wood is good exercise and, traditionally, a great way of working off steam. Incidentally, this isn't just men's work. If you doubt that, let me tell you that my mother, who is eighty-four, still splits her own wood. Tending the stove is most often the woman's job, simply because she is the one who is usually home.

Getting rid of wood ashes is no real problem. They're good for slippery walks and driveways

How Many Cords?

One of the most frequently asked questions is "How many cords of wood will I need to get through the year?" Here's a rule of thumb:

For a fireplace	1–2 cords
For a stove	4–6 cords
For a furnace	6–8 cords

NOTE: This does not mean that you can heat your whole house with a fireplace by burning one or two cords of wood; it means that the average fireplace user actually burns about that much in a year. The stove and furnace figures, on the other hand, refer to how much wood is generally used to actually provide heat. Whether the estimates shown will heat your *whole* house depends on other factors but, everything else being favorable, they should be sufficient.

in the winter and great for the garden in the summer. Wood ashes are also useful for making soap, if you are so inclined.

Coal requires work, too, but less so than wood. You don't need to feed a coal fire more than a couple of times a day, which means hauling several buckets of coal. Ash disposal is a bit of a problem. Coal ashes aren't good for anything that anyone has ever been able to discover, so they just end up adding to the great twentieth-century disposal problem.

Splitting Wood

If you are planning to split your own wood, ease of splitting is obviously an important quality. Here is a guide to easy- and hard-to-split species.

EASY TO SPLIT

Ash	Sugar maple
Basswood	Red oak
White birch	White oak
Cherry	Pecan
Cedar	Southern yellow pine
Cottonwood	White pine
Dogwood	Yellow poplar
Douglas fir	Tamarack
Hemlock	Walnut
Hickory	Willow

HARD TO SPLIT

Elm	Norway spruce
Black locust	Sycamore

NOTE: If you're buying wood and plan to split it, be sure you don't buy any of the "Hard to Split." If you don't know how to recognize the different woods, study the barks of the various trees and ask to see a split log of the kind you are buying. If it is elm or black locust, even a novice will see immediately that the grain is very twisted and the log has not split cleanly. Even experts avoid these woods.

Where to Get Free Wood

WASTE WOOD. Any local industry—a furniture factory, for instance—that uses wood will discard much that is not suitable for its purposes. It may be great for burning, and you are usually welcome to it if you will pick it up.

SLAB WOOD. Lumberyards create slab wood when they process logs into board lumber. This includes bark and it means cutting, but not splitting, on your part. Most people can manage the small chain saw necessary to cut slab wood into firebox size, and the lumberyard is often willing to get rid of it free or for a small delivery charge. If demand for it increases, you may find your local yard selling it instead of giving it away, but it will still be a bargain.

CONSTRUCTION SITES. Builders have to cart away any materials they don't use or that they create in the course of construction. They are often forbidden to use the local dumps for this material, so getting rid of it can be a real headache to them. You can pick up all sorts of wood scrap—from oak flooring to birch and pine. It is usually in small, odd-sized pieces that can be fed directly into your stove, and the builder will be delighted to have you collect it after his working hours.

DRIFTWOOD. Among the many gifts from the sea is driftwood, which is surprisingly dry and burns interestingly, with sparks and crackles. Make sure your stove can handle driftwood; read your owner's manual in case the manufacturer advises against using it in his stoves.

TELEPHONE COMPANY TRIMMING. As part of its ongoing maintenance program, the telephone company routinely checks and trims trees to make sure branches haven't grown in such a way as to present a hazard to their wires. You are welcome to these trimmings. It is your telephone charges that go to pay for this work, so it's nice to know you can get some of your money back in free wood.

Collecting this kind of wood means really being on your toes, because commercial wood dealers will try to get there before you do and sell this wood to you at their usual prices.

ICE, WIND, AND OTHER STORMS. These are some of nature's pruning methods. Much of the wood that falls is dead, so it is fairly dry and can be used fairly soon. Often the branches are large enough to require splitting as well as cutting, but don't disdain the excellent kindling provided by the smaller windfalls.

PARKS AND RECREATION AREAS. As we are learning more about forest management, we are beginning to realize what the forest service has always known, a well-managed forest is one that is culled every so often. Gradually, permission is being given to the public to collect fallen wood and to cut

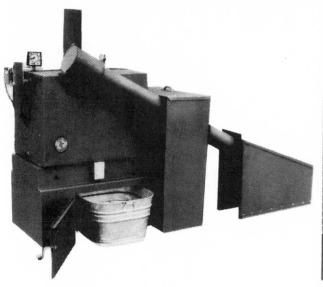

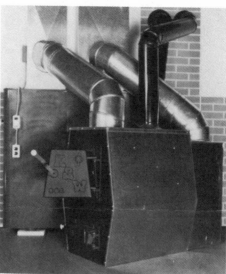

If you want your stove to be your primary source of heat, you should consider a furnace, either to replace your existing heating system or to augment it. The Eshland Coal Gun will operate unattended for up to a week; the D-5 Kickapoo BBR Home Furnace will burn either wood or coal and is a great addition to your current system.

8   down specifically designated trees in public areas. When controlled by experts, this is beneficial both to the forest and to the wildlife in the area.

NEIGHBORS. Trees have a way of taking over and growing more than a homeowner may want. If you are handy with a chain saw, you may do a neighbor a favor by cutting down a tree and taking the wood in payment for your work.

YOUR OWN WOODLOT. Growing your own wood is just as practical as growing your own flowers, vegetables, and lawn. And whatever you grow is free.

STATE FORESTS. You'll have to get in line for this one, but at least you don't have to stand and wait. Put your name on the list for a permit and forget about it until your turn comes.

ROADS. New road construction often requires cutting down trees. So does widening roads and, often, simply repairing them. Bring along your chain saw, ask permission, and bring home all the free wood you can transport.

TOWN DUMP. Sometimes as much as 30 percent of the material that finds its way to the town dump is usable wood fiber in one form or another. Do not turn your nose up at broken-down furniture, and ask where builders dump their material (if they are allowed to use the dump). Also, check your own throw-aways for burnability.

POLLUTION

There's no question that coal is more polluting than wood. You can minimize this to some extent by burning only anthracite (hard coal). Since this is also the best coal for domestic heating, there's no reason not to, unless you live in an area where it's much more difficult to get and where it's much, much more expensive than soft coal. (Hard coal will produce significantly more heat than softer coal, so even if it's a little more expensive, it can still be economical to burn.)

Environmentalists consider wood nonpolluting and more desirable. With modern technology, though, it's possible that the pollutants in coal will be greatly reduced in the future. Most of the horror stories about coal pollution come from the burning of soft coal by utilities, not from domestic burning of hard coal.

WHERE TO PUT A WOOD OR COAL STOVE

Before you go shopping, you have to know where you are going to put your stove.

It depends partly on what you expect from it. If you want the stove to heat your whole house and replace your oil burner, consider a furnace. Your best bet will probably be either a combination furnace or an add-on furnace: in other words, either a furnace that burns two fuels—wood/oil, coal/oil, wood/gas, and so on —or a furnace that can be attached to your current furnace. The advantage of this kind of arrangement is that the two fuels will work in tandem. For instance, if you are heating your house with a wood/oil furnace and go away for a week, the oil part will kick on when the wood part runs out of fuel. You'll run much less risk of coming home to a cold house and frozen water pipes. On the other hand, there are excellent wood furnaces that hold a cord or more of wood and gravity feed it as needed. You can run a furnace for a long time on a cord of wood so with this type of furnace you would not have to worry about all but the longest trips. Gravity-fed coal furnaces, with large storage capacities, are also available.

If you don't want to go this far just yet, you can consider a free-standing stove. For maximum heat this should be located as centrally as possible. Usually the living room is a good location, but it depends on your floor plan. A ranch house is almost impossible to heat with one stove; a house with a wing also presents a problem. A two-story colonial, on the other hand, heats beautifully from a single stove. If natural convection, drawing heat into the second story, isn't sufficient, you can put in registers, louvers, or fans to get the heat where you want it. You may doubt that a small stove can heat a whole house but be warned—the problem most people have with their first stove is that they get one that's too big and produces too much heat.

Appearance is also a factor in stove placement. If a stove standing out in the middle of the room is going to bother you, you may prefer one that sits on the hearth, or even entirely within the fireplace. If you don't want to lose the look of the fireplace, you may want to buy an insert, a unit that fits right into your fireplace and will increase its efficiency. Because heat rises, a fireplace sends most of its hot air right up the chimney. An insert recirculates the heated air into the room.

INSTALLATION

Since the cost of installation can be greater than the cost of the stove, this is a very important subject to consider.

The cheapest way to install a stove is to vent it into an existing fireplace flue. *Under no circumstances can you vent it into the flue that your oil burner uses. It's dangerous and illegal.* The cheapest way to use your fireplace flue is to install a fireplace insert.

The second most expensive installation is for a free-standing stove that must be vented through a specially built flue. This can go up outside of the house or inside the house, through the floors and roof.

The most expensive installation is for a furnace in the cellar. This must be done by a contractor familiar with installing wood or coal furnaces, and the venting duct will have to go through the whole house to the roof.

After obtaining a permit from your local building inspector, get several estimates. Fire-

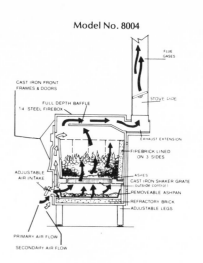

10 place inserts are the only really easy do-it-yourself project; most homeowners will find all other installations a job for an expert.

CAST IRON OR STEEL?

Contrary to what you may have heard, both high-quality cast iron and high-quality steel make outstanding high-quality stoves.

If you like rustic-looking stoves with pictures "carved" into the sides, you want cast iron. That may be about the only difference in appearance, since many steel stoves are black and look very much like cast iron. And many cast-iron stoves, like the Scandinavian cast irons, come in all sorts of pretty colors. If a stove is round or oddly shaped, it is probably steel.

Otherwise it doesn't matter. Cast iron heats up more slowly; holds the heat longer. Steel heats up more rapidly but does not hold the heat quite as long. For the people who build a fire at the beginning of the season and keep it going until the end of the season, such a consideration is unimportant.

Cast iron cracks more easily. Banging it with a vacuum cleaner or a hockey stick, resting an icy or snowy log against it, dropping the stove when moving it, will all tend to crack it. Steel won't crack. On the other hand, theoretically, steel has a shorter life—although I know of at least one steel-stove manufacturer who is still supplying parts for stoves he sold more than forty years ago.

Steel is lighter in weight. Since your stove must sometimes be moved—for the annual flue cleaning, for instance—this is a distinct advantage. Some people like to put their stove out of sight in the summer; with a cast-iron stove that is extremely difficult. Even steel stoves, however, are rather heavy.

Don't let anyone tell you cast iron is automatically better. Many of the top-rated American stoves (such as the Fisher and the Frontier) and many of the fine European stoves (the Petit Godin and the Styria Imperial, for example) are steel.

Steel got a bad name originally because of so-called tin stoves. These are steel stoves in which the metal is very thin. Because of its thinness, there is a tendency for a very hot fire to create thin spots or even to burn through. Stoves of this sort are still made, since they are light in weight and very inexpensive, and therefore ideal for a cabin or garage or for occasional use. If the owner understands the product and doesn't abuse it, a tin stove is good for its purpose. If you check the gauge of the metal used in the stoves you encounter at reputable dealers, you'll see that stoves of this type are not generally offered for regular home heating.

Incidentally, most steel stoves do use some cast iron, doors, for instance, because cast iron usually withstands higher heat than steel. The firebox itself may be lined with firebrick but it isn't practical to put firebrick on the door. Do not assume, however, that steel cannot take a lot of heat. Many quality coal stoves—and coal burns with a hotter fire than wood—are routinely made of steel. In fact, though I haven't done a count, I wouldn't be surprised to find there are more coal stoves made of steel than of cast iron.

HOW TO CHOOSE A STOVE

Once you have decided on the fuel you are going to use and on where you will locate your stove, you're ready to go shopping. At this point, there are several factors that you ought to consider.

1. *Weight.* In general, the heavier the better. With cast iron, check the number of pounds; with steel, check the gauges (steel stoves will have different gauges of steel in different parts of the stove). You don't have to rely on the dealer's knowledge of specific gauges; the manufacturer's brochure will give these specifications. Look and compare.

Don't try to compare cast-iron and steel specifications; they are entirely different from one another. Compare like with like. And, of course, compare stoves of the same size.

2. *Finish.* Sharp or rough edges on doors, draft controls, or any protruding parts are a bad sign. At best, they indicate lack of attention to fine detail. Don't buy any stove that the manufacturer hasn't cared enough about to finish off properly.

3. *Moving parts.* All moving parts should work smoothly. Don't accept the dealer's excuse that it is "stiff and will work in." If it doesn't move smoothly now, it probably never will. A door should fit tightly but open easily, and draft controls should be easy to work.

4. *Check out the firebox.* If it is small, you will have to use logs that are small—which means more work in preparing the wood or greater cost for having it cut small. You'll also have to feed it that much more often. If it is a coal stove, and you intend to use it for wood some of the time, remember that coal-stove fireboxes tend to be smaller than those of wood stoves. All else being equal, a larger firebox will mean less work on your part.

5. *Parts replacement.* Nothing lasts forever. The moment of truth often comes when you have to replace a part. Discuss this with the dealer. If he sees that you are aware of the eventual need for parts and if he gets the idea that you will hold him responsible if this turns out to be a problem, he may steer you away from stove manufacturers with a poor record in this area.

This is particularly important with viewing glass for fireplace inserts (or for any stove that has viewing glass). Here you need to know not only that the glass is available, you also ought to check out how easy it is to replace. It's best if the unit is designed so that you can perform this chore yourself.

6. *Country of origin.* Foreign and American stoves are equally good—or equally bad. If, however, there is a dock strike or some internal

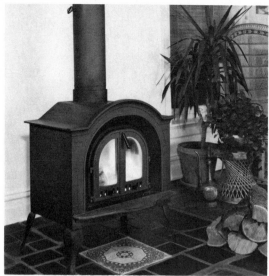
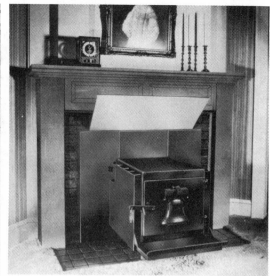

problem in the country of origin, you may have trouble getting delivery or parts. Foreign stoves also tend to be among the most expensive. On the other hand, they usually come from manufacturers who have been making their stoves continuously for hundreds of years. European stove standards are high, and most of the imports are of excellent quality. Styling is generally quite different from American stoves and this may well be the deciding factor in your final choice.

KINDS OF STOVES

Stoves cannot be clearly separated into kinds because there is considerable overlap. A free-standing stove, for instance, may often be suitable for placing on the hearth or within the fireplace, in which case it might be designated a fireplace or hearth stove. Here are four basic kinds you will encounter.

1. *Free-standing stoves.* A stove that can be installed anywhere in the room. It may or may not be vented into a fireplace flue but it doesn't have to be in order to be called free-standing. There are many types of free-standing stoves.

2. *Fireplace stoves.* These are stoves that can sit on or within the hearth. They are usually comparatively small so that they do not come higher than the fireplace opening, although a few manufacturers who recommend their stoves for both free-standing and fireplace use

make them somewhat higher than the opening. They are back-vented, with the vent low enough to go into the fireplace; an elbow directs gasses into the fireplace flue.

3. *Fireplace inserts.* These are designed to slide right into the fireplace with little or none of the unit extending beyond the fireplace opening. They are usually easy for do-it-yourselfers to install and when in place look like a fireplace with glass doors. They are based on the principle of convection so that you get a steady flow of hot air into the room when there is a fire in the unit, producing more heat than you ever thought possible.

Although inserts come in many design variations, the first question is whether the one chosen can be retrofitted. Can it be put into an existing fireplace? If not, a special fireplace must be built.

If you do not have a fireplace and wish to install an insert, one option is to build a fireplace that has the same masonry requirements as a regular fireplace: it must be footed to the ground, even if that means going down through the cellar. This is expensive, but in the process you can also arrange for it to heat upstairs and adjoining rooms.

Another type of insert, which can be used where there is not an existing fireplace, is a "zero clearance" unit. This type does not require masonry or footing and can be put anywhere you choose at considerably less expense than the fireplace varieties. Since it is "zero clearance," you can simply frame it and vent it

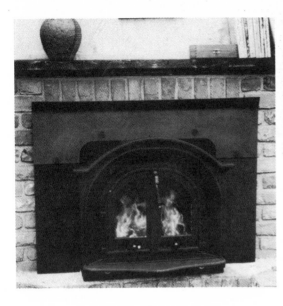

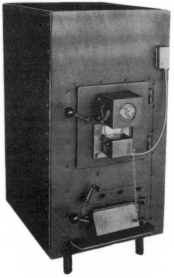

From left to right: free-standing stove (Quaker Stove Co., Inc.); fireplace stove (Liberty Bell); fireplace insert (El Fuego Corp.); furnace (Eshland Enterprises, Inc.).

through triple-walled stovepipe to the roof. This is considered a do-it-yourself project for handy homeowners. The manufacturer's brochure usually contains step-by-step photographs that will give you an idea of what is involved and whether you can handle it.

Inserts produce both radiant heat—heat that warms objects directly in its path—and convective heat—heat that warms the air—but mostly convective heat. Some are ingenious and heat water—enough for domestic use or your hot-water convection system.

If you like the idea of an insert, you'll have to make some decisions. You'll have to balance, for instance, your particular heating needs, the cost of the stove, your style preferences, and fuel requirements. In addition, you'll have to determine whether to go with hot air or hot water, and whether you want a unit that requires a fan, can use a fan or not use a fan, or works entirely without a fan. Some inserts use outside air, which means constructing a duct from the fireplace to an outside wall.

4. *Furnaces.* A wood or coal furnace is the same as any other furnace except for modifications required by the nature of the fuel. There are dual-fuel furnaces that burn a combination of fuels, switching from one to the other automatically. Most can hook into your present central-heating system simply and efficiently and are installed by a contractor, just as are oil- or gas-fired furnaces. Many will require a second flue.

VARIATIONS

These four major kinds of stoves may be further described according to several other variations. Here again, there is considerable overlap. A baffled stove may or may not be automatic, box, or combine radiant and convective heat, and so on. Once you understand that one stove may meet several descriptions, you're on your way to making some sense out of the many different stoves you will encounter.

Box. In its simplest form, a box stove is just a rectangular or round firebox. The firebox is put on legs, vented back or top, and provided a loading door and draft controls.

Baffled box. In this type, the firebox includes a baffle—some sort of horizontal metal panel usually at the top of the inside of the firebox—which deflects the volatiles and smoke so that they stay in the firebox longer than they would if they went directly out the vent. The smoke is "baffled" by not being able to take the direct path to the flue. In theory, this results in more complete combustion. Scandinavian stoves have a special baffle system that causes the logs to burn back to front, rather like a cigar.

Automatic thermostat. There are different materials used, but all automatic thermostats function by controlling the air input. As the fire dies down, more air is added; as the fire heats up, the air is cut down. You set the thermostat for the heat you desire and, as long as fuel is available in the firebox, the stove does

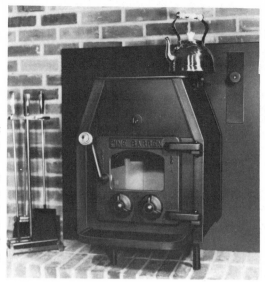

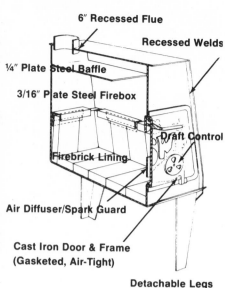

6" Recessed Flue

Recessed Welds

¼" Plate Steel Baffle

3/16" Plate Steel Firebox

Draft Control

Firebrick Lining

Air Diffuser/Spark Guard

Cast Iron Door & Frame
(Gasketed, Air-Tight)

Detachable Legs

Some variations, from left to right: hearth stove (Pine Barren Stove Company, Inc.); baffled box stove (Kickapoo Stove Works Ltd.); automatic thermostat, with arrows showing the path of air through the stove (Defiant Stoves).

14   the rest, increasing or decreasing its heat production as required.

Many European and American stoves come with automatic thermostats, and prices range widely.

Automatic thermostats relieve the homeowner of some of the work involved in tending the fire. Of course, not everyone wants to give up control of the fire, so it's very much a matter of individual preference.

Cabinet.   A firebox with an outside shell or cabinet has many advantages. For example, a stove so insulated doesn't get burning hot on the outside (especially important if there are small children around the house), and it doesn't have to be installed at great distance from combustible surfaces or materials. It also invariably provides a greater volume of convective heat.

Cabinet stoves lend themselves to a greater diversity of finishes—even to beautiful tile surfaces with a wide range of colors and patterns.

These stoves, made both in Europe and in America, come in every price range. Any stove in which the inside wall of the firebox is not the outside wall of the stove is probably a cabinet stove.

Hearth.   A hearth stove sits on a fireplace or within the fireplace. If it is just outside, it often has extension panels that close off the fireplace opening. A hearth stove always vents into the fireplace flue, and since no stove that requires any section of its stovepipe to slant *down* to reach the flue is suitable, the stovepipe

must be level or, preferably, slant slightly upward. Thus, only back-vented stoves are suitable for this purpose.

A stove seated within the fireplace requires less stovepipe and can usually be vented vertically directly up the flue. The fireplace damper must always be removed so that the pipe will fit and the opening can be sealed.

In some ways, there are even more variations in inserts than in other kinds of wood and coal stoves. Do not expect to get any idea

---

SMOKING AND SPARKING OF SELECTED WOOD SPECIES

Wood that produces a lot of smoke is never desirable and should be avoided because it will make for an inefficient fire and a dirty chimney. All wood will smoke more when it is green or wet, so try to burn only wood that is seasoned and dry. Some woods, however, smoke even when seasoned, and it is best to avoid these.

Sparking may make a lively fire in an open fireplace, provided it is well shielded so that sparks do not land on a rug, wood floor, or other combustible surface. Sparks in a wood stove serve no useful purpose and are considered undesirable. Driftwood, regardless of species, sparks most. You should be aware of which woods give off the most sparks.

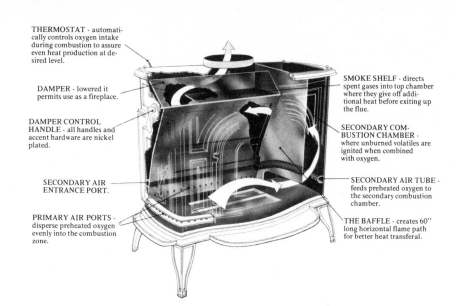

THERMOSTAT - automatically controls oxygen intake during combustion to assure even heat production at desired level.

DAMPER - lowered it permits use as a fireplace.

DAMPER CONTROL HANDLE - all handles and accent hardware are nickel plated.

SECONDARY AIR ENTRANCE PORT.

PRIMARY AIR PORTS - disperse preheated oxygen evenly into the combustion zone.

SMOKE SHELF - directs spent gases into top chamber where they give off additional heat before exiting up the flue.

SECONDARY COMBUSTION CHAMBER - where unburned volatiles are ignited when combined with oxygen.

SECONDARY AIR TUBE - feeds preheated oxygen to the secondary combustion chamber.

THE BAFFLE - creates 60" long horizontal flame path for better heat transferal.

Type of wood	Spark Rating	Heavy Smoke
Apple	few	no
Ash	few	no
Beech	few	no
White birch	moderate	no
Cherry	few	no
Cedar	many	yes
Douglas fir	many	yes
Elm	very few	medium
Hemlock	many	medium
Hickory	moderate	no
Black locust	very few	no
Sugar maple	few	no
Red oak	few	no
Spruce	moderate	yes
White pine	moderate	yes
Willow	few	no

of your options unless you go to several retailers.

STOVE SAFETY

One of the questions I am most frequently asked is, "Just how safe is a coal or a wood stove?" My answer is, "As safe as your oil burner. The difference is that you have more of the responsibility for making and keeping it safe."

Once, when I was doing some radio shows in Boston, a listener called in with a question about a tragic fire in which a middle-aged couple had died. The fire marshal had ascribed the cause of the fire to the family's wood stove. "Doesn't this show," the caller asked, "that wood stoves are dangerous?"

I told the caller that although I wasn't familiar with the facts of this particular fire, I'd be willing to bet that the fire had been caused by the woodburner's carelessness, rather than by any problem with the stove. I said it was like a cigarette, which is not inherently dangerous but which can kill you if you smoke in bed and fall asleep with it in your hand.

As it turned out, I was right on target. The fire had occurred because the homeowner, in preparing the stove for the night, had removed some ashes, inadvertently dropping a few hot coals on a combustible floor. The couple had then gone off to bed. The coals started a fire —just like the cigarette in bed—and people died because of it.

Stove safety requires care and common sense on the part of the homeowner. For this reason, stoves are ever so much safer than automobiles —where one of the danger factors is the other driver. Stove safety is mostly up to you.

KEEPING YOUR STOVE SAFE

There are a number of things you should do to minimize stove-safety problems.

- *Install properly.* Safety starts with proper installation. If your stove is too close to combustibles, you will, sooner or later, have a problem. Your owner's manual will clearly state required distance to combustibles and

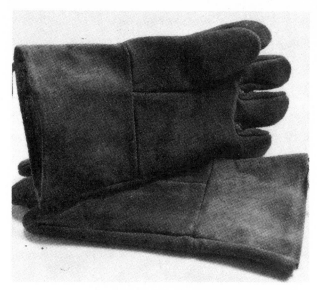

Keep a pair of insulated gloves next to your stove, since you never know when you'll have to grab something fast. (Warming Trend)

16   your building inspector will check to make sure you have complied with local codes. Do not blindly trust the person who installs your stove; unfortunately, many installers are careless and inexperienced. If you do not do it yourself, be sure you know pretty much how it should be done and check it out. Always pay for installation by check so that you can immediately stop payment if you discover it was improperly done.

- *Watch the installation.* In some cases, it is the only way you can know what has been done. Be sure, for example, the stove is not being vented into the oil-burner flue or into any flue used by another heating device. Be sure clearances to combustibles are correct. Be sure the chimney and smoke shelf are clean (ask the installer about the smoke shelf).
- *Get a written estimate with a diagram and specifications.* Unless the stove dealer is installing your stove free, get the estimate in writing and be sure it specifies how it will be done, what gauge stovepipe will be used, etc. A good building inspector will require this and you should, too.
- *Check your owner's manual* for any special instructions and point them out to the installer—he may not be familiar with your particular stove model.
- *Ask questions.* Don't be afraid of asking questions because they may be thought silly. If anything puzzles you or seems contrary to what you may have heard, ask the installer. He may not know what he is doing.

- *Look at labels.* Make sure the type of stovepipe and the gauge of the metal are what has been specified or what is called for in your owner's manual. If the pipe is too thin, if ordinary stovepipe is installed where double- or triple-walled pipe is called for, you may be creating a dangerous situation.
- *Ask to have the stovepipe sections bolted together.* Since pipe is designed for one section to slip into the next, it is possible to put it all together without then bolting it. In the event of a chimney fire, these sections may separate accidentally. For maximum safety, stovepipe should be bolted.
- *Be sure a damper is put on the stovepipe.* The installer may tell you the stove does not require, or use, an outside damper. This may be true, but you should still have a damper installed. In the event of a chimney fire, it's very important in controlling the blaze.
- *Be sure the stove is installed on a noncombustible surface.* Never put a stove directly on a wood floor. Usually the fireproof surface should extend at least 18 inches beyond the front of the stove. Ashes, coals, and clinkers can easily start a fire if you drop some of them on a combustible surface.
- *Keep ashes in a covered metal container and do not place container on a combustible surface.* If your ashes are from coal, take them outdoors as soon as possible. The lack of oxygen in a closed container creates noxious gasses which can be released into the room by seepage or when you open the container.

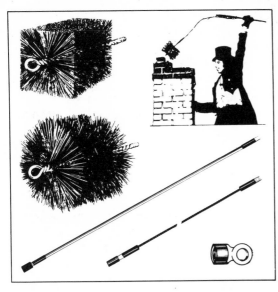

There's still no better way to clean a chimney than with a good stiff brush. Chimney brushes are available in all shapes and sizes to fit any flue or stovepipe. (Schaefer Brush Mfg. Co., Inc.)

Sprinkling Safe-T-Flue over coals will help fight creosote build-up. As it burns, the cleaner forms catalytic gases which cause creosote to flake off the chimney wall and fall under its own weight. (Warming Trend)

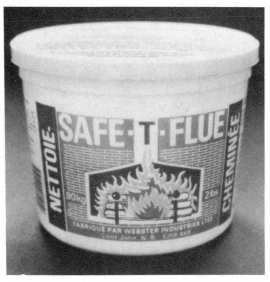

- *Always open air-intake controls for a minute before opening loading door.* This will avoid back-puffing.
- *Burn the recommended fuel.* Do not burn coal in a wood stove unless the owner's manual says it's okay. Even then, be sure you're using the specified type of coal.
- *Keep your chimney clean.* It's usually sufficient to clean a chimney and smoke shelf once a year but, the first year you use a stove, check every couple of months to see how the creosote is building up. Some stoves produce much more creosote than others. Green, wet, or soft wood produces more creosote than dry; frequently banked fires create more creosote than fast-burning ones. An airtight stove has the capability of creating more creosote than a nonairtight because it maintains a low fire for a much longer burn time.
- *Never leave an open fire unless it is properly screened.*
- *Do not run a stove with cracked viewing glass.* The only exception is when it is so well screened that the fire would burn safely with no glass at all.
- *Do not overload the firebox.* You may burn through or crack even a good stove if you build too hot a fire. You will also waste fuel because there will not be enough room in the firebox for proper combustion of volatiles. Many of the heat-producing gasses will simply go straight up the chimney.
- *Reduce creosote buildup by proper management*

of the fire. Once the flue is thoroughly heated, burn the fire hot (about three-quarter level) for at least half an hour. This will burn out the creosote that may have been deposited during the low-burn time, such as overnight.
- *Install smoke and gas detectors.* Smoke detectors are advised for all homeowners and a must for wood/coal stove owners. Gas detectors should be added for those using coal stoves.
- *Have a fire extinguisher handy.*

IF YOU SHOULD HAVE A CHIMNEY FIRE

In the event of a fire in the chimney, follow this procedure.

1. Call the fire department.
2. Close the stovepipe damper.
3. Close the air-intake controls on stove.
4. If a lot of red sparks are coming out of the chimney, hose down the roof and surrounding shrubbery, but *be careful not to get water on the chimney or inside it.*

Depriving the fire of air should help to put it out quickly. Never throw water on the stove while it is hot or you may crack it. If you have had a chimney fire, do not open the stove door until the stove has cooled down completely; if you do, you may cause a flashback that could start the fire all over again.

17

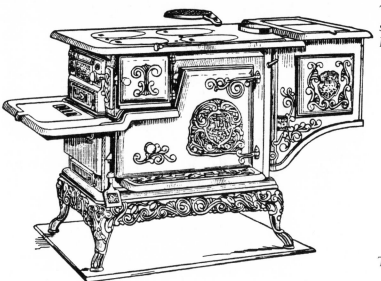

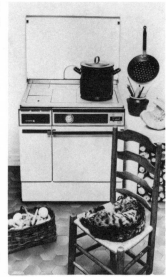

The Star Sunshine cooking stove, from the 1897 Sears Roebuck and Co. Catalog.

The deceptively modern De Dietrich kitchen range.

18 It is estimated that 90 percent of flue fires are caused by improper installation so, with normal care, the odds are you will never have this unpleasant experience.

COOKING ON A WOOD OR COAL STOVE

The slow-simmered stews, the succulent pastries, the aromatic bread that once came out of grandma's—now great-grandma's—kitchen have lived on in legend. We have always believed that no matter how hard we tried, nothing produced on our modern gas and electric cooktops or carefully nursed in our ovens could possibly match these culinary delights of a simpler time.

On the other hand, travelers abroad have often come back with tales of the marvelous food they found all over Europe. What most of them never dreamed was that much of the food they ate was prepared in or on stoves still fueled by wood or coal.

The more sophisticated traveler may know at first hand that his or her favorite small restaurant in Spain cooks in this "primitive" way, but not many realize that even the finest Swiss hotels often have nothing in their kitchens but wood- or coal-burning stoves. Even if you have been so lucky as to get a peek into one of these great hotel kitchens, you might not have been aware of anything unusual; many European kitchen stoves are designed so that they look

exactly like electric stoves—all enamel and gleaming chrome—and you will have to look closely to detect the firebox door or the stove lids that can be lifted to reveal the open fire.

If this fact inspires you to buy a wood- or coal-burning cookstove for your own kitchen, you have a wide range (no pun intended!) to choose from. In the modern mode, there is the De Dietrich kitchen range from France. Made by a company that has been in the wood-stove business since 1684, it will burn wood and coal equally well. It will not only cook, roast, and bake but it will also provide domestic hot water with a built-in water jacket, which may be connected to your existing hot-water-heating system or may simply be used to provide hot water for washing and similar needs.

Other modern-looking ranges include the Styria, which has a baking oven that can turn the novice into an expert baker, the expert into a pastry chef. Made in Austria, it is designed on the principle of the great tile stoves of Europe and Scandinavia, the *kachelofen.* Each stove is handmade and the design is handsomely executed in cast iron, stainless steel, and enameled steel. It can be ordered in a range of colors.

If you prefer to cook on the same stove your great-grandmother probably used, you can still order it—the Queen Atlantic Range, a stove that looks like an antique and is still made in the original foundry from the original 1906 patterns. It comes with a number of options and you will need to talk to the Portland

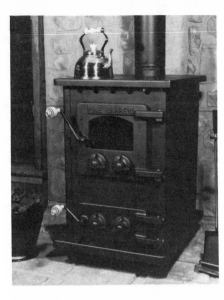

The flat top of a box stove can double as a cooking surface. Just set a pot or kettle on top and enjoy the wonders of heat conduction. (Pine Barren Stove Co., Inc.)

Foundry in Maine to find which they are currently offering. Also ask them how long it will take to get your stove. When wood stoves first became popular again a few years ago, the waiting list was prohibitive, but the foundry subsequently caught up with its orders and you may be lucky enough to get one within a couple of months of your order.

I smell yo' bread a'burnin, turn yo' damper
  down,
If you ain't got a damper, good gal, turn you'
  bread around.

                   Mule Skinner Blues

If you want to hedge your bets, there is a stove, such as the Monarch, which combines a coal- or wood-burning range with an electric range. The model I have seen has two top "burners" for wood or coal, as well as four electric burners, and the oven works on either fuel. One of the major advantages of this type of stove is that, by switching to electric, you can have a cool kitchen in the summer, and, by using wood, a cosy, warm kitchen in the winter.

If, however, you aren't ready to go all the way with a special cookstove, you can easily get a bonus from a wood or coal stove you have bought primarily to provide heat. Most of these stoves—in fact, any that have a flat top—can be used very successfully for cooking. You can even buy a portable oven to place on the top when you want to bake or roast.

European stoves are often specially geared to this extra use. The Weso, for instance, is frequently used as a cookstove in European kitchens, although in this country it is sold primarily for its heat production. Because it has an automatic thermostat, you can take much of the guesswork out of your cooking. And, although you cannot use them simultaneously, you also have two cooking surfaces, which gives you great flexibility in surface temperatures.

Even a simple box stove performs a useful cooking function. A more sophisticated version, the Cawley/LeMay, which is designed with a Scandinavian-type baffle system, provides removable stove lids and a handy tray that positions on the side of the stovetop and is useful for the cook.

Many stoves, such as the Defiant and its smaller versions, have a specially built griddle or gridiron in the top that will turn out the most superb pancakes and other grilled foods. Or you may choose a Franklin-type stove where you can cook over the open fire, with all sorts of options available to make barbecue cooking easy and fun.

If cooking with wood appeals to you, you may be discouraged to find that you will probably burn your first batch of biscuits or will have to watch the stew very carefully to keep it simmering instead of reaching a violent boil. You'll soon realize, though, that cooking with coal or wood isn't so much difficult as it is different. Even with an electric or gas stove, you probably still burn a batch of cookies oc-

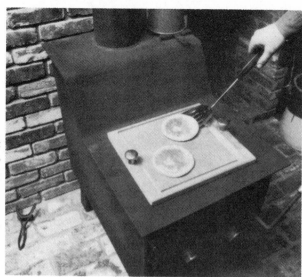

A soapstone griddle will sit on top of your stove, absorb heat quickly, and release it slowly and evenly. It's perfect for pancakes, steaks, and eggs, and it cleans with mild soap and water. (Minuteman International Co.)

20   casionally, and if pots never boiled over, we wouldn't need catchplates under the burners. Time, patience, and experience will soon get you over the initial problems, and the results, when you finally master your medium, will surpass your wildest dreams. You will get all the credit but you will always know down deep that part of it should really go to your wood stove.

TIPS FOR COOKING WITH WOOD

- A wood stove is not just for heating and cooking; it's also great for drying herbs, vegetables, fruits, and spices. Be sure the drying surface doesn't get too hot (you will need to elevate whatever sort of rack you improvise, or else buy a dryer to put on top of the stove). Too much heat will cook instead of drying. Remember, the ideal temperature for oven drying is 150° to 200° F, so you need very little warmth.

- If you've always wanted a stockpot, this is your chance. Keep a large pot, with the equivalent of a flame tamer, on the stove and toss all your vegetable parings, bones from roasts, vegetable water and other good scraps from your kitchen into the pot. It should simmer away steadily, gradually incorporating the flavors into a delicious broth. At some point, whenever it's convenient, taste, add a minimum of seasoning

and cool quickly. You can then freeze the strained broth in ice cube trays. Once frozen, store in your freezer in a plastic bag with some sort of label so you know if fish or some other strong flavor is predominant. You will soon have a store of flavored cubes that can be used for a cup of soup, as the base for a tasty casserole or stew, or the beginning of a gourmet dish. (Japanese soups, those wonderfully light and fragrant clear broths, are often just a little chicken broth with a thin slice of cucumber and a square of seaweed to dress them up and add texture.) With your bags of flavored cubes, you have endless, easy-to-fix dishes at your fingertips.

- If you like to make pancakes, eggs, and so on, you might want to buy a soapstone griddle. It doesn't have to be greased, cooks beautifully evenly, and is a joy to clean. Just be sure to get *real* soapstone. A process now exists for grinding up the stone and binding it together into a processed-soapstone product. I think genuine soapstone would be more satisfactory for cooking.

- Speaking of soapstone, if you have someone in the house who doesn't like flannel sheets but dislikes the icy feel of percale on a winter's night, get a soapstone bedwarmer. You can heat it on your stove and then slide it between the sheets just before the toes go in. An old-fashioned comfort that is worth reviving!

- If you get serious about wood-stove cookery,

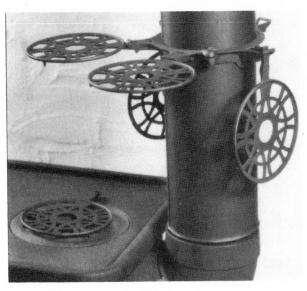

This trivet tree attaches directly to the stovepipe. The trivets swing up straight and lock, providing a warm ledge for rising bread, or they detach to rest on the stove top. (Warming Trend)

you may want to buy some cast-iron pots. They will give excellent results and the bottoms will stay flat, unlike some of the thin aluminum or stainless steel pots, which may warp. Use glass pots with caution, preferably not on too hot a surface.

- Be creative. Many of the dishes you think of for the oven will cook just as well in a covered pot on top of your stove. Stews, braised dishes, and many casseroles fall into this category. If the dish needs a browned topping to finish it off, you can always pop it under the broiler just before serving.

- Three-legged cast-iron trivets used to be a standby for cooking in the fireplace and on wood stoves. You may find one in an antique shop, or you may find that they are actually in production again. With a trivet as a heat buffer, you can keep coffee ready to pour, a meal in a chafing dish bubbly hot.

RECIPES FOR A COAL OR WOOD STOVE

Spanish Olla Podrida. The following is the recipe for the favorite Spanish dish. A superior housekeeper tried it, and it was so much liked that several of her family were harmed *by eating too much.*

Spanish Olla Podrida. Fry four ounces of salt pork in the pot, and, when partly done, add two pounds of fresh beef and a quarter pound of ham. Add two tea-spoonfuls of salt in cold water, and only enough just to cover the meat. Skim carefully the first half hour, and then add a gill of peas, one carrot, one turnip, two leeks, three stalks of celery, three stalks of parsley, two stalks of thyme, two cloves, two onions sliced, two cloves of garlic, ten pepper-corns, and a pinch of powdered mace or nutmeg. Simmer steadily for five hours. When the water is too low, add that which is boiling. Put the meat on a platter, and the vegetables around it. Strain the liquor on to toasted bread in a soup-dish.

From *The Housekeeper's Manual* by Catherine E. Beecher and Harriet Beecher Stowe (New York, 1873).

Libyan Couscous. I throw in lots of fat—this really adds flavor and is usually cut out by Westerners. This dish takes time to make, but it's really worth every minute put into it.

10 large onions, chopped
4–5 lbs. leg or shoulder of lamb, cut in large cubes (I like Australian lamb for this)
1–2 cups olive oil
2 large cans Italian tomatoes
5, 10, or 15 garlic cloves, chopped
1 can Italian tomato paste
2 teaspoons turmeric
2 teaspoons curry
1 teaspoon fresh ground pepper
5–15 crushed cardamon pods (optional)
10 large potatoes, quartered
    handful of pine nuts
2 or 3 cans chick peas
5–10 zucchini or yellow squash, large pieces
2 1-lb. boxes couscous

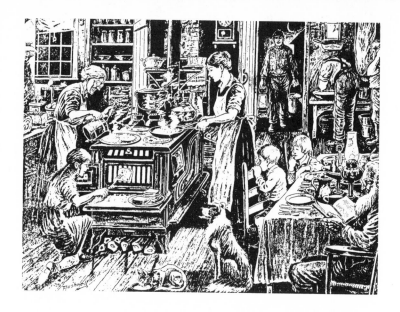

22   At least 8 hours, preferably overnight, are required for the first steps:

1. Brown onions and lamb in lots of olive oil. Add garlic and brown. At the end of browning, add tomato paste, pine nuts, turmeric, curry, and pepper. If you can get it (Middle Eastern food stores carry it), add 1 teaspoon of harissa for mild, 2–3 for hot (and genuine) couscous . . . this stuff is really potent. I didn't include it in the regular list of ingredients because it might be hard to get.

2. Put browned mess into large pot. Add tomatoes, crushed cardamon pods, and enough water to cover everything. Bring to a boil, then turn down low and simmer, covered, either overnight or from about 2:00 P.M. to 6:00 or 7:00 P.M. (Harissa gets hotter the longer it cooks, so if you have used that, better start tasting about 6:00 P.M.)

3. About 3 hours before you plan to finish cooking, add chick peas; 1½ hours, add potatoes; 1 hour, add squash.

4. Follow directions on package for couscous. Or do it my way: takes 3 hours. Wash for 3 minutes in cold water, let stand in bowl for 1 hour. Then put it in strainer or cheesecloth, steam for 1 hour. (If you have room in the pot you are cooking the rest of the stuff in, put couscous in sieve or strainer and steam over that . . . covered.) Take out, wash in cold water, drain. Mix in olive oil with your fingers so you can feel it covering all grains, break up any lumps. Steam for another hour.

5. When couscous is steamed, put in the serving bowls. Mix in 1–3 cups of liquid and fat from stew so it all looks orange red. Do it fast.

6. Pile the stew on top. Then everyone gathers round and eats it with fingers or large spoons—it's meant for gorging on.

From *The College Cookbook* by Geri Harrington (1973).

Sweet Potato Dumplings

1 teaspoon butter
¾ cup flour
¾ cup sweet potatoes, grated
¼ teaspoon nutmeg
⅛ teaspoon allspice
Salt and pepper

Combine butter and flour, blending with pastry blender until crumbly. Stir in sweet potatoes and seasonings.

Add about ½ to ¾ cup water, or enough to make a stiff dough. Blend until dough is of even consistency.

Shape into dumplings. Drop into boiling consommé and simmer 30 minutes. Serve with soup or a cream sauce.

Cod's Hard Roe. Tie a cod's roe in a cloth, place in a pan two quarts of water and two teaspoonfuls of salt; put in the roe, boil gently for one hour, take it out, cut off as much as you require, put it in the dish, pour over parsley and butter, and serve. Or egg sauce, or plain with a little butter and pepper. The remainder, when cold, may be cut into slices and semi-fried, as fish.

From *A Shilling Cookery for the People, Embracing an Entirely New System of Plain Cooker and Domestic Economy* by Alexis Soyer (London, 1854).

Cock-a-Leekie

1 frying chicken, cut in small pieces
4 quarts water
3 tablespoons parsley, chopped
2 onions, chopped
10 leeks
½ cup rice, uncooked
8 pitted prunes, cooked and chopped
2 tablespoons butter
2 tablespoons flour
Salt and pepper to taste

Remove all chicken fat from chicken pieces. Simmer chicken, water, parsley, and onions 1 hour in salted water.

Remove chicken and reserve. Split leeks, cut into 1-inch pieces and wash thoroughly in warm water. Add to chicken broth. Add rice. Simmer for 20 minutes, until rice is tender.

Meanwhile, bone chicken and cut in small chunks. Add chicken and prunes to soup and reheat.

Combine flour and butter, blending thoroughly, and stir briskly into soup. Simmer 2 or 3 minutes, until slightly thickened. Taste to adjust for seasoning. Serve hot.

A WOOD- AND COAL-BURNER'S GLOSSARY

Anthracite coal. Anthracite is by far the hardest and most desirable coal but not every coal stove can handle it, so check your manual. There are different grades of anthracite but you usually have to take what you can get; it will still be better than any other type of coal. If you buy anthracite, be sure to buy the correct size for your grate. Sizes range from large chunks to small, the so-called rice anthracite. Nut coal is the size most commonly called for in domestic coal stoves.

The highest-grade anthracite will burn longer and cleaner than second-grade anthracite, but any anthracite will burn better than soft coal. Unfortunately, most of the anthracite known to exist in the earth comes from a comparatively small area in the state of Pennsylvania, and it will be the first type of coal that we use up.

Bituminous coal. This term covers a number of grades of soft coal but does not extend as low as cannel, lignite, and peat. There is a greater supply in the world of bituminous coal than of any other kind, and it is what we will probably have to fall back on when our supply of anthracite runs out. Meanwhile, it is considered less desirable for home heating because it is more polluting, lower in carbon content, higher in moisture, and will give you less heat for your money than anthracite.

Briquet coal. Coal briquets are a processed

Carrying coals from *Newcastle, 1764.*

24

fuel. They are usually made from coal dust, compressed into square or oval shapes that are uniform in size. They are handy to store and comparatively clean to use but they may be much more expensive than buying coal by the ton. Compare prices.

Brown coal. Often used to describe lignite, brown coal also describes a slightly higher-ranked coal. Its characteristics are so close to that of lignite that it is scarcely more desirable.

Btu. The initials stand for British thermal unit(s). This is the most commonly used measure of heat, the amount required to raise the temperature of one pound of water one degree Fahrenheit.

Carbon. An element found in quantity in diamonds, graphite, and coal. The harder the coal, the more carbon it contains and the more heat it produces. Here is the percentage of carbon found, on the average, in various types of coal:

anthracite	84+%
semibituminous	70–80%
bituminous	50–75%
Texas lignite	41+%
peat	13+%

The higher the carbon content, the less the sulfur and ash content, and the cleaner and more heat producing the coal will be. Unfortunately, anthracite is created at the end of the process that makes coal, and it takes approxi-

mately ten inches of peat and millions of years to make one inch of anthracite.

Cannel coal. Cannel coal is beloved by people with open fireplaces for its long beautiful flame and the cheerful chattering sound it makes when burning. Do not assume, however, that your coal stove will take cannel coal; many manufacturers specifically say not to use it.

Cast iron. A metal commonly used for stoves. It is an alloy of iron, carbon, and silicon that is poured into a mold made from a master pattern.

Chunk wood. Short, thick pieces of wood, rather than whole logs. Usually waste wood and, therefore, cheaper than logs.

Clinkers. Unburned material from a coal fire that has fused into chunks. Handle with care; they are often sharp.

Coal ash. Ash is the noncombustible material in coal. High-rank coal has a lower ash content than low-rank coal. Coal ash is a

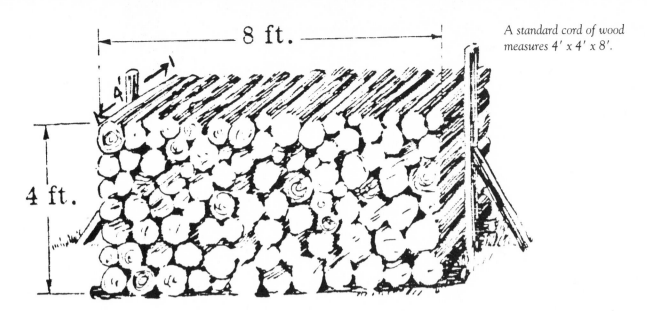

8 ft.

4 ft.

A standard cord of wood measures 4' x 4' x 8'.

bother to dispose of since it cannot be used as a garden fertilizer. Anthracite has the lowest ash content.

Cord. A stack of wood—traditionally 4 feet by 4 feet by 8 feet—that measures 128 cubic feet. Any stack, regardless of log length, that measures 128 cubic feet is a cord. You should know, however, that a cord of 4-foot logs cut into shorter than 4-foot lengths will measure less than a cord of wood, partly due to loss of wood as sawdust. Be sure that you specify a cord, "128 cubic feet," when buying wood or the wood dealer may argue that it was a cord before he cut it, even it it isn't when you stack it. Order your cord of specified length *delivered,* and stack it quickly to make sure you got fair measure.

Creosote. A complex oily substance formed by wood or coal combustion and deposited in a flue or stovepipe by the smoke and gasses of the burning fire. It may appear as black sooty material or as tarry residue. Under certain circumstances, it will also liquify. Chimneys and stove pipe should be cleaned regularly to avoid creosote buildup that could cause chimney fires.

Damper. The draft-regulating mechanism of a chimney or stovepipe. Even if your stove has an automatic thermostat or built-in damper, you should be sure there is an additional damper on the stovepipe, near where it leaves the stove vent. In case of chimney fire, it is important to be able to close this damper.

Firebrick. A special, high-heat-resistant brick that is used to line the firebox, which protects the firebox from direct contact with the flames, lengthening its life. Firebricks are usually set in place, without cement, and must be replaced when they deteriorate—usually after three or four years of constant use.

Fireclay. A high-heat-resistant clay used in the construction of flues, some fireplaces, and so on. It can also be used to mortar firebricks in fireplace construction.

Flue. What most people think of as the chimney, actually, the fire-resistant pipe through which smoke and gasses are carried to the outside. A chimney may contain more than one flue, one for each heat-producing source. For instance, your oil burner and your wood stove should always be vented into entirely separate flues.

Gauge. Sheet metal or steel thickness is measured in terms of gauge. The lower the gauge number (such as 24, 18, etc.), the thicker the metal. Sometimes, as in describing the construction of the stove, thickness will be stated in fractions of an inch or in millimeters. Gauge is usually used, however, to describe stovepipe.

Green wood. Wood that has just been cut from a live tree. Also, any wood that is not at least partly seasoned. Even wood that has been cut for a month would be considered green.

Hard coal. Anthracite is the only truly hard coal. It is the most desirable coal because it burns cleaner, longer, and contains more Btus than soft coal.

25

Hardness (of wood). The denser and heavier the wood, the harder it is and the better it is for firewood. Most trees we think of as "pines" are soft wood. Hard wood will burn longer, leave less ash, and usually spark and smoke less than soft wood.

WHICH WOOD BURNS BEST?

Beechwood fires are bright and clear
If the logs are kept a year.
Chestnut's only good, they say,
If for long it's laid away.
Birch and fir logs burn too fast,
Blaze up bright and do not last.
Elmwood burns like a churchyard mould;
E'en the very flames are cold.
Poplar gives a bitter smoke,
Fills your eyes and makes you choke.
Apple wood will scent your room
With an incense like perfume.
Oak and maple, if dry and old,
Keep away the winter cold.
But ashwood wet and ashwood dry,
A king shall warm his slippers by.

Anonymous

Lignite. A step above peat on the coal scale, lignite is a cheap fuel widely used by utility companies who have a nearby source. It is not practical to transport it any distance since it cracks and crumbles as it dries out, and will actually disintegrate if stored outdoors. Many wood-stove manufacturers claim that their stove will burn lignite. Lignite is satisfac- tory if you live near lignite mines—although it provides comparatively little heat and is a dirty fuel. Of no use to most wood-stove owners.

Nut coal. The size of anthracite coal most commonly used for domestic coal stoves. Chestnut is the nut used in sizing nut coal.

Pea coal. Pea-sized anthracite coal, second in popularity for domestic heating. With some grates, however, pea coal will fall through before being fully burned. With others it will pack down too tightly, extinguishing the fire.

Peat. Peat is the first stage in the process in the transformation of vegetable matter into coal. It is the least efficient of the fossil fuels, and burns very smokily and dirtily. It has long been the native fuel of Ireland and can be collected from bogs throughout North America, as well as in other cold climates. If your stove will burn it and you want to give it a try, ask your local nature center to show you what it looks like and where to find it locally.

Seasoning (of wood). Seasoning is the gradual reduction of the moisture content of wood. If wood is stored under proper conditions, with reasonable air circulation, for nine months to a year, it will reach a moisture content of about 20 percent, which is the most you can hope for. Completely dry wood is possible only under laboratory conditions.

Semibituminous coal. A semisoft coal that ranks between bituminous and anthracite in the hardness scale.

Slab wood. A lengthwise outside piece cut from a log to square it. Lumberyards used to

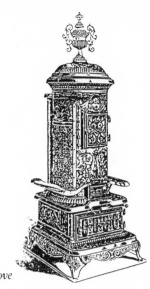

St. Nicholas cast-iron stove

think of such slabs as waste and used them for chips. They may be suitable for wood stoves, depending on the tree they are cut from.

Soft coal. Semibituminous, subbituminous, cannel, and peat are some of the forms of soft coal. Soft coal contains more sulfur, more ash, less carbon than hard coal. It burns more quickly and dirtily than hard coal.

Steel or sheet metal. An iron material distinguished from cast iron primarily by its lower carbon content and the fact that it is much more malleable. There are many grades and gauges of this type of metal, and a manufacturer will tend to mention the fact if the steel in his stove is of a superior grade.

Stove coal. A size of coal larger than nut. In spite of its name, stove coal is generally suitable only for furnaces.

Subbituminous coal. Soft coal that is ranked even lower than bituminous. Not a good idea for the home coalburner.

COAL/WOOD STOVE CATALOG

There are so many fine stoves on the market that it is impossible to mention them all. Here are a few to give you an idea of the variety.

None of the stoves shown is less than $600, so only two categories of price are used: "Under $1,000" and "Over $1,000." Savings of up to $400 may be possible beginning in January. Sometimes, also, preseason sales offer stoves at substantial savings.

Always ask why a stove has been reduced. You need to determine that the reduction is seasonal and not due to any problems.

Esse Dragon. A lovely cast-iron Victorian stove made by a Scottish company that has been manufacturing heating appliances for over 125 years. Described by the *New York Times* as "a cast-iron jewel," the Esse is very decorative with a lustrous midnight or copper finish that gives it a look quite unlike any other stove. In spite of its handsome appearance, however, it is a very efficient and hard-working stove, with front- and side-loading doors, viewing windows of mica (rather than glass), and an ingeniously designed shaker grate with individually removable bars. The top lifts up to reveal a cooking surface, and the stove can be used either free standing or on the hearth. Windrose Corp., 59 River Road, Cos Cob, CT 06807. Over $1,000.

The St. Nicholas. A richly ornamental cast-iron stove from the hundred-year-old Portland Foundry (Maine). The grate is mounted on steel balls, with a draw center and an anticlinker door. The silver nickel-plate bands and foot rails add to the stove's decorativeness, are useful for drying wet socks, warming toes, etc. and can be easily removed if desired. The final top lifts off to reveal an oven for baking or cooktop cooking. Portland Stove Foundry Co., Portland, ME 04104. Under $1,000.

Pacific Princess. Gleaming black cast-iron body and bright nickel trim make this coal/

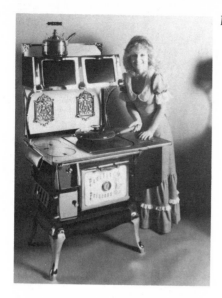

Pacific Princess

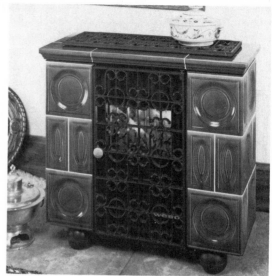

Weso Ceramic Tile Stove

28

wood range handsome enough for any kitchen. There are many noteworthy features such as automatic grease drain-off for the easy-to-use, easy-to-clean griddle. Broil right over the coals, bake in an oven that cleans itself if your berry pie spills over. And you can even add useful options such as a water reservoir that will provide anything from hot compresses to hot spiced cider *on tap;* and warming closets for raising bread dough, drying herbs, keeping food ready to serve, and warming plates. Pioneer Lamp & Stove Co., Box 4173, Seattle, WA 98104. Over $1,000.

Moravian Parlor Stove. A remarkably pretty wood stove from Pennsylvania, the Moravian's graceful lines conceal a firebrick-lined firebox that is fully baffled and holds 25-inch logs. The inside of the arch is finished in porcelain enamel and comes in a choice of colors. I like the cranberry, which looks as if it is reflecting the fire. The body is plate steel; the front, doors, and decorative areas are cast iron. A 6-inch wide ash shelf keeps your floor mat or hearth clean, and the top provides three small cooking surfaces. Quaker Stove Co., Inc., 200 West 5th St., Lansdale, PA 19446. Under $1,000.

Weso Ceramic Tile Stove. A descendent of the famous European *kachelofens,* or tile stoves, the Weso is also a serious cookstove; in Europe, it is often put in the kitchen. The Weso is attractively designed with a decorative wrought-iron grill on top and in front (enameled for easy cleaning) combined with large,

hand-fired, individual tiles. The tiles are available in a wide range of colors and patterns. The tiles act as a heat sink to hold and give off a gentle warmth that lasts long after the fire has gone out. The outer-tile shell contains channels through which air flows and is vented out into the room after being warmed by the double cast-iron heater. There are many more features than space allows listing, but I should mention that this is an automatic-thermostat stove with all the advantages of that useful device. Made in West Germany and imported by Ceramic Radiant Heat, Lochmere, NH 03252. Under $1,000.

Free Heat Machine. If you can get to see the President's study on your tour of the White House (it's usually off limits), you will find this insert ensconced in the fireplace. As with many inserts, it looks, at first glance, like a fireplace with glass doors. But behind the glass is an efficient C-Grate heat exchanger that delivers hot air at the rate of 38,000 Btu per hour with the help of two built-in, two-speed blowers. The Free Heat Machine will actually burn any solid fuel—coal and paper logs, as well as wood—and has a handy, removable ash pan, which eliminates one of the chores of tending a fire in an insert. In spite of its efficiency, the unit is exceptionally lightweight, a boon to the homeowner who wants to be able to manhandle it for maintenance, chimney cleaning, etc. And I don't need to tell you it is attractive when you already know it was considered handsome enough for the White House.

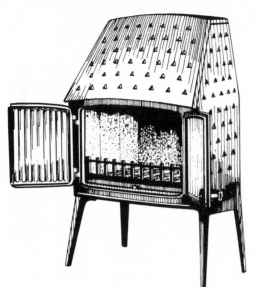

Morso Franklin stove

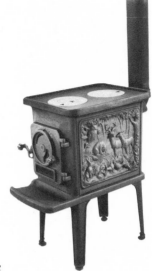

Cawley/LeMay Wood Stove

Aquappliances, Inc., 135 Sunshine Lane, San Marcos, CA 92069. Under $1,000.

Morso 1125 Franklin. With the doors open, this handsome Danish stove is an open fireplace; with the doors closed, it is an efficient heat producer. At all times it is most unusual looking. You can order it not only in black but also in green, charcoal grey, white, and blue enamel. Because of the enamel finish, rust will not be the problem it is with most cast-iron stoves and you will not have the chore of an annual touch-up. Scandinavian stoves have such a fine reputation that it is probably unnecessary to mention how efficient, well constructed, and well baffled the Morso is. It can be had top- or back-vented and the firebox is firebrick-lined. Southport Stoves, Inc., 959 Main Street, Stratford, CT 06597. Over $1,000.

Cawley/LeMay Woodstove. If you don't examine the Cawley/LeMay, it looks just like any other picture cast-iron stove, but it is unique in a number of respects. First of all, the height of the top surface is designed to be comfortable to cook on and even has a shelf to attach to one side. The shelf will hold utensils, an extra pot, seasonings or whatever you like to keep handy; it even has a rail for a dish or hand towel. The firebox has a Scandinavian baffle system. Some models will hold 27-inch logs. There are also a rotating flue collar for easy installation; front and back draft-distribution devices; a reversible baffle, and much, much more. Take a look. There are three

models—one of them a Franklin for those who like to view the open fire. The Cawley Stove Company, Inc., 27 North Wathington Street, Boyertown, PA 19512. Under $1,000.

Franco Belge Coal and Wood Stoves. Here is a rugged stove that is handsome enough for the most elegant living room. The two-tone steel cabinet with its Federal-style gold trim has a large window for seeing the fire within the cast-iron firebox. Between the firebox and the outer shell, hot air is produced by natural convection, with an automatic thermostat regulating combustion air for the fire. There are several designs to choose from and a choice of fuels: wood, coal, and wood/coal. The coal stove gravity feeds the fuel from a coal hopper so that you can leave the fire unattended for a much longer time than if you were dependent solely on the capacity of the firebox. It has cooking capability, a heat exchanger, and many other features worth looking into. Franco Belge Foundries of America, Inc., 15 Columbus Circle, New York, NY 10023. Over $1,000.

Ashley Circulator. An American-made cabinet stove with an automatic thermostat, which has been popular in the United States for over 100 years. The manufacturer is very proud of this record of continuous service and makes it a point to keep parts in stock even for stoves that have long been discontinued. The cabinet never gets burning hot, so this is a particularly safe kind of stove when there are children in the family. The stove produces

Ashley Circulator

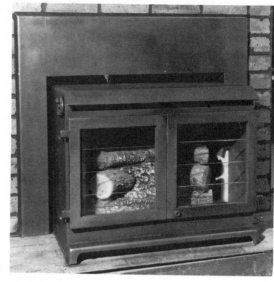

Fire Rite Fireplace Insert

convective as well as radiant heat. Many sizes and models are available but you can't beat the Ashley Imperial, which holds 100 pounds of wood at a time—with that firebox capacity and its automatic thermostat, this is a stove that requires minimum effort on the part of its owner. Coal capability is also available as are coal/wood models. The stove has a heavy-gauge, enameled steel cabinet and a cast-iron firebox. The Ashley Heater Company, P.O. Box 128, Florence, AL 35630. Under $1,000.

Fire Rite Fireplace Insert. The impressive twenty-five-year warranty that comes with this insert is bound to create confidence in the product. As with most inserts, the Fire Rite is easy to install. A panel covers part of the fireplace opening and the insert slides right into the remaining opening. Although the manufacturer suggests venting directly into the fireplace, in order to make it as easy as possible for the homeowner to do the installation, I would strongly recommend you take the additional trouble required to vent it up to the flue. The procedure's not *that* much more trouble and is all around better practice, since it permits much less creosote buildup inside your chimney. You may order the insert with glass viewing panels or with metal panels. As with all other inserts, the Fire Rite produces convective air, but the blower is optional so you can always order it later if you find you want to boost heat production. Fire Rite Stoves, 654 North Colony Street, Wallingford, CT 06492. Under $1,000.

Fuego Fireplaces. The Fuego line includes an insert, a zero-clearance fireplace, and a free-standing stove. No matter which you choose, all produce heat through natural convection and all have wide glass viewing panels in the doors. Heavy-gauge steel construction, no fan needed, slanted grate that keeps the wood away from the glass. El Fuego Corp., 30 Lafayette Square, Vernon, CT 06066. Under $1,000.

Stanley Kitchen Range. Made in Ireland in the same town that gives us Waterford crystal, the Stanley is a compact, cast-iron, wood-burning cookstove that has a generous-sized oven (big enough for a 25-lb. turkey), a three-lid cooktop, and a large hotplate. It will burn for ten to twelve hours on a single load and is rated up to 70 percent fuel efficient. Forshaw of St. Louis, Inc., 825 S. Lindbergh, St. Louis, MO 63131. Over $1,000.

Chubby Coal Stove. A cozy-looking little stove that is only 30 inches high so it can sit within most fireplaces or, if you prefer, on the hearth. The round shape of the firebox means you don't need to line it with firebrick, and it comes with either a manual or a shaker grate. The manufacturer's claims of 80 to 90 percent efficiency cannot be checked, but his claim that it will hold a fire 18 to 70 hours is at least consistent with high efficiency. Even if, by chance, the stove doesn't test out to quite this high rating, it would still seem to be a good buy. Plimoth Coal Stove Works, Route 106, Plympton, MA 02367. Under $1,000.

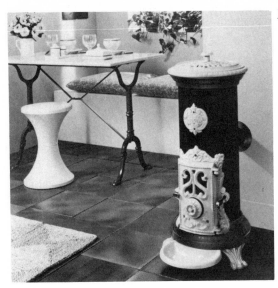

Petit Godin

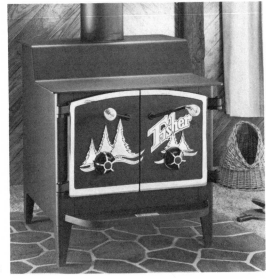

Fisher "Grandpa Bear"
wood stove

Petit Godin. For all its elegant French styling, the Petit Godin is a workhorse. It will burn either wood or coal but is more efficient with coal. Designed and first manufactured in 1889, the Godin still uses mica, rather than glass, for its viewing window—no danger of breakage—and the top lifts up to reveal a surface just right for your fondue pan or hot-chocolate pot. Designed originally as a hall stove, its compact shape fits agreeable into any room, and it comes in two sizes. The body is made of heavy-gauge steel, and the trim, of high-quality porcelain enamel, comes in a sand color and a number of other unusually attractive colors. Bow and Arrow Imports, 14 Arrow Street, Cambridge, MA 02138. Under $1,000.

Defiant. This is, quite simply, a superb stove. It is cast-iron throughout, with an automatic thermostat, interior baffle, primary and secondary air ports, front- and side-loading doors, both coal and wood capability in the two smaller sizes, a removable, specially ground cast-iron griddle, and what is said to be the longest flame path of any stove made. It can be used as an airtight or as a Franklin for viewing the open fire. The only conceivable problem you may have with the Defiant is too much heat. Check out the three sizes and buy the one that is right for your home. Unlike most stoves, the Defiant is currently sold only direct from the manufacturer and, as you might expect, there is usually a waiting list. Vermont Castings, Inc., Prince Street, Randolph, VT 05060. Under $1,000.

Fisher. Oregon seems to be a great state for quality wood stoves and the Fisher is no exception. It has a two-step design, which gives you an efficient firebox with a high rate of combustion, as well as two cooking surfaces of different temperatures, a very handy feature that means an extensive cooking capability. With the doors open and the firescreen in place, you can enjoy an open fire to your heart's content. Close the doors when it starts to get chilly and bask in warmth. Heavy-plate-steel construction, a firebrick-lined firebox, and easy-to-use draft controls on the door come in all three sizes as well as in the fireplace insert. The Grandpa Bear, which is the largest, will hold 24-inch logs, a great time-saver both in cutting and loading your wood. Fisher Stoves, Inc., P.O. Box 10605, Eugene, OR 97440. Under $1,000.

Weso Coalburning Stove. Unlike the Weso's tile stove that burns both wood and coal, this new stove is meant only for coal burning. Instead of tile, it features a surface of enameled cast iron that comes in a beige-and-bronze color scheme. If you burn nut-sized anthracite as recommended, the firebox will hold 38 pounds at one time. A load of this size will burn up to 24 hours and will require shaking approximately every 8 hours. The reason such a small stove (26½ inches high with lid raised, by 24¼ inches wide by 17 inches deep) can hold so much coal is that the firebox is top loaded and gravity feeds into the fire as the bottom coals burn. Primary air intake is ther-

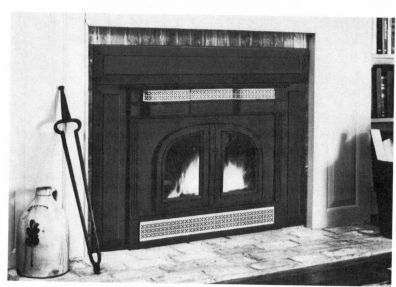

Shelburne Fireplace Stove

EASE OF STARTING

A wood fire needs two kinds of wood, easy starting and long burning. Long-burning wood will be more difficult to start; easy-to-start wood will give a hotter, faster-burning fire. Generally speaking, hardwoods are harder to start and the softwoods, like pines, are easy. Choose from woods rated "excellent" or "good" for kindling. Choose from woods rated "fair" or "poor" for your main fire.

Check the table below for ratings.

	Kindling Quality			
Type of wood	Excellent	Good	Fair	Poor
Apple				X
Ash			X	
Aspen	X			
Basswood	X			
Beech				X
White birch		X		
Cedar	X			
Cherry				X
Elm				X
Douglas fir	X			
Hemlock		X		
Hickory			X	
Black locust				X
Sugar maple				X
Red oak				X
White pine	X			
Norway spruce		X		
Tamarack	X			

mostatically controlled, according to your setting, and, because the stove has a cabinet over the firebox interior, both radiant and convective air are produced. Clearance to combustibles is considerably less than the 36 inches of an ordinary cast-iron box stove. Ceramic Radiant Heat, Pleasant Drive, Lochmere, NH 03252. Under $1,000.

Shelburne Fireplace Stove. This is a new insert with coal and wood capability, as well as a number of unique features. First, it is mounted on four concealed wheels, which may not seem a world-shaking innovation, unless you have tried to move the average insert. The wheels make it both much easier to install as well as to pull out for the annual maintenance check and chimney cleaning. Combustion is unusually complete for an insert because burning volatiles are baffled through a 44-inch system, forced back to the flame path through overhead tubes. Behind the decorative bottom grill is an adjustable damper handle and pullout ash pan, and the andirons are removable—a safety factor for when you want to enjoy the open fire. A blower with variable speed control increases heat production, and an automatic thermostat lets you dial the heat levels you wish. All in all, a technologically interesting unit with a good-looking facade that would go with any decor. You won't find the Shelburne at your local retailer; like the Defiant, it is sold direct to the consumer only. The Vermont Stove Company, Shelburne Road, Shelburne, VT 05482. Under $1,000.

Sir Cyril. A top-loading cast-iron coal stove, the Sir Cyril has a more formal styling than one expects to find in stoves of this type. It is, however, a completely serious coalburner with a top loader with hopper, shaker grates, and the essential ash pan sensibly located above an ash shelf. It is designed to be used as either a free-standing stove or a hearth stove, and is approximately 33 inches high x 18 inches deep x 22 inches wide. The viewing window allows sight of the fire, and you can always switch to wood, if you wish. Quaker Stove Co., Inc., 200 West 5th Street, Lansdale, PA 19446. Under $1,000.

NOT-SO-TRIVIAL TRIVIA FOR THE COAL/ WOOD-BURNER

If all the coal that we estimate exists in the earth at the current time could be mined, we would have enough, at the current rate of consumption, to last at least 2,000 years.

A fireplace is just about the most inefficient heating device you can have in your home. At most, it delivers 10 to 15 percent of the heat potential in the wood you burn. The rest goes to heat the chimney and outdoors. You'd probably be warmer sitting on your chimney than in front of your fireplace.

According to the *New York Times,* a cord of wood has about the same heat-producing power as 200 gallons of heating oil and requires the same amount of space as a grand piano. It is also equal to one ton of coal.

The heat from a pound of coal will brew more than 100 cups of your morning coffee.

As late as the 1940s, America depended on coal for about 90 percent of its fuel.

A cord of green wood will shrink at least 8 percent in volume during seasoning.

The leaves on trees cut in the summer will draw moisture from the wood and dry it more quickly than if you cut off the branches as soon as you cut down the tree.

A cord of hardwood weighs 2 tons.

A dump truck can hold up to 4 standard cords of wood.

Creosote will not condense on the inside of flues or stovepipes until the stack temperature drops below 250°F.

According to a 1980 Gallup poll, more than five million American homes have a working woodburning stove.

The stove Ben Franklin invented in 1816 works on the same principle found today in almost all fireplace inserts and many free-standing stoves.

If your house is so well caulked, insulated, and weatherstripped that very little outside air is coming in, your stove or fireplace fire may go out for lack of oxygen.

Today the United States still has almost 75 percent as much forest land as existed in the time of the pioneers—754 million acres.

Your woodlot can save you money on air conditioning. The combined cooling and humidifying effect of a forest is equal to that of the same area of ocean.

33

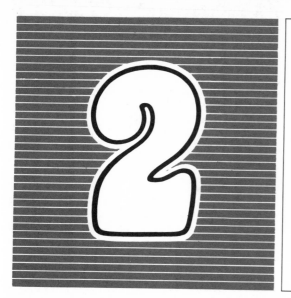

Working Within the System: Conventional Warmth in Energy-Conscious Times

Michael deCourcy Hinds

CUTTING YOUR LOSSES

The first and most important energy-saving "product" to buy for your home is an energy audit. Having skilled technicians cruise through your house looking for leaky windows, sooty heating systems and dripping faucets does more than pinpoint the problems. (You probably knew about most of them yourself and were planning to get around to them some day, right?) What the energy audit does, most importantly, is develop an energy-conservation program, establishing a schedule for repairs. The idea is to start off making the least costly, most effective improvements and, later on, as you have the cash to invest, gradually undertake the more costly repairs that have longer payback periods. The logic is very convincing, and studies show that people who have had their homes audited almost always get gung-ho about making repairs.

In most homes, the list of priorities usually looks like this:

1. Put the heating system and controls in order;
2. Check out the hot water heater and reduce water consumption;
3. Check insulation throughout the house, but especially in the attic;
4. Install storm windows and doors or, at the very least, weatherstrip and caulk around all exterior openings.

After these basic measures, the list continues:

5. Install insulating draperies, shutters, or shades to prevent nighttime heat loss through glass windows and doors;
6. Consider solar improvements when making renovations. A solar greenhouse, for example, will help heat the house as well as grow some very nice flowers and useful vegetables.

HEAT LOSSES IN TYPICAL TWO-STORY HOME

Half the heat produced by the furnace in a typically inefficient two-story home quickly escapes. (The same principle applies to any dwelling.) Here are the basic routes the heat takes and the percentages of this heat loss if no energy-conserving measures are taken:

1. Attic or roof: 27 percent
2. Windows: 25 percent
3. Walls, joints, and cracks: 15 percent
4. Fireplace and flue: 13 percent
5. Doors: 10 percent
6. Electric outlets and switches on exterior walls: 10 percent

FINDING AN AUDITOR

The best auditing bargain in the country is provided by local utilities. Under the National Energy Conservation Policy Act of 1978, large utilities must offer homeowners an audit of their home's energy use for $15 or less.

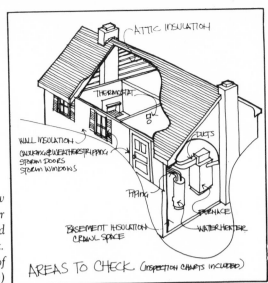

An energy audit will show you exactly where your house is losing heat, and what you can do about it. (U.S. Department of Energy)

In some states, the utilities do that and no more. In others, like New York, Tennessee, and Oregon, the companies do much more. Take Consolidated Edison of New York, for example. The company's auditor will spend a couple of hours going over your house, then he'll make recommendations, supply a list of approved contractors, estimate the costs and paybacks, and even arrange for low-cost financing. If the homeowner desires, the utility will act as the general contractor, arranging and overseeing all the work to make sure it's properly done.

To those skeptics who wonder whether utilities, which make their money selling fuel, will conscientiously advise homeowners on how to save fuel, think about this: the audit only costs you $10 or $15, but it often costs the utility over $125 to perform. And in some states the audit makes you eligible for that nice, cheap loan. (In my experience with a utility energy audit in Brooklyn, N.Y., the auditors did overlook some minor areas but all their recommendations were good.)

To have your heating system's efficiency checked, you may have to specifically request the service and may have to pay another $10–$15. Still, it's an excellent value for the money.

A few words of advice before you take the plunge. The utility audits are good for finding general household energy ills. But the utility auditors are rarely allowed to recommend unconventional energy-saving products or models and brands of replacement equipment for improving the heating system, nor will they suggest ways of using alternative fuels, like solar or wind. For this kind of detailed advice, you have to pay more money. Independent energy specialists, primarily engineers and architects, can help plan major energy-conservation improvements. Heating system specialists—if you're not satisfied with your current dealer or if you want a second opinion—will recommend the most cost-effective improvements for the heating plant. These energy professionals will usually consult on an hourly basis, often ranging from $15 to $50 an hour. They will provide a detailed analysis of the situation and will often design and oversee the recommended work. When handling the complete project, architects and engineers generally charge fees based on a percentage of the project's cost.

Professional consultants can be found by getting in touch with local chapters of professional organizations, such as the American Society of Heating, Refrigerating, and Air Conditioning Engineers (headquarters in New York: 345 East 47 Street, [212]644-7953); the American Consulting Engineers Council (headquarters in Washington, D.C.: Suite 713, 1155 15th Street N.W. 20005, [202]347-7474) and the American Institute of Architects (headquarters in Washington, D.C.: 1730

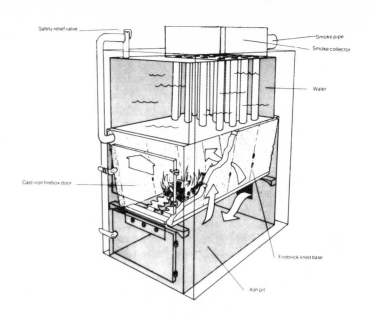

Safety relief valve — Smoke pipe — Smoke collector — Water — Cast-iron firebox door — Firebrick lined base — Ash pit

New York Avenue, [202]626-7300).

For independent heating-system mechanics, look in the Yellow Pages under the type of system you have. An alternative is to call the manufacturer of your heating plant and ask him for the name of a qualified mechanic in your area, as well as the best ways to improve the system.

FINDING THE MONEY

For most energy-conserving improvements, you can claim a federal income tax credit of 15 percent of the cost, up to a maximum of $300. This applies only to your principal residence. Insulation, weatherstripping, storm windows and doors, heating-system improvements, and other conservation measures are included.

Use IRS Form 5695 to apply for the credit. For more information about the credit and eligibility, ask the IRS for Publication 903.

Utilities may also arrange for low-cost loans. And consult the energy office in your state capital for other loan and grant programs. Local governments may also have good programs. In New York City, many homeowners qualify for a program called J-51 that repays 90 percent of the cost of major improvements over a twelve-year period by lowering local real estate taxes on the residence.

THE PLACE TO START: THE HEATING SYSTEM

Before getting down to the nuts and bolts, here's a technical definition of a couple of frequently misused key words. "Boiler" and "furnace" are often used interchangeably. This is incorrect, but we all do it. A boiler, as the word implies, is a heater system in which water or steam is warmed and then sent through the house, typically in radiators. A boiler may also have water coils in which domestic hot water is heated. A furnace is a forced warm air system in which the heated air travels through the house. Both boilers and furnaces use all fuels.

OIL SYSTEMS

A recent government survey began by stating that "a third of the fuel oil delivered to the typical home for heat is wasted, and many dwellings lose as much as half." Inefficiency in oil burners and other systems is primarily due to their being poorly tuned, oversized, or outdated.

A simple tune-up and cleaning may cost only about $75, but it could save you $300 a year on your heating bill. Oil heating systems are the most likely to get out of tune. Normally, one tune-up a year is sufficient, but how does a homeowner know if his system needs additional tuning?

With a few simple instruments, you can monitor the efficiency of the oil burner yourself. Four test instruments—for measuring

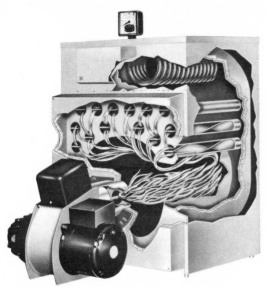

Opposite, a boiler, in this case fueled by coal, heats the water in the upper chamber to produce steam, which is then forced through your heating system. A furnace heats air, which is then channeled through the house. (Boiler, Kerr Controls Limited; furnace, Axeman Anderson)

ZERO COST IMPROVEMENT

Lower the water temperature in the boiler from 200° to 140°F, and you will save as much as 10 percent on your heating bills. According to Brookhaven National Laboratory, a reduction of 35 degrees, say from 185° to 150°F, will save around 5 percent. The reduced temperature, however, will mean that it will take longer for the heating system to warm up the house. If you make manual adjustments several times a year as the climate changes, you can get comfortable results. Homeowners with forced warm air systems should ask their service company whether temperature reductions can be made in their systems in order to reap similar savings.

the draft in the chimney, the temperature of the flue gases, the amount of soot going up the flue, and the percentage of carbon dioxide in the flue gases—will give you exact readings on how efficiently your system is working. Efficiencies of 75 to 80 percent can be achieved; a reading below 70-percent efficiency means you're wasting a third of the money you are spending on oil.

These instruments are generally available at local heating suppliers. If you have any trouble locating a dealer, contact one of these two major manufacturers: Bacharach Instruments, 626 Alpha Drive, Pittsburgh, PA 15238;

Dwyer Instruments, Inc., Box 373-T, Michigan City, IN 46360. Complete kits cost between $150 and $225.

At the very least, buy a flue thermometer ($17–$20). It will alert you to excess heat going up the chimney rather than into your house. In most systems, if the flue temperature goes over 500°F, it means that the boiler is dirty. Dirt and soot on the water coils act like insulation, preventing expensively produced heat from being absorbed by the system's water and allowing it to go briskly up the chimney.

The boiler or furnace is now working efficiently, but is it too big? If so, it's wasting your money. A federal Department of Energy study concluded that most houses built in the past forty years have systems that are too large.

Prior to the oil embargo of 1973, it didn't matter if a Cadillac-sized heating system were hooked up to a Volkswagen-sized home, but now engineers are much more concerned with putting in a properly sized or "rated" burner to heat your fuel. If properly rated, the burner should be operating almost constantly when the thermostat calls for heat. An oversized burner, on the other hand, will kick on, waste a lot of heat warming the furnace up, send a few mighty blasts of heat upstairs, and then shut down, wasting even more heat as the furnace cools down. By derating the burner, you can often save 10 percent, and sometimes as much as 20 percent, of your heating bill.

In derating, you want to make your furnace burn less oil per minute and operate more min-

Considerations When Weighing Alternative Steps for Upgrading an Oil Burner System

Corrective Action Taken	Approx. Cost ($)	Annual Fuel-Saving Possible (%)	Annual Payback Period (Yrs.) [1]	Problems
Replace old burner-boiler unit with a more efficient system (using a matched flame-retention burner or blue flame burner)	1,500–2,000	24[2]	3.3–4.4	None
Replace existing burner with a flame-retention burner	200–350	5–22	0.5–3.7	Boiler may need new combustion-chamber liner
Install a flue economizer	450–650	9–20	1.2–3.9	Heat-transfer surfaces must be periodically cleaned
Install a flue damper	250–350	2–14	1.0–9.3	Possible safety hazard if improperly installed or maintained
Replace oil-burner nozzle with a smaller nozzle that reduces firing rate by 25%	0–30[3]	8[2]	0.0–0.2	Cannot be done unless existing system is oversized
Reduce boiler-water temperature manually by 35°F	None[4]	5	0	Requires seasonal resetting
Tune burner to achieve best combustion	0–30[3]	3	0.0–0.5	None

[1] Based on an assumed current oil consumption of 1500 gallons per year, at $1.25/gallon.
[2] Where the existing system has a dry-base steel boiler with a conventional burner.
[3] The cost may be covered by the homeowner's annual servicing contract for the unit.
[4] This adjustment can be easily done by the occupant.
(Revised Feb. 18, 1981, to adjust for higher oil price.)
Source: Brookhaven National Laboratory

Your Savings for Every $100 Fuel Costs by Increasing Combustion Efficiency

From an Original Efficiency of	To an Increased Combustion Efficiency of:							
	55%	60%	65%	70%	75%	80%	85%	90%
50%	$9.70	$16.70	$23.10	$28.60	$33.30	$37.50	$41.20	$44.40
55%	—	8.30	15.40	21.50	26.50	31.20	35.30	38.90
60%	—	—	7.70	14.30	20.00	25.00	29.40	33.30
65%	—	—	—	7.10	13.30	18.80	23.50	27.80
70%	—	—	—	—	6.70	12.50	17.60	22.20
75%	—	—	—	—	—	6.30	11.80	16.70
80%	—	—	—	—	—	—	5.90	11.10
85%	—	—	—	—	—	—	—	5.60

Source: ABC Sunray Company

utes of each hour. If the furnace takes longer to burn the same amount of oil, less oil is wasted—and the house will probably be more comfortable. Unless you are a devoted do-it-yourselfer, this is definitely an area for the experts—first to determine whether and how much oversized the system is and, second, to do the work. The work involves replacing the original burner nozzle with a smaller one, so that less oil per minute is shot into the burning chamber.

If the burner itself is old and inefficient, it may be worth investing in a new "flame-reten-tion head" burner—to be installed by an experienced technician. Retention burners are more efficient than the older models because they combine high-speed air delivery with a specially shaped flame funnel (which recirculates the fuel and air past the flame) to produce maximum burner efficiency. Normally, these burners cost about $400 installed.

In February 1981, *Consumer Reports* tested and rated six retention head burners. A summary of their findings follows. Ask your dealer about these burners, or contact the company for installers in your area.

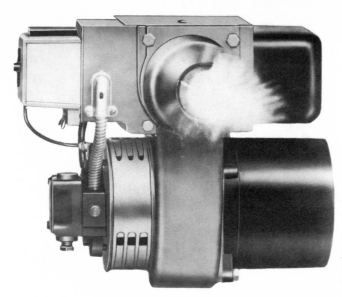

The Sloan Interburner retention-head burner funnels its flame for maximum efficiency. (Sloan Valve Company)

40   *Aero FAFC* (Aero Environmental Limited, 37 Hanna Avenue, Toronto, Ontario, Canada M6K 1X2) had a combustion efficiency of 86 percent. It cost $300 plus installation in February 1981.

Sloan Interburner Mark 1 (Sloan Valve Company, 10500 Seymour Avenue, Franklin Park, IL 60131). Combustion efficiency, 86 percent; cost, $300 plus installation.

Beckett AF (R. W. Beckette Corporation, 38251 Center Ridge Road, Elyria, OH 44036). Combustion efficiency, 83 percent; cost, $250 plus installation.

Carlin 100CRD (Carlin Company, 912 Silas Deane Highway, Wethersfield, CN 06109). Combustion efficiency, 81 percent; cost, $285 plus installation.

Wayne MSR (Wayne Home Equipment Division of Scott & Fetzer Company, 801 Glasgow Avenue, Fort Wayne, IN 46803. Combustion efficiency, 81 percent; cost, $300 plus installation.

ABC-Sunray FCF-234 (ABC Sunray Corporation, 45 South Service Road, Plainview, NY 11803). Combustion efficiency, 80 percent; cost, $320 plus installation.

Gas Systems

Gas burners are extremely efficient, smooth operating, and clean burning. If you have an older unit, you can greatly improve its efficiency by replacing the pilot light with an electronic spark ignition for about $200, thus reaping a savings of up to 8 percent a year.

Other energy-saving products, such as heat exchangers on the flue (which send warm air into the room) can be useful and cost-effective.

Although gas systems can go for three years without a complete tune-up, it is wise—and thrifty in these inflationary times—to have an annual check up:

1. Check the gas valve for leaks (needs pressure gauge).
2. Clean burners.
3. Clean pilot light or replace it; inspect thermocouple.
4. Check and adjust gas pressure.
5. Adjust air mixture until flame is blue.
6. Adjust pilot light.
7. Inspect all connections and wires.

Standing by and asking questions while the serviceman is at his job is a remarkably good way of making sure the tune-up and cleaning are done properly.

When considering a new gas burner, make sure it is a "gas-powered burner"; this controls air intake better than the more common "atmospheric burner." The rule of thumb is the more air used in a burner, the less efficient it is.

Electric Furnaces

These usually require the least maintenance of any system, primarily because they do not have a combustion system to tune up. Still, annual cleaning of fans, humidifier, filters and thermostat are wise procedures.

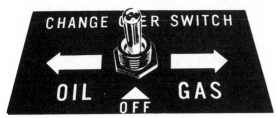

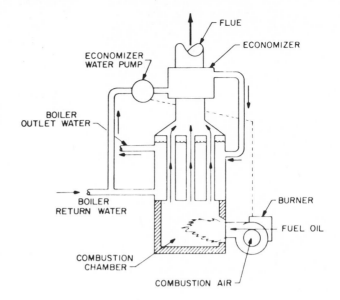

A combination burner—switch to gas or oil. (ABC Sunray)

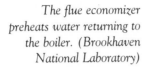

The flue economizer preheats water returning to the boiler. (Brookhaven National Laboratory)

Gas-Oil Combination Conversion Burner

For the ultimate in flexibility, consider installing a system that runs on gas *or* oil, depending on which is cheaper. With a flick of a switch you can go from one fuel to the other. Nationally, gas-conversion burners cost about $800.

For about $100 more, ABC Sunray has a high-efficiency (80 percent with gas/83 percent with oil) combination burner that burns both oil and gas. Two sizes are available. The GC-385 is for larger homes and costs $720 to installers, who will mark up the price and add an installation fee of $200 to $300. The GC-210 is for most residences; it costs $520 wholesale, plus mark up and installation, which will vary from place to place but averages $900. These combination conversion burners are highly efficient (they have retention-head burners). For more information, contact ABC Sunray, 45 South Service Road, Plainview, NY 11803.

More Medium-Cost Improvements

Flue dampers, sold and installed by most dealers and general companies, shut down the flue to prevent heat loss when the burner has cycled off. *They must be cautiously considered.* According to a Department of Energy laboratory at Brookhaven, the devices may create problems, will cost $30 to $50 a year in servicing, and are really effective only in oil systems with older burners. With new retention-head burners, the dampers may only save

2 to 3 percent of your fuel bill. The $300 to $500 these installed dampers cost would obviously be better spent on a new efficient burner. However, if you're considering a damper, keep in mind the information that follows. The DOE laboratory found that odor and smoke problems may result because a few drops of oil may ignite after the burner has shut down. To allow for this, vent damper manufacturers have come up with two solutions. First, they have developed a damper with holes punched in it that closes down within seconds of the burner's cycling off. These holes greatly defeat the purpose of the damper (to seal the flue) but do allow smoke and odor to escape. The second, and better, solution is a solid damper that automatically closes in about three minutes, allowing time for the "afterburn" gases to escape. Servicing these dampers is essential, since a malfunction could cause operational problems.

The *flue economizer,* sometimes called a stack economizer or stack heat reclaimer, is usually used on a hot-water boiler. Water returning to the boiler to be reheated is first passed through the economizer, which is located in the flue pipe. The hot escaping gases pass around the coils of the economizer and preheat the water before it reaches the main boiler. Economizers can run $450 to $650 and may cut fuel consumption by 9 percent, or as much as 20 percent in older systems, according to Brookhaven National Laboratory.

Humidifiers. Sixty-eight degrees Fahren-

41

heit, the recommended energy-conservation home-heating temperature, can cut fuel bills by 20 percent and can be just as comfortable as 75 degrees, as long as the relative humidity is kept at about 45 percent. But in many parts of the country, it is difficult to moisten the air sufficiently without a humidifier. The average northeastern home, for example, needs between 6 and 10 gallons of water added to the air daily to bring humidity up to a comfortable level in winter.

Humidifiers can be centrally installed in warm-air systems; homeowners with other systems must rely on portable humidifiers. See chart for the size humidifier you need. Central systems, which cost $200 to $300, are sold and installed by heating and cooling contractors; often your fuel dealer will do it. Portable units range from the $20 variety sold in drugstores to fancy ones in consoles that cost several hundred dollars.

THERMOSTATS

After nearly a decade of sharp increases in fuel prices, just about every homeowner is aware of the benefits of lowering the thermostat at bedtime and during the day if no one is at home. Depending on variables like local climate and family schedules, the annual fuel bill can be reduced one percent for each degree the thermostat is lowered over an eight-hour period. If the house is empty during the day or if the one or two occupants in the house rely on cost-effective task heating with portable electric

Home Size in Square Feet	Humidity Needs (in gallons per 24 hours)		
	—Weatherproofing of House—		
	Tight[1]	Average[2]	Loose[3]
500	0.1 gallons	2 gallons	2.5 gallons
1,000	2.1 gallons	4.4 gallons	6.9 gallons
1,500	4.2 gallons	7.7 gallons	11.4 gallons
2,000	8.3 gallons	10.9 gallons	15.9 gallons
2,500	8.4 gallons	14.1 gallons	20.4 gallons
3,000	10.4 gallons	17.4 gallons	24.8 gallons

[1] House is well-insulated, has weatherstripped and caulked storm doors and windows.
[2] House has some insulation, but storm doors and windows are loose fitting.
[3] House has little or no insulation and no storm doors or windows.
Source: Association of Home Appliance Manufacturers

Total Warmth

heaters, the savings can be doubled. The same conservation principle works in summer as well, if you have central air conditioning.

Most set back thermostats can be installed for $125, and older thermostats can simply be replaced by the homeowner for $60–$75. But homeowners who want to program the thermostat for set backs during the day and night or for weekends will have to pay a little more. Here are a few good set back thermostats:

Robertshaw/Consumer Products Division, P.O. Box 2222, Corona, CA 91720, makes several models, ranging from $50 to $60. This includes thermostats for heating and cooling, with two set backs. Models T30-1241 has double set back for heating, and model T30-1243 has a double set back for heating and cooling systems. Both cost about $60 and are available from heating supply stores or from dealers the company will refer you to.

Honeywell, Inc., Honeywell Plaza, Minneapolis, MN 55408 (612) 870-5200, makes a line of thermostats, including the Chronotherm, which has one set back. It costs about $65.

Champion Home Builders Company, Dryden, MI 48071, makes the Energy-Dial, which replaces most round-type thermostats. Additional set backs are optional. It costs about $60.

Dynelco, Dynamic Electron Controls Inc., P.O. Box 193, 47 Mill Plain Road, Danbury, CT 06810, makes Therm-O-Guard thermostats that are sensitive to light and have solid-state components. The multisetback ther-

Night Setback—Winter					
Setback:	5°	10°	Setback:	5°	10°
City	%	%	City	%	%
Atlanta	11	15	Milwaukee	6	10
Boston	7	11	Minneapolis	5	9
Buffalo	6	10	New York City	8	12
Chicago	7	11	Omaha	7	11
Cincinnati	8	12	Philadelphia	8	12
Cleveland	8	12	Pittsburgh	7	11
Dallas	11	15	Portland	9	13
Denver	7	11	Salt Lake City	7	11
Des Moines	7	11	San Francisco	10	14
Detroit	7	11	St. Louis	8	12
Kansas City	8	12	Seattle	8	12
Los Angeles	12	16	Washington, D.C.	9	13
Louisville	9	13			

Source: Reprinted from the August 1973 issue of ASHRAE JOURNAL by permission of the American Society of Heating, Refrigerating and Air-Conditioning Engineers, Inc.

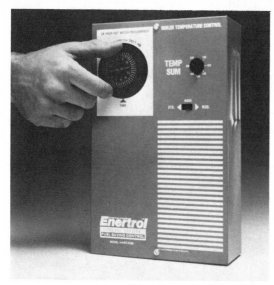

This Enertrol temperature control unit saves energy two ways. Most boilers keep their water at a constant temperature no matter how cold it is. The Enertrol temperature control unit will regulate the water temperature by measuring the outdoor temperature, so your boiler is never hotter than you need it to be. It will also program your hot water system to work at full tilt only during those hours when you need it most. (American Stabilis Inc.)

44

mostats range from $80 to $100 and can be installed by the homeowner.

Control Pak, 44480 Grand River Avenue, Novi, MI 48050, recently introduced the Temp Tron, which allows precise programming of the user's choice of temperature and schedule. The thermostat can program six changes per twenty-four-hour period and plan two different twenty-four-hour periods, as well as a weekend schedule. An outdoor sensor allows the user to see the outdoor temperature displayed on the large-faced thermostat. Price for the unit has not been established yet, and it may not be widely distributed until 1982.

More Advanced Controls

Several companies make controls that relate outside air temperature to the temperature of water circulating in the boiler and radiators. Under ideal circumstances, these controls provide comfort by delivering heat more evenly; by virtue of their sensitivity, they should also eliminate overheating. Claims by manufacturers indicate that the products may save up to 40 percent, but 20 percent is probably a more realistic number. Here are a couple of well-known brands:

Enertrol, made by American Stabilis Inc., P.O. Box 1289, Lewiston, ME 04240, is a control mechanism that keeps hot water continuously circulating at a temperature no higher than that needed to maintain the

Manufacturers' Efficiency Claims

About efficiency claims made by manufacturers: Companies are required to report the "annual fuel utilization efficiency," which reports the company's own tests on their systems, not independent tests. These efficiency ratings, called AFUE, are based on the heating system's efficiency over a nationally averaged heating season. The ratings indicate how much energy is lost when the burner cycles off and cools down—the largest single contributor to lowering efficiency. Because the ratings are based on a national average, the efficiency of any particular heating system will be greater in cold climates like Maine, where the system will be idling less; and will be less than stated in warm climates like Georgia, where the equipment will not be working continuously.

In addition, the AFUE does not include heat losses through the jacket of the furnace or boiler, on the assumption that the heat eventually rises and is used by the house. However, in houses with unheated basements and well-insulated ceilings, these jacket losses are not well utilized, meaning that the rated efficiency will be lower by as much as 6 percent, according to Brookhaven National Laboratory.

house at the temperature indicated on the thermostat. In conventional systems, the

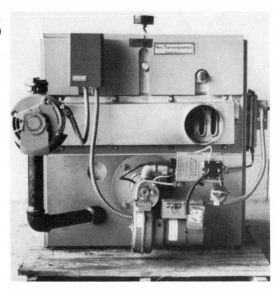

Blueray oil-fired boiler. (Blueray Systems Inc.)

water coursing through the radiators is always at some high preset temperature like 180°F. The makers of the Enertrol and other such devices claim that this preset temperature wastes fuel in mild weather and in summer, when the boiler heats only domestic hot water. The Enertrol automatically regulates the temperature of water inside the boiler or the air inside the furnace to the exact needs of the house. American Stabilis makes four models of Enertrol for all types of systems, and the prices ranges from $150 to $300 installed. The most popular models have a clock timer that also regulates domestic hot water (inside the boiler) on a schedule set by the homeowner. The company does not recommend using the control with warm-air furnaces as the energy savings are very small; however, they do say that comfort is increased.

Honeywell, Inc., Honeywell Plaza, Minneapolis, MN 55408, is another maker of these controls.

REPLACING THE OLD HEATING SYSTEM

You'll probably know it when it's time to buy a new heating system; your fuel bills will tell you. Or your mechanic may start suggesting expensive repairs, providing the impetus to spend the extra money for a very efficient system.

Assuming that you have decided to stick with oil as the fuel, there are a number of very efficient boilers and furnaces on the market. They're likely to cost $1300 to $1500 installed, but a number of the good ones operate annually at over 75-percent efficiency. Here are the leaders in the field:

The Blueray. Tests conducted by the Department of Energy indicate that fuel savings of up to 40 percent can be achieved by replacing a conventional boiler with a Blueray. The Blueray has a special burner that draws combustion back into the ignition chamber to preheat the oil before it enters the flame. Preheating is important because it makes the oil burn hotter, cleaner, and more completely.

Aside from having a high seasonal efficiency—averaging 85 percent and sometimes hitting 90—the Blueray units are better at retaining the heat they generate and thus can send more of it to the house.

The cost for an oil-fired hot-air furnace is about $1600 to $1750 installed. (No gas-fired hot-air system is available yet.) A boiler system, which includes domestic hot water, costs about $2200 to $2400 installed. If you are considering switching to gas, Blueray has a gas system, too. Their gas unit, recently introduced to the market, has about an 84-percent efficiency. It costs about $2000 to $2400 installed. The unit also provides domestic hot water.

For information about local dealers, contact

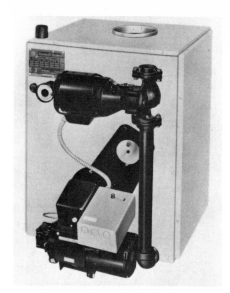

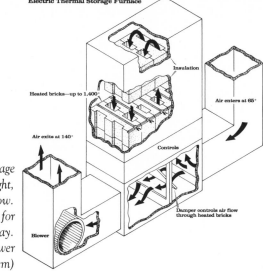

Burnham V-1 oil boiler.
(Burnham Corporation)

An electric thermal storage furnace heats bricks at night, when electric rates are low. The bricks retain the heat for distribution during the day. (American Electric Power System)

Blueray Systems, Inc., 6800 Jericho Turnpike, Syosset, NY 11791.

The Axeman Anderson. Conventional design, but with high efficiency, for the 1980s. The company's leading models are the PO Series, about $1200 installed; and the Custom Mark 3, which has a special fan that induces a constant draft and is more efficient than the PO Series, about $1350 installed. Anderson also makes a coal burner (see coal).

For more information, contact Axeman Anderson, 233 West Street, Williamsport, PA 17701.

The Burnham. Burnham makes excellent conventional equipment. Its V-1 oil system has an efficiency of about 82 percent, and its HE system is rated at 83 percent. Installed, costs range from $1000 to 1400. (Burnham also makes gas systems with 80 percent efficiency; the Series 2 costs around $1000.)

For more information, contact Burnham Corporation, 2 Main Street, Irvington, NY 10533.

New Gas Systems

The Hydropulse. The Hydropulse operates much like an internal-combustion engine and has no burners, no pilot light, and no conventional flue or chimney. Air is pulled into a sealed chamber where it is mixed with gas and ignited by a spark plug. The hot gases are then forced through a heat exchanger that heats water in the system. Exhaust gases are vented through small-diameter plastic pipes. Effi-

ciency is in the 91- to 94-percent range. Installed price, $2800 to $3500, depending on size and regional variations.

For more information contact Hydrotherm, Inc., Rochland Avenue, Northvail, NJ 07647 (201) 768-5500.

The Blueray. Blueray has a gas system as well as an oil. Just introduced to the market, the gas unit is about 84 percent efficient and costs $2000 to $2400 installed. The unit also supplies domestic hot water.

For more information contact Blueray Systems, Inc., 6800 Jericho Turnpike, Syosset, NY 11791.

New Electric Systems

The American Electric Power System. The American Electric Power System, which serves utilities in Virginia, Indiana, Michigan, Kentucky, Tennessee, Ohio, and West Virginia, has introduced a central electric furnace that makes optimum use of off-peak electric rates in these states. The warm-air furnace, called the electric-thermal-storage (ETS) unit, heats a large mass of bricks to 1400°F during the night, when rates are relatively inexpensive. During the day, a fan distributes the warm air through the ductwork into the house. The unit's water heater is similar to conventional heaters, except that it is more heavily insulated and has a capacity of 120 gallons of water, once again taking advantage of low nighttime rates.

This system costs about $1700 installed, is

Underwriters Laboratory listed, and is currently available from the TPI Corporation, P.O. Box T,CRS, Johnson City, TN 37601. The furnace should be considered only in areas where utilities offer discounts for off-peak use.

For more information, contact the American Electric Power System, 2 Broadway, New York, NY 10004.

NEW COAL SYSTEMS

The Axeman Anderson. Axeman Anderson (see address above, under oil systems) produces the Anthratube, a coal-fired hot-water boiler that uses Pennsylvania anthracite coal. This coal is available on the East Coast and west to Ohio; check with Anderson for availability in your area.

The system, first designed in 1947, has been refined and now has an efficiency of 87 percent, according to the U.S. Bureau of Mines statistics cited by the company. It is automatically stoked and costs about $3500 installed. According to the company, one ton of Pennsylvania anthracite usually costs $70 and is the equivalent in heating power of $230 worth of oil (at $1.15 a gallon).

THE HOT-WATER SYSTEM

The hot-water heater is the second largest user of energy in the home, typcially accounting for 18 to 25 percent of the fuel bill. There are several traditional ways to lower the cost of hot water.

1. Insulate the water heater itself. Simpex Company, 115 M Midtown Plaza, Syracuse, NY 13210, is one of many companies that mail order insulation jackets for electric or gas tank water heaters. Their Thermo Saver costs $24.95, and Simpex estimates it will save $147 worth of electricity or $81 worth of gas over a five year period. Clearly, it would be cheaper to buy a foil-backed batt of insulation and do it yourself, but the kit provides convenience.

2. Insulate the hot-water pipes. In new construction this is very easy, but in existing houses about all you can do is insulate the exposed pipes in the basement and under the sink. Plumbing-supply stores carry pipe insulation. If your heater or pipes are warm to the touch, you need insulation.

3. Turn down the thermostat on the water heater from 140° to an energy-saving 120°F and save 18 percent on your fuel bill for hot water.

4. Set the thermostat on a timer, which can save up to 35 percent of operating costs because most families need hot water only four hours a day. Energy House, P.O. Box 4035, 105 West Merrimack Street, Manchester, NH 03108, sells a $39.95 Hot Water Economizer for electric water heaters and guarantees it will pay for itself in four months or it can be returned for a full refund. Installation by an electrician may cost $25 or $30. The Economizer is simply a timer that activates the hot-water heater according to your schedule instead of keeping water hot twenty-four hours a day.

There are many economical ways to save on your hot-water bills. Insulating your water heater will reduce the energy needed to keep the water temperature constant and should pay back the cost of insulation in a year (A). Dishwashers can cause a strain on hot-water systems, since most models require a water temperature of 140° to 150°F. A booster heater (B) will allow you to set your water heater at 120°. When the dishwasher starts, it activates the booster heater to raise the water temperature to the required level. Showers can be fitted with simple flow-restrictors (C) that reduce the flow from 7 gallons per minute to just 2 or 3, or with more elaborate models that not only restrict the flow, but actually heat the water themselves (D). (Insulation: Johns-Manville; booster heater: Instant-Flow, from Chronomite Laboratories, Inc.; flow-restrictor: Resources Conservation, Inc.; water-heating shower head: Orlando Enterprises)

48

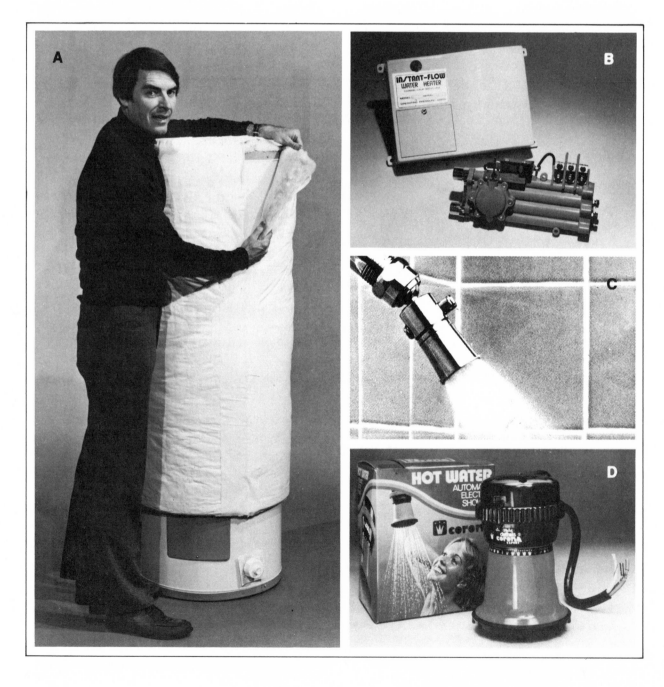

5. On gas heaters, replace the pilot light with an electronic spark ignition. This costs about $185 and could save about 3 percent of the gas bill.

6. Replace leaking washers on water faucets. Steadily dripping hot water from one faucet will annually waste up to 27 gallons of oil, or 3484 cubic feet of gas.

7. Install flow restrictors in shower heads, reducing the flow from 7 to 10 gallons per minute to 2 to 3 gallons per minute with no loss of comfort. Shower restrictors may pay for themselves in a *few hours of use.* The Saver Shower, an excellent series of shower heads, is available from Kalwall Solar Components Division, P.O. Box 237, Manchester, NH 03105, for $7.95. The deluxe model costs $10.95 and has a button that stops water flow while you are lathering up with soap.

Kitchen-faucet aerators cost $1.59 and cut water flow to 2 gallons per minute, paying for themselves in just two hours, according to the company. To save hot water as well as to conserve water in general, install inexpensive flow restrictors on all faucets.

8. A relatively new idea is to install hot-water heaters right where you need the hot water permitting you to turn off your central hot-water heater and storage tank. Kalwall Company's mail order brochure describes an instant "in line" hot-water-heating unit that uses electricity to heat the water as it flows through the pipe. The unit costs $149.95 and requires an electrician to install.

Chronomite Labs, 21011 South Figueroa Street, Carson, CA 90745, makes an Instant Flow model that uses 220 volts or 110 volts. It costs about $165. Your gas utility may be able to recommend a gas-powered in-line heater.

9. Showers can also be retrofitted with hot-water-heating shower heads. Orlando Enterprises, 1874 S.W. 16 Terrace, Miami, FL 33145, sells the Corona Automatic Water Heating Shower Head that restricts the flow of water as well as heating it up. It costs $79.95 and can be used in campers as well as at home.

OIL OR GAS: MAKING THE DECISION

Making a decision about which fuel to use should be one of the last steps in a fuel-conservation program. Reducing overall fuel consumption by installing storm windows, insulating draperies, attic insulation, and the long list of other conservation measures must be the primary concern. You can save money regardless of the fuel you decide to use. And the more energy-conservation steps you take, the less impact the difference in the cost of fuels will have.

The heating system, of course, is the heart of the matter. If you have an old cast-iron monster that was converted from burning coal in the 1930s or if your newer-vintage machine cannot be brought up to an 80 percent efficiency with a flue temperature of under 500°F,

50 you have good reason to consider major repairs or installation of a new heating system. (If the temperature is below 500°F but the efficiency rating is lower than 80 percent, the problem will almost certainly be solved by replacing the burner with a high-efficiency flame-retention burner.) Price the installed costs of both oil-burner repairs and gas conversion; price both oil-burner replacement and installing a new gas system or a combination oil-gas system. Be sure to get all the facts, and remember that you may have to pay for installing a new gas line, removal of the old oil tanks, and other fees.

Some Examples and Alternatives

If it currently costs $1500 to heat your home with oil, it would cost you only $600 to heat it with gas, using national average costs for these fuels. (Bear in mind that deregulation will drive up the cost of gas.)

You could

1. Spend an estimated $800 for a gas-conversion burner and bring the heating bill down to $600.
2. Spend the same $800 on a high-efficiency oil burner and storm windows and bring the heating bill down to $825.

If you need a new heating system, here are your choices:

1. Install a gas system for $1200 to $1900.
2. Install a high-efficiency gas system (Hydropulse, Blueray) for $2800 to $3500.

3. Install a new oil system for $1300 to $1500.
4. Install a high-efficiency system (Blueray) for $1600 to $1750.
5. Install an ABC Sunray combination gas-oil conversion burner for $900 to $1000.

Factors in Selecting Your Fuel

1. **Convenience offered by the fuel. Considerations: Coal is dirty; wood is work; gas is nearly maintenance free; oil isn't.**
2. **Availability of the fuel. Not all fuels are easily available—or if they are now, they might not be later. Amazingly enough, New Yorkers who installed coal stoves couldn't find coal dealers last winter though there's a lot of coal to sell. The shortage may only be temporary, but this kind of problem must be considered.**
3. **Storage space required. Gas and electric are space savers; coal and wood are gluttons.**
4. **Cost of the fuel. To determine the true cost of the fuel, the heating value of the fuel and the efficiency of the heating plant must be related to the sale price of the fuel. (See efficiencies chart on opposite page.)**
5. **Cost of the heating plant.**
6. **Cost of maintenance. Each system has its own maintenance requirements, and these will greatly affect efficiency.**

Heating Efficiencies of Different Fuels	
Fuel	*Maximum Overall System Efficiency*
Bituminous coal (stoker-fired)	65%
Oil	80%
Oil (converted from other fuel) (or vaporizing units)	70%
Gas (all types, all burners)	80%
Electric (room units)	100%
Electric (central system)	90%

Source: The Small Homes Council-Building Research Council, University of Illinois.

FUTURE PRICES

Future costs of gas and oil are the big unknown. The Natural Gas Policy Act deregulated gas prices for newly discovered gas and is intended to bring the price of this new gas up to the price of oil by 1985. But the Act doesn't affect all existing supplies.

The American Gas Association, a trade group for the industry, says that for the next decade gas will be 20 to 50 percent less expensive than oil. This assumption is generally supported by the federal Department of Energy statistics. However, the Consumer Energy Council of America, a public-interest group, contends that the prices of gas and oil will be the same within five to twelve years. Consequently, the council believes that strict conservation measures are the best bet for homeowners, no matter what kind of system they have.

FUEL AVAILABILITY

Coal: **Enough to last hundreds of years. However, transportation to and distribution in any specific area may not be adequate; check with local dealers.**
Wood: **Generally available. Too expensive in urban areas; if you've got some wooded land, harvest your own.**
Oil: **About half the oil used in the United States is imported; domestic supplies may last 100 years at the current rate of use.**
Gas: **Becoming scarce in some places; not available for new construction in many areas in the East.**
Electricity: **Generated from other fuels; universally available.**

HOW TO COMPARE FUELS

Estimating the seasonal cost of fuel for residences is a very complicated business, based on such factors as heat loss of the house, the number of occupants, orientation to the sun, amount of cooking done in the house, and number of appliances and lights used. These sources of energy within a house can affect seasonal cost of operation by as much as 30 percent. In the chart above, which takes into account heating-system efficiencies, you can compare cost of the fuel you use with the cost of other fuels you may be considering.

Table of Equivalent Fuel Costs

Electricity Unit in Room ¢/kwh	Electricity Central System ¢/kwh	LP Gas Propane[1] ¢/gal.	Nat. Gas ¢/Therm or ¢/100 cu. ft.	No. 2 Oil ¢/gal.
0.5	0.55	9.9	10.2	14.3
1.0	1.11	18.9	20.5	28.7
1.5	1.67	28.4	30.7	43.0
2.0	2.22	37.7	41.0	57.4
2.5	2.78	47.3	51.2	71.7
3.0	3.33	56.6	61.5	86.1
3.5	3.89	66.0	71.7	100.4
4.0	4.44	75.4	82.0	114.8
4.5	5.00	84.8	92.2	129.1
5.0	5.56	94.3	102.5	143.5
5.5	6.11	103.7	112.7	157.8
6.0	6.67	113.1	123.0	172.2
6.5	7.22	122.5	133.2	186.5
7.0	7.78	132.0	143.5	200.9
7.5	8.33	141.4	153.7	215.2
8.0	8.89	150.8	164.0	229.6
8.5	9.44	160.2	174.2	243.9
9.0	10.00	169.7	184.5	258.3
9.5	10.56	179.0	194.7	272.6
10.0	11.11	189.5	205.0	287.0

[1] If LP gas sold in your area is butane, use the price of natural gas per therm as the price of butane per gallon.

Source: The Small Homes Council-Building Research Council, University of Illinois

(Note: If the fuel price varies with the quantity used, determine your average cost per unit when using the chart.)

READING LIST

Save Energy, Save Dollars, $1.50
  Distribution Center
  7 Research Park
  Cornell University
  Ithaca, NY 14850

Hickok, Floyd. *Your Energy Efficient Home.*
  (Englewood Cliffs, NJ: Prentice-Hall, 1979) $11.95
Nash, George. *Old Houses: A Rebuilders Manual.*
  (Englewood Cliffs, NJ: Prentice-Hall, 1980) $10.95 softcover

Rothchild, J. and Tenney, F.
    The Home Energy Guide.
    (New York: Ballantine Books, 1978) $1.95
Energy Savers Catalog, 50¢
    Box 99
    New Rochelle, NY 10804
*Rating Your Oil Heating System, Upgrading Oil
    Heating Systems*, free
    Brookhaven National Laboratory
    Building 130
    Upton, NY 11973
Home Heating Systems: Systems, Fuels, Controls
    (Bulletin 2235), 50¢
    U.S. Dept. of Agriculture Document

U.S. Government Printing Office
Washington, D.C. 20402
Small Homes Council—Building Research
    Council—Ask for list of publications; all
    are excellent and inexpensive.
University of Illinois—Urbana-Champaign
One East Saint Mary's Road
Champaign, IL 61820
Consumer Reports magazine; see following is-
    sues in your library
    "Thermostats": October 1977
    "Water heaters": March 1976
    "Fuel-saving devices": January 1977
    "Insulation": February 1978

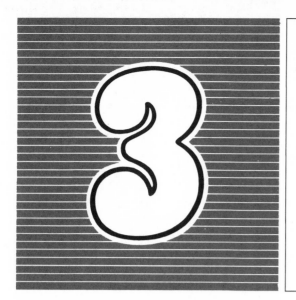

Sun Power: Keeping Warm the Solar Way

Sandra Oddo and Delores Wolfe

OVERVIEW

These are the things that are wrong with solar warmth: You can get a sunburn, a kid can throw a rock and mess up the window or the glass collector cover that lets the sun in. It costs more money than a furnace, and it doesn't come with switches to turn it on or off.

These are the things that are right with it: It will be around for the next six billion years, give or take a few, and mechanical breakdowns aren't expected much before then. It is delivered at about the temperature people like—even in winter. It costs less money than a furnace plus fuel. It doesn't come with fuel-truck routes, supply lines, or monthly bills that are connected to switches. And kid-proof collector covers are available.

You can get it from builders (some of them), architects (some of them), manufacturers (some of them), utilities (some of them), heating ventilating/air conditioning people (some of them), plumbers and sheet-metal people (some of them), and backyard inventors (a lot of them). You can build it yourself. It may look like a series of big black metal boxes with glass fronts, it may look like a greenhouse or it may look like a plain old house with extra windows on the south side (where the sun is) and fewer windows on the north side (where the sun isn't).

A solar energy system can cost as little as $500 or as much as the entire cost of your house. After you get it, your yearly bills for

To find south: (1) Use a compass. This isn't as practical as it might seem, because the sun isn't enormously respectful of the earth's magnetic north pole. (2) Or use a stick and a newspaper. Drive the stick into the ground as near to upright as possible, in the sunlight on what you think is the south side of the house. Check the local newspaper for the times of sunrise and sunset that day. At the moment exactly halfway between them—solar noon—mark the position of the stick's shadow. It will lie north/south. (3) Or use a protractor, a pencil, and the newspaper. Lay the protractor on a sunny windowsill, straight side parallel to the glass. At solar noon, stand the pencil upright in the center of the straight side. The pencil's shadow will fall across the number of degrees by which the window deviates from south. If the deviation is less than 30° passive or active solar collectors mounted on the house will work.

other kinds of heat can range from $0 to exactly what you were paying before—so it makes sense to know what you're doing before you go charging out to get some solar warmth for yourself.

Herewith the accelerated short course in solar energy:

101, PHYSICS, OR WHY IT WORKS
The sun radiates energy in all directions.

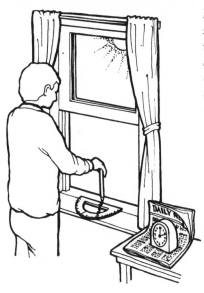

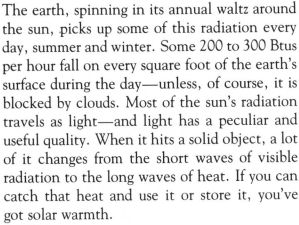

Finding south. If a pencil's shadow at solar noon—the midpoint between sunrise and sunset—is within 30° of perpendicular, a solar collector mounted on that wall will work. (Drawing by Richard Steinbock)

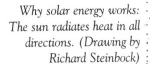

Why solar energy works: The sun radiates heat in all directions. (Drawing by Richard Steinbock)

The earth, spinning in its annual waltz around the sun, picks up some of this radiation every day, summer and winter. Some 200 to 300 Btus per hour fall on every square foot of the earth's surface during the day—unless, of course, it is blocked by clouds. Most of the sun's radiation travels as light—and light has a peculiar and useful quality. When it hits a solid object, a lot of it changes from the short waves of visible radiation to the long waves of heat. If you can catch that heat and use it or store it, you've got solar warmth.

Some radiation gets caught naturally. Trees are excellent collectors, turning sunlight into wood. (By extension, coal, oil, and gas are merely stored and concentrated forms of solar energy—and the rest of this book is unnecessary, or redundant, because every source of heat is ultimately one form or another of solar energy.) Large bodies of water, lakes or oceans, soak up quite a bit, too, holding it long enough to even out the earth's day/night temperature swings. That's why climate tends to have fewer extremes near water. Soil can also hold on to some solar warmth. The coldest days of winter are in January, not around December 21, when there is least sunlight, partly because heat stored during the summer is still slowly draining away in December.

Btu: British thermal unit, a measurement of heat. It takes 180 Btus to heat a pound of water from the freezing water point (32°F) to the boiling point (212°F).

The average household, according to figures assembled by Andrew MacKillop, one of the authors of the Club of Rome's *Blueprint for Survival,* **may use some 200,000 Btus of energy, in various forms, every day to supply its daily demands. A one-story house with a south-facing wall and a roof oriented east/ west might expose 1,000 square feet of surface to the sun every day. If 25 percent of the sunlight that hit that surface could be collected, the house might gain an annual average of 276,750 to 461,250 Btus a day.**

And a lot of heat accumulates accidentally, short term. Beach sand and rocks get hot in the sun. Cars, sitting in the sun with their windows rolled up, get very hot. Blacktopped roads warm up. Tin roofs can get blistering hot while the sun shines.

Solar warmth is slippery, however. Three hundred Btus per hour, per square foot, when it's sunny, are nothing compared to the 12,000 or so Btus packed into a pint of fuel oil. To draw on the earth's solar income, rather than on the capital laid down over millions of years in the world's basements, requires a certain amount of subtlety and sophistication.

102, THE MECHANICS OF SOLAR COLLECTION (PREREQUISITE: 101)

In order to hunt, catch, and use solar heat deliberately, you need an understanding of its simple, law-abiding nature and a little knowl-

Sun Power

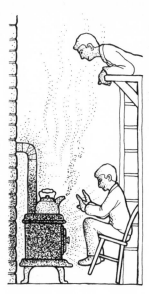

The stove and the teakettle radiate heat. *Convection warms the face in the loft. If the young man were to touch the stove, he'd quickly find out about* conduction. *(Drawing by Richard Steinbock)*

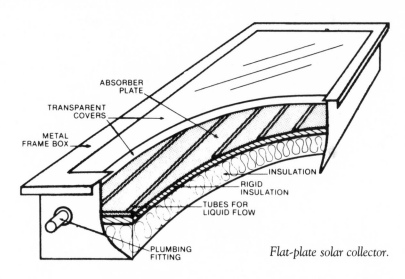

Flat-plate solar collector.

56 edge about materials. These are the laws heat recognizes:

Radiation: Heat moves in waves away from its source.

Conduction: Heat travels through solids from molecule to molecule, each warming the next.

Convection: Heat travels in air by warming the molecules of air, causing them to spread out and—because the air is therefore less dense and lighter—to rise away from the source of warmth; cooler, denser air flows in, establishing a current, and is warmed in turn.

The nature of certain materials makes it possible to exploit those laws. For instance, glass (or transparent plastic or fiberglass) lets the short waves of visible light radiation come through easily but is nearly opaque to the longer waves of heat when they try to get out again. Lightweight materials often have fewer molecules, so they may not conduct heat readily. They insulate. Some heavy materials, like metal, conduct heat quickly; others, like water or rock, conduct heat slowly. So metal is useful for catching a lot of heat quickly, and water or rocks are useful for storing it. Insulating materials can help make heat stay put.

103, ENGINEERING

Put the useful materials together, and you have a basic solar-collecting box, an active solar-energy system. Sunlight sails through the transparent cover and runs headlong into a dark (because dark colors absorb best) metal absorber plate where it changes to heat. The metal conducts the heat quickly to a fluid flowing through tubes imbedded in it (a liquid collector) or to air flowing around it (an air collector). The liquid or air carries the heat off to storage, usually a large mass of rocks or a large tank of water that is warmed by the heat collected in the box. Insulation around the whole thing keeps heat from wandering away en route.

A little less obviously, houses are also passive solar-collecting boxes. Windows let sunlight in. The materials of the house absorb it as heat and—if they have enough weight or thermal mass—store it for appreciable periods of time. The air of the house distributes the heat. Good conservation practices like insulating, caulking, and weatherstripping hold it in. This approach to collecting solar warmth is called, for want of a better term, "passive."

The solar community has made something of a point of dividing solar use into active and passive forms. Active solar collection uses panels, pumps, and plumbing. Passive solar collection uses the natural laws of heat flow. Because of the hardware involved, active solar collection tends to be more expensive, but it can achieve higher temperatures—say, up to 200°F. Also because of the hardware involved, active systems have encountered substantial early problems. Installers need to be carefully trained. Fluids can sometimes freeze, pumps and blowers malfunction.

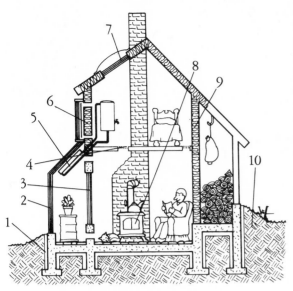

Passive solar houses apply many of the lessons from Physics 101 and Mechanics 102. (1) Insulation is added to the outside of the foundation, adding the weight of the foundation to the thermal mass of the house. (2) The south-facing greenhouse lets light in, catching heat in barrels full of water. (3) A double-glazed wall lights the interior, and vents at top and bottom allow heat to circulate through the house. (4) Floor registers allow the heat to rise to the upstairs rooms. (5) A thermosiphoning water heater collects solar heat from the top of the greenhouse. (6) A double-glazed Trombe wall with vents allows for convection. (7) A triple-glazed skylight lets the sun shine on the chimney for even more heat storage. (8) A wood-burning back-up system feeds its exhaust heat to the chimney, creating still more thermal mass. (9) An insulated north wall with an unheated buffer space protects the house from north winds. (10) A low earth berm borrows more of the earth's insulation value. (Drawing by Richard Steinbock)

A passive solar system, because it is more a matter of design than hardware, might add little to the cost of a house and eliminate most mechanical difficulties. But it cannot often achieve temperatures much higher than those needed to heat your house—say, 80°F to 120°F. Distribution of heat that depends on the vagaries of natural convection may be erratic, and a badly designed passive house may not function at all or may function too well, overloading storage capacity with too much heat.

Current building trends seem to favor hybrid houses, with passive systems for household heat, active systems for hot water, and perhaps a fan or two to help things along.

201, History

Making use of solar energy is not a new idea. Socrates understood and recommended it. The Greeks planned and built passive solar cities to gather winter warmth. Roman baths were solar heated. Incas, Aztecs, and American Pueblo Indians had its principles well in hand. Perhaps the first active solar collector was built in 1767, when Horace de Sassure, a French-Swiss naturalist, made an insulated black-painted box with glass covers and raised the temperature of the air inside to 228°F. (For historical perspective, the kitchen stove was invented by Sir Benjamin Thompson, Count Rumford, an expatriate American, in 1796.)

At the Universal Exposition in Paris in 1878, where some of the first light bulbs were

Solar Cuisine

In addition to drying clothes, heating domiciles and other enclosures, and growing and dehydrating food, solar heat can cook up a batch of brownies, toast hot dogs, or roast a bird. The solar cooker works on the same principle as setting fire to paper with a magnifying glass: if you concentrate solar radiation, the spot you concentrate on gets hotter.

To make a solar cooker requires no great skill. Most of the plans use cardboard boxes cut to specifications and covered with aluminum foil. Or, to get fancier—and also have a more permanent arrangement—cookers can be constructed with sheet metal, or a commercial model may be purchased through an energy supply store.

VITA (Volunteers in Technical Assistance) has developed and tested a model used extensively in tropical countries. This cooker is larger than those made as school projects because it is an alternative to the family stove. For information write to: VITA Publications, 3706 Rhode Island Ave., Mt. Ranier, MD 20822.

Among the VITA publications are Beth Halacy's *Solar Cookery Book* (Peace Press). It takes the mystery out of solar cooking with many tasty recipes. Then, as long as the sun's rays can be kept focused on the food, it cooks.

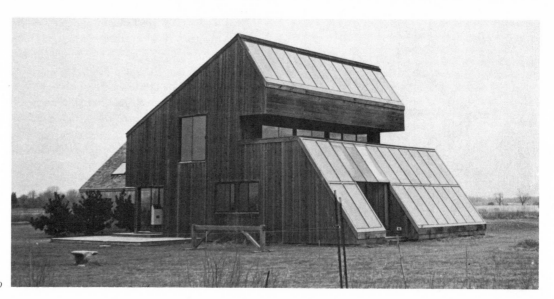

Photo by Sandra Oddo

In 1973, when the Arabs decided to raise our petroleum consciousness, twenty-five solar-heated buildings were constructed in the United States, as near as anyone could figure. "Anyone" was William A. Shurcliff, who for a number of years documented them in *Solar Heated Buildings: A Brief Survey.* By 1977, he decided things had gotten out of hand when he heard about a new solar house nearly every day, and he published his "13th and final edition" with detailed information on 319 houses. In 1980 the Department of Energy estimated there were 80,000 buildings in the United States that used solar energy in some form. Meanwhile, Dr. Shurcliff has gone on to document and inspire a number of other solar phenomena.

Recommended reading: His *Solar Heated Buildings of North America* (1978), *Thermal Shutters and Shades* (1980), and *Superinsulated Houses and Double Envelope Houses* (1981), all published by Brick House, Andover, Massachusetts.

shown, a solar concentrator produced steam to run a printing press. By 1900 one solar water-heater company had 1600 installations in Southern California alone. Between 1935 and 1941 there were an estimated 25,000 to 60,000 water-heating installations in the Miami area.

Recommended Reading. *A Golden Thread. 2500 Years of Solar Architecture and Technology* by Ken Butti and John Perlin, Chesire Books/Van Nostrand Reinhold, 1980.

Immediately after World War II, Libby Owens Ford, makers of the brand-new Thermopane, sponsored a demonstration whereby-leading architects designed solar houses that were built in every state, and for several years *House Beautiful* and other magazines ran frequent articles on solar heating and climate consciousness.

But in 1973, the year of the first Arab oil embargo, fewer than two dozen solar houses were built in the United States. What happened?

202, Economics I

The quick answer to why so few solar-heated buildings is "cheap gas and oil." It's also a true answer. When fuel was cheap, it was easier and less expensive to skimp on house design and materials and to override the ups and downs of climate with furnaces and air conditioners. But there are some other explanations (see below).

203, Politics I

Shortly after he was elected president, Dwight D. Eisenhower appointed a commission to study the energy future of the United States. The Paley Commission made three recommendations in its 1954 report: pay attention to developing oil and gas reserves; push solar energy; continue research in nuclear energy. President Eisenhower implemented the third recommendation—Atoms for Peace—but funds for solar research dried up, and the United States increased its imports of oil.

Between 1950 and 1975, fossil fuel and nu-

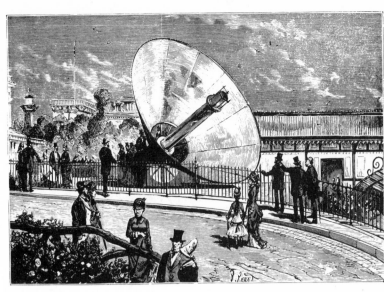

clear energy received some $60 billion in federal subsidies of various kinds. Federal subsidies for solar averaged $100,000 a year.

301, Politics II

With the Arab oil embargo of 1973, energy conservation and—by extension—solar energy were now in the national interest. Plans were made, policies were outlined, and programs were set in motion. Solar was suddenly sexy—at one point the informal group of senators and representatives that called itself the Solar Coalition numbered some fifty members. The Department of Housing and Urban Development sponsored a demonstration program that got several thousand solar-heated houses built. The Department of Energy contracted with major corporations for pilot programs and research. The solar portion of the fiscal 1980 federal energy budget authorization was still in the millions (about $600 million), compared with $1 billion for nuclear fission (research and development alone), $800 million for fossil fuel, and nearly $400 million for magnetic fusion, which is not expected to produce commercially available power until after 2050. After Sun Day (May 22, 1978) the Sun Day organization rearranged itself into the Solar Lobby (1001 Connecticut Avenue NW, Washington, DC, 20036), and solar energy acquired its first political pressure group. Federal tax credits were finally passed. Nevertheless by 1981 solar was again (still) in trouble in Washington.

Sunlight falls everywhere. It works best as energy if you use it close to where you get it. The materials to harness it for household heat are relatively simple but the knowledge to put them to work is sophisticated (details of design and construction matter) although not esoteric. And no one method of collecting solar energy is likely to do all things for all people.

None of this is likely to endear solar to policy makers, dealers in conventional energy, or industry. Established utilities can help (or hinder) the implementation of solar through their policies and actions, but solar shows strong signs of competing with the sale of conventional energy even while it conserves that energy and lessens the need utilities feel to expand their capacity. Big business has found that solar does not seem to conform to established centralized patterns of manufacture and marketing, and some of the major corporations that had begun to acquire solar divisions have recently divested themselves. In the classic development-of-an-industry pattern—invention, research, pilot programs, demonstrations, and final marketing to an aroused set of consumers—solar still shows gaps. It isn't a furnace or a dishwasher; to use it you still have to know something about how it works. This seems to put solar, to the thinking of government administrators, in the do-it-yourself category where constituencies are disorganized and not likely to react badly when funds are cut—as they were in the spring of 1981 when the Solar and Energy Conservation Bank, which was

Form **5695**	**Energy Credits**	**1980**
Department of the Treasury Internal Revenue Service	▶ Attach to Form 1040. ▶ See Instructions on back.	34

Name(s) as shown on Form 1040 | **Your social security number**

Enter in the space below the address of your principal residence on which the credit is claimed if it is different from the address shown on Form 1040.

Part I   Fill in your energy conservation costs (but do not include repair or maintenance costs).

If you have an energy credit carryover from a previous tax year and no energy savings costs this year, skip to Part III, line 16.

A. Answer the following question: Was your principal residence substantially completed before April 20, 1977? . . . ☐ Yes   ☐ No

B. If you checked the "NO" box, you CANNOT claim an energy credit for conservation cost. Do NOT fill in lines 1 through 7 of this form.

1 **Energy Conservation Items:**		
a Insulation	1a	
b Storm (or thermal) windows or doors	1b	
c Caulking or weatherstripping	1c	
d A furnace replacement burner that reduces the amount of fuel used . . .	1d	
e A device for modifying flue openings to make a heating system more efficient	1e	
f An electrical or mechanical furnace ignition system that replaces a gas pilot light	1f	
g A thermostat with an automatic setback	1g	
h A meter that shows the cost of energy used	1h	
2 Total (add lines 1a through 1h)	2	
3 Maximum amount	3	$2,000 00
4 Enter the total energy conservation costs for this residence from your 1978 and 1979 Form 5695, line 2 .	4	
5 Subtract line 4 from line 3 (If line 4 is more than line 3, do not complete any more of this part. You cannot claim any more energy conservation credit for this residence.)	5	
6 Enter the amount on line 2 or line 5, whichever is less	6	
7 Enter 15% of line 6 here and include in amount on line 15 below	7	

Part II   Fill in your renewable energy source costs (but do not include repair or maintenance costs).

If you have an energy credit carryover from a previous tax year and no energy savings costs this year, skip to Part III, line 16.

8 **Renewable Energy Source Items:**		
a Solar	8a	
b Geothermal	8b	
c Wind	8c	
9 Total (add lines 8a through 8c)	9	
10 Maximum amount	10	$10,000 00
11 Enter the total renewable energy source costs for this residence from your 1978 Form 5695, line 5 and 1979 Form 5695, line 9	11	
12 Subtract line 11 from line 10 (If line 11 is more than line 10, do not complete any more of this part. You cannot claim any more renewable energy source cost credit for this residence.)	12	
13 Enter amount on line 9 or line 12, whichever is less	13	
14 Enter 40% of line 13 here and include in amount on line 15 below	14	

Part III   Fill in this part to figure the limitation

15 Add line 7 and line 14. *If less than $10, enter zero.*	15	
16 *Enter your energy credit carryover from a previous tax year*	16	
17 Add lines 15 and 16	17	
18 Enter the amount of tax shown on Form 1040, line 37	18	
19 Add lines 38 through 44 from Form 1040 and enter the total	19	
20 Subtract line 19 from line 18. If zero or less, enter zero	20	
21 Residential energy credit. Enter the amount on line 17 or line 20, whichever is less. Also, enter this amount on Form 1040, line 45	21	

Form **5695** (1980)

Total Warmth

Renewable energy source items include solar, wind, and geothermal energy items which heat or cool your principal residence or provide hot water or electricity for it.

Examples of solar energy items include:

- collectors,
- rockbeds,
- heat exchangers, and
- solar panels installed on roofs (including those installed as a roof or part of a roof).

An example of an item that uses wind energy is a windmill that produces energy in any form (usually electricity) for your residence.

To take the credit for a renewable energy source item, you must:

- be the first one to use the item, and
- expect it to last at least 5 years.

The credit for renewable energy source items cannot be more than $4,000.

Form 5695, the IRS Energy Credit form, with allowable items.

SOLAR AND THE INTERNAL REVENUE SERVICE

Tax credit, to the tune of up to 40 percent of the first $10,000 spent on solar equipment, can be claimed on your annual income tax if the equipment or system is installed before December 31, 1985. The equipment must meet the specifications spelled out in IRS 903, *Energy Credits for Individuals,* available from your local IRS office.

Active solar systems purchased through a dealer are easily defined by the package. This is not true of passive solar devices or site-fabricated systems because parts of these systems also serve as part of the building structure and would have to be erected in any case. If there is any doubt about calculating this incentive, see an accountant experienced in figuring energy credits.

Don't overlook state and local tax rebates or credits for solar-energy-system purchases that further reduce the initial investment. These credits change rapidly. For latest information, consult the National Solar Heating and Cooling Information Center (800-523-2929) or your local tax office.

slated to begin the distribution of $122 million in loan subsidies, died a quiet death. The solar budget for 1982 was scheduled to be cut 67 percent, whereas the nuclear budget was increased 30 percent.

So. Do-it-yourself it is. Individual independence and a pioneering spirit are a little estranged from modern Americans, but still dear to them. If you want solar, you can have it—if you go after it. The popular myths about solar promulgated widely by a couple of large fossil fuel corporations—"Well, maybe by the year 2000" and "It's too expensive"—are just that, myths. But how *do* you figure out the economics? Herewith a couple of concepts followed by a couple of rules of thumb.

Purveyors of solar systems have glommed onto a somewhat peculiar concept called "payback." Under payback, a solar system or a solar device is supposed to "pay back" its cost in the savings for the energy it replaces. If a collector costs $10, for a ridiculous example, it ought to save $10 in fossil-fuel bills over a period of time, and that time is called its "payback period." At $1 saved per year, the collector would have a payback period of ten years. The concept is strange on three counts. First, fossil-fuel savings depend on the cost of fossil fuel and the rate at which it rises—and every government projection from 1973 to date has been wrong. Second, payback period ignores things like interest on loans, inflation, and other peculiarities of money. And third—solar use is a method of ensuring creature comfort and convenience, like a refrigerator. Nobody ever tried to justify the purchase of a refrigerator by figuring up the savings in food that would otherwise have spoiled.

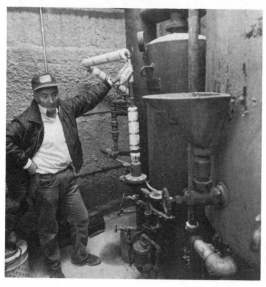

Harry Buck and his magic manure machine. (Photo by R. R. Haines)

HARRY BUCK, THE TWO-FARM FUEL COMPANY

Harry Buck breeds race horses, which may explain why he doesn't like to stand around waiting. So, when he found himself waiting on a gas line one day, he got to thinking about his $3,000 fuel bill for 1975. Between his horses and his neighbor's dairy cows, he had plenty of a particularly pungent renewable resource—manure. Manure can be broken down into methane (gas) and nitrogenous waste (fertilizer), so Harry Buck built a methane digester to produce some 27,000 cubic feet of methane a day. He bubbles it through water to scrub it ("odorless," he swears), then compresses it into tanks that supply his gas-fired household appliances. If there is any left over, he uses it to run an electric generator.

That left the heating system—and the truck and the tractor—so Harry Buck went to a couple of government-surplus auctions and came home with a commercial-size still. Using the silo juice from his neighbor's silos or cracked corn if the silos aren't juicy enough, he can produce up to 200 gallons of 160-proof (fuel-grade) alcohol a day. Heat and vehicle fuel are on tap, and he is now one of the first 100 percent energy self-sufficient farmers in the country. Heat and carbon dioxide, waste products of the still, are piped into a brand-new greenhouse.

He has drawn up a modular plan whereby small cooperatives of farmers could make and even sell energy as a farm product. The United States Department of Energy and the New York State Energy Research and Development Agency have seen it—but Harry Buck still isn't waiting around. He'll share his experience with anybody who'll listen: Whinney Haw Stables, Route 1, Pine Bush, NY 12566.

"Return on investment" is a concept that makes a little more sense. If you invest $10 in a solar system, will it save you more money than the amount you would have earned if you stuck the $10 in a savings bank? Figuring can be tricky (remember to count in such things as tax credits), and the refrigerator analogy still applies.

Therefore, rules of thumb: (1) if you want it, you can figure out a way to do it. (2) A passive system for a new house is likely to add between $1,000 and $6,000 to the cost of the house; a system on an existing house is likely to be more expensive. (3) Active hot-water systems are running around $2,500 each, depending on all sorts of factors; active systems in general are not likely to come down much in price because they use a lot of expensive materials, and they are costly to distribute. (4) Solar systems are more like buildings than they are like furnaces—you can get mortgages and home improvement loans for them.

401, ESTHETICS

Most ways of getting warm have certain esthetics attached. The sensual pleasure of a warm bath, for instance, the satisfaction of a fur coat. But solar? With what other form of warmth can you also enjoy the knowledge that you are benefitting the entire world by using a renewable, pollution-free, environmentally proven source of heat? What other warmth awakens you so to the state of the day—sunny, cloudy, and all the shades between? How else (except, perhaps, by gardening) could you become so sensitized, so involved with the turn of the seasons and the swing of the year? The solstices are friends, and equinoxes major turning points. The sun is noted in its yearly path up and down the southern sky, rising in December behind the lilac bush, perhaps; setting in June over the pear tree. The warmth of stone, the patterns of leaves on a wall, carry messages.

There are always people who can't wait for the future to arrive—they have to go out and meet it head-on. Arcosanti is the creation of Paolo Soleri and the Cosanti Foundations to demonstrate that urban entities using solar energy can be built to save energy and serve their citizens. Progress at Arcosanti is slow, for all funds come from the private sector. But this has allowed experimentation and testing of principles that would not have been possible under government funding.

New Alchemy Institute, working on both the East and West coasts, has been experi-

WEATHER

Ever since man started prowling Mother Earth, weather has been an important topic of conversation. It influences dress, house design, activities, work and leisure, vocabulary and speech idioms, and our general well being—even our behavior. And if solar energy is to be used to keep warm (or cool in the proper season), such bits of data as the number of cloudy and sunny days in a year, wind speed, temperature, and the amount of direct solar radiation falling on our patch of earth becomes interesting. Most of this is not readily available through newspapers, TV or radio weather reports, or almanacs. However, for a small fee that covers costs, this information is available through the National Climatic Center. Request data for the nearest weather station, large city, or major airport. The Superintendent of Documents prints a pamphlet on the data from each state; prices vary according to the size of the publication and printing date.

National Climatic Center
Federal Building
Asheville, NC 28801

Superintendent of Documents
Government Printing Office
Washington, DC 20402

All the houses in The Village, a development in Davis, California, are oriented toward the sun (the south). By owners' choice, about 80 percent are solar-heated. The streets are tree-shaded and narrower than usual because black asphalt soaks up heat, which is undesirable in the desert climate of the Sacramento Valley. Surface runoff water is channeled into streams that water fruit trees, cared for by resident gardeners paid out of Village Association dues. Community gardens edge the playing fields that surround the community center (lower left). Most village residents can get to the center of the fields without crossing a single street.

TOGETHERNESS UNDER THE SUN

The communities of the future are rapidly becoming part of the current landscape. People are banding together in small neighborhood- and town-sized groups, determined to use their wits and ingenuity to solve energy problems and regain control of at least this aspect of their lives.

The County Energy Plan Guidebook, prepared by Alan Okagaki with Jim Benson, serves as a model for community energy assessment and a springboard for creative energy policy (Institute for Ecological Policies, 9208 Christopher Street, Fairfax, VA 22031; $7.50). Oregon, as long ago as 1975, carried out a statewide analysis of its energy resources, then developed and implemented plans to conserve them. Crotched Mountain in New Hampshire has one of the first New England wind farms to be erected, and with private funds at that!

Solar-heated housing developments are becoming more popular. The Village, in Davis, California, was one of the first, but there are a number of others. And urban-redevelopment projects often include residential-scale solar hot-water heaters and passive solar space-heating options in the remodeling package. Urban solar neighborhoods are gradually becoming a reality.

Perhaps surprisingly (or perhaps not,

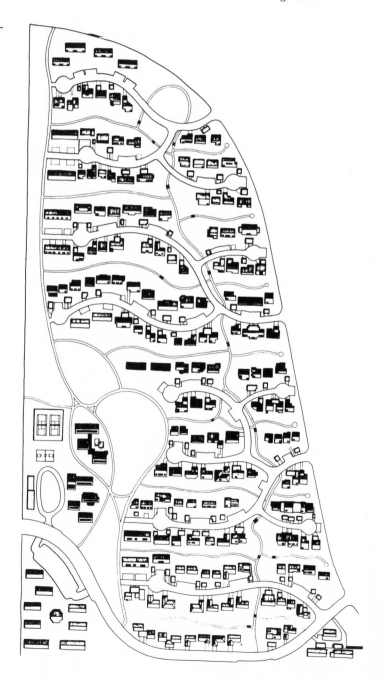

because they feel the pinch first) the poor often take the lead. Under a sweat-equity program in which work is substituted for a cash down payment, a number of buildings on New York's dilapidated Lower East Side have gone solar. One 262-unit housing project in the South Bronx gets most of its hot water from the sun. Under a solar and energy conservation program sponsored in part by the Massachusetts Municipal Association, Cambridge projected energy savings of $7 billion by the year 2000; Chesterfield cut heating oil use for its town garage from 7,500 gallons to 30 gallons per year; and the Agawam school system halved its heating bill. A third of Maine's 498 organized municipalities are engaged in energy prospecting—evaluating their sources of solar, wood, and wind. Burlington, Vermont, generates 7 megawatts of electricity yearly by burning the leftovers of its lumber industry. In the San Luis Valley in Colorado, where 40 percent of the people have incomes below the poverty level, 20 percent of the houses use some form of solar heat. Recommended reading: *Shining Examples: Model Projects Using Renewable Resources* (Center for Renewable Resources, 1001 Connecticut Ave. NW, Washington, DC 20036; $8).

Community solar interests are increasingly concerned with high food costs resulting from energy costs and are constructing community-sized greenhouses where crops are raised cooperatively. Some serve the double purpose of contributing heat to a school or other municipal building, which in turn heightens the awareness of school children in food production and provides part of a learning package on solar energy.

One thing tends to lead to another, and before the community is aware of it, the indirect benefits it reaps may surpass those originally sought.

---

menting for more than ten years on the adaptation of renewable energy resources to everyday living. Recently, at a small conference, the Institute took the next step: the future development of solar communities that would rely on those energy resources indigenous to the site.

Recommended Reading: The Institute's erratically "annual" report, the *New Alchemy Journal* (P.O. Box 47, Woods Hole, MA 02543).

Solar energy also figures heavily in the planning of the first space colonies, the L-5s proposed by Dr. Gerald O'Neill of Princeton University. These colonies will be solar-oriented for maximum access to the sun's light and heat, especially important for production of necessary foodstuffs and power generation. Dr. O'Neill thinks that technology exists to build these colonies now, although they are still in the conceptual stages.

Popularization of solar energy for home

66 heating and power generation will cause a change in our attitudes and in community planning. Renewable energy resources are small scale, lending themselves well to decentralized, local control rather than to corporate rule. Small towns will run their own power companies. Entrepreneurships and small local businesses, using locally produced energy, will manufacture and sell goods within the community. This does not rule out large corporate structures, but it will force them to reconsider the economics of energy when producing a product.

SOLAR SYSTEMS

STORING SOLAR HEAT: THEORY AND PRACTICE

The sun has an unfortunate habit—it goes down at night. It was, in fact, this habit that prompted human beings to investigate stored warmth in the first place. Cavemen started it when they figured out how to burn wood to warm themselves and keep sabertoothed tigers away, a process that now has us fracturing atoms to squeeze out a little extra heat. When you get right down to it, it's probably easier to dream up ways to keep solar warmth around overnight.

Anything heavy will hold onto solar warmth. If the heavy material conducts heat slowly, like clay or rock or water, it will hold onto solar heat longer. The more of the mate-

rial there is, the more heat it will hold. This is, therefore, the concept of *thermal mass*. Thermal mass is good. Every solar house should have some.

Storage Materials	Heat They Hold*	Weight in lbs per ft³
Brick	24.6	123.0
Cement (Portland)	19.2	120.0
Clay	13.86	63.0
Gypsum	20.2	78.0
Sand	18.06	94.6
Stone (quarried)	19.0	95.0
Water	62.4	62.3

* In Btus per cubic foot of material, for each 1°F rise in temperature (Btu/ft³/°F).

Thermal mass, however, is also heavy; very heavy and usually very bulky. This is generally okay in new buildings, where provision for big heavy things can be designed in. Existing houses have problems. A thermal mass of sand or stone is not easily accommodated under the coffee table. Owners of existing houses have three options: (1) Bolster up the house to allow thermal mass somewhere. This can be as simple as doubling up layers of gypsum board (Sheetrock) on walls or as complicated as digging a new basement. (2) Forget storage. Keep warm in the daytime; pay for fossil heat at night. (3) Try another route, like eutectic salts or annual storage.

Anything that freezes releases substantial quantities of latent heat and soaks it up again

Total Warmth

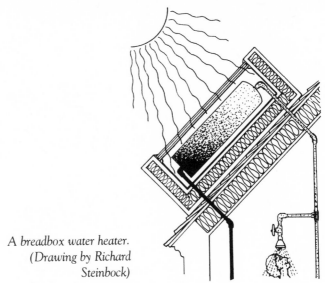

A breadbox water heater.
(Drawing by Richard Steinbock)

when it thaws. When water freezes it's so cold around (32°F) that heat release is hardly noticed—yet it takes 144 Btus added to a pound of ice to turn it back into a pound of ice water, nearly the amount of heat it takes to raise it from ice water to boiling water. *Eutectic salts* are peculiar chemicals that crystalize (freeze) at more or less ordinary temperatures—say, about 72°F depending on the eutectic salt you use. Apply heat—like solar warmth—and the salts melt again, soaking that heat up in the process. They're lighter than other storage materials and more compact. They are also chemically cantankerous. Dr. Maria Telkes first began working with them for solar-heat storage more than thirty years ago and only recently have some of the problems been unkinked enough to permit widespread marketing. So far, eutectic salts are stackable, usable in windows and floor or ceiling tiles, compatible with air or liquid systems, and very expensive.

Annual storage is another possibility. If thermal mass is too much for one house and too unwieldy for overnight or if sunlight in winter is too weak and too infrequent, think big. A complex of houses for the elderly near Toronto has a thermal-storage tank that holds several million gallons of water. All summer it soaks up heat; all winter it releases it. A United States government project called ACES (Annual Cycle Energy Storage) used heat pumps to gradually turn underground water storage to an enormous ice cube during the winter. (Your refrigerator is an example of a heat pump.) The

ice cube took all summer to melt, so it provided cooling as well. Most solar designs can, in fact, be jiggered to exclude, as well as include, solar warmth.

Breadbox Water Heaters

If you leave a container of water outside in the sun, it will get warm. Application of this principle has resulted in the development of a number of simple low-cost solar water-heating systems that range from strategically placed black plastic pipe to water bed mattresses, water pillows, and wood or metal water trays. This is fine if you live in a warm climate or if you fill up the container every morning and empty it every evening, but it is not very practical for regions where days or nights are cool.

In recent years the "breadbox" water heater, originally developed by Steve Baer of Zomeworks, has overcome some of these difficulties. The south-facing side is glazed to allow sunlight to strike the tank. To improve efficiency, the inside of the box is lined with a reflective material that bounces additional light onto the tank. Breadbox heaters may be mounted on the roof, just off the ground, or in attached solar greenhouses, excellent places in cold climates, where the danger of freezing may be great.

The amount of hot water such a system can provide depends on the amount of sunshine available (at least half the days during a year must be clear to partly cloudy), outside temperatures, and the efficiency of the particular system. Since these heaters cannot always supply 100 percent of the 80 gallons of hot water that the U.S. government says a family of four needs daily, they should be plumbed into conventional systems that take over when the solar system is not producing enough.

Breadbox heaters may cost anywhere from nothing to about $500 depending on ingenuity and the cost of labor and materials.

Plans. Breadbox water heaters with no moving parts can be constructed with available building supplies and hand tools. This list is only a beginning. Steve Bear's *Breadbox Water Heater Plans* require one or more 30-gallon hot water tanks (new or recycled) painted a flat black and enclosed in an insulated reflecting box. The south side of the box is translucent —covered with plastic or glass—with an insulated hinged lid that prevents heat loss at night. (Zomeworks, Box 712, Albuquerque, NM 87103.)

Prepackaged Systems. These systems may be installed by the handy homeowner or local plumber. The "Sun Wizard," designed by E.P.I., can produce from 10 to 2000 gallons of hot water per unit in a glass-lined carbon-steel tank. The required 10-foot or larger aperture (window) makes this a big system for the average home. (E.P.I., 1424 West 259th St., Harbor City, CA 90710.)

Another ground-mounted system with an external reflector is offered by SAV Solar Systems. Each unit produces up to 20 gallons of hot water a batch. (SAV Solar Systems, 550 W. Patrice Place, Suite A, Gardena, CA 90248.)

Solar American Corporation's "Summersun" differs from some of the other units in that it may be plumbed parallel to a conventional system to increase storage capacity. Each unit will produce between 30 and 40 gallons of hot water per batch.

Resources. "Solar Hot Water . . . and You!," Paul Shippee in *Alternative Sources of Energy*, No. 34 (107 South Central, Milaca, MN 56353; back issues, $3). The average family of four uses 27,000 Btus of fuel a year to heat water. Shippee discusses the various ways to achieve this with solar energy, including the pros and cons of various systems, sizing the system, and the efficiency to be expected.

"A Comeback for Breadboxes," Bruce Maeda and Bruce Melzer in *Solar Age*, October, 1980 (Church Hill, Harrisville, NH 03450; back issues, $2.50). A review of the development of and recent innovations in the breadbox water heater.

"Breadbox Designs," Jeff Reise and Dave Bainbridge in *Alternative Sources of Energy*, No. 34. Information on basic design principles and installation practices for breadbox water heaters useful to those designing and constructing their own systems, as well as to those purchasing packaged systems.

"Preheating Water in Greenhouses," Rick Schwolsky in *Solar Age*, June 1979. If you have, or are planning, a solar greenhouse attached to the house and live in a cold-winter climate, consider tucking the breadbox water heater near the peak of the roof inside the greenhouse. Schematics plus information on mounting and plumbing are included.

Active Solar Hot Water Systems

Active solar water-heating systems are usually roof-mounted but may be mounted elsewhere since it is not important that the collector be located below the storage tank. The system (composed of one or more flat plate collectors, fans and pumps, a storage tank, and controls) heats a fluid. In a closed-loop system, this heat is pumped to the storage tank where it passes through a heat exchanger (see Thermosiphoning Systems for Heating Water) and the heat is transferred by conduction to the water. Drain-down systems dump the hot water directly into the storage tank. Most active systems are used to preheat the water supply and are plumbed into the regular hot-water-heating system.

Active systems work better if attention is paid to such details as orientation of the collector to the south and collector tilt (equal to the latitude of the location). Shade from trees, such house parts as dormers and chimneys, or

---

In contrast to passive systems, active solar systems include fans, pumps, and other moving parts to transfer heat from the collector to the heat-storage system and from there to the place where it will be used.

---

the neighbor's house and trees can decrease the efficiency of these systems to the point of making them uneconomical.

Leaks caused by improper installation or damage to the collector from weather stresses are important concerns. When planning to purchase an active system or install one, consult Rick Schwolsky's "Solar Installer's Checklist for Domestic Hot Water Systems" in the *Solar Age Resource Book* (Everest House, 1979).

Thermosiphoning Systems for Heating Water

Heat rises. The water at the top of a tank will be warmer than that at the bottom because hot water, like hot air, is less dense. Thus if you make a loop of pipe connecting the top of the tank with the bottom, hot water will flow out of the top of the tank and reenter it at the bottom. There are no moving parts. This is a thermosiphoning system.

This system has been successfully adapted to heat water supplies. It is simple to construct, install, and maintain and costs about half as much as an active solar hot-water heater. First mass-produced back in the 1920s for the Florida and southern California markets, some of these solar hot-water systems are still functioning. Recent improvements have extended their use to cooler climates. While thermosiphoning systems are slightly more complex than breadbox solar water heaters, they require less attention to operate.

Thermosiphoning: the natural transfer of heat in a fluid (air or liquid) caused by currents of rising warm fluid and descending cool fluid.

Thermosiphoning systems are usually mounted near the ground to allow the upward flow of hot water into a storage tank but can be located elsewhere as long as the collector is below the storage. For example, Zomeworks "Big Fin" can be fitted along the bottom of the south-facing glass wall of greenhouses and sunspaces.

Hot water can be supplied directly by these systems, or they can be used to preheat the water entering a conventional hot-water system, reducing the amount of fossil fuels used for heating water. In either case, water can be heated and stored in the tank for future use.

Many of the commercially available thermosiphoning systems use nonfreezing liquids instead of water where there is danger of freezing. In these systems, the liquid is heated in the collector panel and then transported to a heat exchanger located inside the storage tank. The heat in the liquid is conducted to the water, raising the temperature of the water in the tank. This process continues until the water is almost as hot as the collector liquid or until the collector cools below the temperature of the liquid.

A manual and set of blueprints for constructing a thermosiphoning water heater, written by Arnie Valdez and Akira Kawanabe, may be purchased for $7.50 plus $1.00 postage and handling from *The Solar Water Heater Book*, P.O. Box 1014, Alamosa, CO 81101.

Resources. *Handmade Hot Water Systems*, Art Sussman and Richard Frazier, describes the construction of thermosiphoning systems and their integration into wood-fired hot-water systems.

Sources of Plans and Kits. Zomeworks sells plans for a simple-to-construct thermosiphoning water heater and markets the "Big Fins" kit. (Zomeworks, Box 712, Albuquerque, NM 87103.)

Environment/One offers a kit for a ground-mounted prepackaged system. (Environment/One, 2773 Balltown Rd., Schenectady, NY 12301.)

TROMBE WALLS

Felix Trombe, a French scientist, didn't build the first known Trombe (pronounced Trōm) wall. Professor Edward S. Morse probably did, when he glazed the slate south wall of his house in Salem, Massachusetts, in the

Heat exchanger: a device made of metal, usually copper, which readily conducts heat. Car radiators are heat exchangers. The purpose of a heat exchanger is to take heat from one fluid (air or liquid) and transfer it to another.

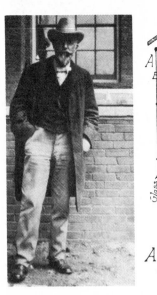
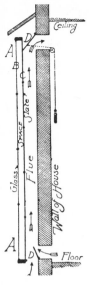

Professor Edward S. Morse built a double-glazed solar air heater on the side of his Salem, Massachusetts, house in about 1882. The system he later built for the Boston Athenaeum saved up to 50 pounds of coal a day. (From Ken Butti and John Perlin, A Golden Thread [Palo Alto: Cheshire Books, 1980], p. 199.)

1880s and punched holes through, top and bottom, to let air circulate between the glass and the warm stone. But Professor Trombe experimented with, measured, and refined the effect on a series of houses near Odeillo, France, and so is immortalized.

A Trombe wall uses all three of the laws of heat movement. The mass wall—brick, stone, concrete, or even water in a metal casing—absorbs heat and lets it migrate slowly through (conduction). When that heat arrives at the other side of the wall, usually some time after the sun has set, it radiates to the room (radiation). To speed things up, if you want heat during the day, vents at the bottom let floor-level cool air into the space between wall and glazing where the air warms and rises (convection). Vents at the top let it spill back into the room.

A few niceties of design improve efficiency. The best thickness for the wall depends on your climate and the material of the wall, but it is usually between 12 and 18 inches. There should be no holes inside the wall (cinder blocks should have their spaces filled with sand or cement) and no insulation on the room side —a fact that may confound construction people with their newly raised awareness of the virtues of insulation. The space between glass and wall should be considered carefully, and so should the seals and the dampers (see TAPs, first cousins to Trombe walls). For further guidance the New Mexico Solar Energy Association offers a *Thermal Storage Wall Design*

Manual ($4.75; P.O. Box 2004, Santa Fe, NM 87501).

Thermosiphoning Solar Air Heaters (TAPs)

Thermosiphoning air panels are inexpensive solar-heat-collection systems, usually mounted on house walls. They work on the basic principle that hot air rises. Cold air enters the bottom of the collector through vents, gains warmth as it passes up the collector between the house wall and the glass or plastic cover, and exits through a second set of vents at the top. There are no moving parts, no thermal storage, and no equipment to operate.

It is easy to add a thermosiphoning air panel to an existing house or to incorporate it into new construction. Costs can be kept minimal if standard sizes of material found in building supply stores are used and if the system is owner installed. A section of the south-facing wall of the house can be lined with metal, perhaps aluminum roofing or siding painted a flat black to absorb heat or metal boxes fitted between the wall studs. Replacement patio-door glass is frequently used as a cover. The absorber panel and light-transmitting cover are framed into a unit, with the cover about ½ to 1 inch in front of the absorber. The unit must be sealed with silicon caulk; otherwise, air infiltration or leakage will reduce the effectiveness of the system. TAPs are vertical, so during the warm season most of the sun's rays are deflected by the cover.

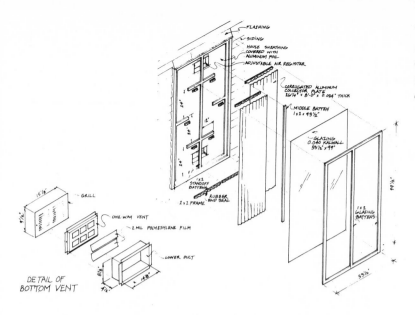

Thermosiphoning air panels (TAPs) produce heat only when the sun is shining on them; they have no storage capacity.

DETAIL OF BOTTOM VENT

72 At night, the bottom vents should be closed to prevent *reverse* thermosiphoning, which could cause heat losses equal to or exceeding daytime heat gains. Simple one-way dampers can be constructed by taping thin, vent-size films of plastic to the top of the ½-inch hardware cloth (screening) cut to fit inside the vents. Cooler daytime air will blow the vents open and set up convection currents. When the system cools down and the convection currents are reversed, the lightweight damper will flop into place and stop the air flow.

TAP plans can be obtained for $1.00 from Bergen County Community Action Program, 8 Romanelli Ave., South Hackensack, NJ 07606.

FIVE QUESTIONS TO ASK YOUR FRIENDLY NEIGHBORHOOD SOLAR SALESPERSON, AND ONE FOR YOURSELF

1. Are the salespeople qualified? The biggest problem is finding a qualified installer, says Rebecca Vories, a partner in Infinite Energy (Denver, Colorado) and the Solar Energy Research Institute's first senior consumer specialist. Check these points:

- If a license is required by state, county, or local government, does the company have one?
- If none is required, how many systems has the company installed? If it's fewer than twenty-five, be particularly alert. The Tennessee Valley Authority, for its solar program, believes that's a bare minimum.

- How many systems have the people who will work on your house installed personally? If it's fewer than ten and there are no mitigating circumstances (like being a master plumber, or having taken an accredited installation course at one of the five or six colleges that offer them), pay close attention.

2. Are the prices competitive? The typical advice to consumers most often ignored, says Ms Vories, is "shop around." Get three bids. The cost for a particular kind of system (an air-heating collector for space heat and hot water, for instance) should not vary more than 20 percent—but this is one area where the lowest bid is not likely to be the best. Several studies have noted that the least experienced installer tends to bid lowest. In solar installation, experience really counts.

Ask for *and check* references on other systems installed. When you call the references, find out whether the job was neatly done, whether the installers cleaned up after themselves, whether there were problems, whether the customer is satisfied, and—especially important—whether service, if necessary, is fast, competent, and cheerful.

3. What are the performance claims? What does the company say the system will do for you? In the north and the midwest, an active system for heating water, for instance, is not likely to deliver more than 60 percent of household needs, says Ms Vories. If a salesperson claims more than 80 percent anywhere in the country, look at those claims very carefully —and if the claim is "100 percent," turn around and walk away.

If the company makes money-saving claims —for instance, "this system will save 35 percent of your fuel bill"—find out what they base the claims on. Is it monthly costs averaged over a year? Winter costs? Savings this year averaged over ten years? Savings plotted against projections of skyrocketing fuel price rises? Judge accordingly.

Watch out for claims made by people who haven't looked at the building involved.

And find out what the warranty covers. There should be a one-year warranty on labor and on parts and materials. Major parts could be covered by a three to five to ten year warranty. And the warranty should include service, even if you have to pay an extra fee for it.

4. Is it compatible with your house and current heating system? If you have forced air, for instance, can the solar system deliver hot air via your present distribution system?

For both active and passive systems, ask for homeowner's operating manuals or instructions (an informed and active user can get a lot more out of a solar system than somebody who sits there passively, rain or shine). Compare the manuals and ask yourself: is the company customer oriented? Does the company know what it's talking about? Check these points:

- What condition is the structure in? Most houses more than five years old have settled enough to need some extra bracing for the weight of an active solar system on the roof, according to Ms Vories. Does the estimate cover that cost? And what, exactly, do the installers plan to do?

- Are there places to put ducts, pipes, and storage? Or might you come home to find some plunging through the middle of the living room?

- If your orientation is not ideal for solar, go back to question 3, and check performance claims again. How did they arrive at the performance figures and how do they intend to get that performance?

5. A question to ask yourself: do you know yourself? The biggest single factor in whether solar will work for you is your style of living. If an installer says that 120 square feet of hot water collector on your roof will provide 80 percent of the hot water for your family of four, it probably will—if you are a water-conservative family. If two of the four are teenagers, however, or if a hot tub is an essential part of your existence, it won't. Do you close doors automatically in winter? Have you thought about (and done) some energy-conservation work on the house? Do you *like* sunlight? Are you open to change?

And 6. What's in the contract? Once you've decided to buy solar, the installation contract becomes very important. It should be a written contract spelling out exactly what the installer will (and won't) do. It should list the permits he or she will get, the materials that will be

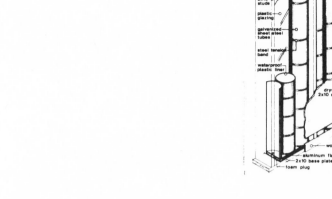

2x10 top wall plates
roof truss
3½" wood trim
plastic liner accessible thru opening
warm air out
selective black absorber
2x10 studs
plastic glazing
galvanized sheet steel tubes
steel tension band
waterproof plastic liner
drywall on 2x10 studs 24"oc
cool air into con't. bottom vent opening
wood base
aluminum flashing
2x10 base plate
foam plug

A tubewall consists of a series of passive solar thermal storage tubes set between the studs of an existing wall. Cool air enters through the bottom vent, hot air exits through the top. (Waterwall Engineering)

74

used, and the bonding and insurance that exists. It should name and describe the system. It should specify what the service contract entitles you to, on what terms. It should set a schedule and mention clean up.

As a final bit of self-protection, says Ms Vories, never pay the full amount until the system is in and has been working for two weeks or so, and you are reasonably sure that you are completely satisfied.

Passive Solar for Existing Houses

Some very general rules of thumb:

- Every square foot of passive solar collector added to a house will replace about 1 gallon

---

Samson's Dog House

Samson, best friend to Don Finkle of Knoxville, Tennessee, contributed considerable expertise on canine dwellings when his new home was designed and built.

An example of the latest information on passive solar techniques, his solar-heated pooch palace features a direct gain window with heat-storing brick floor and an overhang for summer shading. Well-insulated, the small wooden abode is comfortable all year round.

If your pet petitions for similar living quarters, contact the National Solar Heating and Cooling Information Center for a set of do-it-yourself plans.

---

of fuel oil a year, forever (or as long as the house and the collector last).

- The average window, which qualifies as a passive solar collector if it is on the south side of the house, is about 12 square feet in area.
- An installed window costs $10 per square foot, more or less.

Adding insulation will help to save fuel oil (bills drop, then start to rise again as the cost of fuel oil continues to go up). Adding a solar collector can replace fuel oil (the bill for some oil is eliminated, not lessened). After the easier conservation measures have been applied —weatherstripping, caulk, storm windows— solar may make very good sense for an existing house if further conservation means costly ripping out of walls to add insulation, or otherwise wrenching the house into energy-efficient shape. If one wall is within 30° of solar south (see "To find south," p. 54), you can do it.

What kind of solar? It depends first on what kind of space you want, then upon what natural advantages your house already has, then upon what use you make of the solar-heated rooms, and finally upon what kind of money you intend to spend.

Do you want solar heat for existing living space? Add good double-glazed windows or, if you want heat without more light, consider darkening the outside wall (paint? metal for better collection efficiency? rip the siding off and install storage tanks or tubes between the studs?), then glazing it to turn it into a collec-

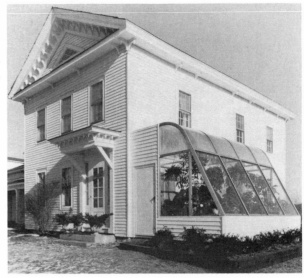

Modular Sunplace solar greenhouse added to 1840s Vermont farmhouse. Note the shadows. It's late morning, and the south wall isn't oriented toward true south. (Sunplace)

tor. If the wall is brick or masonry, you might try a Trombe wall.

Do you want to add a solar-heated-only space that can coast with outside temperatures sometimes and sometimes contribute heat to the house? Glaze a south-facing porch and use a window to let heat into the house (close the window at night). During the day it's extra living space. Or, better, build an attached greenhouse. A solar-heated greenhouse (see Solar Greenhouses, p. 75) can add considerable heat to the house during the spring and fall, some heat during the winter, and some food year-round. In fact, the energy saved by growing food may be even more than the energy saved by adding household heat.

Do you want new living space, at living temperatures twenty-four hours a day? Put provision for thermal storage (see Storing Solar Heat, p. 66) into your new south-facing solar-heated addition. It may produce solar heat to add to the rest of the house or it may not—but it can take care of most of its own needs.

South-facing bedrooms, particularly if they're for children who nap during the day, probably should not have more windows—so use indirect gain. South-facing living rooms may welcome more windows.

On all of these you can spend $50 for materials (scrap lumber, plastic), and do-it-yourself, or you can spend as much as you would for any other construction job. New building costs, depending on the part of the country, are running from $50 to $75 per square foot.

PASSIVE SOLAR JARGON

Solar retrofit: **putting a solar system into an existing house.**

Direct gain: **The sun shines in, as through a window.**

Indirect gain: **The sun shines on, and only the heat moves in, as with a Trombe wall or a TAP.**

Isolated gain: **The sun shines in, but the heat is moved somewhere else, as from a greenhouse to a house.**

Sun-tempered: **The sun warms the house, but nobody bothers to store the heat.**

Sun space: **A greenhouse, usually without plants.**

SOLAR GREENHOUSES

Solar greenhouses are greenhouses heated by the sun. They face south and usually are open to the sun through south-facing windows. Attached to or integrated into the house, they operate on much the same principle as a thermosiphoning air system, pumping extra warm air into living spaces behind them. If thermal mass—for instance, a brick or stone wall—separates the house from the greenhouse, heat will travel through the mass by conduction and then radiate into the living spaces, thus adding to the efficiency of the heating system.

Sunny spaces with lots of windows will lose heat rapidly when outside temperatures drop and the sun does not shine because glass is a

Plans for a solar greenhouse designed by a team led by Barbara Putnam, an architectural designer. Materials cost $1200–$1500. (Drawings by Barbara Putnam; plans are available from her at RFD, Marlborough, NH 03455)

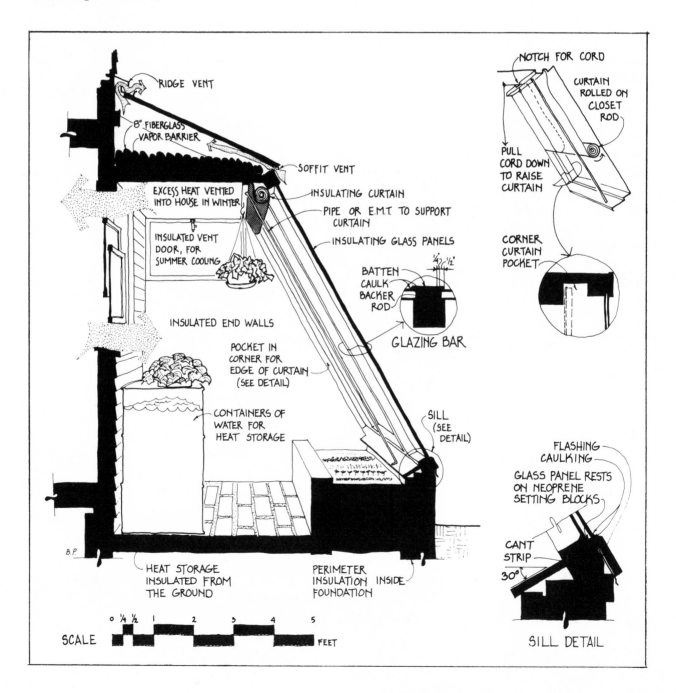

RIDGE VENT

8" FIBERGLASS VAPOR BARRIER

SOFFIT VENT

EXCESS HEAT VENTED INTO HOUSE IN WINTER

INSULATING CURTAIN

PIPE OR E.M.T. TO SUPPORT CURTAIN

INSULATING GLASS PANELS

INSULATED VENT DOOR, FOR SUMMER COOLING

BATTEN
CAULK
BACKER
ROD

½" ½"

GLAZING BAR

INSULATED END WALLS

POCKET IN CORNER FOR EDGE OF CURTAIN (SEE DETAIL)

CONTAINERS OF WATER FOR HEAT STORAGE

SILL (SEE DETAIL)

B.P.

HEAT STORAGE INSULATED FROM THE GROUND

PERIMETER INSULATION INSIDE FOUNDATION

SCALE   0 ¼ ½   1   2   3   4   5   FEET

NOTCH FOR CORD

CURTAIN ROLLED ON CLOSET ROD

PULL CORD DOWN TO RAISE CURTAIN

CORNER CURTAIN POCKET

FLASHING
CAULKING
GLASS PANEL RESTS ON NEOPRENE SETTING BLOCKS

CANT STRIP

30°

SILL DETAIL

Total Warmth

rotten insulator. To reduce heat losses, use double-glazed windows, thermal curtains, insulating draperies, cloth-covered Styrofoam panels, and other means of retaining heat.

Solar greenhouses can be effectively used for food production, another way of conserving energy. If you are attuned to the climates within the greenhouse and understand the needs of the different plants, it is possible to reap bountiful harvests all year long. Growing in the greenhouse will lessen the amount of heat pumped into the house during the coolest time of the year in some locations, but compromises between food and fuel needs can usually be resolved over a good dinner with lots of vegetables. Growing foods in solar greenhouses may, in fact, save more money and energy than using the glass house as a heat source.

Design Books. *The Complete Greenhouse Book*, Peter Clegg and Derry Watkins, Garden Way Publishing Co., Charlotte, VT 05445.

The Solar Greenhouse Book, James C. McCullagh, editor, Rodale Press, 1978, Emmaus, PA 18049.

The Food and Heat Producing Greenhouse, Bill Yanda and Rick Fisher, John Muir Publishing, rev. ed., 1980.

Growing Information. *Growing Food in Solar Greenhouses: Month-by-Month Guide to Raising Vegetables, Fruit and Herbs Under Glass*, Delores E. Wolfe, Doubleday, 1981.

Solar Living and Solar Greenhouse Digest, P.O. Box 2626, Flagstaff AZ 86003. Subscription $10 per year.

The Planter, Hobby Greenhouse Association, Box 951, Wallingford, CT 06492. Subscription $5 per year.

Organizations. Solar Survival, Box 119, Harrisville, NH 03450.

Solar Greenhouse Association, 34 North Gore Ave., Webster Groves, MO 63119.

Plans. Solar Sustenance Team, Route 1, Box 107 AA, Sante Fe, NM 87501.

Prepackaged Greenhouses.

Sun-Ray Solar Equipment Co., Inc.
  4 Pines Bridge Road
  Beacon Falls, CT 06403

General Aluminum Corp.
  P.O. Box 34221
  Dallas, TX 75234

Vegetable Factory
  100 Court St.
  Copiague, NY 11726

Solar Technology Corp.
  2160 Clay St.
  Denver, CO 80211

Brady and Sun LivingRooms
  12 Jacques St.
  Worcester, MA 01603

The Energy Factory
  5622 East Westover, Suite 105
  Fresno, CA 93727

Abundant Energy Inc.
  Newport Bridge Road
  Warwick, NY 10990

Allstate Greenhouse Mfg. Corp.
  P.O. Box 89
  Shoreham, NY 11786

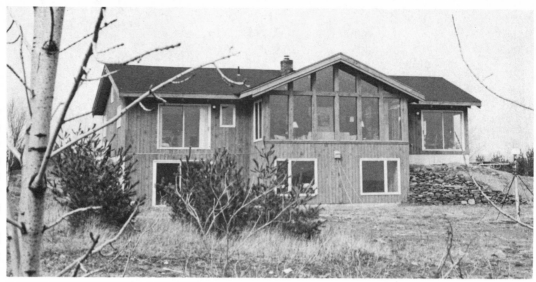

Adirondack Alternate Energy designs solar houses that require very little additional energy. This house, located 30 miles from Albany, New York, has no furnace and uses less than a cord of wood a year, for a total annual fuel bill of $25. (Photo by Sandra Oddo)

78 Solar Resources, Inc.
    Box 1848
    Taos, NM 87571
Four Seasons Greenhouses
    910 Route 110
    Farmingdale, NY 11735
Weather Energy Systems, Inc.
    P.O. Box 968A
    Barlows Landing Rd.
    Pocasset, MA 02559
The Garden Way Solar Greenhouse by Sunplace
    Garden Way Research
    Charlotte, VT 05445

LER

Even among opinionated solar people, Adirondack Alternate Energy (AAE) considers itself a little odd. The company has built more than 200 passive solar Low Energy Requirement® (LER) houses, most of them north of Albany, New York (8,300 degree days), where winters are among the coldest in the country. And those houses break a lot of passive solar "rules." Where fiberglass is the insulation norm, AAE uses a 4-inch rigid foam box around its post-and-beam construction—*outside.* "Fiberglass degrades over twenty or thirty years," says President Bruce Brownell. Where passive solar people use an average of 40 to 50 tons of rock for thermal mass for storing heat, Brownell and his bunch use up to 200 tons, usually of sand. Where the passive solar rule of thumb is ½ square foot of south-facing glass for each square foot of floor area, AAE installations need less than ⅓ square foot on an average. And where building inspectors have just begun to worry about the health hazards of sealing houses too tightly, AAE has been shielding its houses against possible byproducts of indoor pollution like radon gas for twenty years. (Radon gas is a daughter product of natural background radiation from some rocks, sand, etc. Dangerous concentrations could build up in very weather-tight houses.)

Degree Day: **A way of measuring the amount by which indoor temperature (held steady by fossil or solar energy) differs from outdoor temperature. Assume that natural law has decreed a temperature of 65°F for human existence. Yet, perversely, the average temperature outside for one day is 5° cooler —60°F. Those 5° have to be replaced for the day by 5° of heat from some other source. Therefore, that day has accounted for five heating degree days. Add up all the degree days for a year, and you have a rough gauge of the need for heat in any given location. At Key West, Florida, for example, the climate demands fewer than 100 heating degree days (there are, of course, cooling degree days— the amount by which outdoor temperature exceeds that hallowed 65°F—to contend with). At International Falls, Wisconsin, on the Canadian border, folks shiver through some 10,000 heating degree days a year.**

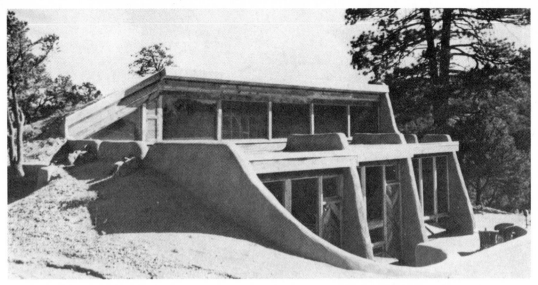

Designed by architect David Wright and built by solar contractor Karen Terry, this underground adobe house in Santa Fe, New Mexico, uses a small fireplace for back-up heat. (Photo by Sandra Oddo)

LER houses seem to need very little energy besides solar heat, perhaps a cord of wood a winter or $100 or so for electric heat. That may be one reason that the six-person staff are up to their ears in design work, even though AAE is one of the very few energy-conservation firms to offer house packages, either for complete houses or for additions. For information, a $5 booklet of details, or a Saturday house tour, write AAE, Edinburg, NY 12134.

A System of Sorts: Hobbit Houses, or Living Comfortably Underground

Twenty thousand years ago, caves and underground houses were all the rage. Cool in summer, warm in winter, easy to heat and maintain, this style of housing lasted many thousands of years.

Tolkien's Hobbit, Bilbo, lived quite comfortably in his below-ground shelter. In fact, the folk tales of most European countries abound with stories of wee folk and giants inhabiting dwellings deep in the earth. Early civilizations, ranging from Greek to North American Indian, used caves and underground rooms in their religious practices.

Now, in the search for more energy-efficient housing, we arrive full circle back at the mouth of the cave and find the prospect pleasing.

What is it that makes an underground house —a Hobbit house—appealing to the modern home buyer? Aside from the fact that the roof may be mowed (or grazed) or snow shoveled off the skylight, these houses require little work to maintain because they are bermed with earth on several sides. And because they are bermed with earth, they require little energy to keep warm or cool. They operate on the principle of thermal lag.

Did you ever notice that if you dig into the earth a few feet on a hot summer day, it will feel cool? That's because the earth has not caught up with the warm season. It takes earth a long time to capture enough heat to warm it up to 55°F, and it takes an equally long time for the earth to cool down. So by the time fall arrives and the trees are shedding their leaves, the earth has finally become as warm as it will get that year, and starts to cool off as winter sets in. But it takes that same patch of earth all winter and into the spring before the cooling trend is reversed. All told, the temperature swing—high to low—may be no more than 10° to 15°F, not much at all when you think about what the outdoor above-ground temperature was doing between summer highs of 95°F to 100°F and winter lows of 0°F to −15°F for a spread of about 100°. Since we feel best at temperatures ranging from 65°F to 75°F, a lot of energy is spent warming us up in winter and then cooling us down in hot weather.

If the ground has a temperature of 50°F to 55°F for most of the winter months, this means we only have to raise the temperature inside 15° to 20°F rather than the 70° to 80°F required for conventional above-ground housing. In summer, the cool earth moderates the heat to the comfortable 70's naturally.

Underground houses make great solar houses. The south-facing wall can be opened to the sun and the house will become a high passive solar collector. Because Hobbit houses are largely masonry, they have built-in thermal storage that naturally interacts with the thermal lag of the surrounding earth. Natural day lighting for most of the rooms is an added bonus, as is the sheltered microclimate found outside in front of the glass wall.

It sounds simple, doesn't it? Just put spade to the earth and dig in! But . . . there are some things to beware of. Not all soils act alike. Some soak up water and are not much good for anything but a batch of mud pies. Other soils will slip under certain conditions and may cause damage to subterranean shelters. Underground springs and waterways may put water where it's not wanted. Water is powerful stuff—it moves mountains—and must be diverted away from the house, or the next thing you know, it will be flowing through the living room. Common sense, good building practice, and care in sealing the structure should avert potential problems caused by the soil and water.

A few years back, when underground housing was still a very new concept, the Underground Space Center at the University of Minnesota published its book on *Earth Sheltered Housing Design*. The material on site selection and soils, financing, zoning, design and construction is still very relevant and goes a long way in helping the average homeowner into his Hobbit house. Minnesota is considered the underground space center of the world because of the pioneering efforts of the university and local builders in promoting this type of building for commercial as well as residential use.

Early underground construction costs more than similar conventional construction for a number of reasons: reinforced concrete is expensive; forms for 12-inch thick walls use more material and require more labor to set up than those for 8-inch walls; and forms must also be stronger to retain the added weight of concrete; the concrete is a special grade mixed to withstand the pressures of the roof and its loads. All in all, the pennies add up. On the bright side, energy savings soon add up to change the debit into a credit.

It's a good idea to find out if Hobbit life is appealing to you before investing in an underground structure. Bilbo's idea of comfort may not be everyone's cup of tea. Visit underground houses nearby, or plan a vacation trip that features them (a tough new challenge for travel agents).

A trip through New England can range from the hills of Lyme, New Hampshire, to Cape Cod and should include a few stops in between. Minnesota offers many varieties of underground buildings from the University of Minnesota bookstore to the Ouroboros House (named for the mythical worm that completes a closed cycle by consuming himself) to single- and multifamily housing. Ohio and Illinois are also centers for subterranean dwellings and should not be bypassed. In Texas and the Southwest, underground houses are a buffer against the intense heat of summer. Once you've made the trip and have no more questions about dampness, the psychological effects of living underground, water, and the like, the decision to go under or stay on top can be made.

Resources. Underground Space Association, Department of Civil & Mineral Engineering, University of Minnesota, Minneapolis, MN 55455.

The Underground Space Center publishes the journal *Underground Space* and a newsletter, sponsors workshops, and acts as a clearinghouse for information on construction underground.

Earth Shelter Digest (WEBCO Publishing, St. Paul, MN 55109; $18 annual subscription) is a bimonthly magazine that is devoted to underground design and construction.

Underground Plans Book 1 by Malcolm Wells and Sam Glenn-Wells (P.O. Box 1149, Brewster, MA 02631; $15). Also by Malcolm Wells, *Gentle Architecture* (McGraw-Hill, 1980) and *Notes from the Energy Underground* (Van Nostrand Reinhold, 1980).

Earth Integrated Architecture, James W. Scalise, editor. Architecture Foundation, College of Architecture, Arizona State University, Tempe, AZ 85281; $10.

Earth Shelters by David Martindale (Hawthorn/Dutton, 1981).

Just a few years ago, the amount of solar-energy information available to the average person could have fit on the head of a pin and still left room for dancing angels. Now the problem is one of having to wade through an overabundance of the stuff to find the nuggets worth pursuing. For the newcomer to the field of solar energy, the task is almost impossible, and an awful lot of bother to go through to save a few bucks.

But don't give up! There are some Helpful People out there who have digested all—or most—of the paper, and can offer you the results. Most are nonprofit and will not charge for the service, although some may ask for a dollar or two to cover their expenses. The solar industry, through various trade associations, also distributes information on products and their installation.

For general information, bibliographies, lists of architects, builders, manufacturers, and the like, and answers to queries, try Conservation and Renewable Energy Inquiry and Referral Service (CAREIRS), P.O. Box 1607, Rockville, MD 20850. Or call one of these toll-free numbers: 1-800-523-2929 except... 1-800-462-4983 in Pennsylvania and 1-800-523-4700 in Alaska and Hawaii.

Local chapters of the American Section, International Solar Energy Association (AS/ISES), are also excellent sources of information pertinent to their area. For a list of chapters and addresses, write AS/ISES, American Technical University, P.O. Box 1416, U.S. Highway 190 West, Kileen, TX 76541 (817-526-1300).

Solar Age and *Solar Engineering* magazines are good sources of continuing information. *Solar Age* is oriented toward the solar professional with enough of a spread that the energy-interested layperson can tag along; *Solar Engineering* is intended for the engineer and the business-person.

Solar Age
Church Hill
Harrisville, NH 03450
$20 per year; free with membership in
AS/ISES

Solar Engineering
8435 Stemmons Freeway
Dallas, TX 75247
$20 per year

Low-cost, low-technology solutions to the energy crisis have been developed by such organizations as AERO (Alternative Energy Resources Organization), the Ecotope Group, and Farallones Institute. You will notice that they are all located in the northern half of the country, where winter sunlight is generally limited. However, the fact that the challenge is great also means that the satisfaction of finding a solution, especially when you've been told there isn't one, is sweet. These helpful people are developing some rather ingenious answers, and offer workshops, seminars, and printed information to spread the word.

AERO
435 Stapleton Bldg.
Billings, MT 59601

Ecotope Group
2332 East Madison
Seattle, WA 98112

Florida Solar Energy Center
300 State Road 401
Cape Canaveral, FL 32920

Farallones Institute
15290 Coleman Valley Rd.
Occidental, CA 95455

Memphremagog Group
P.O. Box 456
Newport, VT 08533

THE LEARNING EXPERIENCE

Whether you're nine or ninety, there are a number of ways to learn all about solar energy. School curricula, workshops, lectures, meetings, seminars, adult-education courses, and more start with kindergarten and follow through adult education.

For those on the teaching end, ERIC, the Educational Resources Information Center, contains computerized annotated bibliographies of material suitable for classroom or course work. Most state colleges subscribe to ERIC and have the materials on hand. Many teacher-training schools offer one or two semester courses in energy education for the elementary and high school teacher.

Sources of Learning Experiences:

A number of organizations across the country offer in-depth, hands-on courses in the design and construction of solar housing for the person interested in doing it on his own.

Cornerstones
    54 Cumberland St.
    Brunswick, ME 04011
Owner-Builder Center
    1824 4th St.
    Berkeley, CA 94710
Heartwood Owner Builder School
    Jackson Rd.
    Washington, MA 01235
Shelter Institute
    Bath, ME 04530
Northern Owner Builder
    Route 1
    Plainfield, VT 05667

The National Solar Energy Education Directory, assembled through the National Solar Energy Information Data Bank (SEIDB) and available from the Superintendent of Documents, lists many of the college-level courses available, as well as some of the vocational-school offerings. (Superintendent of Documents, Government Printing Office, Washington, DC 20402; stock number: 061-000-00368-1). Courses are quite likely to change from semester to semester, so it is best to inquire for the latest listings at any college.

SOLAR ON WHEELS

Solar fairs and traveling solar road shows are family events with a picnicky atmosphere. They are casual—inviting a lot of poking and prodding of displays ranging from Rube Goldberg inventions to futuristic devices. This is the place to pick up practical tidbits of information, meet people who are doing things in the solar field, and spread your own wings a bit.

For those of you who would like to sponsor an energy fair in your neighborhood or at your local school, the Government Printing Office's Superintendent of Documents (see Helpful People) has published *Reaching Up, Reaching Out: A Guide to Organizing Local Solar Events,* an excellent source of ideas and trivia for the organizer.

And when the fair is in the planning stages, consider featuring one or more of the traveling exhibits. Your local solar-energy-association chapter may be able to help you with names and addresses, or contact one of the organizations listed below.

New Western Energy Show, 226 Power Block, Helena, MT 59601. A traveling "medicine show" on energy that tours the northwest United States during the summer months.

Great New England Energy Show, Brattleboro, VT 05301. Exhibits and skits traveling throughout New England.

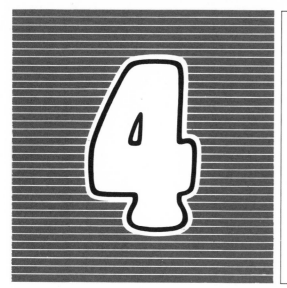

Plugging the Leaks: Insulation and Other Ways of Keeping Heat Where You Want It

L. Donald Meyers

If evil can be defined merely as an absence of good, in the same spirit we can say that cold is merely the absence of warmth. As far as houses are concerned, there is some truth to that. In a completely sealed-off house, using space-age insulation products, it is theoretically possible to heat up a house and have it stay that way for a long time without reheating.

That's theory, though, and assumes a house that is windowless and doorless and has impermeable walls. In real houses, heat is constantly on the move. If there's a cold spot somewhere, any warm air that's around will move in its direction.

Regardless of temperature, heat always flows from warm to cold, so that keeping cold out is theoretically, at least, the same thing as keeping warmth in. Even when it's 68°F inside and 65°F outside, the warm inside air will flow toward the colder air outside (although at a very slow rate), in an attempt to achieve "equalization."

How does this work in a house? Your heating unit pulls in cold air by one method or another, and dispenses it throughout the home as warmed air. The warmed air moves through the house doing its duty, but inexorably it heads for the colder outer regions. When it hits a barrier, such as a wall, it is slowed down for a while, but eventually the warmed molecules transfer their heat to the colder outside air. Since the warmed air does tend to rise over colder air, this is more pronounced in the roof area, but the same process goes on whenever warm air meets a colder or floor area. The warmed air keeps slipping out.

What can be done to halt this loss of heat? If you're building a new house, you can plan wisely and well, using new sources of warmth or constructing with energy efficiency in mind. Most of us, however, are stuck with what we have. Better to suffer the pangs of high heating costs than fly to a new mortgage with interest rates we know not of (among other disadvantages of moving). Thus, for most of us, the problem is how to retrofit an older house for greater comfort and lower fuel bills. This can and should be done, and the overall savings are probably a lot more than you imagined they could be.

CUTTING DOWN ON THERMAL LOSS—AND FUEL EXPENSES

There are many fairly obvious and straightforward ways to cut your consumption of expensive fuel—turning down the thermostat, putting up storm windows, using your fireplace efficiently, installing wood and coal stoves or kerosene or quartz heaters.

The job here is to outline what can be done to make your house thermally efficient, to conserve the heat you're now generating. There's no need to remind you that saving fuel means saving money—a lot of it. It also results in lowering OPEC imports, an improved trade balance, a strong dollar, and an economically

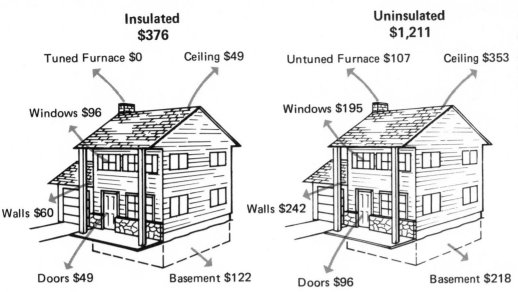

**Insulated
$376**

Tuned Furnace $0   Ceiling $49

Windows $96

Walls $60

Doors $49   Basement $122

**Uninsulated
$1,211**

Untuned Furnace $107   Ceiling $353

Windows $195

Walls $242

Doors $96   Basement $218

The dollar figures represent the cost of energy lost through each part of your house. Since they are based on Department of Energy estimates from several years ago, the savings achieved by insulation are much greater today.

healthier United States (which also results in more money in your pocket).

If you need any more economic incentive than that, the federal government also offers a generous tax break to those who invest in energy-saving home improvements. All forms of insulation, caulking, and weatherstripping—including that for hot-water heaters and pipes—are eligible for a 15 percent federal tax credit. In addition, a number of other energy-savers, such as storm windows and certain furnace modifications, qualify. There are other items which many homeowners feel should qualify—wood and coal stoves, heat pumps and replacement boilers or furnaces, and so on—but which are now ruled out by the IRS. Write your congressman.

Home-energy-conservation credits are allowed for 15 percent of the cost, up to a maximum of $2000 invested ($300 credit) a year. If you invest more than the $2000 maximum, you can carry over the credit balance to the following year. If, for example, the total cost of insulating your house is $3000, take a credit of $300 for expenditures on the first $2000. The next year, you're allowed an additional credit of $150 for the remaining $1000 of the investment.

There are few catches in this legislation. It applies only to your principal residence, not to a summer or vacation home, and homes built since April 19, 1977, are not eligible at all. For other *caveats* and further information, see IRS Form 5695 and the explanation on the

back page of the form. For energy credits see IRS Publication 903; consult Publication 525 for carryovers.

It should be emphasized that these are *credits*, not deductions. A deduction is subtracted from your taxable income, and only available if you itemize. The bottom-line saving is generally small unless you're in a very high tax bracket. A credit is deducted from the tax you owe. If you invest $1000 in insulation, for example, you first calculate what you must pay Uncle Sam, then take an additional $150 (15 percent of $1000) from the tax and put it back in your pocket. Tax credits offer substantial savings. Add the credit to what you can save in fuel costs by increasing thermal efficiency, and it's obvious that there is a great financial gain in making an energy-saving home improvement.

Let's take a look at three important ways of saving fuel—insulation, weatherstripping, and caulking. There are other methods, of course, but these three are among the cheapest and most effective ways to retard the flow of expensive heat from your home to the hostile cold.

Insulation. Briefly, insulation is a material designed to enclose your house in a warm envelope to prevent the flow of warm air to the colder outside. Ideally, it should be placed above all of your ceilings on the top floor, in every exterior wall, and below the ground floor or along basement walls. The home, in other words, should be completely surrounded by a thermal barrier between warm and cold air.

Plugging the Leaks

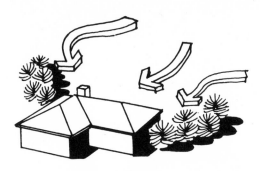

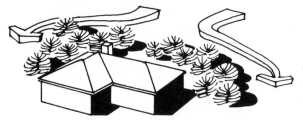

Cool air flows downhill in the evening. Properly placed vegetation can provide a first line of defense, deflecting the flow of cool air rather than channeling it toward your house.

Do-It-Yourself Checklist for Heat Loss

For a nominal fee your local utility can probably perform a complete energy audit which will include all facets of energy use in your home. However, if you wish to per-your own inspection, here's a checklist of where to look and what to look for.

Attic:

- Determine thickness of insulation, if any (check flanges of back of vapor barrier for R-designation, or measure thickness).
- Check for vapor barrier under insulation (is there foil or kraft paper attached or a polyethylene sheet below?).
- Find out whether there's adequate ventilation. There should be one square foot of vent space for every 300 square feet of attic area.
- Depending on construction, look down into wall cavities to determine extent of insulation, if any.
- For finished attics, check insulation behind and above finished area where possible.

Inside:

- Perform hand test, feeling the relative temperatures of the inside and outside surfaces of exterior walls.
- Remove electric outlet covers to check presence and density of insulation.
- Check weatherstripping of all doors and windows, including garage, if attached.

- Remove molding and check insulation around window frames.
- Note insulation level below bottom floor or on basement walls.
- Determine whether band joists (vertical wood framing above the foundation) are insulated.
- Check all openings to outside, where pipes, vents, wiring, and so on protrude, and see whether insulation has been stuffed in.
- See whether there is any insulation in attached garages, and determine its R-value.
- If garage is below living area, check to see whether it's insulated where adjacent to living area (should be covered by gypsum wallboard or paneling).
- Check water pipes and hot-water heater for insulation.

Outside

- Do all windows and doors have double or storm sash?
- Inspect around all doors and accessible windows. Is caulking in place and in good condition?
- Check chimneys, vents, pipes, wiring, and all other openings for caulking.
- Check bottom row of siding or shingles for caulking.
- Inspect caulking wherever two dissimilar building materials meet (such as brick against wood siding).

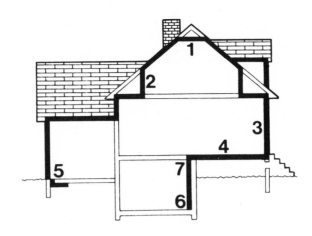

Where to insulate a home

1. Ceilings with cold spaces above
2. Rafters and "knee" walls of a finished attic
3. Exterior walls or walls between heated and unheated spaces
4. Floors over unheated or outside spaces
5. Perimeter of a concrete floor slab close to grade level
6. Walls of finished or heated basement
7. Top of foundation or basement wall

Weatherstripping. While insulation provides an air-encapsulating envelope for the home, weatherstripping (and its sister, caulking) more or less seals the envelope. Unless you're a hermit or a cloistered monk, you regularly leave and return to your home. You also like to see outside and to let in fresh air. That means doors and windows, and every time you open or close one, a lot of heat escapes. As a matter of fact, a lot of heat slips out even when doors and windows are closed. Weatherstripping is designed to prevent heat from escaping and cold wind from entering the cracks and edges of doors and windows.

Caulking. If our homes were built of one huge piece of solid plastic, we wouldn't need caulking. But homes are made of separate pieces of wood, asphalt, brick, stone, and other materials. Each time the small pieces are joined, there is a chance that there will be tiny (sometimes larger) cracks and spaces. Sound house construction eliminates most of these—by the use of overlapping siding and roofing, for example—but it's a little more difficult to eliminate all of these chinks in your house's armor where two dissimilar materials come together.

Some of these vulnerable areas are at the top of the foundation, around the outside of doors and windows, and where pipes and vents penetrate the exterior. There is considerable heat loss through these holes and cracks which can be plugged up with an elastic material called caulking.

How Much Will It Save?

Will insulation, weatherstripping and caulking save money? Does it snow in Buffalo? I live on eastern Long Island, and the only fuel out here is oil. I was just feeding some newspapers into my fireplace and ran across an article in a September 1980 paper. The paper predicted that oil would go up to almost a dollar a gallon by the end of winter. If only it were a dollar a gallon now!

If you think things are going to get better, don't. And natural or propane gas users shouldn't be complacent, either. Gas is being decontrolled by the government and prices are rising fast. Though very expensive now, electric heat may be the conventional choice in the future, since it will be generated by sources such as coal; which is still plentiful, nuclear energy, and plain old water.

So, in general, almost anything we do to cut down thermal waste will result in considerable saving. It is true that a few years ago, contractors were peddling their wares as if anything you did, energy-wise, would save lots of money. That was clearly an exaggeration, at least at the time. Even now the cost of blowing insulation into walls may sometimes outweigh the fuel savings. But the continued rise in fuel costs has proved that even some of those unscrupulous contractors who oversold their products were right.

The instrumental term in thinking about insulation and other coldproofing measures is cost-effectiveness, or how long it will take to

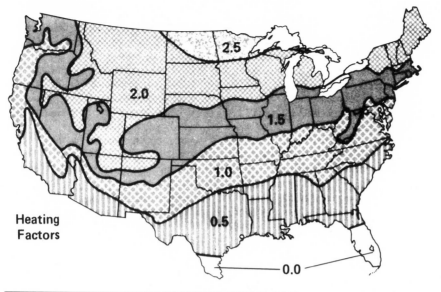

Heating Factors

88

The figures presented here are the sort that strike fear into the heart of the reader, but experience has shown that fuel-cost estimates have generally been on the low, rather than the high side. These numbers are based on a variety of sources and are average for the nation. There is, of course, wide regional variation, but percentage comparisons should be reasonably consistent across the country.

Perhaps the most interesting calculations are those of the Edison Electric Institute (EEI), which show a much slower rate of increase in costs for electricity for the future than oil or natural gas. This may well mean that electricity will be the cheapest form of heat in the future (or that EEI is overly optimistic).

Comparative Costs per Heating Unit (100,000 Btus)			
Year	#2 Heating Oil (gal.)	Natural Gas (120 cu. ft.)	Elec. (30 kws.)
1970	0.18	0.13	1.26
1975	0.30	0.20	1.35
1980	0.90	0.50	1.36
1985	2.00	0.80	1.53
1990	4.50	1.30	1.62
2000	9.75	2.80	1.71

Sources: American Gas Association, Edison Electric Institute, U.S. Department of Energy.

pay back your investment. If you're investigating the wisdom of doing a certain energy-saving improvement, you should make a serious effort to determine the payback period. But it can be fairly safely said that these days it's almost always worthwhile to invest in insulation, weatherstripping, and caulking you can do yourself. With some specific effort, the average home can probably become 25 to 50 percent more fuel-efficient—saving the homeowner a great deal of money to boot.

THE ECONOMICS OF INSULATION

The best way to calculate your thermal losses and to assess potential savings from insulation is to have an energy audit. Many elaborate formulas have also been devised to enable you to estimate reasonably the actual thermal loss in your house yourself and to compute reliably the expected savings from various energy-saving improvements. Those interested should consult the U.S. Department of Energy or state and local energy offices. Several books, including my own *Home Insulating* (New York: Harper and Row, 1978), also provide the necessary formulas.

All these calculations, while reasonably precise, are quite complex. And, in any event, the enormous increases in fuel costs since the publication of most of these formulas have rendered them somewhat obsolete.

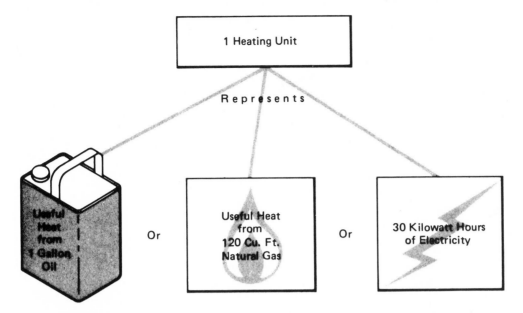

The following charts are an attempt to compromise exhaustive mathematics and a calculated guess. They are intended to give you a simplified, reasonably accurate way to estimate costs, savings, and payback periods.

FUEL-COST FACTOR

The Fuel-Cost Factor is determined by multiplying the Heating-Cost Factor (above) by the Cost Per Heating Unit. The Heating-Cost Factor has been computed on the basis of how many degree days of heat are used in different areas of the United States. Cost Per Heating Unit is equivalent to the useful heat given off by one gallon of oil (above). If you use oil, for example, at a cost of $1.20 per gallon, enter $1.20. If you use gas, use the local cost for 120 cubic feet of gas. For electricity, a heating unit is equal to the cost of 30 kilowatt hours of electricity. Get these figures from your fuel bill or supplier. Better yet, ask for an estimate of the unit cost for the next several years. This will give you a clearer idea of the projected costs and savings.

In our example (p. 92), we used a Heating-Cost Factor of 1.5, multiplied by the projected cost of a gallon of oil over the next few years ($1.50). If electricity costs 3.3¢ per kilowatt hour, multiply by 30, and use 99¢ ($0.99). If gas will cost 1.2¢ per cubic foot, use $1.44 (multiply by 120). With our 1.5 Heating Factor times the Cost Per Heating Unit ($1.50) of oil, we arrive at a Fuel-Cost Factor of $2.25.

FUEL-SAVING FACTOR

The Fuel-Saving Factor is arrived at by first determining how much insulation you want to add. This can be tricky, and depends on area, costs, and so on. The R-levels on page 90 are fairly recent recommendations, but rapidly escalating costs may have already rendered them obsolete. (For example, note the accompanying chart, suggesting possible insulation of up to R-66 when oil costs reach $1.25, which has already been exceeded.) For the moment, though, use this table to determine optimum R-levels or check local sources.

When you have determined how much insulation you wish to add, consult these "Added R" charts. Listed here are figures designating the change in thermal resistance. If you now have an R-value in your ceiling of R-11, for example, and want to insulate up to R-33, subtract 11 from 33 to get R-22. That is the amount of insulation you should add. Following the chart, look for 22 on top and R-11 at the left. The corresponding 0.045, where the figures meet, is the Added-R Factor.

Now determine the square feet of the area to be insulated (1000 sq. ft. in our example). Multiply the number of square feet to get the Fuel-Saving Factor (1000 × 0.045 or 45 in our example).

SAVINGS PER YEAR

Now we get to figures with meaning. Take the Fuel-Saving Factor (45 in the example) and multiply it by the Fuel Cost Factor ($2.25

89

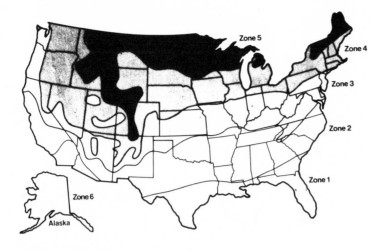

in the example). Adding R-22 insulation to existing R-11 insulation will save $101.25 per year in the sample.

Note that the potential savings get smaller as you add more insulation on top of already existing insulation, until a point of diminishing returns is reached. Determining where that point exists is impossible here, but you may find that the savings calculated are minor. If so, stop here and forget about the rest. But first make sure that you have done your best to reasonably estimate future fuel costs. That could make all the difference.

Also note that the savings are enormous if you have no ceiling insulation at all. Adding only R-11 to an insulationless attic has a high Added-R Factor. If, in our example, there was no existing insulation, the savings in the same house would be $562.50 *each year* (0.25 × 1000 × $2.25).

COST OF IMPROVEMENT

The cost of improvement represents, somewhat obviously, the cost of having a particular improvement done. Adding R-22 insulation, for example, will cost about 32¢ per square

Optimum R-Levels for Ceilings (Depending on Fuel Price)								
Type of fuel:	*Heating Cost*							
Gas (therm)	15¢	18¢	24¢	30¢	36¢	54¢	72¢	90¢
Oil (gallon)	21¢	25¢	34¢	42¢	50¢	75¢	$1.00	$1.25
Electric (kWh)		1¢	1.3¢	1.6¢	2¢	3¢	4¢	5¢
Heat pump (kWh)	1.7¢	2¢	2.6¢	3.3¢	4¢	6¢	8¢	10¢
Zone 1	**R-19**	**R-19**	**R-19**	**R-19**	**R-19**	**R-19**	R-19	R-19
Zone 2	**R-19**	**R-19**	R-19	R-19	R-30	R-30	R-38	R-38
Zone 3	R-19	R-19	R-30	R-30	R-33	R-38	R-44	R-49
Zone 4	R-30	R-30	R-33	R-33	R-38	R-49	R-49	R-57
Zone 5	R-30	R-30	R-38	R-38	R-44	R-49	R-60	R-66
Zone 6	R-38	R-38	R-44	R-49	R-49	R-60	R-66	R-66

Note: Gas and oil are listed using "therms" (one heating unit), equivalent to 120 cubic feet of gas or one gallon oil. Electrical costs are given in kilowatt hours. Multiply by 30 to get one heating unit of electricity. (Zone 6 is Alaska.)

Source: Johns-Manville, based on recommendations of National Bureau of Standards (NBS) and American Society of Heating, Refrigerating & Air-Conditioning Engineers, Inc. (ASHRAE). Air-conditioning criteria not included.

"Added-R" Charts

Use these charts to estimate the effect of adding insulation in various areas of the house. The mathematical factors given measure the thermal effect of added R-values.

Ceilings

Existing R-value	Added R-Value				
	11	19	22	30	38
	"Added-R" Factor				
0	0.23	0.25	0.25	0.26	0.26
R-5	0.084	0.10	0.10	0.11	0.12
R-11	0.033	0.042	0.045	0.050	0.053
R-19	0.024	0.032	0.034	0.037	

Walls

Type of insulating material	Situation		
	1. No information about sheathing	2. Insulated sheathing	3. No insulated sheathing
	"Added-R" Factor		
Fiberglass	0.15	0.13	0.20
Rock wool	0.16	0.14	0.22
Cellulose	0.18	0.15	0.23
U-F Foam	0.19	0.16	0.24

Where it is not known whether the exterior sheathing contains insulation, use the first column. Factors assume 2 × 4 stud walls with no other insulation.

Floors (No Existing Insulation)

R-value to be added	"Added-R" Factor
R-11	0.23
R-13	0.24
R-19	0.26
R-22	0.26

Source: Cornell University Extension, New York State Energy Office

foot in our example, if the homeowner lays it himself. With 1000 square feet to insulate, the total cost will be $320.

The best way to compute this figure, of course, is to check a building-supply dealer or insulating contractor and ask what the cost is. If you just want to make an educated guess right now, use a figure of 1.5¢ per R; R-11, for example, should cost about 16.5¢ per square foot (11 × 1.5).

From the cost, however, you should also deduct the tax credit, to get a true out-of-pocket expense. For $320 invested in insulation, you get a 15 percent credit of $48. Deduct $48 from $320, and the true cost is $272.

PAYBACK PERIOD

This is the most significant figure of all. It tells you how long it will take to recoup your investment. To find this out, simply divide the Cost of Improvement by the Savings per Year. In the example, the true cost (with tax credit) of the insulation was $272. Divided by the projected annual savings of $101.25, we get a payback period of 2.7 years.

CAVEATS

As you surely noticed, many of the figures here are projections. Someone may discover an immense new oil field in Lake Michigan, and prices may drop. But the odds weigh heavily in the opposite direction. In any case, remember that these are just estimates. Use your good judgment before making final decisions. And read the newspapers for further updates on cost estimates.

Also, for our purposes here, we have ignored several other factors, such as cooling costs and savings. If you live in an area where air conditioning is a significant expense, see your local utility about factoring in the cost of electricity for cooling purposes. Savings can be considerable in Sunbelt regions.

Furthermore, if you must borrow money to insulate, interest should also be considered. In general, however, the interest costs should be offset by expected fuel-price increases.

Another important factor not considered here is the effect of insulation on resale value. Although elusive and probably impossible to calculate, this is something to be kept in mind. Already prospective buyers are paying a lot of attention to energy efficiency in a home. The impact should be even greater in the future as fuel prices rise.

Computing the Bottom Line

	Sample House		Your House
Fuel Cost per Heating Unit	$ 1.50		$————
x Heating Factor (p. 89)	x1.5		x————
Fuel-Cost Factor		$ 2.25	$————
Square Footage Insulated	1000		————
x "Added-R" Factor (p. 91)	x.045		x————
Fuel-Saving Factor		x45	x————
Savings per Year		$101.25	$————
Square Footage Insulated	1000		————
x Cost per Square Foot	x16.5¢		x————¢
÷ Cost to Improve (convert cents to dollars)		÷ $320.00	÷ $————
= Payback Period		2.7 yrs.	————yrs.

HOW TO PAY FOR ENERGY IMPROVEMENTS

The wealthy can pay cash, of course. If you are among the poor—working or nonworking—see your local social services department for a variety of federal-assistance plans. Most of us are in the middle and will probably have to borrow. Happily, loans intended for energy-conservation measures are easier to obtain than most other kinds of loans. In many areas, utilities are mandated by law to provide energy-saving loans to their customers at a lower rate of interest than is available otherwise. Some states provide tax credits. Check into these and other government help before trying conventional loan sources below.

FEDERALLY BACKED LOW-INTEREST LOANS

There are several ways you can get loans that have relatively low interest because the payment is guaranteed against default by the federal government. Check local lending institutions for eligibility, rates, and so on.

FmHA (Farmers Home Administration) loans are made to persons in rural areas, not necessarily farmers. Interest rates are very low. Many "suburban" areas are still regarded as rural, so don't assume that you are not eligible just because you don't raise chickens.

HUD (Department of Housing and Urban Development) now the administrator of the old FHA (Federal Housing Authority) loans. Most of the jobs in this chapter fall under the

Title I category, designed to "enhance the livability" of the home. Such loans are made through regular lending institutions and are insured by FHA. Limits and interest rates are relatively generous, FHA insurance costing a half percent above the base rate.

OTHER LOAN SOURCES

Life Insurance Loans are made on the cash value of a non-term policy. It is possible to borrow up to 95 percent of the value of the policy at a low rate—perhaps even 5 percent.

Credit Unions are a good source of funds at reasonable interest. Members are usually given loans without too much difficulty. (They know where to find you.)

"Open-End" Mortgages allow you to borrow up to the full amount of the original principal that has been repaid, usually in $1000 increments. If, for instance, you took out a $30,000 mortgage on your home and have lived there for some time, the principal may now be down to $25,000. You can now borrow up to $5000 more. This type of mortgage is not too common any more. Check your contract, lawyer, or bank.

Refinanced Mortgages involve abandoning a low-interest mortgage for a new one at a no-doubt higher rate. There will also be additional closing costs. If, however, tax credits and pay backs in fuel savings are great enough, the disadvantages may be outweighed.

Secondary Mortgage Loans are available in most states. This is another popular way of

The total R-value of a wall equals the sum of the R-values of its components. Notice that the insulation provides more than four-fifths of the total R-value for this wall.

Interior Surface	.68
3/8″ Gypsum Board	.32
3-1/2″ Blanket Insulation	11.00
3/8″ Plywood	.47
Bevel Siding	.81
Exterior Surface	.17
Overall R = 13.45	

Mineral Wool Insulation (Fiberglass)

Exterior Wall

borrowing on the increased equity of a home. Interest rates are relatively high but better than standard loans.

Other Financing Methods include a personal bank loan, collateral loans (using stocks, bonds, real estate or other assets), or an understanding relative. Some banks offer a discount for energy-saving loans. Contractors may also be able to arrange financing for you.

HEAT TRANSFER

Before getting into the nuts and bolts of insulation, here's a quick definition of what you're fighting in the way of heat transfer.

Radiation is the emission of energy directly from an object, such as the sun. It travels at the speed of light. In the home, radiant heat is the principle involved in portable electric heaters, solar panels, and fireplaces. Radiated heat travels in straight lines only.

Convection is the transmission of heat by the movement of masses of liquid or gas. It is the principle by which many heating systems work. Typically, cold air is drawn into a heating unit, where its temperature is raised, and it is then forced out through pipes or ducts. In general, warm air rises and cold air falls, contributing to the circulation of the heat, but the molecules of air also churn throughout the house, so that an overall warming of the structure occurs.

Conduction is the flow of heat energy through a solid, for example, from one side of a wall to the other. In space travel, esoteric materials reduce this type of heat flow almost to zero. Ceramics, mica, urethane, and other elements are combined to keep the intense heat of space travel outside the vehicle. Even so, there is no material or combination of materials that does not have some conductivity.

K- AND R-FACTORS

Heating engineers use the letter K to stand for the rate of heat flow through a given material. The "K-factor" tells you how much heat energy will pass through one square foot of a given material in terms of Btus per hour at one-degree difference in temperature. The abbreviation Btu means British Thermal Unit, an arbitrary standard based on the energy it takes to raise the temperature of one pound of water by one degree. One Btu is roughly equal to the heat given off by one wooden kitchen match.

We will be more concerned here with the R-factor, which is the opposite of the K-factor. While K represents the heat *transfer* of certain materials, R represents the thermal impedance, or the *resistance* of that material to heat flow. For any given material, R is the inverse of K as expressed in the formula K = 1/R.

In building materials the higher the R-Factor, the better the insulation value. (Conversely, the higher the K, the greater the heat loss.) In more technical terms, the more Rs you have, the better the capacity of the wall, ceiling, or floor to resist the flow of heat mol-

R-Values of House Components

Material	Thickness	R-Value
Air Film and Spaces		
Air space, bounded by ordinary materials	¾″ or more	0.91
Air space, bounded by aluminum foil	¾″ or more	2.17
Exterior surface resistance	—	0.17
Interior surface resistance	—	0.68
Masonry		
Sand and gravel concrete block	8″	1.11
Sand and gravel concrete block	12″	1.28
Lightweight concrete block	8″	2.00
Lightweight concrete block	12″	2.13
Face brick	4″	0.44
Concrete cast in place	8″	0.64
Building Materials (General)		
Wood sheathing or subfloor	¾″	1.00
Fiber board insulating sheathing	¾″	2.10
Plywood	⅝″	0.79
Plywood	½″	0.63
Plywood	⅜″	0.47
Bevel lapped siding	½″ × 8″	0.81
Bevel lapped siding	¾″ × 10″	1.05
Vertical tongue and groove board	¾″	1.00
Drop siding	¾″	0.94
Asbestos board	¼″	0.13
⅜″ gypsum lath and ⅜″ plaster	¾″	0.42
Gypsum board	⅜″	0.32
Interior plywood panel	¼″	0.31
Building paper	—	0.06
Vapor barrier	—	0.00
Wood shingles	—	0.87
Asphalt shingles	—	0.44
Linoleum	—	0.08
Carpet with fiber pad	—	2.08
Hardwood floor	—	0.71
Insulation Materials (Mineral Wool, Glass Wool, Wood Wool, Etc.)		
Blanket or batts	1″	3.70
Blanket or batts	3½″	11.00
Blanket or batts	6″	19.00
Loose fill	1″	3.33
Rigid insulation board (sheathing)	¾″	2.10
Windows and Doors		
Single window	—	Approx. 1.00
Double window	—	Approx. 2.00
Exterior door	—	Approx. 2.00

ecules from the warm side to the cool side. (Of course, even air has a specific R-value.)

Air Infiltration

Warm air will normally be lost through the chinks and cracks of your house even on a calm day. This loss is greatly accelerated, however, when the winds are strong. Winds tend to build up pressure on one side of the house, forcing cold air in and, by natural convection, pushing the heated inside air toward the cold outside air. This is what is commonly called a "draft."

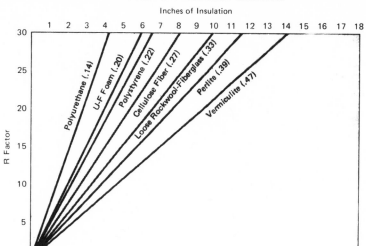

R Factors and Insulation Thickness

Inches of Insulation

The relative efficiency of various insulating materials. The figures in parentheses are the K-factors, measuring the ability to transfer heat. For insulation, the lower the K-factor, the better it is.

96

Research has shown that from 25 percent to 50 percent of heat loss is due to such air infiltration. Much of this loss occurs at windows. Other losses occur through openings at such places as the band joists on the top of the foundations, as well as through chimneys, vents, outside pipes, and electrical outlets.

Related to this is the so-called chimney effect, present in all homes but more prevalent in homes where there are two or more stories, including a basement. Here, the heated air rises naturally, escaping through crevices and low-R materials. At the same time more cold air is being sucked in from below, producing a constant cooling effect.

WHAT EXACTLY IS INSULATION?

Insulation is funny stuff. Its value does not lie in the material itself. Neither urethane, fiberglass, cellulose, nor plastic foam stop heat loss as such.

Fiberglass, for example, is made of glass, a very poor insulator. Fiberglass insulation is quite a different story, however, not because it is chemically altered, but because of the way it is spun into tiny fibers. The fibers are arranged to trap air. The air is, in fact, the insulator.

Air is also used as insulation in storm and thermopane windows, but it should be remembered that air by itself is not an effective insulator. When heated its molecules become agitated, transfering the heat from warm to cold by convection, or movement of heat energy.

What insulation materials do is stratify, or trap, air in minute particles to inhibit its movement. If the air cannot move, it cannot transfer heat energy as quickly. Insulation, therefore, slows down or retards the flow of heat from warm to cooler areas.

The ideal insulator is a vacuum, where there are no air molecules to transmit the heat. A thermos bottle works on this principle to keep your coffee warm or your lemonade cold. If we could design a house like a thermos bottle, we wouldn't need insulation.

Since we can't live in a vacuum, the next best thing is to use building materials with the fewest molecules, so that there is less heat transmission. The elements with the fewest molecules by volume are gases such as hydrogen and helium, which are impractical to use. Air, however, is made up of gases, primarily nitrogen, and it has a fairly low density of molecules. Air is plentiful and cheap. Because air molecules are fairly mobile, however, the air must be partitioned into small enclosures to minimize movement. The partitioning, or insulating, material should be as thin and light as possible. But, remember, the insulating material does not itself stop heat flow. For example, if we squeeze or compress fiberglass until all the air pockets are dissolved, it turns into a solid mass which has virtually no insulating capacity.

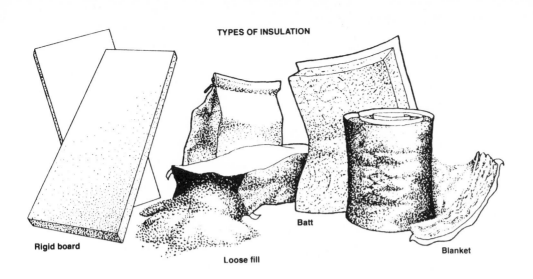

TYPES OF INSULATION

Rigid board

Loose fill

Batt

Blanket

The common types of home insulation are compared in the accompanying chart in terms of K-factors. Polyurethane with a K-factor of 0.14 has the most resistance to heat flow. Vermiculite, with a K-factor of 0.47, has the least heat-flow resistance. To reach R-30, you need only 4¼ inches of U-F foam, whereas 14 inches of vermiculite are needed to attain the same R-value (top of the graph).

In choosing insulation materials, the R-factor is extremely important. Other factors, however, may play an essential role, such as cost, availability, suitability, safety, and ease of installation. Entwined with all of these considerations is another—whether you can install the material yourself. If you can, you'll save a lot of money and in most cases get a much higher R-value per dollar expended and a quicker payback period. No one material is a better insulator in every respect. The most important consideration is the R-value, but other factors such as suitability may play a crucial role. For example, no matter how much you like urea-formaldehyde (U-F) foam, it cannot be used for the ceiling.

Regardless of the other considerations, however, mineral-wool blankets six inches thick will inhibit heat loss exactly the same as about four inches of U-F foam rated at 4.9 per inch. Both add up to R-10. Urea-formaldehyde foam yields more insulating effect per inch and may therefore be a better choice where space is narrow (such as closed walls), but that does not necessarily mean that urea-formaldehyde is a

better insulator. As a matter of fact, it may be the worst choice because of potential health hazards (discussed below).

FEATURES OF INSULATING MATERIALS

Assuming you have decided to add insulation, many factors come into play when you choose which type to use. In some instances, there is little or no choice. Between existing walls, for example, there is only blown-in insulation—unless you want to tear down the walls. This will involve a contractor and greater expense than other types of insulation.

Furthermore, your choice of blown-in materials may be severely limited. Urethane foam is rarely available, and it is very expensive when used this way. Urea-formaldehyde foam is under intense scrutiny by the government as a possible health hazard.

Where a wider choice of materials is available, the intelligent way to choose is to use the cost-benefit ratio. In many cases, this means a simple computation of the cost times the R-factor. If, for example, the R-factor desired is R-30, find out what the cost is to achieve R-30 among the various materials. With one material, the cost may be 20¢ per square foot to bring the R-value up to 30; with another it may be 25¢ a foot. Assuming all other considerations are equal, the clear choice is the less expensive material.

The problem is that all other considerations are not always equal. Take the installation of mineral-wool insulation, for example. Blown-

Comparing Popular Insulating Materials					
Type	*R-Value/Inch*	*Do It Yourself?*	*Where Used*	*Cost*	*Cautions*
U-F foam	4.2–5.4	No	Walls only	High	Questions as to health and shrinkage; choose contractor carefully.
Rigid plastic (various chemicals)	4.6–9.0	Yes	Anywhere	Mod.– High	Cover with gypsumboard or other fire-retardant material.
Blown cellulose	3.2–3.8	No	Walls and ceilings	Mod.	Be sure of fire-retardant treatment; look for UL listing; watch for fly-by-night operators.
Pour cellulose	3.1–3.7	Yes	Walls and ceilings	Low	Be sure of fire-retardant treatment; look for UL listing.
Mineral-wool batts or blankets	2.9–3.6	Yes	Anywhere	Low	Cover any vapor barrier to prevent fire hazard.
Blown mineral wool	2.1–3.2	No	Walls	Mod.	None
Perlite	2.6	Yes	Walls[1]	Mod.	None
Vermiculite	2.1	Yes	Walls[1]	Mod.	None

[1] These materials can be used where wetness is a problem. One common use is for filling the holes in concrete blocks.

in mineral wool might cost 20¢ per square foot. Mineral-wool blankets might cost 25¢ per square foot. But the fact is, it's simple to lay blankets and both difficult and expensive to blow in the mineral wool. If you do your own work, the cost for the blankets might well come in low. If you're at all handy and have the time, you would probably opt for laying the blankets yourself instead of having it blown in professionally.

As you read the following survey of materials, consider the various factors, then decide what's best for you. The materials are listed in order of declining R-Factors.

Urethane Foam. Although this has the highest R-factor (9.0) among the conventional materials, it is generally available only in aerosol cans for small installations around such structural openings as window frames and electrical boxes. The cost is relatively high, and only a handful of contractors are willing to use this high-priced material for general insulation work.

U-F Foam. Well over half a million homes

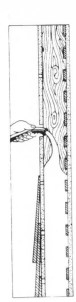

One of the best features of U-F foam is that it fills every nook and cranny of the wall cavity.

Rigid foam boards applied to basement walls to a depth of 4 feet can save up to 10 percent of a home's total heat loss.

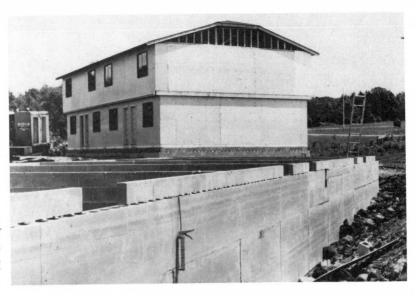

have had this type of insulation installed in their walls. It has a high R-factor (4.8 to 5.6) per inch and is moderately priced. For most homes, U-F foam is the only material suitable for raising wall insulation to the desired R-value.

When properly installed, U-F foam fills every nook and cranny within the wall surfaces, leaving absolutely no voids or dead spots. The key phrase is "properly installed." When insulation became a hot item in the mid-1970s, many incompetent and inexperienced operators caused problems.

There is also a question of shrinkage. A study by the National Bureau of Standards (NBS) showed that some installations shrank as much as 7.3 percent after 20 months. (Manufacturers say that shrinkage should be only 2 to 3 percent.) Such shrinkage would mean that 10 percent or more actual R-value is lost, which means that such an installation would approximate the R-value of cheaper cellulose. Further, as it shrinks, foam is inclined to pull away from walls, and may split and crack, leaving passages for wind, air, and thermal loss.

Another more serious problem with U-F foam is its use of potentially toxic chemicals. There is often an odor problem after its application, although this usually disappears quickly. More seriously, the foam tends to break down, especially in high-heat areas such as attics, and formaldehyde gas may seep into the living areas, causing nausea, difficulty in breathing and other health problems. There is

some evidence, further, that formaldehyde may be a carcinogen. The foam is already banned in several states. In Massachusetts, for example, the product is not only forbidden, but contractors must remove it from homes that already have it. As of this writing, the U.S. Consumer Product Safety Commission has proposed banning U-F foam nationwide, but final action has not yet been taken.

Rigid Plastic Foam. You are probably familiar with plastic foam in the form of take-out coffee cups or Christmas decorations. It is lightweight and easily cut or shaped to fit difficult spaces. For our purposes, it comes as rigid boards in thicknesses from ½ inch to 3 inches. Sizes range from 2 × 4-foot to 4 × 8-foot sheets. Styrofoam (a brand name) and polystyrene are common foam materials.

Plastic foam has a closed-cell construction, with millions of tiny air bubbles contained in such a way that little air passes through, making it a superior insulator. The R-factor varies from 4.6 for polystyrene "beadboard" to 9.0 for isocyanurate, a dense plastic foam, used primarily in exterior sheathing. Styrofoam uses Freon gas instead of air between beads, and has a cost-efficient R-factor of 5.4.

Plastic foam is an excellent choice for tight areas. Rigid urethane foam, for example, is used for thin walls of refrigerators and freezers. It is good for basement walls for similar reasons and can be glued to the concrete with furring strips between. Paneling or other finishing material can be nailed or glued over it. That way,

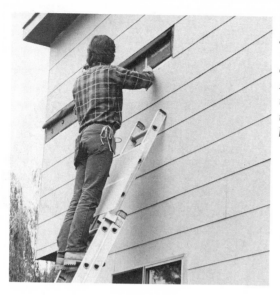

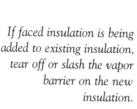

Blown-in cellulose is generally applied through the exterior walls. The contractor removes a row of shingles and drills holes in the sheathing, then blows the insulation through the holes into the wall cavity.

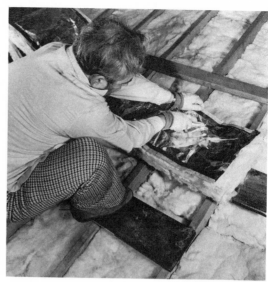

If faced insulation is being added to existing insulation, tear off or slash the vapor barrier on the new insulation.

100 thicker stud walls can be avoided, saving several inches of space all around, which can make the difference between having a usable pool table or not.

Be sure to use a special type of construction adhesive, which will not attack the foam. Rigid panels can be cemented to almost anything, including concrete. Plastic foam cuts easily with a pocket or utility knife. Always cover plastic foam with gypsum wallboard or other fire-resistant material.

Cellulose Fiber. Cellulose insulation is made of paper, usually old newspapers ground up and treated. It is organic vegetable matter and flammable. When properly treated with chemicals such as borax, however, it is safe and effective. Its R-value ranges from 3.1 to 3.8 per inch.

Cellulose fill, a popular choice of contractors for blown-in installation, also comes in bags for pouring. Major manufacturers treat their cellulose properly, but with the boom in insulating materials, some smaller manufacturers may skimp on the proper chemical treatment. This may cause a fire hazard. Watch for a fire rating of less than 0.25 or a UL rating on the bag, and avoid cellulose treated with aluminum sulfate. Some cellulose may have a higher R-value than others, so check specifications on the bag.

Blown-in cellulose is a good choice for walls in older homes, which often have little or no insulation. A typical 3¾-inch "blow" offers about R-19 thermal resistance. Blown-in cel-

lulose does require some covering material to be temporarily removed from the wall. Generally, this is done outside by removing one row of shingles and siding and drilling holes between the studs. The cellulose fiber is blown in with a hose and fills the area between the studs.

Certain sidings, such as plastic, aluminum or steel, are not easily removed without damage, so the contractor may enter the wall through the inside. After the insulation is blown in, a wooden plug is placed in the hole and spackled over.

When properly treated, cellulose is resistant to moisture and should not deteriorate or get soggy. To be on the safe side, however, it is recommended that paint applied to the inside walls be oil based, to act as a form of vapor barrier.

Blown-in cellulose is also used for attics and other areas. Most attics are easy enough to do yourself by pouring the material between (and preferably over) ceiling joists, so it ordinarily would not pay to hire a contractor. If you are already having your walls done, however, it may well be that the contractor can do the attic also for a small additional price. A 6-inch-thick "blow" of cellulose in an attic should yield an R-value of about 22–23.

Mineral Wool. There are two types of mineral wool, fiberglass and rock wool. Both are made by melting inorganic substances and forming them into fibers. Fiberglass, the most commonly used, is manufactured by heating

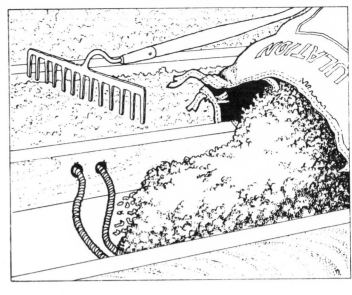

Loose mineral-wool fills well around wiring and other obstructions. (Cornell University Extension Service)

silica sand, the main ingredient of glass, and spinning it into fibers. Rock wool is made by blowing air through molten slag or limestone and forming it into woolly fibers. The fibers are formed into long rolls called blankets, or 4- to 8-foot sections called batts. Sometimes they are chopped up into pellets, forming loose or pour insulation.

Mineral wool is the most commonly available insulating material, and is the choice of most insulators. It is easy to apply, and, being immune to decay, insects, deterioration and fire, is almost indestructible.

Blanket length depends on the thickness of the material. R-11 (3½″) wool, for example, comes in 60-foot rolls, while R-19 (6″) wool comes in 40-foot rolls. The thicker the material, the shorter the length. Many people still use the thickness designations (3½″ and 6″) instead of the R-factors. Other sizes are also available, but are more difficult to find.

Vapor Barriers. These may or may not be attached to mineral-wool batts or blankets. They are usually made of foil or kraft paper. The vapor barrier is intended to prevent moisture from infiltrating the insulation, where it often condenses. Wet insulation is of little value, and the vapor barrier is usually needed.

When insulation containing a vapor barrier has already been installed, use unfaced insulation (without a vapor barrier) over the insulation in place. Two vapor barriers are almost as bad as none at all. If unfaced insulation is not available, slash or pull off the vapor barrier.

Loose Mineral-Wool Fill. This is somewhat difficult to find, and has less R-value per inch than cellulose fill. Occasionally, it can be poured into walls from the attic, depending upon how the house was constructed, or from the top of the wall after the gypsum board or other covering material has been removed. This method is difficult and time consuming, however.

Loose mineral wool can also be used in attics and is especially good for filling between joists when unfaced blankets are being laid on top of existing insulation.

Mineral wool can also be used for blowing in by contractors in attics or between walls. Ordinarily, cellulose is a better buy for walls, although it is a good idea to get a price from a mineral-wool installer and see for yourself. An audit by the Center for Energy Policy and Research (CEPR), New York Institute of Technology, Old Westbury, NY, found that mineral-wool installers charged prices that were slightly to moderately higher than cellulose contractors. But the best R-factor you could get from a 3½-inch-thick mineral-wood blow would be 9.0, compared to an R-factor of about 13.0 for cellulose. Mineral wool by its nature is resistant to "fire, rodents, and vermin," but so is properly treated cellulose.

PERLITE AND VERMICULITE

Perlite and Vermiculite are lightweight minerals that are often used as potting materials for plants. They are found in small bags in nurser-

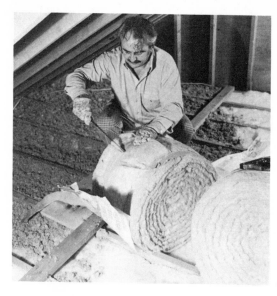

Adding insulation to an attic is easy when there's no floor to go through. Note the loose cellulose that's been added over the old insulation up to the level of the joists.

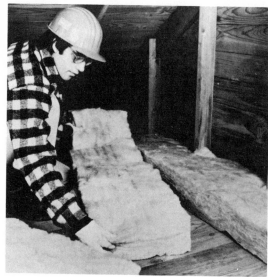

Lay insulation directly over an unused floor in the attic; use unfaced insulation to prevent moisture from collecting in the floorboards.

TIPS FOR CHOOSING INSULATION TYPES

- First and foremost, insulate your home as close to the local recommendations as possible. This is the best way to insure the best value for your dollar. Whatever you pay will be reimbursed in lower fuel costs and tax credits.
- Since prices between the several types are approximately the same per R-value, your main consideration should be the suitability of the material to the type of insulation. Pour cellulose may be a little cheaper, but mineral-wool blankets are easier to lay in an attic, under floors, and in crawl spaces. For use between walls, cellulose usually is the best and safest buy. Plastic foam is easier and quicker for basements, foundations, and where space is limited.
- Often you may have to settle for what is locally available, regardless of cost or use.
- When using a contractor, have him give you a written estimate. He should be able to tell you the cost per R-value. Choose your contractor carefully, and ask for a written warranty.
- Unless the health-hazard picture has cleared by the time you read this, avoid U-F foam altogether.

ies and garden shops. Both are expensive and hard to find in large quantities. Their R-values are not great, but the materials do not settle, and they do filter well between obstacles such as wires, ducts, and outlets.

For special use in areas where access is difficult, you may want to use perlite or vermiculite, but other materials are better and cheaper for bigger jobs.

OTHER MATERIALS

Standard homebuilding materials are poor insulators. Glass, masonry, and most metals are among the worst. There may be times when the standard insulating materials won't do, however. If you simply wish to cover up an area to keep out the wind, for example, wood is probably the best material. Of the various woods, particleboard and fir plywood have the best R-values for the money.

Polyethylene plastic is not an insulating material as such, but makes an effective vapor barrier. It is commonly used in 4-mil or 6-mil thicknesses to cover the ground in a crawl space. For new walls, unfaced insulation laid between framing members and covered with a sheet of polyethylene is the best method. This provides a continuous vapor barrier and also covers the framing.

HOW TO INSULATE YOUR CEILINGS

Ceiling insulation is the most valuable of all energy-saving measures. It is most important

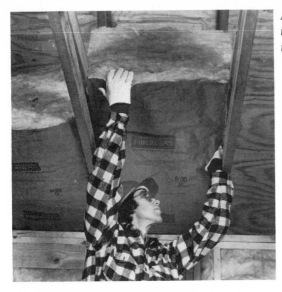

Add insulation to the rafters if you're converting the attic into usable space.

Cathedral ceilings can best be insulated with rigid foam boards. Always cover the boards with gypsum board.

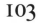

Rigid Foam   Gypsum Board

in cooler climates, because heat rises and escapes through the roof, but it is also of value in warmer regions. On hot days, heat builds up in the attic and penetrates downward, making the rooms below extremely uncomfortable.

Most homes are built with some sort of attic space, and for most of us, ceiling insulating means attic insulation. The attic may be a substantial one, as in older homes, where you can walk around and even build extra rooms. Newer homes are usually built with a small, enclosed area over the top floor, where there is barely room to stand in the center.

INSULATING THE ATTIC

Luckily for most of us, modern attics are usually unused and unfloored, so it's a simple matter for the do-it-yourselfer to insulate one.

Blanket mineral-wool insulation is the usual choice for attic insulation. To find out how much you need, simply find the area of the attic by measuring the perimeters of the rooms below and multiplying the length by the width. If your measurements are a little off, it's usually no problem to purchase a little more, or take back an unused roll for a refund or credit. Unlike wallpaper and paint, there are no subtle differences in batch colors to worry about.

PREPARATION

In addition to the insulating materials, you'll need a folding rule or metal tape for measuring,

103

SPECIAL ATTIC-INSULATING SITUATIONS

When you have a floor or living space in the attic, or if you intend to finish an attic in the future, special insulating techniques must be used. If there is an unused floored storage area (common in older homes), the insulation should be laid directly on top of the floorboards. Use unfaced insulation, since a vapor barrier will cause moisture to collect in the floorboards.

If the attic is used as living space and the walls are already in place, you can usually get in behind the "kneewalls" and put up insulation in the walls from behind. Use the techniques for cathedral ceilings (below) for the roof.

When you plan on converting the attic to usable space in the future, add insulation to the rafters using the same guidelines as for regular ceilings, and the techniques for open walls. Always leave some space for air circulation, though. It is wise to put up the kneewalls before adding insulation. (You can finish them at a later date.)

Cathedral ceilings present an insulating challenge. The most efficient way to increase insulation is by adding rigid board (foam) insulation to the existing ceiling. You may wish to consult a contractor for this, since you will have to cover up any new insulation with new ceiling materials.

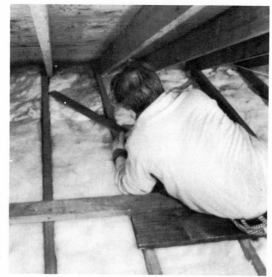

When laying new insulation between joists, shove the end of the blanket as far as you can by hand, then press it down into the cavity with a long board.

104 a sharp knife for cutting the insulation, some long, strong planks to stand or kneel upon, and a long stick for poking the insulation into corners. A trouble light or some other form of illumination is also a must. Get one with a long extension cord, or use several cords.

For your safety and comfort, wear cotton gloves, a long-sleeved loose-fitting shirt and other clothes that expose as little of your skin as possible. Mineral wool can be very irritating to the body. Those who have allergies or respiratory problems should wear a surgical-type mask, since the fibers can irritate throat or lungs. (In fact, they should check with their doctors before undertaking such a job.) It's a good idea, too, to wear goggles to prevent eye irritation, although insulating is a sweaty job even on cold days, and goggles are bound to steam up.

Push up all materials, boards, and tools before you pull yourself up into the attic. Attach all the lights and extensions and extend them as far as you can into the attic. Choose a corner in which to begin, and lay out your boards ahead of you to form a walkway. Try not to let too much board extend unsupported over any joist, because you're bound to step on the unsupported section and thereby become the unwitting principal in a situation comedy. Be careful of the ends of nails sticking through the roof. Wear a hard hat just in case.

INSTALLING YOUR ATTIC INSULATION

Where there is no existing insulation, you will be laying the batts or blankets between the joists. Take the loose end of the roll and shove it toward the eave. Don't cram it in, since a little room should be left for air circulation from the eaves up to the ridge. If there are vents in the eaves, be sure not to cover them.

The insulation should fit rather tightly between the joists, so push down on it gently until it hits the ceiling wallboard. Use your long stick to accomplish this at the edge where you have difficulty reaching. Don't compress the material too much, or you'll destroy its effectiveness.

When the end of the roll is in place, keep unrolling it until you reach the other side, or the end of the roll. To cut the insulation, place your utility knife on the foil or paper side with a board underneath. It should be very easy to cut the vapor barrier. The mineral wool may take several cuts because of its thickness. If you are laying very thick insulation, it is easier to make the first cut with the razor knife and finish the job with a serrated butcher knife.

Try to get the insulation under and around wiring and other obstructions. You may have to cut the insulation to work around bridging, pipes, and so on. Make sure that the insulation stops about three inches from the edge of any recessed fixtures, chimneys or other heat producers.

Double layers of insulation will be required in most parts of the country. Actually, R-factors are additive. Instead of using one R-30 roll, for example, lay one layer of R-19 and one of R-

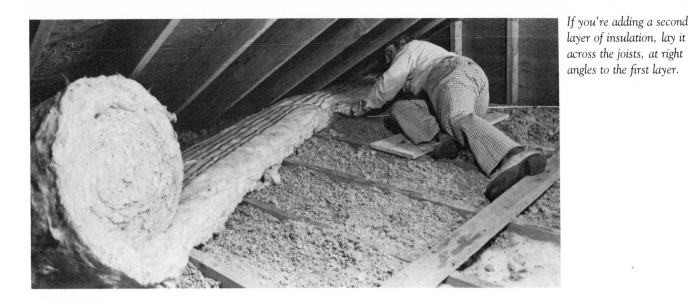

11. If you cross over the joists at right angles with the second layer, you actually get a better overall result than using one layer of R-30, because the joists are covered up. The first layer should always have vapor barrier at the bottom, next to the warm side, and the second layer is always unfaced.

When there is already some insulation installed, but not enough to provide sufficient thermal resistance for your region, a second layer is laid on top of the first. Where the total R-requirements are R-22 or less, the second layer can be laid on top of the first *between* the joists. Otherwise, the second layer should be placed at right angles to the first.

Pour cellulose or mineral wool may also be added to attics to bring the insulation up to the desired R-level. This material is generally most effective when only a few more Rs are needed. It can also be used as an intermediary between two layers of batts or blankets. Cellulose is good for adding to poor or damaged insulation.

There are no special problems with this type of insulation except for keeping an even surface. It is simply poured out of the bag and leveled with a board or rake.

WALL INSULATION

Wall insulation, though a valuable energy saver, usually requires the highest initial investment for existing homes. Unless the house is of "balloon" construction, where the walls are built before the floors, there is no way to pour insulation down into the wall cavity. Newer houses are rarely built that way, but it is worthwhile to check an older house to determine whether you can look down between the studs from the attic. If so, it is not too difficult to pour insulation down between the exterior and interior wall surfaces. This is one of the few instances where perlite or vermiculite might be the material of choice. For most of us, wall insulation calls for the services of a professional.

How do you know whether your home needs more wall insulation? Unless your home was recently built, you can be quite sure that there is little or none in your walls. Even homes built in the past ten years probably need more.

The only way to tell, unless you rip open a wall, is to remove a switch plate from an electrical outlet and try to look inside. Use a flashlight if necessary, and, to be safe, turn off the current to that outlet. Another way to find out, although it isn't foolproof, is to place one hand on an outside wall and another on an interior partition. If there is a noticeable difference in temperature, you can be quite sure that additional wall insulation is in order.

Sometimes the exterior studs are exposed, so it is simple enough to determine whether or not there is insulation, and whether it is adequate. You may find exposed studs in an attached garage or an uncompleted addition or basement.

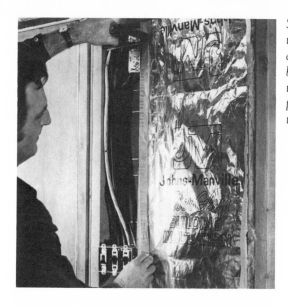

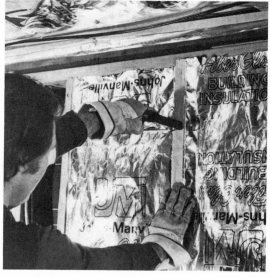

Staple insulation from the top down. Although it's easier to staple the vapor-barrier flanges to the sides of the studs, you'll get better protection if you staple them to the front of each stud.

When stapling the flanges to the front, staple the flange of the next strip of insulation directly over the flange of the first strip.

106   With exposed studs, adding new insulation is simple. In all cases, you should add enough insulation so that the wall cavity is completely filled without compressing the material. Mineral-wool blankets or batts with an R-value of R-11 to R-13 are the usual insulating materials for exposed 2 × 4s. See above for the clothing requirements and tools needed. Be sure that the vapor barrier is on the warm side (facing in), and staple the insulation to the studs on both sides. The vapor-barrier flanges can be stapled to the inside of the sides, but it is better to staple to the face of the studs for gap-free protection. Insert staples about every 6 inches, from the top down, making sure that there are no holes or gaps.

Basement walls can be insulated in the same way if you have 2 × 4 or 2 × 3 stud walls. If not, rigid foam between furring strips is an excellent form of insulation. See above for instructions on putting up plastic foam.

Some of the most neglected wall areas are the spaces around doors and windows. When insulating an exposed wall, stuff scrap pieces of insulation into these spaces. On covered walls, remove moldings and fill in all cavities.

FLOORS AND BASEMENTS

It is interesting to note that the recommended R-value for walls in virtually every part of the country is R-19. Yet in colder climates, floor insulation should exceed wall insulation; and in the Sunbelt, the recommended R-value of a floor is less than that for walls.

Obviously, floor insulation is of greater value for preventing heat loss than cooling loss. One reason for this is that the ground itself is a good insulator. The temperature of the ground beneath the frost level stays about 55°F year-round countrywide. When the ground itself freezes, the basement areas get very cold, and there is considerable heat loss through the floor. In hot weather, the ground stays relatively cool even near the surface.

The best way of insulating floors is to install mineral-wool batts or blankets between the first-floor joists. This is an easy job for the do-it-yourselfer, although just a little more complicated than exposed-wall insulation.

Remember, vapor barriers should always be on the warm side. In this case, the warm side is *above* the insulation. You can't attach the insulation by stapling to the framing, because that will put the vapor barrier on the cool side. The best thing to do is buy special insulation that has a permeable backing material with stapling flanges on the opposite side of the vapor barrier. But this is not readily available. Other methods must be devised to hold the insulation in place. The easiest method is to use "tiger's teeth," bowed wires with pointed ends especially made for this purpose. If these are not available, you can staple chickenwire to the bottoms of the joists and slide the insulation above it.

Another attachment method is to put small

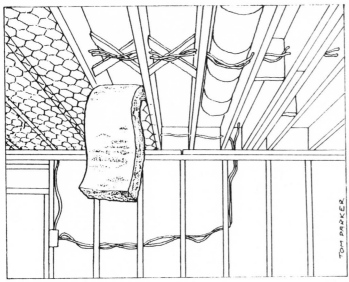

common nails every foot or so into the joists and lace thin wire between the nails. You can also use lath, furring strips or almost anything else that is handy.

THE BAND JOISTS

Band joists are the 2 × 8s or 2 × 10s between the flooring and the wood sill plate that rests on the foundation. The true wood thickness of nominal two-inch lumber is only 1½ inches, which gives an R-factor of only 1.8 or so at this point. In addition, there is quite a bit of air infiltration at the top and bottom of the band joists.

The band joists at right angles to the floor joists are easily insulated by simply bringing the floor blankets down to cover the bands and sill plate. The end band joists are insulated by cutting insulation to size and running it along each joist. Friction will keep this insulation in place without stapling. Remove the vapor barrier, or use unfaced insulation, to eliminate any potential fire hazard.

INSULATING BASEMENT LIVING SPACE

When the basement is to be used for living space, the basement walls and the band joists are insulated rather than the floor above.

For smooth, straight basement walls, when furring strips are attached to the concrete and covered with gypsumboard, rigid plastic foam is installed between the furring strips with construction adhesive. Use a type especially formulated for use with foam. Spread the adhesive on the wall with a caulking gun, then alternate the foam and furring.

When you use standard 2 × 3 or 2 × 4 framing for the basement, mineral wool batts are as good as anything. These are stapled to the studs the same as for any wall, except that the batts should be extended at the top to cover the band joists. Short pieces of furring can be employed to nail the insulation to the band joists. Use long nails, tapping them into the band joists just enough to hold.

If you want more insulation than is possible with 1 × 2 or 1 × 3 furring, use 2 × 2s as furring strips. The space will be just about right to accommodate R-7 batts or 2-inch rigid foam. Foam will extend one-fourth to one-half inch beyond the framing, but the foam itself provides a rigid backing for the finish material, so it does not matter if the nailing strip is a trifle thinner. Two inches of rigid foam will provide about R-13.

You don't have to run foundation insulation all the way down to the basement floor. Just make sure it extends below the frost line, usually about two feet below ground level.

WARNING: In some very cold areas such as Alaska, northern Maine, and the upper Midwest, it may actually be harmful to insulate the basement walls. The thermal difference between the sides of the concrete can cause cracking. Check local recommendations.

107

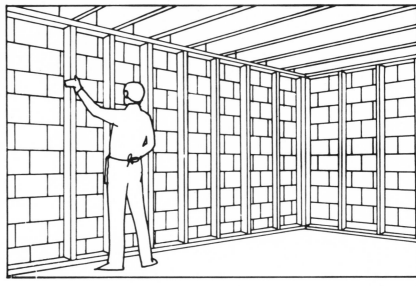

Basement walls of 2x3s or 2x4s can be insulated with mineral-wool blankets. Left to right, simply put up the wall, staple the insulation to the studs, and cover with wallboard or paneling.

108 INSULATING A CRAWL SPACE

The best way to insulate a crawl space is to lay mineral-wool blankets along the walls. The walls are low and do not require much material. Run the blankets down the inside wall and two feet onto the floor of the crawl area. A moisture barrier should cover the ground under the floor space unless you have a concrete floor, which is rare. The moisture barrier is usually made of polyethylene plastic 4 to 6 mils thick, although heavy tar paper will also do the trick.

After the moisture barrier has been put down and smoothed, use rocks or lumber to hold down any loose ends of the insulating material. It is a requirement of some building codes to put a 3-inch layer of ground limestone, sand, or gravel over the moisture barrier. This helps to hold down the plastic. It also provides something to walk on when you have to re-enter the crawl space.

VENTING A CRAWL SPACE

No matter how dry or well insulated the crawl space is, some dampness is bound to be present because the floor is earth. There should be at least two vents to allow cross-ventilation (check local codes). Most vents are the same size as a concrete block (nominally 8″ × 16″) so that they can be easily fitted into a block foundation.

If you are installing new vents, get the clos-

able type. These can be opened up during warmer weather to air out the crawl space and closed up in winter to prevent thermal loss. If the vents you have are not closable, replace them or nail up plywood to cover them during the winter months. Remove the covering, of course, as soon as the cold months have passed.

One caution here—check with your furnace man before covering up any crawl-space vents. Some furnaces may draw their combustion air from the crawl space. If so, the vents must be left open all year.

INSULATING A CONCRETE SLAB

If your home is built on a concrete slab without insulation, it is already too late to do the job properly by using rigid foam between the foundation walls and the slab, and under the bottom of the slab.

You can cut down some of the heat loss, however, with rigid foam placed on the outside of the foundation. To install the foam, dig down around the foundations until you reach the footings. At least 2-inch-thick foam panels should be used, and they should be cemented with compatible adhesive in a caulking gun. It is advisable to cover the foam with exterior siding material to protect it from damage. Decay- and insect-resistant plywood is good for this purpose.

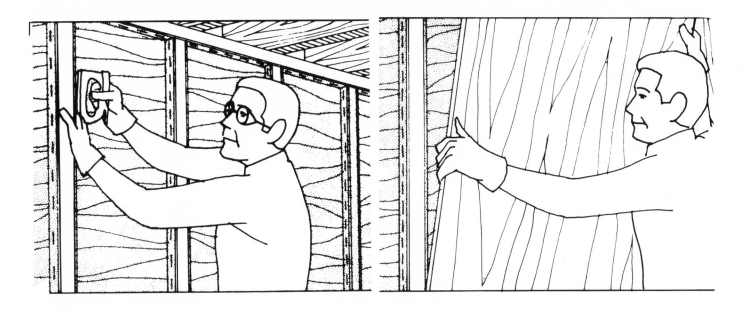

OTHER PLACES TO INSULATE

Insulation is also advisable for all pipes and ductwork in unheated areas. Hot-water heaters should also be insulated, but be very careful not to cover up the heat stack on gas heaters. Kits sell for about $20 and repay their cost in a year. You can also use unfaced R-8 batts. In addition to caulking around pipes and other openings to the outside, it is also helpful to stuff unfaced insulation around the openings from inside.

CARPETING

In homes where it is difficult to install floor insulation, it helps both comfort and heat retention to carpet as much of the downstairs flooring as possible. Even in the kitchen, carpeting can be used to help ward off chilly feet. Thick carpeting with a fiber pad is equivalent to about R-2, which isn't a great deal, but it helps. Even thin carpeting feels warmer to the toes than cold resilient flooring, slate, or hardwood.

WEATHERSTRIPPING AND CAULKING

Insulation helps prevent thermal loss, but it is surely no guarantee against air infiltration. One way to stop air infiltration is by weatherstripping. The other is by caulking.

ECONOMICS OF CAULKING AND WEATHERSTRIPPING

Computing the benefits of adding new caulking and weatherstripping is simpler, if less scientific, than doing such calculations for insulation. First, use the same method of computing the Fuel-Cost Factor as given on p. 92, and enter that figure in the top line of the chart below.

Then skip to the following charts on caulking and weatherstripping to estimate the Fuel-Savings Factor (SF). Windows are assumed to be approximately 3 × 5 feet and doors 3 × 6½ feet. For any great disparity in your own windows and doors, adjust the figures up or down proportionately.

"Fair" caulking or weatherstripping means that it is present, but old and damaged, perhaps missing in spots, causing minor drafts. "Poor" means that there is no caulking and/or weatherstripping, or that it is in such poor condition that there are noticeable drafts.

In addition to the doors and windows shown in the charts, add a factor of 2.0 for fair caulking around a chimney and 5.0 for poor or no caulking. Use the same factors for fair or poor caulking around the top of the foundation. Add 0.5 for any other condition needing caulking.

Our sample house has six windows with fair caulking and weatherstripping, and six with poor conditions for both. We found

Plugging the Leaks

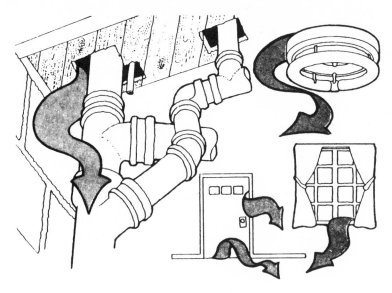

Heat loss occurs whenever there's a break in the exterior of the house. Caulking and weatherstripping will reduce the thermal flow through these gaps. In addition to caulking the pipes at left, insulation should be stuffed into the floorboards.

110

only one door with poor caulking. There was one door with fair, and one with poor weatherstripping. High-quality materials are assumed for all jobs. Costs can be considerably lower with less-long-lasting materials, resulting in much shorter payback. But then you will have to do the job over again in a few years.

The main task of weatherstripping is to plug up the gaps that allow warm air to escape at the perimeter of doors and windows—those parts of the house that are moveable, and therefore must allow some heat transfer when opened.

Types of Weatherstripping

Newer windows and doors usually come with factory-installed weatherstripping. This type of weatherstripping is usually of high quality and should not ordinarily be tampered with. Interlocking metal door channels, for example, give excellent protection. To replace the weatherstripping, the door must be removed and the metal precisely aligned.

Weatherstripping materials available for the homeowner are made by several manufactur-

The Bottom Line for Caulking		
	Sample House	*Your House*
Fuel-Cost Factor (p. 92)	$ 2.25	$————
x Fuel-Savings Factor (below)	x8.1	x————
Savings per year	$18.23	$————
÷ Cost to Improve	÷30.00	÷————
= Payback Period	1.6 yrs.	———— yrs.
	SF per window	*SF per window*
Number of windows with:		
Fair caulking	6 x 0.3 = 1.8	——— x 0.3 = ———
Poor caulking	6 x 0.9 = 5.4	——— x 0.9 = ———
	SF per door	*SF per door*
Number of doors with:		
Fair caulking	0 x 0.3 = 0.0	——— x 0.3 = ———
Poor caulking	1 x 0.9 = 0.9	——— x 0.9 = ———
Total = savings factor for caulking	= 8.1	———

Total Warmth

The Bottom Line for Weatherstripping		
	Sample House	*Your House*
Heating Factor (p. 89)	$ 2.25	$———
x Savings Factor (below)	x<u>72.3</u>	x———
	$612.68	$———
÷ Cost to Improve	÷<u>80.00</u>	÷———
= Payback Period	.5 yrs.	— yrs.
	SF per window or door	*SF per window or door*
Number of windows with:		
Fair weatherstripping	6 x 1.0 = 6	——— x 1.0 = ———
Poor weatherstripping	6 x 8.0 = 48	——— x 8.0 = ———
Number of doors with:		
Fair weatherstripping	1 x 2.0 = 2.0	——— x 2.0 = ———
Poor weatherstripping	1 x 16.3 = <u>16.3</u>	——— x 16.3 = ———
Total = savings factor for weatherstripping	= 72.3	= ———

ers, with the price and quality fairly uniform. The choice lies not much in the brand, but in the type.

Considerations when you are buying are effectiveness, durability and ease of installation. The price is reasonably low no matter what type you choose. The more expensive types usually do a better job and last longer, so the cost is approximately the same in the long run. Most materials come in 17-foot rolls, enough for one door or two standard windows.

Spring Bronze. Spring bronze is probably the most effective and durable of all the weath-

erstripping products. It is a little more difficult to apply than the others, but worth the small extra effort.

Spring bronze forms a tight seal between the door or window and the frame, which becomes even tighter when the wind blows because the pressure against the flexible metal holds it tighter against the sides of the opening. This type of weatherstripping is installed in such a way that it cannot be seen when the door or window is closed. It is relatively expensive, and not recommended for irregular openings or metal windows.

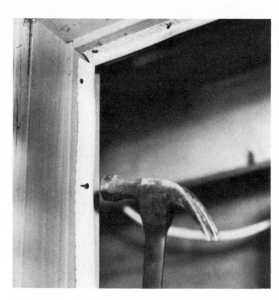

Sponge tubular gaskets consist of a sponge-filled vinyl tube, which can be tacked or stapled so the window or door presses lightly against it when closed. They are as effective as sponge bronze, and more adaptable to uneven gaps.

A new threshold will keep cold air from blowing in under the door. Simply screw in the new aluminum threshold and insert the vinyl bulb (opposite). The door will press against the vinyl when closed, forming a perfect seal against air infiltration.

112

Sponge Tubular Gasket. This is basically a piece of sponge vinyl or rubber inside of a vinyl tube, which is formed with a flange. The flange is nailed or stapled to a door or window so that the tube presses lightly against the opening when the door or window is closed, making a tight seal.

A filled gasket is second only to spring bronze in effectiveness, and may even be better when the gap is not uniform. The better types have a spring-wire flange, which is very durable. This type of weatherstripping is easy to install and can be used almost anywhere. Unlike spring bronze, it can be glued as well as nailed.

Hollow Tubular Gasket. Similar to the filled gasket but without the sponge rubber or vinyl insert. Most hollow gaskets are made without spring wire in the flange, and are not quite as durable as the sponge-filled type. In all other respects, the hollow gasket is similar to the filled type. The price is about one third to one half of its sponge cousin, and a good choice where a lot of weatherstripping must be done on short finances.

Felt. One of the oldest types of stripping, felt is the least expensive and is easy to install. Its chief defect is low durability. Do not use felt where there will be a lot of friction—like the sides of windows. Felt does not weather well, either, so its chief use is at the bottom of windows or on door stops, away from the elements. When used where recommended, felt is effective and has low visibility.

Foam. Easiest of all the weatherstripping materials to install, foam is made of sponge rubber or foam vinyl. Made with an adhesive backing, the strips are simply pressed into place. Sponge rubber is a little more effective than vinyl, but costs a little more. Neither type is very durable, but people use them even along the sides of windows because the foam is easily pulled off and replaced when it wears out. Because of its low durability, the best uses for foam are the same as for felt. Foam weathers better, however, and can be used outside.

Tape. You can't use tape on a door or window you plan to open. But weatherstripping tape is quite effective, cheap, and convenient, if you want to stop drafts at a difficult window which will probably stay closed all winter. The tape is removed when the weather warms up. Special transparent weatherstripping tape is available that is invisible when applied. You can also use duct or even masking tape on basement windows, or other places where appearance doesn't matter. Obviously, tape can't be used for doors.

Specialized Applications. There are several variations of the above materials, such as felt, vinyl, or rubber attached to long wood or aluminum strips. These are more visible than the materials themselves, but they are simple to apply with a few nails through the strips. One problem is that the weatherstripping material itself may wear out relatively quickly, leaving only a useless piece of wood or aluminum.

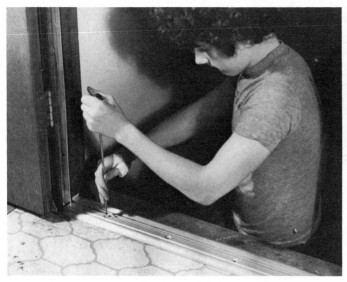

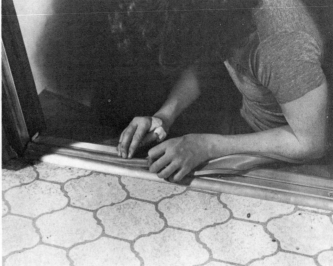

There are also special kits made for uses such as door thresholds (below), casement and louvered windows, and garage-door bottoms and sides (below). Basically, the same materials are used as discussed above.

THRESHOLDS

One of the most vulnerable areas to air infiltration is at the bottom of doors. Yet this is often the most neglected, mainly because the homeowner doesn't know what to do about it. Ordinary weatherstripping materials won't work there.

A weatherstripping threshold is used for this purpose. Sweeps are the most popular and easiest to install. A sweep consists of about an inch of heavy vinyl glued, screwed or nailed to the inside bottom of the door through an aluminum or wooden top piece. When the door is closed, the sweep helps plug the gap between the door bottom and the floor. One problem is that a strong gust of wind may force the sweep open, defeating its purpose. If the room inside is covered with a rug, the sweep may catch on the rug. Although effective to some degree, sweeps are less satisfactory than more sophisticated threshold strippings.

One of the best types of threshold is the vinyl bulb, which has several variations. Some are installed on the bottom of the door, which may necessitate removing and planing the door.

It is usually easier to remove the old threshold (if any) and replace it with a new aluminum threshold-bulb combination, which is almost as effective as the ordinary vinyl bulb. Screw in the new threshold, cut the bulb to size with scissors or knife and push it down into the flanges of the metal. The bulb is flexible enough so that it seals off any space between the door and the metal.

WHERE TO CAULK

- **Between window frames and siding or shingles**
- **Between door frames and siding or shingles**
- **At corners formed by siding**
- **At sills where wood meets the foundation**
- **At water faucets, oil filler pipes, dryer vents, and other breaks in the siding of the house**
- **Between porches and the main body of the house**
- **Where chimney or other masonry meets the siding**
- **Where storm windows meet the window frame (but leave weep holes open at the bottom)**
- **Where pipes and wires penetrate the ceiling below an unheated attic**
- **In heated attics where the wall meets the eaves and at the gable ends**

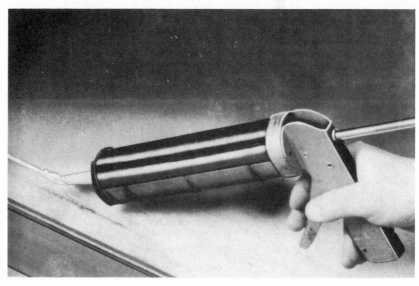

114 GARAGE-DOOR WEATHERSTRIPPING

There is not much point in weatherstripping a detached garage, but it makes good sense to weatherstrip the doors when the garage is attached to the house or located in the basement. The garage in such a case can act as a sort of pressure or decompression chamber between the outside cold and the warm house.

There are several types of weatherstripping kits for garage doors. A thick rubber strip is available which is nailed to the bottom of the door and flattens out when it is closed. Flexible vinyl strips attached to rigid vinyl are also on the market. These are nailed so that the flexible part covers the openings at the top and sides of the garage doors when closed. All can be cut to size with a large shears or metal snips. Wooden strips may also be used for garage door tops and bottoms.

TYPES OF CAULKING

Caulking does for the body of your house what weatherstripping does for the doors and windows. It plugs up cracks and other defects which let heated air escape and cold, drafty air come in.

Many places in your home are subject to air infiltration—where two different materials come together, where a vertical board meets a horizontal one, where holes were made in the siding, etc. Each of these meeting points has a strong potential for thermal loss.

Chemistry has come to our rescue again, this time with caulking compound, a flexible material designed to seal up cracks and niches. Caulking compound is similar to putty or glazing compound. It comes in tubes or cartridges which fit into a tool called—appropriately enough—a caulking gun.

Caulking compounds are usually divided into four groups:

- *Oil- or resin-based.* Lowest in cost and widely available. These bond to almost any surface, but are not as durable as the others.
- *Latex-, butyl- or polyvinyl-based.* More durable than the first group, but also more expensive.
- *Elastomeric caulks.* The most durable and also the most expensive, with guarantees ranging up to twenty years. Some of these are the silicones, polyurethanes, and polysulfides. They can be a little tricky to apply, so read the labels. Silicone caulk is one of the best, but most brands cannot be painted over.
- *Filler or rope caulk.* Similar to other caulks but reinforced with fiber, cotton, or sponge rubber. These are used for wide cracks or as a backup for the elastomeric types. Oakum is a common fiber type often used to fill larger spaces. Rope caulk comes in rolls and is a good choice where it is difficult to use a caulking gun.

How to Caulk

Insert the cartridge into the caulking gun and cut off the end of the cartridge snout at an angle. The compound should come out in an oval shape. Don't cut off the plastic too near the end, or the bead will be too small, but don't cut too far down, either. The size of the bead can vary with the width of the crack, with a ¼-inch width about average.

The rear of the cartridge is a collapsible cardboard plate. The end of the gun "bolt" presses this cardboard in and forces the caulk out the other end. The bolt is pushed in by hand until it won't go any further. Then the "trigger" is pulled, forcing the bolt in by means of a ratchet on the bottom of the bolt. The bolt won't ratchet until it is in the right position, with the handle pointed down.

The caulk will flow until you disengage the ratchet by turning the bolt handle to the up position and pulling it back. Just taking your finger off the trigger won't stop the action.

When you are ready to start, puncture the end of the cartridge with an extra-long nail or a piece of long, stiff wire stuck deep inside the snout.

If you've never caulked before, though, practice a bit on some scrap lumber or even a piece of newspaper, just to get the hang of it.

Before applying the caulk to any cracks, make sure that they are cleaned out. Use a large screwdriver or putty knife to scrape away dirt, deteriorated old caulk, chipped paint, etc. Hold the gun up to the end of the crack and squeeze the trigger. As the caulk begins to flow, move the gun along the crack as rapidly as necessary to lay an even bead. The bead should cover both sides of the crack.

If the caulk doesn't get into the crack just right—and it might very well not, even after you've had some practice—you can smooth it out with a wet finger. Don't, by the way, try to apply caulk when the weather is cold. The temperature should be at least 45°F.

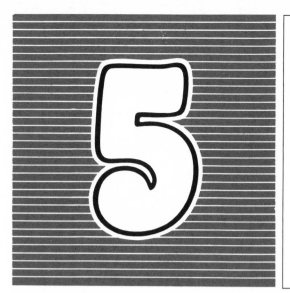

Guarding the Home Front: Temperature Control Room by Room

Carolyn Jabs

If your goal is to feel warm without paying more for the privilege, two indoor strategies can make a tremendous difference. First, choose carefully the territory in which you'll make your stand against cold. Second, eliminate any opportunity for infiltration by the enemy. If the metaphor sounds military, it is. Consider yourself at war with cold, an enemy that regularly uses the draft to win its skirmishes. You must be equally ruthless.

Rather than fighting on every front, choose a few rooms for fortification. Older homes are often so large that you can close off entire sections of the house during the winter without cramping the household. If you don't use the third floor or the "maid's wing," close them up. If you have a choice, shut up rooms on the north side of the house so there will be a barrier of unused space between you and the winter winds. To seal off a room, weatherstrip the door (see below), shutter the windows, and cover the furniture. Close any heating vents and shut off the ducts themselves as close to the furnace as possible. Most important, drain any water pipes servicing the room so they won't freeze and burst.

Of course, many families don't have the luxury of rooms to close. You may, however, find that you can consolidate everyday activities into fewer rooms. For example, if you have a den that is used only once a month for bill paying, consider putting a desk in the bedroom and doing that job there during the winter. If you have a guestroom that is used one weekend a month, don't heat it the rest of the time. If your family eats in the kitchen and uses the dining room for special occasions, install a door so the room can be closed off. For arched doorways and other entranceways in which doors would be difficult to install, hang heavy drapes that can be pulled across the doorway when the room is not in use. Similarly, if your bedrooms are on the second floor, install a door at the bottom of the stairs and keep it closed until an hour before bedtime.

The object of all this is to concentrate the heat you pay for in the rooms you use. Think about it right now. How many rooms in your house are occupied at the moment? How many are you heating? If you can cut one room out of the total being heated, then those you occupy can be that much warmer without costing you a penny more.

CALL IN THE RESERVES

Consolidating your activities in fewer rooms may also mean that you can splurge a little on some heating extras. For example, a portable heater can increase the comfort level significantly—and economically—if used selectively. Try "task heating"—putting the heater where someone needs warmth. Task heating concentrates heat around people so they feel warm even though the room around them may be cool. If you use portable heaters judiciously, you can turn the household heat down without

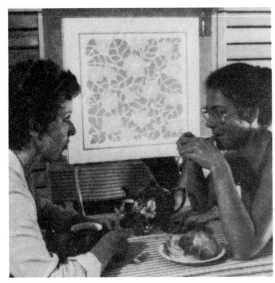

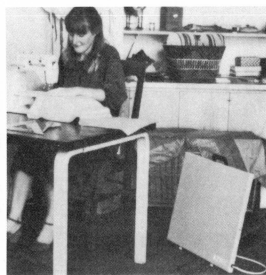

Aztec Radiant Heaters provide heat to a localized area of the house. The wall panel models range from 350 to 500 watts, and come in a variety of decorative styles, or blank white that you can paint yourself. (Aztech International Ltd.)

discomforting the night owl watching the late movie, the student reading at her desk, or the hobbyist working at the kitchen table.

Electric heaters, the usual choice, come in several forms. The standard boxlike heater with a grill on the front produces heat by sending current through a wire which glows red hot. The wire radiates heat to objects in front of the appliance and a fan blows air past the wire, creating convection currents that warm the air in the room. A variation on this theme is the quartz heater, in which the hot wire is enclosed in a quartz tube; this allows it to get much hotter without self-destructing. Quartz heaters don't have fans, so they heat entirely by radiating waves of heat that warm objects in their path. A third type of electric heater is shaped like an old-fashioned radiator. Instead of using water, these heaters are filled with oil, which is heated by the electricity and circulates through the humps in the heater, warming the air around the appliance. Finally, some electric heaters are disguised as flat, decorative panels that hang on the wall and radiate low-level heat.

Box heaters and quartz heaters are widely available in appliance stores. Radiator heaters are harder to find because they are bulky, and panel heaters must usually be ordered directly from companies like Aztech International (2417 Aztec Rd., N.E., Albuquerque, NM 87107). Manufacturers of each type of heater inevitably claim that their product is the cheapest and most efficient, but these claims

are often beside the point. The only way to compare the cost of electric heaters is to know their respective wattages—1500 is typical. Beyond that the cost depends upon the number of hours you run the appliance, which, in turn, depends upon the use to which you put it.

In general, box heaters are the easiest to move around, so they are preferable if you need occasional spot heat in several locations. Quartz heaters focus heat on a narrow area, so they are best for heating a single sitting person or a small tight group of people. Radiator-type heaters warm the air in a room, so they are effective in relatively small closed rooms where the people will be moving from place to place. Panel heaters are stationary and inconspicuous, so they are ideal for locations where you need low-level heat regularly—perhaps above or below a desk or in the bathroom.

Electric heaters do pose some dangers—they can start fires if they are too close to combustibles and they can cause shocks if they are damaged. Still, the heaters are considered safe if used with the same care given to any electrical appliance. The same cannot be said of kerosene heaters. Twenty years ago, many states banned kerosene heaters because they were responsible for fires and deaths by suffocation. Today, the heaters are enjoying renewed popularity largely because manufacturers claim that new technology has made the stoves safer and more efficient. Perhaps, yet a kerosene heater is still a stove without a vent. As the stove operates, it consumes oxygen and gives

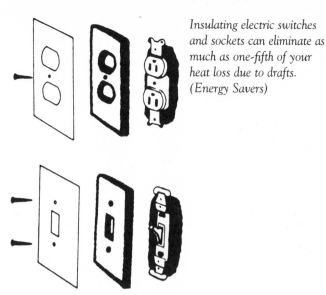

Insulating electric switches and sockets can eliminate as much as one-fifth of your heat loss due to drafts. (Energy Savers)

118 off carbon monoxide. The only way to replenish the oxygen is to ventilate the room, usually by opening a window. That, of course, seems to defeat the purpose of the heater, so people are tempted to use the heaters in closed rooms, creating a dangerous and potentially deadly situation. If you're going to call in the reserves to combat cold, don't count on kerosene heaters.

DRAFT DODGERS

No matter how much heat you pump into a room, the space won't feel warm if there are little eddies of cold air swirling around your ankles or your ears. Drafts have been the bane of householders since the first person thought of putting a partition between a cold space and a warm one. In 1875 the author of a book of household advice complained, "Draughts in the house cause great discomfort and a house is frequently draughty through being constructed on erroneous principles."

Too true. Yet even a well-constructed house can develop drafts through the inevitable process of settling and wear. Quite simply, drafts occur whenever there are holes, gaps, or cracks between cold spaces—like the attic, cellar, garage, or great outdoors—and warm spaces like the one you are sitting in. The obvious solution is to plug the holes, gaps, and cracks. This requires some detective work since every house leaks in different places. Still, there are some predictable trouble spots.

Be suspicious of any hole that has been cut into a wall, ceiling, or floor to accommodate electrical, plumbing, or heating fixtures. Gaps around heating vents may be admitting cold air as well as warm. Small storms may be brewing under the sink, where cold air gushes in around the water pipe. Cold may be seeping into your house around light fixtures and wall sockets. Such problems are easily remedied. Stuff rags into holes around plumbing fixtures. Buy or make little insulation panels to go under the face plates for electrical switches and outlets. Caulk the inevitable cracks that occur where one material meets another.

Caulk, in fact, is the draft dodger's best companion. Once you get the hang of it, caulking cracks is quick, relatively cheap, and very effective. For interior work, you can use an inexpensive oil-base caulk. In the long run, however, you'll probably be happier with a latex caulk because it's less likely to become brittle, cleans up with water, and takes paint nicely. Although you can buy caulk in cans and apply it with a putty knife, most homeowners prefer caulk cartridges which fit into a reusable gun. After locating and cleaning the offending crack, snip the tip off the caulk cartridge and puncture the inner seal. While you move the gun, squeeze the trigger to produce a long and, you hope, even bead of caulk.

Caulk is supposed to flow smoothly at room temperature, but you'll still get blobs and splotches at first. Keep practicing. Since caulk works best if the seal is concave and not con-

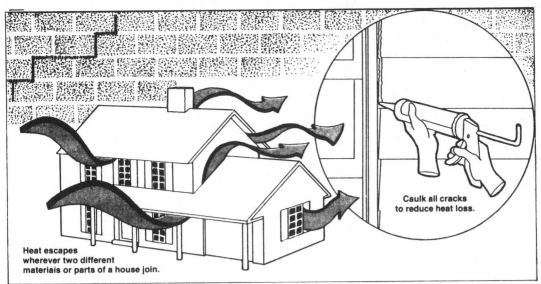

Heat escapes wherever two different materials or parts of a house join.

Caulk all cracks to reduce heat loss.

Cornell University Extension, New York State Energy Office

vex, resist the temptation to run your finger through the caulk to smooth it into the crack. If you have only a few cracks to fill, consider using rope caulk, a less gooey substitute which comes in roles and can be molded to fit all kinds of gaps. Rope caulk can also be removed without difficulty, so it can be used to seal cracks around movable windows.

No matter what kind of caulk you use, wait for a windy day to carry out your search-and-plug mission. To track down drafts, light a candle and take a walk through the house. Watch where the flame flickers. Don't be surprised to find cold air oozing out behind moldings. Moldings, after all, conceal the joint between floor and walls, and that joint may be less than tight. Windows and doors need special attention, too, since both are installed by cutting a hole in the house and slipping in the frame. If the house settles or the frame warps, there may be draft-producing gaps.

WEATHERSTRIPPING TALES

Caulk seals cracks between two immovable surfaces, so it's fine around the frame of a door or a window. But what about the cracks that are necessary if the doors and windows in the house are going to open? Here you need a material that will allow free movement but will still provide a nice tight seal when the door or window is closed. The solution is weatherstripping, a squishy material which compresses a little when the door or window closes against it.

Weatherstripping definitely blocks drafts, so the basic question is not whether but what. A trip to the hardware store reveals a bewildering proliferation of products. The chart on the facing page is not at all comprehensive but it does compare the most commonly available products. Foam and felt are really stopgap measures because they wear out quickly and will have to be replaced in a season or two. The other types can all be effective if they are installed properly. Because weatherstripping has been so widely promoted as an easy do-it-yourself project, many people expect to make quick work of it. Actually, installing weatherstripping properly can be exasperating, so give yourself time to do the job right.

Remember that the object is to have the door or window compress the weatherstripping just a little when closed. If compression isn't firm, you'll still have air leaks. If the weatherstripping presses too tightly on the movable part, you'll have trouble opening and closing the door or window, which will, in turn, wear out the weatherstripping more quickly. The problem is further complicated by the fact that older doors and windows are rarely square, so you must seal a gap that varies in width. The best advice is to do the job on a mild autumn afternoon. Follow the directions on the weatherstripping package and install the strip so the squishy part hangs over the edge of the jamb by just a fraction. Be careful not to twist or stretch the weatherstripping, and use a tack hammer to get into narrow spaces. Check your

		Weatherstripping				
Type	Description	Installation	Visibility	Durability	Price	Comments
Felt	Narrow strips of felt, may have aluminum backing for extra durability	DIY with staples or brads	Varies	NG	Low	Wool is better than other fibers; staples may compress the felt, allowing drafts.
Foam strips	Foam strips in various widths and thicknesses, often with self-adhesive back	DIY—just remove paper and press in place	Varies	NG	Low	Good for sealing cracks that vary in width.
Wood strips	Look like molding edged with felt, foam, or vinyl	DIY—nail molding to door or window jamb	Looks like molding when painted	Varies		Must be painted.
Vinyl tube	Molded vinyl with flat strip for nailing and tube for sealing crack	DIY—nail flat strip to jamb	High	Good	Mod.	Difficult to get a firm fit unless gasket has metal or wood backing.
Spring metal	Aluminum or bronze strip bent just enough to seal gap	DIY—need tin snip, hammer, and nails	None	Good	Mod.	Cannot seal a gap that isn't uniform; may whistle in wind.
V or J strips	Interlocking strips of metal, for doors only; must be installed on door and jamb	Difficult to install—usually best done by a carpenter	None	Good	High	Very good protection but difficult to install on older doors that are worn or warped; often found in new homes.

work as you go by opening and closing the door or window to make sure the seal is tight.

DEFEND YOUR DOOR

Weatherstripping may seal the sides and top of your door, but it's useless on the bottom where scuffling feet will make short work of felt, foam, or even spring metal. Chances are good that scuffling feet have already worn down the threshold in an older home, so you

TYPE		COST	DURABILITY	COMMENTS
Sweep	DOOR / SILL	Least expensive	1 to 2 years.	Visible, for use on flat thresholds. May drag on rug.
Door Shoe	DOOR / SILL	Moderate cost.	Indefinite. Vinyl insert replaceable.	Useful on wood, unworn threshold. Note drip cap to shed rain.
Vinyl Bulb Threshold	DOOR / SILL	Moderate cost	Indefinite. Vinyl insert replacement.	Useful where there is no threshold. With wear, vinyl bubble will flatten and tear. Can be replaced.
Interlocking Threshold	DOOR / SILL	Most expensive	Permanent.	Exceptionally good seal. Should be recommended.

may need to replace it altogether. If you have a carpenter do the job, ask him to install an interlocking threshold. This is a delicate job that requires precise alignment if the hook attached to the bottom of the door is going to catch the tab on the threshold, but when properly installed, the seal on an interlocking threshold is excellent.

For do-it-yourselfers, lumberyards sell specially milled oak for thresholds. Or you can get a vinyl gasket threshold—threshold and weatherstripping in one package. In this setup, you replace the wooden threshold with a metal molding that has a broad vinyl bump running down the center. The door bottom is planed at a light angle so it presses the vinyl when it's closed. A variation is the door shoe, a metal molding with a vinyl gasket that clamps on the bottom of the door. If the gap under your door is very large, you may be able to install the shoe without removing the door. Most doors, however, must be unhinged and planed on the bottom before the shoe is attached. The advantage, of course, is that a gasket on the bottom of the door receives less wear than one on the threshold.

Perhaps the simplest under-door weatherstripping is a "sweep," a metal strip attached to a strip of felt, vinyl, or rubber. The sweep is screwed to the face of the door so the flexible part just brushes the floor and seals the crack. Though the sweep doesn't look particularly good, it can be installed without taking the door down. Install an automatic sweep with a flexible part that retracts when the door opens if you have carpet in your entranceway that might make it difficult for a door with a sweep to open.

Every door that separates a warm space from a cold one needs to be weatherstripped. In addition to the entrance doors, seal doors to the attic, basement, garage, large closets or cupboards, and rooms you don't want to heat. For basement and attic doors consider hanging a packing blanket behind the door as an extra layer of protection. For interior doors that aren't opened very often, elaborate thresholds aren't necessary. Instead, borrow a trick from our inventive ancestors and make "dust puppies." Sew up a narrow tube of fabric as long as the door is wide. Fill the tube with just enough sand so that it's still floppy, and close both ends. Snuggle the dust puppy next to the door so it covers the crack at the bottom. If you don't want to make your own dust puppies, you can probably buy them from crafts shops, where they've enjoyed a revival as a quaint and practical piece of Americana. Last but not least, don't forget to tape or plug unused keyholes.

Even after weatherstripping your doors, you haven't eliminated the threat they pose to your comfort. Every time a door between a cold place and a warm place opens, icy air rushes in. You can minimize the problem if you limit the number of times each door is opened and the amount of time it remains open. Try to have people enter and leave the house in

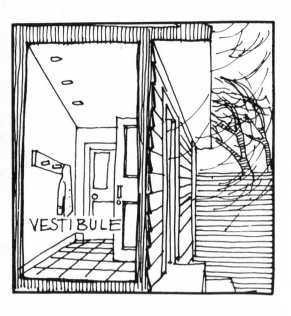

VESTIBULE

An air lock or stormhouse will keep cold winds from blowing directly into the house whenever you enter or exit. (U.S. Department of Energy)

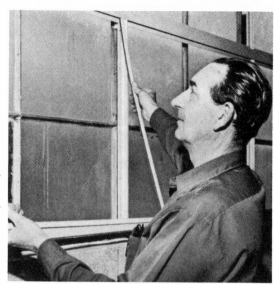

Adding a second layer of glass to your windows creates an insulating layer of dead air between your interior window and the cold. (Thermatrol Energy Systems)

122 groups. Save up errands for the cellar or garage so you don't have to pop in and out several times a day. Consider installing a spring or pneumatic mechanism on exterior doors so they snap shut even if your hands are full of firewood or groceries.

None of these tactics will do much good if the wind has direct access to your entranceway. Hanging a storm door may keep heat inside when the door is closed, but it doesn't help much when the door has to be opened. The best way to hold back the cold air that tries to force its way into the house each time a door is opened is an air lock. An air lock is created by having two entrance doors separated by a space large enough for one and perhaps more people to stand. A person can come into the air lock and close the exterior door entirely before opening the door to the house. Wind and snow may make it through the first door, but they'll never get into the house itself.

Older homes usually have some kind of air lock. Country houses often include a mudroom, ostensibly a place for storing firewood, boots, and other winter paraphernalia. In fact, the mudroom, which is usually uninsulated, is an excellent air lock. Town houses often have a front hall with doors leading to the various rooms. As long as the doors are closed, the hall itself functions as an air lock. An attached garage or an open porch screened for the winter with shutters or sheets of plastic can serve the same purpose.

Unfortunately, newer homes rarely have mudrooms, closed hallways, or porches. In fact, many have a front door flush with the front of the house, an arrangement that gives the wind a straight shot inside. In very severe climates, some people remedy this problem by building a storm house, a small portable plywood structure that resembles a guardhouse outside Buckingham Palace. The storm house fastens right over the house's most used entrance during the winter and can be removed during the summer. A storm house can, of course, be added to a home permanently. Insulation is unnecessary since the space won't be heated. Attach the storm house to the main house with L-brackets and caulk around the juncture with rope caulk. All in all, a storm house is a cumbersome solution to a problem that shouldn't occur in a house built with respect for its surroundings.

If possible, don't locate or use entrance doors on the north or west sides of the house, which are generally colder. Provide an air lock inside the house, and landscape around the doorway to baffle the wind. A dense clump of evergreens or a decorative wall outside the door will, at least, blunt the power of the wind.

Window Tactics

When it comes to the fight against cold, windows are double agents. They admit light, which makes us feel warmer, and solar radiation, which actually can raise indoor temperatures a degree or two. Even the stupidest house cat can tell you how cozy it is to sleep on a

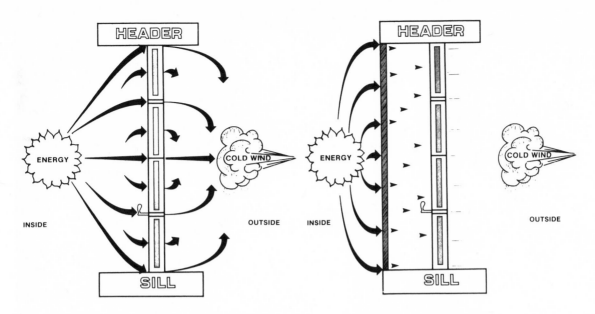

windowsill in a pool of winter sunshine. Let the sun go down, however, and that same window will betray you, letting cold in and heat out with virtually no resistance. The problem, of course, is that glass is a poor insulator, which means that even after you've weather-stripped and caulked, your windows are still robbing you of precious warmth. An insulated wall has an R-value of at least 11, and 19 is recommended (the R-factor represents the resistance of any material to the outflow of heat.) The average double-glazed window, on the other hand, has an R-value of 2, which means that you lose ten times as much heat through the window as through the wall. Furthermore, air that touches the glass cools and sinks, setting up a convection current that can chill the air in an entire room.

So what's a homeowner to do? No one is going to give up windows, though energy experts estimate that you could save 70 percent of your heating bill by living in a house without any openings. Fortunately, contemporary homeowners are being saved from such drastic expedients by some very clever energy inventors who have turned their attention to windows and come up with ingenious solutions.

In the recent past, the most effective way to insulate a window was with dead air space, and that's still a good front-line strategy. To create dead air space, you need an extra layer of glass or plastic fastened over the basic window. Although many people cover windows with sheets of polyethylene fastened down with strips of wood, plastic is, at best, a stopgap. Aside from being difficult to see through, plastic is vulnerable to wind damage and cuts heat loss no more than 10 percent.

A second layer of glass is better protection for a window. In older homes, this means covering double-hung windows with a storm window that must be removed each spring. Although such windows are unwieldy, they are effective when they fit tightly. If you have them, take care of them, painting them periodically and replacing any cracked or broken panels. Every couple of years, check the glazing compound around the panes. When it starts to crack and fall out, it leaves gaps around the glass. To repair the window, clean out the old putty and replace the points which hold the glass if they've come loose. Purchase glazing compound, not putty, and roll a gob of it between your hands until it becomes a long thin rope. Press the rope into the right angle between the glass and the wood frame to make a tight seal.

Many modern windows have the screen and storm window on tracks in one unit. As long as the storm window doesn't rattle in the wind, you can be sure the air between the windows is functioning like insulation. Casement and picture windows usually don't have storm windows because they are made of thermal glass, which has more than one panel of glass separated by a narrow air space. Although double-glazed windows are most common, contractors in very cold climates sometimes recommend

123

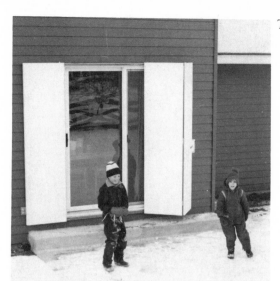

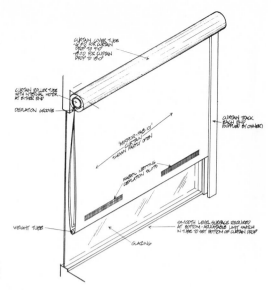

The Self-Inflating Curtain
Wall

124   triple glazing. In addition, some manufacturers now sell clip-on plastic panels to go over double-glazed windows. One product called the Insider is a sheet of acrylic that fastens to the window with an adhesive-backed vinyl track. Also available are interior storm windows made of thermal plastic. Products like Thermatrol (Perkasie Industries, 50 East Spruce Street, Perkasie, PA 18944) or Defender 1 (Defender Energy Corporation, Mahopac, NY 10541) consist of plastic panels which snap into tracks installed directly on the window frame.

The object behind all these strategies is to create a dead air space that will turn back at least some of the warmth that's trying to escape through your windows. Adding a pane of glass or plastic doubles a window's resistance to heat flow, but the total R-value is still only 2, which is pathetic by contemporary standards. Even colonial standards were apparently higher, since early American homeowners regularly used shutters to run windows into walls at night and during storms. Today, too many American homeowners treat shutters as quaint ornaments rather than practical devices for keeping warmth inside the house. Europeans are way ahead of us here. Many of their homes are equipped with functional shutters, including Rolladen shutters which are made of interlocking slats that can be rolled up during the day. As if to prove that Yankee ingenuity still lives, a few American architects are now experimenting with exterior shutters that slide on tracks or open on hinges attached at the top, bottom, or sides of the window. The Thermafold shutter, for example, closes over a glass patio and, like most of the new shutters, can be opened and closed from indoors.

Although exterior shutters can certainly cut the loss of heat through windows, they are expensive and labor intensive, so many homeowners are experimenting with interior window treatments that will make rooms look as well as feel warmer. Most of the new designs marry old ideas like shutters, shades, and curtains to new materials like fiberfill, reflective plastic, and rigid insulation. They also strive to create a layer of dead air space against the window by sealing the edges of the protective material against the window frame. Most traditional window treatments do just the opposite. By leaving space at top and bottom, they create a tunnel which encourages warm air to slip in at the top, slide down the window, losing heat as it goes, and emerge at the bottom as a chilly draft. The new window treatments try to eliminate such convection currents.

They also take advantage of elementary solar theory, using the windows as low-grade solar collectors. In fact, before you rush out to dress your windows in the latest thermal fashions, consider their orientations. Northern windows don't get any direct sun in the winter, and because they are in the shadow of the house, the air outside is always cold. Unless the view is special, consider installing semipermanent protection or even closing up northern win-

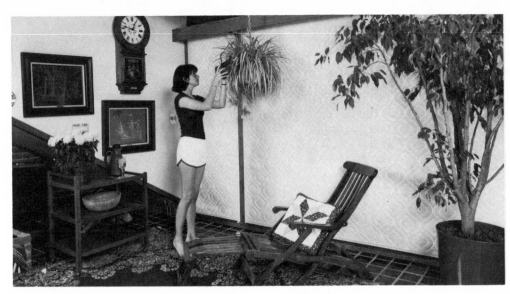

The Window Quilt

dows altogether in the cold months. In contrast, southern windows enjoy full sun during the winter in the northern hemisphere. If you are thinking about replacing leaky old windows, consider enlarging the windows on the southern exposure. If you plan to install some sort of movable insulation that will insulate the windows at night, consider the fact that southern windows can be single-glazed so they will absorb more of the sun's radiation. Eastern and western windows get moderate winter sunlight, so they too can benefit from movable insulation. Protect the west windows first because they are likely to get hit by winter winds.

One of the simplest types of protection is a shade that can be pulled down at night and rolled up during the day. Even the dimestore variety cuts heat loss 25 percent when it is installed one inch from the window and cut to fit the window frame precisely. To maximize its thermal properties, the shade should be mounted inside the window frame so it rolls toward the window. You can further increase its protection value by making tracks for the sides of the shade from slats of wood. Weight the bottom of the shade so it will sit firmly on a strip of weatherstripping you install on the sill, and install a metal V-strip between the roller and the top of the frame. Window shades become even more effective if they reflect heat back into the room. You can create this effect by covering a standard shade with a reflective material like Mylar or Foylon. Or you can purchase special solar shades like those manufac-

tured by Sun Control Products, Inc. (431 Fourth Avenue SE, Rochester, MN 55901).

Several companies have improved upon the conventional window shade by combining layers of insulating material separated by air space or fiberfill. The Window Quilt made by Appropriate Technology Corporation (P.O. Box 975, Brattleboro, VT 05301) consists of a layer of reflective plastic sandwiched between layers of fiberfill and fabric. The five layers are "quilted" together and provide an R-value of about 3.5. The IS High R Shade also consists of five layers, but they are separated by curved plastic strips that hold the layers apart when the shade is down. Made by the Insulating Shade Company (P.O. Box 282, Brandford, CT 06405), the shade has an R-value of over 10. Similar R-values are claimed for the Self-Inflating Curtain Wall available from Thermal Technology Corporation (P.O. Box 130, Snowmass, CO 81654) and the Independence 10 available from Defender Energy Corporation, Route 6, Mahopac, NY 10541.

Some energetic homeowners make their own insulated shades by machine quilting layers of fabric with a layer of reflective plastic like Foylon (made by Duracote) and a layer of fiberfill like Thinsulate (made by 3M). If the shade is to roll smoothly, the total thickness can't be much more than half an inch. Just as important, the sides of the shade must fit snugly against the window frame. Some people use hinged slats of wood that clamp over the edges of the shade when it is rolled down. Oth-

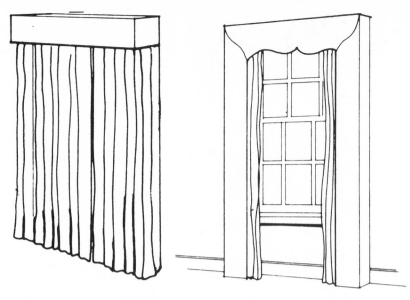

A closed cornice covering the drapery rod will greatly improve the heat retention of drapes (left); a lambrequin (right), by enclosing the drapes from rod to floor, will do even better. (Cornell University Extension, New York State Energy Office)

126 ers finish the edge of the shade by wrapping the material around a cord which moves up and down a sail-track slot (available from Appropriate Technologies). Still others sew Velcro or magnetic tape to the edge of the shade and glue matching strips to the window frame. Detailed instructions for making a quilted window shade are included in *Movable Insulation* by William K. Langdon.

The insulation value of a window shade depends upon its thickness, yet it is difficult to roll thick shades on conventional rollers. For that reason, many homeowners prefer Roman shades made of insulating fabric that is pulled into loose folds at the top of the window. Like the shade described above, the Roman shade starts with an outer layer of decorative fabric and a layer of reflective plastic. The fiberfill, however, can be one to three layers thick. The Roman shade is tied with quilting knots at 8-inch intervals rather than machine quilting. Each knot ties a plastic ring to the back of the shade. When the shade is installed, cords run through the plastic rings so the shade can be raised and lowered. Detailed instructions for building a Roman shade as well as kits come from Creative Energy Products (1053 Williamson Street, Madison, WI 53703).

Even homeowners who install protective shades often want drapes for their decorative value. Although drapes have been touted as an aid to heat conservation, their value is negligible when they are conventionally hung. The easiest way to improve the heat retention of

WINDOW READING

In the average home, windows occupy 10 percent of the surface area and lose 25–50 percent of the heat generated inside. No wonder energy experts are working hard to find new ways to make windows energy efficient. Innovative designs and products are appearing at a rapid rate, and consumers who are contemplating large investments in window protection will want to evaluate as many of them as possible. Two good books on the subject are available: *Movable Insulation* **by William K. Langdon (Rodale Press, 1980) and** *Thermal Shutters and Shades* **by William A. Shurcliff (Brick House Publishing, 1981).**

drapes is to stop air from circulating behind them by installing a closed cornice or valance covering the drapery rod. To carry the idea a step further, build a lambrequin by extending the valance down both sides of the window so the entire frame is enclosed in a decorative box. Although lambrequins can look very elegant when they are painted, papered, or covered with fabric to match the furnishings, they are too stylized for many contemporary rooms. To get similar results, simply tack the drapery fabric to the window frame on either side. It's also important that drapes overlap at the center by at least four inches. You may want to close the center gap by sewing Velcro or magnetic tape to both panels. The bottom of the

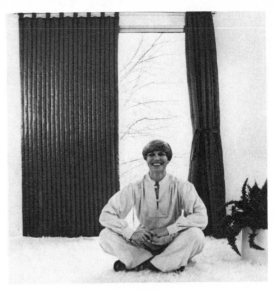

drape is often the most difficult part to seal. If the drape touches the floor, use chain or drapery weights in the hem to hold it firmly in place. Otherwise, use Velcro or magnetic strips to fasten it to the window sill.

After eliminating air currents, you can turn to the more interesting question of fabric. Many so-called thermal drapes are backed with a stiff plastic material that is not very attractive and can, in some cases, crumble after a year or two in the sun. You're better off with a standard lined drape, which will at least produce a layer of still air between the drape and the liner. Or consider lining the drape with one of the new insulating materials such as Astrolon, a reflective fabric. Another possibility is the Warm-in Drapery Liner, which is made from polyethylene bubbles and is available from Conservation Concepts (Box 376, Stratton Mountain, VT 05155). Another attractive idea comes from the Window Blanket Company (Route 7, Lenoir City, TN 37771), which sells a fiber-filled quilt designed to hang like a curtain. For very large expanses of glass in a solar home, consider the Sun Quilt (Box 374, Newport, NH 03772), which was designed for greenhouses and has an R-value of 5.9.

Because specially designed drapes and shades are expensive, many people want window protection that they can make themselves to supplement whatever drapes they may already have. The best solution is insulated pop-in panels. Although some people cut their panels from aluminum-faced beadboard, you'll get a more durable panel if you make a sandwich from quarter-inch plywood fastened with screws to an inner frame of 1 x 2s. The hollow core of the panel can be filled with an insulating material ranging from corrugated cardboard or mineral wool to polystyrene board. The side of the panel that faces the room can be papered, painted, treated as a bulletin board, or covered with a poster.

Some people recommend attaching pop-in panels directly to the window panes with magnetic Night Clips available from Zomeworks (P.O. Box 712, Albuquerque, NM 87103). For most windows, however, it is simpler to prepare a single panel that fits into the window frame. Such a panel must fit precisely and can be held in place with magnetic strips, spring fingers (also available from Zomeworks), or butterfly latches. Most people remove pop-in panels to admit sunlight during the day. Since storing the panels can be awkward, some devise track systems so the panels can slip to the side of the window and others hinge the panels to make attractive shutters. Ready-made shutters can also be purchased from companies like Vermont Thermal Shutter (RD 2, Woodstock, VT 05091). Their wood shutter has a core of insulation so its R-value is 8.

The idea of making windows as resistant to the flow of heat as walls is relatively new, so new products are being developed rapidly. Some are rather dramatic. The Beadwall, created by Zomeworks (address above), consists of

128 two layers of glass separated by several inches. A vacuum system pumps polystyrene beads into the space to insulate it at night and then sucks them out during the day. Exciting as such ideas are, consumers need to be cautious. Some new products suffer from design flaws which make them inconvenient or inefficient. Their inventors usually work out these problems within a year or two but that's small comfort to the homeowner who bought in the first rush of enthusiasm. In other words, check out new products as carefully as possible. Ask for R-values determined by an independent laboratory, and request names of previous customers so you can ask them about the system. If possible, see the system installed so you can try your hand at operating it. Most energy-efficient window treatments require your participation, so you should decide in advance whether you're willing to do what's required.

WARM WALLS AND FLOORS AND FURNITURE

Plugging cracks, weatherstripping doors, and covering windows may win the war against cold, but will they make the house feel warm? Not necessarily. It's no accident that the word "warmth" refers to an emotional as well as a physical condition. To make your house feel warm, you have to consider psychology as well as temperature.

If you doubt that fact, consider a study spon-sored by the American Society of Heating, Refrigerating and Air Conditioning Engineers. Researchers at Kansas State University put subjects in two rooms and asked them to iden-tify the temperature that felt "comfortable." Subjects in a sparsley furnished room decorated with light colors didn't feel warm until the temperature hit 69°F, but subjects in a carpeted room decorated with bright colors, rough tex-tures, and overstuffed furniture felt comfy at 65°F.

To replicate these results in your own home, start with the furniture. Upholstered furniture seems warmer and you should indulge yourself in fuzzy, furry fabrics because the texture traps warm air. Metal, wood, canvas, leather, and plastic feel cold, so consider covering chairs and other seats made of these materials with nubby slipcovers. At the very least, smother such furniture in pillows and throws.

The arrangement of furniture can be as im-portant as its composition. Don't let chairs and sofas block heating vents. In fact, move them away from exterior walls whenever possible. If there's space, group sofas and chairs in conver-sational units at the center of the room. A semicircle of chairs around a stove or fireplace is particularly cozy, especially if you have wing chairs, which catch the heat.

Floors, walls, and ceilings deserve your at-tention, too. Carpets have some insulation value, especially when they are placed over a bonded urethane pad. Remember that the thickness of the fiber is more important than

Is Wetter Warmer? The Question of Humidity

For years, people have believed that a dry house is a cold house because dry air allows moisture to evaporate from the skin, creating a feeling of cold. Today, many researchers dispute that idea, arguing that there is no physiological sensation of cold until the air is much drier than it ever gets inside the average home. Regardless of whether it makes you warmer, humidity does contribute to winter comfort because your furniture, skin, and nasal passages are less likely to dry out.

The simplest way to put moisture into the air is to attach a humidifier to the furnace. The job, which must be done by a professional, costs between $150 and $300. A less expensive and less convenient alternative is a free-standing humidifier. Look for a model that's quiet, easy to fill, and equipped with a humidistat so it will turn itself off when the air is humid enough. Most important, the tank of the humidifier must be easily accessible so it can be cleaned once a week. The warm, moist conditions in the tank encourage the growth of scale, bacteria, and fungi which can then be released into the air. Breathing the contaminated air causes a condition called "humidifier fever" which may result in permanent lung damage.

If you don't like the idea of an energy-consuming humidifier, there are other ways to get moisture in the air. Leave shallow pans of water near heat vents, on the woodstove, or under houseplants. After you finish your bath, leave the hot water in the bathtub to evaporate, and open the bathroom door after a steamy shower. Consider venting your electric clothes drier into the house, or string up a clothesline and hang up some wet clothes to dry indoors. Mist your houseplants, and don't use your kitchen vent when you're boiling soup or steaming vegetables.

its composition—acrylic and wool can be equally warm. For walls, take a tip from sixteenth-century castle owners who hung tapestries to take the chill off their stone walls. Cover the inside of exterior walls with cork, fabric, even carpet. Or use fiber wall hangings, quilts, and "fabrications" as graphic accents. As for ceilings, stand on a chair some winter evening and you'll be shocked at the warmth of the air at the top of the room. High ceilings may be chic, but they aren't conducive to comfort. You may want to take advantage of high temperatures in high places by building a loftbed. Otherwise, consider dropping the ceiling with one of the prefab bracket systems that are so widely available.

Of course, the colors you use in decorating the walls, floors, and ceiling can effect how warm a room feels. Color, however, is prob-

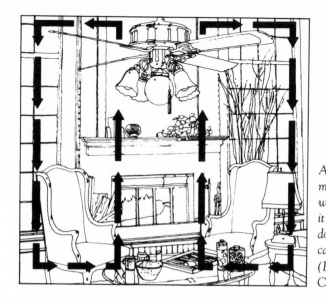

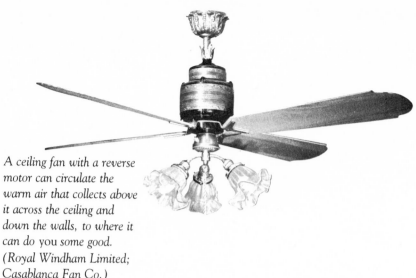

A ceiling fan with a reverse motor can circulate the warm air that collects above it across the ceiling and down the walls, to where it can do you some good. (Royal Windham Limited; Casablanca Fan Co.)

130 lematic. The red, pink, and orange that make you feel comfortable in the winter may seem claustrophobic in the summer. One solution is to keep the permanent parts of the room neutral and to introduce colors appropriate to the season in slipcovers, curtains, throw rugs, and pillows.

Finally, remember a few tricks for directing warm air and deflecting cold air. Heating vents should be cleaned regularly so the heat flows easily. Vents under windows should be equipped with deflectors that will direct the warm air into the room. Folding screens are easy to make and can deflect drafts if they are installed between a door or window and the occupants of the room. And last but not least, don't neglect the lowly footstool—it keeps your feet off the floor where drafts are most likely to lurk.

PIPING HOT PIPES

New heating strategies can mean plumbing problems. If you've figured out how to keep the heat concentrated in your living areas, your cellar may be getting colder than it used to. Water in pipes and pumps will, of course, freeze if the temperature dips below 32°F. At best, this means the inconvenience of rising one frosty morning and having no water for flushing, brushing, or making coffee. At worst, the pipes actually split open because water expands as it freezes.

To spare yourself the large bill and larger mess of frozen plumbing, protect your pipes. In moderate climates, simply insulate any pipes that are isolated from a heat source or located on outer walls. Pipe insulation comes in three common forms—long plastic tubes with "Ziplocs" on one side, narrow rolls of foam faced with foil, and fiberglass which must be wrapped around the pipes and then covered with plastic to keep it from getting wet. The tubes are the easiest to install but the most expensive.

In more severe climates, install heat tape, a ribbon of plastic with an electric heating element inside. Simply wrap the tape around the pipe, using electrician's tape to secure it, and cover it with fiberglass insulation. The number of coils per foot determines the temperature to which you are protected (see the package), and the best tapes have thermostats so they go on only when the temperature drops below 40°F.

If all this sounds like too much work, you might at least hook up an alarm like those greenhouse owners use in the vicinity of the most vulnerable pipes and water pump. That way you'll know when the temperature dips dangerously close to freezing and can move in auxiliary heaters. You'll have to bring in heat of some kind if the pipes do freeze. If you still have a source of water, try wrapping towels around the pipes, setting basins underneath, and pouring boiling water on the towels. Using a propane torch is quick but dangerous. Not only do you risk a fire when you have no water but you may melt the solder between pipes.

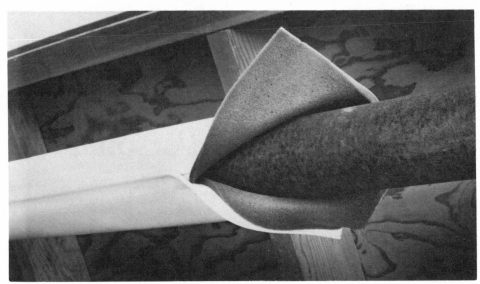

(Obviously, you can't even consider using a torch on plastic pipes!) An effective but slow solution is to warm the pipes with an electrical appliance—a space heater, a heat lamp, a blanket, a heating pad, hot air blown from a hair dryer, or the exhaust end of a vacuum cleaner.

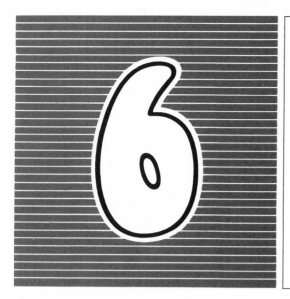

The Cold Warrior: Strategy and Tactics for Personal Warmth

Carolyn Jabs

132   Even after you've installed the most efficient heating system and insulated to the rafters, you still have to set the thermostat. In most homes, lower means savings, higher means comfort. Balance that subjective feeling of "warmth" against cold cash, and the subjective feeling will win hands down. Government researchers drew that conclusion after correlating the amount of fuel used by families with the families' "comfort needs." People who felt comfortable at 65°F used less fuel than those who shivered until the temperature hit 70°F.

It's no use telling people they *should* feel comfortable at 65°F. Comfort is comfort. You have it or you don't. True, your comfort needs can change. The process is called acclimatization, and it occurs gradually after repeated exposure to the uncomfortable temperature. Anyone who doubts that acclimatization is possible only has to look at American homes in the 1930s, when the standard temperature was 65°F and everyone felt just fine. For the past fifty years, we have been adjusting to ever higher temperatures until now many of us don't feel comfortable in rooms under 70°F.

So what do we do while we're waiting for this process to reverse itself? There are two strategies for feeling comfortable in cooler houses. One is to manage our body heat better so we will be warm physically, and the other is to indulge ourselves in small pleasures that make us feel warm psychologically. Hand in hand, these strategies can lower anyone's comfort threshold several degrees.

The most undervalued energy resource in most homes is body heat. The human body is an efficient furnace, keeping itself at a constant 98.6°F by producing approximately 390 Btus per hour if it's male and 330 Btus per hour if it's female. To take advantage of all this heat, we need to insulate our bodies as well as we insulate our houses. Some people object to the idea of personal insulation because they fear that it will make them feel and look like an overstuffed teddy bear. Actually, the object of indoor dressing should be insulation and mobility since activity is the best way to increase the body's heat production.

INDOOR WARMTH

By now everyone knows that you should dress in layers because layers trap air and air insulates your body. What you may not know are the numbers. The Department of Energy estimates that wearing one heavy sweater will allow you to lower the temperature three and a half degrees and still feel comfortable. Wearing two medium-weight sweaters will feel less bulky and will allow you to lower the thermostat a full 5° without feeling any cooler.

How you put your layers together is largely a matter of personal style. Still, scientists have come up with some guidelines about the insulation value of various articles of clothing. Using heated copper dummies, scientists can measure how well different garments trap heat.

To calculate the clo value of an outfit add up the values assigned to each article of clothing.

Briefs or panties	0.05	Cool shirt or blouse, long sleeves	0.21
Warm tights	0.25	Medium-warm shirt or blouse	0.25
Short-sleeved undershirt	0.09	Warm shirt or blouse	0.29
Full slip	0.19	Long-sleeved knit shirt	0.37
Long-underwear top	0.25	Medium-warm trousers	0.29
Long-underwear bottoms	0.25	Warm trousers	0.32
Thermal top	0.35	Medium-warm slacks	0.35
Thermal bottoms	0.35	Warm slacks	0.44
Warm socks	0.04	Medium-warm skirt	0.16
Light socks	0.03	Warm skirt	0.22
Warm knee socks	0.08	Medium-warm vest	0.22
Low shoes or pumps	0.04	Warm vest	0.30
High shoes	0.15	Medium-warm sweater	0.27
Lined knee-high boots	0.30	Warm sweater	0.37
Medium-weight dress	0.48	Jacket or blazer	0.17
long sleeves, below knee		Medium-warm suit coat	0.35
Warm dress	0.72	Warm suit coat	0.49
long sleeves, below knee		Cool shawl	0.30
		Warm shawl	0.40

They express the results in clos, the amount of insulation needed to keep a resting body at 98.6°F in a 70° room. One clo is approximately equal to a man's business suit. As you can see from the chart, clo ratings confirm what common sense told you long ago—a sweater is warmer than a shirt, pants are warmer than a skirt, and so on. Nonetheless, if you know the number of clos required to make you feel warm at a particular temperature, you can decide whether a particular outfit is appropriate by adding up the clo values of its components.

	Clo Comfort Requirements	
	Room Temperature	
Activity	65°–68°F	68°–70°F
Seated quietly: eating, writing, reading	1.6–2.0	1.4–1.6
Light activity: typing, dressing	1.2–1.5	1.1–1.4
Moderate activity: dishwashing, shaving	0.9–1.1	0.6–0.8
Heavy activity: cleaning, laundry	0.5–0.8	0.5–0.5

The clo chart also contradicts popular wis-

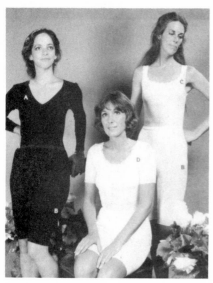

Winter is no time for skimpy underwear. These wool undershirts and knee-length snuggies from Hanro of Switzerland are perfect for women who want to keep warm but don't care for union suits. (Garnet Hill)

134 dom about the superior insulation value of natural fibers, particularly wool. Although wool's absorbency may make it preferable in outerwear, indoors the warmth of the fabric is determined by its ability to trap air. Practically, that translates into thickness and fuzziness. Brushed nylon pajamas are warmer than cotton broadcloth, a flannel shirt is warmer than a cotton one, and a thick acrylic sweater feels just as warm as a wool sweater of equal thickness. Synthetic fibers are, of course, cheaper and easier to clean. Despite this evidence, many people cling to the mystique of wool. Even the United States Department of Energy claims that the "warmest" sweaters are Icelandic, Shetland, and regulation Navy wool (available at surplus stores). If you can afford a wool wardrobe and are convinced that it is warmer, by all means wear it, since believing you're warm is half the battle. On the other hand, clothing made from other fibers can be equally warm if the fabric is springy and thick. Check for loft—does the fabric spring back when you squeeze it—and nap—does the texture of the fabric allow for lots of little air pockets?

The one exception to the any-fabric rule is underwear. Since your body is constantly giving off moisture, you need a skinside fabric to absorb it if you want to maintain your body heat. Cotton, silk, rayon, and wool are preferred. And while we're on the subject of underwear, don't relegate your long johns to the outdoor drawer. Lightweight long underwear is the ideal foundation for an indoor wardrobe.

One-piece union suits are good because they don't gap between shirt and pants, however, they are inconvenient in other ways. Every department store offers a selection of long underwear for people of all ages. Pure-cotton and pure-wool long johns are available from Garnet Hill (Franconia, NH 03580), a company whose catalogue also shows thermal garments which are simultaneously warm and sexy, for women. Women who prefer not to wear such garments can get similar results from a camisole and a pair of heavy tights.

After the long underwear, consider your torso. Because it houses your vital organs, it gets first claim on body heat. If you can keep your torso toasty, your body will be less stingy about sending heat to your arms and legs. Start with a shirt and dickey or a turtleneck. Add a pullover that fits comfortably over the first layers. Top the ensemble off with a cardigan, if necessary—or a vest. Many people find that down vests are as good at keeping the torso warm indoors as out. Remember that sweaters should be hip length and shirts should have long tails so you aren't exposed every time you bend over.

On the lower half of your body, pants are clearly the best bet. Slightly baggy corduroy or wool pants will be warmer than tight cotton jeans. If your legs need further protection, take a tip from professional dancers, who pull on knitted tubes of fabric called leg warmers. Women who insist on wearing skirts around the house should make them as long as pos-

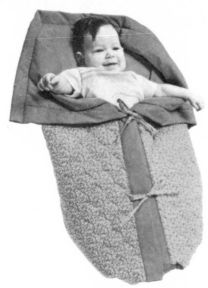

Old-fashioned baby buntings will keep little ones warm and cozy. (Frostline Kits)

BABY, IT'S COLD OUTSIDE (AND INSIDE)

Most doctors agree that small children cope just fine with temperatures between 66° and 68°F. In fact, infants often suffer from overheating because they are bundled too heavily by overprotective parents. Cold hands are not an indication of a cold baby; loss of facial color may be.

Toddlers are a bigger problem because they play on the floor, where the air is likely to be coldest. Dress them in layers, buying clothes in various sizes so they fit comfortably over the underlayers. Look for quilted overalls—cute and warm—and reinforce the knees with iron-on patches inside or out. Tights are a good lining for both boys and girls. At night, a one-piece sleeper is the best way to be sure that little bodies stay covered. Remember that dirt and moisture reduce the insulation value of fabric, so keep the kids' clothes as clean and dry as possible.

There are several devices to keep mittens (warmer and easier than gloves) on small hands, from store-bought clips to homemade strings that attach to one mitten, go up through one sleeve, down through the other, and come out at the other mitten. Most are no match for a determined toddler, so always be watchful.

Coats with hoods are very warm, especially with hats under them. Knot the hood drawstrings a few extra times to keep

them from slipping through the eyelets and disappearing forever. A waterproof fabric is best, and look for tight wrists or internal wristlets. A scarf will keep a tender chin toasty on a cold day.

Boots, again waterproof, should be at least a size too large, to fit over shoes. Nursery school hint: Put plastic bags over shoes to smooth the way into boots.

For infants there are indeed baby buntings —one-piece coveralls that zip or fasten to the neck. And a waterproof cover can be snapped over many baby carriages and strollers.

sible. A floor-length skirt is almost as warm as pants. Similarly, if you like to lounge in a bathrobe, lounge warmly in a floor-length robe.

If you've packaged your torso properly, your extremities should stay warm—unless you smoke, drink, or suffer from circulation problems, which often accompany aging. Even if they are evidence of a warm heart, cold feet are a misery. Eliminate them by layering. Start with socks. You'll need at least two pairs—a thin underlayer and a bulky overlayer. Your ordinary shoes won't fit over two pairs of socks, and you'll defeat your purpose if you slow down circulation by cramming your feet into them. Instead, invest in a pair of winter shoes large enough to fit over the socks you need to feel warm. Better yet, buy slipper socks with leather soles or fleece-lined slippers. A nice

The Cold Warrior

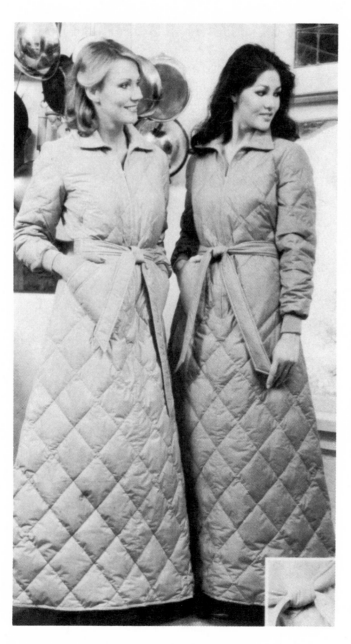

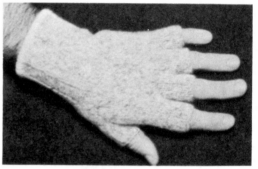

Floor-length goose down robes. (Eddie Bauer)

Fingerless gloves allow for a maximum of warmth and dexterity. (Eddie Bauer)

Undershirt and knee-length briefs, cut to fit easily under any business suit. (L. L. Bean)

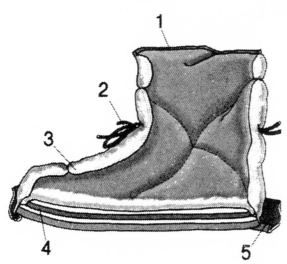

Down booties—quilts for your feet: (1) nylon upper, (2) drawcord closure, (3) goose down insulation, (4) three-layer insole, (5) leather-edged foam sole. (Eddie Bauer)

selection is available from French Creek Sheep and Wool Company (Elverson, PA 19520). For occasions when you simply must wear shoes, try lambswool liners, available from the same source. Finally, if your feet bother you only when you sit down to relax at night, treat yourself to a pair of down booties (available from Down in Vermont, RD 1, Box 162 A, Graniteville, VT 05654) or a double foot warmer with heating pad, which is available in most department stores.

After cold feet, cold fingers are the next most common complaint. Most people need to use their hands in the house, so ordinary gloves and mittens are out of the question. One solution is thin glove liners like those made by Damart Thermolactyl (1811 Woodbury Avenue, Portsmouth, NH 02805). Another alternative—fingerless gloves—is available from Eddie Bauer (P.O. Box 370, Seattle, WA). Some people carry around something warm that they can hold in the afflicted fingers now and then. Colonial schoolchildren used to favor hot boiled eggs; New Englanders like blocks of soapstone, which release heat slowly (available from Woodstock Soap Stone Company, Rt 4, Box, 223, Woodstock, VT 05091). As a last resort, hold your hands in your armpits for a few minutes.

Finally, ignore the old taboo about wearing a hat indoors and cover your head. As much as 25 percent of your body heat goes to your head, where the only thing that keeps it from escaping is your hair. Colonial women understood the problem, so they kept their heads modestly covered with little caps. Today, a stocking cap will do. If you don't like the raffish look, try a scarf, a turban, a hooded sweater, or even a wig.

WARM AT WORK

If your company has really turned the thermostat down to 65°F, there are probably pockets where it's even colder. To keep warm at work, try these tricks:

1. Eat breakfast. Eating raises your body temperature for about two hours while the food is being digested.
2. Wear long underwear. Several companies make underwear thin enough so it can be worn under business clothes. For women, silk snuggies are a particularly luxurious choice. At the very least, men can wear undershirts; women can wear camisoles and tights or a body stocking.
3. Layer your clothes. Layering is both fashionable and sensible since you can remove an outer layer if you move to a different office where the temperature is warmer. Try V-neck sweaters over turtlenecks, vests over shirts. And keep a bulky cardigan in the office that can be worn over anything.
4. Buy boots big enough to go over heavy socks. Women, in particular, should avoid narrow high-fashion boots which cut off circulation in the feet, making them more susceptible to cold. Don't forget liners—

The Cold Warrior

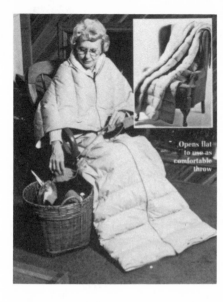

Snug sacks come in full-length and waist-high styles and open flat for use as comforters. You can make your own with this kit. (Frostline Kits)

plain felt or the silver space-age radiant-barrier insulating material used on astronauts' clothing.

5. Defend your desk. Many desks are raised a foot off the floor, exposing your feet to drafts. Close that gap. If you can't get someone to build a skirt for the desk, make your own from cardboard covered with Con-Tact paper or fabric. Fasten it to the desk with double faced tape. If you are still cold, consider a desk-top heater—Braun makes a compact model. Or get yourself a "hot seat," a self-heating cushion used by duck hunters to keep their tails toasty.

AFTER-HOURS WARMTH

What we've described so far will keep you comfortable when you're moderately active. For most people, the chill sets in when they sit down to read, talk, or watch television. No problem. Every home that aspires to be cool but comfortable needs a supply of shawls and afghans, comforters and capes, throws and lap blankets. Whatever you call them, the result is nothing more than an extra layer of fabric that you can wrap around yourself when you need it. A popular variation on this theme is the snug sack, a modified sleeping bag with snaps or zippers that allow you to fasten yourself in a fiberfill cocoon and laugh at the howling winds—until the phone rings. Fortunately, most manufacturers now include foot holes so you can move about without winning an Academy Award for comedy.

Of course, a nation that has turned snug sacks into a craze might be ready to reconsider bundling. Two hundred years ago young couples got acquainted in bed because it was the warmest place in the house. Fully clothed, they could chat in comfort. Today, bed may still be the location of choice on brutal winter nights. Just get yourself a bigger night table so it can hold books, magazines, stationery, a telephone, a snack, and other diversions.

Even if you use your bed only for sleeping, it can be an energy-saving device if it is properly outfitted. It's common knowledge that you can save as much as 15 percent of your energy bill simply by setting your thermostat back 10° at night. Many people sleep more soundly in cool surroundings—within limits. When you reach yours, try these ideas.

Electric bed pads and blankets are one solution, though purists frown on them because they do consume energy. Still, the difference between heating an entire house with the furnace and the bed with an electric blanket can be significant. Electric blankets cost about four cents per person per hour, and electric bed pads cost slightly less because the heat rises around you rather than drifting off into the air. Although electric blankets are perfectly safe for adults—they don't cause shocks or fires unless they are abused—they should never be used to warm infants, invalids, or people with sensitive skin. Also, to avoid futile arguments about what setting is comfortable, occupants of double beds should get dual controls.

Total Warmth

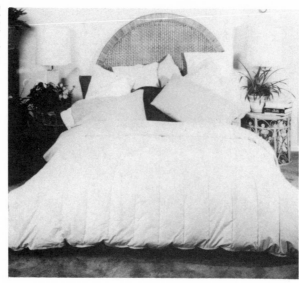

The well-made winter bed —flannel sheets, flannel pillowcases, and a down comforter. (Garnet Hill)

In choosing blankets, follow the same rules that apply to fabrics in clothing. Wool is certainly warm, but not warmer than synthetics or fiber blends of the same texture and thickness. Unfortunately, thick blankets of any fabric are usually heavy. Down comforters are both light and warm, a luxury that many feel justifies their high prices. If you do splurge on a comforter, be sure to buy a washable cover, too, since down is difficult to clean. Both covers and comforters from crib to king size are available from Down in Vermont (RD 1, Box 162A, Graniteville, VT 05654).

A stack of blankets will seal in your body heat once you're in bed, but they do nothing to minimize the icy shock of cold cotton sheets. As an alternative, consider flannel sheets, whose softy, nappy finish traps warmth. A few years ago, you had to order such sheets from Europe, but now they are available in most department stores. Particularly luxurious sheets are sold by Lucy Stewart's Private Stock (P.O. Box 443, Grafton, NH 03240). Before you throw away your cotton sheets, remember that they too can be warmed. Although you are unlikely to have an old-fashioned bed warmer with its long handle and container for coals, there's no reason you can't heat up a brick, wrap it in flannel, and tuck it into the foot of the bed a few minutes before you get in. Soapstone is legendary for its ability to absorb heat, and a specially designed bedwarmer, complete with a convenient handle and a drawstring bag, is available from Minuteman International (8 Nickerson Road, Lexington, MA 02173).

What you wear to bed is your business, but for personal warmth you can't beat one-piece pajamas with feet. Nightgowns and shirts creep up and tangle around your torso; two-piece pajamas can't be trusted not to expose your midriff. A body stocking made of soft and stretchy fabric is unquestionably the best bet. Supplement it as necessary with bed socks, a bed jacket, and a nightcap. The latter is particu-

THE GOOD OLD DAYS

Better, far better, the old houses of the olden time, with their great roaring fires, and their bed-rooms where the snow came in and the wintery winds whistled. Then, to be sure, you froze your back while you burned your face, your water froze nightly in your pitcher, your breath congealed in ice-wreaths on the blankets, and you could write your name on the pretty snow-wreath that had sifted in through the window-cracks. But you woke full of life and vigor, you looked out into the whirling snow-storms without a shiver, and thought nothing of plunging through drifts as high as your head on your daily way to school. . . . Your blood coursed and tingled, in full tide of good, merry real life, through your veins.

—Catherine Beecher, *Housekeeper's Manual* **(1869)**

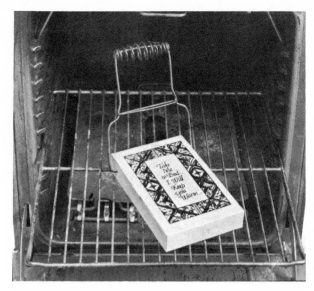

Pop this soapstone bedwarmer into a 300° oven for an hour and slip it between your sheets. It will radiate heat slowly for hours, making it the almost perfect bedtime companion. (Minuteman International)

larly important since your head is the only part of your body that is exposed all night and, as we've mentioned before, up to 25 percent of your body heat ends up there.

If a nightcap seems old-fashioned, you're right. Our forebears slept in rooms where a lid of ice formed in the water pitcher overnight. Though we live under less spartan conditions, we might borrow a few of their tricks. For one thing, they built their beds tall to keep them out of the cold air that settled near the floor. For another, they enclosed their beds in curtains and canopies that kept the body heat, which seeped through their blankets, from dissipating in the room. Finally, they invented quilts whose many layers trapped extra insulating air over their bodies.

SMALL WARM PLEASURES

Although your body can generate measurable heat, your mind helps determine whether that heat will make you feel warm and comfortable. Research indicates that you can change people's comfort levels without changing the actual temperature if you surround them with objects, furnishings, and activities that they associate with warmth. Clearly, winter is a time to indulge in the small pleasures that elicit feelings of warmth and well-being. Each person has different comfort triggers. If you don't already know yours, try some of the suggestions that follow. None, except exercise,

appreciably changes the measurable temperature, yet all have been known to make people feel warmer.

PLANTS

Plants, particularly a flowering plant, are a visual reminder that winter does give way to spring. Many houseplants actually prefer cooler temperatures and full winter sun in a southern window will inspire many plants to bloom. For a sneak preview of spring, try forcing bulbs. Paper white narcissus are particularly easy—just plant in a dish of pebbles and water—and the fragrance alone will raise your mental temperature. If you set your plants in dishes, you'll also benefit from the humidity generated by keeping the water in the dishes.

PROJECTS

It's no secret that our grandparents got through the long winters by making useful things. Today crafts are so popular that it's easy to find books or kits to teach you how to make everything from candles to quilts. So teach yourself a skill like whittling or weaving, refinishing furniture or playing the harmonica. Not only will your craft keep you moving mentally and physically, but if you become sufficiently engrossed, the winter will zip by.

PETS

An affectionate cat who will curl up on your chest while you're lounging in the evening is as good as a small space heater. The same is

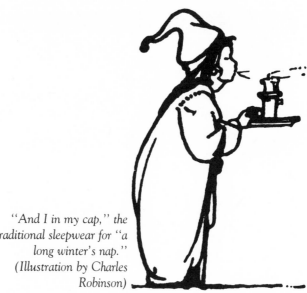

"And I in my cap," the traditional sleepwear for "a long winter's nap." (Illustration by Charles Robinson)

true of a dog with the endearing habit of lying on your feet. A pet, of course, requires more than a seasonal commitment, but there's nothing like snuggling with a furry friend on a winter's evening.

THE WARM TOUCH

With a little forethought, you can warm up the things you use before you use them. Cupboards, for example, are often colder than the kitchen, so think ahead and take out your plates, cups, and bowls in advance. Set them near the stove or actually in the oven so they'll be warm when you're ready for them. Similarly, you can set up a clothes rack near the wood stove or over a register. In addition to drying wet mittens and leggings, use the rack to warm up sweaters, socks, even bath towels. In the morning before you get up, pull your underwear under the covers with you for a few minutes so it's warm when you put it on.

HOT WATER

If you suffer from cold fingers, something as simple as washing your hands in hot water can help, since it will warm your wrist, where your blood is close to the surface of your skin. Similarly, many people like to soak their feet in hot water, perhaps with a soothing dose of Epsom salts. Drape a towel over the top of the basin so the water doesn't cool so fast. Hot-water bottles are turning up in new and whimsical shapes, and many have plush fabric covers so the bottle feels terrific against your tummy

or your toes. So go ahead, get into hot water, and to keep your conscience clear, supplement the insulation of your hot-water tank with an exterior jacket, available in most hardware stores.

141

EXERCISE

Your body produces more heat when it's moving, so the quickest way to sidestep a chill is to leap up and do a few calisthenics. Unfortunately, winter can encourage lethargy, which, in turn, makes you feel colder. If possible, arrange your schedule to alternate periods of activity with periods of inactivity. If you are watching television, get up at the commercial to water the plants or check the fire. If you work at a desk, walk to the other side of it when you talk on the phone. When you are settling in for a long stretch of sitting, wrap yourself up with shawls and lap blankets.

COMPANIONSHIP

Two bodies side by side make more heat than one by itself. Take advantage of that fact to get closer to people you like. Gather your children around you and read them stories. Invite friends over and sit close together to talk. Snuggle on the sofa when you watch television rather than sitting in individual chairs. And so on. The idea of getting close in the winter is not a new one. For years, the months with the highest birth rates have been August, September, and October, which means more children are conceived in winter.

The Cold Warrior

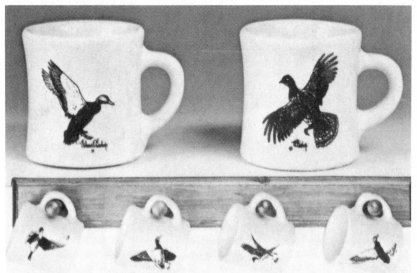

A brimming mug of any hot brew will warm your body, but there's nothing like real hot chocolate to warm the soul. Melt one ounce of bitter chocolate, and add four cups of scalded milk and two tablespoons of granulated sugar for a rich chocolate taste you can't get from powdered cocoa. (L. L. Bean)

Popcorn isn't just for movies. Even the sound of kernels popping madly will make you feel warmer on cold winter nights. These poppers are ideal for fireplace or stovetop. (Hart Fireplace Furnishings)

STEAMING LIQUIDS

Drinking hot liquids is a time-honored warm-me-up, particularly if you serve them in ceramic mugs which will conduct the heat to your fingers. If you've reached your coffee quota, experiment with herbal teas, spiced fruit juices, bouillion broths, and steamed-milk drinks. Stay away from alcohol in the winter. It brings your blood closer to the skin's surface, so after the first flush of warmth, you actually feel cooler.

FOOD

Although your body uses food to produce heat, no particular food will increase your physical temperature. However, favorite foods, particularly those you remember from childhood, may make you feel secure and satisfied. Of course, many traditional winter foods, like raisin-dotted oatmeal, hearty stews, and homemade muffins, are high in calories. The only way to compensate is with more exercise, which will in itself make you feel a great deal warmer.

In short, winter is a time for being both tough and gentle with yourself. Force yourself outside on cold days to chop wood or shovel snow and then welcome yourself indoors with a hot apple turnover. Most of all, surround yourself with the people and objects you love, for, as one wise woman put it, "Winter is the time for comfort, for good food and warmth, for the touch of a friendly hand and for a talk beside the fire: It is the time for home."

For a nice, cozy, warm feeling, there are few snacks that beat popcorn. You don't need anything more than a can of kernels, some butter or oil, and a heavy-bottomed, tightly covered pan, but an old-fashioned popper shaken in a fireplace or on a wood stove seems to make everyone feel warmer. Watch out for scorching.

GETTING OUT

Snug as your house may be, sooner or later, something—your boss, your kids, your empty refrigerator—will force you outdoors. Unfortunately, outdoor clothes that are truly warm make most people look like relatives of the Pillsbury doughboy. That may be fine on a backpacking trip through the Himalayas, but many people still feel self-conscious about stumbling into the office looking like the abominable snowman.

To be both snug and stylish, first analyze your climate and your lifestyle. Are winters in your region rainy, windy, snowy, or subzero? Do your winter expeditions take you from heated garage to car to enclosed shopping mall? Or do you wait on a windy corner for an unreliable bus?

Now, match your coat to the conditions you are likely to encounter. Fur is wonderfully warm, especially if it comes from long-haired (farm-grown!) animals like raccoon, beaver,

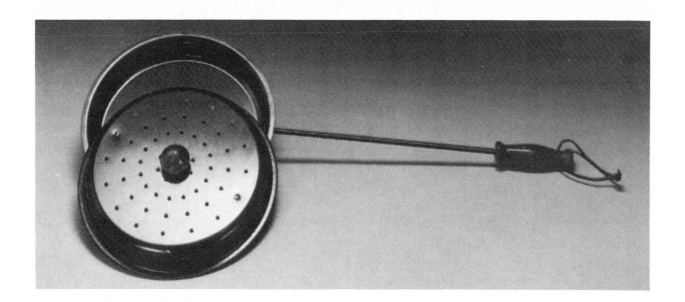

and mink. In rainy weather, however, fur fails, though you can use a plastic poncho to cover up during an occasional storm. Down, for all its popularity, is also inadequate under wet conditions. Down coats do offer extraordinary warmth for their weight, but they are bulky. Other fiberfill materials such as Kodel and Dacron 88 are even bulkier, but they respond better to rain, especially if they are covered with a nylon outer layer. The classic wool coat is perhaps the most versatile material, since it resists winter's snow, wind, and rain reasonably well.

No matter what fabric you choose, examine the design for warmth-conserving features. First, is the coat roomy enough to accommodate layers underneath—perhaps a blazer or sweater or both? Does it have a collar that can be turned up against the wind? Is the coat long enough to cover your kidneys or to reach your boot tops if you wear skirts? Does the coat fit snugly at neck and wrist? (You can always sew wristlet inserts into your sleeves.) Does it have enough fasteners to keep it wrapped around you in the wind?

After getting a coat that suits your habits and climate, protect your head, hands, and feet. Feet are the most difficult because fashionable boots are often tight enough to constrict the flow of blood, making your feet feel cold quicker. For your feets' sake, buy a pile-lined boot that's large enough to accommodate at least one pair of socks without squishing your toes. If the boots are leather, waterproof

them with silicone spray (not wax) or mink oil.

On your hands, wear mittens if possible, since the fingers will warm each other. If you need the dexterity gloves provide, select wool or lined leather. Tight, unlined leather restricts circulation, and plastic leather look-alikes keep perspiration from escaping, so your hands feel clammy and cold. If you do wear gloves, consider carrying a large pair of mittens to slip over your hands when your fingers aren't in use.

Finally, keep your head covered. There are many attractive alternatives ranging all the way from a brightly colored stocking cap to a fur bonnet.

If possible, the hat should cover your ears, though you can always add earmuffs. Earmuffs alone sacrifice 10 percent of your body heat, which just floats off through the top of your head. One especially cozy choice for headgear is the balaclava, a sort of hooded hat that extends down into your coat.

Of course, some people wrap a woven scarf or muffler around their heads, but that limits the potential of that versatile garment. A scarf can tie down your hat in a windstorm, form a pocket of warm air around your face, protect your throat, double as a shawl or lap blanket, and even function as a muff if you loop it loosely around your hands. So when there's no choice and you've just got to go out, don't forget to take your muffler to help you outwit the weather.

144 WARM WHEELS

It's all well and good to keep yourself warm in the winter, but what about your car? All the warmth and well-being created by insulating yourself and your house will vanish quick as a snowflake on a hot stove if you have to contend with a recalcitrant car. Though cars can function in the cold, they don't like to, so you'll get more cooperation from your vehicle if you create the illusion of warm weather. Here are some suggestions:

1. *Conserve your car's "body heat."* A car warms up every time you use it, and you should hold on to that heat as long as possible. An insulated garage is a decided advantage, but if you don't have one, park in a protected spot where a building, a row of trees, or even a snowdrift will keep the prevailing winds away from the car. Whenever possible, back into your parking spot so it will be easier to jump start the car if that's necessary. Cover the hood of the car with old packing blankets—some people tuck them right in around the engine. On bitter nights, consider running an extension cord to the car and leaving a mechanic's trouble light burning under the hood. Just be careful that the bulb doesn't touch any wires or hoses.

2. *Pamper your battery.* Seventy percent of all winter starting problems are caused by a faulty battery. Even a brand-new battery will lose half its power as the temperature approaches zero. Do have the battery checked and, if necessary, recharged before the season begins. Fill the cells with water and clean any corrosion off the terminals with a wire brush. Important as these preventive measures are, most batteries can still use a little outside help during a prolonged cold spell. One possibility is a trickle charger, a plug-in device that provides a sort of energy transfusion. Another alternative is a battery heater, either a hot-plate model that slips under the battery or a blanket model that wraps around it. Both operate off household current and are available for under $20. Under extreme conditions, you can remove the battery and bring it indoors for the night.

3. *Heat your coolant.* Everyone knows that a car's engine is cooled with water which must be mixed or replaced with antifreeze in the winter. Although the antifreeze keeps the coolant from freezing, it does nothing to keep it warm. For that you'll need a coolant heater. One do-it-yourself model connects to the heater's inlet hose and is sold with the appropriate clamps and connectors. Another more permanent heater goes right into the engine block. The in-block heater is available in some new cars but can be installed by any professional mechanic and is probably the single best way to keep an engine warm. One extra advantage is that when the car's coolant is warm, the interior heater warms up quicker.

4. *Keep your oil running free.* Like molasses, oil gets thick and slow in January, not to mention February and December. You can mini-

mize the effects of cold by using a multiweight oil like 10-W-40 or, in very cold climates, 5-W-30. Check the owner's manual for recommendations on your car. Again, under very cold conditions, you may want to turn to a supplementary heater—in this case, an electric dipstick. The dipstick replaces your regular oil stick. When you plug it in, the tip gets hot and keeps the oil warm and runny.

5. *Adjust your starting habits to the season.* It doesn't really matter very much how you start your car in the summer, but if you want to keep on trucking in the winter, follow these directions: Unplug and remove any electrical devices used to keep the car warm overnight. Inside the car, press the gas pedal to the floor and release slowly. Do it again. Turn the key. If the engine starts, then stalls, do it again. Don't crank for more than fifteen seconds because you'll debilitate the battery, and don't pump on the gas pedal because you'll flood the engine.

6. *Buy jumper cables and starting fluid and learn how to use them.* If your engine groans and is reluctant to crank, your battery has failed you, and you'll need help from a friend with a functioning car. (Before it gets cold, arrange an emergency exchange for the winter with a nearby friend whose schedule is similar to yours.) Pull the cars nose to nose and open both hoods. Clip the ends of one cable to the positive terminals of both batteries. For the other cable, clip one end to the negative terminal of the functioning car and one to an unpainted piece of metal in the dead car. Turn on the working car. Within a minute or two, the problem car should start when you turn the key.

If the engine tries to turn over but can't, chances are good that your carburetor is having trouble vaporizing the cold gasoline. Open the hood and locate the air filter. In most American cars it is a large circular container at the center of the engine. (For other cars consult your mechanic—before the winter begins.) Unscrew the wing nut on top and remove the entire filter box, exposing the carburetor, a cylinder with a movable plate inside. Hold the plate open and spray starting fluid into the cylinder. Since the fluid is highly flammable, do not allow anyone to crank the engine while you're spraying. Spray for about three seconds and then ask someone to turn the ignition. The car should start.

7. *Other odd tips.* The back seat of a car is never as warm as the front so provide lap blankets for backseat passengers—just like an old-fashioned sled. Check the weatherstripping around doors so you won't have unwanted drafts. If your lock freezes, heat the key with your cigarette lighter and insert it into the lock until the mechanism thaws. If you don't smoke, carry a small can of de-icer spray in your trunk. Keep your gas tank full and add a can of dry gas now and then. Carry work gloves, an extra jacket, and a pair of snow boots in case you get stuck somewhere and have to get out of the car.

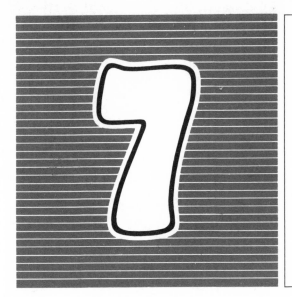

7

The Sporting Life: Keeping Warm in the Great Outdoors

A. T. Perrin

Spring, summer, even fall are considered acceptable seasons for outdoor activities. But winter? Not usually. Most people find it too cold, too wet, and too miserable. If Mother Nature can crawl under a blanket of white to catch forty winks for four months, they ask, why can't I? The bears are sleeping in their caves, there's a blanket of snow covering everything—why not crawl into bed and stay warm for four months?

But there *is* a hardy breed of sportsman which is just getting warmed up to outdoor activity in the fall and doesn't hit full stride until midwinter. Skiing, skating, and a whole host of interesting activities can round out the three-season outdoor person's year of fun. Why sit inside for four months just because it's cold outside? It's entirely possible to be warm and comfortable outdoors during cold weather, so let's have a look at these aspects first and then consider the exciting sport activities you can get involved in.

THE ART AND THEORY OF OUTDOOR WARMTH

Four basic factors affect winter warmth and comfort:

1. *The Person.* Each person has a different tolerance for cold. Physiologists have found that blue-eyed people seem to take to the cold better than dark-eyed ones; women, with their extra layer of fatty tissue, often feel warm in temperatures that would have men shivering. Obviously, much of this is attitude—whether a person wants to be out there or not.

2. *The Terrain.* Is the area you'll be in level, swampy, rocky, hilly, forested. . . ? Different terrains affect what you should wear. For example, the wind-chill factor on a large, open, ice-covered lake will be totally different from that on a heavily forested slope. Soft swampy lowlands call for one kind of footwear, icy rocky hills for another.

3. *The Weather.* Is it sunny, rainy, snowy, cold, windy, or what? The place you live, the time of year, and the terrain all affect the weather. The weather you'll be sporting in dictates the clothing combinations you should have with you so you can adapt to any changes. Everyone knows the weather can change at a moment's notice, but few outdoor types appreciate the importance of this fact. Keeping posted on the weather reports is useful preparation for any outdoor activity.

4. *The Activity.* What's going on? Are you planning to sit on a snowmobile for three hours just riding, or are you going to do heavy snowshoe jogging up a fir-covered slope in deep snow? Are you figure skating or sledding? Each activity requires a different amount of mobility. If your activity requires freedom of movement, cut down on restrictive, binding, and bulky clothing. Don't worry about losing warmth when you strip off these garments; high mobility usually means high activity, and greater body heat will be generated. Put an-

Total Warmth

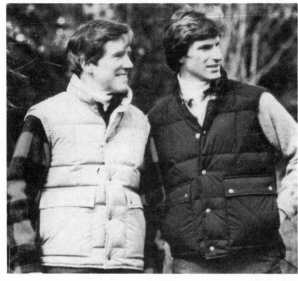

A vest, shirt, and sweater combination is comfortable, flexible, and allows you to move freely: perfect for moderate activity in moderate cold. (Eddie Bauer)

other way, although reducing clothing equals chilling, increased activity equals warming. Your body balances the equation, but it doesn't always work so simply. For example, too much activity will produce not only heat but also perspiration. This wetness will soak into your clothing and destroy its insulation value. The result is that the nice body warmth you've been generating will be sucked right into the cold through the wet clothing.

If you overdo it—whatever you're doing—everything goes out of balance. In any and all outdoor activity the words to heed are *move, but don't sweat.*

When you begin to perspire, you have only two options: slow down or reduce the insulation. Of the two options, slowing down is the wiser because it reduces energy expended and, over the long run, prevents fatigue. Reducing insulation takes you in the opposite direction. Energy expenditure is often increased, not only to maintain the pace of activity but also to keep warm in the face of reduced insulation. This warmth leaks out quickly through the thinned insulation, forcing the body to work harder. The cycle continues until the body collapses in fatigue. Putting on a coat at this point will do very little. The exhausted body is cooling down fast and is just not capable of producing enough heat to warm up the person inside the coat. Hypothermia could result unless the person is brought to a source of warmth.

So always remember that *you are the source of your warmth*—not your coat or your jacket.

Without you inside it, your jacket is as cold as the snow.

DOWN TO BASICS

Armed with this knowledge of the basic factors of outdoor warmth, you can judge what degree of activity your chosen winter sport involves. Each one calls for a certain clothing combination that will balance the need for mobility against the need for warmth. Even within a particular sport, however, there are periods of much exertion and periods of little exertion, and this change may require an adjustment of clothing. Overlay this with a change in the weather, such as the sun suddenly coming out (warming) or the wind unexpectedly picking up (cooling), which may require another modification, and it becomes obvious that the adjustment picture can get somewhat complex.

The answer, of course, is a clothing arrangement that is versatile and easily adapted to the needs of the moment. This calls for layering rather than bulking. In other words, a thermal undershirt, a wool shirt, a sweater, a vest, and a parka will be better than a T-shirt, a wool shirt, and a heavy coat. The former can be adjusted in small units. If you wear the latter, you may be too active to keep on the heavy clothing but not active enough to take it off with only a T-shirt and wool shirt beneath.

Layering is the key to this flexibility, to your ability to retain or release body heat and prevent perspiration and heat loss. The easiest

The Sporting Life

	BODY	Very Cold	FEET	HANDS	HEAD
1	UNDERWEAR Standard	Standard and Fishnet	Cotton or wool socks		
	2ND UNDERWEAR Fishnet, Thermal or wool long johns	Wool long johns or thermal	Wool socks		
2	DRESSWEAR Wool pants, wool shirt		Boots		
3	OVERWEAR Sweater or vest	Sweater		Liner gloves	Knit cap
	2ND OVERWEAR	Vest, or down sweater			
4	OUTERWEAR Jacket, parka			Gloves	Balaclava or toque
	2ND OUTERWEAR Windbreaker jacket and pants or shell parka.	Expedition parka & pants			Hood

approach to layering is to consider your cold-weather attire a uniform made up of four wear levels built up from the inside out: underwear, dresswear, overwear, and outerwear. The under, over and outer layers may be further subdivided if necessary to increase versatility. The following chart will give you a better illustration of the layering concept.

Here are some points to keep in mind regarding layering:

1. The primary function of all layers is to insulate—to prevent the flow of heat to the outside, keeping the body warm but cool enough not to perspire.

2. The under layer's secondary function is to provide air circulation during high activity in order to avoid "hot spots" where heat will accumulate and cause perspiration. During low activity it holds the air still to retain heat. Fishnet underwear is excellent for this because of its large holes. This layer's third function is absorption, sponging up any perspiration that may appear to avoid actual wetness. The process is called "wicking."

With respect to feet, absorption is the secondary function of socks. Feet tend to perspire readily, and after a day's wear socks have pretty well accumulated enough perspiration, body oils, and other matter to transform them from insulators to conductors of heat. This is one of the main reasons for the constant admonition to bring extra socks and change daily.

3. Because it is usually in direct contact with the environment, the dress layer's secondary function is to resist wind and water. Wind blowing through to the air layer within the trousers destroys its insulating quality. Wetness allows the heat of that air layer to directly convect (short-circuit, you might say) to the outside. Water is a conductor of heat.

4. The over and outer layers have as their secondary function resistance of wind and wetness.

A comment about the head, which plays a very important part in keeping the body warm: Blood will always be supplied to the brain first, to keep it warm. If your head is being cooled too fast, blood flow to other parts of the body will be reduced to keep up with the rapid temperature drain at the head; your extremities will begin to feel cold. So always wear a hat to keep your feet warm.

COLD-WEATHER CLOTHING

By breaking down your clothing needs into these four levels discussed above, you can cover the complete range of cold-weather clothing. Here's a descriptive listing with comments regarding design, purpose, use, and approximate prices.

UNDERWEAR

Underwear has two functions: to provide insulation by trapping air next to the skin and to absorb any perspiration produced by the body to prevent wetness.

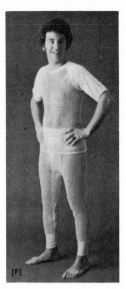

Fishnet underwear takes the worry out of being active. The holes let air circulate across your body, cooling hot spots and slowing perspiration. (Recreational Equipment, Inc.)

If pants cramp your style when you're traipsing up a mountain, try knickers. They won't bind at the knees, and they lend a Tyrolean feel to the whole endeavor. (Ski Hut)

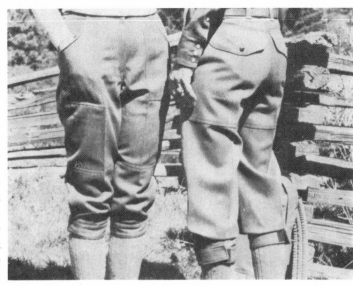

Fishnet Underwear. This underwear has large holes designed to provide dead air spaces for retention of body warmth when you're not too active. When you increase your activity, the large air spaces, together with body motion, provide for air circulation. This circulation cools hot spots and thus reduces the tendency to perspire. Fishnet is the preferred underwear for active winter sports. For comfort look for solid panels at the top of the shoulders and in the crotch. The cost runs about $12 to $15 for a shirt and pants set.

Thermal Underwear. This is quilted underwear with an insulating filler. It definitely provides warmth and absorbs moisture, but a suit of thermals is bulky and will make the dresswear it is worn under tight and binding. Typically, $15 to $18 for a set.

Long Johns. This group includes the old one-piece, flap-in-the-seat union suit, usually of wool, and the more modern two-piece non-itchy synthetics. The two-layer Duofold underwear, with an outer layer of a wool-polyester blend and an inner of 100 percent cotton, has stood the test of time and is popular with outdoor types everywhere. Other versions are available in single and double layers, from the straight 100-percent wool number to exotic ones made of angora, lamb's wool, and a multitude of synthetics. Just about all of them insulate and will absorb moisture, but they won't ventilate like fishnet underwear. Because of this, long johns are best suited to low-activity sports. If you expect to be out in subzero temperatures, the best bet would be long johns over fishnet. Long-john prices vary all over the lot, but Duofold sells for about $25 a set, about average for long johns.

DRESSWEAR

Pants. For openers, forget blue jeans. These are absolutely the worst pants for winter activities. They're too tight, which restricts circulation and movement, and they're too water absorbent—one roll in the snow and they're sopping wet. Bad news all around. The best pants are wool, which repels water naturally and even retains some of its insulating qualities when wet. Second best would be a blend of cotton and polyester that has been treated for water repellency. Pants should be straight leg, without cuffs; cuffs catch debris. A word about belts: They're okay, but since they have to bind to keep your pants up, that's a point against them for cutting circulation. Suspenders are better for winter. Wool trousers range from a low of $35 to a high of $75.

Knickers. These are the standard wear for mountaineering and ski touring. They do not bind at the knee the way long pants do. That's important when you're doing complicated articulations with the old legs. For snow walkers knickers mean no floppy wet cuffs. Knickers should be made of wool or a wool blend and should be reinforced at the crotch and seat. Velcro fasteners at the knees are a bit handier than the belt and buckle arrangement. When getting your knickers, don't forget to pick up

149

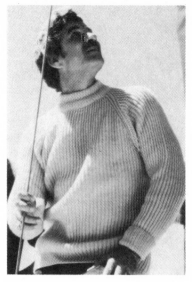

An oiled fisherman's sweater made of unscrubbed wool has much of the sheep's natural lanolin in it to help repel moisture. (Eddie Bauer)

 some knee socks, too. Knickers run about $30.

Shirts. Shirts come in many styles, from turtle-neck pullovers to the standard button-down-the-front collar models. Since a shirt will usually be worn under some kind of overwear, its ability to resist wind and wet is not critical. However, a shirt does play an important role in ventilation, so you should be able to open it at the front and neck. Wool, naturally, is the warmest, but a good second choice would be chamois cloth. Shirts run from $18 to $38.

OVERWEAR

This layer is often the final one for such highly active sports as skating and skiing or for medium-cold environments. As with any layer that comes in direct contact with the weather, it should be wind and water repellent.

Sweaters. Again, wool or a wool and synthetic blend is the warmest. If the sweater is to be the outermost layer, the oiled fisherman's pullover, which has much of the natural lanolin still in the wool, is recommended. When the sweater is not the outermost layer, a button-down-the -front type may offer more versatile ventilation than a pullover. Down sweaters look like and can be used like a light jacket. Sweaters range from $20 to $50.

Vests. These are quite popular. Filled with down or synthetic fillers, they are often worn as the outermost clothing. The idea is to get the best in freedom of movement and warmth from one piece. Vests are excellent sources of additional insulation under outerwear. They allow for versatile layering. Better vests are designed with two Velcro-closured flap pockets in front. Priced at about $25.

Mackinaw. This piece is also known as a shirt-jac, a very heavy shirt worn as a jacket. A mackinaw is all right for late fall or early spring but is not satisfactory for really cold weather, either as an outermost piece or as one to be worn under overwear. Mackinaws cost about $50.

OUTERWEAR

This is the final layer of clothing, the layer normally in contact with the weather. Its function is to keep out snow, rain, and wind and at the same time allow water vapor to breathe out. Until recently this was an almost impossible requirement to meet. If the material was capable of breathing vapor out, it was also capable of leaking rain in. The development of Gore-Tex, though, has changed all this (see "Clothing Materials").

Overalls, Snowsuits. These one-piece suits are very popular with kids for sledding attire and with grown-ups for snowmobiling. However, being one-piece they can hardly fit the layering concept, and thus really not the choice of the serious cold-weather outdoor enthusiast.

Ski Pants. These resemble bib overalls, and though some can be worn over pants, most are designed to be worn over underwear. They're made of nylon with a synthetic filler,

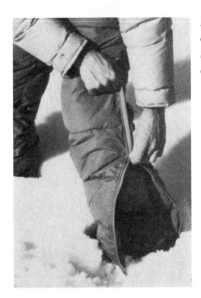

Expedition pants zip down over your regular pants to keep your legs warm in extreme cold. (Ski Hut)

and the better ones have full-length zippers down the outside seam of each leg. This makes it easier to put them on over boots. These pants repel snow and wind fairly well and are light enough to dissipate the extra body heat and vapor generated by the activity of downhill skiing. What this means is that they're good for skiing and, perhaps, ice skating, but not so good for activities that don't generate as much heat. They're not satisfactory for ski touring, because they can cause binding in the legs. Priced in the $40s.

Expedition Pants. These are outerpants designed for subzero weather. "Expedition," incidentally, is the term given to any piece of clothing designed for subzero environments. It's the warmest available. Expedition pants are usually worn over regular ones. They have an inner liner and outer shell of ripstop nylon and are filled with down or one of the newer synthetics. To make it easier to put on and take off boots and to allow for some ventilation, there are full-length zippers on the outside of each leg. These pants are normally available only through mail-order from wilderness outfitters such as Eddie Bauer, Ski Hut, and Recreational Equipment, Inc. Priced at less than $100.

Wind Shells. These are lightweight, non-insulated pants and jackets of closely woven ripstop nylon. The better-quality pants have full-length zippers on each leg to facilitate donning over boots. The others pull on just like sweatpants. The jackets have a front zipper,

pockets, and a drawstring hood. Wind shells have only one function—to windproof the wearer. Wind increases the evaporation of body vapor, which could cool the body too fast. A wind shell acts as a resistor, slowing but not stopping the evaporation. Wind shells are worn over overwear or even outerwear when wind is 10 mph or over. Wind pants run about $20 and jackets about $35.

Jackets, Coats. A jacket comes down to the waist or hips; a coat, to the knees. Coats are not very popular with active winter recreationists because the length interferes with mobility. Jackets, on the other hand, are very popular and come in a multitude of styles and types. What makes for a good jacket?

1. A shell made of an abrasion-resistant material, breathable but water- and windproof.
2. Insulation of down or one of the newer synthetics.
3. Two lower pockets in front with Velcro-closure flaps; pockets should be dual compartmented with an inner insulated hand-warmer section and an outer cargo section.
4. A front closure with a zipper that opens from both the top and the bottom. It should be made of nylon, not metal, which may freeze, and should have an insulated flap beneath and a Velcro-closure wind flap on top.
5. A zippered ventilation opening under arms.
6. Drawstrings at the inside waist and inside

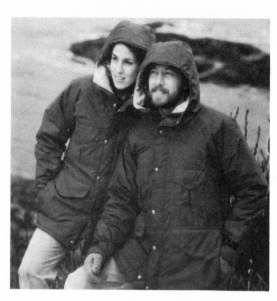

The Silver Lining Ultimo parka has an outer shell of Gore-Tex to keep you dry in rain or snow. (Early Winters Catalog)

152

bottom of the jacket to draw waist and/or bottom closed to prevent drafts.

7. Cuffs with Velcro tabs for adjusting and closing.

8. A collar that is insulated and includes snaps for attaching a hood. Some styles of jacket do not not have a hood as an accessory; check to see which style you're getting.

A word here about buttons, snaps, and Velcro. Buttons are rarely found on cold-weather wilderness recreation clothing nowadays because they're not as easy to work with as snaps and Velcro. Snaps are okay, but they're not as good as Velcro, if you'll be opening and closing a flap a lot. Snaps are often hard to press closed or pull open, and they sometimes require both hands. Velcro is always an easy one-hand operation, and it'll stay closed under normal conditions.

Jacket prices run from $60 to $150.

Parkas. Technically a parka is a hip-length jacket with a permanent hood attached. Without the hood it would be a jacket. Parkas are also supposed to keep you dry against snow or rain; a jacket is not necessarily expected to do that. As can be expected, though, you'll find things called parkas that aren't. A good parka has the same qualities as a good jacket. Parkas are made without insulation (shells), with medium insulation for normal cold, and in expedition grades with enough insulation to keep you warm in temperatures below -50°F. Prices about the same as for jackets.

FOOTWEAR

Socks. Wool. Normally two pairs of socks are worn with boots, not only to absorb perspiration but also to insulate and cushion the foot. If you find wool too itchy, wear an inner sock of cotton or a synthetic and an outer sock of wool. A good pair of thick wool socks runs about $3 to $4. Knee-length ones worn with knickers will run a bit more.

Boots. The main considerations in choosing boots are traction, dryness, and warmth. For traction, the Vibram lug sole has the track record for snow, mud, and rock. Because of their thickness and insulation, winter boots do not breathe well, so your feet will perspire. As long as you change your socks every day, this won't be much of a problem. As far as outside wetness goes, leather is fairly resistant to water unless completely immersed. Alas, this will often happen. But there are many water-repellent compounds on the market, such as Sno-Seal, Leather-Seal, and Snow-Proof, that you can apply to seal the boot against outside wetness. The foot opening and tongue areas are always susceptible to leaks, so check to make sure the tongue flap is sewn to the boot all the way to the top. Lacing is available with speed eyelets or the standard hole eyelets. Speed eyelets are faster and easier. Cold-weather boots run from $80 to $120.

Pac Boots. These are solid rubber or the rubber-lower/leather-upper type that L. L. Bean originally developed as the Maine Hunting Shoe. The leather upper provides a

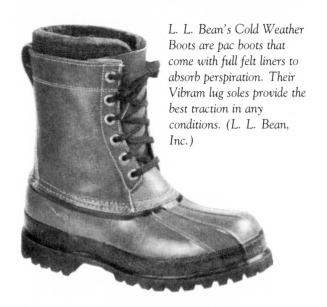

L. L. Bean's Cold Weather Boots are pac boots that come with full felt liners to absorb perspiration. Their Vibram lug soles provide the best traction in any conditions. (L. L. Bean, Inc.)

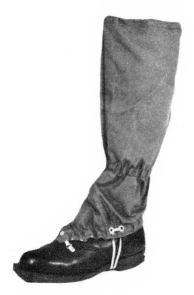

Gaiters: a must for hiking through deep snow. (Ski Hut)

waterproof boot that doesn't have quite the perspiration-condensation problems of a solid-rubber boot. Bean's boot is an excellent product, but you can only get it through their catalog or at their store in Freeport, Maine. The price runs $35 to $60. The only other rubber/leather pac boot on the market, available through sporting goods stores, is the Canadian Sorel boot. Its design is slightly different from Bean's, but it's very servicable and slightly lower in cost. Solid-rubber, foam-insulated boots are readily available. They are quite warm and waterproof, but your feet will perspire heavily in them. Pac boots should always be worn with a felt inner sole (purchased separately) and two or three pairs of socks to provide for the best absorption. Pac boots are also available with a felt inner liner that covers the whole foot, but this means that the boot will be oversize and a bit bulkier than those without the liner. All rubber pac boots sell for about $35.

Gaiters. For anyone trekking in deep soft snow, gaiters are a must. Like the leggings worn by soldiers in World War I, they're designed to protect the ankle area and prevent the boot from picking up snow and debris. Gaiters are made of water-repellent material that resists snow and wetness but allows water vapor to breathe out. They're also made in waterproof material—resulting in sweaty legs. Sizes range from anklet to over-the-calf lengths. Prices range from $15 to $50 depending on the material.

HEADWEAR

Caps, Hats. Baseball-style caps and brim hats are not satisfactory headgear for winter, mainly because they're not really designed to keep the head warm. As far as shading the eyes goes, the sun bounces more brightness off the snow below than it sends from overhead. So much for caps and hats.

Knit Caps. These are standard winter headwear and include the watch cap, ski cap, balaclava, and toque. Knit caps resist moisture, conform to the shape of the head, providing the best insulation, are adjustable for ventilation, and can easily be worn under a hood. A navy creation, the watch cap is a bit "tighter" than the ski cap, which is "looser" and bulkier. Personal preference would dictate the choice here, though if you do choose a watch cap, make sure it's solid wool. Acrylics are okay for ski caps, but after a while a watch cap will lose its resiliency and become somewhat floppy.

The balaclava and toque are about the same, except that the balaclava has a small visor, or bill, and the toque does not. Both are designed to be rolled up and worn like a bulky ski cap. And when it gets cold, you can unroll it and wear it around your head, ears, face, and neck. Really versatile. Prices for knit caps run from $5 to $15.

Hood. A hood is headwear outerwear and is either an integral part of the parka or a jacket accessory. Hoods can be either insulated or uninsulated, depending on the type of parka or

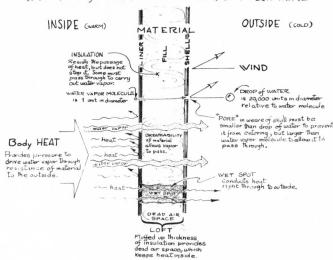

154

jacket they go with. In either case, hoods should have a snug Velcro neck closure and a drawstring face closure with nylon slide locks. These slide on the drawstring and keep it taut —really a lot handier than tying bows with gloved hands.

HANDWEAR

Gloves. Gloves give greater freedom of movement to the fingers than mittens do, but do not provide the same warmth. Two styles are available, the leather and the knit. Leather becomes a problem when it gets wet because it doesn't dry easily. This kills its insulation value. When dried, which takes a while, it becomes stiff and uncomfortable. The knit glove is much more practical. It retains its insulation qualities even when wet, can be wrung out to reduce moisture, and dries easily. When it dries, it's as good as new. The only thing to be sure of with any knit glove is that it has leather sewn to the palms and fingers so it won't be hard to get a grip on things. Cost is about $12.

Liner Gloves. These are knit, silk, or synthetic gloves designed to be worn inside a larger pair of gloves, usually leather, or mittens. The idea is that two are warmer than one. In the case of silk or synthetic liners, they offer short-term (5–10-minute) protection against the cold when you need your fingers to make a fine adjustment, say, to a camera. These liners are so thin that it's like using your bare hands. Liner gloves are sold alone or with

outer gloves. Alone they run about $5 to $10.

Mittens. Mittens provide less versatility since you don't have the use of individual fingers, but they're a lot warmer than gloves because the fingers are all together to keep each other warm. Mittens are made of leather or wool. The wool ones may or may not have leather sewn to the palm and finger areas. Prices range from $8 to $12.

CLOTHING MATERIALS

Outdoor clothing can provide no better protection from cold and wetness than the material from which it is made. It seems sensible to purchase an item of clothing because it *performs* like a parka rather than because it *looks* like a parka. The only way you can reasonably predict performance is to know about the performance of the materials from which a garment is made. Cotton will act like cotton, wool like wool, down like down, and nylon like nylon. But how does wool act in providing warmth and comfort? What are its benefits and drawbacks? If you don't know, it's silly to pick up on wool clothing because *they* say it's good.

As you can see from the drawing showing the dynamics of vapor transmission and water resistance, all cold-weather clothing must keep heat in, keep wind and water out, and allow vapor to pass through. This is a tough act because, until recently, there was no shell material that would pass vapor without also passing

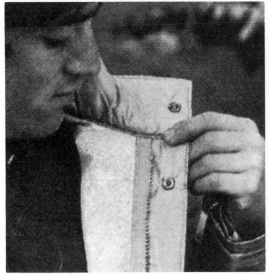

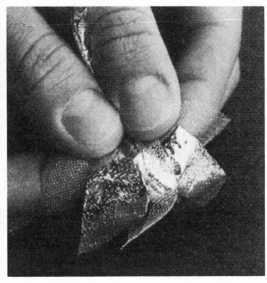

A new insulating material, under the trademark Silver Lining, forms an insulating barrier against radiant heat loss. When added to traditional insulators, Silver Lining will greatly increase warmth with no extra bulk; clothing utilizing Silver Lining is much trimmer than the usual down coat or vest. (Early Winters Catalog)

water. And if it was proofed to the point of stopping water, it would also stop vapor.

One material that almost solved this problem is an extremely close-woven cotton that swelled shut when it became wet, similar to a canvas water bag. However, as with the canvas water bag, capillary action would wick water through and the cloth would become damp on its inner surface. If touched, it would drip. Dripping was prevented, however, by putting a spacer between the cloth and the skin. Jackets made of this cloth, called Ventile, are almost absolutely dry even in heavy rain, yet they still pass vapor.

The problem was solved conclusively in the late 1970s, when W. L. Gore and Associates developed a method of quickly stretching poly-tetra-fluoro-ethylene (PTFE) to produce a microporous film with billions of tiny holes per square inch. How it works is fairly simple. A drop of water is roughly twenty thousand times larger than a hole in PTFE, whereas a water molecule, the smallest component of water vapor, is seven hundred times smaller than a PTFE pore. One fits, the other doesn't. Since PTFE is not strong enough to be used in clothing by itself, it has to be faced and backed with an appropriate material, such as ripstop or taffeta nylon, or polyester. Gore's trade name for the PTFE microporous film is Gore-Tex. Du Pont's trade name for PTFE resin is Teflon. Small world! Gore-Tex is now being used by a number of outdoor clothing manufacturers, and a product called Klimate, which works like Gore-Tex but is chemically different, is also starting to appear in clothes.

After the shell, the fill is the other important part of cold-weather clothing. It lies between the shell and the liner and provides the actual insulation which retains body warmth by trapping and holding air. (In some materials, such as wool, the liner, fill, and shell are all in the same one piece). If the air in the fill cannot move easily because of obstructions such as fibers, then heat cannot be transferred by convection currents; the body stays warm. The thickness of the air space is called "loft," and some fills require more loft than others to provide the required resistance for minimum air movement. As long as the fill remains dry, the air remains to insulate. However, if the fill gets wet, the situation changes. Water causes the fill's fibers to collapse into a soggy mess. With no air space, heat is readily transmitted and chilling results. Even if the fill does not collapse but retains its shape as a sponge does when saturated, insulation may still be lost because water transmits heat twenty times more easily than air.

So the question is will the material absorb or resist absorbing water? If it does absorb water, will it hold it, or will the water drain off easily, leaving only slight dampness? Any material that absorbs and holds water is the worst for wet situations, any material that absorbs but drains easily isn't so bad, and any material that doesn't absorb at all is great.

In summary, the three criteria for satisfac-

156 tory outdoor clothing materials are (1) high vapor conductance, (2) high water resistance, and (3) high heat insulation. With these in mind we can now take a look at the popular materials that go into today's cold-weather clothing and see what can be expected of them.

CLOTHS

Cotton and Cotton Blends. In general, clothing made of 100-percent cotton—denim, corduroy, and khaki—is a bad choice for cold weather because of its high moisture-absorbency-and-retention characteristics. It is cellular and will soak up to four times its weight in water and hold it like a sponge until saturation occurs—then drip, drip, drip. Avoid these fabrics.

On the other hand, cotton poplin (poplin is a tighter than normal weave) blended with some polyester will reduce this high absorbency, and so it is acceptable for pants or jacket shell material for damp, but not wet, environments. Increasing the synthetic decreases the wetness penetration while retaining the good abrasion-resistance qualities of cotton.

Mountain Cloth, also known as Storm Cloth and 65/35 Cloth, is a blend of 65 percent polyester and 35 percent cotton and is a popular shell material for jackets, parkas, gaiters, and so on. It has greater resistance to abrasion than nylon, and its resistance to moisture penetration is fair to good. It will get wet in rain, but unless it's reasonably heavy, it won't leak. It'll dry out easily, too. Vapor conductance is excellent.

The material called 60/40 Cloth is a blend of 60 percent nylon and 40 percent cotton with the cotton woven at right angles to the nylon. This makes you ponder nylon's tendency to stretch against cotton's tendency to shrink. Hmmmmm? Other than that, 60/40, although not as popular as Mountain Cloth, performs about the same.

Ventile (British-made) and Venture Cloth (American-made) are very tightly woven durable cotton fabrics that are highly resistant to moisture penetration. When wet, the tightly woven threads expand and close the pores to any further direct entry of water; however, capillary action will keep the material damp. Touching the damp cloth would produce a drip, but clothing of Ventile is constructed with an inner liner to prevent contact. Vapor conductance is excellent. Apparently this material is not easy to obtain, so only a few manufacturers produce clothing made of it.

Wool and Wool Blends. Wool is a far better natural cold weather material than cotton because of its high insulation, a quality cotton lacks, even when dry. Wool will absorb moisture, but not as readily as cotton. Cotton's fibers collapse when wet, and this is conducive to capillary action, which wicks the moisture through; wool's fibers do not collapse, and this creates high resistance to capillary action. This is also the reason that wool retains its insulating quality when wet. Wool can be wrung out easily and dries from the inside out, which gets the chilling wetness away from the skin first. Wool is also more durable than cotton. About the only major problem with wool is that most people find it very itchy, though not as much when the temperature is really cold. Minor problems are that most wool garments require dry cleaning and moths find it delicious.

Wool is often blended with a synthetic to increase its durability and reduce cost.

Synthetics. Synthetics for outdoor clothing include acrylics, such as Orlon; polyesters, such as Dacron; and nylon. Synthetics resist moisture absorption, and if they get wet, they will dry out quickly. They are very durable—Dacron is particularly abrasion resistant—and when woven into sweaters and caps—in the case of Orlon—provide good insulation even when wet, because the fibers do not collapse. The only problem with Orlon is that it tends to lose its shape after a while, and it's not neat. Sweaters develop little balls of clinging material. But there's no question that synthetics have their place in cold-weather clothing both alone and as blends with cotton and wool.

Nylon. Nylon, in various weights, is probably the most common material used in outdoor gear on the market today, chiefly because it combines strength with lightness. Ripstop and taffeta are the two primary types used in clothing.

Ripstop is woven with an extra large thread every ¼ inch so the material looks as if it has a gridwork of squares on it. This gridwork stops any rip that could develop in the base material. The common weight for shell material is 1.9 ounces per square yard. Lighter weights are sometimes used, but 1.9 ounces is about the lowest you should go if you still want satisfactory strength.

Taffeta does not have larger threads running through the weave. However, it is more tightly woven and usually heavier than ripstop, the most popular weight being about 2.2 ounces per square yard. Taffeta is stronger, more durable, and more wind resistant than ripstop because of its tighter weave. Supernyl is another name for taffeta.

Nylon is a good vapor conductor, resists water absorption, and will retain only 1 percent of its own weight in moisture. This means quick and easy drying. Of course, nylon will leak in rain unless waterproofed. When purchasing down-filled nylon clothes, check for down-proofness to make sure the weave of the nylon is tight enough to prevent down from leaking out; 1.9-ounce material is usually satisfactory, but check anyway, by blowing through the material. If your breath goes through easily, there's a good chance the weave is not tight enough.

Gore-Tex. This microporous film or one of its counterparts, such as Klimate, will soon be as common as nylon in outdoor clothing. As mentioned earlier, it has solved the problem of combining high vapor conductance with high resistance to water penetration. This

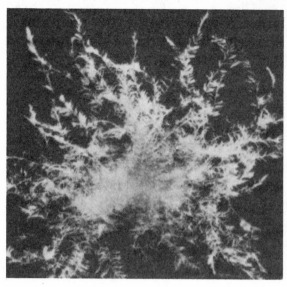

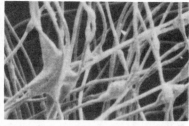

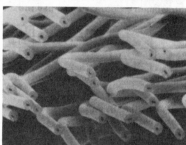

Insulating fillers work by creating air pockets to trap air and prevent heat from escaping. Down (far left) is the natural classic; it's lightweight, it breathes to allow body moisture to evaporate, and it springs back to its full loft after being compressed. New synthetic fibers like PolarGuard by Celanese (top left) and Hollofil II by DuPont (bottom left) are heavier than down and won't spring back as easily, but they're cheaper, and they do a better job of maintaining their insulation value when wet.

158 is the stuff. Look for it when you buy clothes to keep you warm and dry.

FILLERS

Down. Down lies beneath the feathers of geese and ducks and keeps them warm. When these birds are killed for market, the down is removed and through a series of processes ends up as fill in sleeping bags and down clothing. Down's claims to fame are lightness, compressibility, resiliency (it'll fluff right back up after being squashed), insulation value, and vapor conductance. It's the absolutely perfect fill as long as it's dry. This is where the problem starts. Down will absorb moisture on humid days, and this can reduce its warmth. If it ever gets sopping wet, forget it. The fibers collapse and mat, and it's a mess. Drying takes quite a while and, unless it's done properly, still leaves you with a mess, albeit a dry one. So keep it dry. One other tip. Don't store your down jacket in its stuff bag during the summer. Hang it up.

Synthetics. Two polyester synthetics capable of competing with down were developed during the 1970s—Du Pont's Hollofil II, which is a chopped-up fibrous batting, and Celanese's PolarGuard, which is long, continuous filaments. As far as protection against cold weather goes, they're alike. These are their qualities:

1. They occupy less volume per unit of insulation than down but are a bit heavier.

2. They're not quite as compressible as down, but they are as resilient.
3. They absorb very little moisture and can be wrung out or shaken dry in the field.
4. If they do get wet, they will not collapse, they retain insulating qualities.
5. They're much cheaper than down.

Synthetics may lack the aesthetic appeal, lightness, and compressibility of down, but they've sure got the edge when it comes to price and performing in wet conditions.

Within the past year 3M has developed Thinsulate, a polyolefin filler competitive with Hollofil and PolarGuard. Thinsulate promises the same qualities as its competitors, but with more heat retention at less bulk—or twice the warmth with half the loft.

OUTDOOR ACTIVITY

Now that you're familiar with what's available to keep you warm and dry while active in the cold weather, here's a rundown of some of the sports and activities out there in the cold.

By keeping in mind the functions of the clothing and materials mentioned above, and assessing the level of mobility and flexibility required by these activities, you should be able to suit up for total warmth and comfort.

SLEDDING

Of all winter activities, sledding is probably

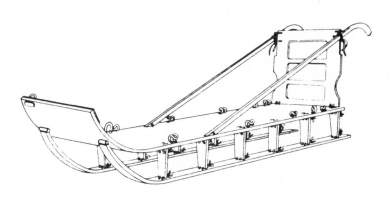

The army has developed this remarkable cross between a sled and a toboggan which is especially useful for carrying gear on winter camping trips. In packed or shallow snow, the sled rides on its runners. In deep snow, it rides on the toboggan floor. The runners also collapse against the floor to make a straight toboggan. (From Calvin Rutstrum, Paradise Below Zero [New York: Macmillan, 1972])

the most common, as well as the oldest means of moving something about on the snow. Sleds with hewn logs for runners were used over fifteen thousand years ago by Neolithic man. Their use as practical winter transportation continued well into the early twentieth century, when the automobile finally took over. By then, of course, kids and even adults had found a more fun use for the sled so that it didn't become an "endangered species."

There are three types of sleds—the rail sled, the toboggan, and the bobsled.

Rail Sled. This sled has two rails or runners, one running along each side of the sled's bed. You steer with a wooden or metal bar attached at right angles to the runners. Pulling on one end of the bar twists the front of the runners in the direction of the turn. You turn the sled by dragging your rear foot on the side of the turn.

The most common position for riding a rail sled is prone, on the stomach facing forward with both hands grasping the steering bar, the legs raised and extended to the rear. This position keeps the center of gravity low and reduces wind resistance. Kids will often lie one on top of the other, sometimes stacking to heights of six bodies, to get a really scary ride. Sitting one behind the other is the second most popular position; depending on the length of the sled, it can fit two or more persons. The recommended sled length for a child is 44 inches and for a teenager, 48.

Sleds rely on a push or gravity to get going.

A sled can really move on the right snow surface, but if the snow's not packed, it just bogs down. In soft powder snow the rail sled with its long thin runners is definitely at a disadvantage. The solution is the toboggan.

Toboggan. This sled is actually a large surface which glides over, rather than sinks into, soft snow. Toboggans are made from long, thin wooden planks joined side by side or from a solid piece of laminated wood. The front curves into a graceful arc to help the sled ride over the snow. Sizes vary from 3 to 8 feet in length and 2 to 3 feet in width. Large toboggans can carry up to eight persons. You steer by pulling one or the other end of a rope bridle attached to the outside tips of the curved front. Through experience, however, I've learned that toboggans do not steer very well, so it's best to aim them where you want to go before starting. Though toboggans are slower than rail sleds, because of the larger surface area they present to the snow, they can get up to 60 mph on a good downhill run.

Bobsled. Thrill-seeking English vacationers playing in Switzerland came up with this one during the late 1800s. They put a set of fixed rails at the back of a toboggan and a set of pivoting ones at the front for steering and had a helluva time racing them down the Alps. The name bobsled comes from the bobbing action of the riders. They'd lie back and quickly sit up in unison over and over again to milk the last bit of speed from the sled on the straightaway.

The Sporting Life

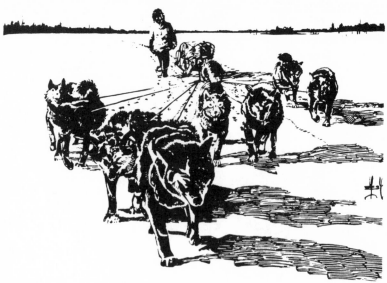

Dogs can be harnessed to sleds in a tandem or fan arrangement. The fan-wise hitch is crucial when the team is traveling over open sea ice; a dog falling through the ice won't pull the others down with him.

160   Modern bobsleds are made of metal frames with wooden beds. At the front they have a metal or fiberglass cowling to protect the riders and reduce wind resistance. Few if any of these sleds are seen in suburban neighborhoods because they require very long, firmly packed snow trenches that descend steep slopes to reach their effective operating speed. In fact, even toboggans are generally a pretty rare sight because of their low maneuverability and the long runs required to really get going.

Sledding doesn't necessarily require a legitimate sled. A large piece of cardboard, a garbage-can cover (without the handle, of course), or anything that slides will do. People have even been known to use aluminum canoes. The hill is the important requirement.

Sledding is definitely a wet activity, with much rolling and tumbling in the snow. Protective clothing should be as water-resistant as possible, and bulkiness would be good for cushioning falls as well as for insulation.

Dog Sledding.   This is a sport usually associated with Eskimos and trappers of the far north. True, but it can also be fun for the average person with a large dog and sled, if he's got the patience to train his dog to the harness.

In standard dog sledding a team of one or more dogs pulls a large rail or flat toboggan-type sled. The driver stands on extended runners at the rear of the sled, from which vantage point he commands the team. Harnesses and hitches for arranging the team vary with the operator's experience and the type of country being crossed.

Today the snowmobile has replaced the dog sled in many areas as the practical means of snow transportation, but sled and dogs are still pulled out on weekends and holidays for racing and competitive events. In Alaska, Wisconsin, and Minnesota, this is one of the really popular winter sports.

Snowmobiling.   For all intents and purposes the snowmobile is a motorized sled. Carl J. Eliason probably put together the first one in 1927, using a 2½-hp outboard motor. Today snowmobiles are propelled by a continuous track or belt in the rear and steered by ski-type runners in the front. They can go up to 60 mph and over and take a person a long way into the wilderness, which means he must be knowledgeable about survival skills in case of a breakdown. Learning to drive a snowmobile is easy enough, but learning to negotiate all snow surfaces is more demanding.

A snowmobile is economical on gas. It can run just about a whole day on its small tank. But in other ways it's not so economical. The initial cost of the machine is high and the season short. Unless you live in the country, you'll have to trailer or truck it to a snowmobile area in a state or national park. During the off season it takes up otherwise useful space in garage or shed.

On the positive side, a snowmobile is an excellent means of winter transportation for those who live in areas of heavy snow. The

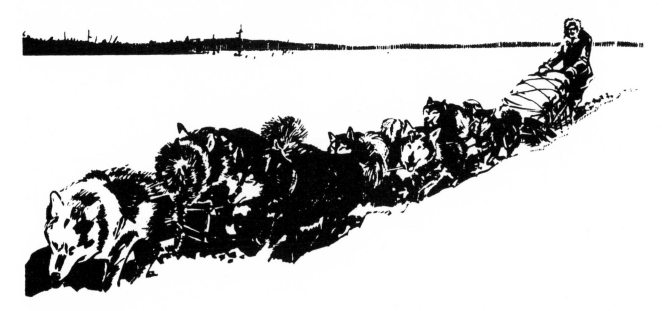

trips that can be taken are only limited by your imagination—exploring, winter camping, ice fishing, a lift for skiers to the top of a mountain, even skijoring, which is like water skiing with a snowmobile, rather than a boat, pulling.

There's a lot of sitting in snowmobiling. This calls for insulation to keep warm—especially for the feet. The sport has developed its own unique attire of overalls and boots to take care of this.

Skiing

Statistics show that the two most popular winter sports are bowling and skiing. So let's take a closer look at the No. 1 outdoor winter activity.

Ski comes from the old Norse word *skith*. It is speculated that the ski developed from the snowshoe more than five thousand years ago in Norway, but skis did not reach the United States until 1840, when the wooden blades were brought over to New England by Norwegian immigrants. There are two types of skiing: Alpine, which is downhill and slalom; and Nordic, which is ski touring, cross-country racing, and ski jumping.

Downhill Skiing. Downhill is what people usually mean when they talk about skiing. Basically, skiing is like sledding in that it uses gravity to slide at high speeds across the snow. But unlike sledding, there are a lot of opportunities to get into trouble on skis. In their haste to get onto higher slopes, many begin-

161

For more information on skiing contact:
American Ski Association
5830 S. Lake Houston Pwky.
Houston, TX 77049
Pacific Northwest Ski Association
3210 So. 176th St.—Apt. 134
Seattle, WA 98188
Eastern Ski Association
22 High St.
Brattleboro, VT 05301
United States Ski Association
1726 Champa St.—Suite 300
Denver, CO 80202

ners graduate themselves to difficult runs far too quickly for their experience. Many pros blame ski lifts for the mishaps of eager amateurs. If there were no ski lifts, you'd have to know how to ski *up* as well as down, and only skiers with experience could climb with ease to the highest peaks.

When starting out in skiing it's best to rent your gear and find out what the sport is all about before investing $350 or so in skis, bindings, poles, and boots. Gear can be rented at ski areas, where lessons can also be arranged. But even before that it's best to get into condition with an exercise program because skiing is an activity that calls on infrequently-used muscles. (This is true of several winter sports.)

Fitting out can be a bit nerve-racking economically, because of the numerous brands and prices—it's really overkill. Best bet is ask lotsa

162 questions and then take three days to sort out all the information. At that point you're ready to go in and buy. Size-wise the proper ski length is from the floor to the palm of your hand stretched overhead. There has been a tendency, though, for many novices to start with shorty skis, 2½ to 3 feet in length because they're slower and make it easier to learn basic techniques. Instructors vary in their opinions about whether this is beneficial, since ultimately most people move on to the longer skis, which means ultimately you'll have to learn how to handle them anyway. *Quien sabe?* As far as materials go, most downhill skis are made of plastics, synthetic laminates of fiberglass, and so forth, which are more durable and flexible than wood.

Bindings are purchased separately, but should be compatible with the ski. They're designed to keep the boot firmly in place, allowing the skier to lean forward without any lateral movement of his foot. Bindings normally have a release that will trip when a skier falls so his boot flies and he avoids a twisted or broken ankle.

Poles should have a strap at the handle and a basket at the lower end to keep the pole from sinking into the snow when it's used for balance or a push-off. Proper length is from the floor to the armpit.

Ski boots, or Frankenstein shoes as some call them, are very stiff and difficult to walk in at first. The reason for this rigidity is that it maintains the foot in an absolute position for balance and control—form. Wear cotton socks with wool ones over when fitting for boots. Your toes should have room to wiggle, but your ankle should be absolutely snug. Your heel shouldn't rise in the boot when you stand or lean forward. It's a good idea to have your skis and bindings on hand when you're buying boots or your boots on hand when you're buying skis and bindings.

Ski suits, parkas, and so forth are many and varied. Far too often, fashion rather than good cold-weather sense dictates choice. Consult the sections on clothing to see what constitutes good protection. Then you'll be equipped to make your own judgment on what brands meet the criteria.

Downhill skiing will seem a difficult and strange technique to the beginner. In the end, however, a person will simply be learning to move across a level surface, stop, turn while in position and while moving, step up a slope, and glide down it. Easier said than done, no doubt about it. Expect awkward moments, falls, and near falls. These are a *necessary* part of learning.

Most ski areas have their courses graded and marked for different levels of proficiency from beginner through intermediate to expert. These grades indicate increasing difficulty and steepness. Remember that it's steepness that affects speed, and speed without experience causes accidents. A 3-degree slope will have you moving at 25 mph, a 5-degree at 35 mph, and a 10-degree at 50 mph. Other hazards are icy spots on a downhill course, which can cause an expert problems in control, and skiing off the regular run, which can land you in traps just beneath the snow's surface, like rocks and stumps.

Competitive Alpine Skiing. The three competitive types of Alpine skiing are downhill racing, slalom, and giant slalom. Downhill racing is skiing as fast as you can down a specified course to beat the clock. The skier with the fastest time wins.

The slalom and giant slalom are basically the same except that the giant is longer and more arduous. The course is set up with a series of flags which the skier must pass through weaving a serpentine course. The competition here is in the style of weaving and the speed with which the course is covered.

Ski Touring. Ski touring is a form of Nordic skiing (some "specialists" classify certain kinds of ski touring as Alpine, but let us not get confused by the facts). It's also a practical means of winter transportation—which cannot be said of downhill skiing. Whereas the downhiller is almost totally concerned with gliding down slopes, the tourer must be much more versatile and ready to traverse level as well as uphill terrain. To him, downhill is the icing on the cake.

Since flexibility is required, the tourer cannot use the same rigid boot and binding arrangement as the downhill skier. Naturally this means he will not have the same degree of built-in control the downhill skier has at high

For more information on ski touring contact:
Ski Touring Council
c/o Rudolf F. Mattesich
W. Hill Rd.
Troy, VT 05868

speeds, but then high-speed downhill skiing is not the real objective of touring. Touring bindings and footwear allow the skier to raise and lower his heel in something like a walking motion while moving on the skis. At first glance the touring "boot" looks exactly like a jogging shoe. Actually it's very similar, though perhaps a bit beefier, and it's designed with a wider welt for the binding to attach to. The toe of the boot is all that is held to the ski, allowing the back of the foot free vertical movement.

Touring skis are lighter and narrower than downhill types. Proper length is measured from floor to overhead-stretched palm. Since touring skis must satisfy the need to ski uphill—that is, slide forward without slipping backward—they must have either a mechanical one-way slip surface, somewhat akin to fish scales, or a surface that will take wax. This means wood is desirable; in touring, wooden skis are more fashionable than plastic.

Waxing the bottom of your skis to provide grip in one direction and glide in the other is an art the tourer must learn because he needs traction on level and rising snow surfaces. A few introductory notes: Different snow surfaces require different ski surfaces to get the most out of your skiing. So first become a student of snow types. With this knowledge try to match the wax to the snow surface.

Touring poles are available in aluminum and cane, cane being the less expensive. Proper length is from floor to armpit.

The ski tourer wears the usual sweaters, windbreakers, and so on as the downhiller on the upper body; however, for the lower body, knickers and knee-length socks will give you maximum freedom of stride.

Ski touring is an easier technique than downhill to learn because of the freedom of the feet; the feel is almost like glide stepping. As with downhill, though, you must learn how to move, stop, turn, and so on with those long awkward "extensions" of your feet.

Outfitting for touring is not that expensive, running about $175 for skis, bindings, boots (all of which should be purchased at the same time), and poles. And for cheap you can learn to ski tour in your own backyard or neighborhood park. This makes it easier and less dear to get into than downhill (travel expense to ski area, lift tickets, etc.). Later during the season, after you've become proficient, there's no reason not to take your touring gear and head for a downhill ski area. All kinds of information on touring can be found in *Ski* magazine's *Cross Country Skiing* annual, which comes out each winter. You can find it on your newstand.

Competitive Nordic Skiing. Ski jumping, the first event in this group, seems to belong in Alpine skiing; however. . . . This sport involves dashing down a straight downhill run that ends in an upswept ramp. Flyaway! The skier gets as much speed up as he can on the downhill run so he can make the greatest distance on the jump. The event is judged on distance; courage; control while on the ramp, in flight, landing, and at the finish; and form.

Cross-country racing also used to be ski touring, but as wilderness recreation grew in popularity more people went on cross-country-ski runs for pleasure rather than competition. So now we have ski touring as a spin-off. A cross-country race is run over a natural terrain of hills and level ground. The most popular length is about 5½ miles, though there are courses as long as 25 miles. Competitors are judged on the basis of strength, endurance, technique, and tactical knowledge.

The Olympic Biathalon is a special cross-country race with military overtones. While doing the cross-country number, the participants, who carry rifles, must stop at certain checkpoints and fire at targets from specified shooting positions. The course is about 12 miles or so. You can imagine how grueling this event is toward the end when a contestant has slogged his way over 10 miles of snow and has to stop and fire at a small target a football field's distance away. Time is valuable on this run, and a missed target can cost the contestant two minutes.

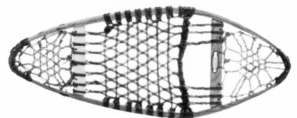

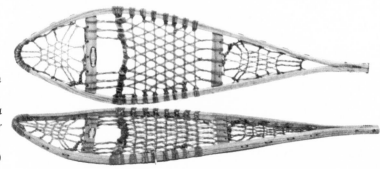

The Bearpaw snowshoe is relatively short and squat and is best for hiking over rough country. (L. L. Bean, Inc.)

The Maine Snowshoe from L. L. Bean (of Freeport, Maine, naturally) is a Beavertail design, for better weight distribution. (L. L. Bean, Inc.)

SNOWSHOEING

Walking through the winter wonderland over a sparkling, fluffy white carpet past snow-laden firs can lose some of its magic when, with each step, you sink up to your middle in snow. The way to rise above this is the snowshoe.

Snowshoes spread the wearer's weight over a larger area so that instead of sinking into the snow's surface he walks on it. Actually, snowshoes do sink, but only about 8 to 10 inches.

The snowshoe is an old winter transportation aid. It was first used on horses in Armenia once upon a time ago. Since men rode more than they walked then, it made sense to wrap the horses' feet with boughs to keep them from sinking.

As far as people go, the design of the snowshoe today is still pretty much the same as it was more than a hundred years ago. It's made of an oval wooden frame, the best wood being New England white ash, with a webbing of rawhide or neoprene stretched across it. The advantage of neoprene over rawhide is that wet snow tends not to cling to it. This keeps the snowshoe light, and mice don't nibble on it

during summer storage in the garage. A harness or the snowshoer's knot attaches the snowshoe to the foot. Though boots are worn with snowshoes, their hard heels tend to chafe the rawhide. Better footwear would be a pair of hightop moccasins.

There are several brands of metal- and plastic-frame snowshoes on the market; of these the Sherpa brand may be worth considering.

There are also many shapes, but, in general, snowshoes fall into the three groups exemplified by the Bearpaw, the Beavertail, and the Alaskan. In some locales (like the state of Michigan) the Beavertail is called the Michigan. Guess where it's called the Maine? The same goes for the other two groups—many names for the same snowshoe.

As to the practical aspects of these three types: the Bearpaw is the easiest to use and excellent for rough country where maneuverability is required; the Beavertail is the most popular, with better weight distribution than the Bearpaw; and the Alaskan, which is long, is best for fast travel over open country where skis would probably do just as well, so its use is limited.

Typically, a pair of snowshoes with harnesses runs about $80.

Using snowshoes isn't too difficult. Some say they're easier to learn than skis. The idea is to step a little higher and wider using a kind of bent-knee stride. Snowshoes do not have the same traction as a pair of boots, so you may have difficulty in climbing or descending a

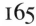 165

For more information on snowshoeing contact:
United States Snowshoe Assn.
RD 1—Box 170
Corinth, NY 12822

The Sporting Life

166 slope. But you can descend by squatting on the snowshoes and "sledding" down.

In case you're wondering how fast you can go on the "webs," 12 mph is not an uncommon pace in snowshoe races.

SKATING

Ice skating is another very old winter activity, which in the past was a means of travel between towns lying on the banks of frozen lakes and rivers. The people of the Netherlands first used polished animal bones as skates. Later they carved blades of hard wood. In 1572, the iron blade came into vogue in Scotland. The steel blade was developed in 1850 by E. W. Bushnell of Philadelphia; the steel blade can hold its edge for a longer time than the iron blades.

Today there are three basic types of skates, each with a different-shaped blade: the figure skate, the hockey skate, and the racing skate.

Figure Skating. This is the skating you see on winter ponds, lakes, and rivers. Though the higher levels of figure skating involve specific skating forms and skills, the lower level just requires moving forward, turn, stopping, and perhaps a little backward skating. (Actually,

---

For more information on skating contact:
United States Figure Skating Association
20 First St.
Colorado Springs, CO 80906

---

these are the basic requirements for any type of skating.)

One needs only the skates for general skating, and these may be either the figure or hockey types.

The figure skate is attached to a high boot and has a medium-length slightly cambered blade, with a serrated front tip. The edge of the blade is hollow on the bottom, giving it inside and outside secondary edges. These make for smooth skating strokes. Incidentally, the inside of a skate blade is toward the wearer's body's centerline and the outside, away from the centerline—two important things to know for serious figure skating.

The hockey skate has a low boot with a shorter but more highly cambered blade. The edge of the blade is flat on the bottom to facilitate quick turns and maneuvers.

The racing skate, with its very long 15- to 17-inch blade, is really not satisfactory for general skating.

Figure and hockey skates are available at large department stores and sporting goods dealers. Costs range from $20 to $80, depending on the quality of the materials.

When trying on skates, bring along a pair of light cotton and heavy wool socks. Skates should be snug at the sides of the foot and ankles, but should have plenty of room for toes to wiggle.

More skaters than ought to complain of weak ankles; after an hour or so of skating their ankles become fatigued and give out. As it

Total Warmth

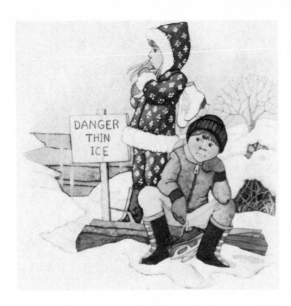

turns out, this is not the skater's fault, but the blade's. The skate blade should be attached to the boot slightly to the inside of the center of the sole, directly over the wearer's center of gravity (for that foot). This aligns the skate with the person's center of balance, and very little stress is placed on the ankle muscles. Unfortunately, mass-produced skates cannot be custom-fitted, so you often end up with skates that are out of balance. Result: weak ankles.

The beginner really ought to start off with an experienced skater to help get his ice legs, so to speak. A steadying hand can be an immense confidence booster in getting accustomed to this totally new way of moving about. After the beginner can stand and move about on his own, the skater should move off and demonstrate what it looks like to skate, turn, and stop properly. The beginner will learn much better by watching and copying—on his own and at his own pace—than by apron-stringing the skater.

A mnemonic on safe ice thickness (in inches):

One—Keep off!
Two—You might.
Three—You may.
Four—Okay.

Formal Figure Skating. This requires the ability to skate proficiently forward and backward while executing specific forms that have been adopted by just about every national skating association. The forms are skated in the shape of figures based on the circle. There are three-circle and two-circle figures like the figure eight. A form consists of skating in a particular manner tracing out the required figure superimposed on itself three consecutive times. That's one form. Another form is skating the same figure in a different manner. There are sixty-four basic (must learn) forms—just to give you an idea of what's involved. In addition to these, there are other techniques, such as the Three Turns, the Spin, the Salchow Jump and so on, that should also be learned.

Hockey. This competitive ice sport is apparently a spin-off of the old stick-ball games. The word hockey itself is believed to be of French origin from *hocquet,* a shepherd's crook, which in a way resembles a hockey stick. The game came to the United States from Scotland via Canada in 1893, and today is quite popular.

Equipment for neighborhood playing is readily available at sporting goods shops and some department stores. In addition to the skates it includes a hockey stick, puck, hockey gloves, shin guards, various body pads, and a helmet.

Racing. Speed skating is done on an oval track over a measured distance against the clock. This type of skating is greatly facilitated by long, straight, noncambered blades. Speeds of over 30 mph on the ice have been achieved by world-class skaters.

ICEBOATING

Iceboating is rare today compared to its popularity at the turn of the century. The winters were colder then, and just about all the lakes and rivers would freeze up for the whole season. Hot spots for the sport were New Jersey and New York state. In fact, the wealthy of that period, the Rockefellers, Vanderbilts, *et al.*, owned and raced large 70- to 100-foot ice yachts handled by professional crews. In addition to racing among themselves, they would also take on the steam trains whose tracks ran along the banks of the Hudson River. Reports of ice yachts attaining speeds of more than 120 mph were not unheard of.

The wealthy were not the only ones into the sport. The early 1900s was the day of the back-yard inventor/mechanic, and many a home-built rig was to be seen skimming along the ice on a breezy winter's day.

The typical design was the T-frame with a mast, sail, and seat for the pilot (never called a skipper). Angle-iron runners were attached to the ends of the three arms of the *T* with one pivoting arm for steering. Another popular design was the Scooter, a shallow, dish-shaped, duck-boat-looking affair with a mast and sail. For all intents and purposes it was a boat hull with runners on the bottom for gliding over snow and ice. If there happened to be a stretch of water to cross, the Scooter went right in, scooted across, slipped back up on the ice and continued on its merry way. Really a fun vehicle. It didn't have a rudder, but was quite

steerable through manipulation of the sail.

Today, iceboating is confined to the north-central United States and Canada, where it's cold enough to provide the ice needed. Boats are small and designed to comply with particular class requirements for racing. Only boats in the same class may race against each other, which puts them all on an equal footing, and the operator's skill is what makes the winning difference. The most popular class is the DN, primarily because the boat is easy to cartop, can be assembled quickly, and is light. Other classes are the Class E, Renegade, Yankee, and Arrow.

Today's boats still follow the T-frame design and are made of tubular aluminum with a fiberglass fuselage, stainless-steel runners, aluminum mast, and dacron sail. Typicallly, a factory-built iceboat will run in the neighborhood of $2000, though kits and partially assembled ones are also available at savings.

Sailing an iceboat is not that different from sailing a softwater boat except that it steers from the front, which can take a bit of getting used to. Also it's a lot hairier than the typical sailboat, because everything happens so fast. Speeds of 100 mph are possible; technically an iceboat can go four times faster than the wind. At first, this statement may not make any sense, but the gimmick is that the iceboat is capable of doing this when sailing *across* the wind, via a phenomenon called the "apparent wind." The iceboat cannot do this when sailing downwind.

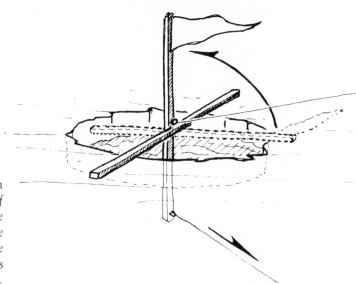

In a tip-up fishing rig, a fish pulling on the line tugs half the frame under water. The flag on the other end of the pole goes flying, telling the lucky ice-fisher that he's got a bite.

As far as outfitting for iceboating goes, the usual accessories are a helmet, goggles, heavy leather gloves, and ice creepers strapped to the boots. Windproof clothing with an emphasis on insulation is called for, particularly for the feet. Though the sport is fast-moving, the pilot is not. He spends all the time sitting in a cramped cockpit which doesn't do much for the circulation and warmth in his legs and feet.

ICE FISHING

It takes a hardy person to sit out on the cold, wind-blown ice two, maybe three, hours waiting to hook a couple of perch or crappies. But who's thinking about the cold? The fisherman is involved with the fish he's going to catch, the rigs he's set up, and how great it is to be far out there on the lake with peace and quiet and no one hassling him. It may well be that ice fishing is the true philosopher's winter sport.

At any rate, there are two kinds of ice fishing, which are based on the catching methods. The tip-up method uses an X-shaped wooden frame to hold the line. When a fish bites and pulls on the line, it pulls on the frame and tips it up, signaling the fisherman he's got a bite. The tip-up method allows several holes to be fished at once. Live bait, such as minnows, is used, and you ought to know at what depth the fish are feeding to set the bait. Tipping works pretty well for larger fish, such as trout, pike, and walleye.

Jigging is the other method. Here the drop line is attached to a jigging rod or just a stick. Jiggling the rod up and down gives the appearance that the bait is alive. This allows the use of lures. This method seems to work best for smaller fish like perch, crappies, and bluegills.

Regardless of the method, you do need to chop a hole through the ice to get to the fish. Specialized tools are available: an ice auger for boring, a spud or chisel for chopping, and a skimmer for clearing floating bits of ice from the water in the hole. Naturally, many home tools could be improvised to do these jobs.

Sitting out on the ice can get to be a cold number even if the fishing mystique is strong. Old timers have developed several methods of contending with this. One is to bring a sled out carrying all the fishing gear and a box to sit on. Put a lantern under the box. Or bring a small hibachi with coal to keep hands and coffee warm. For wind protection, a canvas frame on the sled will do, or if you're really into ice fishing, build a shanty on skids; put all the comforts of home inside. Interestingly enough, the shanty provides an additional benefit. Inside its dark interior it's possible to see to quite a depth into the water through the hole in the ice and watch the fish.

WINTER BACKPACKING

Backpacking in the winter is a whole new ball game to the person familiar only with summer outings. And for the person not even familiar with summer backpacking, only this caveat can be offered: no one should even *think* of attempting a winter backpacking venture,

The Sporting Life

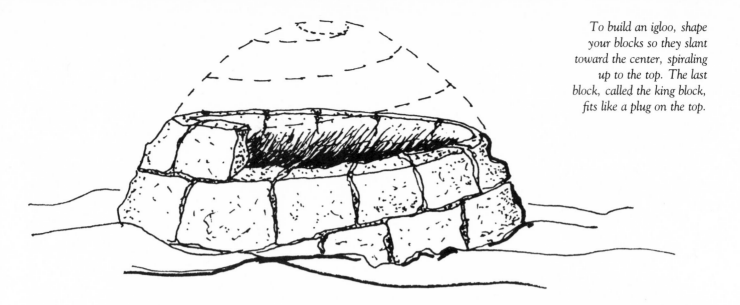

SNOW FUN

Snowflake and Frost Designs. Catching snowflakes on a dark cloth or paper for study can provide an afternoon's entertainment and absolute proof of nature's creativity, for no two snowflakes are alike.

Frost on windowpanes is another delight. Just blow your breath on a window and watch the beautiful patterns that crystallize. For new ones, blow again.

Snow Art. A little imagination leads to a lot of snow art. One popular type is the "snow angel." This is created by lying face up in the snow and moving your extended arms back and forth from hips to head, lightly brushing the snow surface. Stand up and you'll see an angel, wings and all.

Snow Structures. There are a couple of ways to build a snow fort or igloo. The Eskimos use very deep snow that has accumulated for many months and cut blocks with a snow saw. Each is carefully shaped so that when they're put together they form the upward climbing wall that turns into a roof and finally an igloo.

The other way of securing snow blocks is to use orange crates as molds. These blocks can be shaped for building an igloo or used as is for a snow fort. To aid in "cementing" the blocks, use a bucket of snow slush—snow with just enough water added to have a thick plasterlike consistency. Slush doesn't take long to freeze up, so work it in quickly.

Snow Sculptures. Snow sculptures can range from the usual snowman made of three large snowballs stacked on top of one another with a hat, a carrot nose, and a rock or coal mouth, eyes, and set of buttons to intricate carvings like those at winter carnivals which require much more work and a few tools for shaping.

First build a base to support the sculpture. Depending on the design you're executing, this can be a mound or wall of snow, hard packed and sprayed with water to freeze overnight, or a wooden 2-×-4 framework roughly shaped to the design and covered with chickenwire. Snow slush is then packed onto the supportive base, and the design is roughly shaped out by hand. When the slush has frozen solid, a chisel and hammer or axe can be used to finish the shaping. Keep the carving simple, for fine details don't show up very well. Snow sculpturing should be done only when the temperature is well below 32°F.

especially in snow country, until he's had at least a full summer and fall's worth of experience. Amen.

If you already have the basic skills and talent for trip and meal planning, trail navigation, long-distance trekking, setting up camp, and handling general chores like firemaking, cooking, and clean up, then winter packing can be an interesting experience. The snow-bound wilderness is a strange and beautiful place to-tally unlike the summer wilderness. If you thrive on the new and different, winter back-packing is not to be missed.

Backpacking can be combined with ski tour-ing or snowshoeing; in fact, in deep snow country one or the other is a must. When the terrain is mountainous with stretches of rock and ice in some places and large snow fields in

---

For more information on winter backpacking contact:
International Backpackers Association
P.O. Box 85
Lincoln Center, ME 04458
Sierra Club
530 Bush St.
San Francisco, CA 94108

---

others, the technique of ski mountaineering—a composite of hiking, light climbing, and skiing—is often used for travel. For the rocky stretches good heavy-duty climbing or hiking boots with Vibram soles are required. For the ice and small snow patches crampons are use-ful, as well as an ice axe. Crampons are spiked frames strapped to the bottom of boots to pro-vide better traction on ice or hard snow. An ice axe looks like a pickax but is smaller and has a longer handle. It is used as a walking aid, for cutting steps in snow or ice, and to arrest slipping by sinking the handle up to the hilt in snow or the pick into ice and holding on.

For the snow fields, mountain-type skis, which are sturdier and a bit shorter than the touring type, are used. Strap each ski to one side of the backpack when they're not being used. Summer packing gear is suitable for win-ter excursions with the following exceptions. The winter pack should have an inner liner closure that can be rolled or otherwise closed. The standard flap closure is not satisfactory in winter because snow can blow in through it. It's amazing the places you'll find wind-blown snow. Snow can lead to wetness, which is al-ways a danger in cold weather. Your sleeping bag should, of course, be good for the low-tem-perature ranges you expect to encounter. The only satisfactory stove for cold weather is a gasoline model *with pump*. Incidentally, be very careful to avoid spilling gasoline on bare hands—instant frostbite!

Probably the major specialized item required for snow camping is the tent. This does not mean that a summer tent can't be used, but rather that it will not afford the same protec-tion and comfort as a mountaineering tent. A mountaineering tent is light-weight, wedge-shaped, roomy enough for two people with gear, easily pitched and struck (set up and taken down), waterproof but not vapor proof, sturdy and well guyed to stand up to blizzard-force winds, and resistant to blowing snow and debris.

Typically this would be a double-walled nylon tent with a waterproof-coated floor. The floor should curve up at least 10 inches before

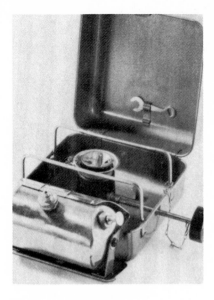

The Optimus 111B gasoline pump stove will burn for two hours on a pint of gas. It weighs just over 3 pounds and will boil a quart of water in under 4 minutes. (Ski Hut)

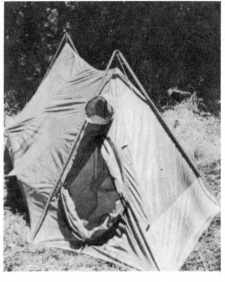

Cold-weather tents should have tunnel entrances rather than flaps to keep out snow and debris. (The Smilie Co.)

172

the wall panels are sewn to it. This keeps the seams high off the ground to prevent leaks—warm bodies inside the tent will cause the snow under the tent to melt. At the front, the tent should have a tunnel or tube-type entrance with a drawstring closure to keep out snow and debris. This is easier to work with than the flap-type in cold, snowy weather. Around the outside bottom perimeter of the tent are sewn wide strips of nylon, called snow flaps. These are piled high with snow to keep wind from blowing under the tent. Shock-cord ties are incorporated with the guys to dissipate wind force. The double-wall feature is really not an extra wall but an extra roof, called a fly. It's set about 4 inches over the tent roof and allows water vapor, given off through breathing and perspiration, to dissipate to the outside rather than condense on the inside and drip back down on the inhabitants. The fly is waterproof, whereas the roof of the tent is merely water resistant, which allows water vapor to pass through. If a hard rain hit the tent and you didn't have a fly, it would leak.

Tents, stoves, packs, and other backpacking gear are best purchased from a wilderness recreation outfitter. If there's none in your town, try a sporting goods store.

Every time you go out on a winter excursion, you learn new ways to make things easier and more comfortable in this hostile environment. I wouldn't want to spoil the fun of self-discovery; however, if you're just starting, a few tips can help speed you on your way.

Survey the area you plan to backpack in the fall. Know what the terrain looks like without all that snow, and avoid unpleasant surprises. Pick a couple of likely looking campsites and squirrel away some decent caches of firewood in a protected and dry place.

Plan meals that are high in calories and easily prepared. Keep them simple—one-pot, if possible.

Candles are handy for warmth (they'll warm up a small tent faster than you think), starting fires, light, and so on.

A whisk broom is very handy for brushing snow off boots and clothes to keep them and the inside of the tent dry.

With all the snow out there, you would think there's not much reason to haul along canteens full of H_2O. Well, as it turns out, it is worth hauling along water. There's not much water in snow—one part to every 10 or 12 of air—so it's definitely wise to bring your own bottle.

And last but not least, keeping dry means keeping warm.

WINTER PHOTOGRAPHY

What can bring out the artist in us more than the soft beauty of a snow-covered scene, especially after the first heavy snowfall of the season? Everything—the ground, the trees, the houses, the roads—is so pristine, so totally different from the dull browns and grays of the late fall. Just makes

you want to grab your 35-millimeter, run outside, and start clicking away.

A relatively quick trip outside to record nature's handiwork of the night past rarely results in any cold-weather problems, other than the standard one always encountered with bright, high-contrast scenes. Whether it's a winter snow scene or a summer beach scene, overexposure is the thing to watch out for, even with today's automatic electronic cameras.

Black and white film is forgiving if you're slightly off the proper setting; however, color film for slides, such as Kodachrome, must be right on or the result could be a washed-out, nothing picture. A good rule of thumb for slides is to close down the aperture a half-stop below whatever f-stop is indicated for a given shutter speed. Another good idea, when your subject is darker than the snow scene itself, is to get a specific closeup meter reading on the subject. When there is a great deal of light in the background and you're not close to the subject, the meter will often read the background only. A shot taken with this reading will result in an overexposed photograph.

Winter photography gets to be difficult when you're outside for extended periods of time—say, all day or over the weekend on a backpacking jaunt.

Cold and wetness, as usual, are the two culprits that get into the woiks and muck it up. Here's what cold does:

1. Slows down all camera parts by thickening the lubrication; shutter speeds will be slower.
2. Reduces the life of batteries. With a weak battery electronic cameras, light meters, and flashes are next to useless.
3. Stiffens the film and makes it very brittle. This means it may crack.
4. Increases static electrical discharges, which can show up as flash streaks on a picture.
5. Freezes moist fingers touching supercold metal to the metal's surface; you may have to leave a little skin behind to get free.
6. Numbs fingers and makes them clumsy.

How about wetness? Any wetness accumulating on the camera will condense on the cold camera as droplets of water, seep into the moving parts, and dilute lubrication, cause rusting, and freeze up solid when the camera is brought back out to the cold.

But there are ways to deal with cold and wetness.

If you really intend to do heavy camera work throughout the winter, it would pay ($50 to $70) to have your camera stripped down, cleaned, and relubricated with a lighter oil; do the same number at the end of the winter season to prep for summer.

As a way around *all* the other cold problems, keep your camera warm in your jacket until you're ready to shoot. This means having a good eye for exposure and composition so that you can adjust settings quickly, snap one off, and put the camera back into the jacket. Silk liner gloves will keep your fingers warm for about 5 to 10 minutes and allow the necessary adjustments should a complicated shot take a little more time. Liner gloves are available from wilderness-outfitting shops for about $5.

To avoid accumulations of falling or windblown snow on the camera, make up a cloth "throw-over" that can be attached to your hat or hood. When shooting, pull the cloth over the camera. It'll not only keep the snow off, but also reduce glare and so facilitate focusing and composing. Other than that, always brush snow off the camera before returning it to the warmth of your jacket. A small good-quality varnish brush from any hardware store serves well for this.

When ducking inside a cabin or wherever for a break, put your camera into a small waterproof baggie and tie it up *before* going in. This will keep the warm air's moisture from reaching the camera. Change film out of doors rather than inside to avoid this same condensation problem.

MAIL-ORDER COLD-WEATHER-CLOTHING SUPPLIERS

These mail-order outlets can supply the outdoor clothing we've been discussing. Most of these places have catalogs. Drop them a card.

Ski Hut
  1615 University Ave.
  Berkeley, CA 94701
Eastern Mountain Sports
  1041 Commonwealth Ave.
  Boston, MA 02215
Holubar
  P.O. Box 7
  Boulder, CO 80302
Synergy Works
  225 Fourth St.
  Oakland, CA 94607
Moor & Mountain
  63 Park St.
  Andover, MA 01810
Early Winters, Ltd.
  110 Prefontaine Place South
  Seattle, WA 98104
Frostline
  Frostline Circle
  Denver, CO 80241
Recreational Equipment, Inc.
  P.O. Box 1685
  Seattle, WA 98111
The Smilie Co.
  575 Howard St.
  San Francisco, CA 94105
L. L. Bean, Inc.
  997 Main St.
  Freeport, ME 04033
Eddie Bauer
  P.O. Box 3700
  Seattle, WA 98124

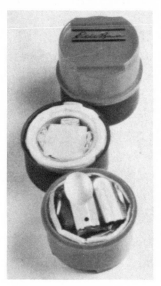

Eddie Bauer makes a combination stove and survival kit that includes almost everything you need in a pinch: a 6-foot tube tent, a windscreen, waterproof matches, a knife, a wire saw, fish hooks and a 20-foot fishing line, all packed into a stove casing that's just 3¾ inches tall and 4¼ inches in diameter! (Eddie Bauer)

SURVIVAL

Survival is basically the ability—the talent—*not* to go into emotional overdrive when confronted with the unexpected. If your mind doesn't run away with panic and projected expectations, it is free for thinking and sorting out what *has* happened and formulating a possible resolution.

The other key to survival is preparation. Read up on cold-weather survival and take along some basic equipment—a kit designed for winter situations (food, flares, waterproof matches), a poncho rolled in a belt pack in case you get wet, candles.

Figuring out a solution to a winter disaster requires knowledge of the way things work in cold weather. How does your body work? How does keeping warm work? How do snow and ice work? You can hardly be expected to solve a problem if you don't know what's involved.

Elsewhere in this book information is given on how the body works in the cold (see Chapter 8, The Body Response). Here we've discussed many of the principles of how to keep warm by keeping dry inside and out. That leaves snow and ice. Here's information that could be useful, plus tips on some basic survival techniques.

SNOW

Skiers are well aware that snow isn't all the same. First there is recently fallen new snow that's fluffy and light; then there's new snow that's dry, very cold, and powdery.

After snow sits on the ground a while, it undergoes changes caused by wind, temperature, sunlight, and humidity and is called old snow. It can take on many forms: settled, granular, crusty, packed, frozen, icy, or wet. Each of these presents different surface conditions for winter travel, and some could contain the makings of a survival situation—for example, icy (injury), wet (chilling, hypothermia), deep and crusty (exhaustion, hypothermia).

Snow can be dangerous in subtler ways, as in snow blindness, which can occur on sunny and even cloudy days. Always take along sunglasses. Symptoms are extreme pain in the eyes, smarting and scratchy eyelids, and headaches. Treatment is getting into a dark place or wrapping a light-proof bandage over the victim's eyes. Time will heal snow blindness, but it can take several days. Bright sun on the snow's surface can also cause sunburn on exposed skin, particularly the face. Try applying a sunscreen if you're going to be outdoors for a long time on a sunny day.

Snow is about 1 part water (the crystal) to 10 to 12 parts air. For this reason, eating snow as a source of water actually provides very little water, but what there is of it will certainly lower your internal body temperature. Better to heat the snow in a pot. Remember to press the snow down

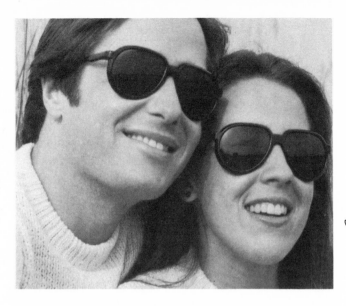

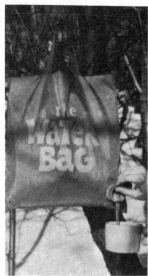

Sunglasses are by no means a luxury. They're crucial for preventing snow blindness from the sharp reflected glare off the white snow-covered ground. (Early Winters Catalog)

Since snow is less than 10 percent water by volume, it's a good idea to travel with a water bag or canteen even when you'll be surrounded by the white, wet stuff. (Moor & Mountain)

176 while it's heating or add some water to get the melting "primed." If you don't, you may burn the bottom of the pot.

The quantity of air in the snow does make it a good insulator, however. Shelters made from snow, such as igloos or snow caves, will keep a person a lot warmer than he'll be out in the open air. An igloo could take a whole day to build, but a snow cave could be built in three hours if you've got a shovel.

If an adverse situation such as a blizzard hits while you're en route, don't keep traveling. It's too easy to get disoriented. Seek shelter immediately. Shelter could be under a big fir tree right next to the trunk. If there's more time, build a lean-to from deadwood and pack the windward side with snow.

After shelter, warmth is normally your second objective. If a fire is practical and materials are available, build one, of course. First think carefully about where you intend to build it, though. In lieu of a fire, light a candle if the shelter is relatively wind-tight —cheer and warmth to a surprising degree. If you're in a shelter that's relatively airtight, like a tent or snow cave, and you're using a stove or even a candle for warmth, make sure some air can escape to prevent carbon monoxide poisoning.

ICE

As winter gains momentum and temperatures dip into the teens, ice forms on ponds then on lakes and finally rivers. Bodies of water freeze from the sheltered shore out toward the center. Ice thickness will vary greatly over an expanse of water, because of wind, feeder streams, water pollution, and so forth. Projections above the ice such as logs and boulders will conduct heat and keep the ice thin or melted in their vicinity. Clear smooth ice forms during periods of slow freezing (about 0°F temperatures) on calm days and nights. If it's windy, however, air turbulence will cause bubbles to be frozen in the water and give the ice a rough and grayish appearance. This does not affect its strength, though.

The safest ice is that formed on still water. The next safest is that on slow-moving rivers. Clear blue lake ice is about 15 percent stronger than clear solid river ice because river ice is constantly subjected to wear and strain from the currents. When walking on safe river ice, you often hear cracking here and there (like bullets ricocheting); lake ice will do this only when the temperature changes. This noise is really nothing to worry about as long as the ice is over 4 inches. Two inches is the absolute minimum thickness for one person—with caution. The problem is variability over the ice surface. Ice formed over swiftly moving water or water that changes levels, as it does in a tidal basin, should be treated with extreme caution, as should sea ice; minimum safe thickness is 6 inches.

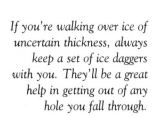

If you're walking over ice of uncertain thickness, always keep a set of ice daggers with you. They'll be a great help in getting out of any hole you fall through.

Ice formed in early winter is new or young ice. It's clear, with a dark blue or black hue —good solid ice (at 4 inches). If, however, it should snow while the ice is still thickening, the freezing process could be retarded, as the snow will insulate the surface against the cold air, so take precautions on early-winter days when it's snowing.

As spring approaches, with a brief thaw here and there, the ice surface will melt slightly and refreeze, taking on a white appearance. As long as the warm periods are short and infrequent, no problem. But as they increase in regularity, we go into the old or rotten ice period. This ice is always unsafe.

Some safety tips on ice travel. Always check the thickness before starting across, especially snow-covered ice. If you're with a group of people and the ice is less than 3 inches thick or it's old ice, space the people 10 or more feet apart. Someone in the group should carry a long pole in the event of a breakthrough. The pole can be used to help pull a person out, or if you're the unlucky one and you've got the pole, it'll straddle the hole and can be used as a self-aid.

If you plan to cross an area with many stretches of questionable ice, a good tool to carry is a pair of wooden "handles" with the business end of a 16-penny nail sticking out of the end of each one about 2 inches. Tie the two handles together with a long lanyard

and drape these ice daggers over the shoulders. There they'll be handy if you need them to get a purchase on the ice should you break through. Without them it's a bit more difficult to claw out of a hole.

If you do fall through the ice, fling your arms out as you break through to keep from going under the ice. Assume, as best as possible, a prone position parallel to the surface of the ice. Frog kick with your arms stretched out in front of you. The idea is to kick and slide your way back onto the ice. The ice edge may break, but keep at it. Once out, roll away. Don't stand up until far away from the hole. Carefully make your way back to the closest point of dry land. If there's snow, roll in it. It will absorb a lot of water from your dripping clothes. Next, pull your poncho from your belt pack, and put it on *over* the wet clothes. This will prevent evaporation and keep you warm enough to gather dry dead branches from trees (overhead, not from the ground, where the wood is wet) and put together the makings of a fire. Pull out your packet of #000 steel wool (wet, of course), shake it out, light a candle with one of the paraffin-coated matches you carry rolled tightly in a baggie or a survival kit and dry the wool. Under the sticks it goes, and soon you've got a toasty fire going. Stand close (not too close) and use the poncho as a tent to catch all that nice rising warm air.

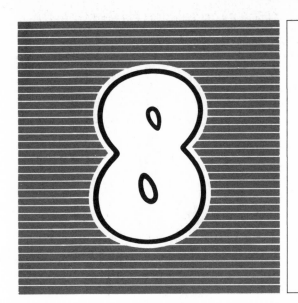

The Body Response: Cold-Weather Physiology and Health

Jonathan Leonard

We human beings are really semitropical creatures. When unclothed and at rest, our bodies crave places where the temperature hovers at around 85°F—places like the forests of Nigeria and the beaches of Acapulco. Our internal thermostat reads 98°–99°F, and unlike the polar bear or walrus we have little insulating fur or blubber, so when we sit around naked at temperatures below about 75°F for any length of time we usually feel the cold.

But not everyone reacts to low temperatures in the same way. Some people detest the cold, and others revel in it. Some even find that an indoor temperature of 60°F can be perilous to life. So it seems reasonable to ask questions like why are babies and older people especially vulnerable to the cold? How do Eskimos survive extreme cold? Why does one hiker die of cold while an identically exposed companion survives? In sum, what accounts for human responses to the cold, and why do those responses vary so?

THE WORKING PARTS

To begin with, how does our temperature-regulating system work? Like all mammals, we human beings are "warm-blooded"—that is, we have the ability to maintain a stable body temperature despite dramatic temperature shifts in the external environment. Responding to the weather, we automatically adjust heat production or heat loss, keeping body temperature at a fairly steady 98.6°F. When it gets hot, we cut heat production, and we remove heat from our bodies by perspiring. Conversely, when it gets cold, we produce heat faster and lose it more slowly. Many creatures —reptiles, amphibians, and insects—cannot do this, but we both can and must, though we're largely unaware of our abilities. Like acrobats, we maintain our thermal balance, practically from birth, and risk all if we lose it.

The machinery that maintains this vital balance controls our response to cold. This machinery has four main cold-regulating elements, corresponding to an ordinary home's outdoor thermometer, thermostat, furnace, and heat-circulation system. Despite this simple plan, the system is complex; indeed, it far more resembles the heating system of the World Trade Center—millions of pipes, thousands of controls—than a home system.

Consider the thermometer. Your body's outdoor cold-sensing thermometer uses multitudes of specialized nerve endings in the skin to register the cold in sophisticated ways. For example, when you step outside in winter, the thermometer immediately tells your brain about the cold, long before your skin temperature has dropped. But when you work outside producing as much heat as you lose—maintaining your thermal balance—the thermometer sends no message of distress, even though your skin is cold. Or in extreme cold the thermometer may have only moments to send an urgent distress call before its nerve endings are

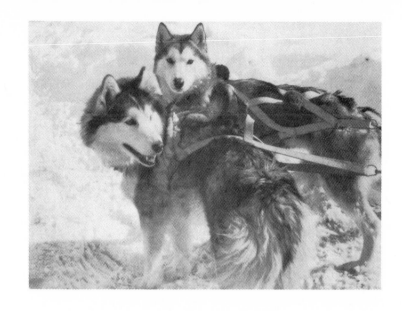

Unlike humans, these sled dogs are covered with insulating fur—quite an advantage when you're trudging through the snow! (Northwest Publishing Co.)

numbed to silence. But it does send a call, and your body gets the information it needs to take preventive action.

The regulator of that action, your body's thermostat, resides in a small central part of the brain called the hypothalamus. Experiments have shown that destroying the back part of the hypothalamus stalls the whole cold-protection system. Even at room temperature, a mouse whose posterior hypothalamus has been destroyed will cool off and die of hypothermia—literally "lack of heat." Similarly, human infants with immature coordination systems and elderly people with weakened systems can get hypothermia.

Normally, though, the hypothalamus responds to cold signals by launching countermeasures. It may stoke the body's furance by making the adrenal glands over the kidneys release adrenaline, causing the heart to beat faster, increasing the flow of oxygen and food to the body's myriad cells, and making the cells generate more heat.

The hypothalamus also cuts heat loss by controlling heat circulation. The body's ductwork of blood vessels carries heat around the system, but the hypothalamus and attendant nerves can contract the arteries to cut both circulation and heat flow. This they do as needed, concentrating on the small arteries in extremities and skin that are exposed to cold. These blood-poor regions then act like insulators, reducing heat loss from the rest of the body even as their own temperature falls. That is why pallor suggests chill; why cold-water swimmers emerge with clammy, pale skin; and why all of us, even when gloved and shod, can get cold hands and feet.

In addition, the hypothalamus activates small muscles attached to body hairs, elevating the hairs and making the little bumps called gooseflesh. This hair-raising act is no use to us nearly hairless humans, but it benefits such creatures as cats and dogs by raising their insulating fur.

If your temperature keeps dropping in the face of all these preventive measures, the hypothalamus will tell your skeletal muscles to get moving. In response they shudder into random motion, causing shivering and using their food stores to make heat. Even if you shiver only slightly, the increased heat, like the heat from an auxiliary furnace set on low, will be significant. And if you shiver violently, running this auxiliary furnace at full tilt, your whole body's heat output can be multiplied several times.

But shivering won't make you warm. All it does is keep your temperature from dropping further. Meanwhile, your body is burning its food reserves in the hope that the situation will improve. Clearly, further action is demanded.

Accordingly, your body makes sure you get the message. This is why cold sensations, especially shivering, make you uncomfortable. This discomfort is your body's way of prodding you into action. Depending on who and where you are, these sensations tell you to put on a

The Body Response

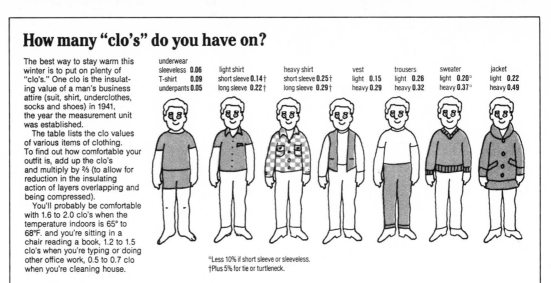

(*From* Changing Times,
November 1979)

sweater, stop making snowballs without mittens, build an igloo, move closer to the campfire, leave the water, or seek shelter. The message is important, because the body's remarkable ability to cope with cold is limited, and real peril may await those who ignore its SOS.

HYPOTHERMIA, THE SILENT KILLER

Consider the case of a young hiker in the Adirondacks who suddenly began to shiver uncontrollably. According to *Outdoor Life* reporter Vin T. Sparano, "As he rested beside the trail, his blue jeans covered with snow, other winter trekkers passed blithely by. Nobody, not even his partner, realized how serious his symptoms were. A few hours later he was dead—a victim of hypothermia" (*National Wildlife*, December 1977, pp. 26–27).

This kind of "exposure" hypothermia can strike people whose cold-sensing systems are working well. It does so by direct assault—exposing the body to so much cold that its defenses are overrun. Drunks who fall asleep on cold sidewalks often get this kind of hypothermia. So do ill-clad or unwary hikers, capsized sailors, cold-water swimmers, and rain-soaked mountaineers.

Another kind of hypothermia, called accidental hypothermia, attacks thousands of infants and elderly people *indoors* every winter.

Many old people, in particular, die of it. No one knows the exact numbers because many die alone, because rectal thermometers reading below 95°F (where hypothermia begins) are not available when needed, or because the cause of death may be hard to trace. But about 10 percent of all people over 65 have some sort of temperature-regulating defect, and between 3 and 4 percent of all hospital patients over 65 are hypothermic. As Dr. Richard W. Besdine of the Harvard Medical School points out, "Fifty thousand to 60,000 elderly people *that we know of* may have hypothermia every year."

This "accidental" hypothermia is very different from the "exposure" hypothermia that threatens Arctic explorers and winter sportsmen. Exposure hypothermia usually strikes healthy adults outdoors—and it can strike very fast. Accidental hypothermia, in contrast, tends to attack slowly indoors, claiming victims whose temperature-regulating systems are very weak.

In both cases, however, hypothermia strikes because the victim cannot maintain his thermal balance in cold surroundings, and so his body cools. If it cools to only 95°F, where hypothermia technically begins, prospects for recovery are bright. But it if cools much further, prospects dim. As hypothermia deepens, the victim's speech and actions slow, drowsiness sets in, and he slips into a coma. Around 85°F—13° below the norm—blood pressure falls, the pulse rate slows, and cardiac irregularities occur. If no one intervenes and body tempera-

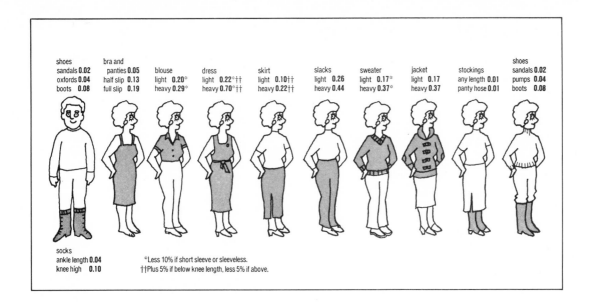

shoes		bra and		blouse		dress		skirt		slacks		sweater		jacket		stockings		shoes	
sandals	0.02	panties	0.05	light	0.20°	light	0.22°††	light	0.10††	light	0.26	light	0.17°	light	0.17	any length	0.01	sandals	0.02
oxfords	0.04	half slip	0.13	heavy	0.29°	heavy	0.70°††	heavy	0.22††	heavy	0.44	heavy	0.37°	heavy	0.37	panty hose	0.01	pumps	0.04
boots	0.08	full slip	0.19															boots	0.08

socks
ankle length **0.04**
knee high **0.10**

°Less 10% if short sleeve or sleeveless.
††Plus 5% if below knee length, less 5% if above.

ture keeps falling, the victim will soon die of fibrillation or cardiac arrest.

Most elderly victims die because their thermal balance systems are defective; many may not even feel cold. Typical victims live alone in badly heated rooms and may be suffering from heart ailments, stroke damage, senility, or other problems in addition to hypothermia. These circumstances help explain why accidental hypothermia often escapes notice until too late and why many victims who are discovered die of heart failure during the rewarming process.

Even so, we know ways to thwart this silent killer. Perhaps the most important thing is simply to be aware of what can happen. Not just doctors but nurses, social workers, people dealing with the elderly, and the elderly themselves should know what can go wrong. Moreover, everyone should recognize that dropping the thermostat to 60–65°F is safe for the young and middle-aged, but can be fatal to the old. Hence, elderly homeowners and homeowners who live with elderly people may wish to reconsider plans for saving fuel. A thermometer in each room will also alert older people and tell them when it's cold enough to put on extra clothes even though they may not feel chilly.

It's also a good idea to know the early signs of an attack, since it's much easier to handle hypothermia before the body temperature has dropped too far. At room temperatures of 50° to 65°F, hypothermia can take hours or days to develop, so there's plenty of time to head off

serious consequences. Shivering, the first early warning sign of outdoor hypothermia, may be absent in old people. Instead, look for signs of abnormal fatigue or profound weakness; victims commonly become confused or sleepy and may lose consciousness.

If you notice these symptoms, take a suspected victim's rectal temperature, provide gentle warmth, and call a doctor. The patient should be put into a warm place and covered with a blanket. (Too-quick rewarming is very risky because it increases the chance of heart failure.) Ideally, the thermometer used to take the patient's temperature should be one that registers to below 95°, though most household thermometers do not. These immediate steps will not ensure recovery, but they should help identify the problem, keep the temperature from falling further, and promote survival.

Besides assailing the elderly, accidental hypothermia can strike babies, especially newborns, because their temperature-control systems are immature. This explains why premature infants must be kept in incubators, newborn infants need around-the-clock warmth for a few weeks, small babies should never be bathed in cold places, all babies should be dressed sensibly, and mothers should check periodically to see whether their babies feel cold. One note: You can't tell whether a baby is cold by touching his hands or feet—they're always cold. Check his body temperature by touching his neck, legs, or arms. As another precaution, if you're nursing a new-

181

COLD MEDICINE

Cold, correctly used, has great preserving and healing powers. Medical workers deep-freeze live vaccines, cell cultures, and tissue specimens to preserve them. Physicians, nurses, and patients use ice packs to soothe everything from aching teeth to sprained ankles. And burn victims find that applying ice water to a burned area immediately for several minutes markedly reduces the ensuing inflammation, pain, and damage.

Beyond all that, medical science has found that red blood cells can survive deep-freezing. In fact, frozen in the presence of the chemical protectant glycerol, these cells can stay alive for many years at $-80°F$ to $-196°F$ and then survive rethawing. Blood banks now preserve rare kinds of red cells in cold storage, and blood suppliers freeze red-cell reserves until they are needed.

Essentially the same technique works fine with sperm, and since it is easier to transport frozen sperm than a several-thousand-pound bull, about half the world's calves are conceived by frozen proxy. Also, human sperm's life at room temperature is brief, but sperm from a potential father can be collected, preserved alive by freezing, and later pooled with more of the father's sperm. Such pooling can help overcome certain kinds of human infertility, and thus far well over 3,000 children have been conceived with frozen sperm.

Cold also helps the surgeon. Freezing the flesh instead of cutting it tends to numb feeling, limit bleeding, and prevent scarring. To achieve these desired effects, surgeons have developed various techniques—from spraying cold liquid (usually liquid nitrogen) on the skin to applying the cold liquid internally through a narrow tube. Surgical application of extreme cold, or cryosurgery, has been successful in removing facial scars, excising warts, extracting cataracts, reattaching detached retinas, curing certain kinds of skin cancer, and giving access to diseased parts of the brain.

Hypothermia has also been enlisted in this cause. Chilled bodies demand less oxygen and chilled hearts pump less blood, so in prolonged operations hypothermia can help reduce tissue damage and blood loss. Naturally, care must be taken to have the equipment needed for overcoming possible fibrillation and cardiac arrest, but hypothermia has by now become standard practice in many major operations. For this reason innumerable survivors of brain, open-heart, cancer, and organ-transplant surgery owe their lives to cold.

born at home, mount a wall thermometer to make sure the room temperature stays above 65°F.

It's distressing, but a baby with hypothermia may not look sick. Danger signs are lack of

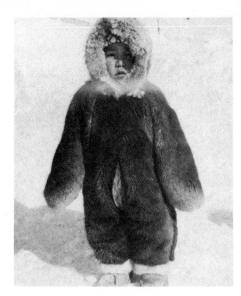

What the well-dressed Eskimo baby is wearing this year. A caribou snowsuit is sensible for the Arctic north; further south, the required degree of bundling varies. (Explorers' Guide, TravelArctic)

interest in food, a whimper instead of a lusty cry, swollen eyelids and extremities, and cold skin that may feel hard in places. These signs mean the baby could be in serious trouble. As with hypothermia of the elderly, the most important thing is to call a doctor. Steps should be taken to keep the baby's temperature from falling further, but immediate rewarming should not be attempted; rewarming is risky and requires a doctor's care, preferably in a hospital.

FROSTBITE, DANGEROUS BUT PREVENTABLE

In extreme cold if all your body's usual ways of staving off hypothermia have failed and too much heat is being lost in particular extremities, your body may have one last desperate card to play. In this case, instead of reducing the blood flow in those extremities to about a fifth of normal, it can cut the circulation altogether, letting one or more extremities freeze so that the rest of you will have a better chance of survival. This physical freezing of the flesh, which can also happen other ways, is known as frostbite.

Like hypothermia, frostbite is bad news. Frostbitten people are usually laid up for months; suffer pain; lose toes, feet, or fingers; and sometimes get gangrene. Virtually all victims survive, but the discomfort and damage done can end their hiking or mountain-climb-

IMMERSION FOOT: A WARRIOR'S CURSE

Immersion foot—also called trenchfoot—generally strikes soldiers who are forced by battlefield conditions to endure wet, cold, and immobility for at least 48 hours. This combination of conditions cuts the blood flow to the surface of the feet, deprives the affected areas of oxygen, and eventually damages nerves and capillary walls. The result: A swollen, numb, and reddened foot that soon becomes pale, mottled, and, finally, blue or black. Later events may include tingling, pain, more swelling, blisters, ulcers, and perhaps gangrene. In rare cases the most effective "treatment" is amputation.

If amputation isn't necessary, the patient generally recovers full use of his foot after an enforced 6 to 10 weeks in bed. However, for months or even years later the foot may be unusually sensitive to weight, cold, or pain.

Many things may increase susceptibility. Wetting or cooling the whole body, wearing inadequate clothing or tight boots, exhaustion, seasickness, dehydration, and starvation can all contribute. But the principal requirement is a wet—or at least a damp—extremity.

From this description it is clear that immersion foot rarely occurs except under conditions of real hardship. Who except the embattled soldier, stranded camper, or shipwrecked sailor would willingly endure

The Body Response

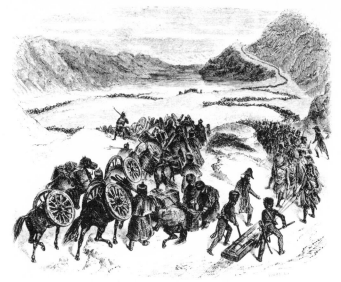

Napoleon's troops struggling through the St. Bernard Pass into Italy in May 1800.

wet feet for the required 48 hours? Furthermore, the main preventive measures are simple: Drying the feet overnight, avoiding tight clothing, moving about, and getting enough rest. So immersion foot generally attacks people who are more concerned about other things—at least until it strikes.

---

ing days forever.

Frostbite, a chronic scourge of war, appears early in recorded history. The Greek historian Xenophon, leading a retreating army across the mountain wilderness of Kurdistan in 400 B.C., reported that soldiers suffered from the cold and their "toes dropped off from frostbite." Frostbite also assailed Napoleon's armies, claimed 100,000 casualties in World War I, and mauled the German invaders of the Soviet Union in World War II.

Not all cases are military, however. Exhausted, stranded, or ill-prepared mountaineers get frostbite. So do drunks on cold benches, skiers on cold slopes, and drivers repairing cold cars. Whoever the victims are, they fall prey for one of two reasons: either they expose some extremity to quick freezing, or they become cold, tired, and vulnerable to gradual frostbite.

Some of the fastest frostbite attacks on record struck U. S. Air Force machine gunners over Germany during World War II. According to Bradford Washburn, then director of Boston's Museum of Science, writing in *The New England Journal of Medicine* (May 10, 1962):

When attacked, the only way that the "waist gunners" of the B-17 and B-24 aircraft could operate their machine guns was to open the large "waist ports" through which the guns were fired, directly into the frigid −25° to −45°F air, rushing by at about 200 miles per hour and swirling around the interior of the airplane.

Starting their work wearing heavy mittens and bulky sheepskin clothing, the gunners often threw away their gloves and even, occasionally, their jackets, working the guns bare-handed to assure better dexterity—which they felt necessary to save their lives. Terrible cases of frostbite resulted from these exposures, some of which [exposures] lasted only a minute or two, but which fulfilled perfectly all the requirements for acute contact.

Gradual frostbite, the kind suffered by Xenophon's men, mountain climbers, and alcoholics, comes on more subtly. Suppose, for instance, that a climber scaling a cold peak becomes exhausted. In this exhausted state his body may have trouble keeping warm, so blood is withdrawn from the extremities to warm his vital core. Of course, some circulation continues, and every so often the constricted blood vessels dilate, sending a fresh flow out to blood-starved extremities. But these efforts may not be enough, and the climber's temperature may continue to fall. More blood will then be withdrawn from his extremities, and some exposed hand or foot may freeze.

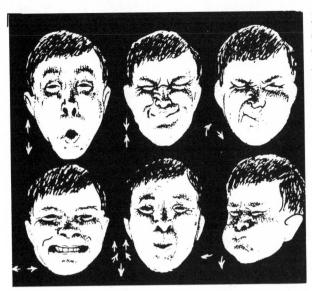

Making faces will keep blood circulating to help ward off frostbite. (From Anthony Greenbank, The Book of Survival [New York: Harper & Row, 1967])

At this point a mountain climber wading through cold snow may have no idea his foot is threatened. Earlier in the day his foot probably felt cold, but as time passed the cold sensors' messages to his brain became less urgent, and his sense of discomfort diminished. Then, just when matters got critical, the climber may have had a twinge of pain or a burning/stinging sensation in his foot.

But if this last call for help went unheeded, there was no further message. Indeed, the afflicted foot, perhaps now frozen hard as stone, is silent, and this lack of complaint registers on the climber's mind as comfort and well-being. So he may trudge on, if he is inexperienced, unaware that his foot has turned into a block of ice.

Actually, this lack of pain may be for the good. It means that the injured member does not need to be rewarmed right away. Thus, the victim can reach safety under his own power and can wait, even several hours, to have his foot properly rewarmed. The alternative, rough-and-ready rewarming somewhere on the slopes, often does irreparable harm. Frozen feet or hands rewarmed against a companion's stomach or in his armpit—the usual last-ditch method—rarely recover well, and those rewarmed near a fire are often damaged. Even if slopeside rewarming is effective, the victim then becomes a litter case; he must be carried to a hospital, and since he is then immobile, generating virtually no heat, the thawed part may refreeze.

In contrast to refreezing, a delay in rewarming does relatively little damage, for freezing alone does not kill the body's cells. Most cells are perfectly able to tolerate ice crystals alongside them temporarily, as long as the cells can get enough oxygen—and at 32°F their demand for oxygen is very low. Cells will die if ice crystals form inside them, as can happen in some cases of rapid frostbite. In cases of gradual frostbite like the one cited here, however, the ice crystals generally form between the cells rather than within them, and so the cells in the hard-frozen foot are alive and well.

The crisis comes when the cells warm up and demand oxygen. When the body made the decision to permit freezing of the foot, it cut the flow of oxygen-providing blood to that suffering extremity. That, together with the freezing, encouraged clots to form in the capillaries serving affected tissues, creating a million tiny roadblocks in the blood vessels. A proper rewarming in a water bath generally allows some detours to be found, but in all places where the blood's path remains blocked, oxygen-starved cells die.

So even when the foot survives, many cells perish. This causes the foot to swell; great blisters form, the flesh discolors, and the skin slowly blackens. The swelling may last a month or more, accompanied by throbbing or shooting pain, and infection and gangrene are common.

Even if all goes fairly well, when the blisters and the dead skin finally slough off, they are

The Body Response

(*From* Explorers Ltd. Source Book, *compiled by* Explorers Ltd., Harper & Row, 1977)

WIND-CHILL CHART

Estimated Wind Speed MPH	ACTUAL THERMOMETER READING °F.											
	50	40	30	20	10	0	—10	—20	—30	—40	—50	—60
	EQUIVALENT TEMPERATURE °F.											
Calm	50	40	30	20	10	0	—10	—20	—30	—40	—50	—60
5	48	37	27	16	6	—5	—15	—26	—36	—47	—57	—68
10	40	28	16	4	—9	—21	—33	—46	—58	—70	—83	—95
15	36	22	9	—5	—18	—36	—45	—58	—72	—85	—99	—112
20	32	18	4	—10	—25	—39	—53	—67	—82	—96	—110	—124
25	50	16	0	—15	—29	—44	—59	—74	—88	—104	—118	—133
30	28	13	—2	—18	—33	—48	—63	—79	—94	—109	—125	—140
35	27	11	—4	—20	—35	—49	—67	—82	—98	—113	—129	—145
40	26	10	—6	—21	—37	—53	—69	—85	—100	—116	—132	—148

Wind speeds greater than 40 MPH have little additional effect	LITTLE DANGER FOR PROPERLY CLOTHED PERSON	INCREASING DANGER	GREAT DANGER
		DANGER FROM FREEZING OF EXPOSED FLESH	

To use the chart, find the estimated or actual wind speed in the left-hand column and the actual temperature in degrees F. in the top row. The equivalent temperature is found where these two intersect. For example, with a wind speed of 10 mph and a temperature of —10°F., the equivalent temperature is —33°F. This lies within the zone of increasing danger of frostbite, and protective measures should be taken.

186 likely to carry off with them the remains of toes claimed by frostbite. Below is new, highly sensitive skin that may itch for many months and may forever after be abnormally sensitive to cold and prone to frostbite.

I have reported here a very serious case of frostbite. Not all frostbite is this severe. Superficial frostbite, when only cells near the skin freeze, tends to cause less damage, though even mild frostbite may require weeks of complete rest, while "deep" frostbite victims can expect to be hospitalized or bedridden for months.

In the face of these very serious and sometimes debilitating consequences, a few words of caution are in order. How can frostbite be prevented? For one thing, avoid barehanded contact with very cold metal objects (crowbars, wrenches, doorknobs, sparkplugs, and so forth); metal can steal body heat very fast and cause freezing. For another, in really cold weather, cover your head well and keep your face out of the wind. According to U.S. Army estimates, air at 0°F blowing at 20 miles per hour can freeze exposed flesh in a few minutes, while air at —25°F blowing at 30 miles per hour can do so in 30 seconds. That means skiers, who create their own wind, must be especially careful in bitter cold, and everybody who confronts winds on subzero days should go out in groups if possible, so that members can watch one another's faces for the sudden blanching of the skin that signals frostbite.

To prevent more gradual frostbite, apply the general rules needed to stay warm. Avoid con-

ENGLAND'S BURDEN: CHILBLAIN AND PERNIO

Few Americans know about chilblain or pernio because they're really English problems. England has the right conditions for these ills—a cool, damp climate and cold homes—while most of the United States does not. Nevertheless, Americans are not immune, as many WACs stationed in England during World War II found out. And since lowered thermostats can make chilblain and pernio more likely, it is worth knowing what causes these ailments and how they act.

Chilblain attacks the hands and feet. A glance at these extremities will show that their palms and soles are well padded, while the back of the hand and top of the foot are not. Instead, the latter are crisscrossed by blood vessels and other working parts just beneath the skin. These are the delicate parts that chilblain strikes.

It turns out that exposing the hands or feet often to dampness and moderate cold (32°–60°F) can interfere with tiny vessels in these areas and disturb the circulation. The eventual result: Swollen reddish-blue patches that itch and burn appear on the back of afflicted hands and the top of afflicted feet. The pain and swelling usually subside in a few days, but continued exposure to humid cold can make them chronic and likely to return spontaneously in cold weather. A

similar affliction that appears on women's unprotected lower legs is called pernio.

The best treatment for pernio and chilblain is preventive—keeping the extremities warm (about 60°F) or away from humid air. Of course, victims rightly claim this may be difficult—especially in England. Nevertheless, medicine can offer nothing better than rewarming the extremity in water or applying corticosteroids and other drugs to diminish the effects. Neither of these treatments is any panacea; and since continued exposure makes matters worse in any case, sufferers are well advised to take preventive measures.

stricting footgear. Wear several layers of loose-fitting dry clothes and mittens. Don't expose yourself to bitter cold for long unless you exercise. When you exercise, adjust your clothes or rate of exercise to minimize perspiration. And, above all, stay dry.

But suppose something goes wrong and frostbite does strike. You can treat a small area of newly blanched skin (frost "nip") by firmly pressing a warm hand on it (do not rub) or by cupping your hands and blowing on the afflicted spot until color returns to the skin. For anything beyond this kind of superficial freezing of the skin, however, you should get to a proper treatment center right away.

Strangely enough, if you walk down a ski slope or mountain on an unbroken but frozen foot, you won't have a real problem. In the 1960s Dr. J. W. Mills, a leading frostbite expert in Anchorage, described in *The New England Journal of Medicine* the results of walking on frozen feet: "We have had a half dozen patients who walked for three or four days with completely frozen extremities—some of whom have sustained no loss at all. Others lost toes only. In no case did any of them lose any more of the foot than toes. There even appears to be an opportunity to preserve all the digits, provided that *as soon as the patient has reached a place where thawing can be managed, it is done by the method of rapid rewarming,* followed by the regular routine of sterile hospital care."

Rapid rewarming, as practiced today, generally involves putting the frozen part of the body into a water bath at 104°–112°F for as long as necessary, usually about 30 minutes. Other details:

- The frozen part should never be rubbed, massaged, or placed in snow.
- The victim should not smoke or drink alcohol before or during treatment. Smoking contracts blood vessels and alcohol expands them; both can do serious harm during rewarming.
- If the rewarming room is cold, the victim's body should be made as warm as possible.
- The warm bath should be deep enough to ensure complete immersion of the afflicted extremity, which should be suspended in it.
- The bath temperature should never exceed

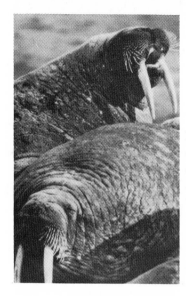

Marine mammals like the walrus have been the essence of survival to the Netsilik Eskimos of Canada's Arctic. The Eskimos eat the meat, wear the skins, and burn the fat in stone vessels for heating and cooking. (Explorers' Guide, TravelArctic)

188   112°F, nor should water over 115°F be added.

- Aspirin should be given to reduce the pain that begins midway through warming.

All this necessitates having a large container, a way of heating water, a thermometer, someone who knows what he is doing, and a safe way of getting the victim to a hospital when rewarming is called for. The results are so good, however, that it is well worth waiting to reach a proper treatment center instead of attempting makeshift rewarming immediately.

None of this should obscure the fact that frostbite need hardly ever happen, except perhaps on Antarctic expeditions or in battle. In one postwar year, the frostbite-conscious U.S. Sixth Army in Korea reduced its cold-related injuries to six, and at McMurdo Sound, America's main Antarctic station, serious frostbite is uncommon. Also, most frostbite happens in deep cold; under less extreme conditions, proper precautions make frostbite very rare.

LEARNING TO LIVE WITH THE ENEMY

Frostbite and hypothermia aren't the whole story of man's relationship with the cold. Indeed, while they had a healthy respect for cold's dangers, our human ancestors generally learned to tolerate the cold rather than avoid it. Many people have learned to live with the cold. So rather than fight the cold with evasive

FAT FACTS AND FANCIES

To stave off winter's chill, it is said, we should stop dieting, stoke our inner fires with food, and eat a lot of fat. These are pleasant thoughts. In fact, for the dieter who endures weight-watching meals all summer or the epicure curbing an enormous appetite, they issue a warm invitation to heavy eating that seems by itself to cheer the soul and loosen winter's icy grip.

Unfortunately, they are just thoughts, nothing more. Diets can even be more important in the winter than in the summer, since many of us are less active in cold weather. Fats do no special service that other foods cannot, and even the need to "stoke our inner fires" depends not on winter's presence but upon our actual physical exposure to the cold.

Consider the value of eating extra fat. Body fat can provide protection. The Greenland whale, which swims in icy waters, has a protective coat of blubber 20 inches thick; some Antarctic seals have 3-inch blubber coats; and even man in cold weather may put a lesser but nevertheless insulating layer of fat beneath his skin. But these useful layers of fat can be made perfectly well by converting starchy food. Their formation depends far more on how much we eat and how our bodies use it than on whether we eat fat.

Eskimos, of course, eat lots of fat, but that

is probably because the animals they hunt have lots of blubber. The Eskimos themselves work hard and burn nearly all this fat within their well-muscled bodies, and so fat Eskimos are very rare. Their clothes, not their fat, provide all the insulation they need.

As for us temperate types, body insulation's slight beneficial warmth should not hide certain facts. Our instincts, like the woodchuck's, may tell us to eat more at the approach of winter, primitive man's season of hardship and starvation. But overeating and obesity today contribute to such dangerous ills as diabetes and heart attacks; we, unlike the woodchuck, face no imminent starvation, and habitual overeating at any season is unhealthful for us all.

On the other hand, if we eat more food and use it, then, like the Eskimos, we are merely eating what we need. Exercising or working in deep cold burns a lot of calories, so hard-working Antarctic soldiers may really need 7,000 calories per day. Even someone living at a "balmy" 50°F around the clock burns 250 to 350 extra calories per day. And campers sleeping on cold ground rest better when they eat a bedtime snack because this food raises their heat output for several hours, delaying the onset of sleep-disturbing cold and shivers.

Nonetheless, careful tests have shown that soldiers in summer and winter settings need the same amount of calories, usually between 3,000 and 4,000, regardless of the temperature outside, and people who live in Greenland usually eat no more than people who live in Atlanta or Miami. Clearly, hard work and actual exposure to the cold, not cold temperatures or the approach of winter, are what justify big meals.

---

action, it seems far more fruitful to explore how we can adapt, how we can acclimate and how we can pace ourselves to take on all kinds of weather.

For instance, we know that sleeping Eskimos, Tierra del Fuego Indians, and Australian aborigines respond differently from ourselves to nighttime cold. The aborigines, many of whom customarily sleep naked on cold ground, have adapted by increasing the insulating power of their body "shell"—that portion between the skin and central organs—so as to lose heat relatively slowly. In contrast, the Eskimos and Tierra del Fuego Indians have adapted by raising their metabolic rate—the rate at which body cells operate—thereby turning out more body heat. Both changes produce the same result—the Aborigines, Eskimos, and Indians sleep comfortably at temperatures at which the rest of us feel cold, shiver, and sleep fitfully at best.

Such acclimatization could have taken many generations to evolve, but there is evidence to show that some kinds of cold conditioning develop fairly quickly. In one interesting experiment eight young Norwegian students were exposed to six weeks of around-the-clock frigidity. During the day they hiked, fished, and hunted; at night they slept naked at 37°F, covered only with light blankets. In the beginning they shivered a lot and didn't sleep much, and their nighttime foot temperature dropped to a painful 56°F.

As time passed, however, this changed. The student guinea pigs still shivered, but they learned how to sleep while shivering, and their foot temperature stayed at a "comfortable" 81°F. That pointed to an Eskimolike adaptation, in which their body cells "learned" to produce more nighttime heat. Even more revealing, when the students returned home six weeks later they no longer liked sleeping in warm rooms and well-covered beds, preferring instead light covers and cold air.

Some animal tests also indicate that moderate cold conditioning can increase a rat's ability to resist frostbite and hypothermia. In one test a group of rats was kept seven weeks at 77°F, while another was kept at 20°F. When both groups were then exposed to 5°F for five hours, all the nonacclimated rats suffered progressive frostbite and hypothermia, while none of the cold-conditioned rats showed any ill effects.

Can cold conditioning have a similar effect on people? We have no proof, but some evidence suggests that it can. For example, during the Korean War thousands of Americans got frostbite while other thousands of their com-

COLD PEOPLE

We can take cold better than we can take heat. A rise in body temperature of 8 or so degrees above normal—say to 107°F—often results in death, but healthy people whose body temperature drops to 90°F, 8 degrees *below* normal, rarely perish. True, body cooling can become life threatening below about 85°F by prompting cardiac arrest or fibrillation—uncoordinated contraction of the heart muscles—but there are recorded cases of people who have been far colder and who have survived.

In the winter of 1951, Dorothy May Stevens was found stone cold and unconscious in a Chicago alley. Her rectal temperature was 64.4°F. Though her heart was beating only twelve to twenty times a minute, hospital treatment revived her and she resumed a normal life.

Even lower temperatures have been reported. In 1955, a woman of fifty-one suffering from terminal cancer agreed to undergo extreme cooling, and her temperature was reportedly lowered to 48.2°F. Several years later, a group of Duke University doctors reported cooling another cancer patient to 39.6°F. Both subjects were said to have recovered fully from the cooling, though both soon succumbed to cancer.

Superficially, these and other examples of prodigious survival might seem to suggest that people could survive actual freezing.

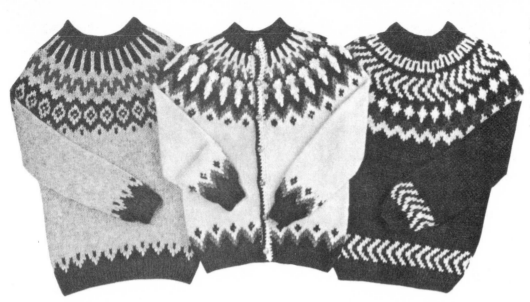

Icelandic sheep have developed a thick, long coat to protect themselves against the cold. Wool from these sheep is soft, strong, and surprisingly light, excellent for cold-weather clothing. (L. L. Bean)

That suggestion has been eagerly embraced by unknowing laymen from time to time, and a number of dead people have actually been frozen—supposedly for thawing and revival after medical science learns how to cure whatever killed them.

Unfortunately, such modern Ponce de Leons stand virtually no chance of cheating death. Even blood and sperm cells, when frozen, are frozen in the presence of glycerol (a chemical protectant) to ensure survival, and medical science has not yet found a way to safely freeze whole organs, much less whole bodies. Therefore, putting a dead body —or even a live one—into long-term suspended animation today seems bound to fail. Someday we may cross this barrier, to the cheers of science-fiction readers, but probably many years stand between us and that time.

---

parably dressed and exposed compatriots did not. Later, Army medical researchers reviewing the record found that men from the colder parts of the United States had far fewer cases of frostbite in the war than men from the warmer zones.

Researchers have also found that men conditioned to 54°F for thirty days showed less tendency to shiver than other men. That could be an important finding, for it suggests their body cells were turning out more heat without any extra muscular gyrations. If so, besides pro-

moting comfort, such stepped-up heat production would presumably reinforce the thermal balance, helping to resist the onslaught of severe cold and hypothermia, and it might partly explain why the cold-seasoned men in Korea resisted frostbite.

The evidence that man acclimatizes to cold weather is convincing; that is, we know people can physically adapt to cold. We know that cold conditioning can increase cold-weather comfort. And we have good reason to suspect that such conditioning can help both animals and man stave off hypothermia and frostbite.

This may be one reason that people from warm climates tend to dislike the cold, being little exposed and ill-adapted to it. It could also be one reason that people who live at 70°F think living at 60°F would be terrible, until they try it and find out it's not so bad. And it could be one reason that you may think 40°F feels colder in October than it does in March, for it's certainly possible that you yourself have become conditioned to the cold.

THERE ARE STILL DANGERS

But even when acclimated, your body's basic cold defenses go only so far. No Maine soldier in shirtsleeves could stand Korea's winter, nor would Maine winter garb equip anyone to confront Antarctic weather. So obviously, how our clothes and bodies interact has a lot to do with how our bodies cope.

This principle applies indoors at 60°F just as well as it applies in the Antarctic. If you feel

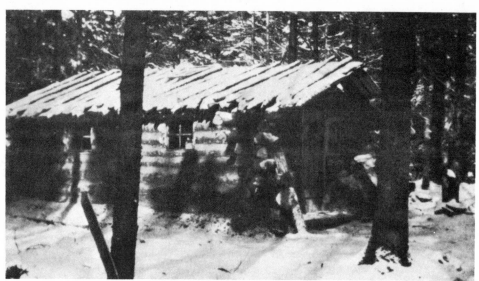

The isolation and restricted activity of winter in the wilds are as much the cause of cabin fever as the cold itself. (From Calvin Rutstrum, Paradise Below Zero [New York: Macmillan Publishing Co., Inc., 1968])

cold and don't want to raise the thermostat, put on more clothes. But if your hands feel cold indoors, you don't need to put on gloves; putting on a sweater can do the job just as well. If your fingers are chilly, the hypothalamus is restricting blood flow to your hands, and if you warm your body's core by putting on a sweater, that will tell the hypothalamus it's okay to restore circulation to your hands. This, by the way, is the principle behind the very popular quilted vests that hardy types sport on frosty days.

Even more surprising, you can warm cold hands by putting on a hat. The head, it turns out, is a privileged extremity, because the massive blood flow to the brain must never be impaired. So the body maintains that flow, even though doing so in cold weather causes a big heat loss. A warm hat helps reduce the loss, enables your core to retain its heat, and so indirectly maintains circulation to the less-privileged extremities. This fact is well known to nightcap wearers, whose quaint bed garment helps prevent cold hands and feet.

Of course, no indoor chill can rival the worst of outdoor weather. Not only do outdoor temperatures fall lower, but the range of possible temperatures is broader. Beyond that, hardy outdoor people must confront a combination of the elements—wind, snow, and water—and any of these, left to its own devices, can do severe if not devastating harm.

Take wind for instance. Wind snatches away warm air and so cools you by a process of con-

WINTER WOES

Some wintry discomforts like chapped lips, flu, and cabin fever relate only indirectly to the cold. For instance, cold does not cause chapped lips. Chapped lips come from dryness—dry wintry winds or dry, heated homes. Nor is cold directly to blame for cabin fever. Nobody talks about "apartment fever," so this affliction is clearly rural. And since it is the rural person whose world shrinks most as the December solstice nears, cabin fever presumably relates at least as much to restricted activity and darkness as to cold.

Nor can cold be entirely blamed for winter ills. Heart attacks do kill more middle-aged people in winter, but most of the "extra" deaths come during or just after snowfalls. This implies that cold does not cause most of these fatalities directly. Instead, prolonged winter inactivity, snow, and the suburban male's lemminglike urge to shovel seem to be the prime forces behind these perennial tragic deaths.

Nor should the common cold and other respiratory ills that plague us in chill times be blamed on cold alone. Much sickness occurs because people clustering indoors and children grouped in a classroom spread cold germs to one another. So it is not really surprising that, as icy times approach, cold and flu epidemics start to spread.

On the other hand, cold does directly

aggravate many medical problems by exposing lungs to cold air and making the body work harder to keep warm—thereby putting stress on the heart, lungs, and other organs. It worsens respiratory problems like bronchitis and pneumonia, and many heart attacks among the elderly arise directly from exposure to the cold.

Whether or not cold is the prime villain, however, knowing its role in these wintry ailments certainly improves our ability to cope with them. Hence chapped-lips sufferers should coat their lips with a thin layer of grease, Chapstick, or Vaseline to prevent drying in winter. Healthy cabin-fever victims should stay active, keep fit, and go out in cold weather. Common-cold sufferers and those seeking to prevent colds should avoid getting chilled, since chilling considerably lowers their resistance to disease.

Everyone with serious respiratory problems should avoid cold air. And nobody who is middle-aged, elderly, inactive, out of shape, or prone to heart attacks should shovel snow—period.

---

vection. It is especially dangerous in bitter cold because a wind of, say, 25 miles per hour can make a temperature like −20°F dangerous to anyone not dressed for Arctic weather, although in still conditions and normal winter gear that temperature is relatively safe.

On the other hand, people who know the wind find it easy to work out some accommodation. Arctic explorers make sure their extremities are not exposed to the wind, taking care to turn their faces from its path. Australian aborigines sleeping in the cold make a small lean-to affair of branches to slow the wind. And everyone properly dressed for winter weather dons some kind of outer garment that will provide protection, or a degree of it, against the wind.

Then there is water. Cold-weather water is far more dangerous than wind. Time after time, drenched or immersed climbers, sailors, and ice skaters come to a sad end. For example, some years back a small sailboat swamped in cold water. The crew, a young man and his fiancée, donned lifejackets and lashed themselves to the hull, expecting to be picked up soon. They were picked up three-and-a-half hours later, but by then it was too late. They were both dead of hypothermia.

Water, it turns out, is almost fiendishly clever at stealing body heat. It does this in three ways. First, it conducts heat nicely. So everywhere it touches you or your clothes it creates an avenue for heat to leave your body. Second, water as it evaporates absorbs a lot of heat. So water (or perspiration) evaporating off your skin or clothes causes rapid cooling. Third, water is very dense compared to air. So increasing the temperature of water—even a small amount of water—takes a lot of heat. This can be immensely helpful, as when we sharply reduce burn damage by immediately cooling the burned place with cold water. But it also means that someone immersed in water at 50°F may not survive three hours, even though that same air temperature would pose no threat.

Besides keeping dry, man in cold weather must know how to deal with water in the form of perspiration. This is a real problem, because clothes designed to protect a person at rest can make the wearer very hot when he becomes active. Then the overheated wearer perspires —wetting the clothes and reducing their power to protect him when he gets tired and wants to rest.

MODERATION IN ALL THINGS

Winter-clothes designers find sweat a source of interminable frustration. They suggest wearing many thin layers, some of which can be removed, as well as using drawstrings, special underarm vents, and retractable hoods for regulating exposure to the cold. None of these worthwhile suggestions is completely satisfactory. Even the Eskimo, true master of the cold that he is, wears limited apparel. His only innovation, besides drawstrings, is wearing his caribou skins loose, so that when he becomes active, the open garments flap, releasing warm air and letting in the cold. Though this is a great help, it is not a total answer.

But the Eskimo goes one step further. Realizing that the problem comes from his body, he maintains a well-paced level of moderate activity. This controls his body's rate of heat production, keeping that rate neither too high nor too low for his clothes. For example, an Eskimo using a dogsled will often ride with one foot on a runner and the other pushing on the ground to help propel the load. If he finds himself cooling down, he gets off the sled and trots behind it; when he's overheated, he stands on both runners and takes a free ride.

This key principle of moderate action— combined with changing pace to cool down or warm up—is a good idea for everyone. The man shoveling fresh snow off his drive can benefit—not just because overexertion will risk a heart attack but because working at an easy pace is the best way to stay cool and comfortable. The same applies to mountain climbers and skiers (not to mention hikers), mailmen on their appointed rounds, North Woods lumberjacks, soldiers on bivouac, stranded motorists, and anyone who wants to effectively endure or enjoy the cold.

Cold lovers also know how to deal with sun. They know there is a world of difference between the weak sunlight at ground level during a northern winter and the fierce sunlight piercing the thin air of the mountains, and they take precautions against sunburn in the mountains. They also know that even a northern sun warms what it strikes, and like the sled-riding Eskimo they use it to adjust their thermal balance, walking in the shade to keep cool or resting in the sun to stay warm; they need

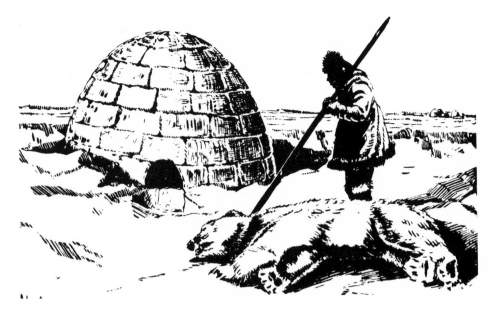

The blocks of ice and snow that form an igloo are a very effective barrier against the cold, trapping and holding the warm air within. (From Calvin Rutstrum, Paradise Below Zero, [New York: Macmillan Publishing Co., Inc., 1968])

nothing more than understanding to exploit this most passive kind of solar heating.

Oddly enough, however, deep snow can counteract such solar heating. For the sun's heat may not penetrate deep snow, leaving the ground in late winter far colder than the air, and so people walking through deep snow should be extra careful. Hikers and mountain climbers in particular should dress their feet for the expected temperature of the snow-covered ground, not the air, and should take special precautions against frostbite.

Massachusetts cranberry growers rejoice, however, when snow tops their low-growing vines. They know a combination of fierce wind and cold can kill cranberry vines, destroying the coming crop. A blanket of insulating snow, however, prevents this.

Besides protecting cranberries, snow can protect people. Cold expert Lucy Kavaler relates this incident in her book *Freezing Point* (John Day, 1972, p. 47):

On a late winter's day in 1967 a sick Eskimo woman and her husband left their home in Agapa above the Arctic Circle in Siberia to go to a hospital 150 miles away. Traveling on dogsled, they were caught in a snowstorm and became lost. The dogs died and the food ran out. At last the husband decided to leave his wife and go for help. He succeeded in reaching a town and a search party set off. But the Arctic storms were so severe that the hunt dragged on for two weeks. During that time

the temperature had dropped to −50°F. When the rescuers finally came upon the Eskimo woman, she was virtually buried in the snow. Nonetheless, she survived this experience. The blanket of snow plus her inherited metabolic adaptation to the cold may have saved her.

Besides being lucky and well adapted, this woman probably knew that snow, like insulating clothes, contains plenty of trapped air, so in some circumstances burying or surrounding oneself with snow provides protection. This is the principle behind the igloo, which is built of blocks of snow, sometimes with a sheet of ice to let in light. So effective is the igloo that sometimes the Eskimos inside need no clothes at all.

The sum total of all these adaptations and adjustments shows that cold, properly handled, can be our friend. That, however, depends largely upon us. If we regard surrounding cold as something to be shunned, we can expect neither our minds nor our bodies to adjust to it. If, on the other hand, we embrace the cold and adapt to it, then, like an athlete in training, we can improve our ability to cope. We may not rescue endangered mountaineers or learn, Eskimolike, to brave the Arctic, but we can deal much more effectively with cold than people who merely shroud themselves in the paraphernalia of cold prevention. And so, in the end, we will come much closer to achieving total warmth.

List of Sources

Chapter 1

Aquappliances, Inc.
135 Sunshine Lane
San Marcos, CA 92069

Ashley Heater Company
P.O. Box 128
Florence, AL 35630

Bow and Arrow Imports
14 Arrow Street
Cambridge, MA 02138

Cawley Stove Company, Inc.
27 North Wathington Street
Boyertown, PA 19512

Ceramic Radiant Heat
Pleasant Drive
Lochmere, NH 03252

El Fuego Corp.
30 Lafayette Square
Vernon, CT 06066

Eshland Enterprises, Inc.
P.O. Box 23
Greencastle, PA 17225

Fire Rite Stoves
654 North Colony Street
Wallingford, CT 06492

Firl Industries, Inc.
321 W. Scott Street
Fond du Lac, WI 54935

Fisher Stoves, Inc.
P.O. Box 10605
Eugene, OR 97440

Forshaw of St. Louis, Inc.
825 S. Lindbergh
St. Louis, MO 63131

Franco Belge Foundries of America, Inc.
15 Columbus Circle
New York, NY 10023

Hart Fireplace Furnishings
2549 Charlestown Road
New Albany, IN 47150

Kemstone Mats, Inc.
420 Quincy Avenue
Shenandoah, WA 22849

Liberty Bell Stove Works, Inc.
162 Reed Avenue
West Hartford, CT 06110

L. L. Bean
997 Main Street
Freeport, ME 04033

Minuteman International Co.
8 Nickerson Road
Lexington, MA 02173

Pine Barren Stove Co., Inc.
P.O. Box 496
Chatsworth, NJ 08019

Pioneer Lamp & Stove Co.
Box 4173
Seattle, WA 98104

Plimoth Coal Stove Works
Route 105
Plympton, MA 02367

Portland Stove Foundry Co.
Portland, ME 04104

Quaker Stove Co., Inc.
200 West 5th Street
Lansdale, PA 19446

Schaefer Brush Mfg. Co., Inc.
117 West Walker Street
Milwaukee, WI 53204

Southport Stoves, Inc.
959 Main Street
Stratford, CT 06597

Vermont Castings, Inc.
Prince Street
Randolph, VT 05060

Vermont Stove Company
Shelburne Road
Shelburne, VT 05482

Wallace Murray Corporation
P.O. Box 372
Nampa, ID 83651

Windrose Corp.
59 River Road
Cos Cob, CT 06807

Chapter 2

ABC Sunray Corporation
45 South Service Road
Plainview, NY 11803
Aero Environmental Limited
37 Hanna Avenue
Toronto, Ontario, Canada M6K 1X2
American Consulting Engineers Council
1155 15th Street, NW, Suite 713
Washington, DC 20005
American Electric Power System
2 Broadway
New York, NY 10004
American Institute of Architects
1730 New York Avenue
Washington, DC
American Society of Heating, Refrigerating, and Air
    Conditioning Engineers
345 East 47th Street
New York, NY 10017
American Stabilis Inc.
P.O. Box 1289
Lewiston, ME 04240
Axeman Anderson
233 West Street
Williamsport, PA 17701
Bacharach Instruments
626 Alpha Drive
Pittsburgh, PA 15238
Blueray Systems, Inc.
6800 Jericho Turnpike
Syosset, NY 11791
Burnham Corporation
2 Main Street
Irvington, NY 10533

Carlin Company
912 Silas Deane Highway
Wethersfield, CT 06109
Champion Home Builders Company
Dryden, MI 48071
Chronomite Laboratories, Inc.
21011 South Figueroa Street
Carson, CA 90745
Control Pak
44480 Grand River Avenue
Novi, MI 48050
Dwyer Instruments, Inc.
Box 373-T
Michigan City, IN 46360
Dynelco, Dynamic Electron Controls Inc.
P.O. Box 193
47 Mill Plain Road
Danbury, CT 06810
Energy House
P.O. Box 4035
105 West Merrimack Street
Manchester, NH 03108
Honeywell, Inc.
Honeywell Plaza
Minneapolis, MN 55408
Hydrotherm, Inc.
Rochland Avenue
Northvail, NJ 07647
Johns-Manville
Ken-Caryl Ranch
Denver, CO 80217
Kalwall Solar Components Division
P.O. Box 237
Manchester, NH 03105
Kerr Controls Limited
9 Circus Time Road
South Portland, ME 04106
Orlando Enterprises
1874 S.W. 16 Terrace
Miami, FL 33145

Robertshaw/Consumer Products Division
P.O. Box 2222
Corona, CA 91720

R. W. Beckette Corporation
38251 Center Ridge Road
Elyria, OH 44036

Simpex Company
115 M Midtown Plaza
Syracuse, NY 13210

Sloan Valve Company
10500 Seymour Avenue
Franklin Park, IL 60131

TPI Corporation
P.O. Box T, CRS
Johnson City, TN 37601

Wayne Home Equipment Division of Scott & Fetzer Company
801 Glasgow Avenue
Fort Wayne, IN 46803

Chapter 3

AAE
Edinburg, NY 12134

Abundant Energy Inc.
Newport Bridge Road
Warwick, NY 10990

AERO
435 Stapleton Building
Billings, MT 59601

Allstate Greenhouse Mfg. Corp.
P.O. Box 89
Shoreham, NY 11786

Alternative Sources of Energy
107 South Central
Milaca, MN 56353

American Section, International Solar Energy Association (ASISES)

American Technical University
P.O. Box 1416
U.S. Highway 190 West
Kileen, TX 76541

Architecture Foundation
College of Architecture
Arizona State University
Tempe, AZ 85281

Bergen County Community Action Program
8 Romanelli Avenue
South Hackensack, NJ 07606

Brady and Sun LivingRooms
12 Jacques Street
Worcester, MA 01603

Buck, Harry
Whinney Haw Stables
Route 1
Pine Bush, NY 12566

Center for Renewable Resources
1001 Connecticut Avenue, NW
Washington, DC 20036

Conservation and Renewable Energy Inquiry and Referral Service (CAREIRS)
P.O. Box 1607
Rockville, MD 20850

Cornerstones
54 Cumberland Street
Brunswick, ME 04011

Earth Shelter Digest
WEBCO Publishing
St. Paul, MN 55109

Ecotope Group
2332 East Madison
Seattle, WA 98112

Energy Factory
566 East Westover, Suite 105
Fresno, CA 93727

Environment/One
2773 Balltown Road
Schenectady, NY 12301

E.P.I.
1424 West 259th Street
Harbor City, CA 90710

Farallones Institute
15290 Coleman Valley Road
Occidental, CA 95455

Florida Solar Energy Center
300 State Road 401
Cape Canaveral, FL 32920

Four Seasons Greenhouses
910 Route 110
Farmingdale, NY 11735

Garden Way Solar Greenhouse by Sunplace
Garden Way Research
Charlotte, VT 05445

General Aluminum Corp.
P.O. Box 34221
Dallas, TX 75234

Great New England Energy Show
Brattleboro, VT 05301

Heartwood Owner Builder School
Jackson Road
Washington, MA 01235

Hobby Greenhouse Association
Box 951
Wallingford, CT 06492

Institute for Ecological Policies
9208 Christopher Street
Fairfax, VA 22031

Memphremagog Group
P.O. Box 456
Newport, VT 08533

National Climatic Center
Federal Building
Asheville, NC 28801

National Solar Energy Information Data Bank
c/o Conservation and Renewal Energy Inquiry and
Referral Services (CAREIRS)
P.O. Box 7607
Rockville, MD 20850

National Solar Heating and
Cooling Information
Center
P.O. Box 1607
Rockville, MD 20850

New Alchemy Journal
P.O. Box 47
Woods Hole, MA 02543

New Mexico Solar Energy Association
P.O. Box 2004
Santa Fe, NM 87501

New Western Energy Show
226 Power Block
Helena, MT 59601

Northern Owner Builder
Route 1
Plainfield, VT 05667

Owner-Builder Center
1824 4th Street
Berkeley, CA 94710

Putnam, Barbara
Marlborough, NH 03455

SAV Solar Systems
550 W. Patrice Place
Suite A
Gardena, CA 90248

Shelter Institute
Bath, ME 04530

Solar Age
Church Hill
Harrisville, NH 03450

Solar Engineering
8435 Stemmons Freeway
Dallas, TX 75247

Solar Greenhouse Association
34 North Gore Avenue
Webster Groves, MO 63119

Solar Living and Solar Greenhouse Digest
P.O. Box 2626
Flagstaff, AZ 86003

Solar Resources, Inc.
  Box 1848
  Taos, NM 87571
Solar Survival
  Box 199
  Harrisville, NH 03450
Solar Sustenance Team
  Route 1, Box 107AA
  Santa Fe, NM 87501
Solar Technology Corp.
  2160 Clay Street
  Denver, CO 80211
Solar Water Heater Book
  P.O. Box 1014
  Alamosa, CO 81101
Sun-Ray Solar Equipment Co., Inc.
  4 Pines Bridge Road
  Beacon Falls, CT 06403
Superintendent of Documents
  Government Printing Office
  Washington, DC 20402
Underground Plans Book 1
  P.O. Box 1149
  Brewster, MA 02631
Underground Space Association
  Department of Civl & Mineral Engineering
  University of Minnesota
  Minneapolis, MN 55455
Underground Space Center
  University of Minnesota
  Minneapolis, MN 55455
Vegetable Factory
  100 Court Street
  Copiague, NY 11726
VITA Publications
  3706 Rhode Island Avenue
  Mt. Ranier, MD 20822
Waterwall Engineering
  Route 1, Box 6
  New Paris, OH 45347

Weather Energy Systems, Inc.
  P.O. Box 968A
  Barlows Landing Road
  Pocasset, MA 02559
Zomeworks
  Box 712
  Albuquerque, NM 87103

Chapter 4

Center for Energy Policy and Research (CEPR)
  New York Institute of Technology
  Old Westbury, NY
Johns-Manville
  Ken-Caryl Ranch
  Denver, CO 80217
U.S. Department of Energy
  Washington, DC 20585

Chapter 5

American Society of Heating, Refrigerating
    and Air Conditioning Engineers
  345 East 47th Street
  New York, NY 10017
Appropriate Technology Corporation
  P.O. Box 975
  Brattleboro, VT 05301
Aztech International Ltd.
  2417 Aztec Road N.E.
  Albuquerque, NM 87107
Casablanca Fan Co.
  P.O. Box 37
  182 South Raymond Avenue
  Pasadena, CA 91105
Conservation Concepts
  Box 376
  Stratton Mountain, VT 05155

Creative Energy Products
    1053 Williamson Street
    Madison, WI 53703
Defender Energy Corporation
    Route 6
    Mahopac, NY 10541
Insulating Shade Company
    P.O. Box 282
    Brandford, CT 06405
Perkasie Industries
    50 East Spruce Street
    Perkasie, PA 18944
Sun Control Products, Inc.
    431 Fourth Avenue, SE
    Rochester, MN 55901
Sun Quilt
    Box 374
    Newport, NH 03772
Thermal Technology Corporation
    P.O. Box 130
    Snowmass, CO 81654
Vermont Thermal Shutter
    RD 2
    Woodstock, VT 05091
Window Blanket Company
    Route 7
    Lenoir City, TN 37771
Zomeworks
    P.O. Box 712
    Albuquerque, NM 87103

Chapter 6

Damart Thermolactyl
    1811 Woodbury Avenue
    Portsmouth, NH 02805
Down in Vermont
    RD 1
    Box 162A
    Graniteville, VT 05654

Eddie Bauer
    P.O. Box 3700
    Seattle, WA 98124
French Creek Sheep and Wool Company
    Elverson, PA 19520
Frostline
    Frostline Circle
    Denver, CO 80241
Garnet Hill
    Franconia, NH 03580
Hart Fireplace Furnishings
    2549 Charlestown Road
    New Albany, IN 47150
L. L. Bean
    997 Main Street
    Freeport, ME 04033
Lucy Stewart's Private Stock
    P.O. Box 443
    Grafton, NH 03240
Minuteman International Co.
    8 Nickerson Road
    Lexington, MA 02173
Woodstock Soap Stone Company
    Route 4, Box 223
    Woodstock, VT 05091

Chapter 7

American Ski Association
    5830 S. Lake Houston Parkway
    Houston, TX 77049
Early Winters, Ltd.
    110 Prefontaine Place South
    Seattle, WA 98104
Eastern Mountain Sports
    1041 Commonwealth Avenue
    Boston, MA 02215
Eastern Ski Association
    22 High Street
    Brattleboro, VT 05301

Eddie Bauer
  P.O. Box 3700
  Seattle, WA 98124
Frostline
  Frostline Circle
  Denver, CO 80241
Holubar
  P.O. Box 7
  Boulder, CO 80302
International Backpackers Association
  P.O. Box 85
  Lincoln Center, ME 04458
L. L. Bean
  997 Main Street
  Freeport, ME 04033
Moor & Mountain
  63 Park Street
  Andover, MA 01810
Pacific Northwest Ski Association
  3210 S. 176th Street Apt. 134
  Seattle, WA 98188
Recreational Equipment, Inc.
  P.O. Box 1685
  Seattle, WA 98111
Sierra Club
  530 Bush Street
  San Francisco, CA 94108
Ski Hut
  1615 University Avenue
  Berkeley, CA 94701

Ski Touring Council
  c/o Rudolf F. Mattesich
  W. Hill Road
  Troy, VT 05868
Smilie Co.
  575 Howard Street
  San Francisco, CA 94105
Synergy Works
  225 Fourth Street
  Oakland, CA 94607
United States Figure Skating Association
  20 First Street
  Colorado Springs, CO 80906
United States Ski Association
  1726 Champa Street Suite 300
  Denver, CO 80202
United States Snowshoe Association
  RD 1 Box 170
  Corinth, NY 12822

Chapter 8

L. L. Bean
  997 Main Street
  Freeport, ME 04033

Index